Evoked Potentials in Clinical Medicine

Third Edition

Evoked Potentials in Clinical Medicine

Third Edition

Editor

Keith H. Chiappa, M.D.

Associate Professor of Neurology
Harvard Medical School
Director
EEG Laboratory
Massachusetts General Hospital
Boston, Massachusetts

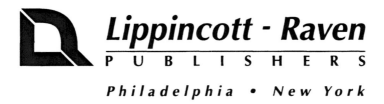

Lippincott - Raven
P U B L I S H E R S

Philadelphia • New York

Acquisitions Editor: Mark Placito
Developmental Editor: Mattie Bialer
Manufacturing Manager: Dennis Teston
Production Manager: Lawrence Bernstein
Production Editor: Tage Publishing Service, Inc.
Cover Designer: Jeanne Norton
Indexer: Tage Publishing Service, Inc.
Compositor: Compset, Inc.
Printer: Maple Press

Printed in the United States of America

9 8 7 6 5 4 3 2 1

Library of Congress Cataloging-in-Publication Data
Evoked potentials in clinical medicine / Keith H. Chiappa, editor.—
    3rd ed.
        p. cm.
    Includes bibliographical references and index.
    ISBN 0-397-51659-2 (hardcover)
    1. Evoked potentials (Electrophysiology)   2. Nervous system—
Diseases—Diagnosis.   I. Chiappa, Keith H.
    [DNLM: 1. Evoked Potentials.   2. Monitoring, Physiologic.   WL 102
E929   1997]
RC386.6.E86E963   1997
616.8'047547—dc21
DNLM/DLC
for Library of Congress

Care has been taken to confirm the accuracy of the information presented and to
describe generally accepted practices. However, the authors, editors, and publisher are
not responsible for errors or omissions or for any consequences from application of the
information in this book and make no warranty, express or implied, with respect to the
contents of the publication.

The authors, editors, and publisher have exerted every effort to ensure that drug
selection and dosage set forth in this text are in accordance with current
recommendations and practice at the time of publication. However, in view of ongoing
research, changes in government regulations, and the constant flow of information
relating to drug therapy and drug reactions, the reader is urged to check the package
insert for each drug for any change in indications and dosage and for added warnings
and precautions. This is particularly important when the recommended agent is a new or
infrequently employed drug.

Some drugs and medical devices presented in this publication have Food and Drug
Administration (FDA) clearance for limited use in restricted research settings. It is the
responsibility of the health care provider to ascertain the FDA status of each drug or
device planned for use in their clinical practice.

Contents

Contributors

David C. Adams, M.D.   *Department of Anesthesiology, College of Physicians and Surgeons, Columbia University, 622 West 168th Street, New York, New York 10032*

David J. Burke, M.D., D.Sc., F.A.A., F.T.S.E., F.R.A.C.P.   *Prince of Wales Medical Research Institute, Department of Clinical Neurophysiology, The Prince Henry and Prince of Wales Hospitals, High Street, Randwick NSW, Sydney 2031, Australia*

Keith H. Chiappa, M.D.   *Associate Professor of Neurology, Harvard Medical School, and Director, and EEG Laboratory, Massachusetts General Hospital, Boston, Massachusetts 02114*

Didier Cros, M.D.   *Department of Neurology, EMG Unit-Bigelow 12, Massachusetts General Hospital, Boston, Massachusetts 02114*

Ronald G. Emerson, M.D.   *Associate Professor of Neurology, Department of Neurology, Columbia-Presbyterian Medical Center, 710 West 168th Street, New York, New York 10032*

Sandra L. Helmers, M.D.   *Assistant Professor, Department of Neurology, Harvard Medical School, Children's Hospital, EEG Laboratory, 300 Longwood Avenue, Boston, Massachusetts 02115*

Richard G. Hicks, M.Sc.   *Prince of Wales Medical Research Institute, Department of Neurology, The Prince Henry and Prince of Wales Hospitals, High Street, Randwick NSW, Sydney 2031, Australia*

Rosamund A. Hill, M.B., Ch.B.   *Neurologist, Neuroservices Unit, Auckland Hospital, Park Road, Auckland, New Zealand*

Lynette Kiers, M.B., B.S., F.R.A.C.P.   *Director, Clinical Neurophysiology, Department of Neurology and Clinical Neurophysiology, Royal Melbourne Hospital, Grattan Street, Melbourne, Victoria 3050, Australia*

Susan R. Levy, M.D.   *Associate Clinical Professor, Pediatrics, Neurology, and Child Study Center, Yale University School of Medicine, 333 Cedar Street, New Haven, Connecticut 06510*

R. Dean Linden, Ph.D.   *Associate Professor, Department of Neurological Surgery, University of Louisville, 210 East Gray Street, Louisville, Kentucky 40202*

Keith J. Nagle, M.D.   *Assistant Professor, Director, Clinical Neurophysiology Laboratory, Department of Neurology, University of Vermont, Fletcher Allen Health Care, 111 Colchester Avenue, Burlington, Vermont 05401*

Barry S. Oken, M.D.   *Associate Professor of Neurology, Oregon Health Sciences University, Portland, Oregon 97201*

Joseph A. Sgro, M.D., Ph.D.   *Associate Adjunct Professor, Department of Neurology, Columbia University, 710 West 168th Street, New York, New York 10032, and Alacron Inc., 71 Splitbrook Road, Nashua, New Hampshire 03060*

Christopher B. Shields, M.D.   *Professor and Vice Chairman, Department of Neurological Surgery, University of Louisville, 210 East Gray Street, Louisville, Kentucky 40202*

Paul C. Stanton, B.S.E.E.   *Alacron Inc., 71 Splitbrook Road, Nashua, New Hampshire 03060*

Con Yiannikas, M.B., B.S., F.R.A.C.P.   *Clinical Neurophysiologist, Department of Neurology, Concord Hospital, Hospital Road, Concord NSW, Sydney 2137, Australia*

R. Zappulla, M.D., Ph.D.   *Professor and Chairman, Department of Neuroscience, Seton Hall University, 65 James Street, Edison, New Jersey 08820*

Preface

The six years since the Second Edition of this book have seen considerable maturation of evoked potentials (EPs) in clinical medicine. This has involved both a contraction produced mainly by magnetic resonance imaging (MRI) and a distillation of experience that has allowed the clinical questions presented to EPs to be more focussed. Economic pressures will also continue to play an increasing role in the clinical utilization of EPs and their cost effectiveness must be documented.

The temporal resolution of EPs (fractions of a millisecond) allows functional imaging that far exceeds positron emission tomography (PET) scan and functional MRI techniques. This, plus the relatively simple technical demands of EPs, result in a useful tool for monitoring function during surgery; and this arena has made significant advances. Therefore, I have added a major section to this book covering this specialty. Multiple authors present different techniques for similar tasks. This was done intentionally to present the range of methods that have been successfully employed in the operating room. The readers should carefully extract those elements most useful in their own context.

Experience gained with the pediatric-age group has allowed a separate exposition of this topic in each modality.

Motor EPs have continued to expand into the clinical and research arenas with dramatic speed and have evolved markedly. Approval by the FDA in the United States should be granted promptly and thus this chapter has been completely rewritten and expanded.

This edition was greatly facilitated by my editorial assistant, my daughter Elizabeth, who performed many difficult and painstaking editorial tasks, including pushing me forward. I have been very grateful for her assistance and company on this project.

It is 16 years since I started work on the First Edition of this book. I have been privileged to be one of the many who have developed the field of EPs and used it to help patients.

Keith H. Chiappa

Evoked Potentials in Clinical Medicine,
3d ed., edited by Keith H. Chiappa.
Lippincott–Raven Publishers, Philadelphia © 1997.

1

Principles of Evoked Potentials

Keith A. Chiappa, M.D.

*Department of Neurology, Harvard Medical School, and EEG Laboratory,
Massachusetts General Hospital, Boston, Massachusetts 02114*

1. INTRODUCTION

1.1. General Considerations

Pattern-shift visual (PSVEPs), brain stem auditory (BAEPs), and short-latency somatosensory evoked potentials (SEPs) are reliable diagnostic tests that yield reproducible results in routine clinical practice. They provide an objective measure of function in their related sensory systems and tracts; they have been studied in large groups of normal subjects and in patients with a wide variety of neurologic diseases. The clinical utility of evoked potentials (EPs) is based on their ability (1) to demonstrate abnormal sensory system function when the history and/or neurologic examination are equivocal; (2) to reveal the presence of clinically unsuspected malfunction in a sensory system when demyelinating disease is suspected because of symptoms and/or signs in another area of the central nervous system (CNS); (3) to help define the anatomic distribution of a disease process; and (4) to monitor changes objectively over time in a patient's status. These tests provide sensitive, quantitative extensions of the clinical neurologic examination. They primarily afford numerical data; sometimes the absence of a wave or an abnormal configuration of its potential field also provides useful information.

An EP is an electrical manifestation of the brain's reception of and response to an external stimulus. For example, the visual EP (VEP) produced by the flash of a strobe light during photic stimulation can often be seen in a routine electroencephalogram (EEG) (Fig. 1–1).

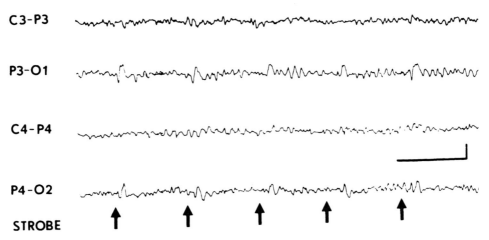

FIG. 1–1. Conventional bipolar EEG recording from a normal subject, eyes open, with some alpha activity still visible. Strobe flashes occur at arrows—note the visible but poorly defined EPs in the occipital areas with peaks at about 150 msec after each stimulus. Electrode locations: C, central, P, parietal, O, occipital; odd numbers, left; even, right. Calibration marks are 1 sec and 50 μV. Relative negativity of the first electrode produces an upward trace deflection. (From Chiappa, 1979, with permission.)

Most EPs, including the three to be discussed here (PSVEPs, BAEPs, and SEPs), cannot be seen in routine EEG recordings. This is because of their low amplitudes [0.1–20 microvolts (μV)] and their admixture with normal background brain wave (e.g., alpha) activity and various artifacts that together are from twenty to several hundred microvolts in amplitude.

Separation of the buried EP waveforms from the other electrical activity is accomplished by signal averaging. Since the electrical response of the brain to the stimulus always comes at the same interval of time after the stimulus, whereas the other activities present are not coupled to the stimulus, simple computers (signal averagers) can be used to extract the desired signal (the EP) from the temporally random background activity (Fig. 1–2). Stimuli are given repetitively and the computer averages the new data acquired after each stimulus (random EEG plus EP) with the averaged results from previous stimuli stored in its memory. The process is continued until the desired waveform becomes sufficiently clarified.

Evoked potentials have been studied in patients with neurologic diseases since the early 1950s, but it was only in the early 1970s that EPs began to have definite clinical utility. This long gestation period resulted in large part from the fact that attention was at first focused primarily on long-latency components—those waveforms appearing more than 75 msec after the stimulus (middle latency = 30–75 msec; short latency = <30 msec). These long-latency potentials have a large amplitude (e.g., 5–50 μV compared to 0.5 μV or less for the BAEP) and so are relatively easy to obtain. However, long-latency potentials often have poor waveform consistency among normal subjects and are easily altered by changes in many psychological variables, such as inattention and drowsiness, which are difficult if not impossible to control, even in normal subjects. Changes thus induced in shape, amplitude, and latency of the waveforms make it difficult to obtain consistent and reproducible results from either normal subjects or patients. Cognitive EPs (e.g., P300) suffer from this problem and currently have no definite clinical utility in individual patients. Brain stem auditory EPs and SEPs are manifestations of activity in brain stem and other subcortical primary sensory tracts and nuclei, recorded from the scalp. As such, despite their low am-

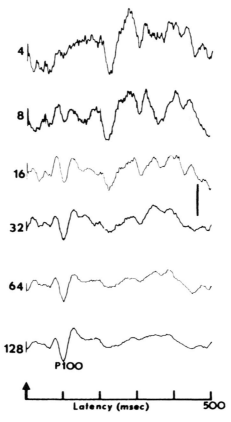

FIG. 1–2. Pattern-shift VEP from a normal subject. The pattern shift occurs at the arrow and the EEG signal is recorded for 512 msec thereafter (*left to right*). Each line displays the contents of the averager's memory after a specific number of stimuli (*left*). The 5-μV amplitude calibration mark applies to each line. After four sweep repetitions a large artifact is present in the middle of the trace at about 225 msec after the stimulus. With increasing numbers of repetitions, this artifact disappears and the normal waveforms appear, with the component of interest, P100, present as a downgoing peak at about 100 msec after the stimulus. Note that after 64 repetitions the amplitude of P100 changes very little but the background continues to become smoother. Recording is a CZ–OZ bipolar derivation (CV and OZ are midline central and occipital electrodes, respectively). Relative positivity at OZ is a downward trace deflection. Calibration mark is 5-μV. (From Chiappa, 1979, with permission.)

plitude, they have a relatively high waveform consistency in normal subjects and are essentially unaffected even by general anesthesia or barbiturate levels sufficient to induce coma and flattening of the EEG. The part of the PSVEP used clinically, the first large positive peak that appears 100 msec or so after the shift of the pattern (the P100 wave—see Fig. 1–2), also has a high degree of waveform consistency and reliability among normal subjects and patients, even though it is a long-latency component. This is probably due to the specific nature of the stimulus itself (compared to a strobe or even pattern flash). Short-latency VEPs, possibly arising in the optic nerve, tract, lateral geniculate body, and optic radiations, have been reported in humans but these findings remain to be confirmed and clinically utilized. Clinical utilization of very low amplitude, short-latency EPs was also aided by advances in transistor technology. In the late 1960s and early 1970s significant improvements were made in physiologic amplifiers. The use of field-effect transistors provided much greater amplification with less instrumental and environmental noise than was possible with vacuum-tube technology. These are critical amplifier features when the biological signals of interest are fractions of a microvolt, as compared with the millivolt levels seen in intracellular microelectrode recordings, for example. These technological advances allowed fast, reliable resolution of waveforms previously obtained only with difficulty, if at all.

1.2. Generator Source Localization

1.2.1. Topographic Mapping Studies and Dipoles

Topographic maps of EP field distributions are used to localize waveform generator sites via application of dipole theory. Although the facts in these studies are solid, the conclusions, of necessity, are usually speculative; they are often based on the assumption that the generators are very small sources, whereas they occupy a significant volume within the bounds of the recording surface (the scalp), have an irregular and asymmetric shape, and may be only partially affected (i.e., inactivated) by lesions. These factors diminish the utility of dipole considerations in EP generator source localization and need to be addressed much more than they are currently. Noncephalic references usually are required and these inject so much artifact that the results are difficult to interpret, or excessive time is required to obtain clear waveforms. Potential-field mapping studies contribute little to the clinical interpretation of EPs, and their contribution to the understanding of generator sources in humans is difficult to ascertain, although they have provided a good source for academic discussions.

1.2.2. Animal Studies

Although animal studies allow a variety of techniques not feasible in humans (e.g., depth electrodes, experimental lesions, and pathologic confirmation of structures involved), the relationship between the findings in the animals and in humans is often difficult to verify. For example, Buchwald and Huang (1975) performed experiments with lesions in cats and found that the fifth EP wave following a click stimulus was abolished by removal of the inferior colliculus. This finding was applied to humans by others despite the fact that the latency separation between the first and fifth waves in the cats is greater by far (5.3 versus 4.0 msec) than it is in humans. Achor and Starr (1980a,b) performed similar experiments and found completely different results. The relevant point is that current ideas about the generator sources for clinical interpretation of EP waveforms in humans come not from the animal studies (or human potential-field mapping studies) but from human clinicopathologic correlations and intraoperative recordings. Presumably the anatomic differences between humans and animals are too great.

1.2.3. Human Clinicopathologic Correlations

Clinicopathologic correlations are the best method for studying human EP waveform generators, but there are pitfalls. Ideally the neuropathology will be available but this is unpredictable. Computed tomography (CT) or magnetic resonance imaging (MRI) scanning is often taken as the final word on anatomic involvement in a disease process, but this is often unreliable and should be used very carefully, certainly more carefully than is the case presently. A careful assessment of clinical evidence of anatomic involvement should supplement the conclusions from the CT/MRI scan evidence. Perhaps a combination of MRI and positron emission tomography (PET) techniques will be able to provide much more reliable anatomic information.

Another confounding factor is the retrograde degeneration that occurs in many CNS systems after tract or nuclear lesions. For example, thalamic VPL neurons show degenerative changes within days to weeks after a purely cortical or centrum semiovale lesion and presumably are functionally paralyzed even earlier. Thus, the SEP studies that correlated waveforms with longstanding lesions (e.g., hemispherectomies) are invalid. The disagreements in human clinicopathologic correlations relative to the generator source of BAEP wave V and its ipsilateral or contralateral lateralization are probably due to differing degrees of retrograde degeneration.

1.3. Clinical Interpretation

1.3.1. Normal Studies and Statistical Considerations

Pattern-shift VEPs, BAEPs, and short-latency SEPs have been well-studied in groups of normal subjects and their variability has proven to be low enough so that they have great clinical utility. Amplitude usually is more variable than latency and has been difficult to use clinically. Also, the amplitude parameters used by different investigators have varied widely. For example, Blumhardt and Halliday (1981) used an amplitude difference of 2 as the upper limit of normal for the difference between the half fields, whereas Haimovic and Pedley (1982a,b) and Chiappa (1983) found a ratio of 4 to 1 in the same measure. On the other hand, Noth et al. (1984) used SEP amplitudes to indicate patients at risk for developing Huntington's disease.

The consensus on statistical levels of limits of normality for clinical use (American Electroencephalographic Society, 1984) is that for EP features with a normal (Gaussian) distribution, a standard deviation level of 2.5 or more should be used for interpreting as abnormal an individual patient's test results. This reflects the stance of clinicians, who usually wish to minimize false positive results.

The statistical evaluation of EP results needs to reproduce the point of view of the clinical neurophysiologist faced with the electrophysiologic tests from an individual patient. Thus, not only are blinded comparisons with conventional techniques necessary, but also prospective studies of patient groups in whom the diagnosis can be established with some certainty. Blumhardt (1984) has reviewed this matter with respect to the role of EPs in multiple sclerosis, but his comments are pertinent here:

> To evaluate the role of a new, potentially diagnostic test, we need to know not only the proportion of patients with a positive result amongst those in whom the disease is established by a "gold standard," but also in equivocal cases of the disease and in patients with other commonly confused conditions. What is the role of the new test in relation to established diagnostic techniques and what are its potential advantages and disadvantages? How reliable and reproducible are the results? How does the new test stand up against the "gold standard"? As the prevalence of the disease in the population will clearly affect the "abnormality rate," we need to know the methods of selection or preliminary screening of patients in studies which evaluate the test. Finally, to determine the benefits for the patient, we need to know the positive and negative predictive abilities of EP's and the subsequent fate of the patients who had either normal or abnormal results.

Furthermore, in evaluating clinical results, a clear distinction must be made between group versus group studies, and group versus individual studies. The latter is the usual situation in a clinical laboratory where a single patient is being compared to "limits of normality" obtained by studying a sample (e.g., 30 normal subjects) from the normal population. In the former case (primarily a research application) a group of patients with a disease is compared statistically with a group of matched normals. The statistical techniques used in this group versus group analysis are very sensitive and often will reveal differences between the two groups, especially when the number of "features" evaluated is in the thousands, as it is with topographic EEG and EP studies. Some of these "significant" findings are merely random fluctuations (Oken and Chiappa, 1986). It is then important to test another group of patients with the same disease to see if they differ from the normal group in the same way. If the findings are valid, they tell us something about the group of patients but not necessarily about a single patient from that group. If the single patient's test results are evaluated using the normal group data for comparison, the single patient may well be indistinguishable from the normals, that is, the patient's data may be within normal limits (e.g., Rowe and Carlson, 1980). This last evaluation, of course, is the one forced upon the clinical neurophysiologist who, faced with the results from a single patient, is trying to determine whether or not the patient's results are within normal limits. Prospective studies are needed to determine the applicability of results obtained from group versus group comparisons to the interpretation of an individual patient's EP data. See Chapter 16 for a further discussion of statistical aspects of EPs.

1.3.2. Physiologic Anatomy

Close correlation between short-latency waveforms and neural anatomy provides a view of "physiologic anatomy" that is as reliable as CT or MRI. Short-latency waveforms in SEPs and BAEPs are unchanged by barbiturate doses sufficient to render the EEG flat and neurologic examination equal to brain death. The same reliability is currently not available in the visual system.

1.3.3. Topographic Analysis

Topographic maps are used as a means of viewing the potential-field distribution of EP activity. They can make a mass of data more comprehensible, and may make it easier to explain the data to a nonneurophysiologist. The topographic map is the neurophysiologists' answer to the CT scan, and it is especially attractive because it is usually in color, but in these circumstances the mapping is not providing new information, and the same end can readily be reached from the original data. Topographic maps potentially are more useful when they are based on statistical data derived from the electrical data, but this technique is so sensitive that artifact recognition is extremely difficult (facial and scalp myogenic reflexes can be easily confused with a cerebral response). In addition, the large number of features (variables) used in the analysis ensures that some will have significant values by chance alone. Proper management of this requires large numbers of normals or other statistical adjustments (Oken and Chiappa, 1986), and prospective studies which have not yet been done.

It has been stated that the eventual aim of topographic mapping must be anatomic localization. However, in the clinical arena, this is much less important now that PET and MRI capabilities are available, and subdural or epidural and depth electrode chronic recordings are performed in epilepsy centers. Evoked potentials give anatomic data (especially short-latency EPs—but these are analyzed most effectively in the time domain), but the generator sites of long-latency components are not well-defined.

The choice of a recording derivation, especially reference site (ipsilateral ears, linked ears, vertex, nose, chin, noncephalic) is a difficult one for topographic studies. These are important considerations, especially with research applications where the actual potential-field distribution is desired. But in the clinical arena such matters can be handled more empirically, so that a bipolar montage might have the advantage of least artifact. The idea that a bipolar derivation does not register far-field activity (because of in-phase cancellation) so that only near-field generator sources are recorded in a bipolar derivation is overly simplistic; BAEPs can be recorded from a bipolar scalp derivation.

In summary, topographic mapping is very useful for research in potential field distribution and dipole studies. Since its clinical application requires the use of complex statistical operations, adequate prospective trials are needed before any statement can be made regarding its clinical utility.

1.4. Clinical Utility

1.4.1. Applications Versus Correlations

There are a large number of published papers that give data on clinical correlations of EPs (for reviews of these, see Chiappa, 1983). It is again pertinent to note that clinical correlations are not necessarily clinical applications, as discussed in Section 1.3.1. For example, Rowe and Carlson (1980) studied 27 patients with postconcussion dizziness and found that their BAEPs were statistically different from the normal control population. However, only three of these patients had BAEP parameters beyond the 99% tolerance limit, that is, in only those three would the test result have been reported as abnormal when interpreted in the conventional, "individual" manner. Thus, the sensitivity of the test in that syndrome is low and would not be useful in differentiating postconcussion syndrome from malingering. However, the group statistics are interesting with respect to the pathophysiology of that syndrome and tell us that those patients do have abnormal brain stem auditory system function, albeit subtle. Prospective studies are the best method for determining the clinical applicability of a test in a specific disease.

1.4.2. Clinical Applications

It is not necessary to discuss individual diseases to understand the clinical applications and limitations of EPs. As was stated above in Section 1.1, they provide a very sensitive, objective extension of the clinical neurologic examination, but no more etiologic information. For example, in a retrospective study of 198 patients with multiple sclerosis (MS) who had had PSVEP testing, Brooks and Chiappa (1982) found that when the PSVEP was normal, there was *never* an abnormality found on the clinical examination, and when the PSVEP was abnormal, clinical examinations were often normal. In those patients with abnormal PSVEPs, the visual fields by usual clinical examination (confrontation) were normal in 96%, formal fields were normal in 55%, pupillary responses were normal in 74%, fundus appearance was normal in 39%, and there was no red color desaturation in 27%. These figures convey the degree of sensitivity that the test can add to the routine clinical ophthalmologic examination, presumably not only in demyelinating disease, but also in most other disorders of the optic nerves. Similar data are available for BAEP and SEP testing.

One clinical application of these EPs is in the evaluation of patients suspected of having demyelinating disease where an abnormal EP in a sensory system not clinically affected can help to define the anatomic involvement in the disease process and thus the disease type itself. One question that arises in this context is whether or not it is "worthwhile" to struggle to make a diagnosis, or quantify an abnormality, when the disease cannot be treated. The alternative—waiting until useful therapies emerge to try to develop better tests for the disease—is itself problematic because the testing of therapies is dependent upon accurate diagnosis and the ability to quantitate abnormalities. Also, the psychological plight of many patients, in diagnostic limbo because their disease is clinically evident in only one CNS locus, can be alleviated by a definitive diagnosis.

In many clinical situations, when the clinical history and sensory examination of a sensory system are equivocal, the objective demonstration of dysfunction provided by EPs is very helpful. For example, in patients with nystagmus, the BAEP can help to differentiate central from peripheral etiologies since the vestibular and auditory systems are so closely approximated for much of their brain stem course (Chiappa et al., 1980).

Evoked potentials have revolutionized the clinical workup in patients in whom acoustic neuroma needs to be ruled out. If the BAEP waveforms are clear and the interpeak latencies are normal, then no further radiologic (MRI) or audiometric tests need to be done since the BAEPs are more sensitive than these (Chiappa, 1983).

1.4.3. Overuse or Misuse of EPs

Cost effectiveness in medicine has understandably been a major focus of attention, especially in recent years. Topics have varied from the approaches to specific diseases [e.g., treatment of acute pulmonary edema (Griner, 1972), coronary care (Martin et al., 1974), and nontraumatic coma (Levy et al., 1981)], to laboratory test ordering practices in general (Griner and Liptzin, 1971; Abrams, 1979; Shuman and Heilman, 1979; Eisenberg and Williams, 1981; Levy et al., 1981; Heilman, 1982; Griner and Glaser, 1982). Martin et al. (1980) even tried to alter medical residents' test-ordering behavior with financial incentives. In articles laden with speculation and inferences drawn from nonexistent, erroneous, or irrelevant data, Menken (1983) and Eisen and Cracco (1983) recently brought this question to evoked-response testing. This topic for EPs was discussed in an editorial (Chiappa and Young, 1985) that was the source for the text of this section.

Menken (1983) said "many of these electrodiagnostic services appear to add little information that cannot be obtained from a careful neurologic history and examination." In a retrospective study of 198 patients with MS who had had PSVEP testing, Brooks and Chiappa (1982) found that when the PSVEP was normal, there was *never* an abnormality found on the clinical examination, and when the PSVEP was abnormal, clinical examinations were often normal. For example, in those patients with abnormal PSVEPs, the visual fields by usual clinical examination (confrontation) were normal in 96%, formal fields were normal in 55%, pupillary responses were normal in 74%, fundus appearance was normal in 39%, and there was no red color desaturation in 27%. These figures convey the degree of sensitivity that the test can add to the routine clinical ophthalmologic examination, presumably not only in demyelinating disease, but also in most other disorders of the optic nerves. Similar data are available for BAEP and SEP testing. Nerve conduction studies and needle electromyography need no further comment in this regard.

Menken uses the word "lucrative" to describe these tests, ignoring the fact that many tests (how many is not known) are performed in university centers by staff who gain no direct financial benefit from the tests. His comments on EP test usage in MS demonstrate an insensitivity to the psychological plight of the patients who are in diagnostic limbo because their disease is clinically evident in only one CNS locus. It is "worthwhile" to struggle to make a diagnosis or to quantify an abnormality when the disease cannot be treated? The alternative is to wait until useful therapies emerge, and then to try to develop better tests for the disease, but how can therapies be tested if the disease cannot be diagnosed or its abnormalities quantitated?

Eisen and Cracco (1983) gave a brief review of clinical EP usage and then stated that "EPs are probably being overused in many clinical laboratories . . . indications for the use of EPs are not understood by many clinicians . . . the indications have not been clearly defined for many disorders." Furthermore, they note that "EPs have been used most extensively in the diagnosis of MS." No data are given to support these statements and harsh judgments, nor are any data available elsewhere in the literature. During the month of March 1983, 94 patients (slightly less than average) had 216 EP tests (PSVEP, BAEP, and SEP) in the EP unit of the Clinical Neurophysiology Laboratory of the Massachusetts General Hospital. Of the tests, 22% were abnormal, 31% of the patients had at least one test abnormal, and in 38% of the patients MS was in the differential diagnosis. A neurologic review of the medical records of all patients revealed that 7% of the tests appeared not to be indicated as far as patient care and/or diagnostic considerations were concerned. All of these figures compare very favorably with the other laboratory tests studied in the articles previously mentioned (wherever comparisons are possible). Nor is clinical involvement of a sensory system always an open-and-shut case, as inferred by Eisen and Cracco. The confirmation of abnormal function in equivocal clinical presentations can be as helpful as the demonstration of a clinically unsuspected malfunction.

Whether, in a specific patient, EPs are overused, underused, or misused must be decided on a case by case basis, and that determination requires the same clinical experience and judgment as is needed for the rest of that patient's medical care. Without this individualized approach, the answer to the question will depend on the criteria used: (1) the patient's desire to know, (2) the physician's desire to know, (3) the bureaucracy's (hospital administrators and third-party payers) desire to decrease expenses, (4) the neurology department chief's desire to increase departmental income, and (5) some academic clinicians' apparent fear (subliminal?) that their clinical opinion (derived from history and physical examination) will be contradicted by objective physiologic tests, that is, mechanized extensions of the routine neurologic examination, although they readily accept "anatomic" tests.

There is no doubt that some EPs are misused. The most blatant example of this occurs with dermatomal SEPs. The techniques, in the proper hands, used in carefully selected cases, can provide useful clinical information. But they are so often abused by inappropriate application, largely driven by financial incentives, that the harm to the medical system so far outweighs the gain for the patients that the use of this test should not be approved. A similar situation is true for "topographic mapping."

Although EP (and other clinical neurophysiologic) tests are not more overused or misused than other laboratory tests, improvement in test utilization can come in (1) screening patients before testing (itself a time-consuming process) and/or restricting testing to patients referred by properly trained physicians, and (2) restricting performance of the tests to qualified (certified) clinical neurophysiologists.

With respect to the latter point, clinical neurophysiologic tests [EEG, electromyelography (EMG), EP] are ordered by neurophysicians or other clinicians for enhancement of the clinical evaluation of the nervous system. Most of these tests need to be modified to fit a given clinical situation, not only at the outset, but also as the test progresses and the results are evaluated. The clinical neurophysiologist supervising the performance of EP tests must review the patient's medical history and examination and the EP test results to determine whether the data collected are sufficient for a clinically useful interpretation, or whether other modifications of stimulating and recording parameters are necessary. Clinical neurophysiologists need to be able to project themselves into the shoes of the neurophysician (or other clinician) who will be receiving the test results and interpretation in order to guide the performance and interpretation of the test to a competent, intelligent conclusion. Furthermore, these tests are of a sufficiently complex nature so that most neurophysicians not specially trained in clinical neurophysiology need some assistance in integrating the test results into a particular clinical situation. Therefore, a laboratory should have a person fully qualified in the three areas mentioned below in order best to serve the patients and their physicians. In addition, an interpretation is only as good as the level of technical expertise used to produce the data. The laboratory director, that is, the person responsible for the quality of work being generated by a laboratory, needs to have intimate knowledge about the technical aspects of the test and be able to train and supervise special technologists.

Therefore, clinical neurophysiology (EEG, EMG, EP) is properly the domain of those with special training in (1) nervous system anatomy, physiology, and diseases; (2) general electrophysiologic principles and techniques; and (3) the particular test in question (EEG, EMG, or EP). The latter two elements can best be achieved by at least 6 months' full-time study in each (a minimum of 18 months for all three tests) after the first element has been attained, usually (and preferably) via a neurology, neurosurgery, or physical medicine residency.

Additionally, journal editors and reviewers routinely abrogate their responsibilities so that the literature is replete with low-quality EP work. These sad examples contributed from major academic institutions by "name" investigators provide a leadership that can only result in erroneous interpretations in practice. Minimal standards for publication (and clinical interpretation) of standard EPs are (1) at least one figure per publication; (2) no redrawn, traced, or otherwise retouched waveforms; (3) at least two test replications (superimposed in figures) of any set of stimulus and recording parameters; (4) sufficient normal controls to reliably define normal variability; (5) use of limits of normality (parametric or other) that exclude at least 98% of the normal population (two standard deviations is insufficient); and (6) unequivocal recording derivation and polarity labels, and amplitude and time calibration marks.

Attention to these matters will automatically result in improvements in any current problems with delivery and utilization of clinical neurophysiologic laboratory tests.

1.4.4. Impact of MRI

Evoked potentials and MRI are largely complementary tests. The former provides a "view" of functional anatomy, whereas the latter mainly registers structure. Clinical studies have reported frequent cases where one test has missed a lesion detected by the other, for example, MRI may miss small lesions in the brain stem revealed by abnormal short-latency EPs (Cutler et al., 1986).

The impact of MRI on EP utilization varies with the specificity of the clinical question. Many clinical problems can be formulated to take advantage of the anatomic specificity and functional sensitivity of EPs (e.g., Is there an acoustic neuroma present?). Evoked potentials can then provide a more cost-effective and accurate answer than MRI. If the clinical question is more nebulous [e.g., Is there a lesion in the posterior fossa (intrinsic or extrinsic to the brain stem)?], then an MRI is indicated. In demyelinating disease, since these patients eventually have an MRI in their clinical course, they may as well have one early. To some extent, the clinical utility of EPs is dependent on the clinical EP experience of the physician, as is true for most medical tests.

There is no doubt that MRI and economic factors have decreased the numbers of EPs performed and this trend may continue, but it will not be to the patient's benefit.

The sensitivity, objectivity, anatomic specificity, and cost-effectiveness of EPs, extended by new applications, test variations, and modalities (motor EPs), will maintain their usefulness as a clinical tool.

2. EQUIPMENT

Most laboratories use equipment assembled commercially and these packages are usually sufficient for clinical purposes. However, in consideration of such equipment it is useful to keep in mind the following basic standards.

2.1. Electrodes

Proper preparation of the electrode–patient interface requires the use of a mild abrasive and cleansing agent to remove skin oils, dirt, and dead cells. Electrode paste should not contain irritants such as calcium chloride because this substance occasionally has caused granulomatous reactions (Schoenfeld et al., 1965; Giffin and Susskind, 1967). Both needle and surface electrodes are acceptable and show no significant differences in test results.

In routine testing, skin/scalp surface electrodes are most commonly used. A technique suitable for routine use is to use cup electrodes with small central holes and cream. The electrode site is prepared by rubbing with a cotton swab dipped in a suitable conductive abrasive compound, and a small amount of electrode paste or cream is applied to the site into which the cup electrode is buried. The area is then covered with cotton wool or adhesive tape. An alternative technique (especially suitable for prolonged testing) is to use cup electrodes and collodion. The electrode is held in place on the skin, and collodion is applied around the rim and dried rapidly with air blown through a tube from a small compressor. Alternatively, a small, single-thickness gauze square is dampened with collodion, the electrode is put in place, the gauze square is plastered over it, and the collodion is blown dry with compressed air (from available lines or compressors). This firmly affixes the electrode with little chance of it being pulled off. A blunt-tip 15-gauge needle or a stub adaptor is then pushed through the hole, being careful not to suddenly push through to the scalp. Saline gel electrode paste (used in electrocardiography) is then injected from the syringe to fill the electrode, by watching until paste appears around the edges. The blunt tip is then allowed to rest against the scalp and the needle rocked back and forth to gently abrade the scalp. This is continued until the electrode impedance is less than 3,000 ohms, as measured by an impedance meter. The needle or stub adaptor is then discarded. Alternatively, the collodion may be simply squeezed out of a collapsible tube onto the electrode to fix it to the skin. The paste tends to dry out over 24 hours but it can be replenished quite simply. These electrodes can be left on for at least 5 days without causing significant skin irritation in most patients, whereas there is a significant risk of infection with needle electrodes left in place for more than a few hours. The collodion is removed by acetone. Note that both collodion and acetone are flammable and fire laws regulate their storage and handling.

Needle electrode application is fast and is recommended in some difficult recording situations (e.g., intensive care units), especially when the patient is comatose. Conventional EEG needle electrodes are used; impedance values with these are slightly higher [5–7 kilo-ohms (K)] than with surface electrodes (2–3 K). Unless anchored, needle electrodes will come out if tension is applied to the connecting wires, so that care must be taken in this regard. There is no truth in the belief, widely held in both EP and EEG work, that needle electrodes produce more artifact than surface electrodes. Studies with surface electrodes overlying needle electrodes showed that one electrode type was not consistently worse than the other in this regard and that the relative amounts of artifact varied between sites and patients (personal observations). Hospitals now employ "universal precautions" (see Section 2.2) and used needles must be handled very carefully and discarded according to set procedures.

In less critical locations, such as over the brachial plexus in SEP testing, stick-on electrodes can be used. These have the advantage of fast application without discomfort.

When recording in difficult situations (e.g., infants in heated incubators) or over a prolonged period of time (e.g., monitoring in the operating room or intensive care unit), a technique must be used which firmly attaches the electrode to the skin surface and the use of collodion as previously described is the most satisfactory.

The state of the electrode–patient interface is critical in obtaining good EPs. Electrically, the interface acts as a complex circuit but it can be simplified as a resistor and capacitor in parallel. The resistance to current flow [termed impedance and expressed in kilo-ohms] is a good measure of the condition of the interface and can be measured by an impedance meter. These generate a known test current of a few millivolts and send it out through one connection with the patient (e.g., the ground electrode); the return path is via another patient connection (e.g., a recording electrode). The drop in voltage during this journey is proportional to the impedance at the two patient connections and is displayed in some fashion (e.g., on a meter). Alternating current is used since the interface has polarizing properties. The frequency of alternating current should be lower than the frequency of the signal of interest since apparent electrode impedance decreases with increasing test signal frequency, for example, it would be an error to use a 1,000-Hz impedance test signal for a PSVEP. The use of impedance meters or similar devices to verify the integrity of the electrode–patient interface is indispensable to EP work. Impedance values must be kept below 5 K or so and amplifier balance must be maintained within broad limits (i.e., the impedance of the two inputs to an amplifier should be approximately the same). If this is not so, excessive artifact (usually mains frequency) will be registered.

Electrode positions are measured carefully using bony skull landmarks and the International 10–20 System of electrode placement (Jasper, 1958). This does not guarantee that electrodes on the scalp overlie specific brain structures, but ensures that, on repeat testing in the same or different laboratories, the same electrode sites will be used. In addition, since the potential-field distribution of EPs varies between subjects, using the same electrode sites is important if intrasubject comparisons are to be reliable.

2.2. Infection Control—Universal Precautions

Universal precautions state that all patients are considered to be potential sources of hepatitis or AIDS virus and hospitals have a set of guidelines for their staff according to their likelihood of coming into contact with infective material. Anyone coming into contact with patients in an EEG/EP laboratory must follow these procedures. Gloves are not worn routinely, although anyone may do so if they wish. Because the patient's skin is likely to be abraded during the application of the electrodes, gloves are necessary if the skin condition of the technologist's hands is less than optimal. Gloves are worn for any procedure which requires needle puncture (e.g., external ear canal electrodes for BAEPs, lumbar needles for SEPs). Gowns, eye shields, and masks are available for special circumstances (e.g., patients vomiting, coughing, sneezing, or spitting, or when the technologist has a cold and the patient is thought to be unusually susceptible). The following procedures are followed routinely by technologists:

Wash hands.

Use gloves if skin condition of hands is not optimum.

If using sandpaper for SEP stimulation site preparation, use new piece for each patient.

Wash paste out of electrodes in hot running water. Soak in bleach for 5 minutes, together with toothbrush used for cleaning electrodes. Rinse in hot water.

Wipe headbox, electrode paste tube, marking pencil, and stimulating electrodes (SEP) with bleach.

Discard tape measure and pencil if the patient has head wounds.

Soak ground bands in bleach for 2 minutes; rinse in hot water.

Discard BAEP ear canal needle electrodes in locked box.

Lumbar needles should be similarly discarded.

Strip bed linen, wash hands, and put fresh linen on bed.

2.3. Electrode Boards and Channel Selectors

The electrodes plug into the amplifiers via a connector panel or electrode board. If the electrode board contains preamplifiers, impedance checking circuitry, or calibration devices, it should not be too bulky. It is usually attached to the averager by a cable and must be placed on or near the patient's bed and is liable to be pushed onto the floor or be difficult to secure if it is too large or heavy. Battery-powered preamplifiers, because of their weight and bulk, are particularly bothersome in this regard. The cable between the electrode board and the averager should be long enough to allow the averager to be stationed outside the patient testing room.

There must be a channel selector mechanism so that, if a given electrode is to provide input to more than one channel, each amplifier channel can be connected to the electrode without the use of jumper wires. These connector and selector panels must accommodate at least 12 electrodes. The selector panel should allow channel input selection to be done remotely at the averaging computer so that the subject is not disturbed. Similarly, remote electrode impedance testing capabilities are useful. The most modern amplifier systems have input electrode channel selection under averager control.

2.4. Amplifiers

Amplification in reasonable steps up to a gain factor of $500,000\times$ is necessary, subject to reduction if there is preamplification and/or amplification in the averaging computer. The amount of amplification used in a given situation depends on the amplitude of the signal of interest and the voltage resolution capabilities of the input (analog-to-digital converter) of the averaging computer.

Appropriate filtering of the amplified signal can shorten the averaging process, but incorrect filtering can distort waveform amplitudes and latencies. Signal-filtering capabilities required depend on the frequency response of the filters used. Approximate values of 1, 5, 10, 25, 100, and 300 Hz should be available as low-cutoff (high-pass) and 100, 250, 500, 1000, and 3000 Hz should be available as high-cutoff (low-pass) filters. A 60-Hz (or mains frequency) notch filter is sometimes useful, but since that frequency is usually included in the range of interest (e.g., for PSVEPs and SEPs), its use is limited. See chapters on methodology for specific bandpasses recommended for each test.

A neck–chest reference system should be available for noncephalic reference during long sweep duration testing. In these circumstances the chance of an electrocardiographic (ECG) QRS complex occurring during the sweep and causing an artifact reject are so high that few sweeps can be gathered from a noncephalic reference until the ECG signals are removed.

The most modern amplifier systems have all of their gain, filter, and input electrode channel selection under averager control. This greatly diminishes operator errors.

Efficient testing in EP clinical practice requires simultaneous registration of a minimum of four channels. This is dictated by (1) normal variations in potential field distribution over the head which require that multiple areas be recorded simultaneously (e.g., with midline PSVEP potentials or partial-field stimulation), and (2) the necessity of following a stimulus-induced volley from peripheral to central generator sites with recordings at several locations (e.g., SEPs). If partial-field PSVEP or spinal EP testing will be done often, then an eight-channel capacity is recommended for similar reasons, although five channels provide a comfortable coverage of required recording sites and derivations.

2.5. Signal Averagers: Seventeen Important Features

In approximate order of importance, the significant features of signal averaging systems are:

1. Number of input channels
2. Vertical (voltage) resolution
3. Horizontal (time) resolution
4. Data points per channel (memory capacity)
5. Stimulus repetition rate allowed
6. Calibration
7. Graphics output
8. Automatic artifact rejection
9. Data manipulation capabilities
10. Time and amplitude cursoring and labeling
11. Parallel (multiple) averaging
12. Automatic parameter set-up
13. Long-term data storage and retrieval
14. Plus–minus reference
15. User interface
16. Network and modem support
17. Report generation

2.5.1. Number of Input Channels

Channel capacity has already been discussed in Section 2.4.

2.5.2. Vertical (Voltage) Resolution

A signal averager is a digital computer. Since digital computers can work only with numbers, the continuously varying (i.e., analog) voltages produced by the differential amplifiers must be converted into sequences of numbers before the computer can perform averaging or any other

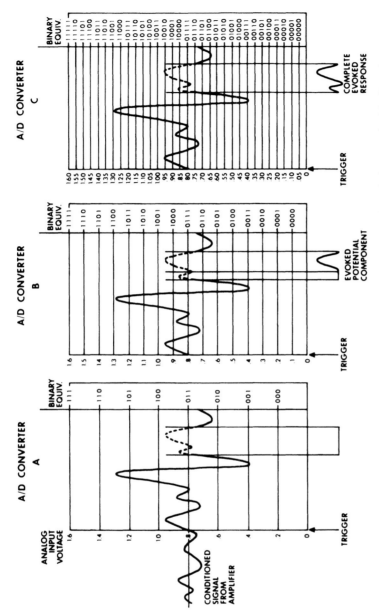

FIG. 1–3. Effect of using different ADC "bits" of resolution (word lengths) on vertical (voltage) resolution. The three ADCs **A**, **B**, and **C** have word lengths of 3, 4, and 5 bits, respectively. In each case diagrammed, the *horizontal lines* represent the voltage levels that can be discriminated by the ADC. Only ADC **C** has sufficiently small voltage increments to allow adequate resolution of the EP. (From Grass and Johnson, 1980, with permission.)

mathematical operation. This process is called analog-to-digital (A/D) conversion and the electronics which does it is called an A/D converter (ADC). The ADC is an integral part of the signal averager and ADC capabilities are important aspects of EP system functionality.

An ADC can differentiate only a finite number of voltage levels over its operating range. The number of levels is usually expressed as "bit" capacity and 2 to the power of "bits" equals the resolving power of the ADC over its operating range. For example, an 8-bit ADC will resolve 256 voltage levels and a 12-bit ADC will resolve 4,096. Effective resolution is also determined by the voltage range over which these levels are spread. For example, if an 8-bit ADC allows input voltages over a range from −5 to +5 V (a 10-V range), then the effective resolution is 10 V divided into 256 levels, or approximately 39 millivolts (mV) per level. This ADC will not be able to discriminate between voltage changes of less than 39 mV, unless a boundary is crossed.

If a physiologic signal of 0.1 µV is amplified 100,000 times, it assumes an amplitude of 10 mV. Therefore, the ADC described above could not discriminate a change in the physiologic signal from 0.1 to 0.3 µV (a 20-mV change at the ADC inputs). Thus, the physiologic signal must be examined carefully and its amplitude related to system amplification and ADC resolution to ensure proper waveform registration. The effects of different voltage resolutions on the shape of the reconstructed waveform seen by the computer are further illustrated in Fig. 1–3.

2.5.3. Horizontal (Time) Resolution

Each voltage measurement (sample) is taken by the ADC at a fixed interval of time from the previous one; this time interval is called the intersample interval (ISI) or dwell time. The shorter the ISI, the faster the sampling rate. Thus, an ISI of 1 msec is a sampling rate of 1,000 samples per second (often, perhaps erroneously, stated as 1,000 Hz). An ISI of 0.5 msec is a sampling rate of 2,000 samples/sec (2 samples/msec). For example, in PSVEP testing, the ISI often used is 0.5 msec and the analysis (sweep) duration is 500 msec. This results in a total of 1,000 samples per channel being taken.

At each sample time, the ADC measures the analog voltage level and outputs a corresponding number which is stored in the memory of the signal averager. The user controls both the ISI and the sweep duration.

The ISIs are set by the user and must match the characteristics of the waveforms of interest. For example, in BAEPs, wave V has a duration of about 1 msec. Therefore, this wave could not be properly resolved using an ISI of 0.5 msec, although that value is suitable for PSVEPs. The BAEP wave V peak would have only two measurements taken of its amplitude, which is insufficient to allow a good reconstruction of the waveform. Figure 1–4 further illustrates the relationship between ISIs and accuracy of waveform representation. There is obviously no constant set of ISIs suitable for EP work; rather, the requirements of waveform resolution must be considered separately in each situation.

2.5.4. Data Points per Channel (Memory Capacity)

As discussed in the preceding section, the number of data points gathered per channel is the product of the sampling rate and sweep duration. There is no consistent minimum number of data points for EP recordings. If it was desired to view only wave I of the BAEP and an ISI of 25 µsec was used (40 samples/msec) with a sweep duration of 4 msec (since wave I usually appears at 1.5–2 msec after the stimulus), only 160 samples would need to be acquired.

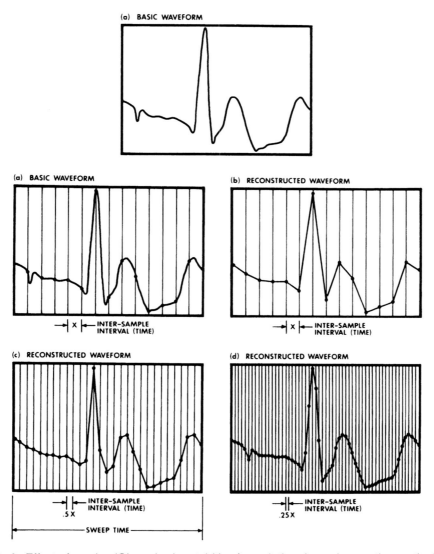

FIG. 1–4. Effect of varying ISIs on horizontal (time) resolution. In each case the *vertical lines* represent the times at which the waveform voltage is read (sampled) by the ADC. Only in case **d** with five samples taken during the major peak is the reconstruction of that waveform adequate. From Grass and Johnson, 1980, with permission.)

In addition, multiple channels require that much more memory capacity. Therefore, the proposed combinations of these factors must be considered to determine whether or not an averaging system has the capacity to perform a given application. For example, it might be proposed to study SEPs by using an ISI of 50 μsec (sampling rate of 20,000 Hz), a sweep duration of 50 msec, and eight recording channels. The ISI and sweep duration result in 1,000 samples per channel being gathered, and, since there are eight channels in use, a total of 8,000 data points will result. Thus, the averager must have a memory capacity of 1,000 samples per channel and 8,000 samples total.

Note that a high capacity of samples per channel and total samples allows resolution of both early and late EP components in the same channel without resorting to different sample rates in different channels to get the same data. For example, an ISI of 100 μsec (10 samples/msec) allows reasonable resolution of BAEP waveforms. If the sweep length is 400 msec, then the long-latency components can be gathered as well. This application requires that the averager have a capacity of 5,000 data points per channel and a correspondingly larger total capacity, depending on the number of channels to be used.

2.5.5. Stimulus Repetition Rate Allowed

Some signal averagers perform the averaging process and artifact rejection after data acquisition for a sweep has been completed. Since these operations take time (anywhere from 10 to 100 msec), the averager may not be able to respond to the next stimulus in the sequence. Usually this is not important since EP shape is not expected to change over these time periods, but it will take significantly longer to complete the given number of stimulus repetitions. Since this is often an important consideration, this factor must be considered in averaging system specifications.

New techniques of stimulation allow acquisition of stimuli at a much faster rate than previously possible [see Picton et al. (1992) and Chapter 17].

2.5.6. Calibration

It should be possible to inject a known calibration signal of approximately the same amplitude as the biological signal of interest at the electrode board, and have the signal processed by the entire amplifier and averager system, and displayed and plotted to provide a comprehensive check of the polarity, amplitude, latency, and filter characteristics of the system. Modern amplifiers are stable enough so that calibration is not required by the user. However, old habits die hard and it is still possible for an amplifier to fail in a fashion that is not easily recognizable from the raw signal monitor channel or the EP waveforms. Therefore, we should continue a practice of intermittent calibration checks, especially if there is anything suspicious or unusual about the EP waveforms. Also, manufacturers could provide an automatic amplifier calibration check on power up.

2.5.7. Graphics Output

For legal, comparative, research, and other purposes, permanent records of EP tracings must be made. Hard-copy (paper) output is a convenient and cheap method of accomplishing the above aims. Very few laboratories at present store EP data on magnetic (tape or disc) media. In addition, although time and amplitude cursoring facilities allow measurements to be made directly on the display screen, it is often necessary to confirm these or measure other aspects of the EP. This is most conveniently and accurately accomplished on 8×11-inch paper, rather than on the small computer cards or paper output used on some averaging systems. The important patient information (name, hospital identification number) and test information (date, time, amplifier, stimulator, and averager parameters in use) should be manually or automatically written onto the paper printout. Every piece of paper generated by the system should have this labeling.

Some graphics output devices use a dot-matrix format in which the resolution is limited by dot density. These may produce a "grain" effect that is not suitable for many purposes and should be carefully evaluated before purchase. Also, paper size is usually limited in these devices.

The EP machine should be able to acquire new data while producing hard-copy output of previous results.

2.5.8. Automatic Artifact Rejection

This feature must be present on a signal-averaging system. Most use a voltage threshold value and if any sample exceeds this, then the sweep is rejected as containing artifact. This can be switched on or off, but in most systems the threshold level cannot be changed. Desirable features of artifact rejection systems are (1) different thresholds allowed on each channel; (2) a display which shows the channel causing the sweep rejection, to allow prompt recognition of the artifact source; and (3) a variable number of samples which can exceed threshold before the sweep is rejected. This latter feature allows a brief artifact to occur without causing the sweep to be rejected. Most systems allow a delay between stimulus and start of sweep; this ensures that stimulus artifact will not be present on graphics output and that the stimulus artifact will not cause the sweep to be thrown out by artifact rejection. It may also be useful for the system to allow a pause after rejecting a sweep so that averaging does not become time-locked to an artifact (e.g., the QRS complex of the ECG) with inclusion of subsequent components of the artifact (e.g., the T wave of the ECG) in the average. There are also other sophisticated methods for minimizing artifact (see Chapter 17).

2.5.9. Data Manipulation Capabilities

A signal-averaging system must be able to store data from an averaging run (a "trial"), acquire another, and then display both (or up to six) together (superimposed) in order that intertrial variability can be determined. In addition, these separate trials must be able to be averaged together, added or subtracted from one another, or undergo some kind of filtering (digital filtering or smoothing). Furthermore, it must be possible to combine different channels in separate trials in the mathematical operations mentioned above, for example, to generate a derivation not recorded from two channels that have a common electrode and the two electrodes involved in the desired derivation (Fig. 1–5).

Effective display of the data often requires a time windowing capability. This allows a restricted section of a sweep to be expanded across the entire horizontal axis for detailed examination and more accurate measurement. Different channels often need to be displayed at different vertical magnifications, and at a high vertical aspect ratio. A channel should not be limited to its own band of display space but should be able to extend to the vertical limits of the screen without being clipped. It is sometimes helpful in creating a desired display if the order of channels on the screen can be mixed, for example, input channel one positioned at the bottom rather than at the top of the screen.

Color is not necessary in EP systems. Its only use is to distinguish between trials when two or more replications are superimposed on the screen, and this is infrequently needed. Manufacturers are compelled to use color to compete in a game of appearances, not functionality.

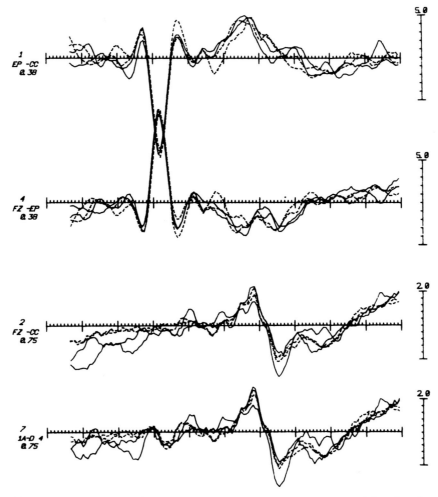

FIG. 1–5. Mathematical derivation of a channel from two channels containing the electrodes desired as inputs for the derived channel (and a common electrode). The upper three traces were all recorded simultaneously. Note that the upper two channels have the Erb's point (EP) electrode in common and also contain CC (central scalp contralateral to median nerve stimulation at the wrist) and FZ. FZ–CC is the desired derived channel, actually recorded as shown in the third trace. The fourth trace shows the result of subtracting trace 2 from trace 1; the contribution from the common electrode EP cancels out, leaving the derived FZ–CC activity. Note the marked similarity with the actually recorded trace 3. *Solid lines* are left-sided stimulation, *dashed lines* are right-sided stimulation of the same subject. Stimulus was an 0.2-msec electrical pulse at the wrist at 5/sec, sweep duration is 50 msec, amplitude values are in microvolts. Stimulus is at 0 msec, with a display delay to ignore stimulus artifact.

2.5.10. Time and Amplitude Cursoring and Labeling

These features are self-explanatory. The accuracy of the amplitude cursor is related to the method and frequency of its calibration. Ease of cursor movement is a major consideration here. Some systems allow labeling of cursor locations with conventional nomenclature and, in addition, keep a list of these labels and their latency values on one side of the screen. The labels and their latencies are written to the hard copy so that subsequent viewers can examine the waveform peak locations chosen by the operator when cursoring. The labels may be stored with the waveform data so that on redisplay the previous cursored points are visible for review. Free text labeling (descriptive) information should be able to be stored with the data.

Automatic machine scoring of EP waveforms has been frequently proposed with obvious implications for consistency of data (e.g., Pratt et al., 1994) but the clinical reliability of these technques has not yet been sufficiently demonstrated.

2.5.11. Parallel (Multiple) Averaging

Conventional signal averagers maintain a single averaging area. In some situations, it is advantageous to be able to maintain several averaging areas simultaneously. For example, in the BAEP different polarity clicks produce different waveform latencies and shapes, and, in some patients, the test may be normal with one click polarity but abnormal with the other (Emerson et al., 1981). If both click polarities are to be used, the test is performed most quickly and reliably (for comparisons) with alternating polarity clicks. The averager keeps the alternate sweeps in separate averaging areas. The separate areas can later be averaged together if a grand average is desired. Another example is in cognitive EPs, such as the P300. Here, different stimuli are intermixed randomly and the EPs to each must be kept separate. This type of work requires a minimum of two averaging areas; one averaging system available maintains up to seven averaging areas for optimum facility in this work.

2.5.12. Automatic Parameter Set-Up (Menus)

Since the same stimulus, recording, and averaging parameters are often used repeatedly, it is very helpful if the averaging system allows storage of complete sets of these "menus." A simple command results in the menu being read in from permanent storage and displayed. The menu can also be used by the system to automatically set amplifier and stimulator controls and to do montage selection, as an alternative to manual set-up by the operator. This greatly shortens set-up time and reduces errors, and most systems allow some degree of this. However, the more this is possible, the less the averaging system can interface with amplifiers and stimulators from a different manufacturer. Often there is a substantial charge for each menu and they can only be generated by the factory, but some systems allow the user to define parameter menus at no extra charge.

2.5.13. Long-Term Data Storage and Retrieval

This is partially discussed in Section 2.5.7 on graphics output. Hard-copy (paper) storage is cheap but may require excessive space. The data are not available for redisplay in different formats, further analysis (e.g., digital filtering), or various group statistical analyses (e.g., grand averaging of a group of normal subjects and variability analysis). Storage on magnetic media (and, soon, video discs) allows all of these but is more expensive. However, this is indispensable for EP research. If the diagnosis, therapy, drug treatment, and test interpretations are suitably encoded with the EP data, then, after a reasonable data base has accumulated, statistical work on such material is relatively easy.

Any such storage should automatically attach the important patient information (name, hospital identification number), test information (date, time, amplifier, stimulator, and averager parameters in use), and calibration information with each data file. When data files are accessed later, all of this information should then be available during the further processing of that data. The data should be compressed as is convenient but unpacking to a standard format should be available for those users wishing to transport the data to other analysis systems.

2.5.14. Plus–Minus Reference

Most averagers work mathematically by continually adding the new data in each sweep to the old data in the averaging area and, when all required sweeps have been added, dividing by the number of sweeps (normalization). If the averager adds the first sweep, subtracts the second, adds the third, subtracts the fourth, and so on, the EP is averaged out instead of the noise; this is a plus–minus average (Schimmel, 1967). Mathematical comparison between the conventional average and the plus–minus reference gives a measure of the signal-to-noise ratio, the amount of noise present, and thus also the reliability of the results (Wong and Bickford, 1980). There are other averaging techniques (e.g., statistical outlier rejection) which have great promise, and filtering techniques that can be used to decrease the amount of noise in an EP; these are covered in Chapter 17, which is largely an expansion of this topic.

2.5.15. User Interface

Most EP systems now are controlled largely via conventional keyboards with keys given special functionality by the software. Careful attention needs to be paid to ease or performance of operations performed repetitively during a test or data analysis. Arcane command strings and file names required to be typed should be minimized.

2.5.16. Networks and Modem Support

The EP machines must provide network and modem support for a variety of functions. In many circumstances the EP machine can acquire patient demographic data from other computer systems, minimizing entry by the technologist. The EP data themselves may be required to be viewed at a distance by a physician (e.g., operating room monitoring situations). Reports produced on the EP system must be transmitted to hospital-wide patient information systems. Service on the EP machines and downloading of new software might be greatly facilitated by modem access for the manufacturer. Fax capabilities directly from the EP machine would allow a cheap solution for remote interpretation of EP data.

2.5.17. Report Generation

In many circumstances the EP report will be best produced on the machine itself. Numerical data could be placed directly into the report, models of interpretation text can be used, and editing capabilities would allow a final report to be produced. This could be printed by the EP machine or transmitted to another system.

2.6. Stimulators

See Chapters 2, 4, and 6 on visual, auditory, and somatosensory EP for details about stimulators and effects of various stimulus parameters on EP waveforms.

3. CONVENTIONS

3.1. Polarity

The differential amplifiers used in neurophysiology record the voltage difference between two electrodes. There are only two possibilities: either Input 1 (I1; from electrode 1) becomes more positive relative to Input 2 (I2; from electrode 2), or vice versa. Another way of saying the same thing is that either I2 becomes more negative relative to I1, or vice versa. (I1 and I2 are often termed G1 and G2.) Both electrodes might be recording a negative potential, but if I1 is less negative than I2 then I1 is also relatively more positive than I2. If both electrodes are recording the same potential then the differential amplifier will see no voltage difference between them.

The direction of trace movement (up or down) is dependent on the way the amplifier and display unit electronics have been constructed to respond to a voltage difference between I1 and I2. If there is no voltage difference the trace does not move. If the electrodes attached to I1 and I2 are simply switched, the trace will move in the opposite direction when the same voltage difference is recorded by the two electrodes. This is a major source of errors in EP work and is the first thing that should be checked when results look familiar yet cannot be identified. A simple check if the EP waveforms are on paper is to hold the sheet in front of a light and rotate the bottom upward until the sheet is upside down and the waveforms are being viewed through the paper. This has the same effect as if the electrodes were switched. Some averaging systems can do this in the computer and reverse the display. Wiring between the averager and the plotter, if accessible, can also be plugged in incorrectly and is another source of the same problem.

The convention in EEG is that if I1 becomes relatively more negative than I2 (I2 more positive than I1), the trace moves upward. There is no universally recognized convention in EP work and attempts to standardize have usually only demonstrated a lack of understanding of the issues. For example, Donchin et al. (1977) stated that "in all published figures the polarity convention would be indicated by a + and − sign by the calibration signal." Since in many EP recording situations (e.g., BAEPs) both electrodes are active at different times, the above convention is inadequate because it does not include specification of which electrode's polarity is to be shown. The simplest procedure is to mark on the figure or state in the legend "Relative positivity of I1 produces an upward deflection" and state which electrodes are I1 and I2 (G1 and G2) for each channel. (Usually the electrode derivations of a channel are stated in order, I1 and I2, e.g., CZ–A1, where CZ is I1 and A1 is I2.)

Furthermore, there is no agreement on how to arrange polarity in specific tests. For example, in the BAEP some investigators have positivity of CZ (relative to the ear electrode) produce an upward deflection while other investigators have an opposite arrangement. These different practices render comparisons more difficult, but if one is attempting to understand results plotted "upside down" relative to one's own, the maneuver outlined above of holding the paper in front of a light, upside down and backward, is helpful.

Since there is no convention in EPs for arrangement of polarity, the most reasonable approach is to copy the method used by most investigators publishing work in that area. This allows one to most easily compare the literature with one's own results. The current recommended conventions are as follows: PSVEP—positivity of the occipital regions (e.g., OZ and inion) relative to distant electrodes (e.g., ears, FZ or CZ) produces a downward trace deflection; BAEP—positivity of the vertex relative to ear electrodes produces an upward trace deflection; SEP—negativity of the parietal scalp electrodes (contralateral to the limb stimulated) relative to distant electrodes (FZ or noncephalic) produces an upward trace deflection.

3.2. Waveform Nomenclature

Waveform nomenclature is most commonly derived from either of two methods: (1) the components are numbered in sequence by polarity, for example, N1, N2, N3, and so forth; or (2) the components are labeled according to their polarity and mean latency in normal subjects, for example, P100, N20. In a variation of the latter method a horizontal bar is drawn across the top of the number to indicate that this is a mean latency as opposed to an actual, individual measurement (which would have no bar). Other methods include using the name of the anatomic source of the waveform, for example, EP (Erb's point) for the name of the activity recorded from the brachial plexus, and using a neutral label, for example, A, B, C, and so forth. The latter method is particularly useful when both electrodes involved in a channel are active and contributing opposite polarity activity to the final waveform; use of a polarity label in this case is only confusing. However, in these cases I now propose a slight modification of the polarity–latency method in which the label reflects the polarity of the activity at G1 and G2, in that order, with the latency following. For example, in SEP recordings the activity registered in the FZ–CII derivation (with a peak at 13 msec after stimulation at the wrist) is contributed by positivity at FZ and negativity at CII; the label used is P/N13 (see figures in Chapters 6 and 7).

Donchin et al. (1977) suggested that a distinction be made between "observational" and "theoretical" nomenclature, the former being actual data and the latter being a more abstract concept. The latter would be distinguished by a mark such as the bar over the numbers, as suggested previously. Thus, one would say that the PSVEP waveform labeled P125 in a trace is P100 (with a bar). However, labeling the waveforms differently according to their observed latencies merely confuses interpretations and comparisons. In addition, the same waveform may appear at a different latency simply because of "technical" factors. For example, most of the SEP potentials produced by stimulation of the median nerve at the wrist can also be evoked by similar stimulation of other nerves in the upper and lower limbs. Although differences in conduction distance account for the supraspinal potentials appearing at different latencies after the stimulus, they presumably are being generated in the same anatomical structures. Different "observational" labels would complicate discussions of analogous waves and hinder the interpretation of the patterns of SEP abnormalities seen following stimulation of the upper and lower limbs of patients with CNS lesions.

Perhaps the best approach is that recommended for polarity arrangement, that is, use of the method employed by the majority of investigators publishing work in that field. In this respect, the suggested nomenclatures would be as follows: PSVEP—first major positive peak at the inion labeled P100; BAEP—vertex positive peaks labeled in sequence with Roman numerals I through VI. Although there is no clear consensus for nomenclature of SEP components, the modification of the polarity–latency method suggested previously (e.g., P/N13) is the least ambiguous (see Chapters 6 and 7).

4. MEASUREMENTS

4.1. Latency

Latency in EP work is usually stated in milliseconds (thousandths of a second). The term "latency" most commonly refers to the time interval between the stimulus and a specific point on the EP waveforms. This time interval is also called "absolute latency" and "implicit time." In EP studies, the waveform peak is most commonly used as the measurement point. This is different from peripheral nerve conduction studies where peak onset (departure from baseline) is most commonly used. The time separation between two peaks is termed "interwave latency" or "interpeak latency." These measurements can be made in three ways: (1) by using cursors in the signal averager; (2) by readout of the latencies directly from the hard-copy printout if it has calibrated time marks; and (3) by calculations based on a few known parameters (this is only necessary when neither of the other two methods is available).

4.1.1. Use of Cursors

Most commercial signal averagers have latency cursors. A cursor is a mark on the screen which can be moved over the waveforms; its position in milliseconds is always displayed on the screen or on a light-emitting diode (LED) numerical display. If two cursors are available, the time separation between them gives interpeak latencies. These values are written on the hard-copy output, either by the signal averager or manually by the operator, or noted in the interpretation. In addition, some systems allow labels to be placed on the screen at the current cursor location; the labels also appear on the hard-copy output in the same place and indicate to other interpreters the point at which that measurement was taken.

4.1.2. Direct Readout of Latencies

Since many interpretations are performed some time after the test was completed, the interpreter does not have the cursor facility available to assist with latency determinations (unless the signal averager is able to store and redisplay the data). If the hard-copy printout has time marks on it which are easily read in milliseconds and, if appropriate, fractions of a millisecond, then there is no difficulty in checking latency values. This is achieved by writing the EP waveforms on graph paper calibrated so that the time correspondence is precise, or by the signal averager writing time marks onto the paper in addition to the EP waveforms.

4.1.3. Calculations from First Principles

If the facilities in Sections 4.1.1 and 4.1.2 are not available, then the latencies must be calculated from "first principles." Four values must be known (Fig. 1–6).

1. Presweep delay: The start of the averaging sweep may be delayed by this amount of time after the stimulus is delivered in order to avoid writeout of stimulus artifact.
2. Sweep duration: The time duration of the entire sweep.
3. Sweep length: The length of the entire sweep.
4. Latency distance: Distance from sweep start to waveform point of interest (for absolute latency), or distance between waveforms (for interpeak latency).

Latency in milliseconds is the desired value, absolute or interpeak. Using simple proportionalities, since:

$$\frac{\text{Latency (msec)}}{\text{Latency distance (mm)}} = \frac{\text{sweep duration (msec)}}{\text{sweep length (mm)}}$$

it follows that:

$$\text{Latency (msec)} = \frac{\text{latency distance (mm)} \times \text{sweep duration (msec)}}{\text{sweep length (mm)}}$$

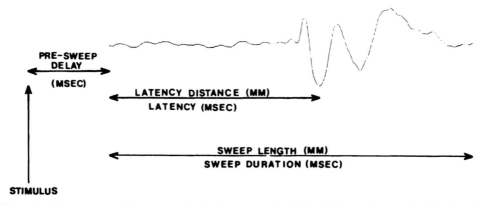

FIG. 1–6. Distances and times used in the latency calculation. Refer to the text for the formula.

but presweep delay, if present, must be added in, thus:

$$\text{Latency (msec)} = \text{delay (msec)} + \frac{\text{latency distance} \times \text{sweep duration}}{\text{sweep length}}$$

The values obtained are rounded off according to the order of magnitude of the numbers and accuracy of measurement.

4.2. Amplitude

Amplitude in EP work is usually stated in microvolts (millionths of a volt). Amplitude of EPs can be measured by three methods: (1) baseline to peak; (2) peak of one polarity to the immediately following peak of the opposite polarity; and (3) area under a peak. The first two of these are most commonly used and the amplitude measurement is sometimes termed "absolute" amplitude. There are no good reasons for using one or the other method except that difficulty in defining the baseline sometimes makes that method more subjective than the peak-to-peak method. However, the peak-to-peak method to some extent "mixes apples and oranges" because the activity producing a peak of one polarity may have nothing to do with the activity producing the immediately following peak of opposite polarity. For example, in the SEP, N20 amplitude is sometimes defined as peak of N20 (a negative peak) to following positive trough (P23); these different polarity activities are produced in different anatomic structures so that the single measure of their peak-to-peak amplitude is confusing.

Area measurements can be done effectively only with computers (Anthony et al., 1979), and practical difficulties in defining the starting points and endpoints of the peak make this approach less useful, at least at present. Theoretically, however, this is the most reasonable technique.

Absolute amplitudes are much less useful interpretive tools than latencies because of much greater variation in results obtained from normal subjects. Also, amplitudes are more likely than latencies to have a non-Gaussian (nonnormal) distribution and so require statistical parameters more complex than standard deviations for definition of normality. As a consequence of these factors, amplitude measures have been most useful when used in comparison with the same measure on the other side of the subject, that is, when subjects serve as their own controls. The amplitude difference is expressed as a proportionality (e.g., percentage) rather than as an absolute amplitude difference. Similarly, waveforms on the same side of a subject may be expressed in terms of their amplitude relationship to one another, rather than as an absolute amplitude difference. For example, in BAEPs recorded in specific conditions, wave I height should not be more than 218% of wave V height. Note that when proportionality comparisons are made it is not necessary to work in terms of microvolts; direct millimeter measurements can be made if all recording and display parameters are equal. This makes the calculations much easier.

The basic technique in amplitude measurement of EPs is to relate waveform height to the height of a known calibration signal, amplification being unchanged between recording of the two signals and the same number of sweep repetitions being used. The only complicating factor is the vertical magnification (sometimes termed "display scale") employed in displaying the waveforms. The waveforms are usually exaggerated in the vertical dimension on display as this makes determination of waveform peaks easier. Obviously, when the display scaling is different for the EP and calibration waveforms (as is usually the case) this must be taken into account in the calculation. If the relationship between the two is not a simple ratio, then proportionality calculations are necessary.

4.3. Determination of Normal Limits

If clinical interpretation of EPs is to be reliable and consistent, there must be some method for determining whether or not a patient's test results fall within the range of normal. In most situations, this requires that each laboratory perform on at least 35 normal subjects the same test that will be used with patients. It must be stressed that exactly the same parameters should be used with the normal subjects as will be used with patients because many of these factors have significant effects on EP latencies and amplitudes. For example, in PSVEPs, small changes in pattern luminance and ambient room illumination will result in P100 latency changes large enough to render a test that was normal with one level of illumination abnormal with another. Thus, it makes no sense to test normal subjects in one room with one stimulator, and to test patients in another room with a different stimulator. It is true that in some areas there is very little difference between results obtained in many laboratories, and one laboratory could use normal results obtained in another. An example of this is BAEP interwave latencies, which differ by scarcely more than two tenths of a millisecond in several published series of normal values. However, testing normal subjects accomplishes two things: (1) a normal data base is gathered, and (2) the technician and physician become familiar and comfortable with the test. The second of these is a very important result of testing normal subjects and is the overriding consideration even when another laboratory's normal values might be used, especially in the case where no one involved has any experience with the new test.

Most EP parameters have a bell-shaped (Gaussian or normal) distribution. In this case, standard deviations (SD) can be used effectively to describe the expected bounds of normal. The standard deviation multiple used as the limit of normal must include at least 98% of the population being tested; most laboratories use 2.5 (98.8%) or 3 (99.7%) SD. It is completely incorrect to use 2.0 or less SD multiples to define the upper limit of normal for purposes of clinical interpretation. Other statistical measures are also used, for example, cumulative frequency distributions and confidence limits, and may provide a more readily understandable picture of the relationship of a given patient's test results to the normal population. Nonparametric (distribution-free) methods are used when the normal values have a non-Gaussian distribution. For example, many amplitude measures demonstrate a steeper curve on the low-amplitude side than on the high-amplitude side. In these cases there is some validity in using the most extreme value seen in normals as the limit of normality, without getting into complex statistical methods.

A distinction must be made between statistically significant differences between groups or populations (e.g., a group of patients versus a group of normal subjects) and between one individual and a group or population. For example, an individual may be within the bounds of normal (within 2.5 or 3 SD, as defined by a group of normal subjects), and yet when his or her group is compared with a group of normals, it may be significantly different from them. For example, the great majority of patients with postconcussion syndrome have normal BAEPs when their tests are compared individually with a group of normal subjects. However, if BAEP results from a group of patients with postconcussion syndrome are compared statistically with BAEP results from the normal group, the two groups are significantly different. Although the latter finding is interesting, in the clinical interpretation situation one is always dealing with an individual patient versus a normal population and such fine distinctions cannot be made with any degree of reliability. See Chapter 12 for a more detailed discussion of statistical considerations in EPs.

5. IN CASE OF DIFFICULTY

5.1. General Considerations

When EPs cannot be recorded, a systematic approach, common to all modalities, most easily resolves methodologic difficulties. First, one must consider whether the EPs are absent because of a conduction defect (lesion) in the patient, or because of a technical error. If some EP waveforms are clearly seen but others are poorly seen or absent, then this is unlikely to be due to a technical error. For example, in BAEP and SEP recordings, if the peripherally generated peaks from the eighth nerve and the brachial plexus, respectively, are present and clearly seen, then absence of later waves is seldom due to a technical error. Conversely, if no waves at all are seen after trial repetition, especially if no stimulus artifact is present, a technical error should be excluded. If a technical error is a possibility, the sections below should be considered in sequence.

5.2. Stimulus

The question here is whether or not the patient is being adequately stimulated. Does the patient see, feel, or hear the stimulus, and/or can you see, feel, or hear the stimulus? If not, the following questions should be asked: (1) Is the stimulator power on? (2) Are the stimulator controls set properly (frequency, duration, intensity, repeat mode)? (3) Is the stimulus turned on at the patient interface (e.g., at an SEP remote stimulus control box)? (4) Is there a break in the wires going to the stimulating electrodes (this is a common problem)? and (5) Is the synchronization pulse getting to the averager?

5.3. Amplifier

The question here is whether or not the signals from the patient are reaching the amplifiers, being amplified and filtered properly, and passed on to the averager. Can you examine the amplified signal just as it reaches the averager to judge its appearance? Does it have a proper appearance or is it all 60-Hz artifact or a flat line? (1) Are the patient electrodes plugged into the electrode interface panel ("headbox")? (2) Is the headbox connected to the amplifiers? (3) Are the channel derivations selected properly? (4) Are the amplifiers "on" (not set to "standby" or "cal")? (5) Are the gain and filter controls set properly? If there is any question, you may want to look at a known calibration signal.

5.4. Averager

Is the averager synchronized properly with the stimulus or is it being controlled by another stimulator or free-running? Was the memory erased before you began the trial? The above steps will reveal the source of the problem in the great majority of cases. If the answer still has not been discovered, then you must average a calibration signal to test the entire system.

REFERENCES

Abrams HL (1979): The "overutilization" of X-rays. *N Engl J Med* 300:1213–1216.

Achor LJ, Starr A (1980a): Auditory brain stem responses in the cat. I. Intracranial and extracranial recordings. *Electroencephalogr Clin Neurophysiol* 48:154–173.

Achor LJ, Starr A (1980b): Auditory brain stem responses in the cat. II. Effects of lesions. *Electroencephalogr Clin Neurophysiol* 48:174–190.

Anthony PF, Durrett R, Pulec JL, Hartstone JL (1979): A new parameter in brain stem evoked response: Component wave areas. *Laryngoscope* 89:1569–1578.

Blumhardt LD (1984): Do evoked potentials contribute to the early diagnosis of multiple sclerosis? In: *Dilemmas in the Management of Neurological Patient*, edited by CH Warlow and J Garfield, pp 18–42. Churchill Livingstone, Edinburgh.

Blumhardt LD, Halliday AM (1981): Cortical abnormalities and the visual evoked potential. *Doc Ophthalmol Proc Series* 27:347–365.

Brooks EB, Chiappa KH (1982): A comparison of clinical neuro-ophthalmological findings and pattern shift visual evoked potentials in multiple sclerosis. In: *Clinical Applications of Evoked Potentials in Neurology*, edited by J Courjon, F Mauguiere, and M Revol, pp 453–457. Raven Press, New York.

Buchwald JS, Huang CM (1975): Far-field acoustic response: Origins in the cat. *Science* 189:382–384.

Chiappa KH (1979): Evoked responses I: Pattern shift visual. In: *Weekly Update: Neurology and Neurosurgery, Vol 2*, edited by P Scheinberg, pp 64–70. Continuing Professional Education Center, NJ.

Chiappa KH (1983): *Evoked Potentials in Clinical Medicine*, 1st ed. Raven Press, New York.

Chiappa KH, Young RR (1985): Evoked responses: Overused, underused, or misused. *Arch Neurol* 42:76–77.

Chiappa KH, Harrison JL, Brooks EB, Young RR (1980): Brain stem auditory evoked responses in 200 patients with multiple sclerosis. *Ann Neurol* 7:135–143.

Cutler JR, Aminoff MJ, Brant-Zawadzki M (1986): Evaluation of patients with multiple sclerosis by evoked potentials and magnetic resonance imaging: A comparative study. *Ann Neurol* 20:645–648.

Donchin E, Callaway E, Cooper R, Desmedt JE, Goff WR, Hillyard SA, Sutton S (1977): Publication criteria for studies of evoked potentials (EP) in man. Report of a committee. *Prog Clin Neurophysiol* 1:1–11.

Eisen A, Cracco RQ (1983): Overuse of evoked potentials: Caution. *Neurology* 33:618–621.

Eisenberg JM, Williams SV (1981): Cost containment and changing physicians' practice behaviour. Can the fox learn to guard the chicken coop? *J Am Med Assoc* 246:2195–2201.

Emerson RG, Brooks EB, Parker SW, Chiappa KH (1982): Effects of click polarity on brain stem evoked potentials in normal subjects and patients: Unexpected sensitivity of wave V. *Ann NY Acad Sci* 388:710–721.

Giffin RG Jr, Susskind C (1967): EEG skin "burn": Electrical or chemical. *Med Res Eng* 6:58–63.

Grass ER, Johnson E (1980): *An Introduction to Evoked Response Signal Averaging*. Grass Instruments Company, Quincy, MA.

Griner PF, Liptzin B (1971): Use of the laboratory in a teaching hospital. Implications for patient care, education, and hospital costs. *Ann Int Med* 75:157–163.

Griner PF (1972): Treatment of acute pulmonary edema: Conventional or intensive care? *Ann Int Med* 77:501–506.

Griner PF, Glaser RJ (1982): Misuse of laboratory tests and diagnostic procedures. *N Engl J Med* 307:1336–1339.

Haimovic IC, Pedley TA (1982a): Hemi-field pattern reversal evoked potentials. I. Normal subjects. *Electroencephalogr Clin Neurophysiol* 54:111–120.

Haimovic IC, Pedley TA (1982b): Hemi-field pattern reversal evoked potentials. II. Lesions of the chiasm and posterior visual pathways. *Electroencephalogr Clin Neurophysiol* 54:121–131.

Heilman RS (1982): What's wrong with radiology? *N Engl J Med* 306:477–479.

Jasper HH (1958): The ten-twenty electrode system of the International Federation. *Electroencephalogr Clin Neurophysiol* 10:371–375.

Levy DE, Bates D, Caronna JJ, Cartlidge NEF, Knill-Jones RP, Lapinski RH, Singer BH, Shaw DA, Plum F (1981): Prognosis in nontraumatic coma. *Ann Int Med* 94:293–301.

Martin AR, Wolf MA, Thibodeau LA, Dzau V, Braunwald E (1980): A trial of two strategies to modify the test-ordering behaviour of medical residents. *N Engl J Med* 303:1330–1336.

Martin SP, Donaldson MC, London CD, Peterson OL, Colton T (1974): Inputs into coronary care during 30 years. A cost effectiveness study. *Ann Int Med* 81:289–293.

Menken M (1983): Consequences of an oversupply of medical specialists: The case of neurology. *N Engl J Med* 308:1224–1226.

Noth J, Engel L, Friedemann HW (1984): Evoked potentials in patients with Huntington's disease and their offspring. I. Somatosensory evoked potentials. *Electroencephalogr Clin Neurophysiol* 59:134–141.

Oken BS, Chiappa KH (1986): Statistical issues concerning computerized analysis of brainwave topography. *Ann Neurol* 19:493–494.

Picton TW, Champagne SC, Kellett AJC (1992): Human auditory evoked potentials recorded using maximum length sequences. *Electroencephalogr Clin Neurophysiol* 84:90–100.

Pratt H, Mittelman N, Geva AB (1994): Machine scoring of somatosensory evoked potentials. *Electroencephalogr Clin Neurophysiol* 92:89–92.

Rowe MJ, Carlson C (1980): Brain stem auditory evoked potentials in postconcussion dizziness. *Arch Neurol* 37:679–683.

Schimmel H (1967): The plus/minus reference: Accuracy of estimated mean components in average response studies. *Science* 157:92–93.

Schoenfeld RJ, Grekin JN, Mehregan A (1965): Calcium deposition in the skin. A report of 4 cases following electroencephalography. *Neurology* 15:477–480.

Shuman WP, Heilman RS (1979): The radiologist as a consultant. *JAMA* 242:1519–1520.

Wong PKH, Bickford RG (1980): Brain stem auditory evoked potentials: The use of noise estimate. *Electroencephalogr Clin Neurophysiol* 50:25–34.

Evoked Potentials in Clinical Medicine,
3d ed., edited by Keith H. Chiappa.
Lippincott–Raven Publishers, Philadelphia © 1997.

2

Pattern-Shift Visual Evoked Potentials: Methodology

Keith H. Chiappa

Department of Neurology, Harvard Medical School, and EEG Laboratory,
Massachusetts General Hospital, Boston, Massachusetts 02114

1. EQUIPMENT

The preferred stimulus for clinical investigation of the visual pathways is a shift (reversal) of a checkerboard pattern (usually black and white). The squares simply reverse without change in total light output (luminance) from the screen. There are two major differences between evoked potentials (EPs) produced in this fashion (without change in luminance) and other visual stimuli that do produce a change in luminance (e.g., strobe light or pattern-flash): (1) greater variation in all EP measures between normal subjects and even in a single normal subject studied at different times with the latter type of stimulus, and (2) greater sensitivity to the presence of conduction defects in the visual paths with the former.

With respect to the first point, in a group of 80 normal subjects tested with strobe (flash) stimulation (Kooi et al., 1965), two waveforms (IV and V) used clinically were missing at least 6% of the time and, when present, had latency values (time from stimulus to wave peak) with 1 standard deviation (SD) equal to at least 10% of the mean value. In contrast, with pattern-shift stimulation in normal subjects, the waveform used for clinical interpretation (P100) is never absent and has latency values with 1 SD equal to 5% of the mean value (Halliday et al., 1973b; Shahrokhi et al., 1978).

With respect to the second point, Fig. 2–1 shows a patient with a normal response to strobe stimulation but an abnormal response to pattern-shift stimulation. If both tests are

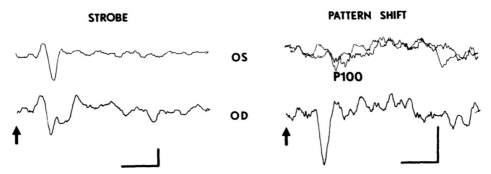

FIG. 2–1. Visual EPs from a patient with multiple sclerosis (MS). Note normal results with strobe stimulus and abnormal results with pattern-shift stimulus in left eye (OS). Recordings taken from OZ to CZ bipolar derivation; each line is the average response to 128 stimulus repetitions; the abnormal test is repeated for verification of P100 latency and amplitude. OZ positivity produces a downward deflection. Calibration marks are 100 msec and 5 μV. (From Chiappa, 1983a, with permission).

done routinely on patients, dissociations like this are not rare (Fig. 2–2 illustrates this effect in a large group of patients). Therefore, strobe (flash) stimulation has clinical utility only in restricted cases: (1) when the question is whether or not at least part of the visual pathways from retina to visual cortex are intact [e.g., following trauma to the orbit (Fig. 2–3), during surgery in the region of the optic nerves, and in various neonatal diseases], and (2) when the patient is unable to cooperate sufficiently for a pattern-shift visual evoked potential (PSVEP) examination to be performed (e.g., during general anesthesia, in coma, or in very young infants) (Taylor et al., 1987b). The information gathered from strobe stimulation is more qualitative than quantitative but in these specific situations is sufficient to answer the clinical questions.

The terms "pattern-reversal" and "pattern-shift" are used interchangeably, although strictly they may not mean the same thing. Pattern-shift stimulators most commonly in use are either electronic [the pattern is displayed on a television screen or array of light-emitting diodes (LEDs) and reversed by the electronics of the display] or mechanical (the pattern is projected from a slide projector, reflected off a small mirror onto the back of a translucent screen, and reversed by electrically rotating the reflecting mirror an amount sufficient to cause the checks to swap places). See Section 8.1.8 for a detailed comparison of stimulator types. All methods stimulate without change in overall luminance and there is no evidence that there is any practical clinical difference between any of these techniques with respect to sensitivity in revealing abnormalities. TV pattern stimulators are easier to use because many different check sizes, stimulus fields, and stimulus rates are readily available.

There is some debate about whether gratings are a better stimulus than checks. The frequency content of gratings can be focused more than that of checks, and to some this implies a more rigorous scientific approach. However, in clinical practice there seems to be no significant difference between the two with respect to sensitivity to abnormal visual system functioning.

Other stimulus parameters which have important effects on PSVEP waveforms are checkerboard pattern dimensions (visual angles subtended by the entire pattern and individual checks) and luminance, and ambient room illumination. See Section 8 for a full discussion of the effects of these and other factors on PSVEP waveforms.

Flash E P

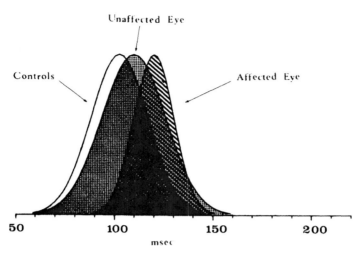

Pattern E P

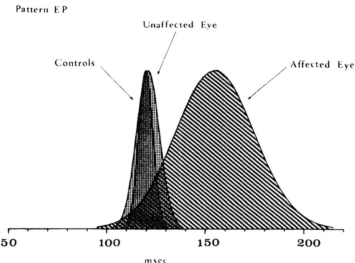

FIG. 2–2. Standardized Gaussian curves for mean latency of the major positivity of the flash (*upper graph*) and pattern VEP (*lower graph*) in normal subjects and the affected and unaffected eyes of patients with acute unilateral optic neuritis from the study by Halliday et al. (1972). Note that the spread of latencies in the control group is much smaller for the pattern EP than for the flash EP and that the mean delay in the affected eye is much larger for the pattern response than for the flash; the separation of normal and abnormal groups is more complete with the pattern EP. (From Halliday et al., 1979b, with permission).

Visual angle is a function of the distance from the subject's eye to the pattern and the width of the pattern (or check). It may be calculated as follows: (1) divide the width (or height) of the pattern (or check) by 2.0; (2) divide that answer by the eye–pattern distance (measured in same units as width); (3) on a calculator or in tables, find the angle that has a tangent value equal to the answer obtained in step 2; and (4) multiply this angle by 2.0. The overall pattern width should be greater than 8° if only full-field stimulation will be used or

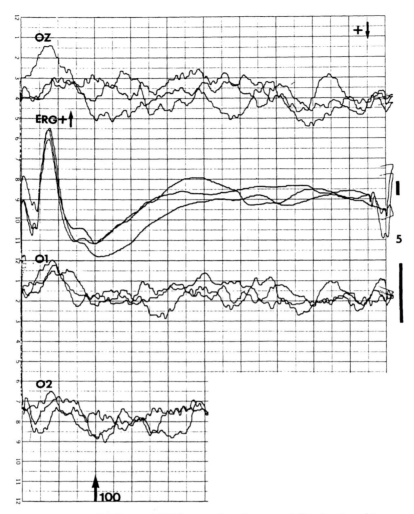

FIG. 2–3. Strobe (flash) ERG and VEP in a patient in coma following head trauma, with or-bital fractures visible radiologically. The posterior scalp channels (OZ, O1, and O2) register no cortical EP, but the ERG is normal, indicating a conduction block central to the retina, pre-sumably a laceration of the optic nerve. The poor prognosis was confirmed when the patient awoke from coma and was blind in that eye. Horizontal divisions are 25 msec (*arrow* is at 100 msec), the calibration bars are 5 μV (small bar is for ERG channel only). Relative posi-tivity of the active electrode causes an upward trace deflection in the ERG channel, down-ward otherwise.

greater than 20° if partial-field stimulation will be used (see Section 8.1.5 for a discussion of partial-field stimulation). Since the screen is usually placed at least 70 cm from the eye, the minimum dimensions above would be 10 cm and 24 cm, respectively. If a large enough screen is not available when partial-field stimulation is performed the subject can be in-structed to focus on the edge of the full screen in order to provide a stimulus of the neces-sary dimensions. The disadvantage of this maneuver is that the half-field response is then not a logical half of the full-field response, both having been produced by the same size stimulus field. However, the potential-field distribution to the half-field stimulation is the most important data and this is most reliable with the larger stimulus size. The check size most commonly used is about 35′ (minutes) (7 mm at 70 cm), although checks as small as 15′ (3 mm) are used. The smaller checks may have greater sensitivity in revealing abnormalities; however, responses obtained with smaller checks are more likely to be affected by visual acuity and luminance changes. At least two check sizes should be tested, and 35′ and 70′ are reasonable. The 12′ to 20′ checks may be used but care must be taken to ensure that poor visual acuity is not the cause of a latency delay.

Luminance (brightness) is not a problem except that it must be very carefully controlled because small changes in luminance produce significant latency shifts in the PSVEP. Television-type devices need to have the variable brightness control removed or otherwise locked. The loss of screen luminance with phosphor aging does not seem to be significant. At present it is not important to be able to quantify screen luminance. The variety of luminance units in use and the widely differing numbers stated in the literature have demonstrated either the difficulty of using or the inaccuracy of available techniques for measuring luminance. However, it is recommended that a high-quality, photographic light meter be used to record the screen luminance, and this reading should be checked once per week to ensure that there have been no major changes. The needle position on the light meter is all that needs to be followed (i.e., this does not need to be translated into a standard measure of brightness such as foot-candles). See also the discussion on luminance in the IFCN recommended standards (Celesia et al., 1993). The same document also discusses pattern contrast, which should be maintained at as high a level as possible without the white checks affecting the black checks. Changes in contrast also cause latency shifts and so this must be kept constant after normal values have been determined.

If partial-field stimulation is to be performed, the greatest reliability is obtained from devices which allow sequential stimulation of the fields to be compared. For example, if the lateral half-fields are being studied, the left half-field is shifted (reversed) and a few hundred milliseconds later the right half-field is shifted. The response to both shifts is recorded on the same sweep of the averager so that they are side by side for comparison (Rowe, 1981). The full-field shift can also be included in the same sweep (Chiappa and Jenkins, 1982). This technique automatically controls for changes in attention which can affect the amplitude of the responses.

Partial-field stimulation is usually accomplished either by the electronics of the display blanking out part of the screen, by physically covering part of the screen (e.g., with cardboard), or by instructing the subject to focus on one edge of the screen. The disadvantages of these techniques are (1) subjects must concentrate their gaze at the edge of a lighted area—this is difficult to maintain; (2) since the results of stimulation of different areas are collected at widely spaced time intervals, the possibility of varying levels of concentration makes amplitude comparisons much less reliable; (3) since the results of each stimulation must be written out before the next can be performed, the patient's presence is required for a longer period of time, and (4) when the half-field is not exactly half the size of the full-field stimulus, the relationship between the two modes of stimulation is partially lost (e.g., the midline amplitude from full-field stimulation is the sum of the two half-field amplitudes when the half-fields subtend half the angle subtended by the full field). All of these objections are overcome by the use of a sequential technique of stimulation (see Rowe, 1981; Chiappa and Jenkins, 1982) in which the pattern is under electronic or computer program control and any part of the pattern can be reversed while other parts are unchanged. For example, the left half-field can be reversed while the right half-field remains unchanged. The important point here is that there is no overall luminance change despite the fact that only a part of the full stimulus field has been altered. Subsequent to the left-field reversal, the right

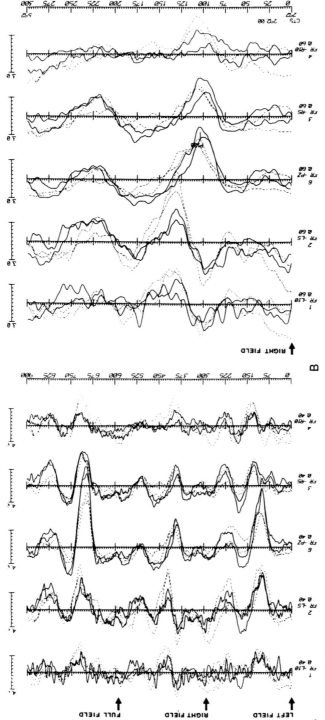

FIG. 2–4. Sequential partial- and full-field stimulation. **A** is the entire 900-msec sweep with all three EPs visible; **B** is the 300-msec time window starting at the instant of right-field stimulation, expanded by the EP computer system for better resolution of the waveforms. The subject is gazing at the center of a checkerboard field (30° diameter, 88′ checks). At the *arrows* the specified part of the field is reversed, other areas being held constant; these stimuli occur about 292 msec apart. Recording is from five electrodes around the posterior scalp; 5 cm above the inion and 5 and 10 cm lateral to the midline on either side. Sweep duration is 900 msec. The averaged responses to two trials of 100 stimuli each for each eye are superimposed (*solid trace*, left eye; *dashed trace*, right eye). The averaging system allows the individual time windows to be expanded across the screen for greater accuracy of latency measurements. Reference is FpZ; calibration marks are in microvolts and milliseconds.

field can be reversed 300 msec later and the entire field 300 msec after that. If a 1,000-msec recording sweep duration is used and the sweep started simultaneously with the left-field reversal, then the responses to all three stimuli (left-, right-, and full-field reversals) will be on the same sweep (Fig. 2–4). This technique answers the three problems stated above: (1) gaze is directed at all times toward the center of the pattern so that eccentric fixation is not a problem, (2) since such a short time separates the three stimuli, factors such as changes in concentration will have no effect on the EPs, and (3) no time is lost writing out the individual stimulations. If the EP machine allows time windowing, the individual stimulations can be displayed and cursored separately (Fig. 2–4B).

The PSVEP equipment is set up so that the subject can be seated at 1 m (eye distance from the screen). Provision must also be made so that the technician can check to see whether or not the subject is watching the pattern. This can be accomplished by having the equipment arranged so that the technician, stationed at the averager, is at an oblique angle in front of the subject as the latter sits watching the screen. Some laboratories use a closed-circuit TV camera on the pattern-shift equipment to accomplish this. Even with these precautions it is still possible for the subject to look just off the edge of the screen and produce a very low-voltage or absent response without the technician's knowledge of the incorrect angle of gaze. Note that although it is difficult for an observer to know the gaze direction of a subject even with reasonably close observation of the eyes, most patients do not know this and the mere act of being closely watched results in much greater compliance with gaze direction instructions. This is especially helpful in poorly cooperative patients.

The pattern electroretinogram (PERG) recorded simultaneously with the PSVEP may be used as an aid to ensure adequacy of fixation in difficult cases. An abnormal PERG raises the possibility of inadequate fixation (as well as the possibility of retinal disease), while a normal PERG can generally be taken to suggest that fixation was adequate and an abnormal P100 is then indicative of postretinal disease. Similarly, the presence of a strobe (flash) electroretinogram (ERG) recorded simultaneously with the flash visual evoked potential (VEP) may be helpful. See Section 8.2.3 for a discussion of psychological parameters, and other sections in this chapter for further discussion of PERGs.

2. PRETEST INSTRUCTIONS

Several pretest instructions need to be given to the patient, the referring physician, and the staff of the ward from which the patient may be coming.

1. The patient should bring eyeglasses used for reading.
2. Hairspray and hair tonics should not be used between the last hair washing and time of test.
3. A patient should not be sent for testing who has had mydriatic (pupillodilator) medication (usually for ophthalmologic examination) within 12 hours of testing, even if meiotic (pupilloconstrictor) drugs were subsequently used. These patients often still have some pupillary dilation that will affect visual acuity and, secondarily, P100 amplitude. Furthermore, the increased pupillary diameter increases retinal illumination and has been reported to decrease P100 latency (Stockard et al., 1979; Hawkes and Stow, 1981).

In the laboratory, corrected visual acuity should be tested using an appropriate chart or test objects (e.g., fingers).

The technician should extract pertinent clinical information from the medical record and/or history of the patient. The results of neuro-ophthalmologic examinations, including visual-field testing, are of particular importance in considerations of clinical correlations. As discussed later, patients with field defects are tested with laterally placed as well as midline electrodes if the midline responses are abnormal, because field defects alter the potential-field distribution of the P100 waveform, shifting the amplitude maximum away from the midline. Thus, it is important to know of the field defect before performing the test if lateral electrodes are not used routinely.

3. ELECTRODE APPLICATION

With the patient seated in a chair, electrodes are applied in appropriate positions. See Section 5 for electrode locations used in PSVEP testing. Any conventional electroencephalography (EEG) technique may be used for attaching the electrodes to the scalp (see Chapter 1 for scalp electrode application techniques).

Several types of electrode are available for recording the ERG. We have found a gold-foil electrode suitable for the PERG (Arden et al., 1979). This electrode is usually tolerated without anesthetizing the cornea and it does not disturb refraction. To apply the electrode the patient is instructed to look straight ahead, the lower eyelid is depressed with the forefinger of one hand, and, by holding the electrode wire with the other hand, the tip of the foil is placed between the eye and the eyelid. The eyelid is released gently and the wire is then fixed to the skin with adhesive tape. We have used a copper-hook electrode to record simultaneously the flash (strobe) ERG and VEP in poorly responsive and comatose patients. The hook electrode is placed between the eye and the eyelid between the midpoint of the lower lid and the outer canthus. A surface electrode on the lower lid may also be used for the flash ERG but it does not provide a satisfactory signal-to-noise ratio for recording the PERG. The Burian–Allen contact lens electrode is excellent for recording the PERG. Although it registers a higher amplitude PERG than the gold-foil electrode, its use requires corneal anesthesia and re-refraction of the patient following insertion (Celesia et al., 1986). Other contact lens and wire electrodes are also available. The eye electrode is referred to an ipsilateral temple electrode since this location contributes the least cortical VEP (compared with ear or vertex). Binocular stimulation may be used for PERG registration since there is very little cross-contamination (see section below on PERG techniques).

The electrodes are then plugged into the proper positions on the electrode board, which connects them to the amplifiers and the averager.

4. AMPLIFIER AND AVERAGER CONTROLS

Different makes of equipment require somewhat different setup procedures for a given EP, and on some systems less operator action is required than on others. Also, it is not always possible either to find the same settings as suggested below (use the closest you can find) or even to ascertain at what values a given piece of equipment is operating (e.g., what total amplification the system is producing). The manufacturer's suggested settings are usually reasonably good and can be used.

PSVEPs are best recorded by using an amplification of 20,000 to 100,000. The filters are 1 to 3 Hz low cutoff (high pass) and 100 to 300 Hz high cutoff (low pass). Testing high-cutoff filter settings of 80, 160, and 320 Hz, Yiannikas and Walsh (1983a) found that P100 latency decreased by about 1.5 msec for each filter step [12 decibels (dB) per octave filter], so this control should be held constant. The averager is set for a total sweep duration of 300 to 500 msec. Shorter sweep durations spread out the P100 and make abnormal responses that may already have a long duration even more difficult to recognize. Each channel should be composed of at least 256 points, sampled with a maximum intersample interval (dwell time) of 2 msec. Note that averager and human interpolation between these points allow latency measurements to a greater accuracy than this interval. The automatic sweep repetition control should be set to 100. It will be necessary sometimes to continue to 200 or 500 sweep repetitions if the patient is "noisy" or the responses are unclear for other reasons (abnormally low amplitude). Also, it is *mandatory* to repeat the trial and superimpose it on the previous trial to test waveform consistency. It may be necessary to repeat the test two to four times to arrive at a good measure of response variability.

5. CHANNELS TO RECORD

Clinical interpretation of PSVEPs is based entirely on latency and, to a much lesser degree, amplitude of the first major positive peak, P100. Thus, recording derivations are chosen which best register P100.

Most normal subjects have a potential-field distribution such that P100 amplitude with full-field stimulation is greatest near the inion and somewhat less at PZ (midline parietal), as seen in Fig. 2–5. The CZ (vertex) and FZ electrodes have a negative peak at the same latency as P100. However, some normal subjects have such a steep potential-field gradient between the inion and the vertex that the polarity reversal occurs between the inion and PZ, as seen in Fig. 2–6, rather than between PZ and CZ, as in Figure 2–5. Other normal subjects have a P100 amplitude maximum at PZ, with only a poorly defined, low-amplitude P100 at the inion. These normal variations are believed to be related to differences in the anatomy

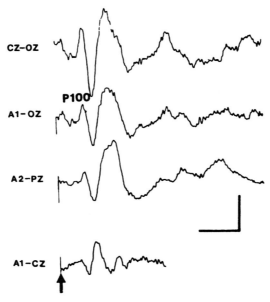

FIG. 2–5. Pattern-shift VEP from one eye of a normal subject. Note the polarity-reversed waveforms registered at CZ and the summation of this with the positivity at OZ in the CZ–OZ channel to produce a P100 of greater apparent amplitude. *N* = 128; sweep duration = 512 msec. Calibration marks are 100 msec and 5 μV. Relative positivity at G2 produces a downward trace deflection. Stimulus at *arrow.* (From Chiappa, 1979, with permission.)

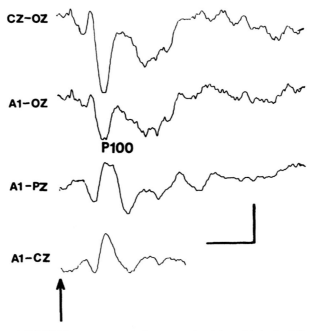

FIG. 2–6. Pattern-shift VEP from one eye of a normal subject. Note that the negative activity, usually seen only at CZ (as in Fig. 2–5), here also involves PZ. If a single, posterior electrode is used and it is placed too high, these inverted-polarity waveforms would be erroneously interpreted. Recording parameters and calibrations as for Fig. 2–5.

of the occipital cortex around the calcarine fissure (see Chapter 3, Section 1). Because of these variations, PSVEPs are recorded from electrodes at both OZ and PZ. Recording from CZ is helpful in understanding the P100 potential-field distribution but is not yet useful for clinical purposes. However, patients have been seen who have marked differences between their two eyes in P100 distribution in the vertical midline electrode array, with P100 shifted toward the vertex in the affected eye, despite perfectly normal latencies (Fig. 2–7). The clinical significance of this finding is still uncertain. An FZ–OZ or a CZ–OZ bipolar derivation can be used to produce a maximum amplitude waveform at P100 latency since activity at the two electrode sites normally is of opposite polarity and is thus summed by the differential amplifier. However, if CZ–OZ is the only channel recorded, the normal variations discussed above will result in some erroneous interpretations, especially when CZ is more active than OZ, as is the case in the patient whose PSVEPs are shown in Fig. 2–7.

Reference sites used are earlobe and forehead. Both are active but to a degree that does not interfere significantly with the posterior midline recordings. Activity in the reference sites has been investigated by recording from those electrodes using a noncephalic reference (Chiappa, 1983b); Spitz et al. (1986) have reported on FZ activity. (The noncephalic reference is not useful for routine clinical testing because of excessive muscle artifact in too many patients.) Forehead sites, especially the one 12 cm above the nasion (e.g., Halliday et al., 1979a), have a negative peak at about the same latency as P100. This has almost the same effect as using CZ in the recording derivation, that is, the apparent amplitude of P100 is increased by the in-phase addition of the opposite polarities by the differential amplifier. However, the negativity at the forehead reference electrode sometimes is out of phase with

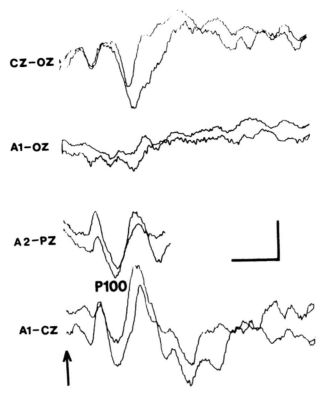

FIG. 2–7. Pattern-shift VEP from one eye of a patient with nonspecific complaints of disturbed vision in that eye. Ophthalmologic examination was normal. Note essentially no potentials registered at OZ, whereas both PZ and CZ have well-formed P100 peaks; the CZ–OZ linkage has "inverted" polarity activity because of the positivity at CZ. If the CZ–OZ or AI–OZ channels were used for interpretation, these responses would be erroneously interpreted. Recording parameters and calibrations as for Fig. 2–5, except that bottom channel calibration is 2.5 μV. Two separate trials of 128 stimulations are superimposed.

the inion positivity, resulting in a broadened or even bilobed appearance of the P100 peak. These observations have been verified and extended by Spitz et al. (1986) (Figs. 2–8 and 2–9). On the other hand, with full-field stimulation the earlobe site has a low-amplitude positivity simultaneous with P100. This results in some in-phase cancellation but not to a significant degree. However, with partial-field stimulation or in patients with visual-field defects, the earlobe site may be more active, especially relative to laterally placed electrodes, and a midline frontal reference should be used. Shih et al. (1988) have discussed the use of a linked mastoid reference.

Asymmetric activation of visual cortex, produced either by changes in the shape of the stimulus (e.g., partial-field stimulation) or by some lesions of the visual pathways, results in lateral shifts of the P100 peak (see Section 8.1.5). In these circumstances, nothing may be recorded from midline electrodes but a normal latency P100 can be recorded from laterally placed electrodes. Thus, if a patient has known visual-field defects, and the midline electrodes show an abnormal response, then it is necessary to confirm the nature of the abnormality by recording from lateral electrodes. If lateral electrodes are used routinely, as recommended below, the horizontal P100 distribution to full-field stimulation may resem-

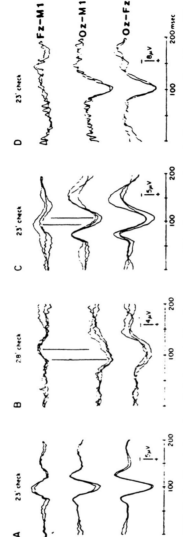

FIG. 2–8. Frontal and occipital mastoid-reference and bipolar recordings in four normal subjects. The latency relationship between frontal N100 and occipital P100 shows that they are closely related but often not identical, and this may affect the shape of the P100 recorded in an FZ–OZ derivation. The FZ N100 is simultaneous with the OZ P100 in **A**, follows it in **B**, precedes it in **C**, and is absent in **D** (as in 15% of normal subjects). Check size 23′ to 28′, field size 12°; M1 is left mastoid. (From Spitz et al., 1986, with permission.)

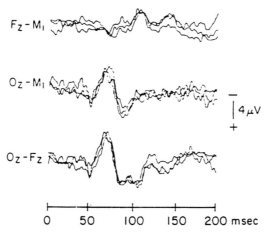

FIG. 2–9. Recordings from a normal subject as in Fig. 2–8, with a W-shaped response in the FZ–OZ derivation produced by the interaction of N100 at FZ and P100 at OZ. (From Spitz et al., 1986, with permission.)

ble a half-field stimulation, suggesting a partial-field defect (Fig. 2–10), and this should be further investigated with half-field stimulation and perimetry. Latency measurements cannot be made at lateral electrode sites with full-field stimulation because of excessive normal variability (Fig. 2–11) (Blumhardt et al., 1982b).

Because of all of the above considerations, it is not practical to perform PSVEP testing with two-channel systems.

A suggested four-channel montage for recording PSVEPs produced by full-field or partial-field stimulation is:

Channel 1: OZ to reference
Channel 2: PZ to reference
Channel 3: L5 to reference
Channel 4: R5 to reference

L5 and R5 refer to electrode locations 5 cm up from the inion and 5 cm lateral to the midline on the left and right, respectively. [Similarly, L10 and R10 (see below) are 10 cm lateral to the midline.] This montage provides some information about the horizontal distribution of P100, thus eliminating the need to repeat the test as is required when midline montages show abnormal responses.

The best montage for recording PSVEPs produced by partial-field stimulation requires at least six channels, and the reference should be FZ since the ears may be asymmetrically active.

Channel 1: L10 to reference
Channel 2: L5 to reference
Channel 3: OZ to reference
Channel 4: R5 to reference
Channel 5: R10 to reference
Channel 6: PZ to reference

If the P100 is abnormal, a binocular PERG may be recorded to assist in differentiating retinal from postretinal disease. If the question is one of adequacy of fixation, the PERG should

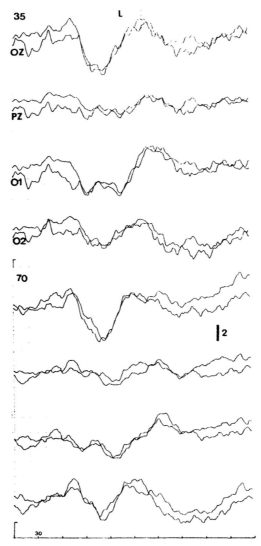

FIG. 2–10. Full-field PSVEP recorded from the left eye of a patient. The O2 channel (5 cm lateral to the midline) has a normal P100, but O1 shows a polarity-inverted waveform at both 35′ and 70′ check sizes. This is the configuration that would be expected with right-hemifield stimulation, suggesting a left-hemifield defect. This was confirmed by perimetry. The upper four channels were obtained with 35′ checks, the lower four with 70′ checks. The time marks are at 30-msec intervals; amplitude calibration in microvolts. The reference was FZ, and relative positivity of the posterior scalp electrodes caused a downward trace deflection.

be recorded simultaneously with the VEP (i.e., monocular stimulation). In the above montage (assuming an eight-channel machine) channel 7 or 8 may be used for the PERG, and, in the four-channel montage, any channel except the OZ to reference channel is suitable. If PERGs are recorded routinely using a four-channel montage, the nature of any abnormal response at OZ should still be verified by recording from PZ and laterally placed electrodes. In other circumstances, monocular or binocular PERGs may be recorded. The best refer-

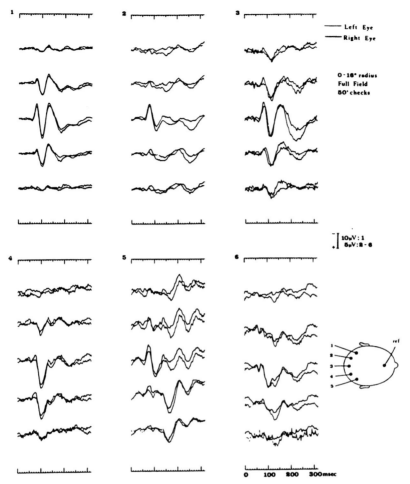

FIG. 2–11. Examples of full-field P100 waveform variation recorded from midline and lateral electrodes (5-cm horizontal interelectrode spacing). Left- and right-eye responses are superimposed. At the 5 cm lateral electrodes subject 2 has low-amplitude or absent responses, subject 4 has a marked asymmetry with the greater amplitude on the right (as is most common in normals), and subject 5 has a 165-msec positive component that could be mistaken for P100 if only these lateral channels were recorded. Sixteen-degree radius stimulus, 50′ checks; relative positivity of posterior electrodes causes a downward trace deflection. (From Blumhardt et al., 1982, with permission.)

ence site for the PERG is the ipsilateral temple, but when adequacy of fixation is being monitored, the reference used for the VEP (ear or frontal) is satisfactory.

6. RUNNING THE TEST

With the preliminaries accomplished, the subject is seated in front of the checkerboard at an eye–screen distance of 70 to 100 cm. At this distance it is more difficult to voluntarily defocus the pattern. The eyes are always tested one at a time (monocularly) and the opposite eye is covered with an eye patch. (Children less than 2 years of age and infants may not tolerate the eye patch, and then binocular testing must be used.) If stroboscopic stimulation is being used, the patch must be constructed of thick, opaque material and attached to the face without light leaks around the edges. Furthermore, if the strobe flash is accompanied by an audible sound (click), this must be masked by placing earphones on the patient and using a white-noise masking sound, otherwise an auditory EP will be indistinguishable from a visual EP.

The pattern stimulator is operated at about two reversals per second. Some EP equipment can be adjusted to average from shifts in one direction only, or both directions, but there are no significant differences between these, and the bidirectional mode, being the fastest, is suggested.

The subject is instructed to gaze at a dot in the center of the pattern being displayed. This dot may be colored or it may be a small light (LED). Although absolutely precise fixation on this point is not important and minor wanderings of gaze do not significantly affect P100 latency or amplitude, it is important that the subject maintain gaze fixation near the center of the screen. If this is not done, P100 amplitude will be diminished and, if partial-field stimulation with fixation at the edge of the pattern is in use, erroneous results will be produced. Patients who have visual-field defects or amblyopia may shift their center of gaze into the good visual field—the eccentric-fixation (sometimes termed "pseudofovea") effect. To offset this, a 1° to 2° blank strip may be inserted on either side of the fixation point when partial-field stimulation is being used.

Special procedures are necessary to test infants since they cannot cooperate or be instructed to watch the pattern. Testing must be scheduled for a time when they will be awake and comfortable (fed and dry). There must be a mechanism by which the technician can start and stop averaging, for example, a switch at the end of a long cable. The infant is held in front of the screen and averaging is allowed to proceed only when it is observed that the infant is looking at the pattern. In this manner, with some patience, good PSVEPs can be recorded from infants of all ages. Some TV stimulators allow superimposition of cartoons on the pattern. This holds the attention of young children and allows PSVEPs to be obtained from that age group.

After the averager memory has been erased, the averaging process is started and will continue until the required number of stimulus repetitions have been accomplished, when it will halt automatically.

If automatic artifact rejection is not available, the raw EEG signal must be monitored on an oscilloscope and averaging halted manually when excessive artifact is present, for example, during coughing, swallowing, and moving. If there is a great deal of artifact, the patient may be uncomfortable (too hot, too cold, or needs bathroom) and the problem should be alleviated.

If no responses are obtained, consideration should be first given to the principles outlined in Chapter 1, Section 5.

If it is recognized from watching the developing average that the responses are of low amplitude, the technician must check that the subject is watching the pattern, and if not, must encourage the subject to do so. Any avoidance must be noted in the technician's report. The presence of a normal PERG recorded at the same time as the VEP can be used in this situation to confirm adequacy of fixation. Although automatic techniques of monitoring fixation (Lavine et al., 1980) are not readily available, the importance of this aspect of PSVEP testing cannot be overemphasized and, hopefully, such equipment and methods will continue to be developed. Unless these techniques are used, the burden of proof that the subject attended properly to the stimulus rests with the person performing the test. Note that patients usually do not know that gaze fixation cannot be determined by an observer, so that the act of observation by the technologist often enforces better cooperation and maintenance of fixation.

When the 100 or so sweeps are finished, most subjects have produced a clean set of waveforms. If this is not so, then the averager should be set to continue to 200 or even 500 sweeps (stimulus repetitions). The responses should be written out or stored, the averager memory cleared, and another 100 or 500 sweeps done. These results are then superimposed on the previous trial's printout. Occasionally three or four separate trials may be necessary. This practice of repetition of trials is extremely important and is the only means of judging waveform consistency. Surprising and instructive results are often obtained (Shors et al., 1986).

If there are no recognizable waveforms, the patient's visual acuity may be too poor to distinguish the checks. The visual angle subtended by the checks must be increased (by making the checks larger or moving the patient closer to the pattern) and another attempt made to record the PSVEP. For example, a 4-mm check subtends 14' at 100 cm, 18' at 75 cm, 30' at 50 cm, 1° at 25 cm, and 2° at 12 cm. (For calculation of visual angle, see Section 1.) At 6.1 m (20 ft) the letters on an eye chart at the 20/20 acuity position (0.9 cm inch height) subtend about 5' at the eye, but the limbs of the letters subtend about 1'. Since it is not necessary to resolve all the limbs of a letter to identify it, the visual angle corresponding to an acuity level is not entirely clear. There is a rough correlation between visual acuity and the check angle at which an easily identifiable P100 can be seen. A visual angle of 5' corresponds approximately to a visual acuity of 20/20, 10' to 20/25, 20' to 20/50, 30' to 20/100, 45' to 20/200, and 1.5° to 20/400. Note that there should be no effective pattern luminance change when the patient–pattern distance is changed (see Section 8). A good amplitude P100 will be registered if the visual system is clearly resolving the checks, so that a clear P100 produced by 30' checks indicates a visual acuity of approximately 20/100. This correlation with standard visual acuity measures is not entirely correct in that overall height of a target character is not the only factor to take into account since individual subcomponents of a letter may be one fifth the overall height and these need to be at least partially resolved before the letter can be recognized. Therefore, check height probably should be compared with letters two to four times higher for visual acuity estimations.

Since the angle subtended by the checks affects P100 amplitude in a predictable manner, P100 being largest with the smallest checks that can be distinguished, this extension of the test can be used to determine visual acuity without subject cooperation and devices have been built specifically to do this. This topic is outside the scope of this text but details can be found in Ludlam and Meyers (1972), Regan (1973, 1977), Millodot (1977), Rentschler and Spinelli (1978), Bostrom et al. (1978), and below in Section 9.

When strobe stimulation is used, recording conditions are often suboptimal (e.g., a young patient or recording in the intensive care unit). Sometimes it is difficult to determine whether a low-amplitude flash VEP is present or whether there is no VEP. In these situations, the following are helpful: (1) The presence of a flash ERG recorded simultaneously confirms correct triggering of the machine and the location of the abnormality behind the eye. Absence of both flash ERG and VEP suggests a technical problem or ocular pathology. (2) Recording two trials with the eyes covered provides a measure of the ambient "noise" which may be compared with the responses obtained with the eye(s) uncovered. (3) Masking the ears with white noise excludes the possibility of recording an auditory EP if the strobe also generates a click with each flash. (4) Trial repetition remains an important means of ensuring reproducibility of the results.

For a further discussion of the effects of stimulus parameters on PSVEPs, see Section 8.1.

7. READING THE RESULTS, NORMATIVE DATA, AND VARIATIONS

Recording from the region of OZ and the inion, three peaks can usually be identified in normal subjects (Fig. 2–5). The peak polarities are negative, positive, and negative, respectively, and the mean peak latencies are 70, 100, and 135 msec. The first negative wave may be difficult to identify in some normal subjects and many patients [although Ghilardi et al. (1991) have reported results from 59 controls and 98 patients with multiple sclerosis (MS); see also Kurita-Tashima et al., 1991], and the second negative peak is too inconsistent in latency and amplitude to be of clinical utility. Only the first, large, positive peak, usually labeled P100 or P2, is seen in all normal subjects and has a variability small enough to make it reliable in clinical situations. In addition, its latency, the measure used for most clinical interpretations, is not significantly affected by parameters difficult to control in patients, for example, level of concentration and visual acuity (with checks larger than 30'). For a further discussion of the effects of these and other factors on PSVEPs, see Section 8.

Thus, waveform identification in the PSVEP test consists of looking for the first, large, inion/OZ positive peak. Depending on the stimulating device in use and the presence or absence of abnormalities, it may be found anywhere from 90 to 250 msec after the stimulus. If the peak is of low amplitude and difficult to locate precisely, it is very important to repeat the test and superimpose an extra three or four trials to allow a more accurate estimation of peak location. P100 is the most persistent of the PSVEP positive peaks and when the EP amplitude is low because of abnormalities P100 is usually the only positive peak present. Rarely, the P100 potential field is shifted markedly toward the vertex and very little positivity is recorded in the region of the inion/OZ, even though a normal latency P100 is present at PZ and CZ (see Fig. 2–7). This demonstrates the importance of recording from PZ as well as inion/OZ.

For full-field stimulation, P100 measurements taken from midline recording derivations are (1) absolute latency, (2) interocular absolute latency difference, (3) amplitude, (4) interocular amplitude difference ratio, and (5) duration. These measurements should not be taken from lateral electrodes because these may show highly anomalous results with full-field stimulation (see Fig. 2–11) (Blumhardt et al., 1982a). When interocular comparisons are made, it is essential to hold the two sheets of paper up to a strong light and to optically superimpose the results from the two eyes. This allows a much more reliable comparison than the use of numbers (latency values) only. Also, superimposition and comparison of the major ascending and descending limbs is often more reliable than attempting to superimpose/compare peaks which may have uneven shapes because of admixed noise.

Difficulty is most frequently encountered in locating the point at which the peak of P100 will be taken for latency measurements. Often the P100 peak will have an irregular shape and will not present a clear, sharp point. In this case, the first (positive-going) and the second (negative-going) sides of P100 are used to interpolate to a point and the measurements made to there (Fig. 2–12). When P100 has two distinct peaks, the so-called W or bifid pattern (see Fig. 3–4), the use of (1) lower half-field stimulation (since the upper field may be contributing inverted polarity, phase-shifted activity at the Fz electrode—see Section 8), and/or (2) left or right half-field stimulation with recording from laterally placed electrodes (see Chapter 3, Section 2.5) will be necessary. Amplitude may be measured from baseline to peak or from preceding negative peak to P100 peak (see Fig. 2–12). When the preceding negative peak is absent, the two measurements are the same. The baseline measurement is

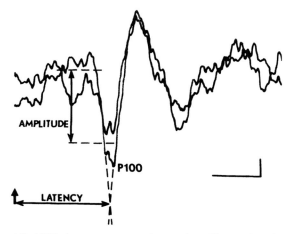

FIG. 2–12. Pattern-shift VEP from one eye of a patient illustrating the lack of a coherent P100 peak, which often presents a problem in making latency and amplitude measurements. Two separate trials of 128 stimulus repetitions each are superimposed. P100 latency is determined by extrapolating from the side limbs of the P100 peak, as shown (latency = 95 msec). Amplitude is measured between estimated baseline and P100 peak. Recording derivation is AI–OZ, OZ positivity producing a downward deflection. Calibration marks are 50 msec and 5 μV.

probably the most consistent and physiologic. Duration may be measured between the two sides of the P100 peak at baseline level.

For partial-field stimulation, recording from laterally placed electrodes (see Section 5), similar measurements are taken at the electrodes 5 cm lateral to the midline on the same side as the field being stimulated. In addition to interocular differences, amplitude difference ratios and interfield latency differences for each eye are calculated and tabulated.

Tables 2–1, 2–2, and 2–3 present data gathered from normal subjects. (Some of these data are presented in greater detail in Shahrokhi et al., 1978.) This is intended to show how such data can be organized and to allow comparisons of variability when a laboratory is inexperienced with this test. Since the absolute values are dependent on many variables not likely to be the same in other laboratories (especially stimulus luminance), the values presented here cannot be used for clinical interpretation other than in the laboratory where they were gathered. However, the interside and interfield latency and amplitude differences should be similar in different laboratories, as should the variability, measured here in standard deviations. PSVEP results from groups of normal subjects have been published and a study of those methods and data is useful (see Asselman et al., 1975; Celesia and Daly, 1977; Hennerici et al., 1977; Matthews et al., 1977; Collins et al., 1978; Kjaer, 1980; Lowitzsch et al., 1980; Shahrokhi et al., 1978; Trojaborg and Petersen, 1979; Shors et al., 1986; Abe and Kuroiwa, 1990). See Section 8.2.3 for a discussion of the consistency of P100 over long periods of recording and recording at repeated intervals for several months. Refer to Chapter 1, Section 4.3 for a discussion of the concepts relating values obtained from normal subjects and those obtained from patients (whose results are possibly abnormal).

When strobe stimulation is used, the information gained is qualitative rather than quantitative. We do not attempt to measure the latency of the strobe responses because of their great latency variability and occasional absence of some components even in normal subjects.

TABLE 2–1. *Full-field PSVEP normal values*

	N	Mean	Range	SD	Mean + 3 SD
Latency of P100	86 Eyes	102.3 msec	89–114 msec	±5.1	117.6 msec
Latency difference between two eyes	43 Subjects	1.3 msec	0–6 msec	±2.0	7.3 msec
Amplitude of P100	86 Eyes	10.1 μV	3–21 μV	±4.2	—
Absolute amplitude difference between two eyes	43 Subjects	1.6 μV	0–5.5 μV	±1.4	5.8 μV
Proportional amplitude difference between two eyes: $\frac{\text{smallest amplitude}}{\text{largest amplitude}} \times 100$	21 Subjects	85.5%	—	±10.5%	53.9%
Duration of P100	86 Eyes	63 msec	47–86 msec	±8.7	89.1 msec
Duration difference between two eyes	43 Subjects	2.8 msec	0–6 msec	±2.9	11.5 msec

Normal values for full-field PSVEP testing using a fixed-luminance device (side projector/rotating mirror), screen size 8.7°, check size 25.8′. Data from 21 normal volunteers and 22 patient controls. (From Shahrokhi et al., 1978, with permission.)

TABLE 2–2. *Partial-field PSVEP normal latencies (msec)*

	Mean ± SD	Range
Absolute latency		
Left field	96.7 ± 5.34	87–107
Right field	95.2 ± 4.61	87–104
Full field	99.2 ± 4.13	92–108
Full-left field	2.5 ± 3.31	−3–10
Full-right field	4.04 ± 3.21	−3–11
Left-right field	1.36 ± 4.88	−9–9
Intereye difference		
Left field	3.7 ± 2.69	0–10
Right field	2.3 ± 1.67	1–7
Full field	2.0 ± 1.68	0–6
Full-left field	3.8 ± 2.42	1–10
Full-right field	3.1 ± 2.68	0–10
Left-right field	5.6 ± 3.99	1–13

Normal latency values for sequential partial- and full-field PSVEPs. For half fields, latency taken at electrode 5 cm from midline ipsilateral to stimulated field; for full field, latency taken at midline electrode 5 cm above inion. Interfield differences are absolute values, except in range data, where a negative value implies that the fields have either preceded or followed one another in different subjects. Intereye difference data are all absolute values. Stimulation sequence was left-right-full fields with 300-msec interstimulus intervals at 1/sec (see Fig. 2–2 and text for methods). Screen size 31.1 (width) by 28.8°; check size 1° 28′ (width) by 1° 13′; video monitor device at constant luminance; 19 normal subjects.

TABLE 2–3. *Partial-field PSVEP normal amplitude ratios*

Ratio	Mean ± SD
Left field/right field	
10 cm Out ipsilateral to field stimulated	1.40 ± 1.03
5 cm Out ipsilateral to field stimulated	1.16 ± .70
Midline	1.44 ± .91
Max amp site	1.16 ± .60
Aver amp	1.26 ± .64
Smallest amplitude/largest amplitude	
10 cm Out ipsilateral to field stimulated	0.58 ± .22
5 cm Out ipsilateral to field stimulated	0.63 ± .19
Midline	0.63 ± .22
Max amp site	0.63 ± .16
Aver amp	0.65 ± .19
Largest amplitude/smallest amplitude	
5 cm Out ipsilateral to field stimulated	
OS and OD	1.79 ± .73
OS	1.78 ± .79
OD	1.81 ± .67
Electrode location	*Max difference between left and right fields*
10 cm Out ipsilateral to field stimulated	5.3
5 cm Out ipsilateral to field stimulated	4.3
Midline	6.7
Max amp site	4.0
Aver amp	4.1

Normal amplitude ratio data for sequential partial- and full-field PSVEPs as described in Table 2–2. "Midline" refers to an electrode in the midline 5 cm above the inion; "max amp site" refers to the electrode with the greatest amplitude (midline, and 5 and 10 cm out ipsilateral to stimulated field)—sometimes different in the two half-fields; "aver amp" refers to the average of the three ipsilateral electrodes. The OS (left eye) and OD (right eye) comparison provides data on the differences seen between the two eyes in homologous fields.

8. NONPATHOLOGIC FACTORS AFFECTING RESULTS

Some technical and patient factors, when altered, produce significant changes in P100. When test results are interpreted clinically, the normal range for each of these parameters must be known as they apply in that test and that patient. Care must be taken that factors not intended to be changed (e.g., pattern luminance) do not, in fact, change between testing normal subjects and patients. This section discusses the effects of changing some of those parameters.

8.1. Technical Factors

8.1.1. Luminance

Pattern luminance is one of the most critical parameters in PSVEP testing and changes in it have marked effects on P100 latency. Pattern luminance is easily changed, especially on many TV-type stimulators which have a continuously variable brightness control. In these devices, this control should be disabled or otherwise locked and/or regular checks made of pattern luminance. Since P100 latency is so dependent on pattern luminance, normal values

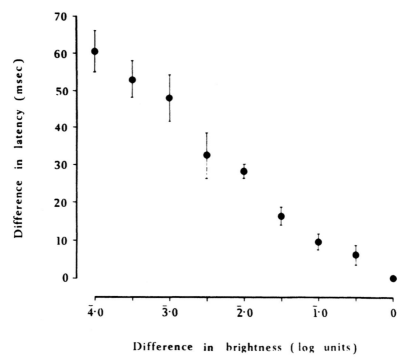

FIG. 2–13. Change in mean latency of P100 with decrease in brightness of the stimulus (via neutral density filters). Mean data for five normal subjects are plotted with the standard deviation. Reduction of brightness by 2 log units (100 to 1) increases P100 latency 20 to 25 msec. Overall initial intensity 60 cd, 32° diameter stimulus, 50′ checks. (From Halliday et al., 1973a, with permission.)

obtained and used for clinical interpretation in one laboratory cannot be used in another. For a discussion of stimulators and luminance, see Section 1.

P100 latency increases as pattern luminance is decreased (Halliday et al., 1973; Cant et al., 1978; Sokol, 1980), as shown in Fig. 2–13. Halliday et al. (1973b) showed that the P100 latency increase is approximately 15 msec per log unit reduction in luminance, with a parallel reduction in amplitude of approximately 15% per log unit intensity reduction. Although van der Tweel et al. (1979) argued that luminance has little effect on amplitude or waveform of the PSVEP, their results were obtained by increasing contrast in the pattern to compensate for successively lower luminance levels.

In patients with MS, Cant et al. (1978) and Camisa et al. (1980) found that lower luminance levels revealed more abnormalities and suggested routine use of more than one intensity level. However, this effect was not observed by others (Diener et al., 1982; Hennerici and Wist, 1982; Waybright et al., 1982) except that Hennerici and Wist did find an increased sensitivity with foveal stimulation at lower luminance levels.

Pupillary diameter has an effect on retinal illumination and thus also on P100 latency (Stockard et al., 1979; Hawkes and Stow, 1981). The latter authors found that an average pupillary diameter constriction of 1.75 mm (SD 0.4) with pilocarpine produced an average latency increase of 4.6 msec (SD 1.8). Thus, gross differences in pupillary diameter need to be taken into account in interpretations. Retinal illumination (in trolands) can be calculated by multiplying the ambient luminance of the pattern [in candelas (cd) per square meter] by the pupil area (in square millimeters).

8.1.2. Contrast

Contrast in percent is calculated by dividing the luminance difference between the light and dark checks by the sum of their luminances, and multiplying by 100.

Reductions in the degree of contrast between the black and white squares of the checkerboard pattern cause increased latency and decreased amplitude of P100 (see Fig. 6C in MacKay and Jeffreys, 1973). However, this effect saturates at a contrast level of about 20% to 40% (Halliday and McDonald, 1981), and since much higher degrees of contrast are most commonly used, this factor has little effect in most situations. For example, among a large group of MS studies, the lowest contrast value used was 74% (Matthews et al., 1977); others have used values as high as 99% (Hennerici et al., 1977). The effect of contrast on PSVEPs has been studied in detail by Wright and Johnston (1982).

It has also been suggested that contrast modulation may be used to separate the magno- and parvocellular components of visual subsystems (Nelson and Seiple, 1992).

8.1.3. Color

The effect of color of checks on the PSVEP has not been well-studied. White et al. (1977) found that colored checkerboard stimuli produced EPs that were "practically identical" to those produced by black and white patterns. Hod et al. (1986) found that red/black, green/black, and red/green LED-generated patterns produced longer-latency P100s than black/white TV-generated patterns. The greater luminance of the black/white checks compared with the colored combinations could explain the differences found. Using red/black and green/black patterns they found abnormalities in only six of eight patients with MS or recent optic neuritis who had abnormalities to black/white checks. As all eight patients had abnormalities to black/white checks, it was not possible to determine whether there might be patients in whom the colored checks showed abnormalities "missed" by the black/white checks. Red/green checks did not elicit EPs in all normal subjects and were not considered useful. Parry-Jones and Fenwick (1979) used black and white and colored patterns to study the relationship between PSVEP amplitude and pattern displacement but, in addition, it can be seen from their data that the colored patterns gave latencies different from the black and white ones. However, the authors doubted that their methods of luminance matching were good enough, and this consideration makes most comparative studies difficult to evaluate. For example, this renders problematic the finding of McInnes (1977) that 6 of 36 patients had PSVEP latencies that were abnormal with colored but normal with black and white pattern stimulation. Klem et al. (1983) studied the effect of color and contrast on VEP amplitudes. Allison et al. (1993) recorded from subdural grids placed for clinical evaluation of epilepsy and studied color function using both EPs and stimulation. Barbato et al. (1994) found that color was more sensitive for revealing conduction abnormalities in Parkinson's disease.

8.1.4. Stimulus Field Size, Distance, and Location

The visual angle subtended by a pattern stimulus is a function of the pattern dimensions and the distance to the subject (see Section 1). Changes in the total stimulus visual angle have marked effects on the horizontal P100 potential-field distribution over the back of the head; these are discussed in Section 8.1.5 below. With posterior midline recordings and full-field stimulation, progressive diminution in field size results in a decline in P100 amplitude but little change in latency. Similarly, patients with progressive, concentric constriction of their visual fields because of retinitis pigmentosa may have a P100 of low amplitude but normal latency down to a few degrees of remaining visual field. However, the greater part of P100 is generated by the central 10° or so of vision, with more peripheral areas contributing much less. The proportions are thought to parallel the relative cortical representations of retinal areas, that is, central areas map to larger cortical areas than do peripheral ones. Thus, (1) Asselman et al. (1975) found that P100 amplitudes with an 18° field were reduced by 50% when the central 5° to 6° were occluded and by 80% when the central 10° were occluded, (2) Blumhardt et al. (1978) using a 32° field found that P100 was completely abolished in three normal subjects and reduced to less than 16% of its maximum value in the other two subjects tested by a 20° radius central scotoma, and (3) Bartl et al. (1978) found that the greatest relative increase in P100 amplitude occurred when field size was increased from 2.5° to 5°. They also noted, as did Douthwaite and Jenkins (1982) and Plant et al. (1983), that the check size which produced the largest response increased as field size increased.

Yiannikas and Walsh (1983) found that at least 80% of the response arose from the central 8°; however, the peripheral 8° to 32° still produced a significant contribution to the P100 amplitude. Figure 2–14 illustrates the contribution of the fovea by plotting the contribution to P100 amplitude per degree of field of the various stimulus annuli. The central 2° contribute 12.5% of P100 amplitude per degree as compared to less than 2% in the 15° to 32° annulus of field. As the figure shows, this correlates well with the curve of the variation of cortical magnification and visual acuity with retinal eccentricity. The variation of the P100 amplitude with the radius of the stimulus field is less pronounced in lateral recording channels. With the smallest fields tested (4° and 8° diameter) P100 latency was also affected (increased). This may be related to a number of factors, including check size, reduction in mean (overall) luminance, and the proportionately larger effect, at narrow visual angles, of small fluctuations in fixation.

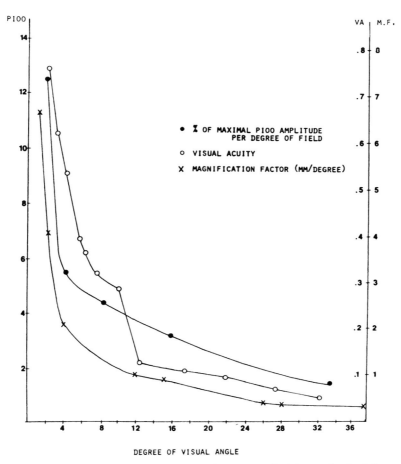

FIG. 2–14. Relative contributions of visual-field areas to P100 amplitude (*closed circles*), determined by changing the diameter of the stimulus field (2°, 4°, 8°, 16°, and 32°) and calculating the change in P100 amplitude produced by that change. Note that the central few degrees have the greatest contribution by far and that this plot closely parallels the magnification factor (X plot and M.F. axis) between retina and visual cortex (i.e., the ratio between a retinal area and the area of visual cortex it projects to), and also parallels the visual acuity changes (*open circles* and VA axis). (From Yiannikas and Walsh, 1983, with permission.)

There has been some suggestion that smaller stimulus fields are more sensitive in revealing abnormalities in an occasional patient (Kriss et al., 1982; Hammond and Yiannikas, 1986). Hammond and Yiannikas (1986) found abnormalities in 75% of MS patients when the central 4° field was stimulated compared with 71% on full-field stimulation. However, there were also cases with normal central-field responses and abnormal full-field responses so that the two techniques were thought to be complementary in detecting abnormalities. Although theoretically an abnormal response secondary to a small central scotoma might be obscured by a normal, larger-amplitude response from the remainder of the visual field, usually this does not occur and even a small scotoma will generate abnormal responses. Note that other studies using small central fields have used a luminance change rather than a pattern-shift stimulus (Hennerici et al., 1977; Rossini et al., 1979; Diener and Scheibler, 1980; Hennerici and Wist, 1982).

8.1.5. Partial-Field Stimulation

The potentials recorded anywhere on the head following full-field stimulation are an algebraic sum of activities generated by the individual half fields (see Figs. 3 and 5 in Blumhardt and Halliday, 1979). For example, half of the P100 recorded at the midline following full-field stimulation is contributed by each individual half field. However, at lateral locations a more complex combination of the activity generated by the two half fields (and occipital cortices) is recorded, due to the variation of striate cortex (Brindley, 1972), which is also reflected in the variability of the "transitional zone" (see below). If one wishes to record from those sites it is most meaningful to use half-field rather than full-field stimulation.

The distribution of activity over lateral portions of the posterior head is related to the cortical projections of the field being stimulated, that is, the central 10° of the visual fields project to the occipital poles and more peripheral field areas project to more medially placed cortex. Thus, stimulus fields which include more peripheral visual areas will produce potential-field distributions different from those of stimulus fields which are restricted to central vision. In addition, the occipital lobes in humans are asymmetric, with the left having a larger mass, more striate cortex which extends further laterally, and more exposed mesial cortex. Furthermore, there is a marked normal anatomic variability, as illustrated in Fig. 2–15, which shows striate cortex distribution in six human brains (Brindley, 1972; also see this report for medial views of the occipital lobes). The result of the interaction of all these factors is such that the potential-field distribution of P100 over the back of the head has a degree of variability that is difficult to define reliably (in addition to the data presented here in Table 2–3, see Abe and Kuroiwa (1990) and Onofrj et al. (1991) for a systematic studies of normal subjects). The most common pattern seen is the "paradoxical" lateralization described first by Barrett et al. (1976). They found that with half-field stimulation P100 is recorded most prominently from those electrodes over the scalp ipsilateral to the visual field being stimulated (see Fig. 2–4). At the same time, electrodes over the scalp contralateral to the field being stimulated record a more variable, negative potential. As the recording site moves from contralateral to ipsilateral posterior head regions (relative to the visual field being stimulated), a polarity reversal takes place. The midpoint of the polarity reversal has been termed the "transitional zone" (Blumhardt et al., 1978). The exact location of the transitional zone varies between normal subjects. Since it may occur at the midline, PSVEPs cannot be recorded only from midline electrodes when partial-field stimulation is being used or if the patient has visual-field defects. In clinical practice, since the latter data may not be known at the time of testing, when a normal response is not obtained from the midline electrodes it is important to add lateral electrodes (if these are not used routinely) and repeat the test. P100 may be present at a normal latency at the lateral electrodes. If more than four recording channels are available, all useful and interesting sites can be recorded from simultaneously (see suggested eight-channel montage in Section 5).

The "paradoxical" localization of P100 is related to the cortical distribution and orientation of the neurons activated by a given visual field. If the field does not map to enough medially placed neurons, that is, when the full-field visual angle is less than approximately 15°, some normal subjects will have half-field responses which have P100 maximal over the posterior scalp contralateral to the field being stimulated. As the field size is reduced this proportion increases so that with an 8° full field about 10% of normal subjects have a contralateral P100 maximal with half-field stimulation. This effect explains apparent discrepancies in P100 distribution noted in some studies, for example, Chain et al. (1982), using a 6.5° stimulus half field, found a contralateral P100 maximum in 15 of 20 normal subjects (one ipsilateral, four midline), whereas Blumhardt et al. (1978), using a 16° stimu-

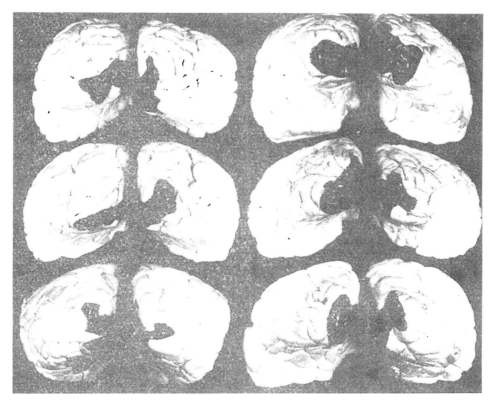

FIG. 2–15. An illustration of the variability of the human striate cortex (area 17). Plaster casts of the posterior poles of six normal brains were made. The intact hemispheres were sliced coronally at 7-mm intervals, the striate cortex identified and marked with India ink on the corresponding casts. Another eight brains showed similar variations. The marked variations shown here in striate cortex distribution were also noted on the medial aspects of the hemispheres. These variations account for the large variability in P100 distribution over the posterior scalp. (From Brindley, 1972, with permission.)

lus half field, found an ipsilateral P100 maximum in all their normal subjects. For practical purposes a full field of at least 20° (half field of at least 10°) should be used to ensure that P100 has a maximum amplitude over the posterior scalp ipsilateral to the field being stimulated.

The fact that P100 and all other components of the PSVEP are being generated in the appropriate occipital lobe despite the "paradoxical" localization of P100 (at the scalp over the opposite side) is illustrated in Fig. 2–16, which shows PSVEP results obtained from a patient who had had a hemispherectomy. Note that Clement et al. (1985) used the source derivation procedure to simplify the interpretation of hemifield pattern stimulation. It is thought that the ipsilateral P100 is generated by more central areas of the visual field, whereas the simultaneous contralateral negativity is generated by more peripheral areas (Blumhardt et al., 1978). Thus, by introducing experimental central scotomata, one can enhance the contralateral negativity while the ipsilateral P100 is markedly diminished in amplitude (Fig. 2–17) (Blumhardt et al., 1978). This effect can be seen in patients with central scotomata, and here the laterally placed electrodes help with test interpretation. If only mid-

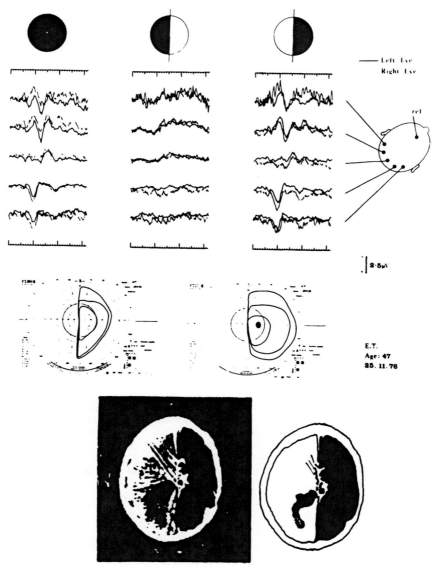

FIG. 2–16. Full- and half-field responses after right hemispherectomy. Perimetry shows macular splitting left homonymous hemianopia. CT scan shows the occipital pole of the left hemisphere in a normal position. No clearly recognizable components are detected above noise level following stimulation of the left half fields. This is confirmed by the virtually identical full- and right half-field responses. Note that the right half-field response has a "transitional" midline waveform due to dominant contralateral components. Note that the ipsilateral complex is recorded from the scalp overlying the excised hemisphere and that all components are at normal latencies. Stimulus diameter 32°, 50′ checks. (From Blumhardt and Halliday, 1981, with permission.)

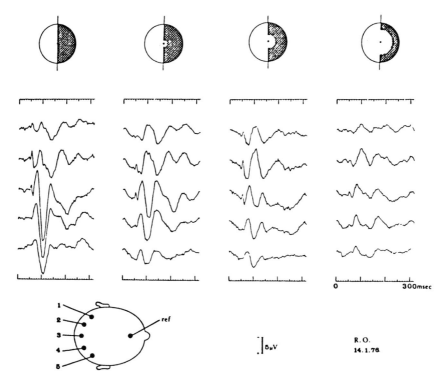

FIG. 2–17. The effect of increasing-radii experimental scotomata on the right half-field response in a normal subject. The P100 is progressively attenuated while the contralateral components, particularly the N105, are initially enhanced. From left to right: intact half-field, 2.5°, 5.0°, and 10.0° scotomata. (From Blumhardt et al., 1978, with permission.)

line recordings are made and P100 is essentially absent, the activity recorded at the midline is primarily that generated by the peripheral parts of the visual field, that is, there is a negativity occurring at the time that should be occupied by P100. The positivities that precede and follow that negativity may be incorrectly interpreted as being P100 if only midline recording channels are available (Fig. 2–18). In these cases, lateral recording channels will demonstrate the fact that P100 is absent and peripherally generated, polarity-inverted components are being recorded at the midline. Conversely, progressive reduction of the stimulus visual angle results in a diminution of the contralateral, polarity-inverted components. Since patients often have central visual-field defects, anomalous full-field waveforms (e.g., W-shaped) are produced and may present interpretive difficulties. The use of half-field stimulation allows better component identification, greater sensitivity to early effects of lesions, and improved detection of masked defects and the ability to distinguish true delays from pseudo delays (Halliday, 1985; Jones and Blume, 1985).

Clinical use of the partial-field aspects of PSVEPs requires a careful study of normals with the particular screen and check sizes to be used for testing patients and a tabulation of latency and amplitude measures, with statistical limits of normality, to utilize in interpretations. There is some disagreement on the consistency of these findings in larger groups of normal subjects. For example, Blumhardt and Halliday (1981) set an upper limit of 1:2 for the amplitude asymmetry ratio between the half-field responses from one eye (32° screen, 50′ checks). Rowe (1981) found that the same ratio included all of his normal subjects, but,

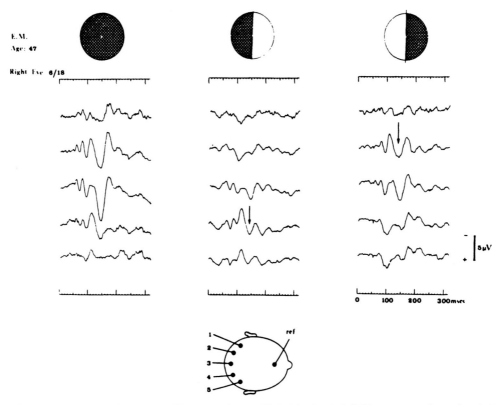

FIG. 2–18. Apparently delayed P100 (major positivity) in the full-field response from the right eye of a 47-year-old patient with MS (*left panel*). Half-field stimulation shows that this positivity is made up by the summation of two contralateral P135 components (*arrows*) within their normal latency range, with the ipsilateral P100 positivity absent, this pattern of components being consistent with a central scotoma (cf. Fig. 2–17). A small, dense, central scotoma was found on visual-field examination. (From Halliday, 1982, with permission.)

interestingly, he did not use amplitude as an interpretive criterion in his report of partial-field stimulation in 250 patients (Rowe, 1982), suggesting that normal variability was a problem. Hammond and Yiannikas (1986) found that a value of 1:3 included all their normal values. As seen in Table 2–3, we have found a 1:4.3 ratio to be the upper limit of normal for the same measure (31° screen, 1.5° checks), a value similar to that seen by Haimovic and Pedley (1982a, b); this suggests that essentially only the complete absence of a response from one field is a reliable indicator of abnormality. Note also that Kuroiwa et al. (1987) and Abe and Kuroiwa (1990) found significantly higher amplitudes on stimulation of the right compared with the left field.

The check size which produces the largest-amplitude response is different for central and peripheral parts of the field; central areas produce larger amplitude with smaller checks and more peripheral fields produce larger PSVEPs with larger checks. See Section 8.1.6 for further discussion of this.

There is much more agreement on interfield latency differences in normal subjects and the means and standard deviations are similar in most studies. In patients, Blumhardt and Halliday (1981) and Plant et al. (1992) did not find this to be of much clinical use, but Rowe

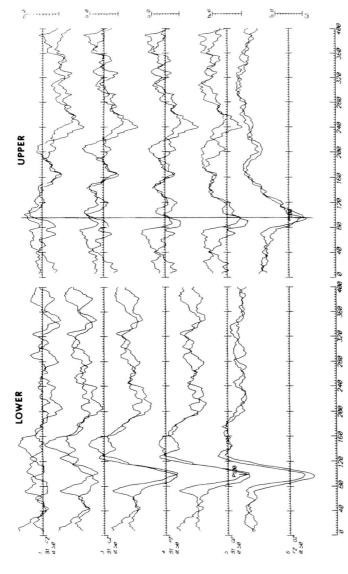

FIG. 2–19. Upper and lower half-field responses in a normal subject. N80 and P100 are well-defined with high amplitudes following lower half-field stimulation, whereas the upper half-field responses are much lower in amplitude posteriorly with a simultaneous, inverted polarity (*negative*) component anteriorly (*top channel*). The cursor in the right (upper) panel is at the P100 latency in the left (lower) panel, facilitating latency comparisons. The channel derivations from the top are FZ, CZ, PZ, and OZ, all referred to a balanced neck–chest noncephalic reference; the bottom channel is FZ–OZ. Relative positivity of the scalp electrodes (OZ in bottom channel) caused a downward trace deflection. Calibration marks are in milliseconds and microvolts. Each trace is the average of 100 stimuli.

(1982) has found a significant increase in PSVEP lesion pickup using these latency measures (see Chapter 3, Section 3.6).

Riemslag et al. (1985) studied interactions between responses to successive presentations of checkerboard patterns occupying different locations in the visual field. They found that the second presented stimulus could be inhibited entirely by the first, providing that the interstimulus interval was less than 40 msec, even when the first occupied only one quarter of the visual field and the second occupied the remainder. This may explain the relative preservation of P100 shape and duration in demyelinating diseases of the optic nerve, and may indicate that function of the fastest-conducting remaining population is being tested.

The majority of P100 is generated by the lower half of the visual field (Fig. 2–19) as noted by Kuba et al. (1982) and Kriss and Halliday (1980). Also, the upper field may generate a negative peak at frontal locations which may be slightly out of phase with the activity in occipital areas (see Fig. 2–19). These differences presumably are related to the location and orientation in the visual cortex of the activated neurons. If the phase difference between the occipital and frontal activities is sufficiently great, the combination of upper-field stimulation and the use of the FZ reference may produce a W-shaped P100. The use of lower-field stimulation may be useful in this circumstance.

8.1.6. Check Size

Smaller checks produce larger-amplitude P100s, as seen in Table 2–4, where the 17' checks have the largest amplitude (compared to 35' and 70'). This relationship is maintained as long as the checks can be clearly perceived, that is, they are not smaller than the visual acuity for the eye. These 30 subjects also had P100 latency for the 35' checks about 4 msec shorter than the 17' checks (significant at $p <0.01$) and 1 msec shorter than the 70' checks (Chiappa et al., 1985; Torok et al., 1992); interocular latency difference did not show significant changes (Table 2–5 and Fig. 2–2). As check size is increased above 2° the contribution of luminance change effects rather than pattern reversal becomes predominant, and this results in excessive variability of P100 latency and shape (Table 2–4 and Figs 2–20, 2–21, 2–22, 2–23). Because of this, the clinical use of checks of 2° or greater is contraindicated, and this may explain some of the check size differences found by Oishi et al. (1985)

TABLE 2–4. *Amplitude values (μV)*

Check size	Absolute Mean ± SD (range)	N	Intereye difference Mean ± SD (range)	ULN	N	Intereye ratio (percent) Mean ± SD (range)	LLN	N
17'	8.34 ± 3.71 (1.6–18.7)	60	1.48 ± 1.19 (0.2–5.2)	5.1	30	83.1 ± 12.2 (48.5–97.6)	46.5	30
35'	7.13 ± 3.68 (1.0–19.1)	58	1.69 ± 2.00 (0–8.6)	7.7	29	80.6 ± 15.5 (42.9–100)	34.1	29
70'	7.95 ± 3.64 (1.8–19.8)	58	1.29 ± 1.16 (0–4.8)	4.8	29	84.4 ± 12.9 (55–100)	45.7	29
144'	7.72 ± 2.95 (1.5–16.1)	58	1.36 ± 1.22 (0–5.4)	5.0	29	83.6 ± 12.6 (52.5–100)	45.8	29
288'	7.31 ± 2.74 (2.6–14)	57	1.10 ± 1.05 (0–3.9)	4.3	28	86.3 ± 9.9 (63.9–100)	56.6	28

Pattern-shift VEP P100 amplitude data for full-field stimulation with five check sizes, using a high-contrast, 15° screen. Stimulus reversal rate was 2/sec. ULN, upper limit of normal (mean plus 3 SD); LLN, lower limit of normal (mean minus 3 SD).

TABLE 2–5. *Latency values (msec)*

Check size	Absolute latency			Intereye difference		
	Mean ± SD (range)	ULN	N	Mean ± SD (range)	ULN	N
17'	106.8 ± 6.4 (96.7–128.8)	126	60	2.73 ± 2.32 (0–8.80)	9.7	30
35'	102.9 ± 7.4 (88.6–121.4)	125.1	58	2.53 ± 2.91 (0–13.4)	11.3	29
70'	103.8 ± 6.9 (88.2–122.5)	124.5	58	2.18 ± 2.59 (0–12.7)	10.0	29
144'	107.3 ± 8.8 (91.1–130.6)	133.7	58	2.44 ± 2.55 (0–12)	10.1	29
288'	113.5 ± 11.8 (91.4–142)	148.9	58	3.95 ± 4.03 (0–15.2)	16.0	29

Pattern-shift VEP P100 latency data accompanying Table 2–4.

in testing a large group of patients with a variety of diseases using 25', 50', and 100' checks. Of 1,006 patients, 32% had abnormal PSVEPs and 16% of these showed a discrepancy between check sizes. The smallest checks showed the only abnormality in 68% and the largest in 28%, the proportions roughly the same irrespective of disease.

Yiannikas and Walsh (1983), using pattern-reversal stimulation, systematically studied the variation in PSVEP amplitude and peak latencies with check size and retinal eccentricity. On stimulating the central 4° of field the maximum amplitude response was obtained by 27' checks, and as greater areas of field were stimulated (32°) the maximal response was

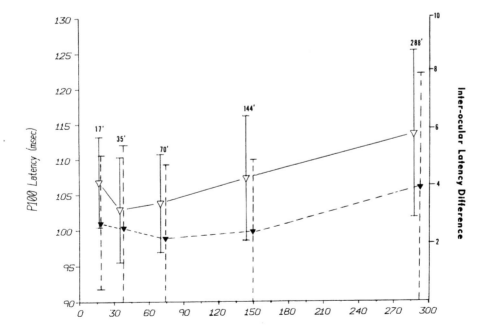

FIG. 2–20. Plots of absolute latency (*solid*) and interocular latency difference (*dashed*) at five different check sizes (from Table 2–5). Mean and 1 SD values are plotted. Stimulus was a high-contrast, 15° screen; reversal rate was 2/sec. Derivation was FZ–OZ.

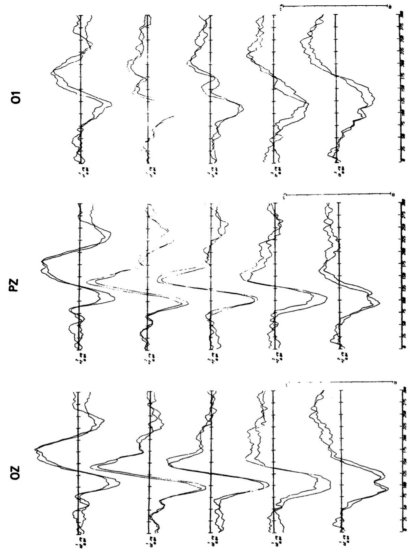

FIG. 2–21. Evoked potentials from one of the normal subjects included in Tables 2–4 and 2–5 and Fig. 2–20. The panels from left to right are OZ, PZ, and O1 recordings, referred to FZ. Traces from top to bottom are responses obtained with 17', 35', 70', 144', and 288' checks. Note the lower-amplitude and more-complex waveforms obtained with the largest checks, and slightly different latencies at each check size. The sweep duration is 300 msec; the amplitude calibration bar in the lower right corner is 17.5 μV. Each trace is the average of 100 stimuli.

OZ   PZ   O1

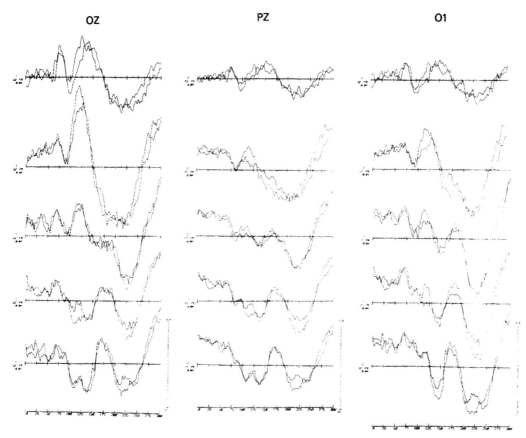

FIG. 2–22. Another normal subject from the same study as in Fig. 2–21, displayed with the same layout. Note that the 144' and 288' check responses are W shaped and apparently delayed, markedly so in the O1 (lateral) channel (*right panel*). The amplitude calibration bars at the lower right of each panel are 6 μV.

obtained from 55' checks (Fig. 2–24). Using a checkerboard reversal stimulus of 18° diameter, Asselman et al. (1975) compared 30' and 57' checks and obtained larger amplitudes with the smaller checks. Erwin (1981) found that the highest-amplitude positive component was obtained from checks subtending an angle between 15' and 30' with attenuation when using larger or smaller checks; his checkerboard subtended 15.6°. Ristanovic and Hajdukovic (1981) (using a 22.6° stimulus field width) found that P100 amplitude measured from preceding negative peak to P100 peak was maximal at a check size of about 60' whereas baseline to P100 amplitude was greatest with slightly larger checks.

Similarly, Meredith and Celesia (1982) studied fields and checks of different sizes in different parts of the visual field and confirmed that visual resolution (i.e., optimal check size) and receptive field size vary across the visual field. Small checks and fields were optimal stimuli at the fovea, larger checks and fields at the periphery. Thus, they suggested that the discrepancies between different studies in regard to the relative contribution to the P100 of different areas of the visual field can be reconciled by correcting for the visual resolution and size of stimuli needed to activate equivalent areas of striate cortex (see also Cowey and Rolls, 1974).

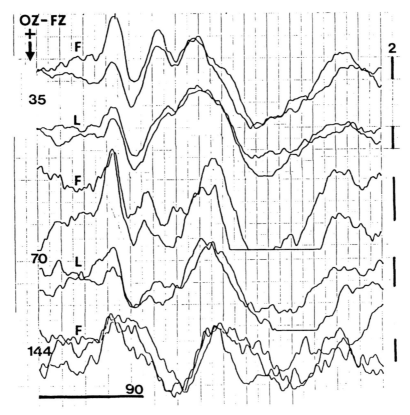

FIG. 2–23. Selected PSVEP results from a patient suspected of having demyelinating disease. The major positivity is apparently delayed with the 144' checks (*bottom channel*), but this is a normal variant (cf. Fig. 2–22). Two sets of traces are shown at the 35' and 70' check sizes; these were obtained with full (F) and lower half-field (L) stimulation. Calibration marks are in milliseconds and microvolts. Each trace is the average of 100 stimuli.

In the study of Yiannikas and Walsh (1983) the peak latency of P100 progressively increased as field size was reduced to below 8° in diameter and was maximal for the largest checks (110') (Fig. 2–24). A moderate amount of intersubject variability in the patterns of responses to different check sizes was also seen, particularly with small stimulus fields. These variations are dependent on visual acuity, with the optimal check size increasing as the visual acuity is reduced (Halliday et al., 1982). Ristanovic and Hajdukovic (1981) also reported that decreasing check size from 60' to 30' produced approximately a 5-msec increase in P100 latency; further diminution in check size produced an exponential increase in P100 latency.

Harding et al. (1980b) found that variations in check size did not affect P100 potential-field distribution. Sokol et al. (1981b) tested 125 normal subjects between 10 and 80 years old with 12' and 48' checks and found that latency increased with age nearly twice as fast for the smaller checks (see also Sokol and Moskowitz, 1981a). Kurita-Tashima et al. (1991) and Torok et al. (1992) have also reported on check-size effects.

Tomoda et al. (1991) have noted that simultaneously recorded PERG and PSVEP spatial frequency functions demonstrated different tuning behavior for cortical and retinal components and that this technique may allow separate analysis of their processing of visual information.

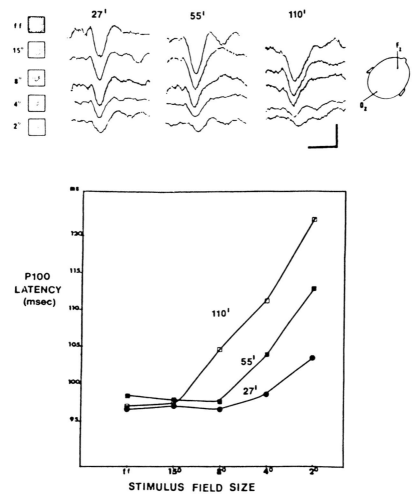

FIG. 2–24. Effect of interaction of check and stimulus field sizes on P100 latency. Note that the smaller fields have significantly longer latencies with larger checks. FZ–OZ recording derivation, OZ positivity produces a downward deflection. Calibration marks are 100 msec and 5 μV, except that top two channels (27′ checks) are 10 μV. (From Yiannikas and Walsh, 1983, with permission.)

Note that, in contrast to changing field size, changing check size does not affect overall luminance; see above.

8.1.7. Reversal Frequency and Direction

The effect of stimulus rate (frequency of pattern reversals) was explored briefly by Stockard et al. (1979) using an LED checkerboard stimulator. They found a P100 latency increase of 4.8 msec when the stimulus rate was increased from 1 to 4 Hz. At faster rates, of course, the waveform becomes less distinct and at about 8 or 10 Hz the waveforms entrain to produce a steady-state EP (see Section 9 below).

Reversal direction has no meaning unless a rotating mirror device is used when the contrast borders move from right to left or in the opposite direction. Asselman et al. (1975) found no difference in the EPs produced by either of these.

With mechanical pattern-shift devices, the checks may not be reversed completely, that is, the displacement may be less than full. Fenwick and Turner (1977) found that P100 amplitude increased in a linear fashion along with the extent of pattern displacement. They also found that with full displacement P100 latency was significantly longer (about 3 msec, $p = 0.003$) than with partial displacements.

Regional cerebral blood flow increased with stimulus rate up to 8 per second and then declined gradually (Fox and Raichle, 1985) for both pattern-reversal and flash stimulation.

8.1.8. Stimulator Type

There are a variety of techniques used to generate pattern reversals without change in overall luminance: (1) back projection onto a translucent screen via a rotating mirror, (2) two synchronized projectors, (3) oscilloscopes, (4) video (TV) monitors, (5) arrays of naked LEDs (Mushin et al., 1984; Lesser et al., 1985), (6) LEDs behind colored squares, and (7) LEDs with optical fibers (Pratt et al., 1984).

The time taken to reverse the pattern has a clear effect on latency of P100. Trojaborg and Petersen (1979) used a mirror system and found that as reversal time increased from 3 to 50 msec, P100 latency increased linearly by 0.6 msec/msec. Video (TV) devices take 20 to 30 msec to completely change the pattern; since most of the P100 is generated by the lower part of the visual field, there can be a delay before that part of the pattern is rewritten. Thus, Stockard et al. (1979) compared TV to LED devices and found longer latencies with the TV. Also, if the pattern reversal with the TV device is synchronized with the start of the raster scan sweep, the blanking pulse (usually close to 60 Hz) produces a prominent artifact. To avoid this, the pattern reversal is usually started at random points on the screen; the uncertainty of synchronization thus engendered may tend to produce a P100 with a slightly broader peak (van Lith et al., 1978), although this is not significant in clinical situations. The intersubject variability is not significantly different between mirror and TV devices (Lowitzsch et al., 1980).

Another matter of interest is whether or not there is a difference in sensitivity to conduction defects between devices which actually move a contrast border across the screen to accomplish the pattern reversal (e.g., mirror devices) and those which do not (e.g., TV devices). The angular velocity of contrast border movement in the former devices is so high when compared to velocities used in classical visual system physiologic investigations that the overall effect is to produce an on–off response. In agreement with this, Lowitzsch et al. (1980) found no consistent differences between mirror and TV devices in patients with retrobulbar neuritis. Andersson and Siden (1994) found longer latencies in normals with a LED array device as compared with a TV monitor and also noted a higher frequency of abnormal findings in patients with MS with the LEDs.

Sinusoidal gratings have been used to study the effect of stimulus orientation (vertical, horizontal, and oblique). The gratings have their spatial frequency component orientation primarily at a right angle to the long axis of the grating, whereas checkerboard patterns have the orientation at an oblique angle. Camisa et al. (1981) found abnormalities in MS patients with gratings in one orientation but not in others, suggesting that stimulation in different planes will increase PSVEP diagnostic sensitivity. However, their waveforms were of irregular outline and repetitions were not shown, so these findings need to be confirmed.

When partial-field stimulation is used, a significant amount of time may elapse between the testing of one field and the next. Since P100 amplitude can be affected by changes in subject concentration, the comparison of amplitudes is then not reliable. This factor is controlled for by the use of sequential stimulation techniques (see Rowe, 1981; Chiappa and Jenkins, 1982; and Section 1).

8.1.9. Potential-Field Distribution

Different midline recording locations do not have significantly different P100 latencies with full-field stimulation. However, the amplitude and polarity of the waveform recorded at a given site can vary greatly between normal subjects (see Section 5). If recordings are made from lateral locations, or if partial-field stimulation is used, then there can be latency differences which must be taken into account (see Table 2–2; also see Sections 8.1.4 and 8.1.5 above). Also note that Towle et al. (1991) have plotted three-dimensional Lissajous trajectories for PSVEPs, in both normal subjects and patients with MS.

8.2. Subject/Patient Factors

8.2.1. Age

Although there have been differing reports in the literature concerning the effect of aging on P100 latency, these may be unified, in many respects, by a consideration of stimulus parameters. For example, age-related effects are more prominent with smaller checks and lower-intensity stimulation. Variations in the methods of data analysis have also contributed to the divergence of results in this area.

Studies by Asselman et al. (1975), Hennerici et al. (1977), Allison et al. (1979), and Stockard et al. (1979) suggested no change in P100 latency until beyond the fifth decade, and then an increase of 2 to 5 msec per decade. In contrast, Celesia and Daly (1977) reported a 2 msec per decade P100 latency increase from the end of the second decade on up.

Sokol et al. (1981) resolved some of the differences in the above studies by showing that check size affected the rate of change of P100 latency with age, and this has been confirmed by others (Celesia et al., 1987). Sokol et al. (1981) found that the rate of increase was nearly twice as fast for 12' as compared with 48' checks (Fig. 2–25). They thought that senile miosis was not the cause of this effect (pupil diameter under low-light conditions decreases with age, from an average of 5 mm at 20 years to 3 mm at 80 years) because (1) previous studies had demonstrated equivalent latency changes for changes in pupillary diameter with the two check sizes, and (2) the change in retinal illumination secondary to the decrease in pupillary diameter is not enough to produce the latency alterations observed in the older subjects. They postulated that the different rate of change between small and large checks as a function of age reflects a differential change in the capacity of the visual system to process spatial frequency information.

Celesia et al. (1987) noted latency increases in the PERG b-wave and in the PSVEP N70 and P100 with 15' checks but changes in the PERG only with 31' checks. The PSVEP latency prolongation with the smaller checks could not be attributed to the PERG changes alone; they found increases in the b-wave to N70 and the b-wave to P100 interpeak latencies (retinocortical times) as well, suggesting that age-related changes occurred both in the retina and in the more rostral parts of the visual system.

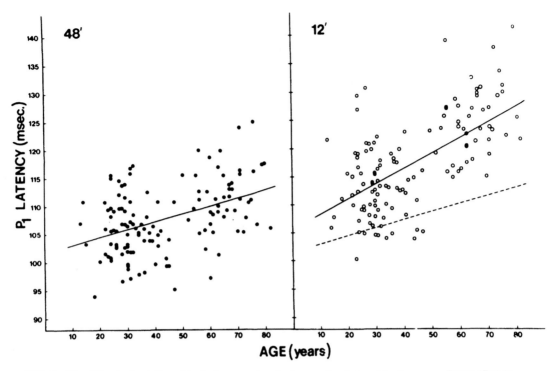

FIG. 2–25. Effect of relationship between check size and adult subject age on P100 (P1) latency. Each data point is the mean latency of the right and left eyes of each subject. Regression lines (*solid lines*) were fit to the data for each check size using a least-squares linear regression procedure. For ease of comparison the regression line for the 48' checks has also been plotted as a *dashed line* on the 12' graph. Stimulus size = 9.5° × 12°, mean luminance = 1.9 log cd/m² , contrast was 0.84. Recording derivation was 1 cm above inion to ear. (From Sokol et al., 1981, with permission.)

Shaw and Cant (1980) found a latency increase beginning in the fifth decade, evident only when patterns of low luminance were used (lowest luminance yielding a clear effect was 7 cd/m²). Brighter patterns gave a slight increase over the age range tested.

Shearer and Dustman (1980) did not find differences among P100 latency means for six decade age groups below 60 years, but they did demonstrate for the 22- to 60-year group an overall correlation between latency increase and age ($p < 0.001$); they also noted increasing standard deviations of older groups' latency values.

Allison et al. (1983, 1984) showed an increase in P100 latency after age 60. However, when their data were subjected to a second-order polynomial regression analysis (Fig. 2–26), increases in P100 latency could be seen from about age 40. Using a simple developmental model, Eggermont (1988) has defined three exponential functions with time constants of 4 weeks, 40 weeks, and 4 years which describe maturational latency changes.

Amplitude of the P100 remains reasonably stable during adult life. In the first decade of life, mean amplitude is almost twice that seen in adults (Snyder et al., 1981; Shaw and Cant, 1981). Beyond the sixth decade there are conflicting data. Shaw and Cant (1981) found a gradual decline, whereas La Marche et al. (1986) found a marked increase in females in the 55- to 70-year group compared with younger (25- to 35-year-old) subjects.

Precise information on normal values for P100 latency in neonates and children is rather scarce. Sokol and Jones (1979) and Moskowitz and Sokol (1983) found that the latency of

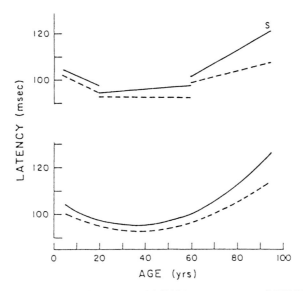

FIG. 2–26. Age-related changes in latency of P100 component of PSVEP. *Solid lines* are results from 130 females, *dashed lines* from 156 males. No significant male–female slope differences were seen. Upper analysis is a linear regression, lower is a second-order polynomial regression. The "S" indicates a male–female difference significant at the $p > 0.01$ level. Check size was 50', left eye only tested. (Adapted, with the publisher's permission, from Allison et al., 1984.)

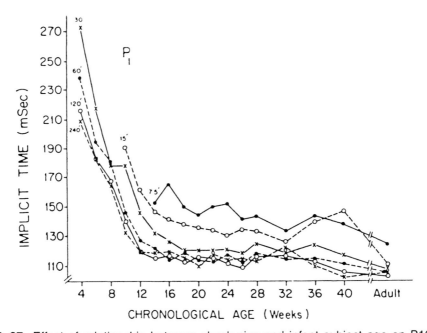

FIG. 2–27. Effect of relationship between check size and infant subject age on P100 absolute latency (implicit time). Stimulus size = $14° \times 18°$, mean luminance = 78 cd/m², contrast was 0.84. Recording derivation was 1 cm above inion to left ear. (From Sokol and Jones, 1979, with permission.)

large checks (>30') reached adult levels by 20 weeks, whereas the latency of smaller checks did not reach adult values until 5 or 6 years, showing the most rapid decrease in the first year (Fig. 2–27). The latter study also found a relation between stimulus rate and age. Sokol et al. (1983) also used PSVEPs to estimate accommodation in infants. Fenwick et al. (1981) found no significant changes in latency or amplitude in 73 children, aged 6 to 11. However, Kjaer (1980) found latencies in the 10- to 19-year age group significantly longer than in adults, and Allison et al. (1984) showed a progressive decrease in latency in the 4- to 19-year age group, suggesting the occurrence of latency changes right up to adult years. Tobimatsu et al. (1993) found similar results and also studied the age effect on multiple check sizes, luminances, and contrasts.

Celesia et al. (1987) found a progressive latency increase of PERG P50 (b-wave) with age for both 15' and 31' checks. Simultaneous PSVEPs showed no age effect for 31' checks, but P100 and N50–P100 latencies for 15' checks did increase. Emmerson-Hanover et al. (1994) studied the combined effects of gender and age.

8.2.2. Visual Acuity

Early results from pattern-flash EP studies indicated a close correlation between EP amplitude and sharpness of the image. Thus, Harter and White (1968) placed a translucent screen in front of the pattern or used +1, +3, and +6 diopter lenses to degrade its appearance and found that the level of acuity determined which check size produced the largest response. Small checks evoked the best responses when refraction was best, but with loss of acuity larger checks were needed to obtain a comparable EP (Harter and White, 1970). These results are in general agreement with what has been found for pattern-reversal stimulation.

With pattern-reversal stimulation the effect of check size accounts for different statements in the literature concerning the relationship between visual acuity and P100 latency. Thus, Collins et al. (1979) using 12' checks found that reducing visual acuity to 20/200 (with a +2 diopter lens) caused a 20-msec increase in P100 latency, whereas Halliday et al. (1973a) using 50' checks found no relationship between visual acuity and P100 latency in patients recovering from optic neuritis. Sokol and Moskowitz (1981) used spherical and cylindrical lenses to study the effects of refractive error and astigmatism (together termed "retinal blur") in cyclopleged and uncyclopleged eyes. They found that P100 latency was shortest when visual acuity was optimal (i.e., when the pattern was least blurred) and that defocusing the retinal image had a greater effect on latency for small checks (12') than for large checks (48'). Blurring in the fundamental frequency component planes of the checkerboard (oblique) produced no change as long as one plane remained in focus. [See also Bobak et al. (1987) for a discussion of the effect of blur and contrast on latency.]

The amplitude–refraction correlation also found by the above investigators has led to the use of the PSVEP for measurement of visual acuity in uncooperative subjects (e.g., infants) and for rapid refraction (see Ludlam and Meyers, 1972; Millodot, 1977; Regan, 1977; Rentschler and Spinelli, 1978). Note that Bostrom et al. (1978) sounded a note of caution in using steady-state EPs for rapid refraction, claiming an accuracy only to about 1 diopter. Millodot and Newton (1981) used the PSVEP to study the amplitude of accommodation.

In the practical use of PSVEPs in neurologic applications, if the diminished visual acuity is not accompanied by a decrease in retinal illumination (as would be the case with a dense cataract) and large-enough checks are used (>35'), even 20/200 visual acuity will not produce P100 latency shifts, a conclusion also generally supported by the careful systematic study performed by Bartel and Vos (1994). For example, Fig. 2–28 (E, F) shows normal latency but decreased amplitude of P100 in a patient with 20/400 visual acuity (lens removed because of cataract) and Fig. 2–29 shows similar P100 latency stability in a patient with 20/800 vision in an eye with a detached retina. However, note that the diminished visual acuity associated with amblyopia-ex-anopsia may be accompanied by P100 latency increases (see Chapter 3, Section 3.8, and Fig. 3–8).

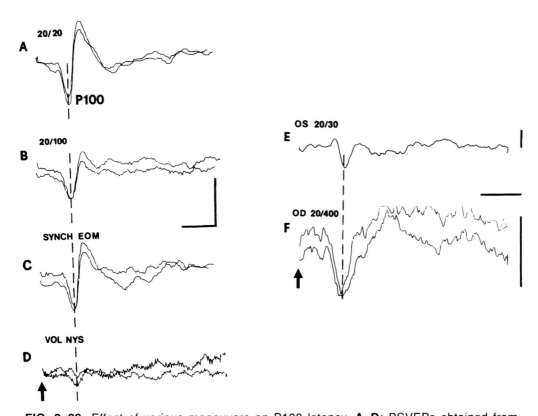

FIG. 2–28. Effect of various maneuvers on P100 latency. **A–D:** PSVEPs obtained from stimulation of one eye of a normal subject under four different conditions; in **A** corrected visual acuity was 20/20; in **B,** without correction, visual acuity was 20/100; in **C** subject attempted to synchronize eye movements with the pattern-shift; in **D** subject produced rapid oscillations of eyes ("voluntary nystagmus") by tonic contractions of all extraocular muscles. Note no change in P100 latency (time from stimulus at *arrow* to P100 peak) with any of these maneuvers. Poor visual acuity and voluntary nystagmus reduced P100 amplitude, however. Calibration marks are 100 msec and 15 μV. **E** and **F** are from a patient after lens removal from right eye (OD) because of a cataract. Even with a visual acuity of 20/400 there is no latency shift of P100 relative to left eye (OS). Amplitude is much lower in right eye; note vertical (amplitude) calibration marks, which are 15 μV in **E** and 5 μV in **F.** Recordings taken from OZ–CZ derivation; each line is the response to 128 stimulus repetitions; each is repeated for verification of P100 latency and amplitude. (From Chiappa, 1983a, with permission.)

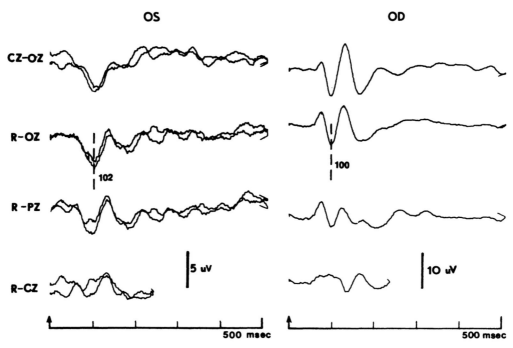

FIG. 2–29. Pattern-shift VEPs from a patient who had a detached retina with a visual acuity in the left eye (OS) of 20/800 (finger counting at a few inches). Note the normal latency, reduced amplitude P100 in that eye. R, linked ears reference; OD, right eye.

8.2.3. Reproducibility–Reliability

A critical element in the utility of any test in clinical neurophysiology is resistance to alteration by changes in the subject's psychological parameters, especially level of attention (or concentration). Meienberg et al. (1979) (24° screen, 60′ checks) tested 10 subjects continuously for up to 17 minutes and found no significant changes in P100 latency. They noted that P100 was the only component that was constantly present and kept its latency, while wave shape and amplitude were more variable. Barber and Galloway (1978) found reasonable consistency in P100 amplitude during a protracted period (about 5 hours) of testing, with amplitude remaining in a 5- to 10-μV range. Uren et al. (1979) studied the effects of accuracy of fixation, degree of concentration, and voluntary defocusing and concluded that only focusing on the corner of the screen instead of the center produced significant latency changes. However, Bumgartner and Epstein (1981) found that 4 of 15 subjects could completely obliterate P100 when instructed to "avoid perceiving the stimulus" and one was able to alter the latency by 15 msec. Tan et al. (1984) found that 7 of 12 normal subjects could deliberately produce abnormal PSVEPs, by near-point accommodation in 6 and eccentric fixation in 1 (remainder unknown). Larger checks and stimulus field partially blocked these changes.

In 11 subjects who performed difficult problem solving during testing, Lentz and Chiappa (1985) found no significant change in the PSVEP and, in fact, a latency decrease in 8 and amplitude increase in 5 (e.g., Fig. 2–30). "Ocular convergence" (an easily detectable maneuver) effectively abolished P100 in three of nine subjects; latencies were stable in the remaining subjects. With near fixation, one of six subjects abolished P100 (restored by use of 136′

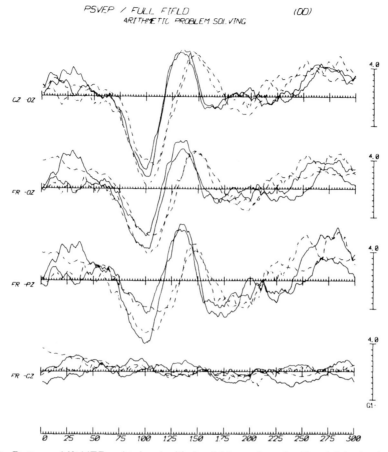

FIG. 2–30. Pattern-shift VEPs obtained with (*solid traces*) and without (*dashed traces*) the normal subject performing mental arithmetic (multiplying two-digit numbers together), gazing at the center of a 30° screen with high contrast, 65' checks. Two trials of each condition are superimposed, the mental arithmetic trials showing a slight but insignificant decrease in latency. The difficulty of the task, with new problems presented aurally as soon as the previous one was completed, was such that the subjects would scarcely recall having viewed the checks during that time. Each trial is the average of 100 stimuli presented at 2/sec. The channels from top down are CZ–OZ, and CZ, PZ, and OZ referred to FZ. Calibration marks are milliseconds and microvolts. (Results reported by Lentz and Chiappa, 1985.)

checks), and another had "abnormal" latency prolongation which was not improved by increasing check size. When instructed to "avoid perceiving the stimulus" (but still maintain gaze direction), using a 21° screen, only 1 of 28 subjects abolished P100 (Fig. 2–31) and 3 had latency prolongations which were at the upper limit of normal for interside differences although within normal limits for absolute latency (Fig. 2–32). Decreasing screen size to 5° or 10° in diameter resulted in 9 of 19 subjects being able to abolish P100. When retested with the large screen P100 returned in all of these but one, and in one of those whose P100 returned it was then abnormal by the interside latency difference measure.

In consideration of possible voluntary (malingering) alterations of PSVEPs in patients, the maneuvers that produce the most marked changes (eyes closed, gaze direction completely off screen, convergence, tip-of-nose fixation) are easily detected by observations. If

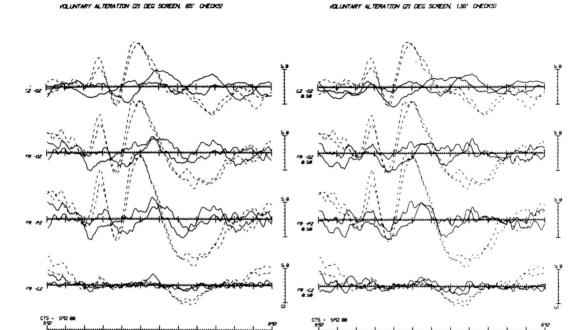

FIG. 2–31. Pattern-shift VEP results from the only normal subject who was able to abolish P100 with purely mental maneuver during testing (close observation revealed good gaze concentration on the center of a 30°, high-contrast screen). *Dashed traces* are control with subject not attempting to affect P100; *solid traces* are with subject employing her mental maneuver (the subject refused to reveal it). With 65' checks (*left panel*) P100 is abolished; with 135' checks (*right panel*) P100 amplitude is markedly diminished but still present. This dramatic result was obtained only after feedback training. Channel derivations as for Figure 2–30; amplitude calibration bars are 5 µV. (Results reported by Lentz and Chiappa, 1985.)

it is recognized from watching the developing average that the responses are of low amplitude, the technician must check that the subject is watching the pattern and if not, must encourage the subject to do so. Although automatic techniques of monitoring fixation (Lavine et al., 1980) are not readily available, the importance of this aspect of PSVEP testing cannot be overemphasized and, hopefully, such equipment and methods will continue to be developed. Note that although it is difficult for an observer to know the gaze direction of a subject even with reasonably close observation of the eyes, most patients do not know this and the mere act of being closely watched results in much greater compliance with gaze direction instructions. This is especially helpful in poorly cooperative patients.

Even with these precautions it is still possible for the subject to look just off the edge of the screen and produce a very low-voltage or absent response without the technician's knowledge of the incorrect angle of gaze. The pattern electroretinogram (PERG) recorded simultaneously with the PSVEP may be used as an aid to ensure adequacy of fixation in difficult cases. An abnormal PERG raises the possibility of inadequate fixation (as well as the possibility of retinal disease), while a normal PERG can generally be taken to suggest that fixation was adequate and an abnormal P100 is then indicative of postretinal disease. See Section 11 for a further discussion of PERGs.

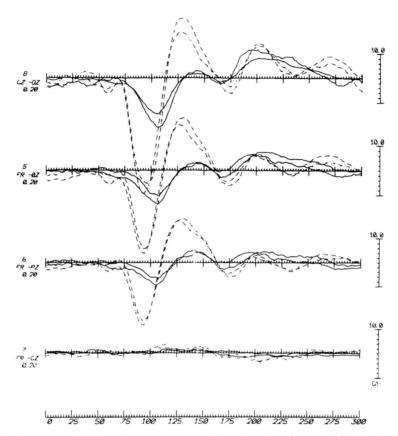

FIG. 2–32. Pattern-shift VEPs from a normal subject showing the usual P100 alteration that was produced by subjects instructed to increase the latency of or abolish P100 with a mental maneuver (without feedback training), while maintaining gaze direction at the center of the screen (parameters as in Fig. 2–31). *Dashed traces* are control. P100 latency is increased by 10 msec or so, and amplitude is diminished by more than half. Channel derivations as for Fig. 2–30; amplitude calibration bars are 10 μV. (Results reported by Lentz and Chiappa, 1985.)

In order to assess the significance of a change in P100 at different recording sessions, a knowledge of the normal variability is necessary. Oken et al. (1987) found P100 latency varied by up to 11 msec and P100 interocular latency varied by up to 9 msec in studies performed on average 6 months apart. There was a large variation in amplitude, the maximum being a decrease by 60. All values remained within normal limits (mean 3 SD), a not-surprising finding. Time since the initial study and check size had no effect on the results. Several other studies have found similar temporal variability while others have found less (Meienberg et al., 1979; Stockard et al., 1979; Diener and Schiebler, 1980; Hammond et al., 1987). Skuse and Burke (1992) showed that over 16 consecutive trials encompassing about

35 minutes, without loss of attention as measured by reaction time, there was a decrease in the amplitude of the N70–P100 without a significant change in the latency, although there was an increase in variability of the latter.

8.2.4. Body Temperature

Raising body temperature in normals has produced no significant change in P100 latency (Matthews et al., 1979; Bajada et al., 1980; Saul and Selhorst, 1981). In patients with MS, Matthews et al. (1979) found no effect on P100 latency from a rise in body temperature, although the short-latency somatosensory evoked potential (SLSEP) showed changes in the cervical component. Bajada et al. (1980) found no changes in five patients with MS, whereas Saul and Selhorst found conduction blocks in some of their patients with conduction delays and previous optic neuritis. However, the waveforms in the latter study were of irregular shape and trial repetitions were not shown, therefore these findings need confirmation.

8.2.5. Gender

Females have usually been found to have slightly shorter P100 latencies than males. Stockard et al. (1979) studied 100 normal age-matched male and female subjects (13 to 67 years) and found the female mean P100 latency to be 2.7 msec shorter. Kjaer (1980) studied 100 normal subjects and, using the means for sex–age groups, found that males had longer P100 latencies in the 20- to 69-year range but females had longer latencies in the 10- to 14- and 15- to 19-year ranges (differences about 3 msec). Allison et al. (1983) also found longer P100 latencies in adult males (20- to 59- and 60- to 95-year age groups) but no sex differences in subjects in the 4- to 19-year group. Celesia et al. (1987) found shorter latencies for females with 31′ checks but not with 15′ checks. Two studies (Shearer and Dustman, 1980; La March et al., 1986) found no gender differences in age-matched normal subjects.

Stockard et al. (1979) suggested that head size might be responsible for the shorter female latencies. The inion–nasion distance in their female subjects was 3.9 cm less on average than the males. They also suggested that higher deep body and brain temperatures in females might be a contributing factor. Allison et al. (1983) used data from Dekaban and Sadowsky (1978) on brain weight (and hence volume) differences between males and females and an estimate by Schmidt-Nielsen (1975) that the length of any brain pathway should vary proportional to the cube root of volume to calculate an expected mean male/female pathway length ratio of 1.034. They found that this value accounted for the differences in P100 latency between their male and female subjects. Guthkelch et al. (1987) found that P100 latency was more highly correlated with head circumference than with gender and that once head circumference was taken into account, gender had little or no effect. Similarly, Erwin et al. (1981) demonstrated in 22 normal volunteers that the transverse (preauricular notch to preauricular notch) head measurement, rather than gender, is a major determinant.

Mean P100 amplitude is usually greater in females than in males (Allison et al., 1984; La Marche et al., 1986; Celesia et al., 1987). The reasons for this are unclear, although hormonal influences may be responsible (Celesia et al., 1987) and Marsh and Smith (1994) have shown shorter latencies in pregnant as compared with nonpregnant women. Emmerson-Hanover et al. (1994) studied the combined effects of gender and age.

8.2.6. Eye Dominance

Seyal et al. (1981) separated normal subjects on the basis of sighting dominance and tested them with a 9.7° screen and 15.6′ checks. They found that P100 amplitudes were higher on average (12 of 14 at OZ) from the dominant eye in right-eye-dominant subjects both in the midline and laterally. Handedness did not appear to influence the amplitude asymmetry. A similar trend was noted in left-eye dominant subjects, but was only significant at O2. The mean latency of the P100 peak was significantly shorter with stimulation of the dominant eye (99.76 versus 99.00, $p < 0.03$).

8.2.7. Eye Movement

There has been no systematic investigation of the effects of eye movements on P100 latency. In one subject who attempted to synchronize eye movements with the pattern-reversal there was no change (see Fig. 2–28C). When the same subject produced voluntary nystagmus (a tonic contraction of the extraocular muscles generating a quivering of the eyes) throughout the recording, P100 amplitude was greatly diminished but latency was unaffected (see Fig. 2–28D). In patients, those with nystagmus caused by problems not associated with optic nerve disease have had normal P100 latencies.

8.2.8. Drugs

There have been few reports of the effects of common therapeutic medications on PSVEPs. Fenwick et al. (1984) reported changes induced by nitrous oxide. Lithium had no effect on latencies, although amplitude changes were seen (Fenwick and Robertson, 1983). Maiese et al. (1992) showed prolonged visual and brainstem evoked responses prior to clinical evidence of optic and otic toxicity in intra-arterial cisplatin use. Bodis-Wollner et al. (1982) reported that PSVEPs became abnormal in 6 of 11 previously untreated schizophrenics who were treated with dopaminergic blocking agents. Chlorpromazine produced changes in the ERG and pattern VEP (Bartel et al., 1990). Bartel et al. (1990) found a small-latency increase with chlorpromazine in both PSVEP P100 and PERG P50, greater with smaller checks (4.7 and 3.0 msec), but no change with oxazepam.

8.2.9. Hyperventilation

Davies et al. (1986) showed a small decrease in mean P100 latency (1.4 msec; range 1 to −3 msec) in seven normal subjects with hyperventilation to a carbon dioxide tension of 13–24 mmHg.

9. STEADY-STATE STIMULATION

When the stimulus repetition rate is sufficiently fast (an interstimulus interval of less than about 200 msec) and the recording sweep is several times the interstimulus interval, a long train of repetitive waves may be seen. For example, the single flashes in the conventional EEG recording shown in Fig. 1–1 produce a visible EP at a latency of about 100 msec. If the strobe flash rate is increased to 8 or 10/sec, the EP waveforms will entrain into a long run of waves with a sinusoidal appearance, the "photic driving" of EEG. This is a steady-state EP;

the averaging process used in EP studies serves to reduce random variation due to artifact. Figure 2–33 shows steady-state PSVEPs from a normal subject.

Each peak of the EP appears at some latency from the stimulus that produced it. This time difference is expressed as phase lag between the stimulus and the EP. The phase lag is usually different for different rates of stimulation; therefore, a phase lag measured at a single stimulus frequency is not equivalent to a transient EP latency. Rather, the phase lag must be measured for at least three stimulus frequencies and the slope of the phase plot (phase versus frequency) determined. "Apparent latency" then equals 1/360 of the slope of the phase plot but note that (1) this measure is not necessarily identical to transient EP latency (Milner et al., 1974), and (2) 180° is the largest phase displacement that can be measured unequivocally, that is, a phase difference of 185° would be seen as a phase difference of 5°. The peak-to-peak amplitude of the EP is also measured and used in amplitude versus stimulus frequency plots. See Milner et al. (1974), Regan et al. (1976), and Spekreijse et al. (1978) for further explanations of these techniques. In addition, the amplitude and phase lag data can be determined continuously by electronic means; this technique has been used while different lenses have been applied to rapidly refract uncooperative subjects (Ludlam and Meyers, 1972; Regan, 1973, 1977; Millodot, 1977; Rentschler and Spinelli, 1978), although Bostrom et al. (1978) have suggested that this method is accurate only to within 1 diopter.

Steady-state EPs have also been used to investigate patients with MS and optic neuritis (Milner et al., 1974; Spekreijse et al., 1978), papilledema (Kirkham and Coupland, 1981),

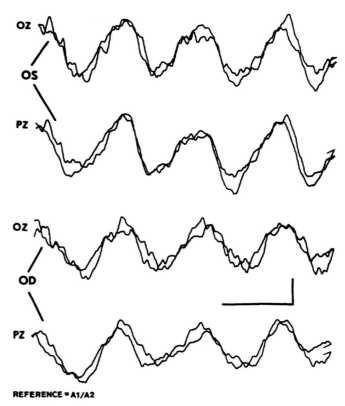

REFERENCE = A1/A2

FIG. 2–33. Steady-state PSVEPs. Checkerboard reversed 20 times/sec. Each trace is the average of 512 stimuli, with a repetition superimposed. Calibration marks are 50 msec and 5 μV.

and visual-field defects (Regan and Heron, 1969; Wildberger et al., 1976; Carlow and Williams, 1980).

The relative difficulty of using steady-state potentials has resulted in transient EPs remaining the primary technique in use.

10. SHORT-LATENCY VEPS

Short-latency VEPs to flash have been reported for many years (Cobb and Dawson, 1960; Ciganek, 1961; Vaughan and Hull,1965; Vaughan, 1966; Allison et al., 1977). These consisted of waveforms starting as early as 28 msec with peak latencies and polarities differing from study to study. Oscillatory potentials starting as early as 35 msec were also reported. Cracco and Cracco (1978) noted oscillatory potentials beginning at 12 msec and persisting for up to 90 msec. It was considered that these were not of myogenic origin since they were unaffected by muscle tension and not of retinal origin because their latency and waveform characteristics were different from those of ERG. Comparison with animal studies suggested a possible origin in optic nerves and tracts. Siegfried and Lukas (1981) found that wavelets recorded between OZ and CZ at 50 msec had different repetition rates and relations to retinal illumination than did the ERG, suggesting a nonretinal origin. Pratt et al. (1982) used a noncephalic reference and concluded that components before 40 msec originate within the eyeball (amplitude maximal periocularly, with appropriate polarity reversals), subsequent components (40–70 msec) in the optic nerves and tracts (latency and polarity characteristics), and later components, more centrally. The consistency of latencies in different scalp locations suggested a possible clinical role.

Harding and Rubenstein (1980, 1982) used a vertex reference and found that 43 of 45 normal subjects had a set of waveforms recordable from just behind T3/T4 with mean latencies of 20.6 (P), 26.2 (N), and 33.8 (P) msec. They found a mean trial–retrial latency variability of 1.06 msec for the P20.6 component over 1 to 12 months. Even more striking were the findings in three patients with unilateral optic nerve lesions; a patient with presumed optic nerve transection (traumatic fracture of orbit and zygoma) with no light perception and a pale and atrophic optic disc had identical ERG in both eyes but the short-latency components at 22 to 33 msec were absent following flash stimulation of the affected eye. They reported similar results in one patient with an optic nerve tumor and another with macular trauma caused by a metallic intraocular foreign body. In two patients with bitemporal hemianopias they found decreased amplitude of these potentials over the hemisphere contralateral to the eye being stimulated, as would be expected. Postchiasmal lesions usually produced diminished amplitudes contralateral to the field being stimulated. However, in six patients with unilateral retrobulbar neuritis there was no latency increase in these components, even though the P100 component with pattern stimulation was delayed. Harding (1985) reported further experience with these potentials.

Whittaker and Siegfried (1983) studied wavelets at 30 to 40 msec and noted that their spectral sensitivity differed from the ERG (greater sensitivity to blue). They found no evidence for ERG activity posteriorly and thought that wavelets recorded from 35 to 70 msec were generated in the occipital pole. These wavelets had a different response to increasing illumination than did P100. Components after 70 msec they related to activity in more distant areas of visual and association cortex.

Perez-Arroyo and Chiappa (1985) used strobe stimulation in normal subjects and found an N50 that was only slightly affected by increasing stimulus rate (1 to 10/sec), whereas later waves had marked configuration changes. Lower stimulus intensities decreased ampli-

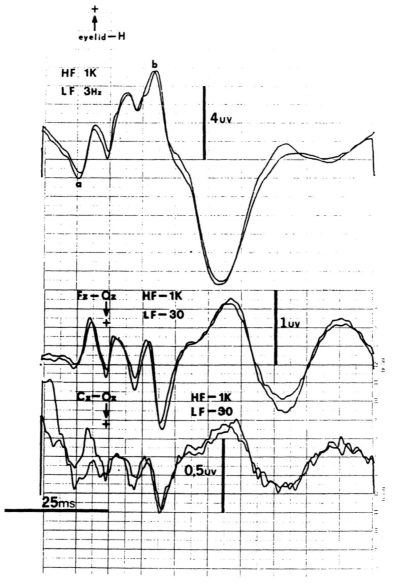

FIG. 2–34. Electroretinogram and VEP following a strobe flash, recorded in a patient who met all clinical criteria of brain death, including no spontaneous respirations. The retinal potentials are visible even in the CZ–OZ bipolar derivation (*bottom channel*), and slow components are visible out to 90 msec (end of sweep). Since the patient was brain dead, a condition characterized by necrosis of all intracranial nervous system structures, no intracranial generator sources could be responsible for any of these potentials. The eyelid electrode was a surface electrode attached to the lower lid, H was an electrode on the dorsum of the hand; relative positivity of the eyelid electrode caused an upward trace deflection (OZ positivity downward for lower two channels). Each trace is the average of 100 stimuli. (Results reported by Perez-Arroyo and Chiappa, 1985.)

tudes of all waves significantly but increased latencies only minimally. N50 amplitude was maximal in occipital and parietal regions; monocular stimulation halved its amplitude. In order to study the scalp distribution of ERG activity, these authors performed similar investigations in brain-dead patients; presumably any EP registered in these patients can only have a retinal origin. The brain-dead patients had 1 to 2 μV of ERG waveforms recordable at the vertex out to 90 msec, and 0.5 to 1.0 μV at occipital and posterior temporal regions; bipolar derivations using these electrodes recorded significant amounts of ERG activity (Fig. 2–34). A comparison between the normal subjects and the brain-dead patients did not show a significant difference in activity until beyond 45 msec and it was concluded that N50 was the first, definite, non-ERG waveform produced by strobe stimulation. A geniculate body origin for N50 was speculated. These conclusions are similar to those of Pratt et al. (1982). Moller et al. (1987) recorded from the optic nerve in humans during surgery and found an initial positivity at 45 msec following a flash stimulus, with a negativity at 60 to 70 msec. Pratt et al. (1994) have suggested the use of high-intensity, goggle-mounted LEDs to improve the consistency of these recordings.

In summary, there has been a moderate amount of investigation in this area but only a few human clinicopathologic correlations are available. Thus, although these findings are interesting and encouraging, the clinical utility of these potentials remains to be clearly delineated.

11. PATTERN ELECTRORETINOGRAPHY

Recording the PERG in combination with the VEP has become increasingly useful in the assessment of the visual pathways. Interest in PERG was stimulated by the demonstration in cats that it was dependent on ganglion cell activity (Maffei and Fiorentini, 1981). The PERG in humans has also been shown to lose amplitude after optic nerve lesions (Dawson et al., 1982; Mashima and Oguchi, 1985). It is still uncertain if there is a contribution from preganglionic sites in humans (Sherman, 1982). Clinically, the PERG has been found useful in evaluating prognosis following optic neuritis (Celesia et al., 1986) and optic nerve compression (Kaufman et al., 1986), and to verify visual fixation in patients with abnormal VEPs (Parsons et al., 1986).

The PERGs may be recorded with gold-foil electrodes (Carter and Hogg, Essex, U.K.) inserted as deeply as possible inside the lower lid in the midline and looped anteriorly to a tape anchor below the eye, with the active side of the foil against the sclera. Local anesthetics are usually not required. Pilot studies with copper wire loops inside the lower lid, and disc electrodes on the skin of the lower lid and medial nose, showed that PERG amplitudes recorded by the gold-foil electrode were consistently at least 20% greater and contained much less movement and muscle artifacts (Tan et al., 1989). Contact lens electrodes are not as practical because it is necessary to use local anesthetics and to refract each eye after lens insertion and apply appropriate corrective lenses during the test, although they register higher amplitudes.

As the PERG is a small response, usually less than 6 μV, artifact rejection during signal averaging is necessary. Froehlich and Kaufman (1992) have described procedures to remove small postsaturation artifacts in an attempt to reduce the variability of PERG amplitudes.

The PERG recorded with a gold-foil electrode (Fig. 2–35) consists of an initial small negativity variably present (N30), followed by larger positive and negative components (P50 and N95) (Holder, 1987). These are usually displayed with relative positivity of the

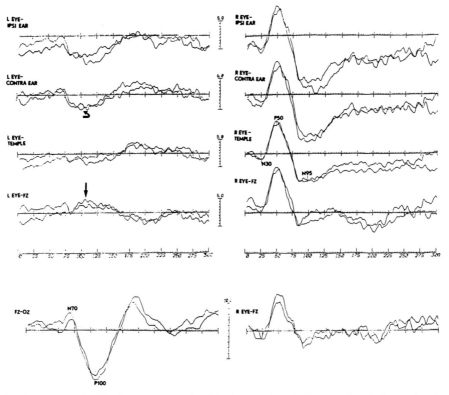

FIG. 2–35. Pattern-ERGs from a normal subject following right-eye stimulation using ipsilateral and contralateral ear, temple, and midfrontal (FZ) references. Simultaneous recordings over the occluded eye are shown on the left. The VEP and PERG in the lowest channels on each side were obtained together but separately from the upper channels (note that this PERG is identical to that shown immediately above). The downward (apparent negative) deflection seen on the occluded side (*curved arrow*) has a latency similar to the VEP P100 and is best seen with ear references (*top and second channels*). A small upward (apparent) positive deflection corresponding to N70 of the VEP is also seen. The Fz reference (*fourth channel*) shows an apparent positive deflection (*arrow*) similar in latency to P100. The temple reference (*third channel*) shows minimal contamination. Each trace is the average of 100 stimuli with two repetitions superimposed. Calibration marks are in microvolts and milliseconds and refer to traces on both sides. Relative positivity at the eye gives an upward deflection (PERG) while relative positivity at OZ gives a downward deflection (VEP). (From Tan et al., 1989, with permission.)

eye causing an upward trace deflection. Some investigators have labeled these the P, Q, and R waves (Kirkham and Coupland, 1983). P50 usually presents an easily identified peak for latency measurements. N95 often has a long duration and an ill-defined peak; its latency is taken at the midpoint of the negative deflection. Measurements are usually not taken for N30 because of its low amplitude and variable presence. P50 amplitude is taken from onset (N30 peak, if present) to P50 peak, and from P50 peak to subsequent trough for N95. Normal values at different check sizes are given in Table 2–6. If the amplifier system is prone to slow recovery from saturation, Froehlich and Kaufman (1992) have suggested procedures to minimize this effect. These same authors (1993) used a nonlinear baseline determination to decrease the variability in N95 recordings.

TABLE 2–6. *Pattern-ERG data from normal subjects*

Check size	Latency	Monocular stimulation				Binocular stimulation			
		Mean (msec)	SD	n	Range	Mean (msec)	SD	n	Range
17 min	P50	55.0	2.0	24	48.9–58.4	54.9	2.2	24	50.2–59.3
	N95	98.0	3.7	24	90.7–106.2	95.9	4.2	24	88.5–105.1
35 min	P50	53.8	2.1	23	48.2–58.5	53.8*	2.1	24	47.7–57.2
	N95	96.0	4.0	23	88.8–104.0	93.9*	5.6	24	85.0–104.0
70 min	P50	—	—			52.1***/***	1.9	24	48.6–55.2
	N95	—	—			91.7***/	4.6	24	85.0–103.8
	Amplitude	Mean (μv)				Mean (μv)			
17 min	P50	3.9	1.4	24	1.8–6.8	4.0	1.4	24	2.0–7.3
	N95	6.2	1.5	24	3.8–9.7	6.0	1.4	24	3.8–10.3
35 min	P50	4.7	1.6	23	2.3–8.2	4.5**	1.5	24	2.8–8.4
	N95	7.1	1.9	23	4.7–12.3	6.4	1.6	24	3.8–10.0
70 min	P50	—	—			4.7***/	1.5	24	2.5–8.7
	N95	—	—			6.4	1.6	24	4.1–10.1
	Amplitude ratio	Mean				Mean			
17 min	P50	0.76	0.14	24	0.52–0.97	0.86	0.08	24	0.71–1.00
	N95	0.76	0.15	24	0.50–1.00	0.84	0.11	24	0.63–1.00
35 min	P50	0.76	0.12	23	0.49–0.94	0.84	0.09	24	0.63–0.98
	N95	0.80	0.16	23	0.36–1.00	0.85	0.11	24	0.56–0.99
70 min	P50	—	—			0.86	0.11	24	0.57–1.00
	N95	—	—			0.86	0.09	24	0.65–0.97

The mean of the two eyes of a subject was used for P50 and N95 latency and amplitude calculations. The amplitude ratio is the smaller amplitude PERG divided by the larger one. Unpaired t-test comparisons between monocular and binocular stimulation showed no significant differences in any parameter. Seventy minute checks were not tested with monocular stimulation. Significance levels of paired t-test comparisons for binocular stimulation are indicated by asterisks (none = NS) following mean values for 35' compared to 17', 70' to 17', and 70' to 35' (to right of /); * = $p < 0.005$, ** $p < 0.001$, *** $p < 0.0005$. (From Tan et al., 1989, with permission.)

Both monocular and binocular stimulation have been used in PERG recording using either contact lens or more commonly gold foil electrodes. Binocular stimulation has several advantages beyond the approximate halving of recording time. Visual fixation is facilitated by the normal eye in conditions where visual acuity is poor unilaterally. Also, since PERG abnormalities are often restricted to a unilateral amplitude reduction, binocular stimulation provides a more reliable interside comparison because identical (simultaneous) recording conditions prevail. Furthermore, inconsistent fixation from drowsiness often results in a loss of amplitude that may lead to interpretive errors; this is more likely to be seen with monocular stimulation when recording session length is essentially doubled.

With binocular stimulation it is imperative that the PERG recorded in one eye not be contaminated by activity from the other eye or other cortical sources. Prominent spread of PERG from one eye to the other has been found during monocular, steady-state stimulation (Peachey et al., 1983; Seiple and Siegel, 1983), and these authors suggest that binocular stimulation should not be used for PERG recording. However, our data (Tan et al., 1989) indicate that most of this apparent cross-contamination is due to the VEP P100 and N100 components being recorded by the ear reference electrodes. The full-field pattern VEP consists of a widespread posterior positivity at about 100 msec, usually encompassing the ears (see Chiappa, 1983b, for a review). This is accompanied by a largely simultaneous negativity at the vertex and frontal regions (Spitz et al., 1986). It is these VEP components which are registered in the occluded eye derivations with apparent opposite polarities and so may augment (ear references) or reduce (midfrontal references) the PERG N95 (Figs. 2–35, 2–36, 2–37). The VEP N70 contributed activity to the reference sites in about half of our normal subjects. As could be predicted from these results in normal subjects, when the P100 is delayed (as in a patient with optic neuritis), these contributions to the recordings in the occluded eye appear at the same (abnormal) latency as the delayed P100 (Figs. 2–36, 2–37). Thus, these VEP components can potentially interfere with interpretation of the PERG N95 and it is not surprising that demyelinating disorders of the optic nerve with delayed VEP P100 often show an amplitude reduction of N95 when an ear reference is used (see Figs. 2–36, 2–37).

In agreement with Berninger (1986), Tan et al. (1989) found the ipsilateral temple to be a better reference site for the PERG since it registers little contaminating VEP activity. In only 2 of 10 subjects did they see a small negative deflection on the occluded side during monocular stimulation using a temple reference. Furthermore, comparison of the two PERG components obtained with both monocular and binocular stimulation (Table 2–6) showed no statistically significant differences. This also indicates little PERG interocular cross-contamination and confirms that binocular testing can be used safely for the advantages outlined above. Comparison of the interside amplitude ratios of the P50 and N95 components showed greater symmetry with binocular stimulation and, similarly, Kirkham and Coupland (1983) found values of 0.65 to 0.75 using monocular stimulation while Holder (1987) reported values of 0.85 to 0.97 using binocular stimulation. The most likely explanation for this difference is loss of visual fixation from drowsiness during the recording, resulting in spurious loss of amplitude. This is less of a problem with binocular stimulation since identical conditions prevail during the test. These findings further emphasize the need to record at least two trials to demonstrate reproducibility when performing PERG.

In a clinical VEP practice aimed at neurologic applications, PERGs need to be performed only when the monocular pattern-reversal VEP is abnormal, and both binocular and monocular stimulation can be used, the latter with simultaneous VEP registration. Pattern ERG testing complements abnormal VEPs by affirming gaze fixation (Parsons et al., 1986) and indicating normal retinal function. Figure 2–38 shows PERG and PSVEPs in a

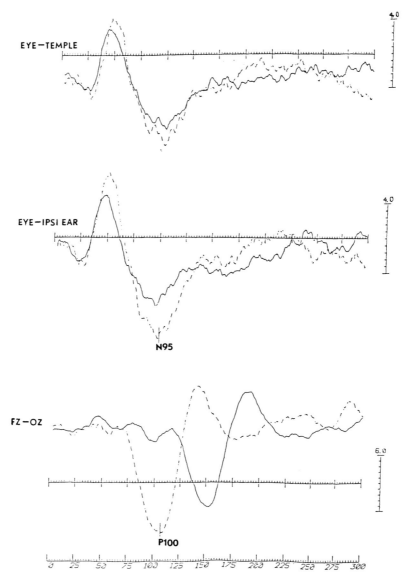

FIG. 2–36. A patient with acute optic neuritis showing a prolonged and lower-amplitude VEP P100 from testing the involved right eye (*solid traces*); the other eye (*dashed traces*) is normal. The PERG shows apparent N95 amplitude reduction on the right with ipsilateral ear reference (*middle channel*) which is not evident with the temple reference (*top channel*). The apparent loss of N95 amplitude is caused by the P100 latency shift because the ear reference contributes much more VEP to the PERG than does the temple. Each trace is the average of two trials each of 100 stimuli. Recording parameters and calibrations are the same as for Fig. 2–35. (From Tan et al., 1989, with permission.)

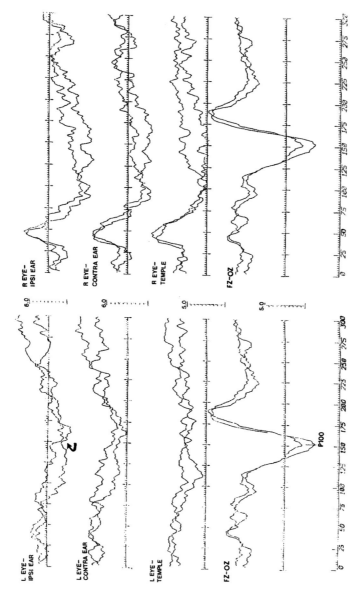

FIG. 2-37. Same patient as in Fig. 2-36, recorded as in Fig. 2-35. The apparent, long-duration (75–100 msec) negativity (*curved arrow*) recorded at the occluded eye (*left*), seen better with ear as compared to temple reference, has a latency corresponding to the prolonged P100. This confirms that the activity recorded from the occluded eye is cross-contamination by VEP P100, not PERG. Recording parameters and calibrations are the same as for Fig. 2–35. (From Tan et al., 1989, with permission.)

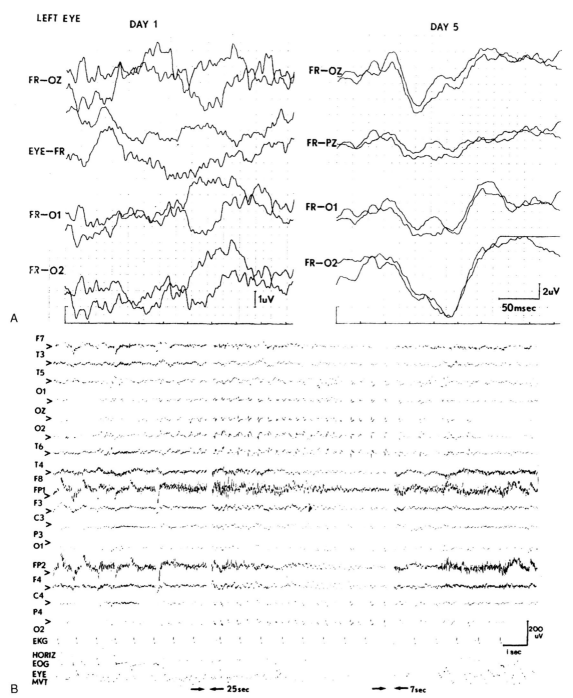

FIG. 2–38. Pattern-ERG/PSVEP (**A**) and EEG (**B**) in a patient who complained of total blindness 8 days postpartum, but who had some clinical features of hysteria-malingering. The presence of a normal PERG on hospital day 1 (*left panel, second channel from top*) simultaneous with an absent cortical P100 provided objective evidence of poor visual function (check size 70′, field size 30°). The EEG showed repeated focal electrographic seizures in both occipital areas; one on the right is shown in **B**. On hospital day 5 the P100 is normal (check size 35′, field size 15°), and visual function had improved markedly. Angiogram and CT scan were normal; MRI showed small occipital lesions. FR is midfrontal reference; relative positivity of the posterior electrode causes a downward trace deflection. EYE is a gold-foil, PERG electrode (see Section 3 on electrode application) with relative positivity causing an upward trace deflection. EYE MVT is a mechanical movement transducer taped over the closed eye. Each trace is the average of 100 stimuli.

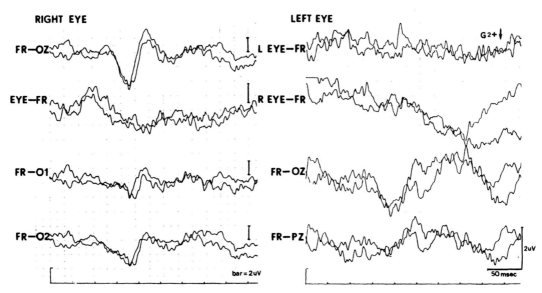

FIG. 2–39. Pattern-ERG/PSVEP results from a patient who claimed to have 20/800 vision in the left eye. The PERG P50 and PSVEP P100 were normal in the right eye, but the P100 latency was abnormal in the left eye and the amplitude was less than half that on the right (see FR–OZ channels). The PERG P50 on the left was of low amplitude (*top channel, right panel*) but present [compared with the lack of a deflection in the recording from the patched right eye (*second channel, right panel*)]. These results in the left could have been produced by poor patient cooperation, but binocular PERG showed that this was not the case (see Fig. 2–40). Electrode nomenclature same as for Fig. 2–38. Each trace is the average of 100 stimulations.

patient who complained of total blindness but had clinical features that raised the possibility of hysteria–malingering. The good PERG on day 1 with absent P100 provided objective evidence of poor visual function; both vision and the P100 had returned 5 days later. Radiologic findings suggested bioccipital infarcts. Figure 2–39 shows normal right-eye P100 and PERG (left panel) in a patient claiming poor vision in the left eye whose PERG and P100 (right panel) are of much lower amplitude. That the low amplitude is not due to poor fixation is shown by binocular PERG testing (Fig. 2–40), where the PERG from the left eye has an amplitude asymmetry compared to the right eye similar to that seen in Fig. 2–39. Since the PERG recordings in Fig. 2–40 are simultaneously generated by the same pattern, and since gaze direction of the two eyes is linked, the lower-amplitude PERG in the left eye cannot be due to poor fixation on the stimulus. Figure 2–41 shows left and right eye results in another patient, with absent P100 on the right. But observation by the technologist suggested that the patient was not attending to the screen during right eye testing. Figure 2–42 shows a similar result with PERG (dashed line) but when the patient was closely observed and "encouraged" (solid line), both the PERG and P100 are markedly enhanced (and normal).

The PERG is also useful in prognostication following optic neuritis (Persson and Wanger, 1984; Serra et al., 1984; Celesia et al., 1986; Ringens et al., 1986; Galloway et al., 1986; Plant et al., 1986) and optic nerve compression (Kaufman et al., 1986), and in the diagnosis of optic atrophies and maculopathies (Kirkham and Coupland, 1981; Sherman, 1982; Arden et al., 1984; Kaufman and Celesia, 1985; Holder, 1987), amblyopia (Sokol

BINOCULAR STIMULATION

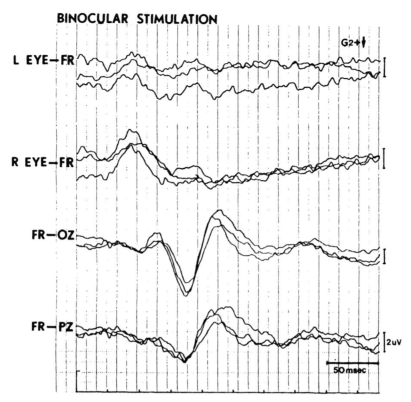

FIG. 2–40. Binocular PERGs in same patient as in Fig. 2–39. The simultaneous recording of a normal PERG P50 on the right (*second channel*) with a much lower amplitude one on the left (*top channel*), similar to the results obtained with monocular testing (see Fig. 2–39), indicated the validity of the abnormal findings from the left eye since the gaze direction of the two eyes and subject stimulus concentration was the same.

and Nadler, 1979; Hess et al., 1985), and glaucoma (Wanger and Persson, 1983; Ringens et al., 1986). Froehlich and Kaufman (1993) used a nonlinear baseline measurement technique to decrease N95 variability and found that maintenance of a normal N95 amplitude at 6 months after onset of optic neuritis was always associated with an excellent clinical recovery, whereas loss of N95 amplitude below laboratory limits of normal was associated with abnormalities in visual function. These same authors (1994) have shown that loss of the PERG N95 component in acute anterior ischemic optic neuropathy can differentiate that disease from optic neuritis, in which the N95 is usually preserved for at least a few weeks.

The relations between check size and PERG amplitude and latency have also been studied. Kirkham and Coupland (1983) found no significant changes in amplitude or latency to four different check sizes (15′, 30′, 40′, and 100′). Trick and Trick (1984) found a relationship between amplitude and check size (comparing their 3.75 per second stimulus reversal data), as did Teping and Groneberg (1984), Berninger and Schuurmans (1985), Schuurmans and Berninger (1985), Tan et al. (1989) and Torok et al. (1992). Sokol et al. (1983) also found similar results for both the PERG and PSVEP. Arden et al. (1982) reported that amplitude increased with increasing check size while latency was unchanged. The largest re-

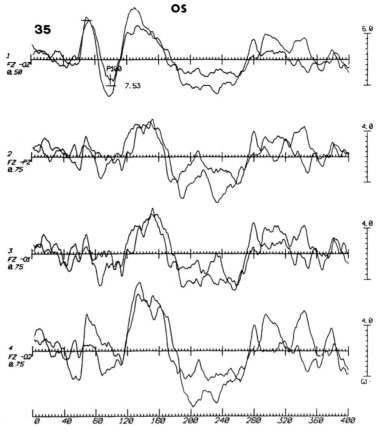

FIG. 2–41. Pattern-shift VEP results from a patient with a normal P100 obtained from the left eye (**A,** *left panel*), whereas the right eye (**B,** *right panel*) had no P100 despite three replications of 100 stimuli each (three traces). The technologist raised a question about the patient's gaze fixation during the test, and a combined PERG/PSVEP was performed (see Fig. 2–42).

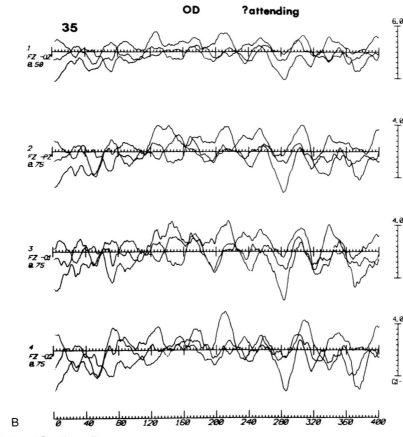

FIG. 2–41. (*Continued*)

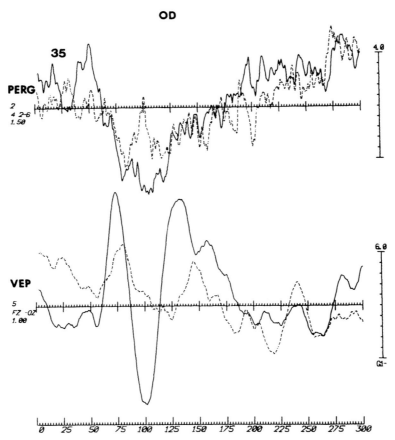

FIG. 2–42. Combined PERG/PSVEP right eye results from same patient as in Fig. 2–41. The first trial (*dashed line*) was obtained with no special instructions to or observation of the patient, and no definite PERG P50 or PSVEP P100 waveforms were seen. The patient was then encouraged to fixate on the center of the stimulus screen and the technologist closely observed the patients' eyes; this second trial (*solid line*) shows a normal P50 and P100. The PERG channel was derived from a gold-foil electrode under the lower lid referred to the ipsilateral temple, the VEP channel was FZ–OZ. Check size was 35'; calibrations are milliseconds and microvolts.

sponse was seen with check sizes between 60' and 30'. They noted that the central 8° produced slightly less PERG than more peripheral areas (out to 16° × 22°), and that the sum of these two was approximately equal to the responses from the whole. As might be expected, PERG amplitude from central areas is much less attenuated as check size is decreased below 30'. Thus, with large stimulus fields, PERG amplitude response to alterations in check size is a complex product of the differential spatial sensitivity of the retinal areas activated, compounded by luminance effects (Spekreijse et al., 1973; Korth, 1983; Riemslag et al., 1985). Refractive errors may also produce important latency shifts in the PERG (Bartel and Vos, 1994) more so than in the PSVEP, and so special care must be taken in that regard.

In conclusion, PERG can be reliably recorded with gold-foil electrode using binocular stimulation. Contamination by VEP is minimized if the ipsilateral temple is selected as the reference site. Binocular stimulation also has the advantage of showing less interside amplitude difference and hence is more sensitive to changes compared to monocular stimulation.

Evoked Potentials in Clinical Medicine,
3d ed., edited by Keith H. Chiappa.
Lippincott–Raven Publishers, Philadelphia © 1997.

3

Pattern-Shift Visual Evoked Potentials: Interpretation

Keith H. Chiappa and °Rosamund A. Hill

*Department of Neurology, Harvard Medical School, and EEG Laboratory,
Massachusetts General Hospital, Boston, Massachusetts 02114; and
°Neuroservices Unit, Auckland Hospital, Auckland, New Zealand*

1. ANATOMIC AND PHYSIOLOGIC BASIS OF PATTERN-SHIFT VISUAL EVOKED POTENTIAL P100

1.1. Human Data

The visual fields as they appear to the subject are mapped onto the retina in reversed format because of the lens properties of the eye. Thus, the right half of the visual field is projected onto the left half of the retina. The retinal areas then map into the lateral geniculate bodies in the thalamus and from there to the occipital cortex in a highly organized manner. Pertinent projections of the visual fields are (1) left visual half field of an eye to right occipital cortex and right field of the same eye to left occipital cortex, (2) macula to occipital poles, (3) more peripheral fields to medial cortex adjacent to the calcarine fissure, and (4) lower fields to cortex superior to calcarine fissure (vice versa for upper fields). The segregation of optic nerve fibers from one eye into the two paths mentioned in (1) above occurs in the optic chiasm; the two paths are (1) temporal half-field (nasal retinal) fibers to contralateral and (2) nasal half-field (temporal retinal) fibers to ipsilateral occipital cortex. (See any standard text of visual system anatomy for a more detailed discussion of this topic.) Consideration of these projection patterns helps to explain the types of

abnormalities seen in pattern-shift visual evoked potential (PSVEP) testing and the potential-field distribution of P100, especially with partial-field stimulus configurations
and visual-field defects.

P100 is generated in striate and prestriate occipital cortex not only as a result of primary
activation but also from subsequent thalamocortical volleys. The exact generator sources of
P100 and the temporal sequence of their activation are not well-defined. Positron emission
tomographic (PET) mapping of human cerebral metabolism showed that both primary and
association visual cortical areas are strongly activated when a reversing-checkerboard pattern is used as a visual stimulus. Furthermore, the metabolic activity produced by the
checkerboard pattern was two to four times greater than with white light (Phelps et al.,
1981). Regional cerebral blood flow increases with stimulus rates up to 8/sec and then gradually declines (Fox and Raichle, 1985) for both flash and checkerboard stimulation.
Noachtar et al. (1993) have recorded from subdural grid electrodes placed for the clinical
evaluation of patients with epilepsy and found well-localized activities in the vicinity of the
calcarine fissure.

Patients with specific lesions of the visual cortex provide some further insight into the
widespread nature of the generator sources of PSVEP activity. There are several case reports of cortically blind subjects studied with PSVEPs: (1) Bodis-Wollner et al. (1977)
found steady-state pattern evoked potentials (EPs) present in a patient who had bilateral
destruction in cortical (association) areas 18 and 19 but preservation in (primary) areas
17, and (2) Celesia et al. (1980, 1982) found essentially normal transient and steady-
state pattern EPs in a patient with bilateral preservation of areas 18 and 19 and destruction of areas 17, and PET scanning showed a preserved island of functioning tissue.
Anatomic verification in these cases was by computed tomography (CT) scan. (Note that
the use of checks smaller than those used in these studies usually reveals abnormalities
in such patients.) These patient data are consistent with the metabolic studies mentioned
above. Experience in similar cases with flash stimulation is noteworthy: (1) Frank and
Torres (1978) found normal VEPs in 30 cortically blind children, (2) Spehlmann et al.
(1977) found present but simplified VEPs in a cortically blind patient subsequently
shown to have extensive infarction of occipital white matter and cortex bilaterally (the
authors suggested an extrageniculocalcarine pathway to secondary visual cortex as the
generator of the VEP), and (3) Corletto et al. (1967) recorded from the occipital cortical
surface of a patient during surgery and found little difference between scalp and cortical
VEP recordings. In the latter case, unilateral occipital lobectomy (for intractable
epilepsy) affected only the components between 45 and 120 msec, causing an amplitude
decrease.

In normal human subjects there have been a large number of EP studies of visual system
physiology. Most of these used flash, pattern-flash, grating, or steady-state stimulation, and
their relationship to transient pattern-reversal stimulation is unclear. Some utilized pattern
reversal as the stimulus (e.g., Michael and Halliday, 1971; Jeffreys, 1971, 1977; Lehmann
and Skrandies, 1979; Lesevre and Joseph, 1979; Blumhardt et al., 1978; Blumhardt and
Halliday, 1979; Haimovic and Pedley, 1982b), with special emphasis on attempting to define the generator sources of the PSVEP. Ducati et al. (1988) recorded flash and pattern-
flash VEPs in awake patients undergoing stereotactic procedures for dyskinetic disorders,
the approach to the nucleus ventralis lateralis thalami being occipital. They concluded that
all components of the VEP recorded from the scalp are generated entirely in cortical layers.
Results from these studies are consistent with, but no more specific than, the sites suggested
by the known anatomic connections, the clinicopathologic correlations mentioned above,
and animal studies.

1.2. Animal Data

There has been a large amount of microscopic anatomic and physiologic investigation of animal visual systems. (See Kandel and Schwartz, 1985, for a recent review, and Hubel and Wiesel, 1977, DeValois et al., 1979, Van Essen, 1979, and Lennie, 1980, for a sample of more detailed discussions.) The relationship of much of this work to checkerboard-reversal stimulation is unclear. For example, Hubel and Wiesel (1965) in their investigations of orientation- and movement-sensitive cells in the visual cortex used contrast border-movement velocities ranging from 1° to 20°/sec. Faster movements did not excite the cells. Goodwin and Henry (1978) also found that most single neurons in the cat striate cortex responded to slower movements (less than 10°/sec). However, the contrast border-movement velocity in a typical mechanical pattern-reversal stimulator is about 100°/sec (complete reversal of a 1° check in 10 msec), a fivefold greater speed. Furthermore, TV-type stimulators, most frequently used, do not have moving contrast borders.

Macroscopically, flash and pattern-flash VEPs have been studied extensively in animals (see Creutzfeldt and Kuhnt, 1973, for a review, and Snyder et al., 1979, and Perryman and Lindsley, 1977, for a sample of more detailed studies), but again the relationship of these studies to pattern-reversal stimulation is unclear. Padmos et al. (1973) did not find a contour-specific component in pattern-appearance VEPs recorded from the scalp in monkeys, but van der Marel et al. (1981) demonstrated that anesthetics abolished the response in those animals. Lieb and Karmel (1974) used pattern-appearance stimuli and depth recordings in awake monkeys. They found initial activation of the parafoveal striate cortex at about 70 msec, followed in succession by activation of foveal striate, foveal prestriate, and inferotemporal cortex. A simple transformation of edge information into VEP amplitude was found in the parafoveal striate region. None of the regions demonstrated long-term habituation of sensitivity to stimulus differences.

Animal data suggest that the visual pathway is composed of several types of cells, each with their own electrophysiologic properties. Briefly, retinal ganglion cells have been classified into X, Y, and W types (for examples of experimental data see Stone and Fukuda, 1974, and for a review see Lennie, 1980). These cell types have been characterized as having the following properties: X, small ganglion cells mediating cone vision via small-diameter axons, with small receptive fields incorporating lateral inhibition, concentration in central visual field, low sensitivity to motion, and providing the substrate for pattern vision via the geniculate pathway; Y, large retinal ganglion cells mediating rod vision without lateral inhibition, via large-diameter axons, with large receptive fields, peripheral retinal location, high sensitivity to motion, and providing one substrate of nonpattern vision possibly via an extrageniculate pathway; W, smallest retinal ganglion cells and axons, projecting exclusively to tectum. One can speculate that the PSVEP is generated by activity in the X system, whereas the strobe (flash) VEP is generated by activity in the Y system.

In summary, animal studies to date have provided little direct information as to the transmission pathways and encoding format, generator sources, and pathophysiology of normal and abnormal responses in the human PSVEP.

2. PATHOPHYSIOLOGY AND CLINICAL INTERPRETATIONS

2.1. Monocular Versus Binocular PSVEP Abnormalities

Since the eyes are tested one at a time (monocularly) and since an eye projects to both occipital lobes, a lesion of the visual pathways posterior to the optic chiasm in one hemisphere does not usually produce an abnormality in P100 as recorded from the posterior midline following full-field stimulation unless there has been a marked lateral shift of the PSVEP potential field. For example, patients with complete homonymous hemianopias from carotid territory infarcts have normal-latency P100s at midline electrodes. The visual pathways in the hemisphere opposite the lesion transmit sufficient impulses to produce a normal latency response. Recording from laterally placed electrodes using full- and half-field stimulation may reveal abnormalities in these circumstances, but the greater normal variability in those conditions renders clinical interpretation more difficult and correlations less definite. (See this chapter, Section 2.4, and Chapter 2, Section 8.1.5, for a discussion of the effects mentioned above.)

Thus, with full-field stimulation, if an abnormality is seen in only one eye (e.g., Fig. 3–1), the lesion producing the abnormality must be anterior to the chiasm. However, it can be in any structure anterior to the chiasm. Glaucoma, retinal degenerations, and compressive lesions of the optic nerve can produce PSVEP abnormalities indistinguishable from those produced by demyelinating disease (see Section 3). These possibilities must be excluded in the clinical situation by the appropriate means. Therefore, the interpretation in the case of a monocular PSVEP abnormality might read: "This abnormality suggests a conduction defect in the left (right) visual pathways anterior to the chiasm." One could add: "Although demyelinating disease is the most common etiology for such a finding, various other possibilities cannot be excluded, for example, retinal disease and compressive lesions of the optic nerve."

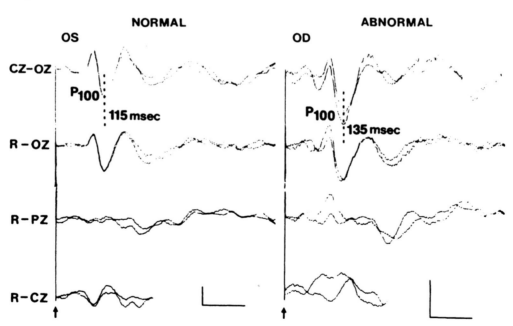

FIG. 3–1. Pattern-shift VEPs recorded from a patient with MS showing a monocular latency abnormality. Left-eye response was normal at 115 msec, right response was abnormal with P100 peak delayed in latency at 135 msec (normal mean plus 3 SD with this pattern-shift stimulator was 117 msec). Each trace is the average of 128 stimuli, with a repetition superimposed. Reference was linked ears; relative positivity at G2 causes a downward trace deflection. Calibration marks are 100 msec and 5 μV. (From Brooks and Chiappa 1982, with permission.)

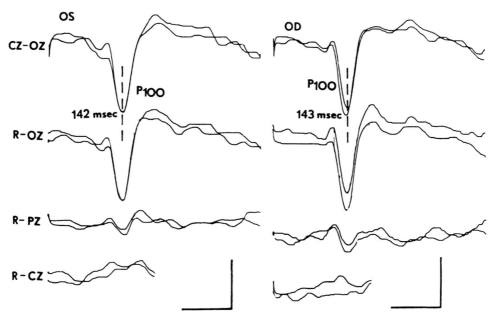

FIG. 3–2. Pattern-shift VEPs recorded from a patient with MS showing binocular latency abnormalities (see Fig. 3–1 legend for normal limits). Each trace is the average of 128 stimuli, with a repetition superimposed. Reference was linked ears. Calibration marks are 100 msec and 10 μV. (From Chiappa, 1983a, with permission.)

If PSVEP abnormalities are found in both eyes with full-field stimulation (e.g., Fig. 3–2), the anatomy of the visual system does not permit one to locate the site of conduction defects in the visual pathways. Thus, binocular abnormalities can be produced by retinal degenerations, tumors in the region of the optic chiasm, central nervous system (CNS) degenerative diseases (e.g., spinocerebellar syndromes), and bilateral optic radiation lesions (e.g., "butterfly" gliomas of the posterior corpus callosum). Therefore, the interpretation in the case of a binocular PSVEP abnormality might read: "These abnormalities suggest conduction defects in the visual pathways bilaterally. However, because of the binocular nature of the findings, the lesion location (retina, optic nerve, tracts, or radiations) cannot be determined."

Presently, with binocular abnormalities, it is not known whether or not there is any significance in the latency difference between the two eyes, that is, is there some degree of asymmetry that tells us that at least one of the conduction defects is located anterior to the chiasm? Patients with bilateral retrochiasmal lesions usually show no greater intereye differences than normal; this suggests that an intereye difference of greater than 3 to 5 standard deviations (SD) (to be conservative) above the normal mean when both eyes have abnormal latencies is clearly indicative of an optic nerve lesion anterior to the chiasm, at least on one side. However, these findings and conclusions need to be extended and confirmed.

2.2. Latency Abnormalities

A very reliable and sensitive measurement in PSVEP interpretation is P100 absolute latency (time interval from stimulus to the first major positive peak over the posterior skull).

The difference in this measure between the two eyes is also very reliable and is even more sensitive, having an upper limit of normal (mean plus 3 SD) in most studies of 8 to 10 msec (see Table 2–1). Figure 3–3 illustrates this abnormality in a patient with multiple sclerosis (MS) (without visual symptoms or signs). Conduction defects in the optic nerve secondary to demyelinating disease most commonly produce latency delays without much change in waveform configuration. This may seem surprising as one might expect latency delays to be accompanied by a broad waveform composed of early responses from relatively normally conducting fibers and late responses from relatively slowly conducting fibers. An explanation for this finding was provided by Riemslag et al. (1985), who investigated the effect of paired pattern-onset stimuli and found that with interstimulus intervals of less than 40 msec the response to the second stimulus was abolished by the first, that is, the response looked the same as when only the first stimulus was delivered. This suggests that (1) the relative preservation of P100 shape in partial optic nerve demyelination is due to the inhibition of late-arriving impulses conducted slowly through demyelinated segments of the optic pathways, and (2) P100 latency reflects function in the fastest group of optic nerve axons. Even when the initial stimulus comprised 25% of the visual field and the latter stimulus 75%, the first suppressed the second, suggesting that the healthiest fibers determine the latency and shape of the response and, if the response if delayed, the majority of the fibers must be involved.

The effects of segmental demyelination have not been well-studied in small myelinated axons such as those in the optic nerves. McDonald (1977) measured the length of 20 optic nerve plaques in 14 patients who died from MS; the length of the individual plaques varied from 3 to 30 mm, with a mean of 10.5 mm. Extrapolating from animal studies, he estimated that a demyelinated plaque of 10 mm in humans would correspond to 50 internodes. Using the conduction velocity of the fastest fibers in the monkey optic nerve (10 m/sec) and fac-

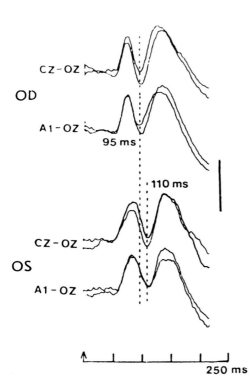

FIG. 3–3. Interocular latency difference abnormality in patient with MS. Absolute latencies were within normal limits in both eyes. The upper limit of normal (normal mean plus 3 SD) for the interocular latency difference was 8 msec; the difference in this patient was 15 msec. The patient had no visual symptoms and no previous history of visual difficulties. The optic discs were "probably slightly pale." Each trace is the average of 128 stimuli, with a repetition superimposed. A1 is left ear. Calibration mark is 10 μV.

toring in a 25-fold slowing of conduction over the demyelinated segment, he arrived at an estimate of 25 msec for an average delay to be expected in MS patients. This is similar to the delays actually seen in the PSVEPs of these patients. McDonald was careful to point out the possible errors in this formulation, but it is an interesting series of speculations. Noel and Desmedt (1980) have suggested that longer delays in the somatosensory system could be attributed to (1) more than one plaque, (2) larger plaques, and (3) the necessity for the low amplitude and desynchronized afferent volley to rely on temporal summation of synaptic potentials for eliciting the response from the next element in the pathway.

Care must be taken in the interpretation of a delay in the major positivity of the PSVEP. Half-field studies show that the delay is usually due to a delayed P100 but it is sometimes due to a delayed P100 interacting with the P135, P135 alone with P100 being absent, or negative components (N105) with little or no positivity (Blumhardt et al., 1982b; Halliday, 1985; Hammond and Yiannikas, 1986). Hammond and Yiannikas (1986) found that the longest major positivity delay due to P100 delay alone was 55 msec. All delays beyond that were shown by half-field studies to be of paramacular (P135, N105) origin (see also Chapter 2, Section 8.1.5). Thus, half-field stimulation is an important part of the evaluation of PSVEPs when the response has any unusual or problematic features.

P100 is not the primary cortical response and delays in conduction through the optic nerve could have more complex effects on the sequence of signal processing along the visual pathways, that is, geniculate bodies, cortex, and thalamus. In this regard, Jacobson et al. (1979) studied diphtheria toxin optic nerve lesions in cats using square wave grating discrimination to follow the time course of recovery of spatial frequency perception. They found a hierarchical progression with medium spatial frequencies returning first (1 to 4 days), then low (1 to 2 months), and finally high (5 to 8 months). These findings suggest that small checks might produce abnormal PSVEPs for a longer time than larger checks. They also found that the recovery time of pupillary reactivity to bright light and the length of recovery to spatial vision testing were both directly related to the magnitude of fiber loss. Furthermore, the anatomic findings suggested that the cat can have a 77% loss of optic nerve fibers and still recover visual acuity and contrast sensitivity.

Axonal loss (e.g., following ischemic lesions) would be expected to produce amplitude changes without latency shifts since the remaining axons will be conducting at normal velocities.

Compressive lesions that produce a mixture of segmental demyelination and axonal loss result in a combination of latency delays and amplitude changes. A complicating factor is the finding of Clifford-Jones et al. (1980) that remyelination occurred during continued optic nerve compression in cats. Since Smith et al. (1979) demonstrated in the spinal cords of cats that central remyelination is capable of restoring the ability of previously demyelinated fibers to conduct trains of impulses, then the rapid recovery of function following decompression might be related to the remyelination mentioned above.

Retinal ischemia does not affect P100 latency, although amplitude is diminished. Kline and Glaser (1982) studied PSVEPs in two patients during attacks of amaurosis fugax, with retinal angiography demonstrating the failure of blood flow. There was little change in PSVEP latency during disappearance and reappearance of P100.

2.3. Interocular Amplitude Abnormalities

The normal interocular variability of PSVEP amplitudes is too great for them to be of much use except occasionally when the two eyes of a single patient can be compared with one another, that is, when patients are used as their own controls. Since PSVEP amplitude is directly related to visual acuity it is affected by any process producing changes in visual acuity (e.g., pupil size, refractive errors, medial opacities, retinal disease, optic neuritis, and optic nerve compressive lesions). Other patient factors that affect PSVEP amplitudes are related to poor fixation on the stimulus screen, for example, nystagmus (involuntary or voluntary, see Fig. 2–28), and excessive blinking or looking away. To control for the latter it may be necessary for the technician to observe the patient's direction of gaze. Note that there is a good deal of variability in interocular amplitude measures, even comparative ratios with full-field stimulation (see Table 2–1). Thus, it is important to pay strict attention to the variability values obtained from the normal subjects (Shors et al., 1986). In most cases with conduction defects in the optic nerve, latency abnormalities accompany and very often precede amplitude abnormalities.

2.4. P100 Distribution Abnormalities

It is important to fully understand the concepts and data on partial-field stimulation (see Chapter 2, Section 8.1.5) before attempting to understand how lesions producing visual-field defects affect P100 distribution.

Since the responses obtained from homonymous half fields of two normal eyes are similar, lesions anterior to the chiasm will be manifest as differences between the responses obtained from the same half field in the two eyes. Lesions posterior to the chiasm will produce the same abnormality in the homonymous fields of the two eyes. Chiasm-splitting lesions will produce the same abnormalities in different fields of the two eyes. These latter abnormality patterns have been termed "uncrossed" and "crossed" asymmetries, respectively (Halliday et al., 1972; Blumhardt et al., 1977; Blumhardt et al., 1978; Halliday et al., 1979a,b; Blumhardt and Halliday, 1979). However, when one takes into account the considerable amount of normal variation, the clinical utility of partial-field stimulation remains small or in dispute. (See this chapter, Section 3.6, for a further discussion of the relationship between lesions and P100 distribution.)

In addition to the effect of half-field defects, there is also the case of scotomata to be considered. Removal of the central-field contribution may allow the peripheral-field, inverted-polarity activity to predominate at the midline (Blumhardt et al., 1978). Recognition of this change in the P100 potential-field distribution can suggest the presence of an unsuspected central scotoma.

2.5. P100 Shape Abnormalities

In normal subjects there is often an initial negative peak at 70 msec or so preceding P100 (see Figs. 2–5, 2–6). This early negativity is lost in most cases when P100 has abnormal latency and/or amplitude features (see Fig. 3–2). There is nothing known about pathophysiologic correlations of this finding.

P100 duration can be reasonably well-defined in normal subjects (see Table 2–1). Increased duration of P100 is almost always associated with abnormal latency and/or amplitude measures and is not used as an interpretive criterion.

P100 sometimes presents as two positive peaks separated by 10 to 50 msec, the so-called W or bifid pattern (Fig. 3–4). This is seen so rarely in normal subjects that its appearance alone suggests that the PSVEP may be abnormal. It is most often produced in one of two ways: (1) the upper visual field contributes inverted-polarity (negative) activity to the inion

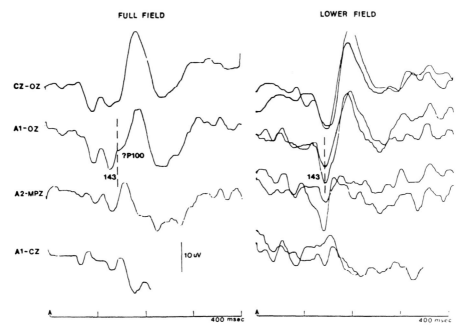

FIG. 3–4. Bifid ("W") P100 waveform (*left panel*), resolved by use of lower field stimulation (*right panel*). The absolute latency of P100 was abnormal (see Fig. 3–2 legend); the first peak seen with full-field testing was at a normal latency. Dashed lines, at 143 msec, indicate the latency of P100 as revealed by the lower-field response. Each trace is the average of 128 stimuli; the lower-field test has a repetition superimposed.

recording site and this may be shifted in latency relative to the positivity at that site so that two peaks are recorded; (2) with visual-field defects, particularly scotomata, the inverted-polarity (negative) activity recorded over the contralateral scalp, contributed mostly by more peripheral visual fields, may predominate or admix with the usual inion positivity (a shift of the "transitional zone") so that two peaks are recorded. In the first case stimulating with only the lower half field will simplify the waveform recorded at the inion. In the second case, perhaps the more common, recording from laterally placed electrodes will show the horizontal potential-field distribution of P100 over the posterior scalp and will reveal the true P100, from which latency measurements can be taken. Figure 3–4 shows a bifid P100 clarified by some of the above maneuvers.

3. CLINICAL CORRELATIONS

3.1. Introduction

Pattern-shift VEPs provide a sensitive extension of the clinical examination and commonly used clinical tests (visual acuity, clinical and formal visual fields, pupillary responses, fundoscopic examination, and red color desaturation). To demonstrate the relative sensitivity of the PSVEP, 198 patients with MS who had had PSVEP testing were studied retrospectively by extracting pertinent aspects of the neuro-ophthalmologic examination from their medical records (Chiappa, 1982; Brooks and Chiappa, 1982). A full comparison of the PSVEP results and clinical findings is given in Table 3–1. When the PSVEP was normal, there was *never* an abnormality found on the clinical examination. Even when the PSVEP was abnormal, various clinical examinations were often normal. For example, in those patients with abnormal PSVEPs, the visual fields by usual clinical examination (confrontation) were normal in 96%, formal fields were normal in 55%, pupillary responses were normal in 74%, fundus appearance was normal in 39%, and there was no red color desaturation in 27% (only 22 patients had this test reported). These figures convey the degree of sensitivity that the test can add to the routine clinical ophthalmologic examination. However, if the formal visual field examination is done carefully a greater incidence of clinical abnormalities can be found even in asymptomatic patients (Patterson and Heron, 1980; Meienberg et al., 1982; van Buggenhout et al., 1982; Nikoskelainen and Falck, 1982; Kupersmith et al., 1983), although it never matches that of the PSVEP.

Despite the sensitivity of the PSVEP, the abnormalities produced by the demyelinating plaques of optic neuritis and MS are indistinguishable from abnormalities produced by

TABLE 3–1. *Pattern-shift VEPs and clinical neuro-ophthalmologic findings in patients with multiple sclerosis*

		MS classification			
	PSVEP	Definite	Probable	Possible	Total
Normal fields (clinically)	Abnl	41/43 (95%)	23/24 (96%)	11/11 (100%)	75/78 (96%)
	Nl	10/10 (100%)	16/16 (100%)	30/30 (100%)	56/56 (100%)
Normal fields (formal)	Abnl	17/30 (57%)	11/19 (58%)	3/7 (43%)	31/56 (55%)
	Nl	5/5 (100%)	4/4 (100%)	11/11 (100%)	20/20 (100%)
Normal pupillary responses	Abnl	48/71 (68%)	33/40 (83%)	14/18 (78%)	95/129 (74%)
	Nl	11/11 (100%)	16/16 (100%)	30/30 (100%)	57/57 (100%)
Normal fundi	Abnl	21/75 (28%)	19/42 (45%)	12/17 (71%)	52/134 (39%)
	Nl	11/11 (100%)	17/17 (100%)	28/28 (100%)	56/56 (100%)
No red color desaturation	Abnl	1/10 (10%)	2/6 (33%)	3/6 (50%)	6/22 (27%)
	Nl	—	1/1 (100%)	1/1 (100%)	2/2 (100%)
Normal eye exam (all above)	Abnl	18/78 (23%)	16/43 (37%)	11/17 (65%)	45/138 (33%)
	Nl	11/11 (100%)	18/18 (100%)	31/31 (100%)	60/60 (100%)
Normal eye exam and no history of optic neuritis	Abnl	16/78 (21%)	16/43 (37%)	10/17 (59%)	42/138 (30%)
	Nl	10/11 (91%)	16/18 (89%)	31/31 (100%)	57/60 (95%)

Correlation of neuro-ophthalmologic examination and PSVEPs in 200 patients with MS. The denominator is the number of patients who had the given PSVEP result [normal (Nl) or abnormal (Abnl)] in that MS classification group, and the numerator is the number of patients who had normal findings on the given aspect of the ophthalmologic examination, e.g., 43 patients with definite MS had abnormal PSVEPs and 41 of them (95%) had normal confrontation fields; 30 patients with definite MS had abnormal PSVEPs and 17 of them (57%) had normal fields by perimetry. Normal values and stimulus parameters for testing as in Table 2–1. (From Chiappa, 1982, with permission.)

many other retinal, compressive, and degenerative diseases. Thus, abnormal findings demonstrated by the PSVEP must be carefully integrated into the clinical situation by a physician familiar with the clinical use of this test. The physician must decide if other procedures (e.g., electroretinography, formal visual fields, radiologic studies, subspecialty consultation) are indicated to differentiate the possible causes of the conduction delay. Blumhardt (1982a) has evaluated the role of PSVEPs in the early diagnosis of MS and has reiterated the point that the test provides a sensitive, objective extension of the clinical neurologic examination but is etiologically nonspecific.

3.2. Optic Neuritis and Multiple Sclerosis

3.2.1. Types of PSVEP Abnormalities

The major change associated with optic nerve demyelination is prolongation of P100 latency. The mean latency in MS patients in a representative study exceeded the normal mean by about 10 msec (possible MS) to 30 msec (definite MS) (Cant et al., 1978), while delays exceeding 100 msec have also been reported (Shahrokhi et al., 1978).

Interocular latency difference is probably the most sensitive indicator of optic nerve dysfunction in the PSVEP and has been used to provide evidence of optic nerve pathology (Duwaer and Spekreijse, 1978; Asselman et al., 1975; Matthews et al., 1977; Collins et al., 1978; Shahrokhi et al., 1978; Hoeppner and Lolas, 1978). Figures 3–3 and 3–5 show examples of this type of abnormality. Failure to utilize this parameter in a comparative study of flight of colors (FOC) testing versus PSVEPs (Swart and Millac, 1980) resulted in erroneously low sensitivity of the PSVEP. Rolak and Ashizawa (1985) used the interocular latency difference parameter and found that although FOC testing compared favorably with PSVEPs, it was less sensitive. Shahrohki et al. (1978) found that 8 of 100 optic neuritis (ON) and MS patients had abnormal PSVEPs based on this parameter alone.

Amplitude of P100 has not proven to be a reliable measure, presumably because of the relatively large normal variability of amplitude. Matthews et al. (1977) reported that 3 of 110 definite MS patients had abnormal PSVEPs on the basis of amplitudes less than 4 μV. Shahrohki et al. (1978) found only 1% of 149 patients who were abnormal in this measure. Halliday et al. (1973b) and Halliday and McDonald (1981) noted that amplitude was correlated with visual acuity, whereas latency was not.

The duration and shape of P100 has also been investigated (Collins et al., 1978; Shahrokhi et al., 1978; Hoeppner and Lolas, 1978). Isolated abnormalities in these parameters are relatively uncommon and when present are usually associated with P100 latency abnormalities. An explanation for the relative preservation of P100 shape (including duration), in spite of absolute latency prolongation, has been provided by Riemslag et al. (1985), who stimulated different segments of the visual field with varying time separations between stimuli. When the stimulus-onset asynchrony was 40 msec or less, no contribution from the second stimulus could be identified in the recorded response. This suggests that the relative preservation of P100 shape and duration in partial optic nerve demyelination is due to inhibition of the late-arriving impulses which had traversed the abnormally conducting segments. In the experimental situation, even when the initial stimulus comprised only 25% of the visual field and the later stimulus comprised 75%, the first suppressed the second. Thus, in the partially demyelinated optic nerve, the healthiest fibers determine the latency and shape of the response and, if the response is delayed, a majority of the fibers must be involved. Sedgwick (1983) has presented some further considerations on the pathophysiologic basis for abnormal EPs.

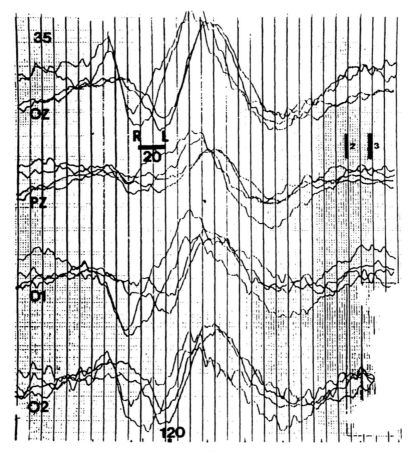

FIG. 3–5. Superimposed right- and left-eye PSVEP results obtained from a patient suspected of having demyelinating disease. The left-eye P100 is within normal limits for absolute latency at about 120 msec, but the interocular latency difference of 20 msec is markedly abnormal, suggesting a conduction defect anterior to the chiasm on the left. Brain stem auditory EPs were also abnormal and an MRI scan showed multiple periventricular lesions. Check size was 35′; 2-μV calibration refers to right-eye traces, 3 refers to left eye; 120 label is at 120 msec from stimulus. Reference was mid-frontal, relative positivity of posterior electrodes caused a downward trace deflection. Each trace is average of 100 stimuli.

3.2.2. Optic Neuritis

A large number of clinical studies attest to the sensitivity of the PSVEP in revealing demyelinating lesions in the optic nerve; about 90% of patients who have a clear history of ON have abnormal PSVEPs (Halliday et al., 1973a,b; Asselman et al., 1975; Hume and Cant, 1976; Mastaglia et al., 1976a,b; Celesia and Daley, 1977; Matthews et al., 1977; Zeese, 1977; Cant et al., 1978; Duwaer and Spekreijse, 1978; Shahroki et al., 1978; Tackmann et al., 1979; Trojaborg and Petersen, 1979; Chiappa, 1980; Diener and Scheibler, 1980; Kjaer, 1980; Wilson and Keyser, 1980; Purves et al., 1981; van Buggenhout et al., 1982; Walsh et al., 1982. Of 438 patients with ON in a group of the above studies, 89% had PSVEP abnormalities. In some studies, the proportion is closer to 100%, as in Fig. 3–6 and Table 3–2. When there was no clinical evidence for optic nerve involvement, the incidence

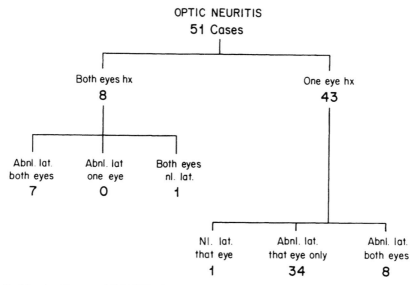

FIG. 3–6. The incidence of PSVEP abnormalites and visual symptoms and signs in patients with optic neuritis. "Hx" refers to whether or not the patient at any time had symptoms or signs suggesting optic neuritis.

of PSVEP abnormalities was 51% (of 715 patients). Recent modifications to magnetic resonance imaging (MRI) techniques (short inversion recovery for suppression of orbital fat signals) were used by Miller et al. (1988) to study 37 patients with recent or past ON. Magnetic resonance imaging revealed abnormalities in 84% of symptomatic and 20% of asymptomatic eyes (mean extent of lesion 1 cm), but PSVEP was even more sensitive than MRI in detecting lesions. Ormerod et al. (1986) studied 35 adults with ON using MRI; 61% showed lesions outside the visual system, indicated by brain stem auditory (BAEPs) or somatosensory evoked potentials (SEPs) in only 30%. Hornabrook et al. (1992) studied 28 patients with clinically isolated ON and showed that 71% had asymptomatic lesions in the white matter corresponding to the optic radiations, the presence of which did not have any relationship to the latency of the VEP. Paraclinical studies often show lesions elsewhere in the CNS and a number of these patients develop clinically definite MS, indicating that ON is a risk factor for MS (Frederiksen et al., 1991; Martinelli et al., 1991).

Kaufman et al. (1988) investigated the use of pattern electroretinography (PERG) in prognosis following ON. Seventeen eyes had gradual and permanent reduction (usually by 16 weeks, occasionally more slowly) of PERG amplitude and all had poor visual outcome. In 29 eyes (various etiologies of the optic neuropathy) the PERG remained normal and in 22 of these the visual outcome was 20/25 or better.

3.2.3. Multiple Sclerosis

When the diagnosis of MS is suspected because of typical symptoms and/or signs referrable to other CNS locations, the demonstration by an abnormal PSVEP of a clinically silent conduction defect in the optic nerve can further delineate the anatomic distribution of the disease process and thus narrow the range of diagnostic possibilities. Optic nerve demyelination is a common finding in autopsy material of MS patients (Lumsden, 1970;

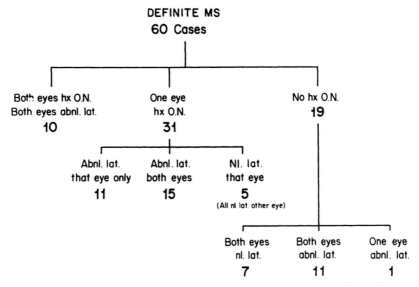

FIG. 3–7. The incidence of PSVEP abnormalities and visual symptoms in patients with definite MS. "Hx" refers to whether or not the patient at any time had symptoms or signs suggesting optic neuritis.

McAlpine et al., 1972), and this is paralleled by the incidence of PSVEP abnormalities, which ranges from a high of 96% (Halliday et al., 1973b) to a low of 47% (Hoeppner and Lolas, 1978). In 26 clinical series (all those mentioned above for ON except Zeese, 1977; Wilson and Keyser, 1980; Walsh et al., 1982; Lowitzsch et al., 1976; Mastaglia et al., 1976a; Hennerici et al., 1977; Collins et al., 1978; Nilsson, 1978; Wist et al., 1978; Rigolet

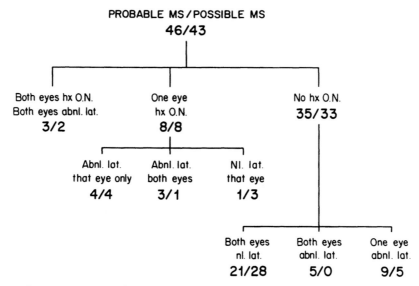

FIG. 3–8. The incidence of PSVEP abnormalities and visual symptoms in patients with probable and possible MS. "Hx" refers to whether or not the patient at any time had symptoms or signs suggesting optic neuritis.

TABLE 3–2. *The incidence of abnormal PSVEP in multiple sclerosis and optic neuritis*

	Definite	Probable	Possible	Total
MS patients with a history of optic neuritis	75/83	21/28	9/17	105/128 (82%)
MS patients without a history of optic neuritis	38/56	38/85	16/80	92/221 (42%)
All patients with MS	113/139 (81%)	59/113 (52%)	25/97 (26%)	197/349 (56%)
Pure optic neuritis group	—	—	—	79/82 (96%)
All patients with a history of optic neuritis				184/210 (88%)

Normal values and stimulus parameters for testing as in Table 2–1.

et al., 1979), encompassing about 1,950 patients with all MS classifications, the average abnormality rate found was 63%. Of 464, 322, and 799 patients classified as possible, probable, and definite MS, the average abnormality rates were 37%, 58%, and 85%, respectively. These figures reflect the greater likelihood of optic nerve lesions with more definite clinical diagnoses. Of 744 patients reported as having no history or clinical findings of ON, 51% had PSVEP abnormalities, ranging from a high of 93% (Halliday et al., 1973b) to a low of 34% (Purves et al., 1981). The differences between studies are best explained by the different definitions of MS used, some studies being composed of a preponderance of one class of patients. Note also that screen and check sizes differed greatly between the studies mentioned above. Contrasts, when reported, were all above 74%. Luminance levels varied so much that the reliability of the measurements has to be doubted. Figures 3–7 and 3–8 and Tables 3–2, 3–3, and 3–4 present the abnormality rates found in groups of patients with various MS classifications, with and without a history of visual symptoms.

Nuwer et al. (1985) studied first-degree relatives of MS patients and found interocular latency difference abnormalities in 6 of 110, although absolute P100 latencies were normal. Shibasaki and Kuroiwa (1982) have found that Japanese patients with MS have a higher incidence of absent PSVEP responses than was seen in series reported from Western countries. Noseworthy et al. (1983) found a greater number of PSVEP abnormalities in

TABLE 3–3. *Evidence of clinically unsuspected lesions revealed by BAEP, PSVEP, and SEP*

	Definite	Probable	Possible	Total
BAEP alone	4/81 (5%)	6/67 (9%)	5/54 (9%)	15/202 (7%)
PSVEP alone	26/79 (33%)	24/67 (36%)	11/54 (20%)	61/200 (31%)
SEP alone	4/16 (25%)	6/21 (29%)	2/14 (14%)	12/51 (24%)
BAEP and PSVEP	0/79	0/67	4/54 (7%)	4/200 (2%)
BAEP and SEP	0/16	0/21	0/14	0/51
PSVEP and SEP	0/16	2/20 (10%)	0/14	2/50 (4%)
All three	0/16	1/20 (5%)	1/14 (7%)	2/50 (4%)

Note that PSVEPs and SEPs are approximately equally useful in revealing "silent" lesions, whereas BAEPs are about one third less sensitive in this regard. "Clinically unsuspected" indicates that there was no history or physical sign suggesting abnormal function in that sensory system, either present or past. For BAEP some nonspecific data (e.g., nystagmus) were taken as indications of "clinically suspected" brain stem lesions (see Chapter 5, Section 3.4, for further explanation). All patients did not have all three tests (see Table 3–4). SEP testing was upper limb only.

TABLE 3–4. *Evidence of clinically unsuspected lesions revealed by PSVEP, BAEP, and SEP in patients who had all three tests*

	Definite	Probable	Possible	Total
PSVEP overall	13 (57%)	11 (41%)	2 (10%)	26 (37%)
BAEP overall	4 (17%)	11 (41%)	2 (10%)	17 (24%)
SEP overall	11 (48%)	12 (44%)	6 (30%)	29 (41%)
PSVEP alone	8 (3%)	6 (22%)	1 (5%)	15 (21%)
BAEP alone	3 (13%)	6 (22%)	1 (5%)	10 (14%)
SEP alone	7 (30%)	8 (30%)	4 (20%)	19 (27%)
PSVEP and BAEP only	1 (4%)	3 (11%)	0	4 (6%)
PSVEP and SEP only	4 (17%)	2 (7%)	1 (5%)	7 (10%)
BAEP and SEP only	0	2 (7%)	1 (5%)	3 (4%)
PSVEP, BAEP and SEP	0	0	0	0
No. patients	23	27	20	70

"Overall" refers to abnormality rate irrespective of clinical suspicion of a lesion. Other data refer to "clinically unsuspected" lesions (see Table 3–3). The number of patients with two and three tests indicating such lesions is much smaller since it is less likely that a patient with MS will not have symptoms or signs in two or three systems.

patients older than 50 years as compared with younger patients. Rolak and Ashizawa (1985) compared PSVEPs with the hot bath test and found only 1 of 50 patients with an abnormal hot bath test and normal PSVEP. Also note that patients with Behçet's disease, a rare multisystem inflammatory, probably autoimmune disorder whose clinical course may mimic MS, have been shown to have abnormal PSVEPs at least 25% of the time (Stigsby et al., 1994).

P100 latency abnormalities are usually present whatever the time interval since the clinical episode of optic neuritis; Shahrohki et al. (1978) reported PSVEP abnormalities 5 years after the clinical episode and Halliday et al. (1973b) reported patients who had abnormal PSVEPs 15 years later. Only about 5% of patients with abnormal PSVEPs have the P100 latency return to normal even when followed for 10 or 15 years after visual acuity has returned to normal following an episode of ON. However, Matthews and Small (1983) found a patient whose PSVEP, although still abnormal 3 years after an attack of ON, had returned to normal after another 3.5 years. They suggested that in some patients a very slow healing process might be at work. Matthews and Small (1983) have reported several other patients whose absolute latencies have returned to normal following ON. Hely et al. (1986) repeated PSVEPs and clinical examinations at 6 to 120 (mean 46) months after the first attack of acute ON in 80 patients. The full-field PSVEP returned to normal in 19% of the 98 eyes that were initially abnormal and 15% of patients had completely normal PSVEPs on follow-up. They concluded that the ophthalmologic examination was a more sensitive index than the PSVEP of past ON in symptomatic eyes, the reverse being the case in asymptomatic eyes.

When the latency difference between the two eyes can be used for interpretation (sometimes patients will have binocular PSVEP abnormalities when first studied), the percentage of patients in whom the PSVEP returns to normal drops further. Thus, if ON is suspected and the patient complains of moderate to severe visual difficulty but the PSVEP is normal, that diagnosis is highly unlikely, especially in the acute situation. Figure 3–9 shows PSVEPs in a patient followed for 7 months after an episode of ON in the right eye. P100 latency returns to within normal limits of absolute latency but remains abnormal when compared to the previously normal left eye (which in the interim has also suffered an attack of ON). N70 has also been investigated in patients with MS (Ghilardi et al., 1991).

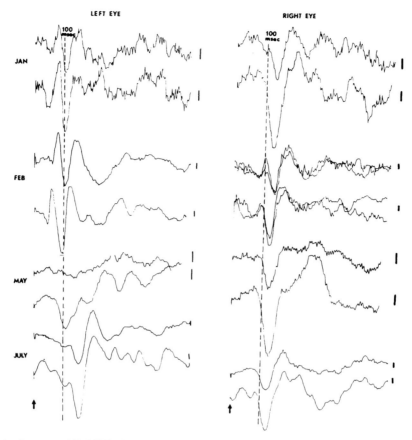

FIG. 3–9. Pattern-shift VEPs from a patient with an attack of optic neuritis (ON) in the right eye initially (Jan). P100 latency is markedly abnormal; over the next 6 months the latency gradually returns toward normal but never reaches a latency such that the latency difference between OD and OS (when OS was normal) is normal. Note that OS in the interim (between Feb and May) has suffered an attack of ON. The two channels displayed are CZ–OZ and Ref–OZ, with relative positivity at OZ producing a downward deflection. Each trace is the average of 128 stimuli. The dashed lines are at 100 msec. Calibration marks are 2.5 μV. (From Chiappa, 1982, with permission.)

3.2.4. Relationship Between Ophthalmologic Findings and PSVEP

As mentioned above, if there is clinical evidence for ON, the incidence of PSVEP abnormalities is very high (average 89% in 438 patients), with some studies above 95%. When there is no clinical evidence for optic nerve involvement, the incidence of PSVEP abnormalities was 51% (of 715 patients). For a retrospective comparative study of clinical neuro-ophthalmologic findings versus PSVEPs (Brooks and Chiappa, 1982), see Section 3.1 and Table 3–1. The striking findings in that series were that when the PSVEP was normal, there were *never* any abnormalities found in the clinical neuro-ophthalmologic examination, and even when the PSVEP was abnormal, the clinical examination was normal to a surprising degree. However, as is indicated by the studies of Patterson and Heron (1980), van Buggenhout et al. (1982), and Meienberg et al. (1982) (using an automated perimeter octopus), if the formal visual-field examination is done carefully, a greater incidence of clinical abnormalities can be found even in asymptomatic patients. Lowitzsch et al. (1976) have also explored the correlation between PSVEPs and clinical examinations. Of their 135 patients, 33 had completely normal examinations and 11 (33%) had abnormal PSVEPs, 8 showing binocular abnormalities. Of a further 27 patients who had normal examinations in one eye, 41% (11) had PSVEP abnormalities in that eye.

The relationship between visual acuity and PSVEP findings is not consistent. Halliday et al. (1973a) stated that increased amplitude was correlated with improved visual acuity, whereas latency was not, remaining abnormal in 90% of cases (Halliday and McDonald, 1981). Asselman et al. (1975) found no relationship between visual acuity and PSVEP latency in a group of patients studied only once. Matthews and Small (1979) reported that 61% of 39 eyes exhibited appropriate parallel latency and acuity improvements over an 18-month period, but they also found 9 eyes which had latency increases into an abnormal range, 6 of which had concurrent improvements in acuity. Diener and Scheibler (1980) noted that only 25% of their patients had PSVEP changes which matched acuity levels.

3.2.5. Relationship Between Clinical Findings and PSVEP

Serial PSVEPs have been recorded in MS patients relative to both disease progression and therapeutic trials. These studies must be interpreted in light of the normal variability seen over time; we have found absolute P100 latency shifts up to 11 msec and interocular latency difference changes up to 9 msec in 20 normal subjects tested 2 to 13 months apart (Oken et al., 1987). Halliday (1981) followed patients with serial recordings over several years, noting steplike increases in latency associated with relapses characterized by visual impairment; if there was no visual system involvement, PSVEPs tended to remain unchanged. Matthews and Small (1979) reported that 61% of 39 eyes exhibited parallel latency and acuity improvements over an 18-month period, but they also found 9 eyes which had latency increases into an abnormal range, 6 of which had concurrent improvements in acuity. Aminoff et al. (1984) found no relationship between changes in nonvisual clinical status and PSVEPs. Smith and Zeeberg (1986) found no PSVEP changes in eight patients treated with 3 days of high-dose methylprednisolone infusions (1 g daily). Gilmore et al. (1985) saw transient PSVEP improvement in some patients given infusions of the calcium antagonist verapamil.

Nuwer et al. (1987) performed EPs annually during a 3-year, double-blind, placebo-controlled study of azathioprine with or without steroids in chronic progressive MS. Treatment-related visual and SEP changes became statistically different 1 year before corresponding differences were seen in the Standard Neurological Examination scores, and the statistical significance of the EP changes was substantially greater than seen for changes in other clinical scales. The degree of significance was increased by using EP latency values, rather than simple criteria for change. Anderson et al. (1987) were less impressed with EP utility in clinical MS trials.

Matthews et al. (1982) followed for 38 months after PSVEP testing 84 patients in whom the diagnosis of MS was under consideration. In 17 of these patients an abnormal PSVEP at initial presentation subsequently proved to be of diagnostic value in that it revealed a separate, clinically silent lesion, indicating a multifocal disease (and the patient on follow-up proved to have MS). This incidence of utility was greater than that of BAEPs or SEPs.

3.2.6. Maneuvers to Increase Diagnostic Yield

There have been various attempts to increase the sensitivity of the test in this clinical area. Phillips et al. (1983) found that hyperthermia increased the incidence of PSVEP abnormalities, although Matthews et al. (1979), Bajada et al. (1980), Persson and Sachs (1981), and Kazis et al. (1982) found no consistent change. Oishi et al. (1985) tested three different check sizes and found abnormalities more common with smaller checks (25'), occasionally only with larger checks (100'), and less often with 50' checks. Spatial vision in MS has been further investigated in MS by Coupland and Kirkham (1982), Regan et al. (1982), Kupersmith et al. (1983), Plant (1983), and Neima and Regan (1984) using sinusoidal gratings and psychophysical techniques. Camisa et al. (1981) and Bodis-Wollner et al. (1987) reported orientation-dependent latency changes in 34% of 74 MS patients, and noted that this was not seen in macular disease. Hammond and Yiannikas (1986) compared full-, half-, and central- (4° field, 27' checks) pattern stimulation and found the techniques complementary. Central stimulation was abnormal in 34% of patients, confirming the preferential involvement of macular fibers in MS, and providing an alternative to half-field stimulation in evaluating full-field responses with abnormal waveforms. Novak et al. (1988) also reported additional abnormalities with hemifield stimulation and different check sizes. Mitchell et al. (1983) studied the recovery cycle of PSVEPs in MS patients and found that there was no good correlation between conditioning (first) responses with abnormal latencies and abnormally delayed test (second) responses. They interpreted this as indicating that the conduction defects are in different locations. Light-emitting diode (LED) array stimulation (Purves and Low, 1976; Nilsson, 1978; Hod et al., 1986) has not shown significant improvement in sensitivity. Cant et al. (1978) and Camisa et al. (1980) found that lower luminance levels revealed more abnormalities and suggested routine use of more than one intensity level. However, this effect was not observed by others (Diener et al., 1982; Hennerici and Wist, 1982; Waybright et al., 1982) except that Hennerici and Wist did find an increased sensitivity with foveal stimulation at lower luminance levels. Intravenous lidocaine, a sodium channel blocker was studied by Sakurai et al. (1992) to unmask subclinical demyelinative lesions.

Kaufman and Celesia (1985) used combined PERGs and PSVEPs to localize the conduction defect in acute ON and patients with MS, usually finding normal PERGs and delayed PSVEPs. Long-standing disease with optic atrophy, presumably with axonal involvement and retrograde degeneration of retinal ganglion cells, may result in absence of PERGs and this has been investigated as a prognostic tool (Celesia et al., 1986).

3.2.7. Spinal Cord Syndromes

Patients with acute transverse myelitis show PSVEP abnormalities in only a small proportion of cases (Ropper et al., 1982; Wulff, 1985). Blumhardt et al. (1982a) studied 31 patients in whom the spinal cord symptoms developed over hours to days (9 of these were classified as transverse myelitis) and found PSVEP abnormalities in 10%. Ropper et al. (1982) found no PSVEP or BAEP abnormalities in 12 patients with acute transverse myelitis. The chronic, progressive myelopathies have a greater incidence of abnormal PSVEPs. The abnormality rates ranged from 76% in the series of Bynke et al. (1977) to 35% in the 100 patients with disease of more than 6 months duration studied by Blumhardt et al. (1982a).

It has been suggested that PSVEP data can be used clinically in the setting of undiagnosed spinal cord disease to help decide whether or not myelography is necessary (Mastaglia et al., 1976b). Bynke et al. (1977) suggested that if the clinical neuro-ophthalmologic examination and the PSVEP are abnormal, and the cerebrospinal fluid (CSF) shows oligoclonal immunoglobulin G (IgG) banding, then radiologic investigations can be limited or avoided. In 42 patients with spinal cord lesions Kempster et al. (1987) found a zero false positive rate for combined PSVEP and CSF oligoclonal banding, although individually the rates were 10% and 12%; the probability of MS, given both tests abnormal, was calculated at 100%, excluding the necessity of myelography. However, the possibility of concurrent diseases dictates very careful assessment of the clinical situation before an abnormal PSVEP (with or without other tests) should be used as presumptive evidence of MS to delay myelography. In fact, Blumhardt et al. (1982a) found five patients with abnormal PSVEPs and abnormal myelograms. Three had only borderline narrowing of the cervical canals and spondylotic changes (two of these have subsequently developed further signs of MS) but two had cord compression caused by prolapsed intervertebral discs. After laminectomy one of these patients had little clinical change but the other had a marked improvement. Paty et al. (1979) looked for MS-related abnormalities in 72 patients with chronic progressive myelopathy (mean duration 10 years) and found abnormal PSVEPs in 44%.

3.2.8. Combined EP Studies

The comparative utility of PSVEPs, BAEPs, and SEPs has been studied in several groups of patients (Mastaglia et al., 1976a; Trojaborg and Petersen, 1979; Chiappa 1980; Green et al., 1980; Kjaer, 1980; Khoshbin and Hallett, 1981; Purves et al., 1981; Matthews et al., 1982; Tackmann et al., 1982; Phillips et al., 1983). As might be postulated on the basis of length of white matter tracts involved, the order of relative utility of the tests in revealing evidence of clinically unsuspected lesions was SEP, PSVEP, and BAEP. These data suggest that there is not a specific differential susceptibility to demyelination in the systems involved in the tests. Rather, it is the length and amount of white matter tracts being tested which determine the likelihood of detection of a lesion in a given system.

Bottcher and Trojaberg (1982) followed patients for 2 to 4 years after PSVEP, SEP, and CSF IgG testing and found that 81% of those in whom both the EPs and the IgG index were abnormal initially had entered a higher MS diagnostic class at the later evaluation. Those patients in whom either the EPs or IgG index were normal initially remained in the same diagnostic class. (See also Paty et al., 1988, and Guerit and Argiles, 1988.) Walsh et al. (1982) followed 56 patients for 2.5 years and found an increased number of abnormalities in multimodality EPs which was paralleled by an increase in overall clinical disability. However, Aminoff et al. (1984) have noted that the correlation between changes in specific clinical features and EPs may be poor.

Noseworthy et al. (1983) have studied PSVEP, BAEP, and blink reflexes in patients presenting after age 50 with suspected MS. They found both the EPs and CSF electrophoresis to have high diagnostic yield in this difficult diagnostic group.

3.2.9. Magnetic Resonance Imaging and EPs

Magnetic resonance imaging is proving to be an invaluable tool in the investigation of patients with suspected demyelinating disease, especially the T_2-weighted images (see Drayer and Barrett, 1984, for a review). Immediate postmortem studies have shown that demyelinated lesions 3 mm in diameter are seen, and that the apparent lesion size on MRI is accurate (Stewart et al., 1986). Where signal intensity varied, so did the degree of inflammation, demyelination, and gliosis, and it was thought that MRI could distinguish gliotic and nongliotic demyelinated lesions. Serial MRI scans show the appearance and evolution of asymptomatic lesions (Paty et al., 1986) and enhancement may afford a measure of activity (Gonzalez-Scarano et al., 1986). Magnetic resonance imaging has been shown to be better than EPs and CT in revealing multiple lesions in the CNS (Kirshner et al., 1985; Gebarski et al., 1985; Cutler et al., 1986b; Ormerod et al., 1986; Paty et al., 1988), including the spinal cord (Maravilla et al., 1985), but MRI is no more specific than EPs with respect to etiology. Note that Guerit and Argiles (1988) found no significant differences between MRI, EPs, and CSF studies. In the brain stem EPs reveal a significant number of conduction defects not seen by MRI (Kirshner et al., 1985; Baumhefner et al., 1986; Cutler et al., 1986b; Farlow et al., 1986; Giesser et al., 1987). Similarly, it can be expected that optic nerve lesions will be detected more reliably by EPs than MRI (Farlow et al., 1986), although Miller et al. (1986, 1988) recently suggested an improved MRI technique for searching for demyelinating lesions in the optic nerve. Thus, although as a general statement it can be said that the overall neurologic workup of the patient suspected of having demyelinating disease is better served by MRI (and most patients with MS will eventually have an MRI scan), in selected cases specific questions are better answered by EPs, and some anatomic areas are better tested by EPs.

3.3. Compressive Lesions of the Anterior Visual Pathways

3.3.1. Papilledema and Pseudotumor Cerebri

Papilledema from lesions not involving the optic nerves does not produce P100 alterations unless severe. Thus, in our and others' (Halliday and Mushin, 1980) experience, patients with pseudotumor cerebri (benign intracranial hypertension) usually do not have PSVEP abnormalities. However, we have followed a patient with pseudotumor in whom P100 latency abnormalities appeared days before significant clinical visual loss became apparent. The PSVEP abnormality resolved with successful treatment but then recurred similarly with a clinical exacerbation. In other such cases the correlation between clinical features and PSVEP abnormalities has been poor. Sorensen et al. (1985) noted a weak correlation between PSVEP latencies and intracranial pressure in 13 patients with pseudotumor cerebri; latencies improved in patients who recovered. Note that Hume and Cant (1976) found PSVEP abnormalities in two patients with benign intracranial hypertension. There has been no systematic study of clinical neuro-ophthalmologic correlates of papilledema (e.g., enlarged blind spot and visual-field defects) and PSVEPs. Kirkham and Coupland (1981) used flash steady-state VEPs to study two patients with chronic papilledema and found abnormal phase lags. Alani (1985) showed improvement in PSVEPs following shunt placement in adult hydrocephalics.

3.3.2. Extrinsic and Intrinsic Tumors

Compression of the anterior visual pathways tends to produce distortion of the PSVEP waveforms, with loss of amplitude but less latency delay than is seen with demyelinating lesions (Halliday et al., 1976; Asselman et al., 1975; Ikeda et al., 1978; Hume and Cant, 1976; Halliday and Mushin, 1980; Kupersmith et al., 1981). Reappearance of an absent PSVEP in one eye and improvement in the other eye was noted 3 hours after aspiration of fluid from an unresectable cystic craniopharyngioma (Gutin et al., 1980).

Halliday et al. (1976) studied 19 cases (4 orbital lesions, 2 sphenoid wing meningiomas, 3 suprasellar meningiomas, 2 craniopharyngiomas, and 8 pituitary tumors) and found abnormalities in all but one (the interocular latency difference was 9 msec in the latter case). Pattern-shift VEP abnormalities were found even when visual acuity, optic discs, and fields were normal; in one patient all three clinical elements were normal but the PSVEP was abnormal. Of nine patients studied postoperatively, three showed a marked improvement in PSVEPs, three were unchanged, two were worse, and one equivocal. The patients with craniopharyngiomas or pituitary tumors did better than those with intracranial meningiomas. Halliday and Mushin (1980) show serial preoperative and postoperative recordings from a patient with an anterior clinoid meningioma, showing apoor correlation between the PSVEP and visual acuity. Gott et al. (1979) found that the PSVEP provided earlier evidence of suprasellar extension of pituitary tumors than did conventional visual tests.

Kupersmith et al. (1981) used steady-state pattern reversal and found amplitude abnormalities in the affected eyes of four patients with chiasmal gliomas. Groswasser et al. (1985) studied 25 young patients with optic nerve gliomas; PSVEPs were absent in the affected eye in 17 (although flash responses were still present in 9 of these) and abnormal in the other 8 (6 of whom had changes indicating involvement of fibers from the fellow eye crossing at the chiasm). Serial recording showed a marked improvement in two patients. Niazy and Lundervold (1982) found PSVEP abnormalities in four patients with chiasmatic tumors and one with a thalamic tumor. The PSVEP has utility as a screening test in neurofibromatosis and Jabbari et al. (1985) found abnormal PSVEPs in 8 of 30 asymptomatic patients; 7 of these had computed tomography (CT) scans, 6 showing enlargement of the optic nerve. No patient had abnormal CT scan and normal PSVEP.

Partial-field stimulation may increase the sensitivity of the PSVEP in this area (Halliday and McDonald, 1981; Muller-Jensen et al., 1981) and Brecelj (1992) reported temporal half-field abnormalities in 85% of patients with compressive lesions of the optic nerve, versus 36% for the nasal half-field and 74% for the full-field.

3.4. Miscellaneous Diseases

Many diseases of the nervous system, some not previously known to affect the visual system, have been found to show PSVEP abnormalities. This section is an accounting of those reports to provide a means for comparing the PSVEP results of a patient at hand with the reported experience in the literature, and to allow easy access to the original reports since techniques and interpretations vary greatly and the original article must usually be studied for an accurate understanding of the findings.

3.4.1. Albinism

Albinism is of interest in partial-field PSVEP work because animal studies show, and it is probably also true in humans, that, in addition to the usual temporal half-field, up to 20% of the nasal half-field for each eye may be projected to the contralateral visual cortex. Because of this, each occipital lobe receives primarily monocular input from the contralateral eye, with only the more peripheral areas of the visual field projected ipsilaterally. Creel (1979), Creel et al. (1981, 1982), Apkarian et al. (1983), and Carroll et al. (1980a,b) have studied PSVEPs in albinism. The latter authors studied 15 subjects and found (1) diminished P100 amplitude without latency abnormalities, and (2) that the full-field P100 showed the same asymmetry as the temporal half-field P100, suggesting that each hemisphere's response was dominated by the crossed fibers from the contralateral eye. In addition, two major types of asymmetry were identified, presumably secondary to different patterns of cortical projection. Creel et al. (1983) also found PSVEP abnormalities in Chediak-Higashi syndrome. Harding et al. (1986) studied both long- and short-latency VEPs in human albinos.

3.4.2. Alcoholism

Chan et al. (1986) studied PSVEPs in 52 chronic alcoholics and found abnormalities in 37% of the patients with and 23% of patients without Wernicke-Korsakoff syndrome. Improvement followed a 6-month period of abstinence.

3.4.3. Alzheimer's Disease

Doggett et al. (1981) studied 15 patients and found normal PSVEPs in all, although the group mean was significantly different from normal. Similar results were reported by Coben et al. (1983) which also parallel our experience in the disease (Rizzo et al., 1992).

3.4.4. Charcot-Marie-Tooth Disease

Although these patients do not usually have optic nerve involvement, Tackmann and Radu (1980) and Bird and Griep (1981) found PSVEP abnormalities in 7 of 17 and 4 of 50 eyes, respectively (using the normal mean plus 3 SD). The PSVEP abnormalities did not seem to be related to the clinical severity of the disease. These findings agree with the occasional optic nerve involvement found clinically. McLeod et al. (1978) studied a family in whom the neuropathy was consistently associated with optic atrophy and found PSVEP abnormalities in the two affected individuals tested but normal responses in a carrier.

3.4.5. Chronic Inflammatory Demyelinating Polyneuropathy

Pakalnis et al. (1988) reported abnormal PSVEPs in 9 of 18 patients with chronic inflammatory demyelinating polyneuropathy, 5 with abnormal MRI scans. Brain stem auditory EPs were abnormal only when the PSVEPs were abnormal.

3.4.6. Diabetes

Puvanendran et al. (1983) reported abnormal PSVEPs in 10 of 16 diabetics and suggested that this could be a confusing factor in the use of PSVEPs to diagnose MS.

3.4.7. Epilepsy

Hammond and Wilder (1985) noted no changes in PSVEPs during gamma-vinyl GABA (inhibitor of the enzyme responsible for GABA catabolism) treatment of epileptics.

Faught and Lee (1984) found that patients with epilepsy and photoparoxysmal responses on stroboscopic stimulation also had P100 latencies significantly shorter than normal. Valproic acid therapy increased P100 latency.

3.4.8. Giant Axonal Neuropathy

Majnemer et al. (1986) found abnormal PSVEPs in three patients with giant axonal neuropathy.

3.4.9. Guillain-Barré Syndrome

Ropper and Chiappa (1986) found normal PSVEPs in 9 of 10 patients with Guillain-Barré syndrome; one patient had pseudotumor cerebri and abnormal PSVEPs which were normal on retesting.

3.4.10. Head Trauma

Gupta et al. (1986) studied 33 patients 6 to 24 months after a head injury severe enough to render them comatose for a few hours to several days. Abnormal PSVEPs were seen in 11; only 1 of 9 patients with mild cognitive impairment had PSVEP abnormalities, compared with 7 of 18 with moderate and 3 of 6 with severe cognitive impairment. Stone et al. (1988) have reviewed EPs in head injury and states of increased intracranial pressure.

3.4.11. Hepatic Disease

Pierelli et al. (1985) used normal mean plus 3 SD as the upper limit of normal and found a 40% PSVEP latency abnormality rate in patients with mild hepatic insufficiency (no clinical symptoms or signs) and a 70% rate in those with moderate insufficiency, suggesting that the test might be useful to evaluate the CNS during the course of this disease.

3.4.12. Huntington's Chorea

P100 latency was normal in 13 patients and 9 clinically unaffected offspring (Oepen et al., 1981). P100 amplitudes were reduced [6 μV (± 2.5) versus 9 μV(-4)] in the patients, normal in five offspring but abnormal in four. However, the actual values were not given and it appears from bar graphs that there was considerable overlap with normal values. Hennerici (1985) studied 55 patients and 55 subjects at risk and noted amplitude abnormalities in 30 of 36 patients and 7% of the at-risk subjects. Latencies were generally normal. Josiassen et al. (1984) also reported reduced PSVEP amplitudes, whereas Ehle et al. (1984) found normal values.

3.4.13. Hypothyroidism

Ladenson et al. (1984) recorded PSVEPs before treatment and after thyroid hormone replacement therapy in 19 patients. Before treatment nine patients had a prolonged P100, and this was unchanged after 1 week of therapy. However, in eight this returned to normal after 12 to 24 weeks of therapy.

3.4.14. Leukodystrophies

Mamoli et al. (1979) studied 10 members of one family, 3 with clinical manifestations of adrenoleukodystrophy. They used a 48° screen with 3° checks. Using the normal mean plus 3 SD as the upper limit of normal (the authors used 2 SD), only the three clinically affected patients had abnormal PSVEPs. There was no apparent relationship between ACTH test and P100 latency. Markand et al. (1982) reported normal PSVEPs in a single patient. Tobimatsu et al. (1985) reported abnormal PSVEPs in adrenoleukodystrophy and adrenomyeloneuropathy.

Pattern-shift VEPs were abnormal in two patients with adult metachromatic leukodystrophy (Wulff and Trojaborg, 1985). Kaplan et al. (1993) showed abnormal PSVEPs in 17% of the men with adrenoleukodystrophy, but no evidence that reduction of very-long-chain fatty acid levels with glycerol trioleate and Lorenzo oil altered visual pathway demyelination.

Markand et al. (1982) found abnormal PSVEPs in all 4 patients with Pelizaeus-Merzbacher disease.

3.4.15. Motor System Diseases

Cascino et al. (1988) reported normal PSVEPs in all 22 patients tested. Group comparisons were made between patients and controls in 13 patients and there was no statistical trend toward abnormality. This is in agreement with the study of Radtke et al. (1986), who found no abnormalities in 12 cases studied. Although Matheson et al. (1986) reported 4 patients out of 32 with abnormal PSVEPs, they conclude that in 3 patients the abnormalities were of such minor degree that they were of doubtful significance. In 3 patients the abnormality was a prolongation of the P100 latency by only 1 msec, using a 2.5-SD upper limit of normal and only one recording channel. The other abnormal patient in their study with normal absolute latencies had an intereye difference of 6 msec, a value which would be considered within normal limits in many laboratories.

3.4.16. Myotonic Dystrophy

Gott et al. (1983) reported abnormal PSVEPs in 10 of 17 patients with myotonic dystrophy, none with obvious retinal disease. In 20 patients with myotonic dystrophy Sandrini et al. (1986) found both abnormal PSVEPs and flash ERGs in 13; 3 had only ERG and 2 had only PSVEP abnormalities.

3.4.17. Neurosyphilis

Lowitzsch and Westhoff (1980) found a 6% abnormality rate in the eyes of 25 patients with "latent" syphilis and a 50% abnormality rate in those with neurosyphilis (16 of 32 eyes). Pupillary abnormalities were found in 62% of the latter patients. Conrad et al. (1983) reported abnormal PSVEPs in 50% of patients with tabes dorsalis and in 18% of patients with general paresis.

3.4.18. Parkinson's Disease

There are significant differences between groups of normals and groups of patients with Parkinson's disease. Bodis-Wollner and Yahr (1978) used sinusoidal grating stimulation and found a normal mean of 116 msec (±9) whereas the patient mean was 139 msec (±22). They also found significant interocular differences (3 msec (±3.5) versus 13 (±17). However, even using 95% confidence limits (about 2 SD), the majority of patients had normal P100 latencies when interpreted on an individual basis. These findings were confirmed for check stimulation by Gawel et al. (1981) and Bodis-Wollner et al. (1980). Bodis-Wollner et al. (1980) and Kupersmith et al. (1982) found a correlation between severity of disease and degree of PSVEP abnormality but Gawel et al. (1981) did not. Gottlob et al. (1987) reported abnormal PSVEPs and flash and pattern ERGs in 24 patients with Parkinson's disease. The response to dopaminergic therapy was varied, although Bodis-Wollner et al. (1980, 1982) found that it reduced interocular differences. Barbato et al. (1994) showed that color was more sensitive to conduction improvements produced by L-dopa. The site of the conduction defect is not known; since interocular differences are a major feature of the abnormalities seen and since the inner plexiform layer of the retina contains dopaminergic cells, this seems a likely site. In agreement with this, Bodis-Wollner et al. (1982) reported that PSVEPs became abnormal in 6 of 11 previously untreated schizophrenics who were treated with dopaminergic blocking agents. Note that Ehle et al. (1982) and Dinner et al. (1985) found normal PSVEPs in patients with Parkinson's disease; although the latter authors used excessively large checks (1.8°), the former used 30' checks.

3.4.19. Phenylketonuria

Although hypopigmentation is often associated with misrouted optic projections and PSVEP abnormalities (see also Section 3.4.1), Creel and Buehler (1982) found normal PSVEPs in 5 of 6 patients with untreated phenylketonuria, all of whom were hypopigmented with blond hair and blue eyes.

3.4.20. Renal Disease

Lowitzsch et al. (1981) used 50' checks and found no PSVEP abnormalities in four chronically uremic patients, either before or after hemodialysis. Two patients were investigated three times each at weekly intervals. However, Rossini et al. (1981) found P100 absent or delayed (using 2.5 SD as the limit of normality) in 12 of 32 (37%) nondialyzed patients and in 6 of 11 hemodialyzed patients. The PSVEP abnormalities were found most often with 15' or 7.5' checks. They postulated a toxic effect of circulating renal factors on the papillomacular bundle. Similarly, Rizzo et al. (1982) found P100 latency abnormalities in 6 of 12 patients on hemodialysis and suggested that etiologic factors might be circulating toxins or demyelination. Cohen et al. (1983) reported PSVEP abnormalities in the majority of 22 patients with chronic renal failure. Brown et al. (1987) followed 18 uremic patients through transplantation. No relationship with blood urea nitrogen was found, but P100 latency shortened following the transplant.

3.4.21. Sarcoidosis

Streletz et al. (1981b) recorded PSVEPs in 50 patients with sarcoidosis. Using the normal mean plus 2.5 SD as the upper limit of normal, they found abnormalities in 15 patients (30%). There was no relationship between clinical visual system involvement and PSVEP findings. An optic nerve biopsy in one patient related the sarcoid lesion to the PSVEP abnormality.

3.4.22. Spinocerebellar Degenerations

About two thirds of patients with Friedreich's ataxia have PSVEP abnormalities (Carroll et al., 1980b; Bird and Crill, 1981; Livingstone et al., 1981b; Pedersen and Trojaborg, 1981;

Wenzel et al., 1982a,b; Nuwer et al., 1983; Ghezzi and Montanini, 1985). In the representative study of Carroll et al. (1980b), increased latencies were found (mean was 7 SD above the normal mean), no significant waveform dispersion was seen, and only 1 of their 22 patients had a significant interocular difference. Partial-field stimulation showed a slightly higher incidence of abnormalities. There was a good correlation between clinical and PSVEP findings, especially temporal disc pallor; note that none of the patients had visual complaints. There was no relationship between latency and duration of illness or between latency and visual acuity, although there was a relationship between amplitude and acuity.

There are a variety of other spinal, cerebellar, and brain stem degenerative diseases which are an uncertain grouping of genetic ataxias and degenerations; incomplete clinical, hereditary, pathophysiologic, and biochemical information renders their precise definition impossible. It is necessary to study each case report in detail to appreciate the similarity with others under study. Overall it seems that only rare PSVEP abnormalities are found, in contrast with the high rate of abnormalities found in the Friedreich's cases mentioned above.

Carroll et al. (1980a) found normal PSVEPs in 16 family members affected with a late-onset, autosomal dominant form of cerebellar cortical degeneration in contrast to the high incidence of PSVEP abnormalities found in their Friedreich's patients. Livingstone et al. (1981b) reported 13 patients with a dominant hereditary spastic paraplegia and 7 sporadic cases. PSVEPs were normal in all the dominantly inherited cases but abnormal in 3 of the 7 sporadic cases. Livingstone et al. (1981a) reported 17 patients with a progressive syndrome of lower limb spasticity and cerebellar ataxia with dysarthria, 10 with a family history suggesting an autosomal dominant pattern of inheritance. Only 3 of these patients had abnormal PSVEPs and only 2 had abnormalities on clinical neuro-ophthalmologic examination. Bird and Crill (1981) studied 19 patients with a variety of hereditary ataxias and degenerations. Three had some form of olivopontocerebellar degeneration (all had normal PSVEPs), two had a Strumpell type of dominant spastic paraparesis (one high normal, the other normal PSVEPs), and one had a dentatorubral degeneration with spinal involvement (normal PSVEPs). Overall six patients with dominant ataxias all had normal PSVEPs, four patients with a nonspecific recessive ataxia all had normal PSVEPs, and nine patients with miscellaneous ataxias had normal or high normal PSVEPs. Ghezzi and Montanini (1985) found PSVEPs delayed in one of eight patients with Strumpell's hereditary spastic ataxia, in two of five patients with cerebellar atrophy, and normal in five patients with Pierre Marie's disease. Nuwer et al. (1983), Hammond and Wilder (1983), Chokroverty et al. (1985), and Nousiainen et al. (1987) reported results in patients with olivopontocerebellar atrophy, hereditary spastic ataxia, and progressive peroneal atrophy.

3.4.23. Vitamin Deficiencies

Troncoso et al. (1979) studied three untreated patients with vitamin B_{12} deficiency (using 48' checks). One patient had P100 latency of both eyes at 2.5 SD above the normal mean, one patient had one eye markedly abnormal, and the other patient had an interocular difference of 15 msec, with the worst eye still within normal limits for absolute latency (taken as the normal mean plus 3 SD). The worst eye of the latter patient had mildly defective color vision but the other patients had no clinical visual abnormalities. Rees (1980) reported two patients with pernicious anemia, Bodis-Wollner and Korczyn (1980) reported one patient, and Hennerici (1985) reported four patients, all of whom had bilateral P100 latency abnormalities. Krumholz et al. (1981) studied seven patients with B_{12} deficiency and found P100 latency abnormalities in the two who were most severely affected clinically, although neither had clinical neuro-ophthalmologic abnormalities. One year later, after treatment, the PSVEPs had returned to normal in both patients. Fine and Hallett (1980) studied three patients with B_{12} deficiency but did not give the statistical level of their limit of normality. Two of their three patients had abnormal P100 latencies with 9- and 15-msec interocular differences; the other patient was at the upper limit of normal in both eyes. Some of these authors investigated other EPs as well and found a higher incidence of abnormalities with SLSEPs.

Severe vitamin B_{12} deficiency eventually produced visual impairment in five of nine rhesus monkeys and autopsy showed degeneration of the peripheral visual pathways in all nine (Agamanolis et al., 1976). Thus, demyelination in the optic nerves may account for the PSVEP abnormalities seen in this disease.

Brin et al. (1986) found abnormal PSVEPs in three of nine patients with abetalipoproteinemia with vitamin E deficiency. Electroretinograms were abnormal in these three and in two others with normal PSVEPs. Messenheimer et al. (1984) saw reversal of P100 latency abnormalities with vitamin E therapy. Kaplan et al. (1988) reported abnormal PSVEPs in 3 of 10 patients with cystic fibrosis and pancreatic malabsorption.

3.5. Spinal Cord Diseases

Patients with acute transverse myelitis show PSVEP abnormalities in only a small proportion of cases. Blumhardt et al. (1982a) studied 31 patients in whom the spinal cord symptoms developed over hours to days (9 of these were classified as transverse myelitis) and found PSVEP abnormalities in 10%. Ropper et al. (1982) found no PSVEP abnormalities in 12 patients with acute transverse myelitis.

The chronic, progressive myelopathies have a greater incidence of abnormal PSVEPs (Halliday et al., 1973b; Asselman et al., 1975; Hennerici et al., 1977; Blumhardt et al., 1982a; Bynke et al., 1977; Paty et al., 1979). The abnormality rates ranged from 76% in the series of Bynke et al. (1977) to 35% in the 100 patients with disease of more than 6 months duration studied by Blumhardt et al. (1982a).

It has been suggested that PSVEP data can be used clinically in the setting of undiagnosed spinal cord disease to help decide whether or not myelography is necessary (Mastaglia et al., 1976b). Bynke et al. (1977) suggested that if the clinical neuro-ophthalmologic examination and the PSVEP are abnormal, and the CSF shows oligoclonal IgG banding, then radiologic investigations can be limited or avoided. However, the possibility of concurrent diseases dictates very careful assessment of the clinical situation before an abnormal PSVEP (with or without other tests) should be used as presumptive evidence of MS to delay myelography. In fact, Blumhardt et al. (1982a) found five patients with abnormal PSVEPs and abnormal myelograms. Three had only borderline narrowing of the cervical canals and spondylotic changes (two of these have subsequently developed further signs of MS), but two had cord compression caused by prolapsed intervertebral discs. After laminectomy one patient had little clinical change but one had a marked improvement.

3.6. Diseases of the Posterior Visual Pathways

It is important to fully understand the concepts and data on partial-field stimulation (see Chapter 2, Section 8.1.5) and P100 distribution abnormalities (see Section 2.4) before proceeding.

As has been discussed in Section 2.1 of this chapter, full-field stimulation and recording from the posterior midline does not usually reveal abnormalities with unilateral posterior visual pathway lesions. Occasionally, the "transitional zone" (see Chapter 2, Section 8.1.5) will shift to involve the midline in these patients and an apparent abnormality may then be seen. Bilateral posterior visual pathway lesions will show binocular abnormalities using midline recordings (Ashworth et al., 1978). However, to best study lesions of the posterior visual pathways, partial-field stimulation with recording from laterally placed electrodes must be used.

3.6.1. Tumors, Infarctions, and Migraine

With partial-field stimulation and recording from laterally placed electrodes, PSVEP abnormalities can be seen in some patients (Blumhardt et al., 1977; Carlow and Rodriguez, 1978; Blumhardt and Halliday, 1979; Halliday and Mushin, 1980; Hoeppner et al., 1980; Lavine et al., 1980; Zschocke and Muller-Jensen, 1980; Halliday and McDonald, 1981; Kuroiwa and Celesia, 1981; Streletz et al., 1981a,b; Holder, 1985), but the clinical correlations in these studies have been disappointing. It is an easy matter to find individual patients whose PSVEP results agree with clinical neuro-ophthalmologic and anatomic data, and the literature contains accounts of such cases. However, systematic studies of series of such patients reveal less consistent relationships. Streletz et al. (1981a,b) studied 20 patients with occipital lobe lesions (18 infarcts, 2 tumors) and 20 normal subjects and concluded that "the presence of asymmetry on VEP alone is not prima facie evidence of occipital lobe damage, since normal subjects have asymmetry in some cases." Kuroiwa and Celesia (1981) studied 23 normal subjects and 16 patients with retrochiasmatic lesions. They noted that "uncrossed asymmetry, defined according to Halliday's group . . . was a poor indicator of retrochiasmatic lesions. It occurred in . . . 2 normal volunteers (8.7% of normals); occurrence in normal persons raises serious doubts about the diagnostic usefulness of this finding." Furthermore, they concluded that "although either steady-state or transient-VEP amplitude distribution and ratios are reliable, neither test has yet proved as sensitive as field perimetry." Blumhardt and Halliday (1981) used a factor of 2 as an upper limit for the amplitude asymmetry between the two half-fields of one eye, that is, the P100 amplitude from one half-field was abnormal if it was less than half the amplitude of the other. Using this measure they found an abnormality rate near 100% in 16 patients with dense hemianopias, but noted that this fell off according to the incompleteness of the field defect so that the detection rate for quadrantic defects was about 50% (overall abnormality rate for patients with visual-field defects was 84%). They found the technique indispensable for identifying abnormal waveform patterns generated by posterior visual pathway lesions, for example, the inverted polarity activity which can be recorded from midline electrodes when a retrochiasmal lesion has caused a lateral shift of the "transitional zone." They further noted that (1) the partial-field PSVEP patterns parallel the type and extent of the visual-field defect; (2) the effect of a cortical lesion appears to depend exclusively on the presence of damage to the primary projection pathways or visual cortical generators; (3) there was no evidence of a transcallosal contribution to the half-field P100; (4) the effects on amplitude and latency appear to be dissociated and few pathologic responses had prolonged latencies; (5) the PSVEP was indifferent to cortical lesions which spared the specific visual pathways; (6) the PSVEP was not as sensitive as perimetry for demonstration of visual-field defects; and (7) although the method did not seem to have wide clinical utility, they find it useful in small groups of patients suspected of psychiatric or mixed organic/psychiatric disease to confirm or exclude a subjectively determined visual-field defect. Celesia et al. (1982) correlated PSVEPs and PET scans (regional CBF or local cerebral glucose metabolism) in 4 patients with hemianopic defects. Celesia et al. (1983) analyzed PSVEP results in 50 patients with homonymous field defects and compared them with results of perimetry; the EPs were absent to stimulation of the affected hemifield in every case with macular splitting but otherwise were abnormal in only 79%.

The use of sequential partial-field stimulation techniques (see Chapter 2, Section 1; Rowe, 1981; Chiappa and Jenkins, 1982) may provide more consistent results and thus allow better clinical interpretation, but this is still being evaluated. Rowe (1982) has found greater utility from latency measurements than suggested in the study of Blumhardt and Halliday, and has documented a significant improvement in the detection rate of retrochiasmal conduction defects using those parameters. Amplitude was not used as an interpretive criterion in this group of patients. Of the 250 patients tested, 205 (82%) had reproducible responses to full- and half-field stimulation. Full-field response abnormalities were seen in 18%, both full- and half-field response abnormalities were seen in 9%, and half-field abnormalities with normal full-field responses were seen in 7% of the patients. Thirty-four of the 71 patients with abnormal PSVEPs (48%) had half-field response abnormalities, suggesting prechiasmal lesions in 25, chiasmal lesions in 3, and postchiasmal lesions in 6. A prolongation of full-field latency was always associated with prolongation of one or both half-field response latencies from the same eye. The interpretation was based on the following assumptions: (1) abnormalities found in both fields of both eyes rendered it impossible to establish the site of the conduction defect, (2) abnormalities only in one field of one eye indicated a probable partial prechiasmal lesion, (3) abnormalities from the same field in both eyes suggested a chiasmal or postchiasmal lesion, and (4) bitemporal half-field response abnormalities suggested a chiasmal lesion. The sequential technique of stimulation used in these studies may account for the improved reliability of the half-field latency measurements.

Haimovic and Pedley (1982a,b) also used a sequential partial-field stimulation technique and studied normal subjects and patients with lesions in various parts of the visual system. They considered a hemifield PSVEP normal if it demonstrated (1) a positivity at the ipsilateral occipital electrode (O1 or O2 in the International 10–20 System) with a latency of less than 110 msec, and (2) either a negativity (latency less than 118 msec) or an isopotential response at the contralateral temporal electrode. A hemifield response was interpreted as abnormal if (1) no consistent ipsilateral P100 wave could be identified in replicated trials; (2) if the expected transition from ipsilateral positivity to contralateral negativity was absent (this seems to be in direct contradiction to the second possibility in point 2 above in the normal definition); or (3) if the interfield amplitude ratio of corresponding P100 waves was greater than 4:1. The latency and amplitude ratio values quoted here are in good agreement with those in Table 2–3, but differ from those of Blumhardt and Halliday (1981). Haimovic and Pedley (1982b) studied the effects of lesions in the retina, optic nerve, chiasm, geniculocalcarine, and parastriate cortex: (1) All of their patients with suprasellar tumors and complete hemianopias had no responses from the affected fields. Evoked potentials were normal in two patients with superior quadrant defects. Only one patient had delay in ipsilateral P100 with hemifield testing; four patients had delayed P100s on full-field stimulation. (2) In the 14 patients with retrochiasmal lesions two types of abnormalities were described. There were no potentials discernible ipsilateral to the field defect in patients with lesions affecting the geniculocalcarine pathway or posteromedial occipital lobe (producing total homonymous hemianopias). Responses in patients with similar dense-field deficits but with lesions located in the posterolateral occipital or parietal lobes were characterized by "gross distortion," with a large positivity over the entire posterior scalp and no contralateral negativity. When the patients with abnormal half-field responses were tested with full-field stimulation, abnormalities (response asymmetry) were seen in only 28%. These authors concluded that half-field stimulation is preferable to full-field techniques in patients with chiasmatic or retrochiasmatic lesions.

Other studies, using similar and/or different techniques, have also been performed to assess and improve the reliability and sensitivity of partial-field stimulation (Celesia and Daly, 1977; Kuroiwa and Celesia, 1981; Streletz et al., 1981b; Maitland et al., 1982; Onofrj et al., 1982; Holder, 1985), with results essentially similar to those covered above.

There are only three brief reports of PSVEPs in patients with migraine (Gawel et al., 1980; Muller-Jensen and Zschocke, 1980; Wenzel et al., 1982a). Abnormalities were found in all studies but since these were in abstract form, little critical evaluation can be done.

3.6.2. Cortical Blindness

Bodis-Wollner et al. (1977) found steady-state pattern EPs present with coarse but absent with fine spatial frequency gratings in a patient who had destruction in cortical (association) areas 18 and 19 but preservation in (primary) areas 17. Celesia et al. (1980, 1982) using 27′ checks found essentially normal transient and steady-state pattern EPs in a patient with preservation of areas 18 and 19 and destruction of areas 17, and made PET scan correlations in this patient and other patients with cortical disease. Anatomic verification in these cases was by CT scan. Bodis-Wollner (1977) reported a patient with probable visual cortical infarction (extent unknown) whose PSVEPs correlated well with visual fields and the patient's subjective visual acuity. Again, the higher spatial frequencies showed greater deficits. Thus, the use of smaller checks (less than 20′) usually reveals abnormalities in such patients, whereas larger checks may produce normal PSVEPs. Note the following experiences with flash stimulation: (1) Frank and Torres (1978) found normal VEPs in 30 cortically blind children; (2) Spehlmann et al. (1977) found present but simplified VEPs in a cortically blind patient subsequently shown to have extensive infarction of occipital white matter and cortex bilaterally (the authors suggested an extrageniculocalcarine pathway to secondary visual cortex as the generator of the VEP); (3) Kooi and Sharbrough (1966) found present but abnormal VEPs in a case of traumatic cortical blindness; (4) Abraham et al. (1975) studied three patients with cortical blindness following basilar artery occlusion and believed that early normal VEPs signified a good prognosis, whereas absent or abnormal VEPs had a bad prognosis; (5) Duchowny et al. (1974) correlated VEPs and prognosis in six children with cortical blindness from trauma or meningitis; (6) Barnet et al. (1970) did the same for six children with various etiologies of their cortical blindness; and (7) Hess et al. (1982) found normal flash but abnormal pattern EPs in four patients with acute cortical blindness secondary to infarction (two of whom had no light perception).

3.7. Hysteria-Malingering

The test can be used to assess visual function in patients suspected of factitious visual loss. The presence of a normal PSVEP in spite of symptoms of moderate to severe visual difficulty strongly suggests that good vision is present. Halliday and McDonald (1981) state that "a visual acuity of 20/120 or less is incompatible with a well-formed pattern evoked potential." Note that to some extent the visual acuity reported by the patient can be correlated with the visual angle subtended by the checks (see the discussion in Chapter 2, Section 6) and check size changed during the test to arrive at a very rough estimate of visual acuity.

However, if the site of possible lesions includes occipital and visual association cortices (cortical blindness), then this does not necessarily apply since patients have been reported

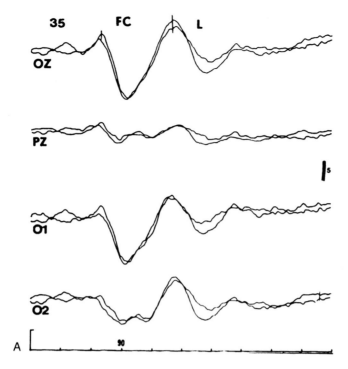

FIG. 3–10. Pattern-shift VEPs obtained from a patient who claimed only finger-counting vision in the left eye (**A,** *left panel*) and no light perception in the right eye (damaged by trauma years previously) (**B,** *right panel*). P100 is normal in the left eye to 35' checks, suggesting visual acuity of 20/100 or better. The right eye has no response to 70' checks (upper four traces), suggesting visual acuity of worse than 20/200, but the good response to strobe flash stimulation (lower four traces) suggests that light perception at least is present in that eye. The reference for all channels is mid-frontal, relative postivity of posterior electrodes caused a downward trace deflection. The 90 label is at 90 msec from the stimulus; calibration bars are 5, 1, and 5 μV for the left eye, right-eye 70' checks, and right-eye strobe stimulations, respectively. Each trace is the average of 100 stimuli.

with reasonably good clinical and radiologic evidence for severe visual impairment on the basis of cortical lesions, who have essentially normal PSVEPs (see above). However, in this regard, if small enough checks are used (less than 20'), these patients also will show PSVEP abnormalities.

Conversely, the demonstration of a definite PSVEP abnormality in a patient considered to be hysterical can be very helpful (see Fig. 10.8 in Halliday and McDonald, 1981). Figure 3–10 shows VEP results from a patient who claimed only finger-counting vision in the left eye and no light perception in the right eye (damaged by trauma years previously). The normal P100 in the left eye to 35' checks suggests good visual acuity (20/100 or better) in that eye, and the good response to strobe flash in the right eye suggests at least light perception in that eye. Thus, the patient was malingering and lowering visual function factitiously in both eyes, although the absent P100 in the right eye to 70' checks (with good patient coop-

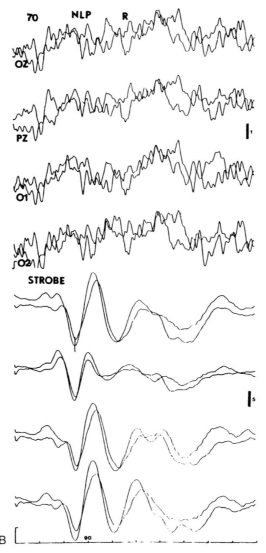

FIG. 3–10. (*Continued*)

eration) indicates a visual acuity of 20/200 or worse. The topic of EPs in hysteria and malingering was reviewed by Howard and Dorfman (1986).

3.8. Retinal and Optic Neuropathies, Amblyopias, and Glaucoma

Ischemic optic neuropathy will affect PSVEP amplitude before latency but most often both are affected, depending on total area of retina involved (Asselman et al., 1975; Hennerici et al., 1977; Ikeda et al., 1978; Wilson, 1978; Robertson and Feldman, 1980; Harding et al., 1980a; Cox et al., 1982; Thompson et al., 1986).

Transient retinal ischemia does not affect P100 latency, although amplitude is diminished. Kline and Glaser (1982) studied PSVEPs in two patients during attacks of amaurosis fugax, with retinal angiography demonstrating the failure of blood flow. There was little change in PSVEP latency during disappearance and reappearance of P100.

Pattern-shift VEPs in toxic amblyopia secondary to tobacco and/or alcohol have been reported by Kriss et al. (1982) and Ikeda et al. (1978). Kriss et al. (1982) studied 23 patients with toxic optic neuropathy. Central-field (0° to 4°) stimulation evoked a grossly abnormal response and full-field stimulation resulted in a pattern consistent with a central scotoma. An increase in amplitude was seen with treatment.

Yiannikas et al. (1983) studied PSVEPs in patients being treated with ethambutol for tuberculosis. In 5 of 14 patients abnormalities were found (associated with clinical findings in only 1) which reversed with cessation of treatment in two. The authors suggested that the PSVEP might be useful for monitoring visual function in such patients. Fledelius et al. (1987) and Petrera et al. (1988) have also investigated this application of PSVEPs.

Deferoxamine is used for treatment of the chronic iron overload in thalassemia major. It has toxic effects on the visual system (site unclear) and Taylor et al. (1987a) found abnormal PSVEP latencies in 21% of 77 patients with improvement while off therapy.

Tropical amblyopia (Asselman et al., 1975; Harding et al., 1980a; Ikeda et al., 1978) and quinine amblyopia (Gangitano and Keltner, 1980) also produce similar abnormalities.

Gross PSVEP abnormalities are usually found in Leber's optic atrophy. Carroll and Mastaglia (1979) investigated a six-generation family with 14 clinically affected members. Pattern-shift VEP abnormalities included increased P100 latency and distortion and decreased amplitude. The PSVEP usually correlated well with clinical severity. Pattern-shift VEP abnormalities were found in some asymptomatic family members, both those at risk of developing the disease and those not. Patients with other hereditary optic atrophies have also been reported (Harding and Crews, 1982).

Selbst et al. (1983) reported abnormal PSVEPs in a patient with optic neuritis following a varicella infection.

Kaufman et al. (1988) investigated the use of PERGs in prognosis of a variety of optic neuropathies. Seventeen eyes had gradual and permanent reduction (usually by 16 weeks, occasionally more slowly) of PERG amplitude and all had poor visual outcome. In 29 eyes (various etiologies of the optic neuropathy) the PERG remained normal and in 22 of these the visual outcome was 20/25 or better. Eidelberg et al. (1988) used recent modifications to MRI techniques (short inversion recovery for suppression of orbital fat signals) to study 20 patients with chronic optic neuropathy of various etiologies and found it to complement PSVEP testing.

Amblyopia-ex-anopsia produces PSVEP latency abnormalities in about half of patients tested (Fig. 3–11) depending on check size used (Arden et al., 1974; Sokol, 1978b; Sokol and Nadler, 1979; Spekreijse et al., 1972). When a range of check sizes is used, a marked attenuation of waveforms in the amblyopic eye is seen with progressively smaller checks and the extent of the abnormality can be diagramed by plotting P100 amplitude against check size (Sokol and Nadler, 1979; Sokol, 1978b). The use of different check sizes is particularly recommended because some check sizes will occasionally evoke larger responses from the amblyopic eye (Sokol and Shaterian, 1976). The presence or absence of a PSVEP latency abnormality is not closely related to the degree of visual acuity impairment. This may be because these patients are a heterogeneous group with respect to etiology of the amblyopia. In true amblyopes, pathophysiology is probably located in the geniculate body or visual cortex, rather than the retina. The clinician must be careful to consider amblyopia when a distant past history suggests optic neuritis and the PSVEP is abnormal.

Pattern-shift VEPs can be used to follow therapy in amblyopia. Wilcox and Sokol (1980) saw amplitude increases with acuity improvement in response to patching.

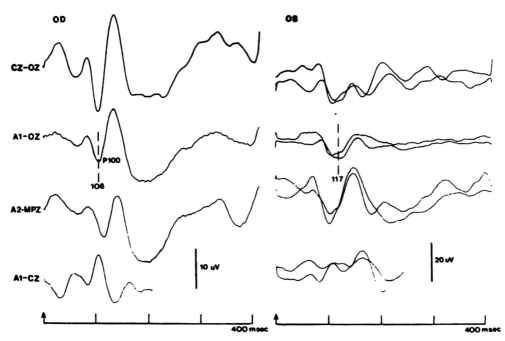

FIG. 3–11. Pattern-shift VEPs from a patient with amblyopia-ex-anopsia. Note the low-amplitude P100 from the left eye, at the upper limit of normal for absolute latency and abnormal for intereye difference (see legends for Figs. 3–1 and 3–3 for normal limits). Each trace is the average of 128 stimuli, with a repetition superimposed for the left eye (*right panel*).

Glaucoma is well known to produce both latency and amplitude abnormalities in PSVEPs (Huber and Wagner, 1978; Cappin and Nissim, 1975; Towle et al., 1983), although the sensitivity of the test in this area is disputed. In certain patients, PSVEPs will detect clinically silent lesions, even when no field defect is found.

3.9. Pediatric Applications

Reliable PSVEPs can be recorded from children of all ages including neonates (Marg et al., 1976; Sokol, 1978a, b, 1980, 1983; Dobson and Teller, 1978; Sokol and Jones, 1979; Banks, 1980). (See Chapter 2, Sections 6 and 8.2.1 for discussions of testing routines and normal variability with age.) Clinically, PSVEPs are used to follow development of the visual system (Sokol, 1978a; Marg et al., 1976; Moskowitz and Sokol, 1980). Sokol (1978a) extrapolated from the check size eliciting maximum P100 amplitude to zero amplitude by regression analysis and found improvement from 20/150 at 2 months of age to 20/20 by 6 months of age. These results were in agreement with Marg et al. (1976), who used a different EP technique, but indicate significantly better acuities than had been found with behavioral acuity measures (preferential looking and optokinetic nystagmus). In addition, the PSVEP is used to assess efficacy of treatments for amblyopia and corneal opacities (Sokol, 1978b, 1980, 1983), and as an aid in infants with normal ophthalmoscopic findings but abnormal visual behavior (Gittinger and Sokol, 1982). This topic is given more detailed treatment in Chapter 4.

3.10. Strobe (Flash) VEPs

This technique has clinical utility (1) when the question is whether or not the visual pathways from retina to visual cortex are intact (e.g., following trauma to the orbit, during surgery in the region of the optic nerves, and in various neonatal diseases), and (2) when the patient is unable to cooperate sufficiently for a PSVEP to be performed [e.g., during general anesthesia, in coma, or in very young infants (Taylor et al., 1987)]. The information gathered from this test is more qualitative than quantitative but in those situations is sufficient.

3.11. Electroretinography

In general, flash ERG abnormalities indicating retinopathy or other conditions involving the retina are correlated with reduced PSVEP amplitudes. Ikeda et al. (1978) found this relationship in patients with compressive and ischemic optic neuropathies, MS, idiopathic optic neuropathies, and toxic amblyopia. Harding et al. (1980a) also reported abnormal results for both tests in ischemic optic neuropathy.

The use of PSVEPs and flash ERGs in tandem is suggested as a means of determining whether or not PSVEP abnormalities have a retinal origin (Armington, 1980; Mustonen et al., 1980). This is a legitimate endeavor. However, the complexity involved in performing and interpreting the flash ERG properly usually demands the attention of a physician specially trained for at least 1 year. Unless such personnel are available with the proper equipment, more mistakes will be made than assistance gained.

(See Chapter 2, Section 11, for a discussion of PERG and its utility in PSVEP testing.)

Evoked Potentials in Clinical Medicine,
3d ed., edited by Keith H. Chiappa.
Lippincott–Raven Publishers, Philadelphia © 1997.

Pattern-Shift Visual Evoked Potentials

References

Abe Y, Kuroiwa Y (1990): Amplitude asymmetry of hemifield pattern reversal VEPs in healthy subjects. *Electroencephalogr Clin Neurophysiol* 77(2):81–85.

Abraham FA, Melamed E, Lavy S (1975): Prognostic value of visual evoked potentials in occipital blindness following basilar artery occlusion. *Appl Neurophysiol* 32:126–135.

Agamanolis DP, Chester EM, Victor M, Kark JA, Hines JD, Harris JW (1976): Neuropathology of experimental vitamin B-12 deficiency in monkeys. *Neurology* 26:905.

Alani SM (1985): Pattern-reversal visual evoked potentials in patients with hydrocephalus. *J Neurosurg* 62:234–237.

Allison T, Matsumiya Y, Goff GD, Goff WR (1977): The scalp topography of human visual evoked potentials. *Electroencephalogr Clin Neurophysiol* 42:185–197.

Allison T, Goff WR, Wood CC (1979): Auditory, somatosensory and visual evoked potentials in the diagnosis of neuropathology: Recording considerations and normative data. In: *Human Evoked Potentials: Applications and Problems*, edited by D Lehman and E Callaway, pp 1–16. Plenum Press, London.

Allison T, Wood CC, Goff WR (1983): Brain stem auditory, pattern-reversal visual, and short-latency somatosensory evoked potentials: Latencies in relation to age, sex, and brain and body size. *Electroencephalogr Clin Neurophysiol* 55:619–636.

Allison T, Hume AL, Wood CC, Goff WR (1984): Developmental and aging changes in somatosensory, auditory and visual evoked potentials. *Electroencephalogr Clin Neurophysiol* 58:14–24.

Allison T, Begleiter A, McCarthy G, Roessler E, Nobre AC, Spencer DD (1993): Electrophysiological studies of color processing in human visual cortex. *Electroencephalogr Clin Neurophysiol* 88(5):343–355.

Aminoff MJ, Davis SL, Panitch HS (1984): Serial evoked potential studies in patients with definite multiple sclerosis. *Arch Neurol* 41:1197–1202.

Anderson DC, Slater GE, Sherman R, Ettinger MG (1987): Evoked potentials to test a treatment of chronic multiple sclerosis. *Arch Neurol* 44:1232–1236.

Andersson T, Siden A (1994): Comparison of visual evoked potentials elicited by light-emitting diodes and TV monitor stimulation in patients with multiple sclerosis and potentially related conditions. *Electroencephalogr Clin Neurophysiol* 92(6):473–479.

Apkarian P, Reits D, Spekruijse H, Van Dorp D (1983): A decisive electrophysiological test for human albinism. *Electroencephalogr Clin Neurophysiol* 55:513–531.

Arden GB, Barnard WM, Mushin AS (1974): Visually evoked responses in amblyopia. *Br J Ophthalmol* 58:183–192.

Arden GB, Carter RM, Hogg C, Siegel IM, Margolis S (1979): A gold foil electrode: Extending the horizons for clinical electroretinography. *Invest Ophthalmol Vis Sci* 18:421–426.

Arden GB, Vaegan, Hogg CR (1982): Clinical and experimental evidence that the pattern electroretinogram (PERG) is generated in more proximal retinal layers than the focal electroretinogram (FERG). *Ann NY Acad Sci* 388:580–601.

Arden GB, Carter RM, Macfarlan A (1984): Pattern and Ganzfeld electroretinograms in macular disease. *Br J Ophthalmol* 68:878–884.

Armington JC (1980): Electroretinography. In: *Electrodiagnosis in Clinical Neurology*, 1st ed. edited by MJ Aminoff, pp 305–347. Churchill Livingstone, New York.

Ashworth B, Maloney AFJ, Townsend HRA (1978): Delayed visual evoked potentials with bilateral disease of the posterior visual pathway. *J Neurol Neurosurg Psychiatry* 41:449–451.

Asselman P, Chadwick DW, Marsden CD (1975): Visual evoked responses in the diagnosis and management of patients suspected of multiple sclerosis. *Brain* 98:261–282.

Bajada S, Mastaglia FL, Black JL, Collins DWK (1980): Effects of induced hyperthermia on visual evoked potentials and saccade parameters in normal subjects and multiple sclerosis patients. *J Neurol Neurosurg Psychiatry* 43:849–852.

Banks MS (1980): Infant refraction and accommodation. In: *Electrophysiology and Psychophysics: Their Use in Ophthalmic Diagnosis*, edited by S Sokol. *Int Ophthalmol Clin* 20 (1). Spring 1980, pp 205–232. Little Brown, Boston.

Barber C, Galloway NR (1978): Adaptation effects in the transient visual evoked potential. In: *Human Evoked Potentials: Applications and Problems*, edited by D Lehman and E Callaway, pp 17–30. Plenum Press, London.

Barbato L, Rinalduzzi S, Laurenti M, Ruggieri S, Accornero N (1994): Color VEPs in Parkinson's disease. *Electroencephalogr Clin Neurophysiol* 92(2):169–172.

Barnet AB, Manson JI, Wilner E (1970): Acute cerebral blindness in childhood. Six cases studied clinically and electrophysiologically. *Neurology* 20:1147–1156.

Barrett G, Blumhardt LD, Halliday AM, Halliday E, Kriss A (1976): A paradox in the lateralization of the visual evoked response. *Nature* 261:253–255.

Bartel P, Blom M, Robinson E, Van der Meyden C, Sommers DS, Becker P (1990): Effects of chlorpromazine on pattern and flash ERGs and VEPs compared to oxazepam and to placebo in normal subjects. *Electroencephalogr Clin Neurophysiol* 77(5):330–339.

Bartel PR, Vos A (1994): Induced refractive errors and pattern electroretinograms and pattern visual evoked potentials: implications for clinical assessments. *Electroencephalogr Clin Neurophysiol* 92(1):78–81.

Bartl G, van Lith GHM, van Marle GW (1978): Cortical potentials evoked by a TV pattern reversal stimulus with varying check sizes and stimulus field. *Br J Ophthalmol* 62:216–219.

Baumhefner RW, Tourtellotte WW, Ellison G, Myers L, Syndulko K, Cohen SN, Shapshak P, Osborne M, Waluch V (1986): Multiple sclerosis: Correlation of magnetic resonance imaging with clinical disability, quantitative evaluation of neurologic function, evoked potentials and intra-blood-brain-barrier IgG synthesis. *Neurology* 36:283.

Berninger T, Schuurmans RP (1985): Spatial tuning of the pattern ERG across temporal frequency. *Doc Ophthalmol* 61:17–25.

Berninger TA (1986): The pattern electroretinogram and its contamination. *Clin Vis Sci* 1:185–190.

Bird TD, Crill WE (1981): Pattern-reversal visual evoked potentials in the hereditary ataxias and spinal degenerations. *Ann Neurol* 9:243–250.

Bird TD, Griep E (1981): Pattern reversal visual evoked potentials. Studies in Charcot-Marie-Tooth hereditary neuropathy. *Arch Neurol* 38:739–741.

Blumhardt LD, Halliday AM (1979): Hemisphere contributions to the composition of the pattern-evoked potential waveform. *Exp Brain Res* 36:53–69.

Blumhardt LD, Halliday AM (1981): Cortical abnormalities and the visual evoked response. *Doc Ophthalmol Proc Series* 27:347–365.

Blumhardt LD, Barrett G, Halliday AM (1977): The asymmetrical visual evoked potential to pattern reversal in one half field and its significance for the analysis of visual field defects. *Br J Ophthalmol* 61:454–461.

Blumhardt LD, Barrett G, Halliday AM, Kriss A (1978): The effect of experimental "scotomata" on the ipsilateral and contralateral responses to pattern-reversal in one half-field. *Electroencephalogr Clin Neurophysiol* 45:376–392.

Blumhardt LD, Barrett G, Halliday AM (1982a): The pattern visual evoked potential in the clinical assessment of undiagnosed spinal cord disease. In: *Clinical Applications of Evoked Potentials in Neurology*, edited by J Courjon, F Mauguiere, and M Revol, pp 463–471. Raven Press, New York.

Blumhardt LD, Barrett G, Kriss A, Halliday AM (1982b): The pattern-evoked potential in lesions of the posterior visual pathways. *Ann NY Acad Sci* 388:264–289.

Bobak P, Bodis-Wollner I, Guillory S (1987): The effect of blur and contrast on VEP latency: Comparison between check and sinusoidal grating patterns. *Electroencephalogr Clin Neurophysiol* 68:247–255.

Bodis-Wollner I (1977): Recovery from cerebral blindness: Evoked potential and psychophysical measurements. *Electroencephalogr Clin Neurophysiol* 42:178–184.

Bodis-Wollner I, Korczyn AD (1980): Dissociated sensory loss and visual evoked potentials in a patient with pernicious anemia. *Mt Sinai J Med* 47:579–582.

Bodis-Wollner I, Yahr MD (1978): Measurements of visual evoked potentials in Parkinson's disease. *Brain* 101:661–671.

Bodis-Wollner I, Atkin A, Raab E, Wolkstein M (1977): Visual association cortex and vision in man: Pattern-evoked occipital potentials in a blind boy. *Science* 198:629–631.

Bodis-Wollner I, Yahr M, Thornton J (1980): Interocular VEP latency differences and the effect of treatment in Parkinson's disease. *Electroencephalogr Clin Neurophysiol* 50:220P.

Bodis-Wollner I, Yahr MD, Mylin L, Thornton J (1982): Dopaminergic deficiency and delayed visual evoked potentials in humans. *Ann Neurol* 11:478–483.

Bodis-Wollner I, Feldman RG, Guillory SL, Mylin L (1987): Delayed visual evoked potentials are independent of pattern orientation in macular disease. *Electroencephalogr Clin Neurophysiol* 68:172–179.

Bostrom C, Keller EL, Marg E (1978): A reconsideration of visual evoked potentials for fast automated ophthalmic refraction. *Invest Ophthalmol Vis Sci* 17:182–185.

Bottcher J, Trojaberg W (1982): Follow-up of patients with suspected multiple sclerosis: A clinical and electrophysiological study. *Neurol Neurosurg Psychiatry* 45:809–814.

Brecelj J (1992): A VEP study of the visual pathway function in compressive lesions of the optic chiasm. Full-field versus half-field stimulation. *Electroencephalogr Clin Neurophysiol* 84:209–218.

Brin MF, Pedley TA, Lovelace RE, Emerson RG, Gouras P, MacKay C, Kayden HJ, Levy J, Baker H (1986): Electrophysiologic features of abetalipoproteinemia: Functional consequences of vitamin E deficiency. *Neurology* 36:669–673.

Brindley GS (1972): The variability of the human striate cortex. *J Physiol* 225:1P–3P.

Brooks EB, Chiappa KH (1982): A comparison of clinical neuro-ophthalmological findings and pattern shift visual evoked potentials in multiple sclerosis. In: *Clinical Applications of Evoked Potentials in Neurology*, edited by J Courjon, F Mauguiere, and M Revol, pp 453–457. Raven Press, New York.

Brown JJ, Sufit RL, Sollinger HW (1987): Visual evoked potential changes following renal transplantation. *Electroencephalogr Clin Neurophysiol* 66:101–107.

Bumgartner J, Epstein CM (1981): Voluntary alteration of visual evoked potentials. *Ann Neurol* 12:475–478.

Bynke H, Olsson JE, Rosen I (1977): Diagnostic value of visual evoked response, clinical eye examination and CSF analysis in chronic myelopathy. *Acta Neurol Scand* 56:55–69.

Camisa J, Bodis-Wollner I, Mylin L (1980): Luminance-dependent pattern VEP delay in human demyelinating disease. *Soc Neurosci Abstr* 6:596.

Camisa J, Mylin LH, Bodis-Wollner I (1981): The effect of stimulus orientation on the visual evoked potential in multiple sclerosis. *Ann Neurol* 10:532–539.

Cant BR, Hume AL, Shaw NA (1978): Effects of luminance on the pattern visual evoked potential in multiple sclerosis. *Electroencephalogr Clin Neurophysiol* 45:496–504.

Cappin JM, Nissim S (1975): Visual evoked responses in the assessment of field defects in glaucoma. *Arch Ophthalmol* 93:9–18.

Carlow TJ, Rodriguez M (1978): Localization of cerebral dysfunction by visual evoked response. *Ann Neurol* 4:176.

Carlow TJ, Williams RH (1980): Localization of visual field defects with a steady state visual evoked potential (SS-VEP). *Neurology* 30:414.

Carroll WM, Mastaglia FL (1979): Leber's optic neuropathy: A clinical and visual evoked potential study of affected and asymptomatic members of a six generation family. *Brain* 102:559–580.

Carroll WM, Jay BS, McDonald WI, Halliday AM (1980a): Pattern evoked potentials in human albinism. Evidence of two different topographical asymmetries reflecting abnormal retino-cortical projections. *J Neurol Sci* 48:265–287.

Carroll WM, Kriss A, Baraitser M, Barrett G, Halliday AM (1980b): The incidence and nature of visual pathway involvement in Friedreich's ataxia. *Brain* 103:413–434.

Cascino GD, Ring SR, King PJL, Brown RH, Chiappa KH (1988): Evoked potentials in motor system diseases. *Neurology* 38:231–238.

Celesia GG, Daly RF (1977): Visual electroencephalographic computer analysis (VECA). *Neurology* 27:637–641.

Celesia CG, Archer CR, Kuroiwa Y, Goldfader PR (1980): Visual function of the extrageniculo-calcarine system in man. Relationship to cortical blindness. *Arch Neurol* 37:704–706.

Celesia GG, Polcyn RD, Holden JE, Nickles RJ, Gatley JS, Koeppe RA (1982): Visual evoked potentials and positron emission tomographic mapping of regional cerebral blood flow and cerebral metabolism: Can the neuronal potential generators be visualized? *Electroencephalogr Clin Neurophysiol* 54:243–256.

Celesia GG, Meredith JT, Pluff K (1983): Perimetry, visual evoked potentials and visual evoked spectrum array in homonymous hemianopsia. *Electroencephalogr Clin Neurophysiol* 56:16–30.

Celesia GC, Kaufman D, Cone S (1986): Simultaneous recording of pattern electroretinography and visual evoked potentials in multiple sclerosis. *Arch Neurol* 43:1247–1252.

Celesia GC, Kaufman D, Cone S (1987): Effects of age and sex on pattern electroretinograms and visual evoked potentials. *Electroencephalogr Clin Neurophysiol* 68:161–171.

Celesia GG, Bodis-Wollner I, Chatrian GE, Harding GFA, Sokol S, Spekreijse H (1993): Recommended standards for electroretinograms and visual evoked potentials. Report of an IFCN committee. *Electroencephalogr Clin Neurophysiol* 87:421–436.

Chain F, Lesevre N, Pinel JF, Leblanc M (1982): Spatio-temporal study of visual evoked potentials in patients with homonymous hemianopia. In: *Clinical Applications of Evoked Potentials in Neurology*, edited by J Courjon, F Mauguiere, and M Revol, pp 453–457. Raven Press, New York.

Chan Y-W, McLeod JG, Tuck RR, Walsh JC, Feary PA (1986): Visual evoked responses in chronic alcoholics. *J Neurol Neurosurg Psychiatry* 49:945–950.

Chiappa KH (1979): Evoked responses I: Pattern shift visual. In: *Weekly Update: Neurology and Neurosurgery* 2:64–70, edited by P Scheinberg. Continuing Professional Education Center, New Jersey.

Chiappa KH (1980): Pattern shift visual, brainstem auditory, and short-latency somatosensory evoked potentials in multiple sclerosis. *Neurology* 30:(7, part 2):110–123.

Chiappa KH (1982): Physiologic localization using evoked responses: Pattern shift visual, brainstem auditory and short latency somatosensory. In: *New Perspectives in Cerebral Localization*, edited by RA Thompson and JR Green, pp 63–114. Raven Press, New York.

Chiappa KH (1983a): Evoked potentials in clinical medicine. In: *Clinical Neurology*, edited by AB Baker and LH Baker, Chapter 7. JB Lippincott, Philadelphia.

Chiappa KH (1983b): *Evoked Potentials in Clinical Medicine*, 1st ed. Raven Press, New York.

Chiappa KH, Jenkins GM (1982): A new method of registration of partial field pattern-shift evoked potentials. *Electroencephalogr Clin Neurophysiol* 53:39P.

Chiappa KH, Gill EM, Lentz KE (1985): Effect of check size on P100 latency. *Electroencephalogr Clin Neurophysiol* 61:29P–30P.

Chokroverty S, Duvoisin RC, Sachdeo R, Sage J, Lepore F, Nicklas W (1985): Neurophysiologic study of olivopontocerebellar atrophy with or without glutamate dehydrogenase deficiency. *Neurology* 35:652–659.

Ciganek L (1961): The EEG response (evoked potential) to light stimulus in man. *Electroencephalogr Clin Neurophysiol* 13:165–172.

Clement RA, Flanagan JG, Harding GFA (1985): Source derivation of the visual evoked response to pattern reversal stimulation. *Electroencephalogr Clin Neurophysiol* 62:74–76.

Clifford-Jones RE, Landon DN, McDonald WI (1980): Remyelination during optic nerve compression. *J Neurol Sci* 46:239–243.

Cobb WA, Dawson GD (1960): The latency and form in man of the occipital potentials evoked by bright flashes. *J Physiol* (Lond) 152:108–121.

Coben LA, Daniziger WL, Hughes (1983): Visual evoked potentials in mild senile dementia of alzheimer type. *Electroencephalogr Clin Neurophysiol* 55:121–130.

Cohen SN, Syndulko K, Rever B, Kraut J, Coburn J, Tourtellotte WW (1983): Visual evoked potentials and long latency event-related potentials in chronic renal failure. *Neurology* 33:1219–1222.

Collins DWK, Black JL, Mastaglia FL (1978): Pattern reversal visual evoked potential. *J Neurol Sci* 36:83–95.

Collins DWK, Carroll WM, Black JL, Walsh M (1979): Effect of refractive error on the visual evoked response. *Br Med J* 1:231–232.

Conrad B, Benecke R, Musers H, Prange H, Behrens-Baumann W (1983): Visual evoked potentials in neurosyphilis. *J Neurol Neurosurg Psychiatry* 46:23–27.

Corletto F, Gentilomo A, Rosadini G, Rossi GF, Zattori J (1967): Visual evoked potentials as recorded from the scalp and from the visual cortex before and after surgical removal of the occipital pole in man. *Electroencephalogr Clin Neurophysiol* 22:378–380.

Coupland SG, Kirkham TH (1982): Orientation-specific visual evoked potential deficits in multiple sclerosis. *Can J Neurol Sci* 9:331–337.

Cowey A, Rolls ET (1974): Human cortical magnification factor and its relation to visual acuity. *Brain Res* 21:447–454.

Cox TA, Thompson HS, Hayreh SS, Snyder JE (1982): Visual evoked potential and pupillary signs. *Arch Ophthalmol* 100:1603–1607.

Cracco RQ, Cracco JB (1978): Visual evoked potential in man: Early oscillatory potentials. *Electroencephalogr Clin Neurophysiol* 45:731–739.

Creel D (1979): Luminance-onset, pattern-onset and pattern-reversal evoked potentials in human albinos demonstrating visual system anomalies. *J Biomed Eng* 1:100–104.

Creel D, Buehler BA (1982): Pattern evoked potentials in phenylketonuria. *Electroencephalogr Clin Neurophysiol* 53:220–223.

Creel D, Spekreijse H, Reits D (1981): Evoked potentials in albinos: Efficacy of pattern stimuli in detecting misrouted optic fibers. *Electroencephalogr Clin Neurophysiol* 52:595–603.

Creel D, Collier LL, Leventhal AG, Conlee JW, Prieur DJ (1982): Abnormal retinal projections in cats with Chediak-Higashi syndrome. *Ophthalmol Vis Sci* 23:798–801.

Creel D, Boxer LA, Fauci AS (1983): Visual and auditory anomalies in Chediak-Higashi syndrome. *Electroencephalogr Clin Neurophysiol* 55:252–257.

Creutzfeldt OD, Kuhnt U (1973): Electrophysiological and topographical distribution of visual evoked potentials in animals. In: *Handbook of Sensory Physiology,* edited by R Jung, 7/3B, pp 595–646. Springer-Verlag, Berlin.

Cutler JR, Aminoff MJ, Brant-Zawadzki M (1986a): Comparative value of MRI and evoked potential studies in multiple sclerosis. *Neurology* 136:156.

Cutler JR, Aminoff MJ, Brant-Zawadzki M (1986b): Evaluation of patients with multiple sclerosis by evoked potentials and magnetic resonance imaging: A comparative study. *Ann Neurol* 20:645–648.

Davies HD, Carroll WM, Mastaglia FL (1986): Effects of hyperventilation on pattern-reversal visual evoked potentials in patients with demyelination. *J Neurol Neurosurg Psychiatry* 49:1392–1396.

Dawson WW, Maida TM, Rubin ML (1982). Human pattern-evoked retinal responses are altered by optic atrophy. *Invest Ophthalmol Vis Sci* 22:796–803.

Dekaben AS, Sadowsky D (1978): Changes in brain weights during the span of human life: Relation of brain weights to body heights and body weights. *Ann Neurol* 4:345–356.

DeValois KK, DeValois RL, Yund EW (1979): Responses of striate cortex cells to grating and checkerboard patterns. *J Physiol* 291:483–505.

Diener HC, Scheibler H (1980): Follow-up studies of visual potentials in multiple sclerosis evoked by checkerboard and foveal stimulation. *Electroencephalogr Clin Neurophysiol* 49:490–496.

Diener HC, Koch W, Dichgans J (1982): The significance of luminance on visual evoked potentials in diagnosis of MS. *Arch Psychiatr Nervenkr* 231:149–154.

Dinner DS, Luders H, Hanson M, Lesser RP, Klem G (1985): Pattern evoked potentials (PEPs) in Parkinson's disease. *Neurology* 35:610–613.

Dobson V, Teller DY (1978): Visual acuity in human infants: A review and comparison of behavioral and electrophysiological studies. *Vision Res* 18:1469–1483.

Doggett C, Harding GFA, Orwin A (1981): Flash and pattern evoked potentials in patients with presenile dementia. *Electroencephalogr Clin Neurophysiol* 52:100P.

Douthwaite WS, Jenkins TCA (1982): Visually evoked responses to checkerboard patterns: Check and field size interactions. *Am J Optometry Physiological Optics* Vol 59, No 11:894–901.

Drayer BP, Barrett L (1984): Magnetic resonance imaging and CT scanning in multiple sclerosis. *Ann NY Acad Sci* 436:294–314.

Ducati A, Fava E, Motti EDF (1988): Neuronal generators of the visual evoked potentials: Intracerebral recording in awake humans. *Electroencephalogr Clin Neurophysiol* 71:89–99.

Duchowny MS, Weiss IP, Majlessi H, Barnet AB (1974): Visual evoked responses in childhood cortical blindness after head trauma and meningitis. A longitudinal study of six cases. *Neurology* 24:933–940.

Duwaer AL, Spekreijse H (1978): Latency of luminance and contrast evoked potentials in multiple sclerosis patients. *Electroencephalogr Clin Neurophysiol* 45:244–258.

Eggermont JJ (1988): On the rate of maturation of sensory evoked potentials. *Electroencephalogr Clin Neurophysiol* 70:293–305.

Ehle AL, Stewart RM, Lellelid NE, Leventhal NA (1982): Normal checkerboard pattern reversal evoked potentials in Parkinsonism. *Electroencephalogr Clin Neurophysiol* 54:336–338.

Ehle AL, Stewart RM, Lellelid NE, Leventhal NA (1984): Evoked potentials in Huntington's Disease. *Arch Neurol* 41:379–382.

Eidelberg D, Newton MR, Johnson G, MacManus DG, McDonald WI, Miller DH, Halliday AM, Moseley IF, Heng GS, Wright J (1988): Chronic unilateral optic neuropathy: A magnetic resonance study. *Ann Neurol* 24:3–11.

Emmerson-Hanover R, Shearer DE, Creel DJ, Dustman RE (1994): Pattern reversal evoked potentials: gender differences and age-related changes in amplitude and latency. *Electroencephalogr Clin Neurophysiol* 92(2):93–101.

Erwin CW (1981): Pattern reversal evoked potentials. *Am J EEG Technol* 20:161–165.

Farlow MR, Markland ON, Edwards MK, Stevens JC, Kolar OK (1986): Multiple Sclerosis: Magnetic resonance imaging, evoked responses, and spinal fluid electrophoresis. *Neurology* 36:828–831.

Faught E, Lee SI (1984): Pattern-reversal visual evoked potentials in photosensitive epilepsy. *Electroencephalogr Clin Neurophysiol* 59:125–133.

Fenwick PBC, Robertson R (1983): Changes in the visual evoked potential to pattern reversal with lithium medication. *Electroencephalogr Clin Neurophysiol* 55:538–545.

Fenwick PBC, Turner C (1977): Relationship between amplitude of pattern displacement and visual evoked potentials. *Electroencephalogr Clin Neurophysiol* 43:74–78.

Fenwick PBC, Brown D, Hennessey J (1981): The visual evoked response to pattern reversal in "normal" 6–11-year-old children. *Electroencephalogr Clin Neurophysiol* 51:49–62.

Fenwick PB, Stone SA, Bushman J, Enderby D (1984): Changes in the pattern reversal visual evoked potential as a function of inspired nitrous oxide concentration. *Electroencephalogr Clin Neurophysiol* 57:178–183.

Fine EJ, Hallett M (1980): Neurophysiological study of subacute combined degeneration. *J Neurol Sci* 45:331–336.

Fledelius HC, Petrera JE, Skjodt K, Trojaborg W (1987): A case report with electrophysiological considerations and a review of Danish cases 1972–1981. *Acta Ophthalmol* 65:251–255.

Fox PT, Raichle ME (1985): Stimulus rate determines regional brain blood flow in striate cortex. *Ann Neurol* 17:303–305.

Frank Y, Torres F (1978): Visual evoked potentials in the evaluation of "cortical blindness" in children. *Ann Neurol* 6:126–129.

Frederiksen JL, Larsson HBW, Olesen J, Stigsby B (1991): MRI, VEP, SEP and biothesiometry suggest monosymptomatic acute optic neuritis to be a first manifestation of multiple sclerosis. *Acta Neurol Scand* 83:343–350.

Froehlich J, Kaufman DI (1992): Improving the reliability of pattern electroretinogram recording. *Electroencephalogr Clin Neurophysiol* 84(4):394–399.

Froehilch J, Kaufman DI (1993): The pattern electroretinogram: N95 amplitudes in normal subjects and optic neuritis patients. *Electroencephalogr Clin Neurophysiol* 88(2):83–91.

Froehlich J, Kaufman DI (1994): Use of pattern electroretinography to differentiate acute optic neuritis from acute anterior ischemic optic neuropathy. *Electroencephalogr Clin Neurophysiol* 92(6):480–486.

Galloway NR, Tolia J, Barber C (1986): The pattern evoked response in disorders of the optic nerve. *Documenta Ophthalmol* 63:31–36.

Gangitano JL, Keltner JL (1980): Abnormalities of the pupil and visual-evoked potential in quinine amblyopia. *Am J Ophthalmol* 89:425–430.

Gawel MJ, Kennard C, de M Rudolf N, Clifford Rose F (1980): Pattern reversal VEPs in migraine. In: *Electroencephalography and Clinical Neurophysiology*, edited by H Lechner and A Aranibar, p 75. Excerpta Medica, Amsterdam.

Gawel MJ, Das P, Vincent S, Rose FC (1981): Visual and auditory evoked responses in patients with Parkinson's disease. *J Neurol Neurosurg Psychiatry* 44:227–232.

Gebarski SS, Gabrielsen TO, Gilman S, Knake JE, Latack JT, Aisen AM (1985): The initial diagnosis of multiple sclerosis: Clinical impact of magnetic resonance imaging. *Ann Neurol* 17:469–474.

Geisser BS, Kurtzberg D, Arezzo JC, Vaughan HG, Aisen ML, Smith CR, Scheinberg LC (1986): Trimodal evoked potentials compared with magnetic resonance imaging in the diagnosis of multiple sclerosis. *Neurology* 36:158.

Ghezzi A, Montanini R (1985): Comparative study of visual evoked potentials in spinocerebellar ataxia and multiple sclerosis. *Acta Neurol Scand* 71:252–256.

Ghilardi MF, Sartucci F, Brannan JR, Onofrj MC, Bodis-Wollner I, Mylin L, Stroch R (1991): N70 and P100 can be independently affected in multiple sclerosis. *Electroencephalogr Clin Neurophysiol* 80:1–7.

Giesser BS, Kurtzberg D, Vaughan HG, Arezzo JC, Aisen ML, Smith CR, LaRocca NG, Scheinberg LC (1987): Trimodal evoked potentials compared with magnetic resonance imaging in the diagnosis of multiple sclerosis. *Arch Neurol* 44:281–284.

Gilmore RL, Kasarskis EJ, McAllister RG (1985): Verapamil-induced changes in central conduction in patients with multiple sclerosis. *J Neurol Neurosurg Psychiatry* 48:1140–1146.

Gittinger JW, Sokol S (1982): The visual-evoked potential in the diagnosis of congenital ocular motor apraxia. *Am J Ophthalmol* 93:700–703.

Gonzalez-Scarano F, Grossman RI, Galetta SL, Atlas S, Silberberg DH (1986): Enhanced magnetic images in multiple sclerosis. *Neurology* 36:285.

Goodwin AW, Henry GH (1978): The influence of stimulus velocity on the responses of single neurones in the striate cortex. *J Physiol* 277:467–482.

Gott PS, Weiss MH, Apuzzo M, Van Der Meulen JP (1979): Checkerboard visual evoked response in evaluation and management of pituitary tumors. *Neurosurg* 5:553–558.

Gott PS, Karnaze DS, Keane JR (1983): Abnormal visual evoked potentials in myotonic dystrophy. *Neurology* 33:1622–1625.

Gottlob I, Schneider E, Heider W, Skrandies W (1987): Alteration of visual evoked potentials and electroretinograms in Parkinson's disease. *Electroencephalogr Clin Neurophysiol* 66:349–357.

Green JB, Price R, Woodbury SG (1980): Short-latency somatosensory evoked potentials in multiple sclerosis. Comparison with auditory and visual evoked potentials. *Arch Neurol* 37:630–633.

Groswasser Z, Kriss A, Halliday AM, McDonald WI (1985): Pattern- and flash-evoked potentials in the assessment and management of optic nerve gliomas. *J Neurol Neurosurg Psychiatry* 48:1125–1134.

Guerit JM, Argiles AM (1988): The sensitivity of multimodal evoked potentials in multiple sclerosis. A comparison with magnetic resonance imaging and cerebrospinal fluid analysis. *Electroencephalogr Clin Neurophysiol* 70:230–238.

Gupta NK, Verma NP, Guidice MA, Kooi KA (1986): Visual evoked response in head trauma: Pattern-shift stimulus. *Neurology* 36:578–581.

Guthkelch AN, Bursick D, Sclabassi RJ (1987): The relationship of the latency of the visual P100 to gender and head size. *Electroencephalogr Clin Neurophysiol* 68:219–222.

Gutin PH, Klemme WM, Lagger RL, MacKay AR, Pitts LH, Hosobuchi Y (1980): Management of the unresectable cystic craniopharyngioma by aspiration through an Ommaya reservoir drainage system. *J Neurosurg* 52:36–40.

Haimovic IC, Pedley TA (1982a): Hemi-field pattern reversal visual evoked potentials. I. Normal subjects. *Electroencephalogr Clin Neurophysiol* 54:111–120.

Haimovic IC, Pedley TA (1982b): Hemi-field pattern reversal visual evoked potentials. II. Lesions of the chiasm and posterior visual pathways. *Electroencephalogr Clin Neurophysiol* 54:121–131.

Halliday AM (1981): Visual evoked potentials in demyelinating disease. In: *Demyelinating Disease: Basic and Clinical Electrophysiology,* edited by SG Waxman and JM Ritchie, pp 201–215. Raven Press, New York.

Halliday AM (1982): The visual evoked potential in the investigation of diseases of the optic nerve. In: *Evoked Potentials in Clinical Testing,* edited by AM Halliday, pp 187–234. Churchill Livingstone, London.

Halliday AM (1985): The value of half-field stimulation in clinical visual evoked potential testing. In: *Evoked Potentials. Neurophysiological and Clinical Aspects,* edited by C Morocutti and PA Rizzo, pp 293–313. Elsevier Science Publishers B.V. (Biomedical Division), New York.

Halliday AM, McDonald WI (1981): Visual evoked potentials. In: *Neurology I: Clinical Neurophysiology,* edited by E Stalberg and RR Young, pp 228–258. Butterworths, London.

Halliday AM, Mushin J (1980): The visual evoked potential in neuroophthalmology. *Int Ophthalmol Clin* 20:155–183.

Halliday AM, McDonald WI, Mushin J (1972): Delayed visual evoked responses in optic neuritis. *Lancet* 1:982–985.

Halliday AM, McDonald WI, Mushin J (1973a): Delayed pattern evoked responses in optic neuritis in relation to visual acuity. *Trans Ophthalmol Soc UK* 93:315–324.

Halliday AM, McDonald WI, Mushin J (1973b): Visual evoked responses in the diagnosis of multiple sclerosis. *Br Med J* 4:661–664.

Halliday AM, Halliday E, Kriss A, McDonald WI, Mushin J (1976): The pattern-evoked potential in compression of the anterior visual pathways. *Brain* 99:357–374.

Halliday AM, Barrett G, Blumhardt LD, Kriss A (1979a): The macular and paramacular subcomponents of the pattern evoked response. In: *Human Evoked Potentials: Applications and Problems,* edited by D Lehmann and E Callaway, pp 135–151. Plenum Press, London.

Halliday AM, Barrett G, Halliday E, Mushin J (1979b): A comparison of the flash and pattern-evoked potential in unilateral optic neuritis. *Wiss Zeit Ernst-Mortiz-Arndt-Universitat,* 28:89–95.

Halliday AM, Barrett G, Carroll WM, Kriss A (1982): Problems in defining the normal limits of the visual evoked potential. In: *Clinical Applications of Evoked Potentials in Neurology,* edited by J Courjon, F Mauguiere, and M Revol, pp 1–9. Raven Press, New York.

Hammond EJ, Wilder BJ (1983): Evoked potentials in olivopontocerebellar atrophy. *Arch Neurol* 40:366–369.

Hammond EJ, Wilder BJ (1985): Effect of gamma-vinyl GABA on human pattern evoked visual potentials. *Neurology* 35:1801–1803.

Hammond SR, Yiannikas C (1986): Contribution of pattern reversal foveal and half-field stimulation to analysis of VEP abnormalities in multiple sclerosis. *Electroencephalogr Clin Neurophysiol* 64:101–118.

Hammond SR, MacCallum S, Yiannikas C, Walsh JC, McLeod JG (1987): Variability on serial testing of pattern reversal visual evoked potential latencies from full-field, half-field and foveal stimulation in control subjects. *Electroencephalogr Clin Neurophysiol* 66:401–408.

Harding GFA (1985): Flash evoked cortical and subcortical potentials in neuroophthalmology. *Acta Neurol Belg* 85:150–165.

Harding GFA, Crews SJ (1982): The VER in hereditary optic atrophy. In: *Clinical Applications of Evoked Potentials in Neurology*, edited by J Courjon, F Mauguiere, and M Revol, pp 21–30. Raven Press, New York.

Harding GFA, Rubinstein MP (1980): The scalp topography of the human visually evoked subcortical potential. *Invest Ophthalmol Vis Sci* 19:318–321.

Harding GFA, Rubinstein MP (1982): The visually evoked subcortical potential to flash stimulation in normal subjects and patients with lesions of the visual pathway. In: *Clinical Applications of Evoked Potentials in Neurology*, edited by J Courjon, F Mauguiere, and M Revol, pp 31–39. Raven Press, New York.

Harding GFA, Crews SJ, Good PA (1980a): VEP in neuro- ophthalmic disease. In: *Evoked Potentials*, edited by C Barber, pp 235–241. University Park Press, Baltimore.

Harding GFA, Smith GF, Smith PA (1980b): The effect of various stimulus parameters on the lateralization of the VEP. In: *Evoked Potentials*, edited by C Barber, pp 213–218. University Park Press, Baltimore.

Harding GFA, Boylan C, Clement RA (1986): Visual evoked cortical and subcortical potentials in human albinos. *Doc Ophthalmol* 62:81–88.

Harter MR, White CT (1968): Effects of contour sharpness and check size on visually evoked cortical potentials. *Vision Res* 8:701–711.

Harter MR, White CT (1970): Evoked cortical responses to checkerboard patterns: Effect of check-size as a function of visual acuity. *Electroencephalogr Clin Neurophysiol* 28:48–54.

Hawkes CH, Stow B (1981): Pupil size and the pattern evoked response. *J Neurol Neurosurg Psychiatry* 44:90–91.

Hely MA, McManis PG, Walsh JC, McLeod JG (1986): Visual evoked responses and ophthalmological examination in optic neuritis. *J Neurol Sciences* 75:275–283.

Hennerici M (1985): Dissociated foveal and parafoveal visual evoked responses in subacute combined degeneration. *Arch Neurol* 42:130–132.

Hennerici M, Wist ER (1982): A modification of the visual evoked response method involving small luminance decrements for the diagnosis of demyelinating disease. In: *Clinical Applications of Evoked Potentials in Neurology*, edited by J Courjon, F Mauguiere, and M Revol, pp 433–441. Raven Press, New York.

Hennerici M, Wenzel D, Freund H-J (1977): The comparison of small-size rectangle and checkerboard stimulation for the evaluation of delayed visual evoked responses in patients suspected of multiple sclerosis. *Brain* 100:119–136.

Hennerici M, Homberg V, Lange HW (1984): Evoked potentials in patients with Huntington's disease and other offspring. II. Visual evoked potentials. *Electroencephalogr Clin Neurol* 62:167–176.

Hess CW, Meienberg O, Ludin HP (1982): Visual evoked potentials in acute occipital blindness. *J Neurol* 227:193–200.

Hess RF, Baker CL, Verhoeve JN, Keesey UT, Frances TD (1985). The pattern evoked electroretinograms: Its variability in normals and its relationship to amblyopia. *Invest Ophthalmol Vis Sci* 26:1610–1623.

Hod Y, Pratt H, Schacham SE (1986): Comparison of fiber optical and video monitor stimulators in normals and multiple sclerosis. *Electroencephalogr Clin Neurophysiol* 64:411–416.

Hoeppner T, Lolas F (1978): Visual evoked responses and visual symptoms in multiple sclerosis. *J Neurol Neurosurg Psychiatry* 41:493–498.

Hoeppner T, Bergen D, Morrell F (1980): Visual evoked potentials after partial occipital lobectomy. *Electroencephalogr Clin Neurophysiol* 50:184P.

Holder GE (1987): Significance of abnormal pattern electroretinography in anterior visual pathway dysfunction. *Br J Ophthalmol* 71:166–171.

Holder GE (1985): Pattern visual evoked potential in patients with posteriorly situated space-occupying lesions. *Documenta Ophthalmologica* 59:121–128.

Hornabrook RS, Miller DH, Newton MR, McManus DG, du Boulay GH (1992): Frequent involvement of the optic radiation in patients with acute isolated optic neuritis. *Neurology* 42:77–79.

Howard JE, Dorfman LJ (1986): Evoked potentials in hysteria and malingering. *J Clin Neurophysiol* 3(1):39–49.

Hubel DH, Wiesel TN (1965): Receptive fields and functional architecture in two nonstriate visual areas (18 and 19) of the cat. *J Neurophysiol* 28:229–289.

Hubel DH, Wiesel TN (1977): Functional architecture of macaque monkey visual cortex. *Proc R Soc Lond (B)* 198:1–59.

Huber C, Wagner T (1978): Electrophysiological evidence for glaucomatous lesions in the optic nerve. *Ophthalmol Res* 10:22–29.

Hume AI, Cant BR (1976): Pattern visual evoked potentials in the diagnosis of multiple sclerosis and other disorders. *Proc Austr Assoc Neurol* 13:7–13.

Ikeda H, Tremain KE, Sanders MD (1978): Neurophysiological investigation in optic nerve disease: Combined assessment of the visual evoked response and electroretinogram. *Br J Ophthalmol* 62:227–239.

Jabbari B, Maitland CG, Morris LM, Morales J, Gunderson CH (1985): The value of visual evoked potential as a screening test in neurofibromatosis. *Arch Neurol* 42:1072–1074.

Jacobson SG, Eames RA, McDonald WI (1979): Optic nerve fiber lesions in adult cats: Pattern of recovery of spatial vision. *Exp Brain Res* 36:491–508.

Jeffreys DA (1971): Cortical source locations of pattern-related visual evoked potentials recorded from the human scalp. *Nature* 229:502–504.

Jeffreys DA (1977): The physiological significance of pattern visual evoked potentials. In: *Visual Evoked Potentials in Man: New Developments,* edited by JE Desmedt, pp 134–167. Clarendon Press, Oxford.

Jones DC, Blume WT (1985): Aberrant wave forms to pattern reversal stimulation: Clinical significance and electrographic "solutions." *Electroencephalogr Clin Neurophysiol* 61:472–481.

Josiassen RC, Shagass C, Mancall EL, Roemer RA (1984): Auditory and visual evoked potentials in Huntington's Disease. *Electroencephalogr Clin Neurophysiol* 57:113–118.

Kandel ER, Schwartz JH, Editors (1985): *Principles of Neural Science,* 2nd edition. Elsevier, Amsterdam.

Kaplan PW, Rawal K, Erwin CW, D'Souza BJ, Spock A (1988): Visual and somatosensory evoked potentials in vitamin E deficiency with cystic fibrosis. *Electroencephalogr Clin Neurophysiol* 71:266–272.

Kaplan PW, Tusa RJ, Shankroff J, Heller J, Moser HW (1993): Visual evoked potentials in adrenoleukodystrophy: A trial with glycerol trioleate and Lorenzo oil. *Ann Neurol* 34:169–174.

Kaufman D, Celesia GG (1985): Simultaneous recording of pattern electroretinogram and visual evoked responses in neuro-ophthalmologic disorders. *Neurology* 35:644–651.

Kaufman DI, Wray SH, Lorance R, Woods M (1986): An analysis of the pathophysiology and the development of treatment strategies for compressive optic nerve lesions using pattern electroretinogram and visual evoked potential. *Neurology* 36(suppl 1):232.

Kaufman DI, Lorance RW, Woods M, Wray SH (1988): The pattern electroretinogram: A long-term study in acute optic neuropathy. *Neurology* 38:1767–1774.

Kazis A, Vlaikidis N, Xafenias D, Papanastasiou J, Pappa P (1982): Fever and evoked potentials in multiple sclerosis. *J Neurol* 227:1–10.

Kempster PA, Iansek R, Balla JI, Dennis PM, Biegler B (1987): Value of visual response and oligoclonal bands in cerebrospinal fluid in diagnosis of spinal multiple sclerosis. *Lancet* 769–771.

Khoshbin S, Hallet M (1981): Multimodality evoked potentials and blink reflex in multiple sclerosis. *Neurology* 31:138–144.

Kirkham TH, Coupland SG (1981): Abnormal electroretinograms and visual evoked potentials in chronic papilledema using time-difference analysis. *Canad J Neurol Sci* 8:243–248.

Kirkham TH, Coupland SG (1983): Pattern ERGs and check size: Absence of spatial frequency tuning. *Current Eye Res* 2:511–521.

Kirshner HS, Tsai SI, Runge VM, Price AC (1985): Magnetic resonance imaging and other techniques in the diagnosis of multiple sclerosis. *Arch Neurol* 42:859–863.

Kjaer M (1980): Visual evoked potentials in normal subjects and patients with multiple sclerosis. *Acta Neurol Scand* 62:1–13.

Kline LB, Glaser JS (1982): Visual evoked response in transient monocular visual loss. *Br J Ophthalmol* 66:382–385.

Klemm WR, Goodson RA, Allen RG (1983): Contrast effects of the three primary colors on human visual evoked potentials. *Electroencephalogr Clin Neurophysiol* 55:557–566.

Kooi KA, Sharbrough FW (1966): Electrophysiological findings in cortical blindness. Report of a case. *Electroencephalogr Clin Neurophysiol* 20:260–263.

Kooi KA, Guvener AM, Bagchi BK (1965): Visual evoked responses in lesions of the higher optic pathways. *Neurology* 15:841–854.

Korth M (1983): Pattern-evoked responses and luminance-evoked responses in the human electroretinogram. *J Physiol* 337:451–469.

Kriss A, Halliday AM (1980): A comparison of occipital potentials evoked by pattern onset, offset and reversal by movement. In: *Evoked Potentials,* edited by C Barber, pp 205–212. MTP Press, Lancaster.

Kriss A, Carroll WM, Blumhardt LD, Halliday AM (1982): Pattern- and flash-evoked potential changes in toxic (nutritional) optic neuropathy. In: *Clinical Applications of Evoked Potentials in Neurology,* edited by J Courjon, F Mauguiere, and M Revol, pp 11–19. Raven Press, New York.

Krumholz A, Weiss HD, Goldstein PJ, Harris KC (1981): Evoked responses in Vitamin B-12 deficiency. *Ann Neurol* 9:407–409.

Kuba M, Peregrin J, Vit F, Hanusova I (1982): Visual evoked responses to reversal stimulation in the upper and lower half of the central part of the visual field in man. *Physiologia Bohemoslova* 31:503–510.

Kupersmith MJ, Siegel IM, Carr RE, Ransohoff J, Flamm E, Shakin E (1981): Visual evoked potentials in chiasmal gliomas in four adults. *Arch Neurol* 38:362–365.

Kupersmith MJ, Shakin E, Siegel IM, Lieberman A (1982): Visual system abnormalities in patients with Parkinson's Disease. *Arch Neurol* 39:284–286.

Kupersmith MJ, Nelson JI, Seiple WH, Carr RE, Weiss PA (1983): The 20/20 eye in multiple sclerosis. *Neurology* 33:1015–1020.

Kurita-Tashima S, Tobimatsu S, Nakayama-Hiromatsu M, Kato M (1991): Effect of check size on the pattern reversal visual evoked potential. *Electroencephalogr Clin Neurophysiol* 80(3):161–166.

Kuroiwa Y, Celesia G (1981): Visual evoked potentials with hemifield pattern stimulation. Their use in the diagnosis of retrochiasmatic lesions. *Arch Neurol* 38:86–90.

Kuroiwa Y, Celesia GC, Tohgi H (1987): Amplitude difference between pattern-evoked potentials after left and right hemifield stimulation in normal subjects. *Neurology* 37:795–799.

Ladenson PW, Stakes JW, Ridgway EC (1984): Reversible alteration of the visual evoked potential in hypothyroidism. *Am J Med* 77:1010–1013.

La Marche JA, Dobson WR, Cohn NB, Dustman RE (1986): Amplitudes of visually evoked potentials to patterned stimuli: Age and sex comparisons. *Electroencephalogr Clin Neurophysiol* 65:81–85.

Lavine R, Morgan S, Parker J, Architowska M, Racy A (1980): A method for recording visual evoked responses to partial field pattern-reversal while monitoring visual fixation in patients with cerebral dysfunction. *Electroencephalogr Clin Neurophysiol* 49:27P.

Lehmann D, Skrandies W (1979): Multichannel evoked potential fields show different properties of human upper and lower hemiretina systems. *Exp Brain Res* 35:151–159.

Lennie P (1980): Parallel visual pathways: A review. *Vision Res* 20:561–594.

Lentz KE, Chiappa KH (1985): Non-pathologic (voluntary) alteration of pattern-shift visual evoked potentials. *Electroencephalogr Clin Neurophysiol* 61:30P.

Lesevre N, Joseph JP (1979): Modifications of the pattern-evoked potential (PEP) in relation to the stimulated part of the visual field. *Electroencephalogr Clin Neurophysiol* 47:183–203.

Lesser RP, Luders HL, Klem G, Dinner DS (1985): Visual potentials evoked by light-emitting diodes mounted in goggles. *Cleveland Clin Q.* 52, No 2:223–228.

Lieb JP, Karmel BZ (1974): The processing of edge information in visual areas of the cortex as evidenced by evoked potentials. *Brain Res* 76:503–519.

Livingstone IR, Mastaglia FL, Edis R, Howe JW (1981a): Pattern visual evoked responses in hereditary spastic paraplegia. *J Neurol Neurosurg Psychiatry* 44:176–178.

Livingstone IR, Mastaglia FL, Edis R, Howe JW (1981b): Visual involvement in Friedreich's ataxia and hereditary spastic ataxia: A clinical and visual evoked response study. *Arch Neurol* 38:75–79.

Lowitzsch K, Westhoff M (1980): Optic nerve involvement in neurosyphilis: Diagnostic evaluation by pattern-reversal visual evoked potentials (VEP). *EEG EMG* 11:77–80.

Lowitzsch K, Kuhnt U, Sakmann CH, Maurer K, Hopf HC, Schott D, Thater K (1976): Visual pattern evoked responses and blink reflexes in assessment of MS diagnosis. *J Neurol* 213:17–32.

Lowitzsch K, Rudolph HD, Trincker D, Muller E (1980): Flash and pattern-reversal visual evoked responses in retrobulbar neuritis and controls: A comparison of conventional and TV stimulation techniques. In: *Electroencephalography and Clinical Neurophysiology*, edited by H Lechner and A Aranibar, pp 451–463. Excerpta Medica, Amsterdam.

Lowitzsch K, Gohring U, Hecking E, Kohler H (1981): Refractory period, sensory conduction velocity and visual evoked potentials before and after haemodialysis. *J Neurol Neurosurg Psychiatry* 44:121–128.

Ludlam WM, Meyers RR (1972): The use of visual evoked responses in objective refraction. *Trans NY Acad Sci* 34:154–170.

Lumsden CE (1970): The neuropathology of multiple sclerosis. In: *Handbook of Clinical Neurophysiology* 9:175–234.

Mackay DM, Jeffreys DA (1973): Visually evoked potentials and visual perception in man. In: *Handbook of Sensory Physiology, Vol VII/3, Part B*, edited by R Jung, pp 647–678. Springer, New York, Berlin, Heidelberg.

Maffei L, Fiorentini A (1981): Electroretinographic responses to alternate gratings before and after section of the optic nerve. *Science* 211:953–955.

Maiese K, Walker RW, Gargan R, Victor JD (1992). Intra-arterial cisplatin-associated optic and otic toxicity. *Arch Neurol* 49:83–86. 1992.

Maitland CG, Aminoff MJ, Kennard C, Hoyt WF (1982): Evoked potentials in the evaluation of visual field defects due to chiasmal or retrochiasmal lesions. *Neurology* 32:986–991.

Majnemer A, Rosenblatt B, Watters G, Andermann F (1986): Giant axonal neuropathy: Central abnormalities demonstrated by evoked potentials. *Ann Neurol* 19:394–396.

Mamoli B, Graf M, Toifl K (1979): EEG, pattern-evoked potentials and nerve conduction velocity in a family with adrenoleudodystrophy. *Electroencephalogr Clin Neurophysiol* 47:411–419.

Maravilla KR, Weinreb JC, Suss R, Nunnally RL (1985): Magnetic resonance demonstration of multiple sclerosis plaques in the cervical cord. *Am J Rad* 144:381–385.

Marg E, Freeman DN, Peltzman P, Goldstein PJ (1976): Visual acuity development in human infants: Evoked potential measurements. *Invest Ophthalmol* 15:150–153.

Markand ON, Garg BP, DeMyer WE, Warren C (1982): Brain stem auditory, visual and somatosensory evoked potentials in leukodystrophies. *Electroencephalogr Clin Neurophysiol* 54:39–48.

Marsh MS, Smith S (1994): Differences in the pattern visual evoked potential between pregnant and non-pregnant women. *Electroencephalogr Clin Neurophysiol* 92(2):102–106.

Martinelli V, Comi G, Filippi M, Poggi A, Colombo B, Rodegher M, Scotti G, Triulzi F, Canal N (1991): Paraclinical tests in acute-onset optic neuritis: basal data and results of a short follow-up. *Acta Neurol Scand* 84:231–236.

Mashima Y, Oguchi Y (1985): Clinical study of the pattern electroretinogram in patients with optic nerve damage. *Doc Ophthalmol* 61:91–96.

Mastaglia FL, Black JL, Collins DWK (1976a): Evoked potential studies in neurological disorders. *Proc Austr Assoc Neurol* 13:15–23.

Mastaglia FL, Black JL, Collins DWK (1976b): Visual and spinal evoked potentials in the diagnosis of multiple sclerosis. *Br Med J* 2:732.

Matheson JK, Harrington HJ, Hallett M (1986): Abnormalities of multimodality evoked potentials in amyotrophic lateral sclerosis. *Arch Neurol* 43:338–340.

Matthews WB, Small DG (1979): Serial recording of visual and somatosensory evoked potentials in multiple sclerosis. *J Neurol Sci* 40:11–21.

Matthews WB, Small DG (1983): Prolonged follow-up of abnormal visual evoked potentials in multiple sclerosis: Evidence for delayed recovery. *J Neurol Neurosurg Psychiatry* 46:639–642.

Matthews WB, Small DG, Small M, Pountney E (1977): Pattern reversal evoked visual potential in the diagnosis of multiple sclerosis. *J Neurol Neurosurg Psychiatry* 40:1009–1014.

Matthews WB, Read DJ, Pountney E (1979): Effect of raising body temperature on visual and somatosensory evoked potentials in patients with multiple sclerosis. *J Neurol Neurosurg Psychiatry* 42:250–255.

Matthews WB, Wattam-Bell JRB, Pountney E (1982): Evoked potentials in the diagnosis of multiple sclerosis: A follow up study. *J Neurol Neurosurg Psychiatry* 45:303–307.

McAlpine D, Lumsden CE, Acheson ED, Editors (1972): *Multiple Sclerosis: A Reappraisal.* Churchill Livingstone, Edinburgh.

McDonald WI (1977): Pathophysiology of conduction in central nerve fibers. In: *Visual Evoked Potentials in Man: New Developments,* edited by JE Desmedt, pp 427–437. Clarendon Press, Oxford.

McInnes A (1977): The visual evoked responses to a red and white checkerboard pattern in patients with suspected multiple sclerosis. *Electroencephalogr Clin Neurophysiol* 43:286.

McLeod JG, Low PA, Morgan JA (1978): Charcot-Marie-Tooth disease with Leber optic atrophy. *Neurology* 28:179–184.

Meienberg O, Kutak L, Smolenski C, Ludin HP (1979): Pattern reversal evoked cortical responses in normals. *J Neurol* 222:81–93.

Meienberg O, Flammer J, Ludin HP (1982): Subclinical visual field defects in multiple sclerosis. *J Neurol* 227:125–133.

Meredith JT, Celesia GG (1982): Pattern-reversal visual evoked potentials and retinal eccentricity. *Electroencephalogr Clin Neurophysiol* 53:243–253.

Messenheimer JA, Greenwood RS, Tennison MB, Brickley JJ, Ball CJ (1984): Reversible visual evoked potential abnormalities in Vitamin E deficiency. *Ann Neurol* 15:499–501.

Michael WF, Halliday AM (1971): Differences between the occipital distribution of upper and lower field pattern-evoked responses in man. *Brain Res* 32:311–324.

Miller DH, Johnson G, McDonald WI, MacManus D, du Boulay EPGH, Kendall BE, Moseley IF (1986): Detection of optic nerve lesions in optic neuritis with magnetic resonance imaging. *Lancet* 1490–1491.

Miller DH, Newton MR, van der Poel JC, du Boulay EPGH, Halliday AM, Kendall BE, Johnson G, MacManus DG, Moseley IF, McDonald WI (1988): Magnetic resonance imaging of the optic nerve in optic neuritis. 38:175–179.

Millodot M (1977): The use of visual evoked potentials in optometry. In: *Visual Evoked Potentials in Man: New Developments,* edited by JE Desmedt, pp 401–409. Clarendon Press, Oxford.

Millodot M, Newton I (1981): VEP measurement of the amplitude of accommodation. *Br J Ophthalmol* 65:294–298.

Milner BA, Regan D, Heron JR (1974): Differential diagnosis of multiple sclerosis by visual evoked potential recording. *Brain* 97:755–772.

Mitchell JD, Hansen S, McInnes A, Campbell FW (1983): The recovery cycle of the pattern visual evoked potential in normal subjects and patients with multiple sclerosis. *Electroencephalogr Clin Neurophysiol* 56:309–315.

Moller AR, Burgess JE, Sekhar LN (1987): Recording compound action potentials from the optic nerve in man and monkeys. *Electroencephalogr Clin Neurol* 67:549–555.

Moskowitz A, Sokol S (1980): Spatial and temporal interaction of pattern-evoked cortical potentials in human infants. *Vision Res* 20:699–707.

Moskowitz A, Sokol S (1983): Developmental changes in the human visual system as reflected by the latency of the pattern reversal VEP. *Electroencephalogr Clin Neurophysiol* 56:1–15.

Muller-Jensen A, Zschocke S (1980): Pattern-induced visual evoked responses in patients with migraine accompagnee. *Electroencephalogr Clin Neurophysiol* 50:37P.

Muller-Jensen A, Zschocke S, Dannheim F (1981): VER analysis of the chiasmal syndrome. *J Neurol* 225:33–40.

Mushin J, Hogg CR, Dubowitz LMS, Skouteli H, Arden GB (1984): Visual evoked responses to light emitting diode (LED) photostimulation in newborn infants. *Electroencephalogr Clin Neurophysiol* 58:317–320.

Mustonen E, Sulg I, Kallanrouta T (1980): Electroretinogram (ERG) and visual evoked responses (VER) studies in patients with optic nerve drusen. *Acta Ophthalmologica* 58:539–549.

Neima D, Regan D (1984): Pattern visual evoked potentials and spatial vision in retrobulbar neuritis and multiple sclerosis. *Arch Neurol* 41:198–201.

Nelson JI, Seiple WH (1992): Human VEP contrast modulation sensitivity: separation of magno- and parvocellular components. *Electroencephalogr Clin Neurophysiol* 84(1):1–12.

Niazy HMA, Lundervold JA (1982): Correlation of evoked potentials (SEP and VEP), EEG and CT in the diagnosis of brain tumors and cerebrovascular diseases. *Clin Electroencephalogr* 13:71–81.

Nikoskelainen E, Falck B (1982): Do visual evoked potentials give relevant information to the neuro-ophthalmological examination in optic nerve lesions? *Acta Neurol Scand* 66:42–57.

Nilsson BY (1978): Visual evoked responses in multiple sclerosis: Comparison of two methods for pattern reversal. *J Neurol Neurosurg Psychiatry* 41:499–504.

Noachtar S, Hashimoto T, Luders H (1993): Pattern visual evoked potentials recorded from human occipital cortex with chronic subdural electrodes. *Electroencephalogr Clin Neurophysiol* 88(6):435–446.

Noel P, Desmedt JE (1980): Cerebral and far-field somatosensory evoked potentials in neurological disorders involving the cervical spinal cord, brainstem, thalamus and cortex. *Prog Clin Neurophysiol* 7:205–230.

Noseworthy J, Paty D, Wonnacott T, Feasby T, Ebers G (1983): Multiple sclerosis after age 50. *Neurology* 33:1537–1544.

Nousiainen U, Partanen J, Laulumaa V, Paakkonen A (1987): Involvement of somatosensory and visual pathways in late onset ataxia. 67:514–520.

Novak GP, Wiznitzer M, Kurtzberg D, Giesser BS, Vaughan BS, Jr (1988): The utility of visual evoked potentials using hemifield stimulation and several check sizes in the evaluation of suspected multiple sclerosis. *Electroencephalogr Clin Neurophysiol* 71:1–9.

Nuwer MR, Perlman SL, Packwood JW, Kark RAP (1983): Evoked potential abnormalities in the various inherited ataxias. *Ann Neurol* 13:20–27.

Nuwer MR, Visscher BR, Packwood JW, Namerow NS (1985): Evoked potential testing in relatives of multiple sclerosis patients. *Ann Neurol* 18:30–34.

Nuwer MR, Packwood JW, Myers LW, Ellison GW (1987): Evoked potentials predict the clinical changes in a multiple sclerosis drug study. *Neurology* 37:1754–1761.

Oepen G, Doerr M, Thoden U (1981): Visual (VEP) and somatosensory (SSEP) evoked potentials in Huntington's chorea. *Electroencephalogr Clin Neurophysiol* 51:666–670.

Oishi M, Yamada T, Dickins S, Kimura J (1985): Visual evoked potentials by different check sizes in patients with multiple sclerosis. *Neurology* 35:1461–1465.

Oken BJ, Chiappa KH, Gill E (1987): Normal temporal variability of the P100. *Electroencephalogr Clin Neurophysiol* 68:153–156.

Onofrj M, Bodis-Wollner I, Mylin L (1982): Visual evoked potential diagnosis of field defects in patients with chiasmatic and retrochiasmatic lesions. *J Neurol Neurosurg Psychiatry* 45:294–302.

Onofrj M, Bazzano S, Malatesta G, Fulgente T (1991): Mapped distribution of pattern reversal VEPs to central field and lateral half-field stimuli of different spatial frequencies. *Electroencephalogr Clin Neurophysiol* 80(3):167–180.

Ormerod IEC, McDonald WI, Du Boulay GH, Kendall BE, Moseley IF, Halliday AM, Kakigi R, Kriss A, Peringer E (1986): Disseminated lesions at presentation in patients with optic neuritis. *J Neurol Neurosurg Psychiatry* 49:124–127.

Padmos P, Haaijman JJ, Spekreijse H (1973): Visually evoked cortical potentials to patterned stimuli in monkey and man. *Electroencephalogr Clin Neurol* 35:153–163.

Pakalnis A, Drake ME, Barohn RJ, Chakeres DW, Mendell JR (1988): Evoked potentials in chronic inflammatory demyelinating polyneuropathy. *Arch Neurol* 45:1014–1016.

Parry-Jones NO, Fenwick P (1979): Coloured pattern displacement and VEP amplitude. *Electroencephalogr Clin Neurophysiol* 46:49–57.

Parsons T, Mishra J, Kaufman DI (1986): The use of a simultaneous pattern electroretinogram to determine whether volitional manipulation of the visual evoked potential has occurred. *Neurology* 36(suppl 1):232.

Patterson VH, Heron JR (1980): Visual field abnormalities in multiple sclerosis. *J Neurol Neurosurg Psychiatry* 43:205–208.

Paty DW, Blume WT, Brown WF, Jaatoul N, Kertesz A, McInnis W (1979): Chronic progressive myelopathy: Investigation with CSF electrophoresis, evoked potentials and CT scan. *Ann Neurol* 6:419–424.

Paty DW, Isaac CD, Grochowski E, Palmer MR, Oger J, Kastrukoff LF, Nord BB, Genton M, Jardine C, Li DK (1986): Magnetic resonance imaging in multiple sclerosis: A serial study in relapsing and remitting patients with quantitative measurements of lesion size. *Neurology* 36:177.

Paty DW, Oger JJF, Kastrukoff LF, Hashimoto SA, Hooge JP, Eisen AA, Eisen KA, Purves SJ, Low MD, Brandejs V, Robertson WD, Li DKB (1988): MRI in the diagnosis of MS: A prospective study with comparison of clinical evaluation, evoked potentials, oligoclonal banding, and CT. *Neurology* 38:180–185.

Peachey NS, Sokol S, Moskowitz A (1983): Recording the contralateral PERG: Effect of different electrodes. *Invest Ophthalmol Vis Sci* 24:1514–1516.

Pedersen L, Trojaborg W (1981): Visual, auditory and somatosensory pathway involvement in hereditary cerebellar ataxias, Friedreich's ataxia and familial spastic paraplegia. *Electroencephalogr Clin Neurophysiol* 52:283.

Perryman KM, Lindsley DB (1977): Visual responses in geniculo-striate and pulvino-extrastriate systems to patterned and unpatterned stimuli in squirrel monkeys. *Electroencephalogr Clin Neurophysiol* 42:157–177.

Persson HE, Sachs C (1981): Visual evoked potentials elicited by pattern reversal during provoked visual impairment in multiple sclerosis. *Brain* 104:369–382.

Persson HE, Wanger P (1984): Pattern-reversal electroretinograms and visual evoked cortical potentials in multiple sclerosis. *Br J Ophthalmol* 68:760–764.

Perez-Arroyo M, Chiappa KH (1985): Early visual evoked potentials in normal subjects and brain-dead patients. *Electroencephalogr Clin Neurophysiol* 61(3):S38.

Petrera JE, Fledelius HC, Trojaborg W (1988): Serial pattern evoked potential recording in a case of toxic optic neuropathy due to ethambutol. *Electroencephalogr Clin Neurophysiol* 71:146–149.

Phelps ME, Mazziotta JC, Kuhl DE, Nuwer M, Packwood J, Metter J, Engel J (1981): Tomographic mapping of human cerebral metabolism: Visual stimulation and deprivation. *Neurology* 31:517–529.

Phillips KR, Potvin AR, Syndulko K, Cohen SN, Tourtellotte WW, Potvin JH (1983): Multimodality evoked potentials and neurophysiological tests in multiple sclerosis. *Arch Neurol* 40:159–164.

Pierelli F, Pozzessere G, Sanarelli L, Valle E, Rizzo PA, Morocutti C (1985): Electrophysiological study in patients with chronic hepatic insufficiency. *Acta Neurol Belg* 85:284–291.

Plant GT (1983): Transient visually evoked potentials in sinusoidal gratings in optic neuritis. *J Neurol Neurosurg Psychiatry* 46:1125–1133.

Plant GT, Zimmern RL, Durden K (1983): Transient visually evoked potentials to the pattern reversal and onset of sinusoidal gratings. *Electroencephalogr Clin Neurophysiol* 56:147–158.

Plant GT, Hess RF, Thomas SJ (1986): The pattern evoked electroretinogram in optic neuritis. *Brain* 109:469–490.

Plant GT, Kermode AG, Turano G, Moseley IF, Miller DH, MacManus DG, Halliday AM, McDonald WI (1992): Symptomatic retrochiasmal lesions in multiple sclerosis: Clinical features, visual evoked potentials, and magnetic resonance imaging. *Neurology* 42:68–76.

Pratt H (1981): Evoked potentials in the operating room: Three examples using three sensory modalities. *Isr J Med Sci* 17:460–464.

Pratt H, Bleich N, Berliner E (1982): Short latency visual evoked potentials in man. *Electroencephalogr Clin Neurophysiol* 54:55–62.

Pratt H, Schacham S, Barak S (1984): A pattern reversal stimulator using optical fibers. *Electroencephalogr Clin Neurophysiol* 59:172–174.

Pratt H, Martin WH, Bleich N, Zaaroor M, Schacham SE (1994): A high-intensity, goggle-mounted flash stimulator for short-latency visual evoked potentials. *Electroencephalogr Clin Neurophysiol* 92(5):469–472.

Purves SJ, Low MD (1976): Visual evoked potentials to a reversing-pattern light-emitting diode stimulator in normal subjects and patients with demyelinating disease. *Electroencephalogr Clin Neurophysiol* 41:651–652.

Purves SJ, Low MD, Galloway J, Reeves B (1981): A comparison of visual, brainstem auditory, and somatosensory evoked potentials in multiple sclerosis. *Can J Neurol Sci* 8:15–19.

Puvanendran K, Devathasan G, Wong PK (1983): Visual evoked responses in diabetes. *J Neurol Neurosurg Psychiatry* 46:643–647.

Radtke RA, Erwin A, Erwin CW (1986): Abnormal sensory evoked potentials in amyotrophic lateral sclerosis. *Neurology* 36:796–801.

Rees JE (1980): Visual evoked responses in pernicious anemia (letter). *Arch Neurol* 37:397.

Regan D (1973): Rapid objective refraction using evoked brain potentials. *Invest Ophthalmol* 12:669–679.

Regan D (1977): Speedy assessment of visual acuity in amblyopia by the evoked potential method. *Ophthalmologia* 175:159–164.

Regan D, Heron JR (1969): Clinical investigation of lesions of the visual pathway: A new objective technique. *J Neurol Neurosurg Psychiatry* 32:479–483.

Regan D, Milner BA, Heron JR (1976): Delayed visual perception and delayed visual evoked potentials in the spinal form of multiple sclerosis and in retrobulbar neuritis. *Brain* 99:43–66.

Regan D, Bartol S, Murray TJ, Beverley KI (1982): Spatial frequency discrimination in normal vision and in patients with multiple sclerosis. *Brain* 105:735–754.

Rentschler I, Spinelli D (1978): Accuracy of evoked potential refractometry using bar gratings. *Acta Ophthalmol (Copenh)* 56:67–74.

Riemslag FCC, Spekreijse H, Van Wessem ThN (1985): Responses to paired onset stimuli: Implications for the delayed evoked potentials in multiple sclerosis. *Electroencephalogr Clin Neurophysiol* 62:155–166.

Rigolet MH, Mallecourt J, LeBlanc M, Chain F (1979): Etude de la vision des couleurs et des potentiels evoques dans diagnostic de la sclerose en plaques. *J Fr Ophthalmol* 2:553–560.

Ringens PJ, Vijfvinkel-Bruinenga S, van Lith GHM (1986): The pattern-elicited electroretinogram. I. A tool in the early detection of glaucoma? *Ophthalmology* 192:217–219.

Ristanovic D, Hajdukovic (1981): Effects of spatially structured stimulus fields on pattern reversal visual evoked potentials. *Electroencephalogr Clin Neurophysiol* 51:599–610.

Rizzo PA, Pierelli F, Pozzessere G, Verardi S, Casciani CU, Morocutti C (1982): Pattern visual evoked potentials and brainstem auditory evoked responses in uremic patients. *Acta Neurol Belg* 82:72–79.

Rizzo JF, Cronin-Golomb A, Growdon JH, Corkin S, Rosen TJ, Sandberg MA, Chiappa KH, Lessell S (1992): Retinocalcarine function in Alzheimer's disease. *Arch Neurol* 49:93–101.

Robertson E, Feldman RG (1980): Pattern shift visual evoked response in carotid occlusion. *Clin Electroencephalogr* 11:67–71.

Rolak LA (1985): The flight of colors test in multiple sclerosis. *Arch Neurol* 42:759–760.

Rolak LA, Ashizawa T (1985): The hot bath test in multiple sclerosis: Comparison with visual evoked responses and oligoclonal bands. *Acta Neurol Scand* 72:65–67.

Ropper AH, Chiappa KH (1986): Evoked potentials in Guillain-Barré syndrome. *Neurology* 36:587–590.

Ropper AM, Miett T, Chiappa KH (1982): Absence of evoked potential abnormalities in acute transverse myelopathy. *Neurology* 32:80–82.

Rossini PM, Pirochio M, Sollazzo D, Caltagirone C (1979): Foveal versus peripheral retinal responses: A new analysis for the early diagnosis of multiple sclerosis. *Electroencephalogr Clin Neurophysiol* 47:515–523.

Rossini PM, Pirchio M, Treviso M, Gambi D, Di Paolo B, Albertazzi A (1981): Checkerboard reversal pattern and flash VEPs in dialysed and non-dialysed subjects. *Electroencephalogr Clin Neurophysiol* 52:435–444.

Rowe MJ III (1981): A sequential technique for half field pattern visual evoked response testing. *Electroencephalogr Clin Neurophysiol* 51:463–469.

Rowe MJ III (1982): The clinical utility of half-field pattern reversal visual evoked potential testing. *Electroencephalogr Clin Neurophysiol* 53:73–77.

Sandrini G, Gelmi C, Rossi V, Bianchi PE, Alfonsi E, Pacchetti C, Verri AP, Nappi G (1986): Electroretinographic and visual evoked potential abnormalities in myotonic dystrophy. *Electroencephalogr Clin Neurophysiol* 64:215–217.

Sakurai M, Mannen T, Kanazawa I, Tanabe H (1992): Lidocaine unmasks silent demyelinative lesions in multiple schlerosis. *Neurology* 42:2088–2093.

Saul RF, Selhorst JB (1981): Thermal effects on VEP. *Neurology* 31(4, part 2):88.

Schmidt-Nielsen K (1975): Scaling in biology: The consequences of size. *J Exp Zool* 194:287–307.

Schuurmans RP, Berninger T (1985): Luminance and contrast responses recorded in man and cat. *Doc Ophthalmol* 59:187–197.

Sedgwick EM (1983): Pathophysiology and evoked potentials in multiple sclerosis. In: *Multiple Sclerosis: Pathology, Diagnosis and Management,* edited by JF Hallpike et al. Williams & Wilkins, Baltimore.

Seiple WH, Siegel IM (1983): Recording and pattern electroretinogram: A cautionary note. *Invest Ophthalmol Vis Sci* 24:796–798.

Selbst RG, Selhorst JB, Harbison JW, Myer EC (1983): Parainfectious optic neuritis. *Arch Neurol* 40:347–350.

Serra G, Carreras M, Tugnoli V, Manca M, Cristofori MC (1984): Pattern electroretinogram in multiple sclerosis. *J Neurol Neurosurg Psych* 47:879–883.

Seyal M, Sato S, White BG, Porter RJ (1981): Visual evoked potentials and eye dominance. *Electroencephalogr Clin Neurophysiol* 52:424–428.

Shahrokhi F, Chiappa KH, Young RR (1978): Pattern shift visual evoked responses: Two hundred patients with optic neuritis and/or multiple sclerosis. *Arch Neurol* 35:65–71.

Shaw NA, Cant BR (1980): Age-dependent changes in the latency of the pattern visual evoked potential. *Electroencephalogr Clin Neurophysiol* 48:237–241.

Shaw NA, Cant BR (1981): Age-dependent changes in the amplitude of the pattern visual evoked potential. *Electroencephalogr Clin Neurophysiol* 51:671–673.

Shearer DE, Dustman RE (1980): The pattern reversal evoked potential: The need for laboratory norms. *Am J EEG Technol* 20:185–200.

Sherman J (1982): Simultaneous pattern reversal electroretinograms and visual evoked potentials in diseases of the macula and optic nerve. *Ann NY Acad Sci* 388:214–225.

Shibasaki H, Kuroiwa Y (1982): Pattern reversal visual evoked potentials in Japanese patients with multiple sclerosis. *J Neurol Neurosurg Psychiatry* 45:1139–1143.

Shih P, Aminoff MJ, Goodin DS, Mantle M (1988): Effect of reference point on visual evoked potentials: Clinical relevance. *Electroencephalogr Clin Neurophysiol* 71:319–322.

Shors TJ, Ary JP, Eriksen KJ, Wright KW (1986): P100 amplitude variability of the pattern visual evoked potential. *Electroencephalogr Clin Neurophysiol* 65:316–319.

Siegfried JB, Lukas J (1981): Early wavelets in the VECP. *Invest Ophthalmol Vis Sci* 20:125–129.

Skuse NF, Burke D (1992): Sequence-dependent deterioration in the visual evoked potential in the absence of drowsiness. *Electroencephalogr Clin Neurophysiol* 84:20–25.

Smith KJ, Blakemore WF, McDonald WI (1979): Central remyelination restores secure conduction. *Nature* 20:395–396.

Smith T, Zeeberg I (1986): Evoked potentials in multiple sclerosis before and after high-dose methylprednisone infusion. *Eur Neurol* 25:67–73.

Snyder EW, Beck EC, Dustman RE (1979): Visual evoked potentials in monkeys. *Electroencephalogr Clin Neurophysiol* 47:430–440.

Snyder EW, Dustman RE, Shearer DE (1981): Pattern reversal evoked potential amplitudes: Life span changes. *Electroencephalogr Clin Neurophysiol* 52:429–434.

Sokol S (1978a): Measurement of infant visual acuity from pattern reversal evoked potentials. *Vision Res* 18:33–39.

Sokol S (1978b): Patterned elicited ERGs and VECPs in amblyopia and infant vision. In: *Visual Psychophysics and Physiology,* edited by JC Armington, J Krauskopf, and BR Wooten, pp 453–462. Academic Press, New York.

Sokol S (1980): Pattern visual evoked potentials: Their use in pediatric ophthalmology. In: *Electrophysiology and Psychophysics: Their Use in Ophthalmic Diagnosis,* edited by S Sokol, pp 251–268. Little Brown, Boston.

Sokol S (1983): Abnormal evoked potential latencies in amblyopia. *Br J Ophthalmol* 67:310–314.

Sokol S, Jones K (1979): Implicit time of pattern evoked potentials in infants: An index of maturation of spatial vision. *Vision Res* 19:747–755.

Sokol S, Moskowitz A (1981): Effect of retinal blur on the peak latency of the pattern evoked potential. *Vision Res* 21:1279–1286.

Sokol S, Nadler D (1979): Simultaneous electroretinograms and visually evoked potentials from adult amblyopes in response to a pattern stimulus. *Invest Ophthalmol* 18:848–855.

Sokol S, Shaterian ET (1976): The pattern-evoked cortical potential in amblyopia as an index of visual function. In: *Orthoptics: Past, Present, Future,* edited by S Moore, J Mein, and L Stockbridge, pp 59–67. Symposia Specialists, New York.

Sokol S, Moskowitz A, Towle VL (1981): Age-related changes in the latency of the visual evoked potential: Influence of check size. *Electroencephalogr Clin Neurophysiol* 51:559–562.

Sokol S, Hansen VC, Moskowitz A, Greenfield P, Towle VL (1983): Evoked potential and preferential looking estimates of visual acuity in pediatric patients. *Ophthalmology* 90:552–562.

Sorensen PS, Trojaborg W, Gjerris F, Krogsaa B (1985): Visual evoked potentials in pseudotumor cerebri. *Arch Neurol* 42:150–153.

Spehlmann R, Gross RA, Ho SU, Leestma JE, Norcross KA (1977): Visual evoked potentials and postmortem findings in a case of cortical blindness. *Ann Neurol* 2:531–534.

Spekreijse H, Khoe LH, van der Tweel LH (1972): A case of amblyopia; electrophysiology and psychophysics of contrast. *Adv Exp Med Biol* 24:141–156.

Spekreijse H, Estevez O, van der Tweel LH (1973): Luminance responses to pattern reversal. *Doc Ophthalmol Proc Series* 2:205–211.

Spekreijse H, Duwaer AL, Posthumus Meyjes FE (1978): Contrast evoked potentials and psychophysics in multiple sclerosis patients. In: *Human Evoked Potentials: Applications and Problems,* edited by D Lehman and E Callaway, pp 368–381. Plenum Press, London.

Spitz MC, Emerson RG, Pedley TA (1986): Dissociation of frontal N100 from occipital P100 in pattern reversal evoked potential. *Electroencephalogr Clin Neurophysiol* 65:161–168.

Stewart WA, Hall LD, Berry K, Churg A, Oger J, Hashimoto SA, Paty DW (1986): Magnetic resonance imaging (MRI) in multiple sclerosis (MS): Pathological correlation studies in eight cases. *Neurology* 36:320.

Stigsby B, Bohlega S, Al-Kawi MZ, Al-Dalaan A, El-Ramahi K (1994): Evoked potential findings in Behcet's disease. Brain-stem auditory, visual, and somatosensory evoked potentials in 44 patients. *Electroencephalogr Clin Neurophysiol* 92(4):273–281.

Stockard JJ, Hughes JF, Sharbrough FW (1979): Visually evoked potentials to electronic pattern reversal: Latency variations with gender, age and technical factors. *Am J EEG Technol* 19:171–204.

Stone J, Fukuda Y (1974): Properties of cat retinal ganglion cells: Comparison of W-cells with x- and y-cells. *J Neurophysiol* 37:722–748.

Stone J, Ghaly RF, Hughes JR (1988): Evoked potentials in head injury and states of increased intracranial pressure. *J Clin Neurophysiol* 5:135–160.

Streletz LJ, Bae SH, Roeshman RM, Schatz NJ, Savino PJ (1981a): Visual evoked potentials in occipital lobe lesions. *Arch Neurol* 38:80–85.

Streletz LJ, Chambers RA, Bae SH, Israel HL (1981b): Visual evoked potentials in sarcoidosis. *Neurology* 31:1545–1549.

Swart S, Millac P (1980): A comparison of flight of colours with visually evoked responses in patients with multiple sclerosis. *J Neurol Neurosurg Psychiatry* 43:550–551.

Tackmann W, Ettlin T (1982): Blink reflexes elicited by electrical, acoustic and visual stimuli. II. Their relation to visual-evoked potentials and auditory brain stem evoked potentials in the diagnosis of multiple sclerosis. *Eur Neurol* 21:264–269.

Tackmann W, Radu EW (1980): Pattern shift visual evoked potentials in Charcot-Marie-Tooth Disease, HMSN Type I. *J Neurol* 224:71–74.

Tackmann W, Strenge H, Barth R, Rojka-Raytscheff A (1979): Diagnostic validity for different components of pattern shift visual evoked potentials in multiple sclerosis. *Eur Neurol* 18:243–248.

Tackmann W, Ettlin Th, Strenge H (1982): Multimodality evoked potentials and electrically elicited blink reflex in optic neuritis. *J Neurol* 227:157–163.

Tan CT, Murray NMF, Sawyers D, Leonard TJK (1984): Deliberate alteration of the visual evoked potential. *J Neurol Neurosurg Psychiatry* 47:518–523.

Tan CT, King PJL, Chiappa KH (1989): Pattern ERG: Effects of reference electrode site, stimulus mode and check size. *Electroencephalogr Clin Neurophysiol* 74:11–18.

Taylor MJ, Keenan NK, Gallant T, Skarf B, Freedman MH, Logan WJ (1987a): Subclinical VEP abnormalities inpatients on chronic deferoxamine therapy: Longitudinal studies. *Electroencephalogr Clin Neurophysiol* 68:81–87.

Taylor MJ, Menzies R, MacMillan LJ, Whyte HE (1987b): VEPs in normal full-term and premature neonates: Longitudinal versus cross-sectional data. *Electroencephalogr Clin Neurophysiol* 68:20–27.

Teping C, Groneberg A (1984): Physiological basis and clinical application of pattern electroretinogram. *Dev Ophthalmol* 9:74–80.

Thompson PD, Mastaglia FL, Carroll WM (1986): Anterior ischaemic optic neuropathy. A correlative clinical and visual evoked potential study of 18 patients. *J Neurol Neurosurg Psychiatry* 49:128–135.

Tobimatsu S, Fukui R, Kato M, Kobayashi T, Kuroiwa Y (1985): Multimodality evoked potentials in patients and carriers with adrenoleukodystrophy and adrenomyeloneuropathy. *Electroencephalogr Clin Neurophysiol* 62:18–24.

Tobimatsu S, Kurita-Tashima S, Nakayama-Hiromatsu M, Akazawa K, Kato M (1993): Age-related changes in pattern visual evoked potentials: differential effects of luminance, contrast and check size. *Electroencephalogr Clin Neurophysiol* 88(1):12–19.

Tomoda H, Celesia GG, Toleikis SC (1991): Effect of spatial frequency on simultaneous recorded steady-state pattern electroretinograms and visual evoked potentials. *Electroencephalogr Clin Neurophysiol* 80(2):81–88.

Torok B, Meyer M, Wildberger H (1992): The influence of pattern size on amplitude, latency and wave form of retinal and cortical potentials elicited by checkerboard pattern reversal and stimulus onset-offset. *Electroencephalogr Clin Neurophysiol* 84(1):13–19.

Towle VL, Maskowitz A, Sokol S, Schwartz B (1983): The visual evoked potential in glaucoma and ocular hypertension: Effects of check size, field size, and stimulation rate. *Ophthalmol Vis Sci* 24:175–183.

Towle VL, Witt JC, Nader SH, Reder AT, Foust R, Spire JP (1991): Three-dimensional human pattern visual evoked potentials. II. Multiple sclerosis patients. *Electroencephalogr Clin Neurophysiol* 80:339–346.

Towle VL, Witt JC, Ohira T, Munson R, Nader SH, Spire J (1991): Three-dimensional human pattern visual evoked potentials. I. Normal subjects. *Electroencephalogr Clin Neurophysiol* 80:329–338.

Trick GL, Trick LR (1984): An evaluation of variation in pattern reversal retinal potential characteristics. *Doc Ophthalmol Proc Series* 40:57–67.

Trojaborg W, Petersen E (1979): Visual and somatosensory evoked cortical potentials in multiple sclerosis. *J Neurol Neurosurg Psychiatry* 42:323–330.

Troncoso J, Mancall EL, Schatz NJ (1979): Visual evoked responses in pernicious anemia. *Arch Neurol* 36:168–169.

Uren SM, Stewart P, Crosby PA (1979): Subject cooperation and the visual evoked response. *Invest Ophthalmol Vis Sci* 6:648–652.

van Buggenhout E, Ketelaer P, Carton H (1982): Success and failure of evoked potentials in detecting clinical and subclinical lesions in multiple sclerosis patients. *Clin Neurol Neurosurg* 84:3–14.

van der Marel H, Daguelie G, Spekreijse H (1981): Pattern evoked potentials in awake rhesus monkeys. *Invest Ophthalmol Vis Sci* 21:457–466.

van der Tweel LH, Estevez O, Cavonius CR (1979): Invariance of the contrast evoked potential with changes in retinal illuminance (letter). *Vision Res* 19:1283–1287.

Van Essen DC (1979): Visual areas of the mammalian cerebral cortex. *Ann Rev Neurosci* 2:227–263.

van Lith GHM, van Marle GW, van Dok-Mak GTM (1978): Variation in latency times of visually evoked cortical potentials. *Br J Ophthalmol* 62:220–222.

Vaughan HG (1966): The perceptual and physiologic significance of visual evoked responses recorded from the scalp of man. In: *Clinical Electroretinography (Suppl, Vision Res)*, pp 203–223. Pergamon Press, Oxford.

Vaughan HG, Hull RC (1965): Functional relation between stimulus intensity and photically evoked cerebral responses in man. *Nature (Lond)* 206:720–722.

Walsh JC, Garrick R, Cameron J, McLeod JG (1982): Evoked potential changes in clinically definite multiple sclerosis: A two year follow up study. *J Neurol Neurosurg Psychiatry* 45:494–500.

Wanger P, Persson HE (1983): Pattern-reversal electroretinograms in unilateral glaucoma. *Invest Ophthalmol Vis Sci* 24:749–753.

Waybright EA, Selhorst JB, Saul RF (1982): The effect of neutral density filters on visual evoked potentials. *Ann Neurol* 12:112.

Wenzel D, Brandl U, Harms D (1982a): Visual evoked potentials in juvenile complicated migraine. *Electroencephalogr Clin Neurophysiol* 53:59P.

Wenzel W, Camacho L, Claus D, Aschoff J (1982b): Visual evoked potentials in Friedreich's ataxia. In: *Clinical Applications of Evoked Potentials in Neurology*, edited by J Courjon, F Mauguiere, and M Revol, pp 131–139. Raven Press, New York.

White CT, Kataoka RW, Martin JI (1977): Colour-evoked potentials; development of a methodology for the analysis of the processes involved in colour vision. In: *Visual Evoked Potentials in Man: New Developments*, edited by JE Desmedt, pp 250–272. Clarendon Press, Oxford.

Whittaker SG, Siegfried JB (1983): Origin of wavelets in the visual evoked potential. *Electroencephalogr Clin Neurophysiol* 55:91–101.

Wilcox LM, Sokol S (1980): Changes in the binocular fixation patterns and the visually evoked potential in the treatment of esotropia with amblyopia. *Ophthalmology* 87:1273–1281.

Wildberger HGH, van Lith GHM, Wijngaarde R, Mak GTM (1976): Visually evoked cortical potentials in the evaluation of homonymous and bitemporal visual field defects. *Br J Ophthalmol* 60:273–278.

Wilson WB (1978): Visual-evoked response differentiation of ischemic optic neuritis from the optic neuritis of multiple sclerosis. *Am J Ophthalmol* 86:530–535.

Wilson WB, Keyser RB (1980): Comparison of the pattern and diffuse-light visual evoked responses in definite multiple sclerosis. *Arch Neurol* 37:30–34.

Wist ER, Hennerici M, Dichgans J (1978): The Pulfrich spatial frequency phenomenon: A psycholophysical method competitive to visual evoked potentials in the diagnosis of multiple sclerosis. *J Neurol Neurosurg Psychiatry* 41:1069–1077.

Wright MJ, Johnston A (1982): The effects of contrast and length of gratings on the visual evoked potential. *Vision Res* 22:1389–1399.

Wulff CH (1985): Evoked potentials in acute transverse myelopathy. *Dan Med Bull* 32:282–287.

Wulff CH, Trojaborg W (1985): Adult metachromatic leukodystrophy: Neurophysiologic findings. *Neurology* 35:1776–1778.

Yiannikas C, Walsh JC (1983): The variation of the pattern shift visual evoked response with the size of the stimulus field. *Electroencephalogr Clin Neurophysiol* 55:427–435.

Yiannikas C, Walsh JC, McLeod JG (1983): Visual evoked potentials in the detection of subclinical optic toxic effects secondary to ethambutol. *Arch Neurol* 40:645–648.

Zahn JR, Matthews P (1983): An early peak of the pattern reversal evoked potential. *Invest Ophthalmol Vis Sci* 24:793–795.

Zeese JA (1977): Pattern visual evoked responses in multiple sclerosis. *Arch Neurol* 34:314–316.

Zschocke S, Muller-Jensen A (1980): Visual evoked responses to homonymous hemifield stimulation in the diagnosis of hemispheric cerebral lesions. *Electroencephalogr Clin Neurophysiol* 50.

Evoked Potentials in Clinical Medicine,
3d ed., edited by Keith H. Chiappa.
Lippincott–Raven Publishers, Philadelphia © 1997.

4

Visual Evoked Potentials in Pediatrics

Susan R. Levy

*Departments of Pediatrics, Neurology, and Child Study Center,
Yale University School of Medicine, New Haven, Connecticut 06510*

The visual evoked potential (VEP) is a neurophysiologic technique that can provide objective information about the function of the visual system in the preverbal infant and young child who cannot communicate visual symptoms or cooperate for standard assessment of visual function. The VEP is used to supplement the neurologic examination in the assessment of visual function and to assist in the diagnosis of specific disorders associated with involvement of the sensory visual pathways.

1. MATURATIONAL CHANGES

The VEP can be elicited by a patterned or luminance (flash) stimulus. The flash stimulus may be produced by a stroboscopic lamp or light-emitting diode (LED) goggles. Developmental changes occur with both techniques as a consequence of maturational changes in the structure and cortical organization of the occipital lobes.

Light-emitting diode flash VEPs can be recorded in premature infants at about 24 weeks gestational age. At this time, there is a single large negative peak recorded at 300 msec (N300) (Taylor and McColloch, 1992; Taylor et al., 1987). Within several weeks a positivity occurs at a longer latency and by term a positivity at 200 msec (P200) is evident (Mushin et al., 1984). Post-term the VEP continues to mature. Between birth and 4 weeks, the P200 latency decreases and the waveform becomes bifid. By 6 months of age, these waveforms merge to form a single positive component, P100. There are no significant maturational changes occurring after 6 to 12 months of age.

The stoboscopic flash VEP also shows maturational changes during the preterm period and during the first several months of life. The VEP response evolves from a predominantly surface negative response to a positive response between 36 and 38 weeks postconceptual age. The latency of the positive component decreases during the first 3 months of life. Adult morphology, characterized by a biphasic negative–positive waveform with the positive component at about 100 msec, is achieved by 6 months of age (Hrbek et al., 1973; Kurtzberg and Vaughan, 1986; Pryds et al., 1989; Stanley et al., 1987).

Rapid maturational changes occur in the response to both types of flash VEPs. There are differences in the maturational patterns and high variability of each type of response, with a wide range of normal. It is important to use stimulus-specific normative data with each type of test (Hrbek et al., 1973; Pryds et al., 1989; Taylor and Farrell, 1987).

The pattern-reversal VEP has been recorded in premature infants from 33 weeks gestation (Harding et al., 1989) and can be reliably recorded in children of all ages (Marg et al., 1976; Dobson and Teller, 1978; Sokol, 1978; Fenwick et al., 1981; Allison et al., 1984; Aso et al., 1988). During the first 4 to 5 years of life, the morphology and latency of the pattern-shift visual evoked potential (PSVEP) change as a consequence of the continuing development of the visual system after birth (Sokol and Jones, 1979; Moskowitz and Sokol, 1983; McColloch and Scarf, 1991). The latency of all PSVEP components decreases with increasing age. At 1 month of age, the PSVEP to large check sizes is a simpler waveform than that of the adult and consists of a slowly rising positive response. No response is recorded to small checks. The latency of the large positivity decreases rapidly at a rate of about 10 msec/week between birth and 5 months of age (McCulloch and Skarf, 1991). At 2 months of age, the positive response to large checks is preceded and followed by negative potentials and there is a small-amplitude response to small checks. By 3 months of age, a late positive wave emerges which decreases in latency with increasing age. Therefore, with advancing age, there is an increase in complexity and shortening of the latency of the PSVEP components. These changes occur more quickly for larger checks than for small checks with both monocular and binocular testing. Pattern-shift VEPs recorded monocularly have slightly longer latencies than those recorded binocularly. Age has not been shown to have a significant effect on the monocular–binocular latency difference (McCulloch and Skarf, 1991). By 5 years of age the PSVEP resembles that of the adult.

2. SPECIAL METHODOLOGY

It is important to consider several factors when performing VEP testing in infants and young children to obtain reliable and reproducible results. In neonates, electrodes should be applied with nonirritating tape and saline jelly. In older infants and young children, electrodes can be applied using paste and gauze or collodion and gauze. The former method is preferred as the application process is less distressing to the child and the electrodes can be more easily removed following the procedure. If electrodes fall off during the testing, they are easily reapplied. If the child is so active that the electrodes do not stay on with paste, it is unlikely that the testing will be completed.

During flash VEP testing the infant should be securely positioned to minimize artifacts. The patient may sleep or be quietly relaxed unless premature. The amplitude of the cortical components can be decreased in quiet sleep in the premature infant (Whyte et al., 1987). Premature infants should be alert or in active sleep during recordings.

In infants flash VEPs are recorded with a stimulus rate of 0.5/sec with a 1000-msec sweep. In children 12 months of age or older, a stimulus rate of 1.9/sec with a sweep of 500 msec is suggested. A band-pass of 1 to 100 Hz is used. Twenty to 30 trials may be adequate for premature infants.

The testing room should be devoid of extraneous auditory or visual distraction during PSVEP testing. The child may be held on the parent's lap or sit independently in the chair in front of the screen. Fixation on the stimulus should be carefully monitored. Averaging should only occur when the child is attending to the pattern. The observer can help maintain focus on the screen by placing small toys in front of the stimulus or by making noise in the direction of the screen. A video cartoon superimposed on the pattern VEP stimulus has been used to enhance children's cooperation (Shors et al., 1987). P100 amplitudes have been noted to decrease with this technique, however, latencies are not altered. Pattern VEPs were recorded from 10 patients ages 4 to 21 months with amblyopia and normal vision using chloral hydrate sedation (80 to 100 mg/kg) (Wright et al., 1986). The results were similar to those obtained in an awake state. These data were reproduced by Cai and Wang (1992), who recorded PSVEP in sleep under chloral hydrate sedation in 20 children ages 3 to 12 months and in 22 children ages 13 months to 6 years. P100, recorded in all cases, was prolonged but closely related linearly to the latency during wakefulness.

The optimal check size to elicit the VEP varies during the first 6 months of life. Optimal check sizes include at 1 month, 120'; at 2 months, 60'; 3 to 5 months, 30'; and at 6 months and older, 15'. If no response is elicited at these check sizes then the check size should be

TABLE 4–1. *P100 latency normative data*

AGE months	120' Check		60' Check		30' Check		15' Check	
	Latency	S.D.	Latency	S.D.	Latency	S.D.	Latency	S.D.
Monocular stimulation								
1	209	—	203	—	185	—	—	—
2	150	—	171	—	154	—	166	—
3	123	10	125	8.9	135	8.9	142	11.7
4	116	5.4	116	4.9	122	9.8	136	12.1
5	113	4.5	116	7.1	118	5.5	128	6.7
6	111	4.4	115	2.5	118	5	126	8.9
7	111	4.3	114	5.8	116	7.9	122	9.1
8	110	5.7	113	6.3	118	4.6	124	5.5
9	108	3.5	112	2.8	114	5.7	122	3.6
10	109	6.1	111	5.5	118	6.2	122	3.9
12	114	8.1	102	8.3	113	4	115	6.5
14	112	3.4	112	3.7	117	4.8	120	4.6
18	112	7.5	112	6.4	120	5.1	121	6.7
22	111	4.1	113	3.2	115	4.6	119	5.1
Binocular stimulation								
1	214	40.3	218.9	23.4	221.5	21	210.5	—
2	156.8	23.4	162.8	20.4	171.2	14.3	182.5	—
3	115.5	7.4	122.4	7	129.7	9.1	145	10.5
4	111.4	5.2	112.8	4.6	120.3	9.2	128.3	7.4
5	114	16.9	111.4	5.5	119.9	18.1	125.3	6.9
6	107.9	1	108	1.5	114	3.2	123.3	5.6
7	106.5	4.4	109.4	4.2	114.4	7.1	123	5.5
8	107.4	5.9	109	5.4	115	6.6	120.7	8.8
9	104.6	2.1	106.6	1.7	113	5.5	120.6	5.2
10	103.4	3.4	105.6	4.9	112.1	8.8	122.7	8.7
12	106	8	106.9	6.7	117.3	6.1	124.9	4.9
14	105	2.7	109.6	3.3	115.9	5.5	119	4.9
18	108.2	4.5	109.6	6.8	116.7	4.5	119.8	6.7
22	106.8	5.4	110	5.7	114	6.5	118.1	5.2

Visual EP latency normative data from McCulloch and Skarf (1991). Recording technique included reversing checkerboard pattern at 1.88 Hz; mean luminance of 16 ft lamberts; 95% contrast between black and white checks; 0.1- to 30-Hz band-pass; 400-msec sweep; 20 to 40 trials averaged.

increased by a factor of 2 (Sokol, 1986b). Age-matched normative data specific for the pattern size must be used for interpretation of results (Table 4–1).

Binocular testing is usually performed in children younger than 6 months. When monocular testing is performed in infants older than 6 months, it is best to first test the better eye while patching the "bad" eye. This sequence will allow the child to become accustomed to the patching before the better eye is occluded. Usually 30 to 50 trials are required to obtain reproducible responses in infants, and in older children 50 to 100 trials are necessary. The band-pass used is 1 to 100 Hz, although 1 to 30 and 1 to 50 Hz have also been used.

3. CLINICAL APPLICATIONS

3.1. Estimation of Visual Acuity

There are several methods used to assess visual acuity in the nonverbal child. These techniques include opticokinetic nystagmus, the preferential looking test, and the VEP. For a comparison of these techniques refer to Fulton et al., 1981, 1989; Hoyt et al., 1982; Sokol et al. 1983; Sokol, 1986a; Moskowitz et al., 1987; Friendly, 1993. Sokol et al., (1983) obtained PSVEP and behavioral acuity measured with forced preferential looking techniques (FPL) in children 4 months to 10 years. In children younger than 2 years, monocular testing was completed more often with PSVEP than with FPL methods. Pattern-shift VEP results agreed with Snellen, Allen, and "E" acuity measures more often than did FPL results in children who completed both tests. The pattern VEP can be recorded from birth and can therefore provide an objective assessment of visual function in infants and preverbal children. Visual acuity can be estimated by determining the smallest check size that elicits an identifiable waveform. It should be possible to obtain reproducible VEPs to check sizes as small as 15′ in children 3 months of age or older with normal vision. Children who have visual impairment demonstrate VEPs only to larger checks or the VEP response is absent. Sokol (1978) estimated visual acuity using the VEP and extrapolating the VEP amplitude versus pattern size function to zero. Infant VEP acuity is equivalent to adult Snellen acuity of 20/20 by 6 months of age. P100 latencies are symmetrical at any age and interocular differences are invariant with age. Significant interocular differences indicate abnormal vision in one eye (McCulloch and Skarf, 1991).

3.2. Detection of Amblyopia

The VEP can be used to detect amblyopia and to monitor occlusion therapy. The amplitude of the PSVEP is sensitive to refractive errors. The amblyopic eye produces smaller-amplitude VEPs or absence of VEPs to smaller pattern stimuli. Sokol et al. (1983) used measurements of interocular VEP amplitude and latency differences to detect amblyopia. The amplitude difference between eyes has been shown to be smaller after occlusion therapy. Visual EPs become equal and symmetrical when visual acuity is equal in the two eyes (Sokol, 1986b,c).

3.3. Cortical Blindness and Developmental Delay

When an infant demonstrates inadequate visual function, it is necessary to determine if the cause is of retinal or cortical origin. In these cases, it is helpful to record the electroretinogram (ERG) and PSVEP. If the ERG is normal and the PSVEP is abnormal, then the visual disturbance can be attributed to pathology of the visual pathways and/or visual cortex and retinal pathology is excluded. It is, however, difficult to differentiate cortical blindness from developmental delay. Delayed visual development causes a child to exhibit reduced visual responsiveness that improves as the child matures. The PSVEPs reflect this delay with prolonged latencies for age. Recording serial PSVEPs may be helpful. If the amplitude and latency improve with time, then developmental delay is more likely. Pattern-shift VEPs have been recorded in infants who appeared to be blind by clinical examination. Several of these cases have been found to have congenital motor apraxia (Gittinger and Sokol, 1982). Taylor and McCulloch (1991) found flash VEPs to be helpful in predicting visual outcome in children with acute-onset cortical blindness due to multiple causes, including trauma, surgery, infection, and hypoxia. Sixteen of 17 children with normal VEPs during acute cortical blindness recovered normal visual function. Pattern VEPs were useful in monitoring the course of recovery in these patients.

3.4. Neonatal Asphyxia

A number of studies (Whyte et al., 1986; Muttitt et al., 1991; Taylor et al., 1992; Whyte, 1993) have studied serial VEPs in full-term infants with documented birth asphyxia. A total of 211 term infants had serial flash VEPs and were followed for 6 to 24 months. Ninety-two infants had abnormal VEPs, defined as absent potentials any time or waveform abnormalities that persisted. All these infants had severe neurologic sequelae or died. The infants with normal or transiently abnormal VEPs had normal examinations on follow-up. McCulloch et al. (1991) found a strong association between normal, abnormal, or absent VEPs and long-term visual outcome.

3.5. Demyelinating Disease

Although demyelinating disease is less common in the pediatric population compared to the adult, there are various clinical presentations in which it is considered part of the differential diagnosis. Evoked potential testing can be helpful in these situations. Visual EPs have been found to be abnormal in central nervous system disorders such as Devic's disease, acute disseminated encephalomyelitis, multiple sclerosis, and optic neuritis. In a group of 12 children with definite multiple sclerosis, Taylor and McCulloch (1992) found 10 children with abnormal VEPs (delayed latency or loss of cortical component) and 2 with abnormal somatosensory evoked potentials (SEPs). In cases of optic neuritis, the VEPs were always abnormal and other EPs tended to be normal. The magnetic resonance imaging scan may be normal. Visual EPs may show improvement after the acute phase of the illness. Some VEPs return to normal, although a significant number of children may continue to have abnormal VEPs despite a clinical recovery (Halliday et al., 1986; Matsubara et al., 1990).

3.6. Neurodegenerative Disease

Visual EPs may be helpful when used in conjunction with other EP modalities to assess various degenerative diseases in childhood. The VEP may assist in the diagnosis and monitoring of a particular disease. Visual EPs can help differentiate the hereditary ataxias of childhood (Taylor and Logan, 1983; Taylor et al., 1985). Eleven of 13 patients with ataxia telangiectasia were found to have low-amplitude or absent VEPs and 10 of 14 patients with

Friedreich's ataxia had normal-amplitude VEPs at increased latencies. Visual EPs can help monitor progression of these disorders. The ERG and VEP are important studies in the diagnosis of ceroid lipofuscinosis. Although the disease can only be confirmed by biopsy, the pattern of the VEP and ERG results may help determine the need for a biopsy. The ERG is abnormal in all cases. The ERG is small in early stages of infantile onset and absent in later stages and in the juvenile form of the disease. A normal ERG excludes the diagnosis. Visual EPs are usually abnormal and deteriorate as the disease progresses (Harden and Pampiglione, 1982). Flash VEPs were abnormal in 6 of 13 patients with mucopolysaccharidoses who had normal neurologic examinations (Perretti et al., 1990).

The VEP can also be useful in the early detection and differentiation of the leukodystrophies of childhood, a group of inherited white matter degenerative diseases. These disorders can present at several months of age to mid-childhood and their clinical presentation is quite variable. Markand et al. (1982) recorded VEPs, brain stem auditory EPs (BAEPs), and SEPs in 12 patients with Pelzaeus-Merzbacher disease (PMD), in 3 with adrenoleukodystrophy (ALD), and in 3 with metachromatic leukodystrophy (MLD). All three EPs were abnormal in all patients except one patient with early ALD who had normal VEPs and SEPs. Of seven patients who had PSVEP, in four no response was recorded, in one the response was normal (early ALD), and in one with PMD responses were absent unilaterally and prolonged on the other side and in one patient with PMD there was a bilateral prolongation of the response. Flash VEPs were done in 17 patients. The VEPs were normal in four patients (two PMD, two ALD) and absent in three patients (two PMD, one mild MLD), and in 10 patients the response was markedly delayed (seven PMD, one ALD, two MLD). In a study utilizing multimodality EP studies, characteristic EP profiles were seen (Demeirleir et al., 1988). Visual EPs were abnormal in most (five of seven) children with MLD and in five of six children with PMD, absent in Canavan's disease (two of two), and progressed in Krabbe's disease (two of two). Visual EPs were normal in multiple sulfatase deficiency (three of four) and in mild cases (two of two) of ADL and Alexander's disease (two of two).

3.7. Coma

Somatosensory EPs are the most reliable predictors of outcome in comatose children. Visual EPs are less helpful than SEPs, however, they do correlate with outcome. If SEPs cannot be recorded in the comatose child because, for example, of brachial plexus injury or lesion, VEPs should be completed. Abnormal LED flash VEPs predicted a poor prognosis in a group of comatose children with various etiologies (Taylor and Farrell, 1989). Visual EPs should be repeated during the first several days of coma, as they are more likley to change than VEPs in comatose adults. Improvements and deteriorations in the VEP correlate reliably with prognosis.

3.8. Neurofibromatosis

Pattern VEPs have been found to be abnormal in patients with neurofibromatosis and optic nerve gliomas large enough to affect visual acuity (Groswasser et al., 1985). Patients may have small subclinical tumors or be visually asymptomatic. Taylor and McCulloch (1992) recorded EPs in 28 such patients (age 1 month to 16 years) and 53% had abnormal VEPs. Visual EP abnormalities were present in some very young patients without clinical findings referable to the visual system. The VEP abnormality is usually a delayed latency of the P100. Jabbari et al., (1985) reported abnormal VEPs in 8 of 30 asymptomatic patients with normal visual acuity and visual fields. Seven of these patients had computed tomography scans, six of which showed abnormally large optic nerves on the side of the VEP abnormality. North et al., (1994) performed PSVEP in 10 children with neurofibromatosis type I and optic gliomas and in 20 children with neurofibromatosis type I and normal visual pathways to determine if the PSVEP is a sensitive method for the detection of asymptomatic optic gliomas. Nine of 10 children with optic gliomas had abnormal VEPs, resulting in a sensitivity of 90%. Eight of 20 children with neurofibromatosis type I and normal visual pathways had abnormal PSVEP, resulting in a specificity of 60%. These data suggest that an abnormal PSVEP provides a stronger indication for neuroimaging that is currently not recommended until optic nerve gliomas are symptomatic. Earlier detection allows for monitoring of tumor progression and timely interventional therapies to avoid visual loss.

3.9. Hydrocephalus

Visual EPs to flash stimulation have been reported in children with hydrocephalus. Sklar et al. (1979) found flash VEPs to be abnormal (prolonged latencies, waveform asymmetries) in 10 patients with hydrocephalus. These abnormalities improved following shunting. A deterioration in the VEPs correlated with clinical progression of hydrocephalus. These results reflect those of Ehle and Sklar (1979), who studied 15 infants with hydrocephalus. Visual EPs and SEPs were recorded in 60 hydrocephalic infants and children at the time of presentation and following a shunting procedure. Infants less than 10 weeks of age had abnormal flash VEPs and less than half had abnormal median SEPs. The EPs improved after successful shunting. Evoked potentials did not improve when complications of shunting occurred. In children 4 months to 17 months EP findings did not correlate with the degree of hydrocephalus but improvement was seen after shunting. Visual EPs remained abnormal after shunt revision and posterior tibial SEPs usually showed improvement in the older children 5 to 17 years of age (George and Taylor 1987a,b). Therefore, these studies found EPs to have limited value in the diagnosis of hydrocephalus but to be helpful in monitoring patients after shunting and on long-term follow-up.

3.10. Systemic Disease

Monitoring VEPs may be helpful in assessing neurologic side effects of various therapies for systemic illnesses in the young child. Neurologic sequelae have been more apparent as children with previously fatal disorders have longer life expectancies. Verity et al. (1990) performed VEPs on leukemic children and found them to be frequently abnormal. Visual EPs may be helpful in determining toxicity of cancer treatment. Seth et al. (1991) performed VEPs in children with tuberculosis treated with ethambutal. The VEP latencies did not vary significantly during therapy and between 3 and 6 months after discontinuation of therapy. These findings indicate that children are not at greater risk for developing ethambutal-induced optic nerve damage. Taylor et al. (1987) found that VEPs varied with the administration of the iron-chelating agent deferoxamine used in the chronic anemias when repeated transfusions are required. Visual EPs were found to be sensitive to the neurotoxic effects of this medication, as one third of children without clinical symptoms had VEP abnormalities. Brinciotti (1994) studied eight epileptic children who had chronically high serum levels of phenobarbital (>40 mg/L), three of whom had no clinical signs or symptoms of drug intoxication. Flash VEPs were obtained during a period of high phenobarbital levels and again when levels were in a normal range. A delay in the latency of the major positive peak (P2) was seen in all but one patient with high phenobarbital levels. The latency of P2 decreased significantly in seven patients when phenobarbital levels were normal.

CONCLUSION

The VEP is a sensitive, noninvasive technique to study the sensory visual pathways in infants and young children who cannot communicate visual symptomatology or cooperate for standard visual testing. The VEP can detect subclinical lesions causing dysfunction of the visual pathways, confirm functional visual loss, provide a means of monitoring patients at risk for visual impairment from various disease processes or therapeutic interventions, contribute information for differential diagnosis, and provide prognostic data for visual and systemic recovery in asphyxiated neonates and comatose children.

REFERENCES

Allison T, Hume AL, Wood CC, Goff WR (1984): Developmental and aging changes in somatosensory, auditory and visual evoked potentials. *Electroencephalogr Clin Neurophysiol* 58:14–24.

Aso K, Watanabe K, Negoro T, Takaetsu E, Furane S, Takahashi I, Yamamoto N, Nomura K (1988): Developmental changes of pattern reversal visual evoked potentials. *Brain Dev* 10:154–159.

Brinciotti M (1994): Effects of chronic high serum levels of phenobarbital on evoked potentials in epileptic children. *Electroencephalogr Clin Neurophysiol* 92:11–16.

Cai F, Wang Z (1992): Comparing study for norms of pattern VEP recorded in wake and sleeping under chloral hydrate sedation in infancy. *Pediatr Neurol* 8:349.

DeMeirleir LJ, Taylor MJ, Logan WJ (1988): Multimodal evoked potential studies in leukodystrophies of children. *Can J Neurol Sci* 15:26–31.

Dobson V, Teller DY (1978): Visual acuity in human infants: a review and comparison of behavioral and electrophysiological studies. *Vision Res* 18:1469–1483.

Ehle A, Sklar F (1979): Visual evoked potentials in infants with hydrocephalus. *Neurology* 29:1541–1544.

Fenwick PBC, Brown D. Hennesey J (1981): The visual evoked response to pattern reversal in "normal" 6–11 year-old children. *Electroencephalogr Clin Neurophysiol* 51:49–62.

Friendly DS (1993): Development of vision in infants and young children. *Pediatr Clin North Am* 40:693–703.

Fulton AB, Hansen RM, Manning KA (1981): Measuring visual acuity in infants. *Surv Ophthalmol* 25:325–332.

Fulton AB, Hartmann EE, Hansen RM (1989): Electrophysiologic testing techniques for children. *Doc Ophthalmol* 71:341–354.

George SR, Taylor MJ (1987a): Somatosensory evoked potentials in children with hydrocephalus. *Can J Neurol Sci* 14:234.

George SR, Taylor MJ (1987b): VEPs and SEPs in hydrocephalic infants before and after shunting. *Clin Neurol Neurosurg* Suppl I: 96.

Gittinger JW, Sokol S (1982): The visual evoked potential in the diagnosis of congenital ocular motor apraxia. *Am J Ophthalmol* 93:700–703.

Groswasser Z, Kriss A, Halliday AM, McDonald WI (1985): Pattern and flash evoked potentials in the assessment and management of optic nerve gliomas. *J Neurol Neurosurg Psychiatr* 48:1125–1134.

Halliday AM, Kriss A, Cuendent F, Francis D, McDonald WI, Taylor D (1986): Childhood optic neuritis: a study of pattern and flash visual evoked potentials. In: *Maturation of the CNS and Evoked Potentials*, edited by V Gallai, pp 41–50. Elsevier Science Publishers, Amsterdam.

Harden A, Pampiglione G (1982): Neurophysiological studies (EEG/ERG/VEP/SEP) in 88 children with so-called neuronal ceroid lipofuscinosis. In: *Ceroid Lipofuscinosis (Batten's Disease)*, edited by D Armstrong, N Koppang, and JA Rider, pp 61–70. Elsevier Science Publishers, Amsterdam.

Harding GFA, Grose J, Wilton A, Bissenden JG (1989): The pattern reversal VEP in short gestation infants. *Electroencephalogr Clin Neurophysiol* 74:76–80.

Hoyt CS, Nickel BL, Billson FA (1982): Ophthalmological examination of the infant. Developmental aspects. *Surv Ophthalmol* 26:177–189.

Hrbek A, Karlberg P, Olsson T (1973): Development of visual and somatosensory evoked responses in preterm newborn infants. *Electroencephalogr Clin Neurophysiol* 34:225–232.

Jabbari B, Maitland CG, Morris LM, Morales J, Gunderson CH (1985): The value of visual evoked potential as screening test in neurofibromatosis. *Arch Neurol* 42:1072–1074.

Kurtzberg D, Vaughan HG (1986): Preterm and post-term regional maturation of flash and pattern ERPs. In: *Maturation of the CNS and Evoked Potentials,* edited by V Gallai, pp 9–15. Elsevier Science Publishers, Amsterdam.

Marg E, Freeman DN, Peltzman P, Goldstein PJ (1976): Visual acuity development in human infants: evoked potential measurements. *Invest Ophthalmol* 15:150–153.

Markand ON, Garg BP, DeMyer WE, Warren C, Worth RM (1982): Brain stem auditory, visual and somatosensory evoked potentials in leukodystrophies. *Electroencephalogr Clin Neurophysiol* 54:39–48.

Matsubara K, Suzuki K, Itoh M, Ohta S, Maeoka Y, Inagaki M, Ohno K (1990): Retrobulbar optic neuritis in a two-year old boy. *Brain Dev* 12:795–797.

McCulloch DL, Skarf B (1991): Development of the human visual system: monocular and binocular pattern VEP latency. *Invest Ophthalmol Vis Sci* 32:2372–2381.

McCulloch DL, Taylor MJ, Whyte HE (1991): Visual evoked potentials and visual prognosis following perinatal asphyxia. *Arch Ophthalmol* 109:229–233.

Moskowitz A, Sokol S (1983): Developmental changes in the human visual system as reflected by the latency of the pattern reversal VEP. *Electroencephalogr Clin Neurophysiol* 56:1–15.

Moskowitz A, Sokol S, Hansen V (1987): Rapid assessment of visual function in pediatric patients using pattern VEPs and acuity cards. *Clin Vision Sci* 2:11–20.

Mushin J, Hogg CR, Dubowitz LMS, Skouteli H, Arden GB (1984): Visual evoked responses to light emitting diode (LED) photostimulation in newborn infants. *Electroencephalogr Clin Neurophysiol* 58:317–320.

Muttitt SC, Taylor MJ, Kobayashi JS, MacMillan L, Whyte HE (1991): Serial visual evoked potentials and outcome in term birth asphyxia. *Pediatr Neurol* 7:86–90.

North K, Cochineas C, Tang E, Fagan E (1994): Optic gliomas in neurofibromatosis type I: role of visual evoked potentials. *Pediatr Neurol* 10:117–123.

Perretti A, Petrillo A, Pelosi L, Balbi P, Parenti G, Riemma A, Strisciuglio P (1990): Detection of early abnormalities in the mucopolysaccharidoses by the use of visual and brainstem auditory evoked potentials. *Neuropediatrics* 21:83–86.

Pryds O, Trojaborg W, Carlsen J, Jensen J (1989): Determinants of visual evoked potentials in preterm infants. *Early Hum Dev* 19:117–125.

Seth V, Khosia PK, Semwal OP, D'Monty V (1991): Visual evoked responses in tuberculous children on ethambutal therapy. *Indian Pediatr* 28:713–717.

Shors TJ, Erikseon KJ, Wright KW (1987): Superimposition of a cartoon program as an aid in recording pattern visual evoked potentials in children. *J Pediatr Ophthalmol Strabismus* 24:224–227.

Sklar FH, Ehle AL, Clark WK (1979): Visual evoked potentials: a noninvasive technique to monitor patients with shunted hydrocephalus. *Neurosurgery* 4:529–534.

Sokol S (1978): Measurment of infant visual acuity from pattern reversal evoked potentials. *Vision Res* 18:33–39.

Sokol S (1986a): Alternatives to Snellen acuity testing in pediatric patients. *Am Orthoptic J* 36:5–10.

Sokol S (1986b): Visual evoked potentials. In: *Electrodiagnosis in Clinical Neurology,* edited by MJ Aminoff, pp 441–466. Churchill Livingstone, New York.

Sokol S (1986c): Clinical applications of the ERG and VEP in the pediatric age group. In: *Evoked Potentials,* edited by RQ Cracco, and I Bodis-Wollner, pp 447–454. Alan R. Liss, New York.

Sokol S, Jones K (1979): Implicit time of pattern evoked potentials in infants: an index of maturation of spatial vision. *Vision Res* 19:747–755.

Sokol S, Hansen VC, Moskowitz A, Greenfield P, Towle VL (1983): Evoked potential and preferential looking estimates of visual acuity in pediatric patients. *Opthalmology* 90:552–562.

Stanley OH, Fleming PJ, Morgan MH (1987): Developmental wave form analysis of the neonatal flash evoked potential. *Electroencephalogr Clin Neurophysiol* 68:149–152.

Taylor MJ, Farrell EJ (1987): Latency, morphological and distributional changes in VEPs with various stimuli. *Can J Neurol Sci* 14:244.

Taylor MJ, Farrell EJ (1989): A comparison of VEPs and SEPs as prognostic indicators in comatose children. *Pediatr Neurol* 5:145–150.

Taylor MJ, Logan WJ (1983): Multimodal electrophysiological assessment of ataxia telangiectasia. *Can J Neurol Sci* 10:261–265.

Taylor MJ, McCulloch DL (1991): Prognostic value of VEPs in young children with acute onset of cortical blindness. *Pediatr Neurol* 7:111–115.

Taylor MJ. McCulloch DL (1992): Visual evoked potentials in infants and children. *J Clin Neurophysiol* 9:357–372.

Taylor MJ, Chan-Lui WY, Logan WJ (1985): Longitudinal evoked potentials in the hereditary ataxias. *Can J Neurol Sci* 12:100–105.

Taylor MJ, Keenan NK, Gallant T, Skarf B, Freedman MH, Logan WJ (1987): Subclinical VEP abnormalities in patients on chronic deferoxamine therapy: longitudinal studies. *Electroencephalogr Clin Neurophysiol* 68:81–87.

Taylor MJ, Menzies R, MacMillan LJ, Whyte HE (1987): VEPs in normal full-term and premature neonates: longitudinal versus cross-sectional data. *Electroencephalogr Clin Neurophysiol* 68:20–27.

Taylor MJ, Murphy WJ, Whyte HE (1992): Prognostic reliability of somatosensory and visual evoked potentials of asphyxiated term infants. *Dev Med Child Neurol* 34:507–515.

Verity CM, Morgan H, Mott M, Oakhill A (1990): Do visual evoked potentials detect neural damage in children treated for cancer? *Dev Med Child Neurol* 27: 223–225.

Whyte HE (1993): Visual-evoked potentials in neonates following asphyxia. *Clin Perinatol* 20:451–461.

Whyte HE, Taylor MJ, Menzies R, Chin KC, MacMillan LJ (1986): Prognostic utility of visual evoked potentials in term asphyxiated neonates. *Pediatr Neurol* 2:220–223.

Whyte HE, Pearce JM, Taylor MJ (1987): Changes in the VEP in preterm neonates with arousal states as assessed by EEG monitoring. *Electroencephalogr Clin Neurophysiol* 68:223–225.

Wright KW, Eriksen J, Shors TJ, Ary JP (1986): Recording pattern visual evoked potentials under chloral hydrate sedation. *Arch Ophthalmol* 104:718–721.

Evoked Potentials in Clinical Medicine,
3d ed., edited by Keith H. Chiappa.
Lippincott–Raven Publishers, Philadelphia © 1997.

5

Brain Stem Auditory Evoked Potentials: Methodology

Keith H. Chiappa

Department of Neurology, Harvard Medical School, and EEG Laboratory, Massachusetts General Hospital, Boston, Massachusetts 02114

1. EQUIPMENT

1.1. Stimulator Features

The preferred stimulus for clinical neurologic investigation of the cochlear (eighth) nerve and brain stem auditory pathways is a click, produced by delivering an electrical square wave of 100 to 200 μsec duration to an audiologic earphone. (See Section 8.1.2 for a discussion of the sound characteristics of the click.) The intensity of the click is varied according to a decibel (log) scale and appropriate stimulator controls are necessary to accomplish this, with smallest steps of 5 dB. Maximum intensity necessary is 110 to 130 peak equivalent sound pressure level (peSPL). Peak equivalent sound pressure level is a standard measure of the "loudness" of a sound and is determined with sound level meters (see following). Stimulus presentation rate should be selectable from 0.5 to 100/sec. The initial movement of the earphone diaphragm is either away from the tympanic membrane (rarefaction click) or toward it (condensation click). The polarity of the click (rarefaction or condensation) affects both latency and shape of the brain stem auditory evoked potential (BAEP) waveforms (see Section 8.1.4), so it must be known. This is particularly bothersome when constructing a stimulator since earphones may be wired "backwards" by the original manufacturers. Commercial auditory stimulators have usually been calibrated for this factor and it is difficult to check without special equipment (see Section 1.2). Although a single click polarity is usually used for obtaining BAEPs, alternating click polarity may be used occasionally to diminish stimulus artifact, or to differentiate wave I from cochlear microphonics (the latter reverse polarity with inversion of click polarity, whereas the former does not), so that this is a useful capability in an auditory stimulator. White noise must be available for masking the unstimulated ear because monaural testing is most commonly used and loud clicks may cross-stimulate the opposite ear and produce confusing waveforms. It must be possible to control the white-noise intensity on a decibel scale and switch the click and white noise from ear to ear without disturbing the patient. Brain stem auditory EPs may also be used to approximate the behavioral audiogram, and in that application frequency-specific stimuli are needed. Presently in use are (1) tone pips which possess a more focused sound pressure wave frequency content and (2) filtered white noise mixed with the clicks or pips (see Section 9). Thus, the ability to produce (1) tone pips and bursts of a variety of frequencies (500, 1,000, 2,000, and 4,000 Hz at a minimum) with variable rise, plateau, and fall times (e.g., 2, 1, 2 cycles) and (2) white noise that can be notch or high- and low-pass filtered at steep slopes (24 to 48 dB/octave) and mixed with the clicks or pips are functions in an auditory stimulator that might prove useful if audiologic investigations will be performed. Cognitive EPs are currently under intensive investigation with respect to their possible clinical utility, especially in dementia. The modality most commonly used is auditory, and thus it should be possible to externally control the stimulator so that tone frequency can be altered automatically to generate the required sequence of frequent and rare ("oddball") stimuli. Electrical shielding of the earphone (usually with μ-metal) and patient comfort are considerations. The coupling or "fit" of the earphones affects the frequency and intensity characteristics of the sound delivered to the ear (Coats and Kidder, 1980), so that a consistent system must be used. Infant recordings require the use of earphones which do not cause external ear canal collapse; a hand-held single earpiece is the simplest solution (Starr et al., 1977; Schulman-Galambos and Galambos, 1979; Marshall et al., 1980; Picton et al., 1986). Vestibular nerve testing (Elidan et al., 1984) remains a research endeavor.

1.2. Stimulator Calibration

Earphones and stimulating equipment are calibrated using sound-level meters. These are used with an artificial ear to simulate actual conditions. The meter reads directly in decibels and it may be necessary to compare the sound of interest to a reference signal. If clicks are being calibrated, it is useful to have a meter option that allows it to hold the peak value recorded (peak hold module), since the click is a very brief signal. Many audiology laboratories have such equipment and the manufacturer supplying the EP device may provide a calibration service. It is suggested that the earphones be calibrated at least every 6 months. However, note that the relationship between the sound output of the earphone and the amount of cochlear basilar membrane (i.e., neural) stimulation is dependent on so many subject variables (shape of external canal, amount of cerumen in external canal, state of tympanic membrane, mechanical properties of ossicles and oval window, to name a few) that a slavish attendance to earphone calibration is, to a great extent, unnecessary. This is especially true when BAEPs are used primarily for neurologic applications where interpeak separations, which are largely un-affected by changes in stimulus intensity, are used for interpretive purposes.

1.3. Stimulus Intensity Measures

Apparent intensity of a sound is related to its frequency, since hearing sensitivity varies with frequency. Stimulus intensity can be defined in any one of four ways. There are minor differences between these but, for most clinical purposes, any one can be derived from any other given properly calibrated instruments, and there is no real difference between them. (1) The base standard scale, dB SPL, is the root mean square pressure of a sound relative to the lowest intensity sound that can be heard by the most sensitive ear [in absolute terms about 20 microPascals (μPa)]. Peak SPL is the maximum sound intensity. (2) Peak equivalent sound pressure level (peSPL) is the intensity of a long-duration sound that has the same amplitude as the peak SPL of a short-duration sound whose intensity is the measure desired. This is deter-mined by using a sound-level meter, often with comparison made to a reference. The maxi-mum intensity sound which can be safely delivered to an ear for extended periods of time is about 110 to 120 dB peSPL, according to government standards. In audiologic practice, inten-sities up to 130 dB peSPL may be used for brief periods. Many auditory stimulators will not deliver more than 105 dB peSPL or so, and thus are much less likely to cause damage. (3) The scale relative to normal hearing level for a particular stimulus is dB HL (sometimes referred to as dB NHL). This is based on the average hearing threshold for that stimulus of a group of normal-hearing subjects. For example, with a particular stimulator and stimulus, a group of such subjects might have an average click hearing threshold (the intensity level at which they can just barely hear the click) of 20 dB peSPL (the normal hearing threshold is about 30 dB peSPL). (This value, even with the same subject, may change slightly between different stim-ulators and earphones.) Zero dB HL is then defined as the normal group's average threshold. If another subject or patient is stimulated at 60 dB peSPL, when the threshold of the normals was 20 dB peSPL, the stimulus intensity is (60 −20) 40 dB HL. (4) Another relative stimulus intensity scale is dB sensation level (SL). Here the click hearing threshold for the specific ear wearing the earphone is determined. This is 0 dB SL (for that ear only). If the threshold was 30 dB peSPL and the stimulus intensity applied during BAEP testing is 90 dB peSPL, then the stimulus intensity is (90 – 30) 60 dB SL. Note that SL is applicable to that one ear only.

2. PRETEST INSTRUCTIONS

2.1. Medical History

The technologist should extract pertinent clinical information from the medical record and/or history of the patient. The clinical examination of brain stem function, the audio-gram and results of electronystagmography (ENG) are of particular importance in consider-ations of clinical correlations.

2.2. Conventional Audiometry

In neurologic applications, a conventional audiogram is generally only helpful in inter-pretation of BAEPs when (1) wave I (eighth nerve activation potential) is absent or (2) am-plitude ratios (waves I:V) are being used. Interpeak latencies, the sole measures used for in-terpretation in most cases, are not altered enough by audiogram shape to affect neurologic interpretations (see Section 8.2.4). However, in those occasional cases in which wave I cannot be registered, the audiogram can help to correlate absolute (stimulus to peak) latencies with the degree of hearing loss to allow making a judgment as to whether or not a prolongation of latency is consistent with a peripheral etiology. If the prolongation is greater than that expected from the degree of hearing loss present, then a retrocochlear lesion is suggested. If amplitude ratios are being used for interpretive purposes, a normal audiogram is important because the ratios change with changes in stimulus intensity.

2.3. Determination of Click Hearing Threshold

Knowledge of the click hearing threshold is helpful because it provides an indication of the stimulus intensity necessary to produce good BAEP waveform resolution. Click threshold is the intensity at which the subject can barely hear the clicks. It is determined (1) by decreasing intensity in 5-dB steps until the subject can no longer hear the clicks, and (2) by then increasing intensity in 5-dB steps until the clicks can be heard. Click threshold is taken as the midpoint between the intensities at which the clicks can and cannot be heard. This maneuver may be repeated a few times to ensure reliability. A typical use of this threshold value would be to increase stimulus intensity 65 or 70 dB above it (this would then be a stimulus intensity of 65 or 70 dB SL for that ear) and do the initial BAEP testing at that intensity. This provides a stimulus which will most likely generate BAEP waves of good amplitude and clarity for neurologic interpretations.

3. ELECTRODE APPLICATION

With the patient seated in a chair, electrodes are applied in appropriate positions. (See Section 5 for electrode locations used in BAEP testing.) Any conventional EEG technique may be used for attaching the electrodes to the scalp. (See Chapter 2, Section 3 for a discussion of recommended techniques.)

3.1. Surface Versus Needle Electrodes

Needle electrodes are completely satisfactory for recording BAEPs and are recommended in comatose patients. There is no significant difference in latencies or amplitudes when BAEPs are recorded simultaneously with needle and surface electrodes. (See also Chapter 1, Section 2.1.) Needles are not recommended (1) in monitoring situations, such as the intensive care unit, because of the risk of infection, and (2) in operating room monitoring, unless firmly anchored, because they tend to fall out easily. Technologists must take care not to stick themselves with the needle, and it is our practice to discard the needles after use. The electrodes are then plugged into the proper positions on the electrode board which connects them to the amplifiers and the averager. Impedance must be maintained below 5,000 ohms. Note, however, that needle electrodes usually have a slightly higher impedance than this.

3.2. Special External Ear Canal Electrodes

In neurologic applications of BAEPs, interpeak separations are the only latency parameters used for interpretive purposes, except in special circumstances. These time differences are related to the state of conduction in eighth nerve and brain stem auditory pathways.

Since wave I is generated primarily by activity in the eighth nerve close to the cochlea, it provides a reference point for latency measurements; conduction times between wave I and later waves (III and V) accurately represent the state of conduction in those segments of the auditory pathway. With good resolution of wave I, changes in stimulus intensity and pathology of the middle ear and cochlea can be largely ignored. Thus, clear registration of wave I is integral to clinical neurologic interpretation of BAEPs. However, an occasional patient with normal hearing and some patients with varying degrees of hearing loss (especially in high frequencies) do not have a wave I that can be recorded easily from earlobe or mastoid electrode locations. The degree of the hearing loss and audiogram shape are not always reliable indicators of whether or not a wave I can be recorded. Conversely, the combination of a near-normal click hearing threshold and absent or difficult-to-record wave I almost always indicates a high-frequency hearing loss. This is because most of wave I is generated by the high-frequency components of the click (which are absent), whereas the normal click recognition threshold is produced by lower-frequency components (Fig. 5–1). Various tech-

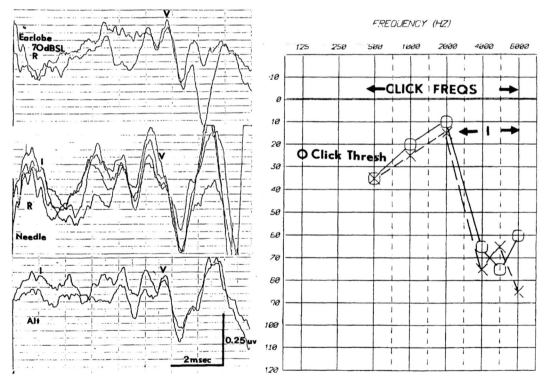

FIG. 5–1. Brain stem auditory EPs and pure-tone audiogram in a patient with a low-amplitude wave I. Rarefaction clicks at 70 dB SL (*upper channel*) show no recognizable wave I. An external ear canal needle electrode with rarefaction clicks (*middle channel*) revealed a presumed wave I (*at I*) but also cochlear microphonics. Use of alternating click polarity (with the needle electrode) to cancel the cochlear microphonics showed a low-amplitude wave I (*lower channel at I*). The click hearing threshold in this ear (*O on audiogram*) was only slightly elevated, corresponding to the near-normal hearing levels from 500 to 2000 Hz, but there was a 40- to 50-dB hearing loss in the high tones (4,000 to 5,000 Hz), the frequencies primarily responsible for wave I generation. Each trace is the average of 500 stimuli. Earlobe or needle electrode was referred to vertex.

niques have been used to record the eighth nerve activation potential in these circumstances, including promontory recordings as performed in electrocochleography (e.g., Morrison et al., 1976) and other methods of placing electrodes close to the tympanic membrane in the external canal (Coats, 1974; Montandon et al., 1975a; Montandon, 1976; Stone et al., 1986). These require varying degrees of technical skill, may be quite uncomfortable for the patient, and may not provide satisfactory results. Another technique, utilized successfully in our laboratory (Chiappa et al., 1980; Chiappa, 1980b, 1983; Goldie et al., 1981; Chiappa and Parker, 1984) is fast, simple, and minimally uncomfortable, and results in registration of wave I in more than three quarters of those patients who have no wave I recorded from the earlobe or mastoid locations. A conventional, small, thin-wire, sterile electroencephalography (EEG) needle electrode is used. The easily visible portion of the anterior wall of the external auditory canal (EAC) (viewing from behind the ear with an ordinary flashlight) is cleaned with a cotton swab moistened with alcohol. The needle is held so that its hub lies flat on the pinna with the tip pointing at the cleansed anterior wall of the EAC, wire extending backwards (Fig. 5–2). The patient is warned to expect a pin-prick and the needle point is jabbed 2 to 3 mm into the anterior wall of the EAC. Electrode impedance is usually around 5,000 ohms. A towel roll is sometimes placed under the lower edge of the earphone to support it away from the needle. The electrode is well-tolerated and records very little stimulus artifact. Figure 5–3 shows a patient who had no wave I visible from the earlobe (panel B), whereas a large, clear wave I is seen with the EAC recording (panels C

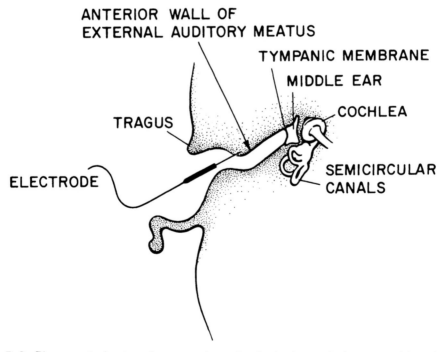

FIG. 5–2. Placement of external ear canal needle electrode used when wave I is not registered from the conventional earlobe site. Top view of horizontal section through ear and external canal showing relative positions of needle, wire, external canal, tympanic membrane and cochlea. (From Chiappa and Parker, 1984, with permission.)

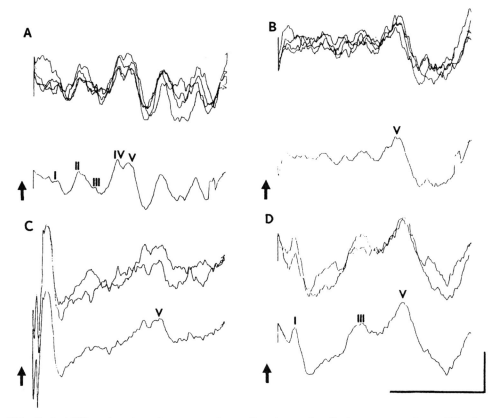

FIG. 5–3. Utility of external ear canal needle electrode. Brain stem auditory EPs from monaural stimulation of each ear of a patient with an acoustic neuroma. **A** is the unaffected AS showing the normal waveforms, labelled I through V, although I is often seen as a more discrete peak than is the case here. **B, C,** and **D** are all from the affected ear (AD). **B** was obtained by conventional recording from the earlobe (and vertex)—note the absence of all waves except V. **C** was obtained by recording from a needle electrode in the external ear canal—note the large stimulus artifact which partially obscures wave I. In **A, B,** and **C** click polarity was constant, whereas in **D** click polarity was alternated—note loss of stimulus artifact which leaves wave I as a discrete peak. Both the I–V and I–III separations are markedly abnormal, suggesting a lesion between peripheral eighth nerve and lower pons; the CT scan was normal but a posterior fossa contrast study showed a tumor, and a 15-mm acoustic neuroma was found at surgery. The superimposed trials have 1,024 clicks each; the single trace below each set of superimposed trials is the average of the superimposed trials. The recording derivation was earlobe ipsilateral to monaural stimulation referred to vertex (CZ); relative positivity of the vertex is an upward trace deflection. The calibration marks are 5 msec and 0.25 μV. (From Chiappa, 1980, with permission.)

and D). The abnormal I–V separation prompted a posterior fossa contrast study despite a normal computed tomography (CT) scan, and a 15-mm acoustic neuroma was found.

4. AMPLIFIER AND AVERAGER CONTROLS

Different makes of equipment require somewhat different setup procedures for a given EP, and some systems need less operator action than others. Also, it is not always possible either to find the same settings as suggested below (use the closest you can find) or even to ascertain at what values a given piece of equipment is operating (e.g., what total amplification the system is producing). The manufacturer's suggested settings are usually reasonably good and can be used.

Brain stem auditory EPs are best recorded by using an amplification of 200,000 to 500,000. The filters are 50 to 150 Hz low cutoff (high pass) and 3,000 Hz high cutoff (low pass) (see Section 8.1.6 for further discussion). The averager is set for a total sweep duration of 10 to 12 msec. Each channel should be sampled with a maximum intersample inter-

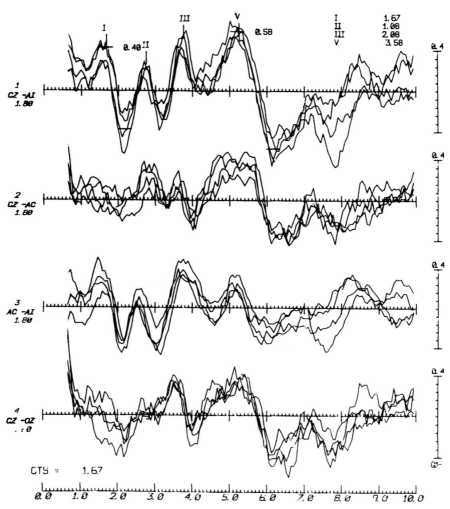

FIG. 5–4. Brain stem auditory EPs recorded from a normal subject using most commonly employed derivations. Note the absence of wave I, lower amplitude and shorter latency of wave III, and shorter latency of wave IV (although its resolution is poor) in the Cz–Ac derivation compared with the conventional Cz–Ai derivation. The Ac–Ai derivation shows wave I about the same as Cz–Ai, but wave V appears to be absent (the wave present has a latency closer to IV than V). In the Cz–inion derivation (*bottom trace*) waves I and II are absent and wave V is not as well-defined as in the Cz–Ai derivation. Each trace is the average of 1,024 clicks, with four separate trials superimposed.

val (dwell time) of 0.1 msec (100 μsec). Note that averager and human interpolation between these points allow latency measurements to a greater accuracy than this interval. The automatic sweep repetition control should be set to 1,000. It will be necessary sometimes to continue to 2,000 sweep repetitions if the patient is "noisy" or the responses are unclear for other reasons (abnormally low amplitude). With a great deal of experience, the waveforms can be examined after 500 stimulus repetitions and, if they are of sufficient clarity, that trial can be deemed complete. Another should then be performed and superimposed (see Section 6.9). The overlapped trials should be examined and reliability estimated from the difference between them. Trials should be repeated until the degree of variability is known. An example of a normal BAEP test performed in this manner is shown in Fig. 5–4.

5. CHANNELS TO RECORD

The electrical activity recorded at the scalp following a click stimulus is generated in the cochlear nerve, pons, and midbrain. The electrical potential field spreads through the conducting medium of the brain, meninges, spinal fluid, skull bone, and scalp at close to the speed of light and appears at the scalp as a potential difference between different areas. Thus, despite the distance between generator and recording sites, there is no appreciable time delay involved in the registration of the activity at the scalp.

The action potential volley in the cochlear nerve (wave I) appears at and around the ear as a negativity. The other waves (II through V) appear at all scalp locations, including the ear, as positivities (see Section 8.1.8 for further details). Thus, if one records from the earlobe using a noncephalic derivation, all waves can be seen, but wave I points in an opposite direction from waves II through V. This is not a useful recording derivation for BAEPs because (1) waves III through V are usually better recorded from the vertex than from the ear, and (2) the noncephalic electrode contributes a great deal of muscle artifact, which makes it much more difficult to obtain good resolution of BAEP waveforms. Since waves II through V are of good amplitude at the vertex and there is little muscle artifact present at that site, the vertex is a good location for one of the recording electrodes. The location of the other electrode is governed by two requirements: (1) wave I amplitude must be at a maximum, and (2) there must be as little ambient muscle artifact present as possible. Wave I amplitude has been shown to be maximum on average at the earlobe, rather than at mastoid locations (Stockard et al., 1978b), and the earlobe has less muscle artifact than does the mastoid. Therefore, the BAEP recording montage most commonly used is a bipolar, earlobe-to-vertex linkage.

There is some enthusiasm for recording a second channel, earlobe contralateral to the ear being stimulated referred to the vertex (Stockard et al., 1978b). This channel characteristically has no wave I negativity and waves IV and V tend to be separated rather than fused. Thus, this recording channel may provide some assistance in waveform recognition (see below). However, we have found the maneuver of decreasing click intensity to be of much greater utility in waveform recognition. In any case, since most averaging systems have two channels, there is no reason not to record the contralateral channel.

Studies of wave I potential-field distribution have suggested that it may be enhanced by recording from one earlobe to the other. Although this may be a useful recording derivation in infants and children, as can be seen in Fig. 5–4, we have not found it helpful in adults. Again, if extra channels are available, there is no reason not to record this channel.

In special circumstances other recording derivations are used. For example, when the binaural interaction waveform is recorded, instead of using an electrode on the earlobe ipsilateral to the ear being stimulated, an electrode in the region of the inion (in the midline) is used (Fig. 5–4). The ears are stimulated monaurally and the waveforms from the two tests summed and subtracted from the waveform obtained with binaural stimulation. The difference is the binaural interaction waveform (see Section 8.1.5 for a more detailed discussion of this).

Although only one channel is essential to BAEP clinical interpretation (channel 1 below), it is easy to record the "interesting" channels mentioned above since most EP systems have a four-channel capability. Thus, the recommended four-channel montage for recording BAEPs is:

Channel 1: Ai–Cz
Channel 2: Ac–Cz
Channel 3: Ai–Ac
Channel 4: Inion–Cz

Ai and Ac refer to earlobe ipsilateral and contralateral to the ear being stimulated, respectively. In this montage, relative positivity of G2 is assumed to produce an upward trace deflection. The unnecessary channels (2, 3, and 4) may be omitted. Figure 5–4 shows a normal subject recorded using this four-channel montage.

6. RUNNING THE TEST

6.1. Subject Relaxation

The test must be performed with the patient supine on a bed with pillows and towels available for head propping to minimize neck muscle tone. The room should be reasonably quiet and sound attenuated. Unless hearing threshold determinations are being done routinely, the room need not be soundproof. The signal-averaging apparatus should be outside the room with a closed door between the averager and the patient. This allows test results to be plotted and discussed without arousing the patient, who, hopefully, has fallen asleep during the test. It is also very helpful if the electrode selection and stimulator controls are outside the room so that no entry is necessary during the test.

The most common problem encountered with the test is excessive muscle activity. If head propping in various ways does not solve this, other factors must be considered: Is the patient too cold or hot? Does the patient need to go to the bathroom? Is the supine position too uncomfortable (lying on the side may help)? Are the earphones uncomfortable? If the problem persists despite consideration of these factors, a mild hypnotic may be given (chloral hydrate, diphenhydramine, or benzodiazepine, or combination) to induce drowsiness and sleep. Note that the patient should not drive immediately following hypnotic/sedative use, and this may make their use impractical in unaccompanied outpatients. In the most difficult cases it may be necessary to plan the study as for an EEG sleep study; the patient is instructed to stay up 2 hours later at night than normal, take no stimulants with breakfast, and have the study in the morning.

6.2. Stimulus Intensity

When BAEPs are performed for a neurologic application, click intensity is set initially at 65 dB (SL or HL) or greater. Since waveform resolution is usually poor with low stimulus intensities, there is no advantage to starting at lower intensities. If the waveforms of interest are not clearly defined, click intensity is increased 10 dB or more, often with better peak resolution.

However, when waveform resolution is poor, it may be as helpful to decrease click intensity as it is to increase it (Chiappa, 1984) (Fig. 5–5). Figure 5–6A shows results from a patient with a click threshold of 30 dB HL, initially tested at 60 dB SL (90 dB HL—maximum for the stimulator). Wave I is not clearly defined and the differentiation of waves V and VI is difficult. Figure 5–6B shows the results obtained by decreasing click intensity 15 dB. All waves become well-defined and an abnormal I–III separation is easily seen. A 15-mm acoustic neuroma was present. Presumably, the utility of this maneuver is related to the fact that higher click intensities stimulate more of the cochlear basilar membrane. Since the traveling wave generated by the sound takes 2 to 6 msec to traverse the entire cochlea, a set of waves may be generated from each area of the basilar membrane, separated in time by a few milliseconds. This would result in peak prolongation and dispersion, and perhaps multiple peaks. This may account for the occasional "bifid" appearance of wave III, and peaks identified as wave VI may sometimes be another wave V. Diminished click intensity lessens this effect. Also, waves II, IV, and VI are more susceptible to loss of amplitude from decreased click intensity, and these are the waves used least often in clinical interpretation. Their removal may also clarify the responses for interpretation.

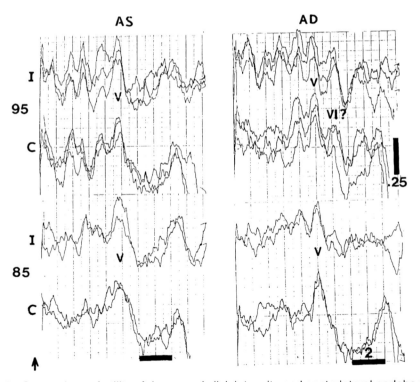

FIG. 5–5. Comparison of utility of decreased click intensity and contralateral earlobe recording in wave V identification. At high click intensity (*top two channels*, 95 = 80 dB HL) in the right ear (*right panel—*AD) there is some uncertainty about wave V recognition since the presumed wave VI (VI?) has a configuration similar to wave V. The earlobe contralateral (C) to the stimulus shows waveforms very similar to those recorded from the ipsilateral (I) earlobe and so is not helpful. With the stimulus intensity decreased 10 dB (*bottom two channels*) the presumed wave VI disappears and there is no doubt about wave V location. Each trace is the average of 500 stimuli.

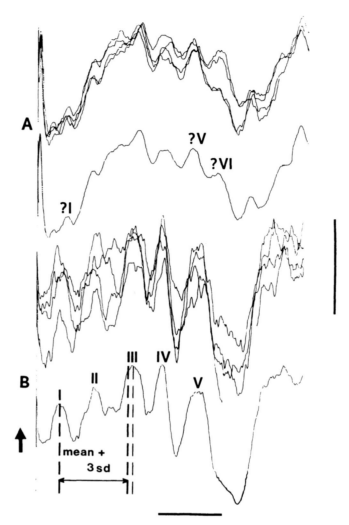

FIG. 5–6. Utility of decreasing click intensity. BAEPs recorded from the left ear of a patient with a 15-mm acoustic neuroma. Pure tone audiogram was 10, 45, 50, 55, and 60 dB down at 500, 1,000, 2,000, 4,000, and 8,000 Hz, with speech discrimination 48%. **A** was recorded at 60 dB SL, **B** at 45 dB SL. Note poor resolution of wave I and difficulty of differentiating waves V and VI at this (higher) click intensity. With reduced click intensity (B) the peaks become distinct and easily recognizable. Wave VI has disappeared. The I–III latency separation is abnormal, contrast-enhanced CT scan was normal, and an acoustic neuroma was found. Each superimposed trace is the average of 1,024 clicks, the line below each is the grand average of the four separate trials. Click rate 10/sec, filter band-pass 100 to 3,000 Hz. Vertex to ipsilateral earlobe with relative positivity of vertex producing an upward deflection. Calibration marks are 2.5 msec, 0.4 and 0.2 μV for A and B. (From Chiappa, 1982, with permission.)

6.3. Monaural Stimulation

The stimulus is applied to one ear at a time, since many BAEP abnormalities are seen following stimulation of only one ear, the other ear producing perfectly normal results. For example, in multiple sclerosis (MS), almost half of the patients with abnormal BAEPs have an

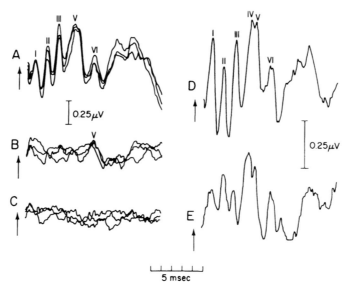

FIG. 5–7. Brain stem auditory EPs recorded from a subject with one nonfunctioning ear showing cross-stimulation and hiding effect of binaural stimulation. Panels **A, B,** and **C** were obtained with monaural stimulation; each trace is the sum of 1,024 responses. Panel **A** was obtained by stimulating and recording from the good ear; panels **B** and **C** were obtained by stimulating and recording from the nonfunctioning ear, panel **B** without masking the good ear (wave V present), panel **C** with masking of the good ear (no wave V can be seen). Panels **D** and **E** were obtained with binaural stimulation; lines are the sum of 3,072 responses. Panel **D** was recorded from the good ear and panel **E** from the nonfunctioning ear (all waves are clearly recognizable). Amplitude calibrations were equal in panels **A** through **C**; panels **D** and **E** were equal and were displayed at twice amplification used in **A** through **C**. (From Chiappa et al., 1979, with permission.)

abnormality in only one ear (Chiappa et al., 1980; Prasher and Gibson, 1980). If binaural stimulation is used, the normal waveforms generated by the "good" ear mask the abnormality in the "bad" ear. For example, Fig. 5–7 (panels D and E) shows normal recordings obtained from both the normal and nonfunctioning ear with binaural stimulation. The only use for binaural stimulation in BAEP testing is for derivation of the binaural interaction waveform. See further discussion of stimulus mode in Section 8.1.5.

6.4. Click Rate

Because BAEP waveform amplitudes are so low, it is necessary to use 1,000 or more stimulus repetitions to ensure waveform clarity. The faster the stimulus rate, the less time is taken in performing the test. However, there is a progressive loss in waveform resolution with rates much above 10/sec (see Table 5–5), so that rate is the preferred one. Faster rates only very rarely reveal abnormalities not evident at slower rates. See Section 8.1.3 for further discussion.

In some audiologic applications (e.g., screening at-risk infants for hearing deficits), the data sought are (1) the lowest stimulus intensity at which wave V can be recognized, and (2) the slope of the curve produced by plotting wave V absolute latency at several stimulus intensities. In these two situations, the information can be effectively generated by using fast click rates (70–90/sec) (Picton et al., 1986).

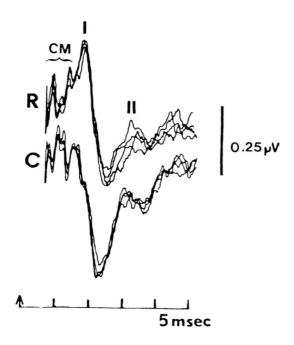

FIG. 5–8. Earlobe recordings in a normal subject following click stimulation (C, condensation, R, rarefaction clicks) showing relationship among click polarity, wave I, and cochlear microphonics. Note the small latency and shape changes in waves I and II with the change in click polarity (wave I peak 0.3 msec earlier and the appearance of a step in the wave I downslope with condensation clicks). The series of small peaks preceding wave I are cochlear microphonics which all reverse polarity with the change in click phase. Each trace is the average of 1,024 stimuli with four separate series superimposed.

6.5. Click Polarity

Different click polarities (rarefaction or condensation) produce many minor changes in BAEP waveforms of normal subjects. Wave I amplitude tends to be greater with rarefaction clicks (Stockard et al., 1978a) and, since recognition of this wave is critical to the clinical neurologic interpretation of the test, that click polarity is usually employed. If waveform

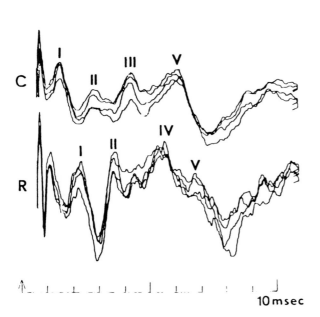

FIG. 5–9. Effect of changing click polarity in some patients with peripheral hearing loss. Brain stem auditory EPs recorded from a patient with a moderate peripheral hearing loss. Note the marked change in waveform latencies and shape with change in click phase. Initially it might appear that wave I has inverted polarity but remained at the same latency when clicks were changed from rarefaction to condensation, but wave I has actually prolonged its latency by 0.8 msec. Recordings from Cz–Ai with each trace the average of 1,024 responses; four separate series are superimposed in each set. Calibration marks: condensation, 0.5 µV; rarefaction, 0.25 µV.

resolution is poor, the opposite polarity can be tried. Occasionally, recognition of wave I will be difficult and the possibility of cochlear microphonics being erroneously identified as wave I can be resolved by switching to the opposite click polarity. Cochlear microphonics reverse polarity when stimulus polarity is reversed, whereas wave I does not (Fig. 5–8). A confusing element here is that in subjects with hearing loss a change in click polarity may result in a latency shift of wave I sufficient to make it appear that wave I reversed polarity (Fig. 5–9). This seems to be especially true with high-tone hearing losses, as was the case in this patient, who had a normal pure tone audiogram at 2,000 Hz, but a 40-dB loss at 4,000 and 8,000 Hz, with normal speech discrimination in both ears.

In rare cases where stimulus artifact or cochlear microphonics are excessive (see Fig. 5–3), alternating click polarity can cancel the unwanted activity. This is not recommended on a routine basis because the different peak locations generated by the small latency shifts seen with the different click polarities will sum to produce composite wave peaks of longer duration than those generated by a single click polarity. This renders peak localization for latency determinations more difficult.

See Section 8.1.4 for a discussion of polarity-specific BAEP abnormalities in patients.

6.6. Contralateral White-Noise Masking

The click stimulates not only the ipsilateral ear but also travels by bone and air conduction to stimulate the contralateral ear at an intensity 40 to 50 dB less than that delivered to the ipsilateral ear. Thus, even if the stimulated ear is nonfunctional, BAEP waveforms can be recorded because of the cross-stimulation of the opposite ear (see Fig. 5–7, panels B and C). When hearing is essentially normal bilaterally, this is probably not important since the ipsilateral ear potentials are earlier and of greater amplitude, and set up inhibitory influences at the level of the cochlear nuclei for the impulses coming later in time from the contralateral ear, thus blocking the incoming contralateral activity. However, where gross abnormalities of function are present, this cross-stimulation may be a confusing factor.

The contralateral ear is therefore masked with white noise at an intensity 30 to 40 dB less than that of the click stimulus.

6.7. Infant Testing

Special procedures are necessary to test infants (Picton et al., 1986; Picton and Durieux-Smith, 1988). Testing must be scheduled for a time when they will be comfortable (fed and dry) and asleep. Conventional earphones cannot be used because they may apply too much pressure to the external ear, causing the external ear canal to collapse. This results in an apparent moderate to severe conductive hearing loss. (See also Chapter 5, Section 3.11.1.) Testing is performed at 10/sec for optimum waveform resolution for assessment of central conduction, and at 50 to 70/sec for assessment of peripheral hearing. In the latter case, the lowest click intensity at which wave V can be identified (the wave V recognition threshold) is the desired information. If wave V is present at a click intensity of 30 to 35 dB above the average normal adult threshold (i.e., at 30 dB HL or NHL) this is considered normal. If there is doubt about the presence of wave V the test should be replicated and higher intensities employed, in 10-dB steps. In difficult cases it may be necessary to progressively decrease click intensity starting at a high level (60 to 70 dB HL) and follow wave V out as it increases in latency with decreasing click intensity. Note that wave V latency may exceed 10 to 12 msec at lower intensities in infants, so that it may be necessary to use a sweep duration of 20 msec. See Picton and Durieux-Smith (1988) for a further discussion of this application.

Because of the frequency of middle effusions in this age group, abnormal tests indicating a peripheral hearing deficit must be replicated after an interval of several weeks before further action is taken.

6.8. Artifact Rejection

As discussed above, the major factor interfering with registration of good BAEPs is ambient muscle artifact, and time spent diminishing this is well-repaid in clarity of results. However, there are transient bursts of artifact that cannot be anticipated and there needs to be a mechanism for excluding these from the average. On the simplest level, the technician watches the ongoing, raw EEG signal (and artifact) on a monitoring oscilloscope set for a sweep speed of 10 msec/cm with automatic triggering. Whenever excessive artifact appears on the screen, the technician manually halts averaging. There is obviously room for error here since there may be a significant lag between artifact appearance and averaging being stopped. Most averaging systems now in use have some form of automatic artifact rejection, and this should certainly be used when recording BAEPs. (See Chapter 1, Section 2.5, for a discussion of automatic artifact rejection techniques.) Recently, more advanced techniques of artifact removal have been described (see Emerson et al., 1982, Chapter XX).

6.9. Trial Repetition

It is *mandatory* in BAEP testing to repeat the first trial and superimpose it on the previous one to test waveform consistency. The overlapped trials should be examined and reliability estimated from the difference between them. Trials should be repeated until the degree of variability is known. It may be necessary to repeat the test two to four times to arrive at a good measure of response variability (e.g., Fig. 5–6, panel B). Rowe (1981) recommends that intertrial variability should be less than 0.1 to 0.2 msec for interpeak latency measurements before the test can be considered technically satisfactory. Stockard et al. (1978a) recommended 0.08 msec, but this is too stringent a level. Although at least 1,000 stimulus repetitions are usually recommended, with a great deal of experience the waveforms can be examined after 500 stimulus repetitions and, if they are of sufficient clarity, that trial can be deemed complete. At least one other should still be performed and superimposed to verify waveform reliability.

6.10. Resolution of Unclear Waveforms

When the BAEP waveforms registered using all of the above-recommended procedures are unclear for any reason, operations that can be tried are (1) increasing stimulus repetitions to 2,000; (2) performing multiple trials; (3) increasing click intensity if waveforms have low amplitude and poor definition; (4) decreasing click intensity if too many or poorly defined peaks are present; (5) switching to the opposite click polarity; and (6) use of special electrodes. These parameter modifications have been discussed in more detail above in their separate sections. Also see Chapter 1, Section 5.

7. READING THE RESULTS, NORMATIVE DATA, AND VARIATIONS

7.1. Waveform Identification

It is difficult to provide a written method for identification of BAEP waveform peaks. The following rules apply reasonably well with normal results but will be increasingly difficult to apply as the degree of abnormality increases.

1. Wave V is usually the most prominent peak after 5.5 msec. With a filter band-pass of 100 to 3,000 Hz it starts above the baseline and the immediately following trough is maximum below the baseline. With progressive decreasing of stimulus intensity wave V is the last peak visible in this area. In an abnormal BAEP with wave V absent, wave IV (if still present) has the shape of an isosceles triangle with its base sitting on the baseline; the fact that there is no subsequent trough below the baseline helps to indicate that the peak in question is not wave V (usually its absolute and postwave III latencies are too early also).

    Waves IV and V interact to present a variety of patterns (see Fig. 5–1 and Table 5–1). For purposes of latency and amplitude ratio measurements, if a consistent wave V can be identified either as a separate peak or as a step, then that point is taken to be the wave V peak. When waves IV and V are completely fused (e.g., D in Fig. 5–10), the resultant peak is taken as wave V. Recording from the contralateral ear has been suggested as an aid to the identification of wave V (Stockard et al., 1978b) because waves IV and V tend to be separated in that derivation rather than fused, as is the case with the ipsilateral ear derivation. I have found that contralateral recordings are less helpful in wave V recognition than decreasing click intensity (see Figs. 5–5 and 5–6).

2. Wave I appears more than 1.4 msec after the stimulus and, in contrast to the cochlear microphonic, does not reverse polarity with reversal of the click polarity, as discussed above. (Note, again, that hearing loss may cause a large phase shift of wave I when click polarity is reversed to give the superficial appearance of wave I changing polarity.) External ear canal recordings show the wave I peak of higher amplitude than earlobe recording sites. Decreasing click intensity leaves wave I as the last peak in this area. The wave I negative peak is absent or of very low amplitude in a vertex-to-contralateral ear derivation, so that comparison with the ipsilateral ear derivation may also help.

3. Wave III appears between waves I and V, approximately equidistant unless abnormalities are present. It is the last wave present in this area with decreasing click intensities. Contralateral recordings are suggested as helpful because wave III may be markedly attenuated in that derivation (Stockard et al., 1978b); I have not found this particularly

TABLE 5–1. *IV–V Complex patterns—frequencies of occurrence*

IV–V complex pattern	Percent of 104 ears with that pattern	Percent of subjects with both ears having same pattern
A	14	4
B	38	27
C	33	21
D	4	2
E	10	4
F	1	0
Total	100	58

See Fig. 5–8 for the IV–V complex patterns **A** through **F**. (From Chiappa et al., 1979, with permission.)

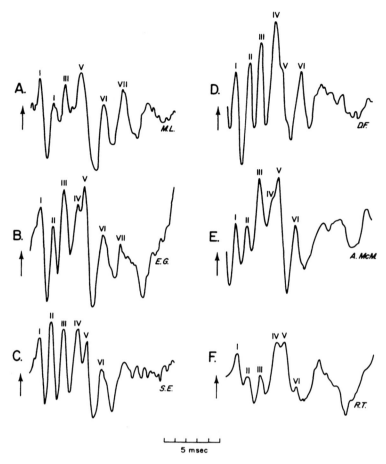

FIG. 5–10. Different shapes of the waves IV–V complex seen in normal subjects. All are normal variations; the order of most to least frequent occurrence is **B, C, A, E, D,** and **F.** Each trace is the sum of 2,048 to 4,096 responses from a single ear of a normal subject. (From Chiappa et al., 1979, with permission.)

useful. Wave III may present two peaks, in which case a midpoint may be taken for latency determinations by visual interpolation and estimation.

4. Waves II, IV, and VI are not commonly or easily used in clinical interpretations of BAEPs. Their removal by decreasing click intensity greatly facilitates identification of waves I, III, and V.

7.2. Interpeak Latencies, Interear Differences, and Amplitude Ratios

Measurements and calculations performed include (1) interpeak latencies (I–III, III–V, and I–V), (2) interear interpeak differences, and (3) amplitude ratios (I/V or I/IV–V). Only where (1) wave I cannot be registered or (2) an intensity–latency curve is being constructed (see Section 8.2.4) are the absolute latencies of waves III and V used in clinical interpretation. The clinical utility of further data analysis and manipulations (e.g., Stockard et al., 1978a; Galbraith, 1984) is uncertain. Picton et al. (1988) have suggested "dynamic time warping" of BAEPs as an automatic method of waveform identification and latency determination.

The only difficulties encountered with latency measurements are when the peaks are poorly defined. In this case, with several trials superimposed, one estimates a point at which to take the measurement. When the peak shape allows some subjective latitude, the preferred technique is to use a point that is more rather than less normal. When making interear comparisons it is essential to hold the two sheets of paper up to a strong light and optically superimpose the results from the two ears. This allows a much more reliable comparison than the use of numbers only since there may be variability in exact peak location between trials and ears. The proper procedure is to superimpose the major ascending and descending limbs of the waves being compared; the differences in their latencies help to judge the reliability of peak latency differences, especially when the peaks may be variable because of superimposed noise. Ogleznev et al. (1983) have also suggested use of these points for latency determinations.

Absolute amplitudes are too variable to be of any clinical use, even in interear comparisons. Amplitude ratios have been suggested as a measure with clinical utility. Since wave I is generated outside the CNS, it can be compared with wave V (generated at the midbrain level) to determine whether or not the expected signal amplitude relationships are present. It is not necessary to calculate the absolute amplitudes in microvolts in order to arrive at this mathematical relationship; the heights in millimeters can be used. The result can be expressed as a percentage or a ratio. The following ratios are usually calculated and used together for interpretation: (1) I:V, and (2) I:IV–V (highest peak of the IV–V complex). The major difficulties with the technique are (1) the ratios change with different click intensities, so that they are reliable only at intensity levels for which normal values have been determined, and (2) they are less reliable when there is peripheral hearing loss because they are affected in different ways by different shapes of abnormal audiograms.

Tables 5–2 through 5–4 present data gathered from normal subjects in our laboratory. These are intended to show how such data can be organized and to allow comparisons of variability when a laboratory is inexperienced with this test. Since the absolute values are dependent on many variables not likely to be the same in other laboratories, those values as presented here cannot be used for clinical interpretation other than in the laboratory where they were gathered. However, interpeak and interear interpeak latency measures show only minor differences between laboratories, as does the variability, measured here in standard deviations. In this test, the major purpose of the development of normal standards in each laboratory is to provide experience for the technicians and physicians who will be involved in the clinical application of this highly sophisticated tool. Brain stem auditory EP results from groups of normal subjects have been published and a study of those methods and data is useful (Starr and Achor, 1975; Rowe, 1978; Stockard et al., 1979; Wielaard and Kemp, 1979; Noseworthy et al., 1981; Oh et al., 1981; Purves et al., 1981; Salamy, 1981). See Section 8.2.6 for a discussion of the consistency of BAEPs over long periods of recording and when recording at repeated intervals for several months. Refer to Chapter 1, Section 4.3, for a discussion of the concepts relating values obtained from normal subjects and those obtained from patients (whose results are possibly abnormal).

TABLE 5–2. *Brain stem auditory EP normal values at 10/sec*

	Absolute latencies (msec)				Interwave latencies				Interear interwave differences		
Wave	Mean	SD	Mean + 3 SD	Waves	Mean	SD	Mean + 3 SD		Mean	SD	Mean + 3 SD
I	1.7	0.15	2.2	I–III	2.1	0.15	2.6		0.10	0.09	0.37 (0.4)
II	2.8	0.17	3.3	I–V	4.0	0.23	4.7		0.13	0.10	0.43 (0.5)
III	3.9	0.19	4.5	III–IV	1.2	0.16	1.7		0.12	0.14	0.54 (0.6)
IV	5.1	0.24	5.8	III–V	1.9	0.18	2.4		0.10	0.11	0.43
V	5.7	0.25	6.5	IV–V	0.7	0.19	1.3		0.15	0.14	0.57 (0.8)
VI	7.3	0.29	8.2	V–VI	1.5	0.25	2.3		0.22	0.19	0.79 (0.8)

	Absolute amplitudes (μV)				Mean amplitudes as %		
Wave	Mean	SD	Range	Waves	Mean	SD	Mean + 3 SD
I	0.28	0.14	0.06–0.85	III/V	50	23	119
III	0.23	0.12	0.03–0.55	I/IV (pre)	132	75	357
IV (pre)	0.25	0.12	0.04–0.63	I/IV (post V)	75	39	191
IV (post V)	0.40	0.13	0.08–0.88	IV	73	48	218
IV/V (highest peak)	0.47	0.16	0.14–0.88	I/IV–V	62	30	152
V	0.43	0.16	0.15–0.86				

	Amplitude difference between ears		
V	20	17	71

Normal values for BAEPs obtained from 50 normal subjects (15 to 51 years old, mixed gender) at 10 clicks/sec. Latencies were measured to the wave peak; where a peak was not well-defined, a midpoint of the wave was estimated. When waves IV and V were fused into a single peak, the latency was taken to the point of final inflection before the negative limb of wave V, and this was recorded as a wave V only. If either wave appeared as a distinct step on the other, this step was taken as the wave peak. Amplitudes were measured from the peak to the following trough except that wave IV amplitude was measured from its peak to both the preceding trough (pre-IV) and the trough following wave V (post-V). The number in brackets after the mean + 3 SD is where the range exceeds the mean + 3 SD. Square wave duration was 0.1 msec, click intensity 60 dB SL, constant polarity. (From Chiappa et al., 1979, with permission.)

TABLE 5–3. *Brain stem auditory EP normal values at 70/sec*

Absolute latencies (msec)					Interwave latencies				Interear interwave differences		
Wave	(%)	Mean	SD	Mean + 3 SD	Waves	Mean	SD	Mean + 3 SD	Mean	SD	Mean + 3 SD
I	76	1.8	0.21	2.3 (2.7)	I–III	2.3	0.29	3.0	0.18	0.13	0.51
II	61	2.9	0.19	3.4	I–V	4.3	0.24	4.9	0.18	0.14	0.53 (0.6)
III	68	4.2	0.35	5.1	III–IV	1.3	0.28	2.0 (2.3)	0.23	0.20	0.73 (0.8)
IV	51	5.4	0.30	6.2 (6.3)	III–V	2.0	0.26	2.7 (2.8)	0.19	0.19	0.7
V	79	6.2	0.30	7.0	IV–V	0.8	0.24	1.4 (1.5)	0.15	0.08	0.35
VI	34	7.8	0.42	8.9	V–VI	1.7	0.39	2.7	0.35	0.24	0.95

Absolute amplitudes (μV)					Wave V latency increase (10/sec–70/sec)		
Wave	Mean	SD	Mean + 3 SD	Range	Mean	SD	Mean + 3 SD
I	0.13	0.09		0.01–0.38	0.48	0.20	1.08
III	0.10	0.08		0.10–0.45			
IV/V	0.37	0.14		0.08–0.73			

Mean amplitudes as %			
Waves	Mean	SD	Mean + 3 SD
IV	40	31	133
III/V	29	22	95

	Mean	SD	Range
% Ear diff. wave V	23	20	0–93
% Change 10–70/sec	−25	33	−129–69

Normal values for BAEPs obtained from 40 normal subjects (15 to 51 years old, mixed gender) at 70 clicks/sec. See legend for Table 5–1 for methods. (From Chiappa et al., 1979, with permission.)

TABLE 5–4. *Brain stem auditory EP gender and click polarity differences*

	Mean ± SD		Range		p Values for sex difference	
	R	C	R	C	R	C
Wave I latency M & F	1.7 ± 0.14	1.8 ± 0.16	1.4–2.1	1.5–2.3		
Wave I latency F	1.7 ± 0.14	1.8 ± 0.17	1.4–2.1	1.5–2.3	ns	ns
Wave I latency M	1.7 ± 0.12	1.7 ± 0.15	1.5–2.0	1.5–2.0		
Wave III latency M & F	3.8 ± 0.16	3.9 ± 0.17	3.5–4.3	3.5–4.2		
Wave III latency F	3.8 ± 0.14	3.9 ± 0.17	3.5–4.1	3.5–4.2	p < 0.005	ns
Wave III latency M	3.9 ± 0.17	3.9 ± 0.17	3.7–4.3	3.5–4.2		
Wave V latency M & F	5.8 ± 0.22	5.8 ± 0.23	5.3–6.3	5.4–6.4		
Wave V latency F	5.7 ± 0.20	5.7 ± 0.21	5.3–6.1	5.4–6.4	p < 0.001	p < 0.005
Wave V latency M	5.9 ± 0.20	5.9 ± 0.22	5.6–6.3	5.5–6.3		
I–III Latency M & F	2.1 ± 0.14	2.1 ± 0.12	1.9–2.5	1.7–2.4		
I–III Latency F	2.1 ± 0.12	2.1 ± 0.11	1.9–2.5	1.7–2.4	p < 0.005	p < 0.025
I–III Latency M	2.2 ± 0.15	2.2 ± 0.13	1.9–2.5	1.9–2.4		
III–V Latency M & F	1.9 ± 0.18	1.9 ± 0.17	1.5–2.4	1.6–2.3		
III–V Latency F	1.9 ± 0.17	1.9 ± 0.16	1.5–2.2	1.6–2.3	ns	ns
III–V Latency M	2.0 ± 0.18	2.0 ± 0.14	1.7–2.4	1.7–2.3		
I–V Latency M & F	4.1 ± 0.19	4.0 ± 0.20	3.6–4.5	3.4–4.6		
I–V Latency F	4.0 ± 0.18	4.0 ± 0.20	3.6–4.4	3.4–4.3	p < 0.001	p < 0.001
I–V Latency M	4.2 ± 0.14	4.2 ± 0.15	3.9–4.5	3.9–4.6		

Normal values for BAEPs at 10 clicks/sec in 35 normal subjects (17 to 54 years old) showing differences due to gender and click polarity. M, males, F, females, R, rarefaction clicks, C, condensation clicks. Square wave duration was 0.1 msec, click intensity was 70 to 80 dB SL. (From Emerson et al., 1982 with permission.)

8. NONPATHOLOGIC FACTORS AFFECTING RESULTS

8.1. Technical Factors

8.1.1. Click Intensity

Changes in click intensity produce marked changes in the absolute latency and amplitude of all BAEP waves (Jewett et al., 1970; Salomon and Elberling, 1971; Elberling, 1973, 1974; Hecox and Galambos, 1974; Picton et al., 1974; Picton et al., 1981). Amplitude is diminished and absolute latency is increased with decreasing click intensity (Fig. 5–11). The

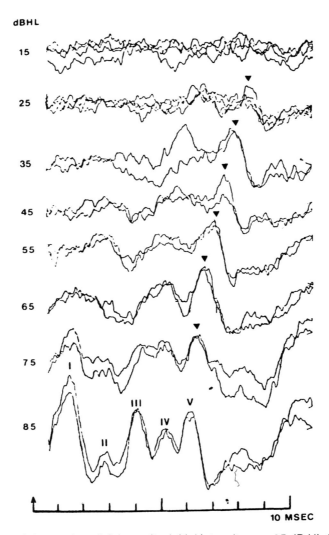

FIG. 5–11. Effect of decreasing click intensity. Initial intensity was 85 dB HL (*bottom*) with all waves visible. At 75 dB HL waves II and III are difficult to identify, and at 65 dB HL only wave V remains (with a poorly formed wave IV). Wave V is still recognizable at 25 dB HL but is absent below that. The wave V absolute latency increases linearly with decreasing click intensity. Each trace is the average of 500 stimuli. The recording derivation was earlobe to vertex.

latency increase is roughly linear at 0.03 msec/dB decrease in stimulus intensity (Fig. 5–12). The latency changes are different for stimuli with different frequency contents (Elberling, 1973, 1974; Coats et al., 1979; Bauch et al., 1980). Eggermont and Don (1980) found that the absolute latency–intensity curves for wave V were parallel (but slightly different) with different center frequencies of the stimulus, but Coats et al. (1979) have found that these curves diverge as intensity diminishes.

Because the latencies of all the BAEP waves shift by roughly the same amounts, there is very little change in interpeak latencies (IPL) (Figs. 5–12 and 5–13) (Terkildsen et al., 1973; Pratt and Sohmer, 1976; Fabiani et al., 1979; Eggermont and Don, 1980). Stockard et al. (1979) found mean IPL differences between 30 and 70 dB SL of 0.19, 0.16, and 0.34 msec for I–III, III–V, and I–V separations, respectively, with the lower intensities having the shorter IPLs. (In one normal subject they found a 0.73 msec difference in the I–V separation.) Much of this effect they attributed to changes in wave I shape. Wave I is a manifestation of activity in two eighth nerve neuronal populations which have different

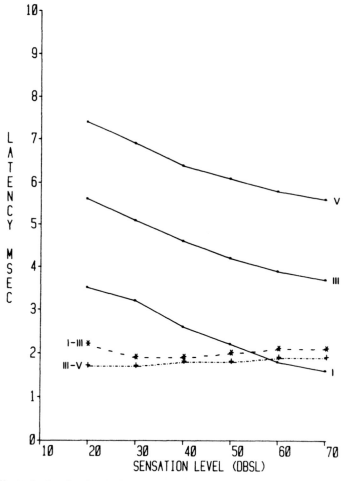

FIG. 5–12. Effect of stimulus intensity on absolute and interpeak latencies. Note that the absolute latency plots are parallel, so that, as would be expected, the IPL plots are flat with very little change until low intensities are reached. Pooled results from seven normal subjects.

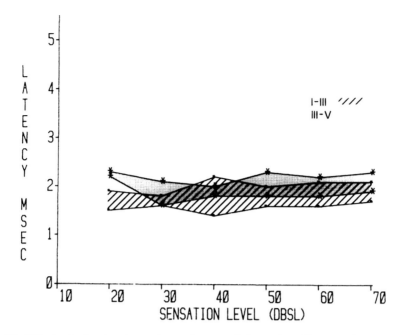

FIG. 5–13. Effect of stimulus intensity on interpeak latencies. This graph shows the maximum–minimum IPL seen in any of seven normal subjects at any intensity, i.e., these are the "worst" cases.

thresholds for activation, and whose activation ranges overlap at stimulus intensities between 40 and 60 dB SL (Elberling, 1973). The shift from predominance of one to the other with the accompanying change in wave I peak emphasis results in the "apparent" IPL changes. Ultimately, this change in wave I shape is due to the fact that wave I components originate in different sections of the cochlear partition (Elberling, 1974), depending on intensity and frequency of the stimulus. The base of the cochlea, close to the oval window, which subserves the highest frequencies (8 to 20 kHz), is activated by higher intensities, and the apex of the cochlea (0 to 500 Hz) is activated by the lower intensities. Since there may be a 5- to 7-msec difference in activation of these areas, their sum (the wave I peak) will have different shapes depending on the relative contributions from the different areas.

As mentioned above, Eggermont and Don (1980), using the "derived responses" technique, found no IPL differences with clicks of different center frequencies, but Coats et al. (1979), using filtered clicks, found that the I–V IPL got shorter with decreasing click intensity, an effect that became more marked as click frequency was decreased (4, 2, 1 kHz). Since the same discrepancy characterizes the wave I results in these studies (i.e., parallel versus divergent trends with intensity changes), the stimulus differences in the two sets of experiments may account for the disagreement.

Pratt and Bleich (1982) used clicks mixed with notch-filtered masking noise and found no absolute or IPL differences with different center frequencies of the notches. The lack of absolute latency change with changes in frequency, which indicates an independence of component latency from cochlear "traveling wave" propagation time, they attributed to the possibility that the clicks in notched noise were activating a low-threshold cochlear apparatus. They believed that the potentials they recorded might be representative of only one subset of BAEP constituent waveforms, as seen with wide-band unmasked clicks.

Stockard et al. (1979) also noted click phase and rate interactions with intensity. Masking the unstimulated ear seems to have little effect (Boezeman, 1983b).

For purposes of clinical interpretation, the relative constancy of the IPL measurements (see Figs. 5–12 and 5–13) in the face of changes in stimulus intensity is a very important factor, since effective stimulus intensity is difficult, if not impossible, to control accurately even in normal subjects. The nature of the earphone fit, the shape and contents of the external auditory canal, the mechanical properties of the ossicles, and fluid properties of the cochlea all contribute to altering the delivery of stimulus energy to the basilar membrane. These unknown quantities render absolute latencies of BAEPs almost useless in neurologic applications of BAEPs. Various sensorineural hearing losses may affect IPLs (see Section 8.2.4) but this is in a direction that tends to produce false negative results, a preferred error in most clinical situations.

8.1.2. Click Frequency Contents

The sound pressure wave produced by the earphone in response to a brief (<200 μsec) electrical pulse has the approximate appearance of a rapidly decaying sine wave. Frequency analysis usually shows a broad-band spread of power from 500 Hz to more than 4,000 Hz, depending on pulse duration and model of earphone. As long as these latter two parameters are not changed, it can be assumed that click frequency contents are a constant.

The frequency characteristics of the effective stimulus can be altered by (1) changing pulse duration, (2) filtering the click, (3) mixing filtered white noise with the click, and (4) using tone pips. As described in the preceding section, changes in stimulus frequency produce changes in latency and amplitude of all waves and alter their behavior when stimulus intensity is changed. Since the unaltered click contains energy at a variety of frequencies, it will tend to stimulate larger areas of the cochlea than stimuli that have more focused frequency contents (Picton et al., 1981). "Derived potential" studies (e.g., Don and Eggermont, 1978) indicate that the waveforms seen with usual click intensities (60 to 70 dB HL) are being generated primarily from the 2,000- to 4,000-Hz region of the cochlea. At higher intensities significant activation of other areas of the cochlea can occur. Since the traveling wave takes 2 to 6 msec to stimulate the entire cochlea, this can produce more than one of each BAEP component; these then blend to result in an unclear set of waveforms which are rendered more distinct by decreasing click intensity (see Section 6.2 and Fig. 5–6). The use of stimuli with more focused frequency contents, for example, tone pips, can also help in this regard.

8.1.3. Click Rate

Increasing click rate results in increased absolute latency of all BAEP waves and decreased amplitude (and thus recognizability—see Table 5–5) of most (Thornton and Coleman, 1975; Hyde et al., 1976; Zollner et al., 1976; Don et al., 1977; Weber and Fujikawa, 1977; Rowe, 1978; Salamy et al., 1978; Stockard et al., 1978b, 1979, 1980b; Chiappa et al., 1979; Harkins et al., 1979; van Olphen et al., 1979; Picton et al., 1981; Shanon et al., 1981a; Suzuki et al., 1986). Interpeak latencies increase slightly at higher stimulus rates (Hyde et al., 1976; Rowe, 1978; Salamy et al., 1978; Stockard et al., 1978b, 1979, 1980b; Chiappa et al., 1979; Harkins et al., 1979; Stockard et al., 1979; Picton et al., 1981; Pratt et al., 1981). Sand (1986) noted that rate affected shape and amplitude of waves I, III, and V.

TABLE 5–5. *Frequency of recognizability of individual waves (%)*

Wave	10/sec (N = 100 ears)	30/sec (N = 36 ears)	70/sec (N = 80 ears)
I	97	97	76
II	96	92	61
III	100	97	85
IV	88	67	57
V	100	97	99
VI	84	67	34

(From Chiappa et al., 1979, with permission.)

Increasing stimulus rate (above 30/sec) will often worsen an abnormality seen at 10/sec. However, it is not clear how often in routine clinical applications a BAEP is normal at the lower rate and abnormal at a faster rate (even 70/sec). The faster rate increases the yield of abnormalities (Hecox et al., 1981; Pratt et al., 1981; Stockard and Stockard, 1982; Gerling and Finitzo-Hieber, 1983), although the incidence of this is not clear. For example, Pratt et al. (1981) found that the abnormality rate in the I–V interval decreased from 34% to 27% when the stimulus rate was increased from 10 to 50/sec, whereas the interear I–V IPL difference abnormality rate increased from 27% to 55%. Chiappa et al. (1980) tested 57 patients with MS at 10 and 70 clicks/sec and found none who were normal at the slower rate but abnormal at the faster rate.

Conversely, one might expect there to be some incidence of apparent normalization with faster stimulus rates. The refractory period of demyelinated axons might be such that they would fail to follow at the higher rates; the loss of their delayed contribution would produce apparent normalization of the BAEPs. Chiappa et al. (1980) searched for this effect in MS patients but did not find it, although, as mentioned above, Pratt et al. (1981) in a mixed group of patients found fewer abnormalities in the I–V IPL at faster rates than at slower rates.

8.1.4. Click Polarity

In normal subjects, Maurer et al. (1980b) and Maurer (1985) found that rarefaction stimulation resulted in shorter wave I latencies, longer I–III interwave latencies, and more distinct waves IV and V. Ornitz et al. (1980) and Ornitz and Walter (1975) noted that rarefaction produced earlier absolute latencies of waves I and V. Stockard et al. (1978b) found that wave V absolute latencies did not vary with stimulus polarity, but that the absolute latencies of waves I through IV were shorter with rarefaction stimulation. Elberling (1974) also noted shorter latencies with rarefaction clicks. Emerson et al. (1982) found small differences, with rarefaction stimulation generally producing larger wave I and smaller wave V amplitudes and separating waves IV and V (Fig. 5–14), slightly shorter absolute latencies, and slightly longer interwave latencies (see Table 5–4). However, they noted that many subjects did not conform to the typical pattern. For example, (1) I–V interwave latencies were longer with condensation clicks in 14 of 90 ears studied, (2) wave I amplitude (peak to following trough) was lower with condensation clicks in 75% of the ears, higher in 18%, and unchanged in 7%, and (3) wave V amplitude was higher with condensation clicks in 66%, lower in 30%, and unchanged in 4%. Sand and Sulg (1984) investigated the influence of click rate and phase, Coutin et al. (1987) compared vector analysis of different phase stimuli, and Chan et al. (1988) investigated the interaction between sex and click polarity in control subjects of Asian and Caucasian origin.

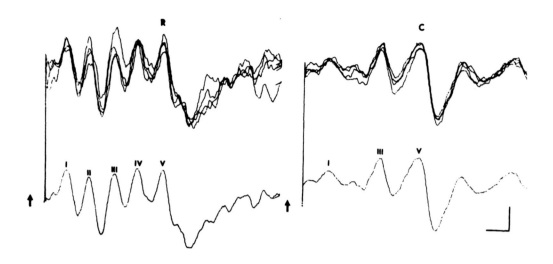

FIG. 5–14. Brain stem auditory EPs obtained from one ear in a single normal subject show-ing clear waves IV and V following rarefaction clicks (*left panel*), and fusion of waves IV and V following condensation clicks (*right panel*). Both panels show four superimposed trials of 1,024 clicks each with the grand average underneath. Derivation is the earlobe ipsilateral to monaural stimulation to the vertex, with relative positivity of the vertex producing an upward trace deflection. Calibration marks are 0.25 μV and 1.0 msec. The arrow indicates the time of stimulation. (From Emerson et al., 1982, with permission.)

The interpolarity latency differences for interwave separations have mean values of 0.02 to 0.04 msec (standard deviations of 0.1 msec), ranging up to 0.4 msec either way (rarefac-tion or condensation with longer or shorter latencies). See Emerson et al. (1982) for more details. Sand (1986) reported changes in the configuration of waves I, III, and V related to click polarity and rate.

Maurer et al. (1980b) and Scherg and Speulda (1982) present patients who had changes in waveform shapes with different click polarities. Emerson et al. (1982) reported 20 pa-tients (of 600 consecutively studied) who showed a selective loss of wave V with one stim-ulus polarity but not the other. In 17 of the 20 patients (85%), wave V was seen with con-densation but not with rarefaction clicks (Fig. 5–15). In all 20 cases, the recordings were otherwise normal and wave V, when obtained, fell within normal latency limits. Complete audiometric examinations were obtained in five patients; they were normal in two and ab-normal in three. Among the patients for whom audiograms were not obtained, eight had normal click hearing thresholds and the remaining six had mild losses (mean −11 dB; worst −23 dB). Seven of these 20 patients were tested at diminished click intensities (usu-ally 15 dB down), and this resulted in the reappearance of wave V in all seven patients (see Fig. 5–15). In normal subjects, when stimulus intensity is decreased, wave V amplitude decreases and its absolute latency increases. It is not definitely known whether the sensi-tivity of wave V to stimulus polarity in patients, and its paradoxical reappearance with di-minished stimulus intensity, represents an abnormality or a normal variation. Since this was seen in 20 of 600 patients and in none of 45 normal subjects (Emerson et al., 1982), it may be either a true abnormality or an infrequently occurring normal variant. Whether these phenomena are mediated by the brain stem, eighth nerve, or cochlea remains to be

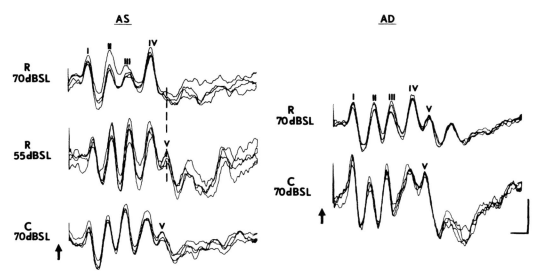

FIG. 5–15. Brain stem auditory EPs obtained from the left and right ears of a single patient following monaural stimulation, showing intensity and polarity sensitivity of wave V. Left ear (AS) shows absence of wave V following rarefaction clicks at 70 dB SL (*top trace*); however, wave V appears when the click intensity is decreased 15 dB with the same polarity (*middle trace*). Wave V is present at 70 dB SL following condensation clicks in that ear (*bottom trace*). Right ear (AD) shows a normal ear with all waves present regardless of polarity. In all cases, four superimposed trials of 1,024 clicks each are shown. Derivation is the earlobe ipsilateral to monaural stimulation to the vertex, the positivity of the latter producing an upward deflection. Calibration marks are 0.25 μV and 1.0 msec. (From Emerson et al., 1982, with permission.)

discovered, although the presence of a normal audiogram in some of these patients suggests that it may be a central effect. The central origin of this phenomenon is further supported by the fact that Rosenhamer et al. (1981), Coats and Martin (1977), and Coats (1978) did not observe it in 110, 29, and 37 ears, respectively, with cochlear hearing loss. Schwartz et al. (1990) studied polarity effects in 92 normal-hearing subjects and 78 patients with varying degrees of cochlear hearing loss; their final recommendations were similar to those given below. Hammond et al. (1986) found click polarity-related differences in BAEPs in 24% of 25 patients with Wernicke-Korsakoff syndrome and in 40% of 20 MS patients.

In view of the sensitivity of wave I to stimulus polarity and intensity, it is not surprising that subsequent waveforms whose generation is logically contingent upon the existence of wave I are similarly sensitive. However, the relationship between polarity-dependent wave I behavior (Peake and Kiang, 1962; Kiang et al., 1965; Antoli-Candela and Kiang, 1978) in cat acoustic nerve fibers and the wave V variations seen in patients is speculative.

Since waves II through V represent structures in the auditory pathway central to the eighth nerve, alterations in the configuration of wave V may be due to a brain stem abnormality. It is equally plausible, however, that alterations in the sequential activation of hair cells in the cochlear membrane might produce a cancellation of wave V and other odd effects since the responses to different polarity stimuli may be so dissimilar (Fig. 5–16).

The binaural interaction waveform (see Section 8.1.5) is thought to represent central neural interaction. The demonstration of abnormalities in this feature of the BAEP may help

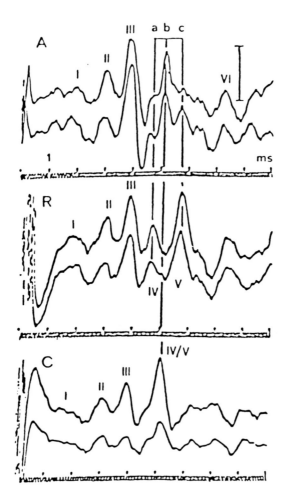

FIG. 5–16. A patient who demonstrates that the BAEP waveforms obtained with alternating click polarity (*upper panel*—A) are a simple and sometimes confusing sum of the responses obtained with rarefaction clicks alone (*middle panel*—R) and condensation clicks alone (*bottom panel*—C). This patient had a high-tone decay and shows a marked difference in BAEP waveform latencies and configurations between rarefaction and condensation clicks (see also Fig. 5–9). The amplitude calibration bar is 0.3 μV. Each trace is the average of 1,000 stimuli presented at 10/sec and 80 dB. (From Maurer, 1985, with permission.)

to determine whether or not the polarity dependence of wave V in the patients is of central or peripheral origin. Ultimately, histopathologic demonstration of a minimum necessary anatomic lesion would resolve the question.

Ideally, one would consistently use both rarefaction and condensation stimulation when recording BAEPs, but in the clinical setting this may not be practical. It is recommended that if one is to use only a single stimulus polarity, rarefaction clicks should be used. This will produce the clearest waveforms in most cases. Furthermore, the greatest number of cases with a polarity-sensitive wave V will be revealed. Condensation can be used in those patients in whom rarefaction does not produce clear waveforms, or when wave V appears absent. The use of alternating polarity clicks as the only mode of stimulation is discouraged because of the possibility of phase cancellations.

Although polarity-dependent disappearance of wave V has not been seen in normal subjects, it remains to be demonstrated whether this is an abnormality or an infrequently occurring normal variant. At present, the clinical interpretation should reflect this uncertainty.

8.1.5. Stimulus Mode—Monaural Versus Binaural

The response to clicks delivered simultaneously to both ears, recording from a midline nuchal to vertex derivation, is about the same as the sum of the responses obtained by testing one ear at a time. The minor difference between the two modes of stimulation is called the binaural interaction waveform (BIW) (Dobie and Norton, 1980; Decker and Howe, 1981; Hosford-Dunn et al., 1981; Levine, 1981; Wrege and Starr, 1981). The main peak of the BIW occurs at about 6 msec, at the same time as the middle of the post-wave V downslope. Note that Decker and Howe (1981) used a slightly different procedure for calculating the BIW and found no difference in four of eight normal subjects.

Levine (1981) and Dobie and Norton (1980) found no intensity effect in the BIW, although Wrege and Starr (1981) did. Hosford-Dunn et al. (1981) found the BIW present in neonates shortly after birth. Although some workers believe that the BIW is due to acoustic cross-talk, Levine (1981) found that this could be a factor only above 50 dB HL. He also found no contribution of the middle-ear reflex to the BIW. Dobie and Wilson (1985) also found binaural interaction waveforms at intensities well below levels at which crossover could occur, and noted that those were not affected by contralateral masking in the monaural trial.

Although Levine (1981) and Wrege and Starr (1981) are hopeful of clinical utility for the BIW, its low amplitude suggests that it will not be possible to register it reliably in patients. Its potential utility lies in its presumed generation in central auditory pathways so that when abnormal it may then definitely indicate a central lesion. Its sensitivity relative to the usual BAEP waveforms is not known.

The use of only binaural stimulation in patients is an error because normal responses generated by a good ear will mask abnormal responses from a bad ear (Fig. 5–7, panels D and E). This will result in significant loss of sensitivity since in patients with MS, for example, almost half have BAEPs with an abnormality in one ear only (Chiappa et al., 1980; Prasher and Gibson, 1980).

8.1.6. Recording Band-pass

Filtering will always affect amplitude and latency of EP components to some degree, depending on the relationship between the filters and the frequency content of the waveforms. Energy in BAEP waveforms is concentrated in the area of 15 to 2,000 Hz (Elberling, 1979; Kevanishvili and Aphonchenko, 1979). Lowering the high-cutoff filter from 3,000 to 1,500 Hz does not have significant effects on latency (Cacace et al., 1980).

The BAEP waveforms are superimposed on a slow wave with a duration of 3 to 4 msec (frequency contents down to 15 to 20 Hz), which can be seen if the higher frequencies are removed by lowering the high-cutoff filter to 150 to 200 Hz. The low-cutoff filter most commonly used, 100 Hz, removes (1) this "slow" activity, for which at present there is no recognized clinical utility, and (2) a great deal of "artifact" (e.g., alpha activity) which would otherwise interfere with the recording. There appears to be no utility in raising the low cutoff filter to 300 Hz in "noisy" subjects (Chiappa et al., 1979) since it does not improve the clarity of the waveforms and causes a 20% reduction in wave V amplitude.

If low-frequency tone pips are the stimulus, the EPs contain significant amounts of activity below 100 Hz so that low-cutoff filters of 20 Hz are then recommended.

The effects of digital and analog filters on BAEPs have been studied (Suzuki and Horiuchi, 1977; Boston and Ainslie, 1980; Cacace et al., 1980; Moller, 1980, 1988; Doyle and

Hyde, 1981). As long as the filter settings in the equipment are held constant, there will be no problem with these effects.

8.1.7. Stimulus Delivery Apparatus

The mechanical and acoustic properties of earphone transducers, and hence the frequency and energy content of the generated sound waves, are dependent on many factors of design and materials [e.g., shielding with μ-metal to reduce stimulus artifact (Coats et al., 1979)]. As these change, so will the characteristics of the recorded BAEPs (see above). In addition, new components may be revealed. For example, Hughes and Fino (1980) used a piezoelectric earphone to eliminate stimulus artifact; this allowed resolution of a wave peak 0.7 msec before wave I (1.1 versus 1.8 msec absolute latency) which they postulated might be a cochlear summating potential or an auditory nerve potential.

The coupling between earphone and ear can also significantly change BAEP waveforms. Coats and Kidder (1980) found that circumaural cushions produced clicks with significantly less energy above 6 kHz than did conventional audiometric earphones or free-field stimulation. They also noted a 0.1-msec difference in the I–V separation above 50 dB HL and a 0.2-msec difference below that stimulus intensity, between circumaural and audiometric cushions.

The auditory stimulus can also be delivered via bone (Mauldin and Jerger, 1979; Boezeman et al., 1983b). This produces BAEPs with absolute latencies an average of 0.46 msec longer than with air-conducted clicks of the same intensity level above behavioral threshold for that ear. This was attributed to the different frequency content of the bone-conducted click. Mauldin and Jerger suggested that the application of a correction factor of 0.5 msec to the bone-conducted results would allow an estimation of the air–bone gap.

8.1.8. Potential-Field Distribution

Since wave I is important as a "reference point" for interwave latency separation measurements, consideration of its amplitude distribution may suggest the most useful recording techniques. Picton et al. (1974) showed that wave I was negative with a localized distribution maximal at the earlobe and mastoid ipsilateral to the stimulated ear. Using a larynx reference which he considered inactive, Barratt (1980) also found that wave I was a negative wave largest at the ipsilateral mastoid, and of inverted polarity and lower amplitude at the contralateral mastoid. Terkildsen and Osterhammel (1981) had similar findings using neck references and recommended an ipsilateral to contralateral ear derivation as the best for registering wave I. However, in routine clinical neurologic application of the test, we have not found this technique to be helpful. Starr and Squires (1982), using a nape of the neck (C7) reference electrode, showed that wave I had a wide distribution of positive activity, with the negativity confined to the region of the ipsilateral ear. They noted that the in-phase addition of the negativity at the ear and the positivity at the vertex in the vertex to ipsilateral ear derivation optimized detection of wave I. Stockard et al. (1978b) studied high- and low-mastoid and medial earlobe recording sites; they found that the medial earlobe site provided the highest-amplitude wave I (due mainly to an increase in amplitude of the subsequent trough). Of course, sites even closer to the cochlear nerve provide even higher amplitudes, and these special techniques are invaluable when wave I cannot be recorded from the sites mentioned above. (See Section 3.2 for a further discussion of these techniques.)

Wave II is positive at all scalp locations, maximum at the vertex, minimum in the contralateral ear region (Starr and Squires, 1982). Thus, wave II is clearly seen in the ipsilateral to contralateral ears and vertex to contralateral ear derivations (Terkildsen and Osterhammel, 1981). The latter feature may help to distinguish wave II from wave I, which is not seen well at the contralateral ear site (Stockard et al., 1978b).

Wave III has a maximum amplitude at the vertex but its distribution is markedly lateralized to the contralateral scalp (Picton et al., 1974; Starr and Squires, 1982), so that it is poorly seen at the ipsilateral ear (where it may be negative) with a noncephalic reference or in the vertex to contralateral ear derivation. The lower amplitude of wave III in the contralateral ear derivation may help with waveform identification (Stockard et al., 1978b). The latency of wave III is slightly shorter in the contralateral ear derivation, as compared with the ipsilateral.

Wave IV has no significant amplitude asymmetry but its mean latency was 0.24 msec earlier at ipsilateral versus contralateral sites (Starr and Squires, 1982).

Wave V is positive at both the vertex and ipsilateral earlobe sites (Chiappa et al., 1979; Starr and Squires, 1982). In seven normal subjects, using a noncephalic reference, the mean amplitude of wave V at the earlobe was 0.15 (SD 0.07) μV, at the vertex it was 0.45 (SD 0.13) μV, and in an earlobe to vertex derivation it was 0.36 (SD 0.09) μV. Thus, there is a 20% loss in wave V apparent amplitude in the earlobe to vertex derivation because of differential amplifier cancellation of in-phase activity at the two sites. However, the fact that much less muscle and other artifact is seen in the "bipolar" vertex to earlobe derivation outweighs the loss of wave V amplitude, so that it is the preferred derivation for clinical use. Wave V latency was found to be either earlier (Stockard et al., 1978b) or later (Starr and Squires, 1982) in the ipsilateral derivation, although a possible difference is that the former study used earlobe recording sites and the latter used mastoids.

There is some enthusiasm for recording a second channel, earlobe contralateral to the ear being stimulated referred to the vertex (Stockard et al., 1978b; Mizrahi et al., 1983). This channel characteristically has no wave I negativity, and waves IV and V tend to be separated rather than fused. Thus, this recording channel may provide some assistance in waveform recognition. However, we have found the maneuver of decreasing click intensity to be of much greater utility in waveform recognition. In any case, since most averaging systems have two channels, there is no reason not to record the contralateral channel. Levine and McGaffigan (1983) found differences between the two ears of normal subjects, with mean amplitudes of some waves larger for right-ear stimulation.

Three-channel Lissajous trajectories of BAEPs have been studied (Pratt et al., 1985a, 1986; Martin et al., 1986; Kaminer and Pratt, 1987; September, 1987 issue of *Electroencephalogr Clin Neurophysiol* 68:323–414; Polyakov and Pratt, 1994) but their contribution to the understanding of generator sources and clinical utility is uncertain. Neonatal three-channel Lissajous trajectories of BAEPs have also been used to gain insight into the developmental aspects of the auditory system (Hafner et al., 1994).

8.1.9. Signal-to-Noise Ratio

The resolution of BAEP waveforms is, to a large extent, dependent on the amount of ambient "artifact" present during recording. The artifact consists primarily of muscle activity. Wong and Bickford (1980) attempted to quantify the signal-to-noise (S/N) ratio by comparing the BAEP averaged in the usual manner with a plus–minus reference (see Chapter 1, Section 2.5.14) and producing a single number, an "estimate" of the S/N ratio (the variance between the two). They suggested that this value could be used as a predictor of the accuracy or reproducibility of a BAEP: a low value would prompt rejection of the BAEP and performance of a repeat with lower ambient "artifact" levels.

Gott and Hughes (1989) presented click stimuli with broadband noise and noted differential effects on the latencies of waves I and V which they interpreted as a central phenomenon.

8.2. Subject/Patient Factors

8.2.1. Age

With increasing age after childhood, there are increases in absolute and peak latencies of BAEP waves (Rowe, 1978; Jerger and Hall, 1980; Kjaer, 1980d; Rosenhamer et al., 1980; Allison et al., 1983, 1984; Thivierge and Cote, 1987; Mitchell et al., 1989). Beagley and Sheldrake (1978) did not observe this effect in their 70 normal subjects. These IPL increases were on the order of 0.1 msec between young and old subjects, both with groups of mixed gender (Rowe, 1978) and when male and female groups were considered separately (Rosenhamer et al., 1980); for example, Rowe (1978) found a mean I–V IPL in young subjects (mean age 25.1 years) of 3.94 msec, versus 4.00 msec for older subjects (mean age 61.7 years) (60-dB SL clicks at 10/sec). Kjaer found a greater difference, but in males only: a mean I–V IPL of 4.1 msec in the 20- to 29-year decade versus 4.51 msec in the 50- to 69-year decade for men, with essentially no change between these age groups in women. Rowe noted that an increase in the I–III separation was responsible for most of the prolongation of the I–V IPL in older subjects, whereas Rosenhamer et al. found the III–V separation increase was predominant. As a general rule, these increases are too small to change an individual's BAEP results from normal to abnormal (or vice versa) when a mixed-gender group of normals was used in determination of the normal range for a laboratory. In clinical practice, one would not use such fine distinctions on a routine basis without incurring more false positives than is acceptable. Allison et al. (1984) have constructed a histogram of age changes over the 18- to 95-year range (Fig. 5–17). Using a simple developmental model,

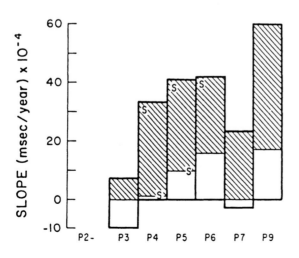

FIG. 5–17. Slopes of age-related changes (18 to 95 years) in BAEP interpeak latencies (cross-hatched, male; clear, female), e.g., the 40 level on the vertical axis is an increase in interpeak latency of 4 msec/year. Slopes which differ significantly from zero ($p \leq 0.01$) have an S in the upper left of the bar, and slopes which differ significantly between males and females have an S at the border between the areas. The 4- to 17-year age group (not shown) showed slight but insignificant increases with age. Total number of subjects for 4 to 95 years is 130 males, 156 females. P2 through P9 are waves I through VII (P6 is wave V). (Adapted from Allison et al., 1984, with permission.)

Eggermont (1988) has defined three exponential functions with time constants of 4 weeks, 40 weeks, and 4 years which describe maturational latency changes.

Older subjects have also been noted to have greater increases in IPLs when stimulus intensity is decreased (Rosenhamer et al., 1980), although Rowe (1978) did not observe this effect.

Jerger and Hall (1980), Kjaer (1980d), and Psatta and Matei (1988) noted that increasing age results in lower amplitude of BAEP waveforms. Rowe (1978) found the opposite effect and noted the large variance in amplitude measures at any age.

The contrast between infant and adult BAEPs is much more dramatic. The waveforms in infants are often higher in amplitude than in adults, presumably on the basis of smaller head size and greater proximity of the recording electrodes to BAEP generators (Stockard et al., 1978b). The relative amplitudes of waves I and V are different in infants and adults, with

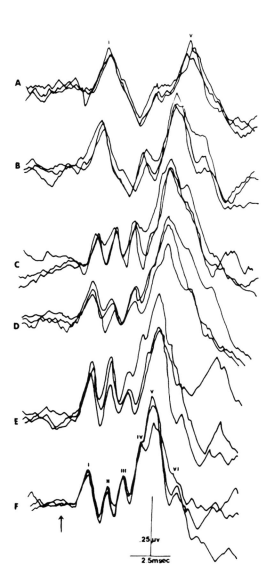

FIG. 5–18. Maturational changes in BAEP waveforms as a function of age: **A,** newborns; **B,** 6-week olds; **C,** 3-month olds; **D,** 6-month olds; **E,** 1-year olds; **F,** adults. Each trace represents an average of 2,400 stimulations obtained from a different subject. Note also the decreases in absolute latency with increasing age. Derivation was vertex to ipsilateral ear. Relative positivity at the CZ electrode produces an upward trace deflection. (From Salamy and McKean, 1976, with permission.)

wave I larger in infants, so that their I:V amplitude ratio is smaller than in adults (Salamy, 1984). In prematures and neonates the waveforms are more variable than adults (Salamy, 1984; Krumholz et al., 1985), often have a simpler appearance, with waves II, IV, and VI less well-resolved (Fig. 5–18), and the contralateral components are alternated (Salamy et al., 1985); an adult configuration is reached by 3 to 6 months of age (Hecox and Galambos, 1974; Salamy and McKean, 1976; Mochizuki et al., 1982). Ken-Dror et al. (1987) found a good correlation between gestational age and BAEP measures of peripheral and central conduction and suggested that these might provide an estimation of developmental age. Collet et al. (1987) found a greater effect of stimuli intensity on neonates than adults. Salamy (1984) has reviewed BAEP changes during maturation, and Salamy et al. (1985) studied maturation of contralateral components in preterm infants.

Absolute and interpeak latencies are markedly prolonged relative to adult values in the youngest prematures. There is then an approximate 0.2-msec/week decrease in wave V absolute latency and 0.14-msec/week decrease in the I–V IPL over the 26- to 40-week gestational age period (Fig. 5–19), with the greatest change earlier (Hecox and Galambos, 1974; Hecox, 1975; Schulman-Galambos and Galambos, 1975; Starr et al., 1977; Salamy et al., 1982; Salamy, 1984). During infancy and early childhood all latency measures continue to decrease more slowly until adult values are reached at 1 to 2 years of age (Fig. 5–19) (Hecox and Galambos, 1974; Salamy et al., 1975; Salamy and McKean, 1976; Salamy et al., 1978; Fabiani et al., 1979; Gafni et al., 1980; O'Donovan et al., 1980; Mochizuki et al.,

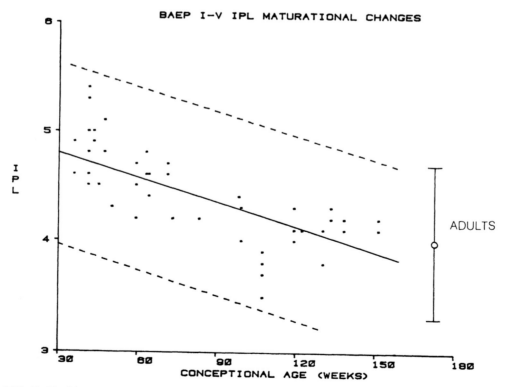

FIG. 5–19. Maturational changes in BAEP I–V interpeak latency. Conceptional age is gestational age at birth plus chronological age.

1982). These rapid changes necessitate the use of age-specific normal values; suggested intervals are every 2 weeks before normal term (40 weeks), then at 3 weeks, 6 weeks, 3 months, 6 months, and 1 year. Note that there is also much greater variability in the youngest age groups, so that the normal range can be expected to be much wider than in adults.

There is some disagreement on the interaction of age and stimulus rate. Hecox (1975) found no change in BAEPs in infants with rates from 20 to 66/sec. Salamy et al. (1975) found that waveform resolution was better at 5/sec than at 15/sec in infants less than 6 weeks old, whereas older children did not show this effect. Fujikawa and Weber (1977) and Lasky (1984) noted that infants and older subjects had greater prolongation of wave V absolute latency with increasing stimulus rate than did young adults. Salamy et al. (1978) noted the same effect in newborns and children for absolute latencies of waves I, III, and V and for the I–V IPL.

The central BAEP changes observed in the early months of life have been ascribed to myelination (Hecox, 1975; Starr et al., 1977), increasing fiber diameter (Hecox, 1975), and increasing synaptic efficiency (Starr et al., 1977).

Age-related changes in childhood have been studied by O'Donovan et al. (1980) and Fabiani et al. (1979).

8.2.2. Gender

There is general agreement on the fact that females have shorter absolute and interpeak latencies than males (Beagley and Sheldrake, 1978; Stockard et al., 1978b, 1979; McClelland and McCrea, 1979; Jerger and Hall, 1980; Kjaer, 1980d; Michalewski et al., 1980; O'Donovan et al., 1980; Rosenhamer et al., 1980; Allison et al., 1983, 1984; Thivierge and Cote, 1987; Mitchell et al., 1989). In addition, amplitudes of most BAEP waves tend to be greater in females (Jerger and Hall, 1980; Kjaer, 1980d; Michalewski et al., 1980). There appears to be no significant sex difference in prematures, newborns, and young children (McClelland and McCrea, 1979; Stockard et al., 1979b), with the divergence occurring at about 8 years of age (O'Donovan et al., 1980). Picton et al. (1974) have noted I–V IPL changes during the menstrual cycle, the mean value being 3.81 msec between days 12 and 26 and 3.92 msec on the other days. They believed that this was related to changes in body temperature during the cycle. They noted that temperature differences cannot explain the overall difference between males and females since males have a slightly higher core temperature than females. However, Stockard et al. (1979, in PSVEP bibliography) have noted that females have higher core body temperatures than males and suggested that this might be a contributing factor in causing PSVEP latencies in females to be shorter than those in males. Allison et al. (1983) suggested that brain stem auditory pathway length varies as the cube root of brain volume (from Schmidt-Nielsen, 1975) and, correlating thus with age- and sex-related variations in brain weight (Dekaben and Sadowsky, 1978), calculated that the male:female ratio should be 1.034 ± 0.008. Comparing this with their normal data they found that latency sex differences were within predicted limits. Mitchell et al. (1989) found correlations using regression analyses between the head diameter and latency of wave V and the I–V interval.

Most authors attribute the male–female difference to different body and brain sizes. However, there is no relationship between height and interpeak latencies within a gender group or across groups (Brooks, *unpublished data*).

8.2.3. Body Temperature

There is an increase in absolute and interpeak latencies with progressive lowering of body temperature. Picton et al. (1974) noted a 0.17-msec increase in wave V absolute latency per degree centigrade decrease in temperature, so that below 32.5°C (90.5°F) the values are abnormal relative to normothermic normal subjects (Stockard et al., 1978a). Markand et al. (1987) found an exponential relationship between body temperature and BAEP latencies, with a 7% increase for each 1°C drop. Below 27°C the waveforms became difficult to identify (Stockard et al., 1978a) or disappeared (Kaga et al., 1979; Takiguchi et al., 1979; Dorfman et al., 1981).

Marshall and Donchin (1981) found that circadian alterations in BAEP latencies could be correlated with changes in body temperature (0.2 msec/°C); the major temperature changes occurred during sleep. Picton et al. (1974) also noted this effect. Changes in BAEPs with hypoglycemia probably result from changes in body temperature (Durrant et al., 1991).

8.2.4. Peripheral Hearing Disorders

To a large extent, this topic has been covered already in this chapter (see Sections 8.1.1, 8.1.2, and 8.1.7). In general, much of BAEP behavior in conductive and sensorineural hearing losses is the same as with diminished stimulus (click) intensity, with some interaction by differential involvement of some frequencies over others. The critical question is whether or not any disorder of the peripheral hearing apparatus alters the interpeak latencies used in clinical neurologic interpretations (I–III, III–V, and I–V). If not, then as long as these waves are identifiable, the interpreter can proceed with confidence even in the face of hearing diminished by peripheral hearing disorders. The available evidence indicates that these IPLs, following a click stimulus, are not significantly affected by peripheral hearing disorders. Eggermont et al. (1980) studied 70 normal-hearing subjects and 43 subjects with unilateral hearing loss of cochlear origin (mostly Meniere's disease) and found essentially no difference in the I–V IPL between the two groups. Rosenhamer et al. (1981) studied 11 ears with rising, 22 ears with flat, and 77 ears with sloping audiograms (etiologies consisted mostly of Meniere's disease, noise-induced hearing loss, and previous sudden hearing loss), and concluded that IPLs were not significantly affected by cochlear hearing loss. Coats (1978) and Coats and Martin (1977) studied 37 and 29 ears, respectively, with cochlear hearing losses and noted that there was a slight shortening of the I–V IPL, especially evident at lower stimulus intensities and frequencies and for the ears with the most severe hearing losses. At higher intensities there was very little difference from normal hearing. In clinical neurophysiology the preferred tendency is to err on the side of interpreting a test as normal when it may be abnormal; since cochlear hearing losses tend to shorten the I–V IPL, errors in interpretation are thus automatically made in the "correct" direction.

Not only are absolute latencies affected by peripheral hearing disorders, but also the shape and slope of the intensity versus latency curve of wave V is altered, producing patterns which can help to distinguish conductive and sensorineural hearing losses. In conductive hearing loss (external canal obstruction, tympanic membrane perforation, fluid in the middle ear) the latency–intensity function is parallel to, but displaced from, that of normal hearing subjects by an amount approximately equal to the degree of hearing loss (Galambos and Hecox, 1977). In sensorineural hearing loss (noise damage, Meniere's disease), the latency–intensity function shows the equivalent of recruitment, that is, at low stimulus intensities there is a large difference in wave V absolute latency between the patient and normal subjects, whereas at high intensities the difference is much less (Galambos and Hecox, 1977). Thus, in the latter situation the normal and patient curves converge at higher-stimulus intensities. The exception to this is in recruiting ears with a steep high-frequency hearing loss (Galambos and Hecox, 1977). Other studies in this area are McGee and Clemis (1982) (conductive hearing loss), Sohmer et al. (1981) (sensorineural), Chisin et al. (1983) (sensorineural, conductive and mixed), and Picton and Durieux-Smith (1988).

Conversely, gross BAEP abnormalities are often accompanied by completely normal behavioral hearing parameters, as is seen in patients with MS (Chiappa et al., 1980). However, these patients usually show abnormal auditory localization and interaural time discrimination (Hausler and Levine, 1980; Levine et al., 1993a,b) perhaps suggesting that BAEP waveforms are more closely related to nonhearing functions of the auditory system. Brain stem auditory EPs are normal in cortical deafness (Bahls et al., 1988).

8.2.5. Drug Effects

Interpeak latencies of BAEPs are not significantly affected by therapeutic doses of central nervous system depressant drugs. Cohen and Britt (1982) found no significant changes in cats exposed to anesthetic doses of pentobarbital, ketamine, halothane, and chloralose. Sutton et al. (1982) found no latency changes in cats at therapeutic coma levels of pentobarbital. The small changes observed are usually accounted for by lowered body temperature. Furthermore, essentially normal BAEPs are seen in patients in whom the EEG has been rendered isoelectric and who have the clinical appearance of brain death following administration of high doses of barbiturates for therapy of increased intracranial pressure. Similarly, Stockard and Sharbrough (1980) reported a case of barbiturate overdose (with isoelectric EEG for 18-minute periods and clinical brain death) with normal BAEPs. However, Drummond et al. (1985) have shown small but statistically significant increases in IPLs with high dose thiopental infusions. Garcia-Larrea et al. (1988) have reported BAEP abolition in a comatose patient with infusion of high doses of lidocaine and thiopental; responses returned to normal after discontinuation of the drugs. Nor do variations in intrinsic metabolic factors (blood urea nitrogen, ammonia, pH, oxygen tension or carbon dioxide tension electrolytes) significantly affect BAEPs. Thus, in situations where the clinical question relates to function or nonfunction of brain stem tracts, these considerations will not affect the clinical interpretation. If fine distinctions need to be made (i.e., slight changes in IPLs), then the following information may be pertinent.

Alcohol in intoxicating doses has small but significant effects on BAEP latencies (Chu et al., 1978; Squires et al., 1978a, 1978b; Church and Williams, 1982), probably caused by lowered body temperature (Stockard et al., 1978a) and phase of the blood alcohol level (Lee et al., 1990). Begleiter et al. (1981) studied 17 alcoholic subjects, abstinent for at least 3 weeks, and found marked I–V IPL prolongations (mean increase 0.95 msec). They suggested demyelination or edema as the mechanism.

There were no BAEP IPL changes seen with acute diphenylhydantoin (phenytoin) levels greater than 50 μg/ml (Stockard et al., 1977a). However, Green et al. (1982) noted small increases in I–V IPL (on the order of 0.1 msec) with therapeutic levels, discernible only with group statistical methods; the difference between these sets of findings may be related to chronic rather than acute administration. Hirose et al. (1986) found absent BAEPs in a patient with phenytoin intoxication, and confirmed the relationship in rats. Chan et al. (1990) reported both peripheral and central effects of phenytoin.

With thiopental anesthesia a small decrease in amplitude has been noted (Goff et al., 1977), but no change in latency (Goff et al., 1977; Sanders et al., 1979). Halothane produces no changes (Sanders et al., 1979), nor does isoflurane (Stockard et al., 1977a), but enflurane, an epileptogenic anesthetic, altered later components at concentrations producing spike-wave activity in the EEG (Stockard et al., 1977a, 1978b; Thornton et al., 1981).

Stockard et al. (1977a) reported that no effect on BAEP IPLs was seen with phenothiazines, benzodiazepines, or short-acting barbiturates in humans or cats receiving therapeutic or toxic doses, but Rumpl et al. (1988) found delayed IPLs in four of five patients with overdose of amitryptyline, barbiturate, meprobamate, and nitrazepam (without hypothermia).

There are isolated reports of cholinergic and serotonergic drugs affecting BAEP amplitudes (Bhargava and McKean, 1977; Bhargava et al., 1978) in rats. Furlow et al. (1980) reported BAEP changes in rats that received infusions of phentolamine and propranolol.

Effects of aminoglycoside antibiotics on BAEPs have been studied with the idea of developing a means of following the ototoxicity of those drugs (Guerit et al., 1981). With rapid intravenous injection in humans, amplitude loss and then increased wave I latency were seen, returning to normal 4 hours after the injection. Minor changes in wave I appearance were seen with slower intravenous injection. With oral administration, latency changes and even disappearance of components were noted, with subsequent improvement following cessation of medication. Animal work by Schwent et al. (1980) and Osako et al. (1979) has extended these studies. Martin (1982) reported that intravenous gamma aminobutyric acid (GABA) significantly reduced the amplitude of waves 2–5 in the cat.

Hypoglycemia has been studied in rats and cats (Deutsch et al., 1983) and found to have little effect on BAEPs even at severe levels.

Born et al. (1989) have reported small latency changes with hydrocortisone.

8.2.6. Psychological Parameters

As one would expect from the previous discussions relating to the minimal effects on BAEPs produced by general anesthesia, there are no changes in BAEPs with differing levels of attention or consciousness (Amadeo and Shagass, 1973; Picton and Hillyard, 1974; Sohmer et al., 1978; Hellekson et al., 1979; Edwards et al., 1982), or sleep (Campbell and Bartoli, 1986), although Bastuji et al. (1988) reported significant I–V IPL increases during nocturnal sleep. Szelenberger (1983) reported a correlation between some BAEP waves and personality, whereas Bolz and Giedke (1982) found none.

8.2.7. Reproducibility–Reliability

Amadeo and Shagass (1973) found little change in BAEP IPLs after 8 hours of continuous testing. Chiappa et al. (1979) tested eight subjects on two occasions (mean interval 4.8 months) and noted no significant changes in latency or amplitude measurements ($p > 0.10$). Edwards et al. (1982) tested 10 subjects on two occasions (mean interval 146 days) and also noted no changes. Thus, as one would expect from the persistence of BAEP waveforms under anesthesia, these EPs demonstrate a remarkable consistency over long periods of time. Lasky et al. (1987) found that low intensity and fast repetition rate stimuli elicited more variable responses than loud, slow stimuli and that wave I was more variable than other measurements. They also noted rapid changes in BAEPs immediately following birth.

8.2.8. Ear Dominance

One study found that half of normal subjects have a binaural interaction waveform, whereas the other half do not (Decker and Howe, 1981). Those who do are said to be exhibiting "auditory tract preference." (See also Section 8.1.5.)

9. FREQUENCY-SPECIFIC TESTING

As mentioned before in this chapter, there is a great deal of interest in using BAEPs to approximate the behavioral audiogram and provide threshold information about specific frequencies. Tone pips and bursts, with and without notched noise masking, and "derived potentials" are all being used in various laboratories. There is not complete agreement on techniques and interpretation of BAEPs in this application and an extensive discussion of these matters is beyond the scope of this text. The following references should be consulted as a starting point: Coats and Martin (1977), Sohmer et al. (1977), Coats (1978), Jerger and Mauldin (1978), Coats et al. (1979), Davis and Hirsch (1979), Hicks (1980), Worthington and Peters (1980), Davis (1981), Picton et al. (1981, 1986), Prasher and Gibson (1981), Rosenhamer et al. (1981), Sohmer et al. (1981), Kinarti and Sohmer (1982), and Picton and Durieux-Smith (1988).

Evoked Potentials in Clinical Medicine,
3d ed., edited by Keith H. Chiappa.
Lippincott–Raven Publishers, Philadelphia © 1997.

6

Brain Stem Auditory Evoked Potentials: Interpretation

Keith H. Chiappa and °Rosamund A. Hill

*Department of Neurology, Harvard Medical School, and EEG Laboratory,
Massachusetts General Hospital, Boston, Massachusetts 02114; and
°Neuroservices Unit, Auckland Hospital, Auckland, New Zealand*

1. ANATOMIC AND PHYSIOLOGIC BASIS OF BRAIN STEM AUDITORY EVOKED POTENTIALS

1.1. Human Data

1.1.1. Anatomy

Neural elements within the auditory pathway are the cochlea, the spiral ganglion and eighth nerve (with segments in the petrous bone and subarachnoid space and entry into the brain stem at the pontomedullary border), the cochlear nucleus (in the low pons), the superior olivary nucleus (in the upper part of the lower one third of the pons), the lateral lemniscus tracts and nuclei (in the mid to upper pons), the inferior colliculus (in the midbrain), and the medial geniculate body (thalamus). Pontine auditory structures are situated in more posterior and lateral regions of the tegmentum. Input from each eighth nerve ascends both ipsilaterally and contralaterally and there are crossing fibers at each level as far rostrally as the colliculus. All of these structures are packed into a relatively small area—the distance between the entry point of the eighth nerve into the brain stem and the inferior colliculus is 2.5 to 4.0 cm (facial colliculus to inferior colliculus about 2.5 cm). Thus, the difficulty which has been encountered in differentiating the origins of the four waves (II–V) being generated in this region is not surprising. However, since the original descriptions of brain stem audi-

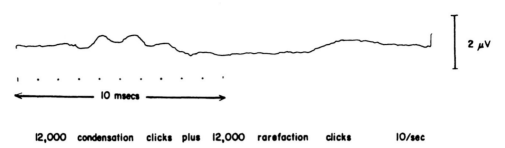

Average of click responses recorded from a scalp electrode placed behind the pinna of a human subject just short of the hairline. In this case, the responses to 12,000 condensation clicks were added to the responses to 12,000 rarefaction clicks. Intensity of clicks: —40 db re 4.4 V across a PDR-10 earphone. The significance of these potentials is unknown; however, they are unlikely to be microphonic potentials and the latencies are too long for auditory nerve potentials. Reference electrode on nose.

FIG. 6–1. First demonstration and report of human BAEPs. (From Kiang, 1961, with permission.)

tory evoked potentials (BAEPs) in humans (Fig. 6–1) (Kiang, 1961; Jewett et al., 1970), the amount of data on this subject has grown.

1.1.2. Clinicopathologic Correlations

Wave I

Wave I of BAEPs is a negative wave recorded at the ear being stimulated, appearing simultaneously with the AP waveform (also called N1) of electrocochleography (ECochG) seen in transtympanic needle recordings from the promontory (near the round window). Both wave I and N1 are manifestations of the volley of eighth nerve action potentials generated by the click stimulus in the segment of the nerve close to the cochlea. Consequently, when wave I cannot be recorded from the earlobe in the conventional manner, it is recommended that ECochG or external ear canal recordings be made to adequately resolve the eighth nerve action potential volley. The latency value for wave I obtained in this manner can then be used in the calculation of the I–III and I–V interpeak latencies (IPLs) (Coats, 1974; Elberling, 1978; Eggermont et al., 1980; Chiappa et al., 1980; Parker et al., 1980; Goldie et al., 1981; Chiappa and Parker, 1984). Moller et al. (1994b) recorded directly from the nerve intraoperatively and calculated the conduction velocity in the eighth nerve at 15.0 to 22.0 meters/sec.

Waves II and III

The working hypothesis in most BAEP work has assigned waves II and III to the cochlear nucleus and superior olivary complex, respectively. Moller and Jannetta (1982a,b), Moller (1988), Moller et al. (1981, 1994c), and Hashimoto et al. (1981), recorded directly from the eighth nerve during surgery and found activity in the intracranial portion of the nerve close to the brain stem at a latency corresponding to the time of appearance of wave II at the scalp. They reasoned that the delay in appearance of the action potential volley was due to the conduction time between the cochlea and the intracranial portions of the nerve (1 to 1.5 cm at 10 to 20 m/sec = 1 to 2 msec). Moller et al. then hypothesized that the activity registered as wave II at the scalp was the same as the activity they had recorded from the intracranial portion of the eighth nerve and they concluded that wave II is generated by that structure. As additional evidence for this they presented the fact that in an occasional patient who is brain-dead, wave II is apparently preserved (Stockard et al., 1980b; Goldie et al., 1981). However, it may be that the activity recorded from the earlobe is not the same as the activity that can be recorded from the intracranial portion of the eighth nerve (i.e., the latter activity may not be seen at the earlobe) and, with respect to the brain-dead patients,

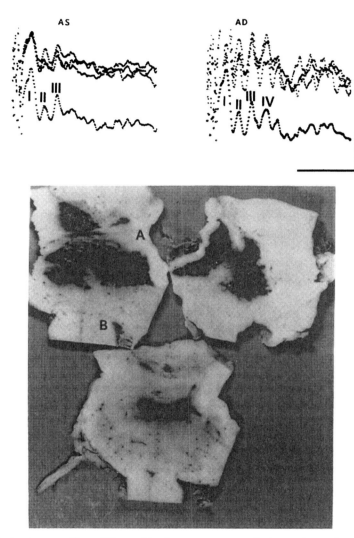

FIG. 6–2. Brain stem auditory EPs and brain stem neuropathology of a patient with a pontine hemorrhage. Both ears had normal waves I–III, only AD (shown above) had a subsequent wave (probably IV). Frontalcoronal sections of pons (A is at pontomesencephalic border, B is at pontomedullary border) show a hemorrhage transecting the pons, sparing the lower one third wherein lie the superior olivary nuclei. Three superimposed trials of 1,024 clicks are superimposed, with the grand average beneath. Recording derivation was vertex to earlobe ipsilateral to monaural stimulation, with relative positivity at the vertex producing an upward trace deflection. Calibration marks are 0.25 µV and 5 msec. (From Chiappa, 1982a, with permission.)

there is no pathologic evidence that the cochlear nucleus is not functioning in those patients. Garg et al. (1982) recorded BAEPs in three patients with hereditary motor-sensory neuropathy, type I, and found the I–II IPL prolonged, but III–V normal. They concluded that (1) the I–II prolongation in this disease (which affects only peripheral nerves), (2) the occasional preservation of wave II in brain-dead patients, and (3) preservation of only waves I and II in the leukodystrophies suggest that wave II might be generated in the intracranial extramedullary portion of the eighth nerve. Hashimoto et al. (1981) also recorded from the surface midline of the dorsal pons at the level of the facial colliculus during surgery and registered high-amplitude waves at approximately the same latency as surface waves II, III, and IV, whereas recordings at the inferior colliculi revealed very little of this activity, suggesting that these waves are generated caudal to that structure.

Similarly, Moller and Jannetta (1982b) found a high-amplitude wave corresponding to III when recording from a site overlying the superior olivary complex. There has been no report of BAEPs in a patient with a lesion that isolated a functioning cochlear nucleus. Starr and Hamilton (1976) reported a case with midbrain and pontine obliteration by a dysgerminoma and hematoma, with waves I–III intact but later waves absent. Similarly, in patients with pontine hemorrhages that spare the lower one third of the pons, waves I–III are left intact (Chiappa, 1982a) (Fig. 6–2). These correlations support the presumed origin of wave III, in the superior olivary complex, but whether wave II is generated in the cochlear nucleus or eighth nerve remains to be proven, although the latter seems the most likely. The presence of a medial nucleus of the trapezoid body in humans suggests that some of wave III might be generated there (Richter et al., 1983), as is the case in animals (Buchwald and Huang, 1975).

Waves IV and V

There are even fewer human data bearing on the generator sites of waves IV and V. Lesions in the mid and upper pons produce abnormalities in both waves (Lev and Sohmer, 1972; Sohmer et al., 1974; Starr and Achor, 1975, 1979; Starr and Hamilton, 1976; Stockard et al., 1976b, 1977b; Stockard and Rossiter, 1977; Boller and Jacobson, 1980; Epstein et al., 1980; Brown et al., 1981b; Chiappa, 1982a). Figure 6–3 shows data from a patient with a restricted midbrain–upper pontine hemorrhage, and Figs. 6–4 and 6–5 are from patients with pontine tumors, all showing waves IV and V absent or at abnormal latency separations from wave III (see Section 1.1.4 below for further details of these cases). Epstein et al. (1980) reported a patient with acute onset of vertigo, vertical diplopia, left-sided sensory loss, right-sided incoordination, palatal myoclonus, and normal computed tomography (CT) scan and vertebral angiogram; waves IV and V were absent. Starr and Achor (1979) reported a case with a restricted collicular lesion and essentially normal waves V. However, this case is not altogether convincing since that lesion was a pinealoma and pathology was not obtained until some time after BAEP testing. Hashimoto et al. (1981) and Hashimoto (1982) recorded during surgery from electrodes situated between the inferior colliculi and registered a large-amplitude positivity that reached a maximum slightly later than wave V at the scalp, followed by a larger negativity peaking at 10 to 11 msec. They postulated that both the positive and negative activities were generated in the inferior colliculus. Moller and Jannetta (1982b, 1983) also recorded the same activities directly from the surface of the inferior colliculus during surgery but thought that the positivity at about 7 msec was generated in the fiber tract of the lateral lemniscus, while the subsequent negative activity was generated in the inferior colliculus. They pointed out that the inferior colliculus was unlikely to be the neural generator of BAEP components that have a shorter latency than the earliest potentials that can be recorded in the inferior colliculus. They concluded that wave V is generated primarily in the lateral lemniscus. Moller et al. (1994c) recorded from the midline of the floor of the fourth ventricle and concluded that the sharp tip of the peak of wave V is generated by the termination of the lateral lemniscus in the inferior colliculus. Curio and Oppel (1988) recorded from an electrode stereotactically implanted along a pontomesencephalic path and concluded that wave V was generated from contralateral sources in upper pons/midbrain Picton et al. (1981) have summarized evidence in the literature and in their experience as indicating that wave V is independent of the inferior colliculus. Although it has been argued that there are contributions to waves IV and V from the generators of earlier waves, especially III, this is difficult to maintain in cases where there is a nor-

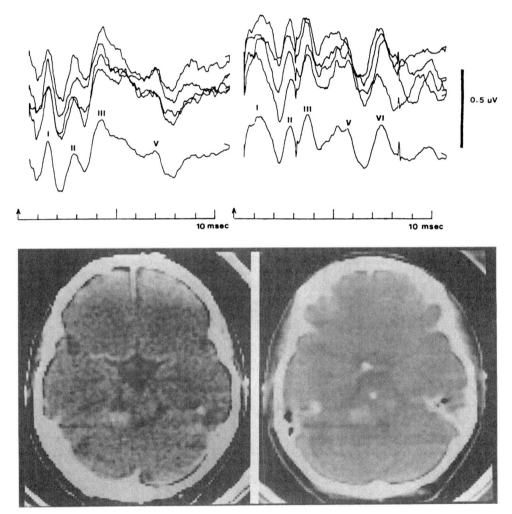

FIG. 6–3. Brain stem auditory EPs and CT scan from a patient with an upper pontine–midbrain hemorrhage. Note that the hemorrhage is primarily left-sided and the BAEPs show an abnormality only in AS (*left panel*), with the III–V separation markedly abnormal and the I:V amplitude ratio at the limits of normality. Each panel has four superimposed trials of 512 clicks each with the grand average beneath.

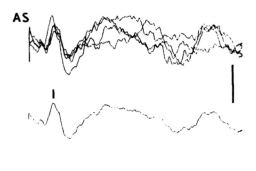

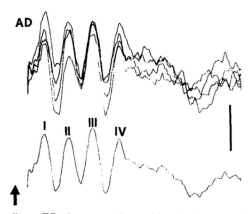

FIG. 6–4. Brain stem auditory EPs from a patient with a brainstem glioma. At the time of testing the left corneal reflex was absent, there was numbness of the entire left face (max. in V2), and the jaw deviated to the left on opening, in addition to other nonlateralized clinical findings (see text). Note the marked asymmetry in BAEPs between the two ears. Clinical, radiologic, and subsequent neuropathologic findings consistently demonstrated a marked asymmetry of tumor involvement with the left brain stem most severely affected, corresponding to the asymmetry of the BAEPs. Calibration mark is 0.25 µV. Each panel has four separate trials of 512 clicks each superimposed with the grand average beneath. (From Chiappa, 1982a, with permission.)

mal III and absent IV and V (e.g., Fig. 6–2) or absent III and normal V (Figs. 6–6 and 6–15). In summary, the available human evidence suggests that wave V is generated in the high pons or low midbrain (lateral lemniscus or inferior colliculus), with no complete answer yet available. In terms of clinical interpretation there is no difference between the two possibilities since they are so close to one another.

Waves VI and VII

It is speculated that waves VI and VII arise in the medial geniculate body and auditory radiations, respectively, but there are few data on this point. Recordings from intrathalamic

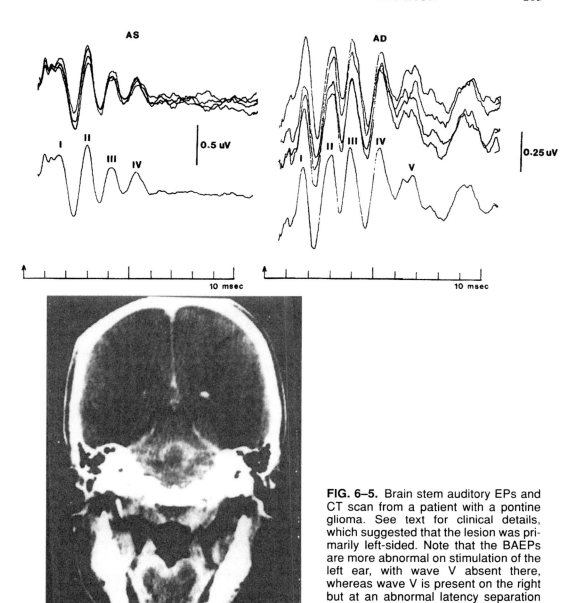

FIG. 6–5. Brain stem auditory EPs and CT scan from a patient with a pontine glioma. See text for clinical details, which suggested that the lesion was primarily left-sided. Note that the BAEPs are more abnormal on stimulation of the left ear, with wave V absent there, whereas wave V is present on the right but at an abnormal latency separation from wave III. Each panel has four separate trials of 512 clicks each superimposed, with the grand average beneath.

depth electrodes in humans have thus far not been helpful (Hashimoto et al., 1981; Chiappa, 1982a; Velasco et al., 1982). Since these waves are unreliable in appearance, they are not used in clinical interpretation. The slow negative peak at about 9 to 10 msec appears to originate in the midbrain and may be postsynaptic activity in the inferior colliculus (Hashimoto, 1982).

1.1.3. Potential-Field Distribution Studies

Potential-field mapping studies have provided the source for a great deal of speculation concerning the generator sites of BAEP waveforms (Ino and Mizoi, 1980; Kevanishvili, 1980; Robinson and Rudge, 1981; Starr and Squires, 1982; Scherg and von Cramon, 1985). However, they have added nothing concrete to the above clinicopathologic correlations.

1.1.4. Lateralization

Human and animal anatomic studies and animal microelectrode studies suggest that the major functional part of the brain stem auditory system ascends contralateral to the active ear. However, the majority of human clinicopathologic correlations indicate that the BAEP waveforms are generated ipsilateral to the active ear, except perhaps for wave V. Preliminary findings in patients indicated the possible ipsilateral generation of BAEP waveforms (Chiappa et al., 1980). Brown et al. (1981a) reviewed all BAEP and clinical records of patients with posterior fossa lesions seen in this laboratory between 1977 and 1980. In 56 cases (Table 6–1) clinical and radiographic data permitted firm diagnosis and anatomic localization of the posterior fossa pathology. Twenty-four patients had intrinsic brain stem lesions without hearing deficits (see Table 6–2 for the diagnostic categories). Nineteen patients with lesions rostral to the pontomedullary junction and at least partially within the pontomesencephalic tegmentum had abnormal BAEPs. In the majority (17/19), the clinical lesions were either strongly unilateral (6), or bilateral with a predominant laterality of involvement (11). In 13 of these 17 cases with lateralizing lesions the monaural BAEP was most abnormal on stimulation of the ear ipsilateral to the lesion. In none was the monaural BAEP most abnormal on stimulation of the ear contralateral to the lesion. In the remaining four cases, interpretation required caution as all BAEPs were absent on stimulation of the ear ipsilateral to the lesions. For example, the patient whose BAEP and CT scan data are shown in Fig. 6–3 had sudden onset of left facial hypesthesia and hyperpathia, a left Horner's syndrome, left-sided cerebellar function abnormalities, and right-sided hyperreflexia. Computed tomography scan showed an upper pontine–midbrain hemorrhage primarily localized on the left. BAEPs from AD were normal, but AS showed a markedly delayed and low-amplitude wave V (wave IV was absent). (The short-latency somatosensory evoked potentials (SEPs) from stimulation of the median nerve at the wrist were normal bilaterally.) Figure 6–4 shows BAEPs from a 25-year-old patient with a history of 11 weeks of numbness of the left face, tongue, and gum and 4 weeks of progressive dysphagia and incoordination. Examination showed horizontal nystagmus on left lateral gaze, up-and-down beat nystagmus, absence of the left corneal reflex, diminished left facial pin-prick sensation, and an up-going right toe to plantar stimulation. Computed tomography scan showed a low-density lesion in the left pons with slight compression of the fourth ventricle, consistent with a brain stem glioma. The BAEP was bilaterally abnormal, but predominantly so on

TABLE 6–1. *Evaluation of documented posterior fossa lesion cases for study. N = 56*

Extrinsic brain stem lesions		Intrinsic brain stem lesions	
Acoustic neuromas	Other	With poor hearing	Accepted for study
25	4	3	24

TABLE 6–2. *Diagnoses of intrinsic brain stem lesion cases. N = 24*

Cases with BAEP normal	
Locked-in syndrome	2
Lateral medullary syndrome	3
Total	5

Cases with BAEP abnormal	
Pontine hemorrhage	4
Brain stem glioma	4
Lateral medullary syndrome	1
Locked-in syndrome	2
Other ischemic brain stem strokes	5
Thalamic glioma	1
Brain stem cyst	1
Unidentified brain stem mass	1
Total	19

stimulation of the left ear, which produced normal waves I and II but no recognizable peaks thereafter. Stimulation of the right ear produced normal waves I, II, III, and IV and no peak for wave V. The patient received 5,000 rads of radiotherapy but expired 2 years later. At autopsy the rostral pons was grossly disfigured by an infiltrating glioma. The tumor infiltrated the pons bilaterally but was clearly much more extensive on the left side. It extended rostrally to involve the caudal mesencephalon on the left; its margin was limited caudally by the pontomedullary junction. Figure 6–5 shows BAEPs from a 40-year-old patient with a 7-week history of left-sided dysmetria, ataxia with falling to the left, and facial numbness (bilateral); there was bilateral lateral gaze nystagmus but the remainder of the cranial nerves were normal. Computed tomography scan showed an enhancing ring lesion in the pons, more prominent on the right. Brain stem auditory EPs had wave V absent in AS (the side indicated by the clinical features) and the III–V separation in AD was abnormal. Presumably in this case the CT scan is not indicating the area of major functional impairment. These cases indicate that, in most clinical situations, for waves I through V the BAEP pattern is most abnormal on monaural stimulation of the ear ipsilateral to the brain stem lesion. As an empirical observation this conclusion is of importance in the clinical interpretation of abnormal BAEPs. With respect to generator sites the data suggest that: (1) the inputs to the generators of waves III and IV ascend the brain stem predominantly ipsilaterally to the ear stimulated. Otherwise, in Fig. 6–4, waves III and IV should be absent on stimulation of the right ear in the presence of an infiltrating left pontine lesion. It could be objected that caudal extension of the left pontine tumor impaired high medullary decussation of input from the left ear to the right pons, thereby obliterating the response to left monaural stimulation. Brown et al. thought that this was not tenable as it would imply that monaural stimulation on the right was able to produce normal BAEPs III and IV from generators in the left pons, despite heavy tumor infiltration. Oh et al. (1981) reported similar findings although their recordings were of poor quality. Hashimoto et al. (1979) focused on recording from the ear contralateral to the one being stimulated but examination of their results also shows predominantly ipsilateral abnormalities. Ebner and Brinkmann have seen a case of a tumor infiltrating the left cerebellar hemisphere, mesencephalon, and quadrigeminal region, with the aqueduct and fourth ventricle displaced to the right. Brain stem auditory EPs were normal on the right and grossly abnormal on the left (*unpublished data*). York (1986) reported ipsilateral BAEP wave V absence in a patient with a strictly unilateral pontine–midbrain lesion, and Scaioli et al. (1988) also had a patient with an inferolateral dorsal pontine lesion on magnetic resonance imaging (MRI) (presumably demyelination) with absent wave V ipsilaterally. Musiek and Geurkink (1982) had a few patients with lateralized brain stem lesions and never found a purely contralateral correlation. Zanette et al. (1990) found ipsilateral correlation except for wave V, which was absent contralateral, in a patient with a brainstem hemorrhage.

With respect to wave V laterality, the only abnormality seen in Fig. 6–4 on stimulation of the right ear was loss of wave V (as seen also by Zanette et al. (1990) in a unilateral pontine hemorrhage). This could have been produced by tumor infiltration across the midline at higher levels to involve the right side or it could reflect diminished wave V generation from a (contralateral) left midbrain or high pontine structure, the impulses having ascended on the right and then failed either to cross or to activate the contralateral generator at the higher levels. Similarly, the loss of wave V on stimulation ipsilateral to the tumor may reflect loss of input to the right wave V generator from compromised pathways on the left. Available data in this case do not allow us to distinguish between these possibilities. The gross unilateral abnormality in Fig. 6–3 with a high pontine and lower midbrain lesion could similarly be explained by failure of either ipsilateral or contralateral inputs to an upper pontine or lower midbrain generator of wave V. The solution would be to find a patient with an isolated, small midbrain lesion, which would not be expected to interfere with crossing paths at mid or upper pontine levels as might have occurred in the patients whose data are shown in Figs. 6–3 and 6–4. Such a case might be that of Epstein et al. (1980); they reported a patient with acute onset of vertigo, vertical diplopia, left-sided sensory loss, right-sided incoordination, and palatal myoclonus. Waves IV and V were absent stimulating and recording from the ear contralateral to the (clinical) location of the lesion. Unfortunately this was not isolated palatal myoclonus and no lesions were seen on CT scan or vertebral angiogram, so that direct anatomic evidence of lesion location was not available. Anderson et al. (1988) recorded BAEPs before and after development of a CT-visualized traumatic midbrain syrinx and found a contralateral wave V abnormality. This case raises the question of retrograde degeneration in the brain stem auditory system, and the loss of wave V is not necessarily directly related to the midbrain syrinx. Jabbari et al. (1982c) found no BAEP abnormalities in three patients with isolated palatal myoclonus. Zanette et al. (1990) studied a patient with a restricted midbrain hemorrhage; initially waves II–V were absent ipsilaterally and V contralaterally, but later when the ipsilateral waveforms had normalized the contralateral wave V was still abnormal. Similarly, Fischer et al. (1995) have reported a patient with a left unilateral lesion involving the inferior colliculus (and higher structures) that produced a delayed and reduced wave V on the right.

In summary, the available evidence cannot conclusively settle the question of laterality. For purposes of clinical interpretation lesions affecting the middle and upper parts of the pons primarily produce BAEP abnormalities on the same side. Occasional cases with a restricted, high locus may produce abnormalities more marked contralaterally for wave V only.

The fact that some inputs to BAEP generators ascend the brain stem ipsilaterally implies that the pathways mediating BAEPs may be distinct from those predominantly crossed pathways which subserve normal hearing. In addition, patients with gross central abnormalities of BAEPs almost always have normal hearing as tested with conventional behavioral techniques. This may mean that there is a large safety factor in the brain stem auditory system or that BAEP waveforms are being generated in a part of the system not concerned with behavioral hearing. The latter idea was underscored by the finding of abnormal interaural time discrimination and auditory localization functioning in a group of multiple sclerosis (MS) patients with central BAEP abnormalities (Hausler and Levine, 1980; Levine et al., 1993a). The latter study also made a detailed comparison of waveform abnormalities and lesion location as determined by MRI scans. However, it seems unlikely that the MRI-detected lesions could be mapped to the brainstem auditory neuroanatomy of a particular patient with such millimeter precision, given the known variability in human neural structures.

1.2. Animal Data

There have been detailed studies in animals related to BAEP waveform generators (Jewett, 1970; Lev and Sohmer, 1972; Plantz et al., 1974; Buchwald and Huang, 1975; Berry et al., 1976; Stockard et al., 1976a; Huang and Buchwald, 1977, 1978; Allen and Starr, 1978; Achor and Starr, 1980a,b; Cazals et al., 1980; Huang, 1980; Rossi and Britt, 1980; Williston et al., 1981; Sohmer et al., 1982; Creel et al., 1983a; Hinman and Buchwald, 1983b; Martin and Penix, 1983; Maurer and Mika, 1983; Wada and Starr, 1983b; Church et al., 1984; Katayama, 1985; Moller and Burgess, 1986; Caird and Klinke, 1987), comparisons with humans (Corwin et al., 1982; Fullerton et al., 1987), maturation (Doyle et al., 1983), and effects of hypothermia (Marsh et al., 1984; Rossi and Britt, 1984; Doyle and Fria, 1985), and hyperthermia (Mustafa et al., 1988). Although these data have provided a source for much speculation, it has not added to or clarified the human data presented above.

1.3. Summary

Although there is no strong primary evidence in humans to define the presumed generator sources of BAEP waveforms, there is also no evidence to suggest that the assumptions listed above are incorrect. The localization errors are probably on the order of 1 cm, at worst, an accuracy level which is more than sufficient for most clinical purposes. The suggested generator sources are as follows: wave I—distal eighth nerve; wave II—proximal eighth nerve or cochlear nucleus; wave III—lower pons (possibly the superior olivary complex); wave IV—mid or upper pons (possibly the lateral lemniscus tracts and nuclei); wave V—upper pons or inferior colliculus.

It is not known whether BAEPs are being generated at synapses in gray matter nuclei or by volleys in white matter tracts, or by some combination of these. It is also postulated that the waveforms may be the result of summation of electrical activity from more than one nucleus.

2. PATHOPHYSIOLOGY AND CLINICAL INTERPRETATIONS

2.1. Relationships Between Hearing and Central BAEP Abnormalities

There seems to be no clinically important effect of peripheral hearing disorders on central BAEP interpeak latencies (see Chapter 4, Sections 8.1.1 and 8.2.4). Therefore, if waves I, III, and V are clearly visible, definitive statements can be made in the test interpretation concerning the state of central conduction in the brain stem auditory pathways. If wave I is not discernible, then that section of the pathway between the peripheral eighth nerve and the lower pons cannot be commented upon. For this reason great effort is expended in resolving wave I when it is not registered with the conventional earlobe recording technique (see Chapter 4, Section 3).

If wave I cannot be registered despite all maneuvers, the behavioral audiogram may be helpful in estimating whether or not wave V latency is appropriate for the degree of hearing loss. Selters and Brackmann (1977) proposed correction factors for wave V absolute latency related to the degree of hearing loss. If wave V latency still falls outside of the normal range despite the correction factor, this suggests the possibility of a retrocochlear conduction delay, although this evidence is much less firm than an abnormal I–III IPL.

The relationship between abnormalities of BAEP waves II–V and functional hearing as tested by conventional behavioral audiometry is not clearly understood. Gross central BAEP abnormalities are usually associated with normal hearing (e.g., in patients with MS and pontine gliomas). Only when auditory localization performance is tested in detail can another manifestation of the lesion producing the abnormal BAEP be seen (Hausler and Levine, 1980). These facts suggest that BAEP waveforms may be related to activity in regions of brain stem auditory pathways more involved with sound source localization than with hearing as usually defined. Another explanation is that minor changes in conduction velocities produce enough desynchronization of the volley so that the potentials cannot be resolved, whereas there is a considerable safety margin for functional hearing. Furthermore, diseases in the peripheral vestibular system do not affect BAEPs. For example, 21 patients with labyrinthine diseases (Meniere's disease, labyrinthitis, and vestibular neuronitis) had no BAEP interpeak latency abnormalities (Chiappa et al., 1980). In 43 patients (most with Meniere's disease), the largest difference between normal and affected ears in the I–V separation was 0.5 msec (mean 0.2 msec) (Eggermont et al., 1980), which is at the upper limit of normal for that measure. Note that BAEPs are normal in cortical deafness (Bahls et al., 1988).

2.2. Latency Abnormalities

Because exact generator sources of BAEP waveforms are not known (synaptic versus tract potentials or both), the pathophysiology of abnormalities is also speculative. In experimental animals, unilateral and bilateral focal brain stem cooling produced BAEP amplitude and latency abnormalities, respectively (Stockard et al., 1976a). However, the variety of diseases in which BAEP abnormalities are found suggests that multiple factors can be involved, presumably including segmental demyelination and axonal and neuronal loss. See Chapter 3, Section 2.2, for a discussion of the effects of demyelination on conduction velocities; the axons of the visual and auditory systems presumably respond to similar lesions in a similar fashion.

Since wave I is generated primarily by that portion of the eighth nerve that is contiguous with the spiral ganglion in the mastoid bone, when there is a conduction defect in the eighth nerve near its entry to the brain stem (e.g., acoustic neuroma, meningitis), wave I is affected only if the cause of the conduction defect also interferes with the blood supply to more distal portions of the nerve or if sufficient time has elapsed for retrograde degeneration to occur.

With acoustic neuromas the interwave separation abnormalities have been attributed to differential involvement of low- and high-frequency fibers in the eighth nerve (Eggermont et al., 1980; Eggermont and Don, 1986). The latter fiber type is situated peripherally in the nerve and is the most affected by the tumor. However, in some patients with acoustic neuromas there is a low-frequency hearing loss with the same BAEP abnormality (Parker et al., 1980), indicating that other processes are at work.

Thus, when waves I, III, and V are clearly seen, the final part of the interpretation of abnormal IPLs might read: (1) When there is an abnormal I–III IPL: "This abnormality suggests the presence of a conduction defect in the brain stem auditory system between the eighth nerve close to the cochlea and the lower pons." (2) When there is an abnormal III–V IPL: "This abnormality suggests the presence of a conduction defect in the brain stem auditory system between the lower pons and the midbrain." (3) When wave I is absent and the III–V separation is normal: "Wave I (the eighth nerve activation potential) could not be recorded. This is usually due to a peripheral hearing disorder. Because of this, the state of conduction in the segment of the brain stem auditory pathway between peripheral eighth nerve and lower pons could not be determined. Lower pons to midbrain conduction was normal."

2.3. Amplitude Ratio Abnormalities

The amplitude ratio of waves I/V varies with effective stimulus intensity and with the shape of the audiogram. Thus, this parameter can be used only when the click-hearing threshold is normal. If there is any doubt, an audiogram is necessary. Also, the values obtained from normals are only applicable to the stimulus intensity (dB SL) used in testing the normal subjects.

The loss of amplitude is presumably caused by (1) fewer fibers conducting the volley and (2) desynchronization of the volley secondary to widely different conduction velocities (demyelination causing very slow conduction).

It is best to be rather conservative about the use of this parameter and to wait until wave V is of markedly low amplitude and poorly defined before making the determination of abnormality. Thus, when waves IV and/or V are absent or of abnormally low amplitude, the interpretation might read: "This abnormality suggests the presence of a conduction defect in the brain stem auditory system rostral to the lower pons."

2.4. Laterality of Abnormalities

Using monaural stimulation and recording, patients frequently have BAEPs that are normal from one ear but abnormal from the other (e.g., Fig. 6–4). Of 64 patients with MS who had abnormal BAEPs, 45% had these abnormalities from only one ear (Chiappa et al., 1980), and patients with intrinsic brain stem tumors or infarcts may show the same pattern (Brown et al., 1981b). Furthermore, when the site of the lesion is known, it is almost always on the same side of the brain stem as the ear producing the more abnormal BAEPs (see above, Section 1.1.4, for a complete discussion). Therefore, when the BAEP abnormality is seen only on testing one ear, in addition to the text suggested in the above two sections, a phrase indicating the probable side of the brain stem lesion (conduction defect) is added.

3. CLINICAL CORRELATIONS

3.1. Introduction

Clinical utility of BAEPs stems from the close relationship between the EP waveforms and specific anatomic structures. This specificity allows localization of conduction defects in the brain stem to within a centimeter or so. In addition, BAEPs are very resistant to alteration by anything other than structural pathology in the brain stem auditory tracts. For example, barbiturate doses sufficient to render the electroencephalogram (EEG) "flat" (isoelectric) and general anesthesia do not significantly affect BAEPs. These factors of anatomic specificity and physiologic and metabolic immutability are the basis of the clinical utility of BAEPs.

Brain stem auditory EPs offer a look at "physiologic anatomy." They provide a sensitive tool for assessment of brain stem auditory tracts and nearby structures. Abnormalities demonstrated by BAEPs are etiologically nonspecific and must be carefully integrated into the clinical situation by a physician familiar with the clinical use of this test. The physician must decide if other procedures (e.g., conventional audiometric studies, ECochG, electronystagmography, radiologic studies, subspecialty consultation) are indicated to differentiate the possible causes of the conduction delay. Brain stem auditory EPs are used to test (1) the peripheral hearing apparatus in conductive and sensorineural hearing disorders and (2) the brain stem auditory tracts in central nervous system (CNS) disorders. The different techniques and interpreter backgrounds required for most accurate clinical correlation of test results in each application usually dictate that a single laboratory not attempt to provide testing in both areas.

3.2. Ototoxic Drugs

The ototoxicity of aminoglycoside antibiotics may be difficult to follow in some patients (e.g., in infants and comatose patients). Therefore, the effects of these antibiotics on BAEPs have been studied with the idea of developing a means of following their ototoxicity. Guerit et al. (1981) followed BAEPs in five patients who were administered the antibiotic via different routes: (1) with rapid intravenous (IV) injection, amplitude loss and then increased wave I latency were seen, returning to normal 4 hours after the injection; (2) with slower IV injection, minor changes in wave I appearance were seen; and (3) with oral administration, latency changes and even disappearance of components were noted, with subsequent improvement following cessation of medication. Kovnar et al. (1986a) found BAEPs useful in screening for cisplatin ototoxicity in young or uncooperative patients. These preliminary observations indicate that BAEPs may have a role in this clinical problem.

3.3. Cerebellopontine Angle Tumors

Brain stem auditory EP findings have been reported in almost 600 patients with acoustic neuromas and other cerebellopontine angle (CPA) tumors (Sohmer et al., 1974; Starr and Hamilton, 1976; Clemis and Mitchell, 1977; Rosenhamer, 1977; Selters and Brackman, 1977; Thomsen et al., 1978; Clemis and McGee, 1979; Glasscock et al., 1979; Hashimoto et al., 1979; House and Brackman, 1979; Salomon et al., 1979; Wielaard and Kemp, 1979; Eggermont et al., 1980; Parker et al., 1980; Shanon et al., 1981b; Zappulla et al., 1981; Maurer et al., 1982; Robinson and Rudge, 1983; Eggermont and Don, 1986; Legatt et al., 1988). The large majority of these studies used as BAEP diagnostic criteria the absolute wave V latency or the interside difference in that same parameter. Because of the known effect of decreased effective stimulus intensity and hearing loss on wave V latency, various correction factors have been devised to increase the accuracy of the test. For example, Selters and Brackmann (1977) subtracted 0.1 msec from the observed wave V latency for every 10 dB or fraction thereof of loss of the 4-KHz pure-tone threshold over 50 dB.

Hyde and Blair (1981) suggested that this correction was excessive when the hearing loss was flat and insufficient with steep high-frequency hearing loss. Selters and Brackmann reported false negative and positive rates of 6% and 12%, respectively, and Hyde and Blair reported a 14% false positive rate using these same criteria. The latter authors suggested a two-step correction, first for the conductive part of the loss and then for the sensory portion; they believed that a correction of 0.1 msec for every 5 dB of loss over 55 dB was better and noted that it lowered the false positive rate in Selters and Brackmann's series by about a half while increasing the false negative rate by a much smaller amount.

However, since BAEP IPLs are not significantly affected by conductive or sensorineural hearing losses, these parameters are by far the most accurate (Salomon et al., 1979; Wielaard and Kemp, 1979; Eggermont et al., 1980; Parker et al., 1980; Zappulla et al., 1981; Eggermont and Don, 1986). Although Hyde and Blair stated that wave I could not be recorded in 42% of 400 patients with noise-induced cochlear hearing loss and concluded that this diminished the utility of the IPL parameters, this need not be the case. Elberling (1978) and Salomon et al. (1979) suggested the combination of ECochG (for wave I registration) and BAEPs (for waves III and V). Others have used external ear canal spring electrodes (Coats, 1974) and needle electrodes (Chiappa and Parker, 1984; Goldie et al., 1981) to increase the identification rate of wave I. When care is taken in the performance of the test and these techniques are used, wave I can be successfully recorded in a large majority of cases and the I–III, III–V, and I–V intervals can be used in interpretation, resulting in marked improvement of the false negative and positive detection rates. (See Chapter 4, Section 8.2.4, for a full discussion of the effects of hearing disorders on BAEP interpeak latencies.) For example, in the study of Parker et al. (1980), in 28 of 41 patients with CPA tumors (acoustic neuromas and meningiomas) who had either wave III or wave V (or both) visible, wave I was registered in 27 using either earlobe or external auditory canal (EAC) needle techniques (the 28th patient was done before the needle method was developed). When wave I cannot be registered despite use of an external ear canal electrode, the tumor is usually large enough so that clinical or radiologic diagnosis should not be a problem. Occasional exceptions to this have been where small tumors have abolished all waves, presumably because of early interference with the eighth nerve blood supply.

Using the normal mean plus 3 SD as the upper limit of normal for the I–V latency separation, Eggermont et al. (1980) had false negative results in 2 patients and borderline results in another 2 patients from a group of 42 patients with acoustic neuromas. In 43 patients with unilateral hearing loss of cochlear origin (mostly Meniere's disease) they had no false positives. In a later study Eggermont and Don (1986) had essentially the same results, and also showed that acoustic neuromas in the internal auditory meatus affect the cochlea and mainly higher frequencies, possibly by interfering with auditory nerve fibers adjacent to the vestibular nerve, originating in the basal cochlea. [Also, Chiappa et al. (1980) found no BAEP IPL abnormalities in 21 patients with various labyrinthine diseases.] Similarly striking results were obtained by Parker et al. (1980) also using IPL parameters; in a group of 41 patients with acoustic neuromas and 9 with CPA meningiomas, BAEPs were abnormal on the side of the tumor in all, including 9 with normal CT scans and 3 with normal standard audiometry (not all of these patients had stapedial reflexes tested but in one of those who did have that test, it was also normal). For example, Fig. 6–6 is from a patient referred for testing because of progressive hearing loss in the left ear. Pure-tone audiogram and speech discrimination were abnormal in the left ear, normal in the right ear. Computed tomography scan was normal. Brain stem auditory EPs from the left ear had normal interwave separations despite abnormal absolute latencies secondary to the peripheral hearing disorder. Brain stem auditory EPs from the right ear had an abnormal I–V separation and a posterior fossa contrast study revealed an unsuspected, incidental acoustic neuroma on that side.

Brain stem auditory EPs are the most sensitive screening test when an acoustic neuroma is suspected. They may be abnormal when routine audiologic tests and CT scans are normal

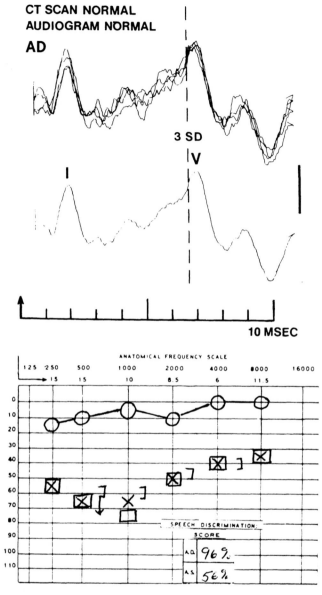

FIG. 6–6. Brain stem auditory EPs and audiogram from a patient tested because of progressive hearing loss in the left ear. AS pure-tone audiogram showed a 40-to 50-dB loss with 56% speech discrimination; BAEPs (not shown) reflected the peripheral hearing loss but IPLs were completely normal. AD pure-tone audiogram and speech discrimination were normal but the BAEPs (above) showed a marked I–V IPL abnormality at 5.0 msec (normal mean plus 3 SD = 4.7 msec). Computed tomography scan was normal but posterior fossa contrast study showed a tumor. (From Chiappa, 1982a, with permission.)

(Figs. 5–6 and 6–6), whereas the converse has not been found. The I–III separation is the most sensitive measure (Fig. 5–6, AD in Fig. 6–7), and the interear difference in this parameter may help to convince the interpreter of the abnormality (Fig. 6–8). There is a small incidence of false positive tests, that is, a markedly abnormal I–III or I–V separation without a tumor on posterior fossa contrast study. The nature of the conduction defect in these latter patients is as yet unknown. For practical purposes, if the BAEP IPL measures are within 2 SD of normal, an acoustic neuroma is not present. Only very small, usually asymptomatic acoustic neuromas break this rule, as in the patient whose BAEPs and gas CT scan are shown in Fig. 6–7. This patient was completely asymptomatic and came to neurologic attention only because of a family history of dominantly inherited, bilateral acoustic neuro-

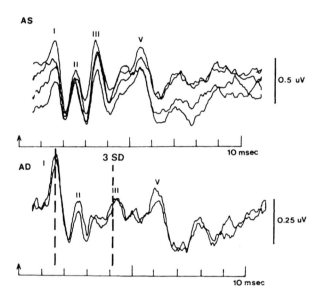

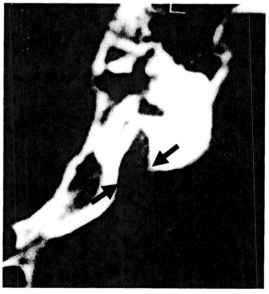

FIG. 6–7. Brain stem auditory EPs from a patient with dominantly inherited bilateral acoustic neuromas. The patient was completely asymptomatic and came to medical attention because of the family history. Audiograms and contrast-enhanced CT scan were normal. The abnormal BAEP from AD prompted a gas CT scan, which revealed a 1-cm acoustic neuroma on that side (removed surgically with preservation of hearing). Despite the completely normal BAEPs from AS, the gas CT scan on that side (figure) revealed a small tumor on the left (the arrows mark the mouth of the internal auditory canal with the irregular shape of the tumor within). Note the normal I–II separation in AD, despite the markedly abnormal I–III IPL. Each trace is the average of 512 clicks.

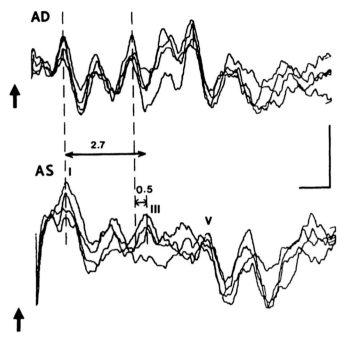

FIG. 6–8. Brain stem auditory EPs from a patient with an AN and normal CT scan. Note that the I–III separation is at the upper limit of normal (mean plus 3 SD) but the interear difference for that measure is greater than the normal mean plus 3 SD, helping to confirm the abnormality of the BAEPs. Each trace is the average of 512 clicks. Calibration marks are 0.25 µV and 1 msec.

mas. Audiograms and a contrast-enhanced CT scan were normal. Brain stem auditory EPs showed a clear I–III IPL abnormality in the right ear (AD in Fig. 6–7A); because of the family history of bilateral acoustic neuromas, a gas CT scan was performed which showed a 1-cm acoustic neuroma on the right; on the left side, despite the normal BAEPs, a small acoustic neuroma was visualized (gas CT scan). The tumor on the right was removed surgically, with preservation of hearing. Whether or not much is lost clinically when a tumor of this size is missed by BAEPs is open to debate, unless the patient is lost to follow-up because of the normal BAEP. If clinical suspicion remains despite a normal BAEP, the test should be repeated in a few months or so. Legatt et al. (1988) have also found normal BAEPs with small tumors, but noted abnormal latency–intensity functions in these patients; they suggested that a latency–intensity function should be obtained if the IPLs are normal and the suspicion of acoustic neuroma is high.

Patients with peripheral hearing disorders do not show clinically significant changes in IPLs (see Chapter 4, Section 8.2.4). Thus, central BAEP abnormalities in a patient with an apparent peripheral problem should trigger further investigation. Figure 6–9 shows the pure-tone audiogram and speech discrimination in a patient who presented with hearing difficulty in the right ear. Eight months later the audiogram deficit had resolved and the initial diagnosis was Meniere's disease. However, the BAEP (Fig. 6–10) showed a markedly abnormal I–V separation, incompatible with a diagnosis of Meniere's disease, and MS was considered. A CT scan was normal. One year later the patient began to have exacerbations of her symptoms with her menses, and a repeat CT (Fig. 6–10) showed evidence of an acoustic neuroma.

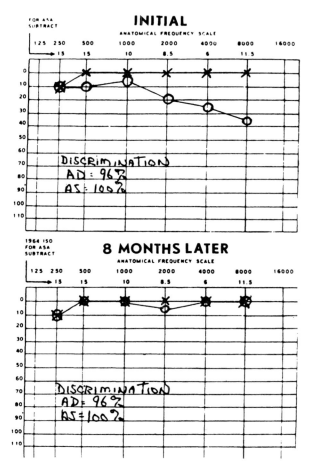

FIG. 6–9. Pure-tone audiogram and speech discrimination in a patient who presented (*top panel*) with hearing difficulty in the right ear. Eight months later (*bottom panel*) the audiogram abnormality had resolved and the clinical impression was Meniere's disease.

Some patients with acoustic neuromas have a good wave I but no subsequent waves (Fig. 6–11), or have no waves at all despite fairly good hearing (Parker et al., 1980). The significance of these patterns is not understood. Patients with large CPA tumors (acoustic neuromas and meningiomas) may have a variety of BAEP abnormalities following stimulation of and recording from the opposite ear. Of 41 patients with these tumors studied by Parker et al. (1980) (see below for breakdown), 6 had contralateral BAEP abnormalities, in addition to the universal ipsilateral abnormalities. One patient each had a wave I–III IPL abnormality, all waves absent except wave I, all waves absent except waves I and II, all waves absent except I, II, and III, and two patients had an abnormal III–V IPL (Fig. 6–12). The latter finding has also been reported by Selters and Brackmann (1977), Wielaard and Kemp (1979), Stockard and Sharbrough (1980), and Zappulla et al. (1981). These abnormalities, thought to be caused by distortion and cross-compression of brain stem structures, have been seen to improve after tumor removal (Fig. 6–12) (Parker et al., 1980). Zappulla et al. (1982) found a correlation between degree of abnormality in the ear contralateral to the tumor and tumor

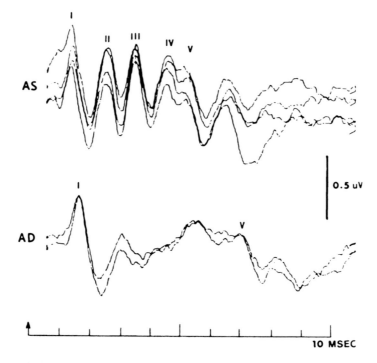

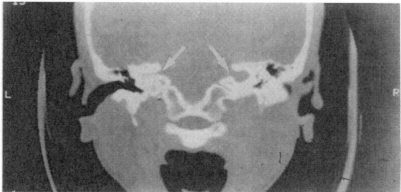

FIG. 6–10. Brain stem auditory EPs from same patient as in Fig. 6–9. The left ear is normal, but the right ear has no identifiable wave III and a marked I–V IPL abnormality of over 5 msec. This is incompatible with Meniere's disease and MS was considered. A CT scan at this time was normal. One year later the patient began to have exacerbations of her symptoms with her menses, and a repeat CT scan (shown here) demonstrates evidence of an acoustic neuroma with erosion of the bony canal (*arrow*).

size. Maurer (1985) has reported rarefaction–condensation differences in patients with acoustic neuromas.

In the study of Parker et al. (1980) (updated statistics) involving 31 patients with acoustic neuromas and 10 with CPA meningiomas, 13 patients (11 and 2 from the acoustic neuroma and CPA meningioma groups, respectively) had no BAEP waves at all, 9 (7 and 2) had I–V IPL abnormalities, 9 (7 and 2) had I–III IPL abnormalities, and 9 (7 and 2) had only wave I

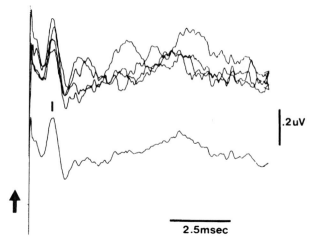

FIG. 6–11. Brain stem auditory EPs from a patient with an acoustic neuroma (visible on CT scan) showing preservation of wave I despite absence of all other waves. Each trace is the average of 512 clicks, with the grand average beneath.

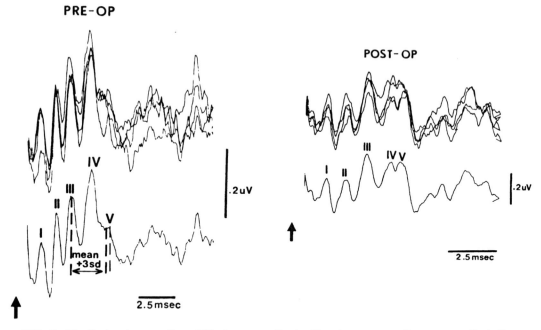

FIG. 6–12. Brain stem auditory EPs from a patient with a large acoustic neuroma that distorted and compressed the brainstem. The tumor was on the opposite side from the ear whose BAEPs are shown here. Note the abnormal III–V separation and low wave V amplitude, both of which improve postoperatively. Each trace is the average of 1,024 clicks, with the grand average beneath.

present. Three patients (two and one) had no wave I present and their BAEPs were judged abnormal and suggesting a retrocochlear lesion on the basis of an abnormal interear wave V absolute latency difference. One patient with a meningioma had waves IV and V missing (Fig. 6–13). One patient with an acoustic neuroma had a I–III interear IPL difference as the only abnormality. Nine of these patients had normal CT scans and, therefore, small tumors. Three of these had no waves, three had a I–V IPL abnormality, two had a I–III IPL abnormality, and one had a I–III interear difference as the only abnormality. In all of these patients the abnormal BAEPs resulted in a posterior fossa contrast cisternogram being done. Three patients had entirely normal pure-tone and speech audiograms and two others had very mild auditory abnormalities. One patient with an abnormal I–III separation (Fig. 6–7) had normal stapedial reflexes (all patients did not have this test).

Cerebellopontine angle tumors which are not attached to the eighth nerve (e.g., petrous ridge and tentorial meningiomas) may grow to a much larger size before affecting conduction in the eighth nerve and brain stem auditory structures. They may be brought to medical attention by symptoms and signs referrable to other structures and are then usually large enough to be evident on CT scans. Thus, in these CPA tumors the utility of BAEPs is not as dramatic as in acoustic neuromas. However, we have yet to see normal BAEPs with a CPA meningioma, despite the paucity of abnormal audiograms [7 of 10 patients in one group (Parker et al., 1980) had symmetric audiograms]. Later waves (IV–V) may be affected before earlier waves (Fig. 6–13) in some cases, helping to make a distinction as to point of origin of the tumor (eighth nerve versus elsewhere).

In summary, BAEP IPLs, especially the I–III separation, are the most sensitive screening test for acoustic neuromas. When this test is available and performed well and the only clinical question relates to the presence or absence of an acoustic neuroma, no radiologic procedures need be done if the BAEP test is completely normal and there is no other strong

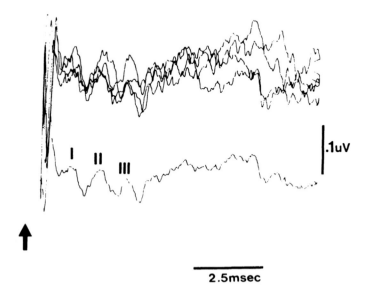

.1uv

2.5msec

FIG. 6–13. Brain stem auditory EPs from a patient with a large posterior fossa meningioma. Waves I–III are preserved but later waves are lost; this would be an unusual pattern for an acoustic neuroma. Each trace is the average of 1,024 clicks, with the grand average beneath.

evidence suggesting the possibility of an acoustic neuroma (e.g., hereditary) or CPA mass. Magnetic resonance imaging compares favorably with combined IV and gas contrast CT (House et al., 1986) and may be the preferred initial test in some patients, but the BAEP is less expensive and can be used with a lower index of suspicion and more frequently for follow-up.

3.4. Multiple Sclerosis

In demyelinating disease, BAEPs are potentially useful in three ways: (1) in patients with a non-brain stem locus of CNS involvement, an abnormal BAEP signals the presence of another clinically unsuspected lesion, thus helping to define the disease process; (2) when the clinical findings are equivocal or otherwise uncertain, an abnormal BAEP provides objective evidence of disturbed function; and (3) various treatments can be monitored objectively by following abnormal BAEPs.

There has been a large number of studies of BAEPs in patients with MS (Robinson and Rudge, 1975, 1977a,b, 1980; Stockard et al., 1977b; Lacquanti et al., 1979; Mogensen and Kristensen, 1979; Chiappa et al., 1980; Green et al., 1980; Hausler and Levine, 1980; Kjaer, 1980a,c; Maurer et al., 1980a, 1981; Prasher and Gibson, 1980; Stockard and Sharbrough, 1980; Tackmann et al., 1980; Fischer et al., 1981; Khoshbin and Hallett, 1981; Parving et al., 1981; Purves et al., 1981; Shanon et al., 1981d; Barajas, 1982; Elidan et al., 1982; Green and Walcoff, 1982; Prasher et al., 1982; Tackmann and Ettlin, 1982; van Buggenhout et al., 1982; Hutchinson et al., 1984; Kayamori et al., 1984; Koffler et al., 1984). Of 1,006 patients with varying classifications of MS from some of the above studies, 466 (46%) had abnormal BAEPs. Of 351, 180, and 206 patients classified as definite, probable, and possible MS, the average abnormality rates were 67%, 41%, and 30%, respectively. Of 326 patients reported as having no history or brain stem findings, 38% had BAEP abnormalities; abnormality rates varied from 21% to 55%. Thus, in one fifth to one half of MS patients without brain stem symptoms or signs, BAEP testing will reveal evidence of clinically unsuspected lesions. Differences in definitions of MS, patient populations, and techniques account for the variations between studies. For example, Noseworthy et al. (1983) have found a higher incidence of BAEP abnormalities in MS patients over 50 years of age as compared with younger patients. Hammond and Yiannikas (1987) found a correlation between BAEP abnormality rates and disability. Nuwer et al. (1985) did not find BAEP abnormalities in first-degree relatives of MS patients.

The following study from our laboratory exemplifies the findings that can be expected when using BAEPs to test patients with (or suspected of having) MS. In a consecutive series of 614 patients tested (Chiappa et al., 1980), 202 were diagnosed as having MS (81 definite, 67 probable, 54 possible) and 18 as having pure optic neuritis (ON) (Table 6–3). Other groups of interest seen were labyrinthine diseases (21), cerebellar disorders (13), trigeminal neuralgia (15), cervical transverse myelitis (14), amyotrophic lateral sclerosis (9), and other diagnostic classifications (226). In 92 of the 614 patients no neurologic diagnosis could be made in spite of adequate information; records were not available on 4 patients. We compared some of the clinical data from our group of MS patients with Kurtzke's Army series which included approximately 2,000 patients (Kurtzke, 1970). Seventy-three percent of those patients had no optic signs, 62% had no sensory symptoms in the limbs, and 19% had diplopia, as compared with 67%, 51%, and 14% in our MS group. On the basis of these clinical findings our group of MS patients seemed to consist of a reasonably typical cross-section of MS patients with respect to these elements of the disease. Fifty-eight percent of

TABLE 6–3. *Incidence of abnormal BAEPs in MS*

	No. (%) of patients			
	Definite	Probable	Possible	Total
With symptoms and/or signs of brain stem lesion	34/60 (57)	8/38 (21)	7/33 (21)	49/131 (37)
Without symptoms and/or signs of brain stem lesion	4/21 (19)	6/29 (21)	5/21 (24)	15/71 (21)
All patients	38/81 (47)	14/67 (21)	12/54 (22)	64/202 (32)

Some nonspecific data (e.g., nystagmus) were taken as indications of "clinically suspected" brain stem lesions. See Section 3.4 for further explanations of this patient group and data. (From Chiappa et al., 1980, with permission.)

their patients had no brain stem symptoms as contrasted with 35% in our group—this difference appears to be due to our (intentionally) more liberal definition of which symptoms or signs might constitute evidence of a brain stem lesion (see below).

The reliability of BAEP techniques was demonstrated by the fact that all parameters in the MS patients with BAEPs interpreted as normal (the BAEP-normal MS group) showed no statistical differences from the normal values. Those MS patients who had BAEPs with abnormal interwave separations had latency values which were a mean of 4.9 SD above the normal mean and those MS patients who were determined to have abnormal BAEPs on the basis of an abnormal I/V amplitude ratio (17% of the BAEP-abnormal MS group) had ratios which were a mean of 5.5 SD above the normal mean. These facts, and the higher incidence of abnormalities in the definite MS group (see Table 6–1), suggest that the BAEP is a reliable test for clinical usage.

Although the normal mean plus 3 SD was used as the upper limit of normal, the BAEP-normal MS patients (including those in the definite MS group) had values for both interwave latency and amplitude parameters which were essentially identical to the normal values. The fact that the values for the MS patients had a bimodal distribution [also noted for absolute wave V latency by Robinson and Rudge (1980)], being either completely normal or markedly abnormal, suggests that the smallest MS plaques in this part of the auditory system are sufficient to produce a marked conduction abnormality. A majority of the BAEP abnormalities (Table 6–4) in our MS patients were wave V amplitude abnormalities (absence or abnormally low amplitude of wave V was seen in 87% of the BAEP-abnormal MS patients). Figure 6–14 shows the progression of abnormalities from normality to complete

TABLE 6–4. *Incidence of types of BAEP abnormalities in MS*

	No. (%) of patients			
Abnormality	Definite	Probable	Possible	Total
Interwave	5 (13)	2 (14)	1 (8)	8 (13)
Wave V amp.	20 (53)	8 (57)	7 (58)	35 (55)
Both	13 (34)	4 (29)	4 (33)	21 (33)
Only I–III present	3 (8)	3 (21)	1 (8)	7 (11)
Only I–II present	3 (8)	0	2 (17)	5 (8)
Only I present	0	1 (7)	1 (8)	2 (3)
No responses	2 (5)	0	1 (8)	3 (5)

(From Chiappa, 1980b, with permission.)

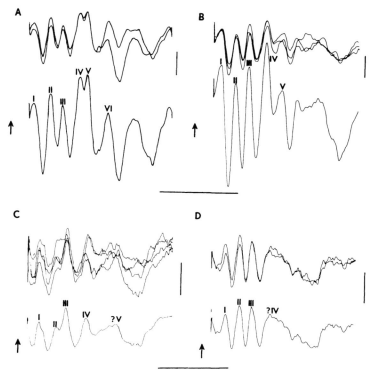

FIG. 6–14. Spectrum of IV–V complex abnormalities seen in MS. **A** and **B** are following stimulation of the same ear of the same patient, **B** 2 months after **A**. The IV–V separation increased from 0.5 msec to 1.1 msec and the I/V amplitude ratio percentage went from 90% to 204%; both measures in **B** are at the upper limit of normal. **C** and **D** are from different patients, showing further progression of the abnormality. In **C** wave IV is clearly visible but wave V is difficult to recognize—note poor reproducibility in repeated trials. In **D** wave V is absent and wave IV is not present as a distinct peak. In **A**, **B**, and **C** the superimposed trials have N=1,024 clicks each; in **D**, N=2,048 clicks each. The single trace below each is the sum of the superimposed trials. Calibration marks are 0.25 μV and 5 msec. (From Chiappa et al., 1980, with permission.)

loss of waves IV and V. The next most frequent abnormality, increased III–V IPL, was seen in 28% of the BAEP-abnormal MS patients. The presumed generators of waves III and V are the superior olivary complex and inferior colliculus, respectively, and thus the majority of the conduction abnormalities were found to occur between them, as would be expected since this is the longest segment of white matter in the tracts being tested. However, in those patients who had recognizable waves V, there was no significant correlation between the III–V separation and the wave I/V amplitude ratio, contrary to our expectations. In fact, in 17% of the BAEP-abnormal MS patients the III–V separation was normal and the I/V amplitude ratio was abnormal. In addition, three patients had the unusual combination of no wave III, a recognizable wave V of normal amplitude, and an abnormal I–V separation (Fig. 6–15). The disparity between these different kinds of abnormalities is not easily resolved merely by consideration of the known conduction deficits in demyelinated axons such as slow conduction across the demyelinated segment and increased refractory period. Multiplicity of lesions, possible contributions to the BAEP waveforms from conduction in sepa-

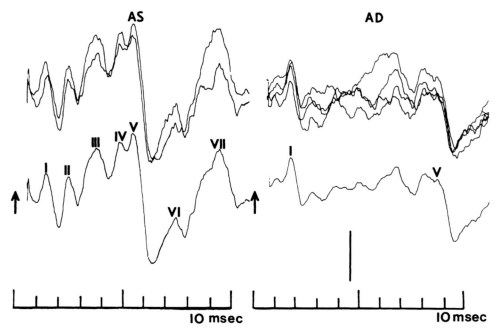

FIG. 6–15. Brain stem auditory EPs from stimulation of each ear of one patient showing the marked asymmetry which can be present with monaural stimulation. This also shows another abnormality type seen in MS with lack of wave III and markedly abnormal I–V separation in AD of 6.7 msec—AS is normal. AS superimposed trials have N=1,024 clicks each; in AD, N=2,048 clicks each. The single trace below each is the sum of the superimposed trials. Calibration marks are 0.25 μV. (From Chiappa et al., 1980, with permission.)

rate but parallel tracts, and possible synchronous activation of different auditory tract structures need to be considered.

The importance of monaural stimulation was evident here since 45% of the BAEP abnormalities were seen with stimulation of one ear only (Table 6–5 and Fig. 6–15) (Chiappa et al., 1980). The prevalence of monaural abnormalities suggests that, with respect to the BAEP waveform generators, there is relatively little bilateral conduction, although the anatomy had suggested otherwise (see also Section 1.1.4). Contralateral recordings have not been especially helpful in MS (Hammond and Yiannikas, 1987).

TABLE 6–5. *Incidence of BAEP abnormalities in MS with respect to laterality (monaural stimulation)*

Laterality	No. (%) of patients			
	Definite	Probable	Possible	Total
Unilateral	16 (42)	4 (29)	9 (75)	29 (45)
Bilateral same abnormality	14 (37)	5 (36)	2 (17)	21 (33)
Bilateral different abnormality	8 (21)	5 (36)	1 (8)	14 (22)
Bilateral total	22 (58)	10 (71)	3 (25)	35 (55)

(From Chiappa, 1980b, with permission.)

Faster rates of stimulation alter all BAEP parameters, including interwave separations. It has been noted previously by Stockard and Rossiter (1977), Stockard et al. (1977b), and Robinson and Rudge (1977a,b) that increased click repetition rate (Robinson and Rudge used paired clicks) revealed a higher incidence of abnormalities in the BAEPs of MS patients. However, in our group of MS patients, more BAEP abnormalities were not seen with 70 clicks/sec, although abnormalities seen at 10/sec were sometimes worse at 70/sec (Chiappa et al., 1980). Elidan et al. (1982) and Jacobson and Newman (1989) have reported similar findings. The relative difficulty of waveform recognition at 70/sec, with increased waveform duration and indistinct peaks, restricted the clinical utility of that stimulus rate. In a few patients with diseases other than MS we have noted the reverse situation, that is, the I–V separation was abnormal at 10/sec and normal at 70/sec. This "normalization" may be due to complete failure of conduction in the abnormal fibers at the faster rate, possibly due to an increased refractory period. With their abnormal contribution removed from the resultant waveforms the activity manifest is only that from the normally conducting fibers, hence the normal appearance. Although this effect was sought in the MS patients, it was not found. Phillips et al. (1983) used hyperthermia but increased the yield of BAEP abnormalities by only one patient.

Emerson et al. (1982), Maurer (1985), and Hammond et al. (1986) have noted that some patients with MS show BAEP abnormalities with only one click polarity, usually rarefaction clicks (Figs. 5–14 and 6–16). The abnormality usually consists of a complete absence of wave V with one click polarity and a normal wave V with the other. Decreasing click intensity results in a reappearance of wave V and this might suggest a peripheral origin of the phenomenon. However, some of these patients have completely normal hearing on conventional audiometric tests and this effect is not seen in normal subjects or patients with any type of peripheral hearing disorder, so that it is presumably due to central conduction abnormalities although firm human clinicopathologic evidence for this is lacking. See Chapter 4, Section 6.5, for a more detailed discussion of this. Sand (1991) has reported a relationship between click polarity and clinical findings in patients with MS.

In spite of obvious abnormalities in the BAEP, none of the MS patients studied here had clinical complaints of hearing difficulties, and click thresholds were essentially normal (formal audiograms were rarely obtained but those which were obtained were normal). This is consistent with the findings of routine audiologic testing in MS patients (Le Zak and Selhub, 1966) but detailed auditory and vestibular testing (Noffsinger et al., 1972) and interaural time discrimination and auditory localization testing (Hausler and Levine, 1980) may reveal functional abnormalities in MS patients. In the latter study almost all MS patients with abnormal BAEPs also had abnormal interaural time discrimination. Interaural time and level discrimination has been correlated with MS lesions localized by MRI mapping and BAEPs (Levine et al., 1993a), although the anatomic accuracy suggested in the study is probably excessive. Occasionally MS patients do have symptomatic hearing difficulties and abnormal BAEPs apparently related to the disease (Lederman et al., 1978; Jabbari et al., 1982b; Daugherty et al., 1983; Hopf and Maurer, 1983; Fischer et al., 1984), but none were seen in our group. The occurrence of grossly abnormal BAEPs in conjunction with subjectively normal hearing may reflect the production of BAEP abnormalities by temporal dispersion of the click-induced volley as it ascends the affected tracts. It may be that, although these asynchronous potentials do not sum to generate a discrete peak of activity discernible at the scalp, the integrity of conduction, albeit deranged, is sufficient to sustain functionally normal hearing. However, this does not explain those cases where the amplitude and waveform shape are essentially normal and there is an abnormally large interwave separation. Perhaps in these cases the demyelination involves a majority of the fibers equally. Also, of

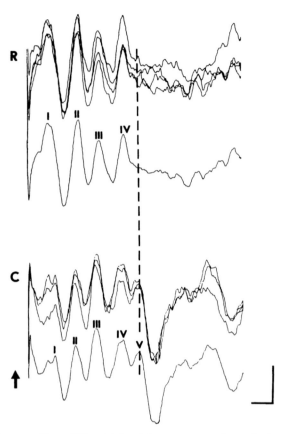

FIG. 6–16. Brain stem auditory EPs obtained from one ear in a single patient showing the complete absence of wave V following rarefaction clicks, but completely normal BAEPs with condensation clicks. The behavioral pure-tone audiogram and speech discrimination were normal. Each trace is the average of 1,024 clicks, with the grand average beneath. Calibration marks are 0.25 μV and 1.0 msec. (From Emerson et al., 1982, with permission.)

course, BAEP waveform generation might have little to do with functional hearing. Satya-Murti et al. (1983) found preservation of late auditory potentials in three patients with grossly abnormal BAEPs.

The consistency of the BAEP when followed over time in normals suggests that it could be used to follow the activity of lesions affecting these tracts and might possibly provide assistance in evaluating the effectiveness of therapeutic measures, as suggested by Stockard and Rossiter (1977). Kjaer (1980a) studied 121 patients with MS and found a significantly increased incidence of BAEP abnormalities with increasing duration and severity of symptoms. In addition, he repeated the testing at least once in 34 patients at intervals of 1 to 20 months and found BAEP alterations in clinically stable patients (none in 10 normal subjects). He concluded that the main value of BAEPs in patients with MS was to indicate clinically silent lesions and that its value in monitoring the clinical condition of the individual patient was less. Matthews et al. (1982) followed for 38 months after BAEP testing 84 patients in whom the diagnosis of MS was under consideration. In nine of these patients an abnormal BAEP at initial presentation subsequently proved to be of diagnostic value in that it revealed a separate, clinically silent lesion, indicating a multifocal disease (and the patient on follow-up proved to have MS). Aminoff et al. (1984) noted a significant increase in variability in the BAEP between tests in patients with clinical exacerbations of brain stem or cerebellar disease, but they also occasionally found a marked discrepancy between clinical and BAEP changes. Smith et al. (1986) found no BAEP changes in MS patients following high-dose methylprednisolone therapy, whereas Gilmore et al. (1985) noted some shortening of IPLs following infusion of the calcium antagonist verapamil. Nuwer et al. (1987) found no relationship between treatment and BAEP latencies in a 3-year, double-blind, placebo-controlled study, although pattern-shift visual EPs (PSVEPs) and SEPs showed statistically significant changes. Anderson et al. (1987) have demonstrated limitations of BAEP testing in follow-up situations, although Nuwer et al. (1988) have suggested a parametric scale for BAEP latencies for use in these circumstances.

In MS patients BAEPs can be very useful in those who do not have clinical evidence of brain stem involvement since the demonstration of a clinically unsuspected lesion helps to define a multifocal disease process (i.e., the only other neurologic symptom might be in the visual system). In order to be conservative about this area of BAEP utility in the analysis of clinical data from our group of MS patients, in addition to indisputable signs and symptoms of past or present brain stem involvement such as cranial nerve abnormalities and diplopia, the following were also taken as evidence of (possible) brain stem involvement—a clear history of dizziness (even if it could not be further characterized), nystagmus, gait disturbance (not due to a lesion which could be located elsewhere by other findings), cerebellar signs, and sensory or motor abnormalities whose vertical position in the CNS could not be determined by other neurologic findings. The symptoms and/or signs were not necessarily present at the time the BAEP was performed. We believed that this definition most clearly defined that group of patients in whom an abnormal BAEP would be useful to the clinician. However, it is recognized that (1) a large part of the clinical utility of the BAEP lies in its ability to document an abnormality when the history and/or neurologic examination are equivocal, (2) some of these symptoms and signs are frequently produced by lesions outside the brain stem, and (3) these factors therefore produce possibly "conservative" figures for the clinical utility of BAEPs in MS.

Our data showed no significant differences between the three MS groups in the number of clinically unsuspected lesions revealed by the BAEP (see Table 6–1) with the overall "find" being 21% of those without symptoms and/or signs of brain stem lesions (7.4% of the entire MS group). The BAEP abnormality rates irrespective of clinical findings were 47%, 21%, and 22% in the three MS groups, respectively. This compares favorably with CT abnormality rates of 49%, 11%, and 0% (Herskey et al., 1979); data with respect to the number of clinically silent lesions revealed were not available in the CT study. To some extent the CT and the BAEP are complementary, since the latter tests a section of white matter not well-defined by the former. These data indicate that the BAEP is a useful clinical diagnostic test in the evaluation of patients suspected of having MS, even if judged only on the number of clinically silent lesions revealed. Almost all of our MS patients also had PSVEPs (79, 67, and 54 in the diagnostic groups, respectively) and some had median nerve SEPs (16, 21, and 14). Tables 3–3 and 3–4 present the comparative incidence of response abnormalities in the three EP tests in this group of MS patients. Note that not all patients in Table 3–3 had all three tests. The PSVEP had the highest overall abnormality rate and also had proportionally the highest incidence of demonstration of clinically unsuspected lesions; these results are consistent with the high frequency of lesions found in the optic nerves of MS patients at autopsy (Lumsden, 1970). As might be expected because of the length of white matter tracts involved in the median nerve SEP, that test had results almost as significant as the PSVEP, while the BAEP ranked third. Purves et al. (1981) have reported similar findings; they also found that combining the three tests significantly increased the percentage of MS patients with abnormal findings to 97%, 86%, and 63%, respectively, in definite, probable, and possible groups.

It should be reiterated here that a large part of the clinical utility of the BAEP lies in its ability to not only reveal unsuspected, and thereby multiple, lesions, but also document clinically equivocal findings. For example, some of our patients with MS initially presented with symptoms and/or signs which could have been produced by disease in the labyrinths. Other than absence of wave I in three of the patients with Meniere's disease, no abnormalities of interwave separations or amplitude ratios in the BAEP were seen in those 21 patients with labyrinthine diseases. Thirty-seven percent of the MS patients who presented with nystagmus at the time of testing had BAEP abnormalities (Table 6–6). Similarly, van Buggenhout et al. (1982) found BAEP abnormalities in half of their patients who had vestibular lesions. Thus, the BAEP can be helpful in this setting: if abnormal, then the lesion is clearly centrally rather than peripherally located. Conversely, 56% of the patients with an internuclear ophthalmoplegia (INO) at the time of testing (Chiappa et al., 1980) had abnormal BAEPs, so that the BAEP does not help to distinguish MS from the other causes of an INO [infarction and tumor (Cogan and Wray, 1970)] which might also affect both medial longitudinal fasciculus and auditory tracts. Table 6–4 presents statistics relating clinical findings to BAEP abnormalities.

The BAEP is abnormal in some patients with system disorders affecting cerebellar function, particularly those who have spasticity, and thus is not helpful in differentiating possible MS in that setting.

Amyotrophic lateral sclerosis (ALS) sometimes presents initially with symptoms and/or signs which might be suggestive of MS; in our patients with ALS there were none with abnormal BAEPs (see Section 3.6.5). Thus, the presence or absence of BAEP abnormalities can be helpful in clinical considerations during the initial presentation of patients with these diseases when MS is part of the differential diagnosis.

Optic neuritis and cervical transverse myelitis may have etiologies closely related or identical to that of MS; all of the patients in those groups had normal BAEPs, and the ON patients tested also had normal SEPs (the cervical transverse myelitis patients all had abnormal SEPs). Also, in a different study 12 consecutive patients with inflammatory acute transverse myelitis (virtually or completely transverse lesions) had normal BAEPs (Ropper et al., 1982), as was also the case in Wulff's 9 patients (Wulff, 1985).

Trigeminal neuralgia has also been associated with MS, 8% (Chakravorty, 1966) and 2% (Rushton and Olafson, 1965) of patients with trigeminal neuralgia having been found to

TABLE 6–6. *Incidence of abnormal BAEPs in MS with respect to various symptoms and/or signs of brain stem lesions*

	No. (%) of patients			
	Definite	Probable	Possible	Total
Internuclear ophthalmoplegia	14/20 (70)	1/6 (17)	1/4 (25)	16/30 (53)
Diplopia	16/28 (57)	2/12 (17)	2/14 (14)	20/54 (37)
Nystagmus	17/32 (53)	5/20 (25)	2/17 (12)	24/69 (35)
Other	15/31 (48)	5/15 (33)	2/8 (25)	22/54 (41)

All patients did not have these symptoms and/or signs when the test was performed. See Secton 3.4 for further explanations of this patient group and data. (From Chiappa et al., 1980, with permission.)

have MS. Iragui et al. (1986) followed a patient with trigeminal neuralgia who had abnormal BAEPs with the attack which disappeared in a delayed fashion after the clinical symptoms had subsided. In our 15 patients with trigeminal neuralgia there was none with abnormal BAEPs. Thus, as is also the case clinically, at the time of onset of ON, cervical transverse myelitis, and trigeminal neuralgia there may be no EP evidence of lesions elsewhere in the CNS.

3.5. Other Demyelinating Diseases

3.5.1. Central Pontine Myelinolysis

Stockard et al. (1976b) and Wiederholt et al. (1977) studied BAEPs in two patients who had central pontine myelinolysis (CPM) by clinical criteria and who subsequently recovered. The I–V IPL showed a clear correlation with the clinical state of the patient. In the first patient, as the quadriparesis developed the I–V IPL was normal, but at the peak of the illness it was 7.0 msec. In the second patient, the I–V IPL was 8.4 msec at the clinical peak of the illness. In both patients this markedly prolonged latency returned to normal during a 6- to 12-week period in parallel with the clinical improvement. Ingram et al. (1986) also found abnormal BAEPs in a patient with CPM which resolved as the patient improved clinically.

3.5.2. Leukodystrophies

Brain stem auditory EP abnormalities have been reported in metachromatic leukodystrophy (MLD) (Ochs et al., 1979; Markand et al., 1980, 1982a; Brown et al., 1981a; Davis et al., 1985). Brown et al. found BAEP abnormalities in one 4-year-old symptomatic patient and in that patient's 14-month-old brother who was asymptomatic but had the disease by enzyme assay. Their 5-year-old asymptomatic sister was a carrier but had normal BAEPs. Another 8-year-old patient with juvenile onset had essentially normal BAEPs. Hecox et al. (1981) found abnormalities in one patient with MLD. Dhuna et al. (1992) reported serial EPs in a patient following bone marrow transplantation, with most results remaining stable or improved.

In 16 of 17 patients with adrenoleukodystrophy, BAEPs were abnormal with prolonged IPLs or absence of all components after wave II (Ochs et al., 1979; Garg et al., 1980; Markand et al., 1980, 1982b; Grimes et al., 1983; Tobimatsu et al., 1985). Black et al. (1979) found normal BAEP waves I through V in a 7-year-old boy with symptomatic disease. In the above studies two of seven carriers had prolonged I–V IPLs, Garg et al. (1983b) found abnormal BAEPs in two of seven family members, and Moloney and Masterson (1982) reported abnormal BAEPs in all three obligate and in one of four possible carriers.

Seven patients with Pelizaeus-Merzbacher disease (PMD) all had abnormal BAEPs, with no waves present after wave II; 10 known carriers of PMD all had normal BAEPs (Ochs et al., 1979). Similar findings were seen by Markand et al. (1982a) in 12 patients and by Davis et al. (1985) and Garg et al. (1983b) in one patient each.

Garg et al. (1982) recorded BAEPs in three patients with hereditary motor-sensory neuropathy, type I, and found the I–II IPL prolonged, but III–V normal. They concluded that (1) the I–II prolongation in this disease (which affects only peripheral nerves), (2) the occasional preservation of wave II in brain-dead patients, and (3) preservation of only waves I and II in the leukodystrophies suggest that wave II might be generated in the intracranial extramedullary portion of the eighth nerve.

3.6. Other Degenerative Diseases

3.6.1. Charcot-Marie-Tooth Disease

Satya-Murti and Cacace (1982) reported on four patients with Charcot-Marie-Tooth (CMT) disease, all of whom had abnormal BAEPs with prolonged I–III IPLs. Pierelli et al. (1985) found normal BAEPs in five patients with CMT disease.

3.6.2. Friedreich's Ataxia

Satya-Murti et al. (1980) studied four patients with Friedreich's ataxia and found that all had poorly defined BAEP waveforms, whereas two patients with olivopontocerebellar degeneration had normal-appearing BAEPs. They thought the BAEP abnormality was secondary to degeneration in the spiral ganglion, a homolog of the dorsal root ganglion. Results of audiometric tests also indicated a disorder of the eighth nerve. Conversely, Jabbari et al. (1983) recorded wave I in all five children with Friedreich's ataxia, usually with wave V absent or abnormal, and conventional auditory studies also indicated central (brain stem) dysfunction. A further confusing element is that Nuwer et al. (1983) reported normal BAEPs in 20 patients. Satya-Murti et al. (1983) found preservation of late auditory potentials in two patients with absent BAEPs.

Hecox et al. (1981) found BAEP I–V IPL abnormalities in two of five patients with Friedreich's ataxia. Other brief reports of BAEPs in Friedreich's ataxia have been published (Pederson and Trojaborg, 1981; Shanon et al., 1981c; Jabbari et al., 1982a; Nuwer et al., 1982; Davis et al., 1985; Pelosi et al., 1985; Pierelli et al., 1985).

3.6.3. Hallervorden-Spatz Disease

Markand et al. (1980) reported one probable case of Hallervorden-Spatz disease with normal BAEPs.

3.6.4. Huntington's Disease

Pierelli et al. (1985) (5 patients) and Ehle et al. (1984) (12 patients) found normal BAEPs in Huntington's disease, in agreement with our occasional experience.

3.6.5. Motor System Diseases

Cascino et al. (1988) found normal BAEPs in 22 of 23 patients with motor system diseases. The one abnormal study was in a patient with moderate clinical hearing impairment and it had changes usually found in patients with cochlear lesions. The absence of waves I and III did not allow central conduction to be assessed. These findings were consistent with our previously reported nine normal cases (Chiappa et al., 1980) and are supported by the study of Tsuji et al. (1981), who found no BAEP abnormalities in 13 Guamanian and 7

Japanese patients with ALS, and Pierelli et al. (1985) who found normal BAEPs in five ALS patients. Matheson et al. (1983, 1986) reported BAEP abnormalities in 4 out of 32 ALS patients. One patient had a mild abnormality only (I–V IPL prolongation by 0.1 msec on one side). Another patient had all waves absent bilaterally, including wave I. This case is similar to the abnormal case in our study. Absence of all waves is usually seen in patients with cochlear pathology and central conduction cannot be assessed. Radtke et al. (1986) found BAEP abnormalities in 2 out of 12 patients but in one case the abnormality was mild (I–V IPL prolongation by 0.1 msec). Statistical group comparisons for patients with motor system diseases compared with controls reveal IPLs differ only by the smallest measurable amount (Cascino et al., 1988) even without an age correction (Allison et al., 1984) and therefore cannot be interpreted as being significantly different. This suggests that there is no tendency for brain stem auditory pathways to conduct abnormally. Thus, if a patient suspected of having a motor system disease (e.g., ALS or bulbar palsy) has an abnormal BAEP, this should prompt a search for coexisting disease or alternative diagnosis.

3.6.6. Neurolipidoses

Markand et al. (1980) reported three patients with Batten's disease who had normal BAEPs. A patient with Gaucher's disease had wave V absent (Lacey and Terplan, 1984).

3.6.7. Parkinson's Disease

Gawel et al. (1981) performed BAEPs on 21 patients with Parkinson's disease and found no delay in wave I but a large delay in wave V (mean delay 0.22 msec). No illustrations were shown and apparently trial repetition was not performed. None of the 13 individuals for whom data were given had a wave V latency greater than the normal mean plus 3 SD.

Tsuji et al. (1981) reported BAEPs in 16 patients with Parkinson's disease and found no abnormalities, nor did Pierelli et al. (1985). In our experience also, patients with Parkinson's disease do not show BAEP abnormalities.

Tsuji et al. also studied patients with Guam Parkinson-dementia disease and found delayed III–V separations or absent response in 11 of 16.

3.6.8. Progressive Supranuclear Palsy

Tolosa and Zeese (1979) found normal BAEPs in seven patients with typical progressive supranuclear palsy, four with moderate and three with severe symptoms of brain stem dysfunction, as did Pierelli et al. (1985). However, we have found BAEP abnormalities in two patients with progressive supranuclear palsy.

3.6.9. Spinocerebellar–Brain Stem Ataxias/Degenerations

There are several reports of BAEPs in cerebellar–brain stem ataxias/degenerations; the diversity of these syndromes and the quality of the work are such that the reports themselves must be read for details before meaningful conclusions or comparisons can be made on clinical and technical grounds.

Fujita et al. (1981) found normal BAEPs in 11 patients with predominantly cerebellar involvement and 9 with pyramidal, extrapyramidal, or autonomic symptoms alone or in combination with cerebellar signs. Pedersen and Trojaborg (1981) found BAEP abnormalities in 3 of 11 patients with hereditary cerebellar ataxia. Gilroy and Lynn (1978) (three patients) and Nuwer et al. (1982) (four patients) found abnormal BAEPs in all patients with olivo-pontocerebellar degeneration (OPC). Satya-Murti et al. (1980) found normal BAEPs in two patients with OPC, Hammond and Wilder (1983) found BAEPs normal in one and abnormal in another, and Pierelli et al. (1985) found abnormalities in three patients. Nuwer et al. (1982) tested one patient with ataxia telangectasia and an unspecified number with a com-bined cerebral–cerebellar atrophy and found that BAEPs were "present and normal in most." Nuwer et al. (1983) reported abnormal BAEPs in all five patients with OPC, and also mentioned findings in a variety of other inherited ataxias. Pedersen and Trojaborg (1981) found abnormal BAEPs in 1 of 13 patients with hereditary spastic paraplegia, Pierelli et al. (1985) in 3 of 3 patients. Garg et al. (1982) found abnormal I–II IPLs in three patients with hereditary motor-sensory neuropathy, type I. Pierelli et al. (1985) found BAEP abnormalities in 7 of 10 patients with cerebellar ataxia.

3.6.10. Wilson's Disease

Fujita et al. (1981) reported six patients with Wilson's disease. Only the three patients who had neurologic symptoms had abnormal BAEP IPLs. In a study of 20 patients,

3.7. Intrinsic Brain Stem Lesions

In the lesions discussed below it is evident that the BAEP abnormality usually indicates both the side and vertical location of the lesion. The worst BAEP abnormality is usually seen when testing the ear ipsilateral to the brain stem lesion and there is a close correlation between preserved/damaged brain stem anatomy and normal/abnormal BAEPs. See Sec-tions 1.1.2 and 1.1.4 for a complete discussion of these subjects, with presentation of some case material (Fig. 6–4).

3.7.1. Tumors

Chiappa (1982a) and Brown et al. (1981b) (five patients) and Stockard and Sharbrough (1980) (one patient) found abnormal BAEPs in all cases of brain stem gliomas (Fig. 6–4 shows BAEPs from one case of Brown et al.). Kjaer (1980b) had two patients with brain stem tumors, both with abnormal BAEPs. Stockard et al. (1977b) found abnormal BAEPs in four patients with brain stem gliomas, in one of two patients with fourth ventricular ependymomas, and in one of three patients with cerebellar tumors. In one of their patients with a brain stem glioma, a posterior fossa contrast study suggested an Arnold-Chiari mal-formation whereas the III–V IPL BAEP abnormality suggested a more rostral lesion. Stockard and Rossiter (1977) tested a patient with a tumor in the upper one third of the pons who had an abnormal III–V separation. Starr and Hamilton (1976) reported one patient with a pinealoma invading the upper brain stem and two with brain stem gliomas, all with abnor-mal BAEPs. Oh et al. (1981) had a patient with a midbrain–pons metastatic tumor with ab-normal BAEP on that side. Lynn et al. (1981) had one patient with an invasive pinealoma, one with a thalamic glioma, one with a cerebellar hemangioblastoma, and one with a later-alized pontine glioma, all with abnormal BAEPs. Jerger et al. (1980) reported two patients with brain stem gliomas and abnormal BAEPs, and one with a pinealoma who had normal BAEPs.

Hashimoto et al. (1979) had three patients with brain stem gliomas, with BAEPs abnormal in all. Green and McLeod (1979) reported one patient with a thalamic tumor and one with a cerebellar tumor with abnormal BAEPs, and two patients with cerebellar tumors who had normal BAEPs. Starr and Achor (1979) reported a case with a restricted collicular lesion (pinealoma) and essentially normal waves V. However, the pathology was not obtained until some time after BAEP testing.

Thus, most patients with intrinsic brain stem tumors have abnormal BAEPs. No adult patient with a pontine glioma has yet had normal BAEPs, although the nature and clinical features of that disease suggest that such a case will be found.

3.7.2. Infarctions and Ischemia

If there is a brain stem infarct, BAEPs will be abnormal only when the infarct involves the auditory pathways. For example, patients with "locked-in" syndrome may have normal BAEPs. This is because the infarcted territory is most commonly in the ventral pons where the motor tracts lie, whereas auditory tracts are found more dorsally and laterally in the pontine tegmentum. Patients with lateral medullary infarcts have normal BAEPs, as would be expected since the structures involved are below the level of entry of auditory tracts; wave I may be missing in some of these patients, probably because in some patients the posterior inferior cerebellar artery supplies structures more rostrally in the brain stem, that is, pontomedullary junction and low pons.

Brown et al. (1981b) reported four patients with locked-in syndrome, two of whom had normal BAEPs. Five other patients with brain stem strokes rostral to the medulla all had abnormal BAEPs. Of four patients with lateral medullary syndrome, three had normal BAEPs and one had no waves at all; this latter finding was believed to be due to interference with the blood supply to the eighth nerve and cochlea, rather than pontine involvement. Hammond and Wilder (1982) found normal BAEPs in a locked-in patient, as did Towle et al. (1985). Stockard and Rossiter (1977) had two patients with lateral pontomedullary junction infarcts in the region of the cochlear nucleus, both with BAEPs abnormal after wave I. Kjaer (1980b) found BAEP abnormalities in 13 of 15 patients with brain stem infarcts, and in only 1 of 9 patients with brain stem transient ischemic attacks (TIAs).

Starr and Hamilton (1976) reported one patient with locked-in syndrome who had normal but low-amplitude BAEPs on one side and no waves (including wave I) on the other; four other patients with anoxic changes secondary to systemic anoxia had wave I present but no other waveforms clearly seen. Neuropathology in Starr and Hamilton's five cases usually showed extensive pontine infarction. Oh et al. (1981) reported two cases with lateral medullary infarcts, one with normal BAEPs and one with no waves including wave I. In two patients with a right Weber's syndrome they found a prolonged I–V IPL ipsilaterally in one and a prolonged wave V absolute latency ipsilaterally in the other; in a patient with left Weber's and Benedict's syndromes they found a prolonged wave V absolute latency ipsilaterally. In a patient with locked-in syndrome they found low-amplitude BAEPs with wave V absent on one side; the other side was normal. Two other patients with pontine infarcts had abnormal BAEPs.

Maurer et al. (1980b) reported a patient with "vascular brain stem disease" who had abnormal BAEPs enhanced by changing click polarity. Hashimoto et al. (1979) reported 15 patients with "vascular lesions of the brain stem," all with abnormal BAEPs. Green and McLeod (1979) reported four patients with "brain stem stroke," all with abnormal BAEPs. Gilroy et al. (1977) and Seales et al. (1981) each had one patient with locked-in syndrome who had abnormal BAEPs. Epstein et al. (1980) reported a patient with acute onset of vertigo, vertical diplopia, left-sided sensory loss, right-sided incoordination, palatal myoclonus, and normal CT scan and vertebral angiogram; waves IV and V were absent. Cascino and Adams (1986) and Lanska et al. (1987) found BAEP abnormalities in patients with brain stem auditory hallucinosis secondary to infarctions and hemorrhages. Ragazzoni et al. (1982) studied 26 patients with TIAs in the vertebrobasilar territory at least 7 days after the last attack, when they were asymptomatic. They found that 8 of 15 patients had BAEP IPL abnormalities. Of their 11 patients who had had a definite stroke but recovered, 6 had abnormal IPLs. However, they used the normal mean plus 2.5 SD as the upper limit of normal and since the actual values were not given a correction to 3 SD could not be performed. Rossini et al. (1982) recorded BAEPs in a patient who suffered a spontaneous cardiorespiratory arrest after testing had begun. During the arrest BAEPs initially decreased in amplitude and then could not be recorded. After restoration of cardiac activity, all waves reappeared immediately; however, waves III–V did not recover their original peak latencies during the 50 minutes following the arrest.

Factor and Dentinger (1987) found abnormal BAEPs in all eight patients with vertebrobasilar TIAs, performed 1 to 16 days after the TIA at a time when the clinical examination was normal. Six of these patients were followed and five returned to normal, one to near normal. They suggested that BAEPs might be helpful in differentiating TIAs from nonbrain stem syndromes. Fischer et al. (1982), Maurer et al. (1979), Rossi et al. (1983), and Ferbert et al. (1988) have reported BAEPs in a variety of brain stem ischemic conditions and infarctions, and Wada et al. (1988) hypothesized brain stem ischemia as the cause of changes in the III/V amplitude ratio in patients with subarachnoid hemorrhage or supratentorial tumor showing increased intracranial pressure (ICP) or hydrocephalus. Stern et al. (1982) followed 35 patients with recent ischemic brain stem strokes and noted that abnormal BAEPs were found in 79% of patients with an unstable course (progression, remission, or relapse), whereas 44% of patients with a stable course had abnormal BAEPs.

In general, in our experience, patients with TIAs of brain stem structures have normal BAEPs unless there are permanent deficits. The length of time needed to perform a BAEP test makes it difficult to complete during an ischemic episode. However, Factor and Dentinger (1987) found abnormal BAEPs in all eight patients with vertebrobasilar TIAs performed 1 to 16 days after the TIA at a time when the clinical examination was normal. Six of these patients were followed and five returned to normal, one to near normal. They suggested that BAEPs might be helpful in differentiating TIAs from nonbrain stem syndromes (e.g., labyrinthine dizziness). Also, Morocutti et al. (1985) found a correlation between BAEP abnormalities and the clinical duration of the ischemic episode, and increasing BAEP abnormalities with increasing severity of residual defects. Baldy-Moulinier et al. (1984) found group differences between patients with vertebrobasilar TIAs and normals.

3.7.3. Hemorrhages

Brown et al. (1981b) and Chiappa (1982a) found BAEP abnormalities in all four of the patients they studied with pontine hemorrhages (see Figs. 6–2 and 6–3).

Stockard and Rossiter (1977) showed a patient in whom the hemorrhage had destroyed the caudal pons and cochlear nuclei bilaterally; only wave I could be recorded in this patient. They also had three patients with hemorrhages in the caudal pontine tegmentum with abnormalities in wave III and subsequent waves. One patient with a hemorrhage in the rostral pons had abnormalities after wave III. Oh et al. (1981) reported a patient with a right pontine–midbrain hemorrhage who had a normal left BAEP but wave V absent on the right. A similar case was reported by Hammond et al. (1985).

Thus, patients with pontine hemorrhages have abnormal BAEPs but, unless the lower pons is involved, waves I–III are preserved. The preservation of BAEP waveforms closely parallels the brain stem structures preserved.

3.7.4. Vascular Malformations

It has been suggested that facial spasm, trigeminal neuralgia, or facial paresis may be caused by malformations or misroutings of arteries or veins in the posterior fossa, and that surgery may ameliorate the problem. Buettner et al. (1983) studied 32 such patients and found BAEP abnormalities in 12, confirmed by CT scan in 5, although the exact findings were not given or unconvincing.

3.8. Coma

Use of BAEPs to assess brain stem integrity in comatose patients is, to some extent, limited by the anatomic specificity of the test. As mentioned above, BAEPs can be normal in patients completely paralyzed from brain stem infarction. Thus, there can be major brain stem lesions without involvement of the auditory tracts and therefore normal BAEPs are not indicative of functional integrity of the entire brain stem. Since BAEPs are generated by structures mostly below midbrain levels, progressive space-taking lesions in the cerebral hemispheres will not produce BAEP changes until structures in the low midbrain or below are involved. Impressions of clinical utility of BAEPs in comatose patients have varied according to whether or not these factors were taken into account, the statistical limits of normality used in interpretation, and the time of BAEP testing in relation to the cerebral insult (Greenberg et al., 1977; Uziel and Benezech, 1978; Seales et al., 1979; Tsubokawa et al., 1980; Goldie et al., 1981; Narayan et al., 1981; Rappaport et al., 1981a,b; Sanders et al., 1981; Hall et al., 1982; Karnaze et al., 1982; Klug, 1982; Stern et al., 1982; Goitein et al., 1983; Hall et al., 1983; Newlon et al., 1983; Lutschg et al., 1983; Taylor et al., 1983; Yagi and Baba, 1983; Anderson et al., 1984; Rosenberg et al., 1984; Facco et al., 1985; Frank et al., 1985; Klug and Csecsei, 1985; Cant et al., 1986; Ottaviani et al., 1986; Ganes and Lundar, 1988).

Uziel and Benezech (1978) found BAEPs normal in 10 patients in coma with lesions at or above the thalamic level. In 10 others they noted a good correlation between the pattern of BAEP abnormalities and the level of coma. However, they used absolute amplitude as part of their criteria of abnormality. In addition, they found that "flaccidity which appears in brain stem lesions involving the inferior pons, always corresponded with a loss of the last 3 waves." If their case material had included patients with locked-in syndrome, they would have noted that normal BAEPs can also accompany flaccidity of pontine origin.

Starr and Achor (1975) studied 37 patients in coma and found that BAEPs were usually normal when the coma had a toxic or metabolic etiology. They commented that the finding of normal BAEPs in a comatose patient suggested a toxic or metabolic etiology or a diffuse cortical process sparing the brain stem. Rumpl et al. (1988) found delayed IPLs with drug overdose, but normal IPLs at therapeutic drug plasma levels.

Tsubokawa et al. (1980) studied BAEPs in 64 patients in coma from severe head injury, using waveform absence or latency prolongation as criteria of abnormality (the statistical measure used for the latter was not stated). They found a progressively greater abnormality rate as more caudal levels of the CNS were involved: (1) of 18 patients without clinical signs of brain stem dysfunction, 14 (78%) had normal BAEPs; (2) of 7 patients with diencephalic syndrome or third-nerve palsy, 3 (43%) had normal BAEPs; (3) of 17 patients with midbrain to lower pontine syndromes, all but one had lost waves I through V. Patients who lost waves III to V all died or remained in a vegetative state. Ahmed (1980) noted BAEP changes with clinical signs of brain stem compression from herniation in three patients, two of whom had reversal of the changes with steroid treatment. Ropper and Shafran (1984) also found BAEP abnormalities accompanying clinical signs of brain stem compression.

Klug and Csecsei (1985) found increasing BAEP abnormalities during acute stages of decerebration syndromes; in improving patients BAEP normalization began rostrally. Garcia-Larrea et al. (1987) noted a simultaneous latency increase of all components with a decrease in cerebral perfusion pressure. Seales et al. (1979) studied 17 comatose blunt head-injury patients using a 2-SD limit of normality for latency and 3 SD for absolute amplitude. Three patients who were clinically brain-dead had no BAEP waveforms. Two patients with abnormal BAEPs, both initially and at follow-up, died of their brain injuries. Twelve other patients with normal follow-up BAEPs recovered, regardless of whether their initial BAEP had been abnormal (three patients) or normal (nine patients). Seales et al. noted the weak correlation between BAEPs performed in the early critical period (2 to 3 days) and patient outcome. Following this period, however, they believed that BAEPs had a good correlation with outcome which often preceded the clinical prognosis, by several days in some cases. They thought that the test would be of greatest prognostic utility in patients in whom neurologic and other signs do not permit a clear prognosis for weeks following the injury.

Karnaze et al. (1982) studied 26 comatose head-injury patients using the 95% tolerance level as the limit of normality for interpeak latencies and a V/I amplitude ratio of 0.5. Nineteen patients had normal BAEPs and all survived, six with a good recovery, nine with a moderate disability, two with a severe disability, and two in a vegetative state (Glasgow Outcome Scale). Six had abnormal BAEPs; three died and three had unfavorable outcomes. Brain stem auditory EPs were abnormal in only 5 of 12 patients with decerebration.

Goldie et al. (1981) studied 50 patients who were poorly responsive but had some preservation of brain stem and CNS function clinically. Twenty-six (52%) had BAEPs within normal limits bilaterally. Three (6%) had bilateral and seven (14%) had unilateral absence of all waves. All but eight (16%) had wave I on at least one side. Five patients had ill-defined and low-amplitude IV–V complexes on one side, earlier waves being normal (Fig. 6–17, panel D). Two patients had no recordable responses because of unacceptable levels of artifact. In this group of 50 patients there was no consistent relationship between BAEP results and clinical outcome. For example, in the 26 patients with normal BAEPs bilaterally, 4 died, 10 remained in coma or vegetative state, and 12 regained some function. However, patients who had bilaterally absent BAEP waves (not thought to be due to peripheral hearing loss) or who had no waves IV and/or V were less likely to survive. Cant et al. (1986) also found the BAEP to be of little prognostic significance. However, in a study of 66 patients with severe head trauma, Ottaviani et al. (1986) found that the BAEP was better at predicting outcome of severe head injury than the Glasgow Coma Scale, CT scan, or EEG, and Facco et al. (1985), from a study of 40 similar patients, suggested the hypothesis that 95% of survivors have a I–V IPL of less than 4.5 msec.

Anderson et al. (1984) studied 39 head-injured patients and had similar findings but also noted that the EPs were more reliable than pupillary or motor clinical examinations. Rosen-

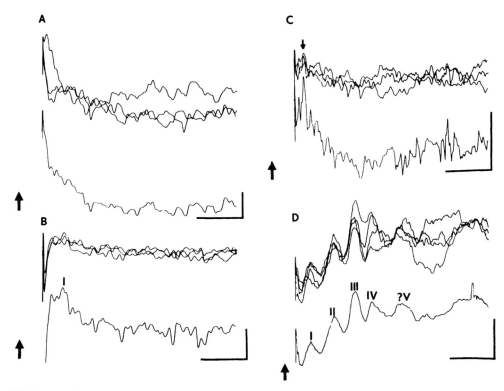

FIG. 6–17. Brain stem auditory EPs obtained from brain-dead patients (**A** through **C**) and a comatose but not brain-dead patient (**D**). **A** and **D** were obtained using conventional earlobe electrodes, and **B** and **C** were obtained using external auditory canal (EAC) needle electrodes. **A** lacks any recognizable waves. **B** shows a small wave I, which was obtained only using the EAC needle electrode. **C**, displayed at higher magnification than **A** or **B**, shows an early cochlear microphonic (at arrow) but no wave I. **D** shows normal waves I–III, distorted IV and absent V. Each trace is the average of 1,024 clicks, with the grand average beneath. Calibration marks are 2.5 msec and 0.25 µV. (From Goldie et al., 1981, with permission.)

berg et al. (1984) in a group of patients comatose from mixed etiologies found that preservation of just middle-latency and/or BAEPs did not correlate with survival, although the head trauma patients did show a good correlation [all patients showed a relationship between survival and preservation of long-, middle-, and short-(BAEP) latency AEPs]. Hall et al. (1983) found a relationship between acute BAEPs, middle-latency auditory EPs, CT scan, neurologic status, and rate of recovery; auditory EPs 4 days after injury were also correlated with long-term outcome of diagnostic speech audiometry. Stern et al. (1982) studied 35 patients with recent brain stem strokes and noted that abnormal BAEPs correlated with an unstable clinical course and a poor prognosis in the presence of pontomesencephalic infarction. Ropper and Miller (1985) correlated abnormal BAEPs with acute traumatic midbrain hemorrhage. Brunko et al. (1985) found absent BAEPs but normal SEPs and brain stem reflexes in two patients in coma following cardiac arrest; neuropathology revealed anoxic damage in Sommer's sector and Purkinje cells. Garcia-Larrea et al. (1992) continuously monitored BAEPs and ICP and found that the stability of BAEPs despite apparently significant (>40 mmHg) acute rises in ICP was associated with a high probability of survival as opposed to prolongation of central latency in response to raised ICP.

Sanders et al. (1981) studied 17 pediatric patients in coma from diverse etiologies using the normal mean plus 2 SD as the upper limit of normal (absolute latency, latency intervals, and absolute amplitude) for the interpretation of "mildly abnormal"; "grossly abnormal" was an absent wave V. Of five patients with normal BAEPs, one died and four recovered, of four patients with mildly abnormal BAEPs, one died and three recovered, and all seven patients with grossly abnormal BAEPs died. Lutschg et al. (1983) investigated 43 comatose children (head injury and hypoxic–ischemic encephalopathy) and found a good correlation between loss of BAEP components and poor outcome, but a weaker correlation with latency changes. Goitein et al. (1983), Strickbine-Van Reet et al. (1984), Frank et al. (1985), and Rappaport et al. (1985) have also studied BAEPs in comatose children.

Patients with persistent vegetative state usually have normal BAEPs (Pollack and Kellaway, 1980; Karnaze et al., 1982; Hansotia, 1985).

To summarize the experience with BAEPs in coma, although there is a limited relationship between BAEP results and clinical outcome, these statistical facts are not particularly useful in the clinical situation, where one is faced with an individual patient, that is, there is no way of knowing into which statistical group the individual patient will fall except in the patients who are also the worst clinically. In these patients the clinicians do not need prognostic help. However, if damage to the peripheral hearing apparatus can be ruled out, then the absence of BAEPs is strongly correlated with a poor outcome. The addition of these data to other prognostic indicators, none of which by themselves are conclusive, may be helpful in assigning a patient to a poor prognosis category with a high degree of certainty. In the area of therapeutic interventions, Nagao et al. (1987), relating wave V abnormalities to upper brain stem compression, have suggested that immediate medical or surgical decompression of ICP should be performed when ICP approaches 30 mmHg with significant prolongation of wave V latency. Stone et al. (1988) have reviewed the relationship between BAEPs and clinical findings, lesion localization, ICP and herniation, and prognosis in head-injured patients.

3.9. Brain Death

Absence of BAEP waves II through V despite a normal wave I indicates a significant lack of function in brain stem auditory tracts. Furthermore, the metabolic and physiologic immutability of BAEPs provides a safety margin for use of the test in comatose patients. For example, in a case of barbiturate overdose sufficient to produce a clinical appearance of brain death and an almost isoelectric ("flat") EEG, BAEPs were essentially unchanged (Stockard et al., 1977a; Stockard and Sharbrough, 1980b; Stockard et al., 1980). Similarly, high doses of anesthetic agents do not significantly alter BAEP components (Sanders et al., 1979; Stockard and Sharbrough, 1980b). Thus, this test can be an indicator of preserved brain stem function in difficult clinical situations (e.g., patients in an intensive care unit being treated with high-dose barbiturates for increased ICP and in the operating room during general anesthesia).

The functional integrity of the brain stem has been studied in brain-dead patients using BAEP testing (Trojaborg and Jorgensen, 1973; Starr and Achor, 1975; Starr, 1976; Stockard and Sharbrough, 1980b; Goldie et al., 1981; Klug, 1982; Klug and Csecsei, 1985; Ganes and Lundar, 1988; Machado et al., 1991). Goldie et al. found that 27 of 35 brain-dead patients (77%) had no identifiable BAEP waveforms, including wave I, even though in nine patients EAC needle electrodes were used (Fig. 6–17). Eight patients (23%) had at least wave I present on one side (Fig. 6–17). Two of these (6%) had low-amplitude but definable

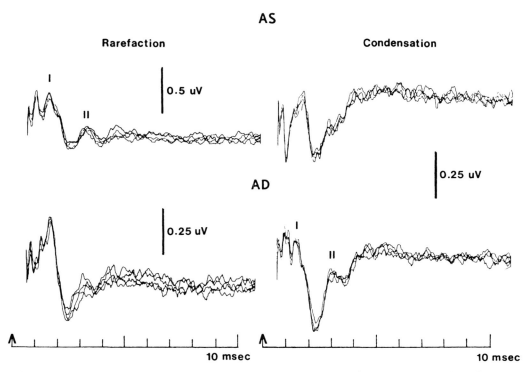

FIG. 6–18. Brain stem auditory EPs from a brain-dead patient showing preservation of wave II bilaterally.

wave I's bilaterally, four (12%) had low-amplitude, but definable wave I's with stimulation of and recording from only one side, the other showing no responses, and two (6%) had waves I and II present bilaterally (Fig. 6–18). Three patients had no recordable BAEPs because of an unacceptable level of ambient noise or muscle artifact. Wave I was present in 11 of 27 (41%) of Starr's cases (Starr, 1976). Six of those 11 cases had only unilateral preservation (22%) and 5 had bilateral preservation (18.5%). Goldie et al. showed wave I preservation in only 8 of 35 cases (23%), but those data were all obtained between the first and second flat EEGs, with a clinical state of no brain stem function already established for several hours, whereas the duration of the clinically brain-dead state was not reported by Starr. Starr (1976) had a patient who showed a progressive neurologic and BAEP deterioration with parallel levels of dysfunction at each stage (Fig. 6–19). Klug and Csecsei (1985) studied 55 brain-dead patients and found none with waves after I; 25 had wave I on both sides, 10 on one side only (65% of the patients had a wave I at least on one side).

Without wave I present, no inferences can be made as to the localization of the interruption of the auditory signal since the integrity of the peripheral apparatus in any individual patient is often not known. For example, a traumatic transverse fracture of the temporal bone might have damaged the cochlea, or, in a case where the clinical history is poor, the patient might have had a pre-existing deafness in the only ear available for BAEP testing. Wave I absence in these patients is thought to be secondary to interference with the eighth nerve and cochlear blood supply, which is derived primarily from intracranial circulation via the anterior cerebellar and internal auditory arteries. Brunko et al. (1985) have suggested that absence of BAEP components following anoxic episodes may be due to a direct effect on the cochlea so that in-

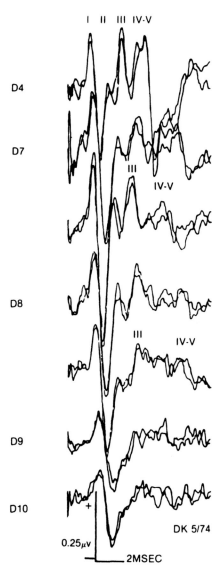

FIG. 6–19. Brain stem auditory EPs in a 19-year-old patient in coma following an anoxic episode. The designations on the left, D4, D7, etc., refer to the hospital day; on days 7 and 8 the two traces represent recordings taken in the morning and afternoon, respectively. On day 4 (D4) all the components were of normal amplitude and latency, and the patient had preserved brainstem reflexes. On the seventh day all interpeak latencies had increased and the amplitude of the IV–V complex was diminished; the patient had lost pupillary, corneal, and oculocephalic reflexes. On the eighth day the EEG contained only low-amplitude delta activity and the BAEP interpeak latencies and amplitudes were more abnormal. On the tenth day the patient was brain-dead, the EEG was isoelectric, and only wave I remained. Monaural clicks presented at 65 dB HL and 10/sec, vertex to earlobe derivation. Each trace is the average of 2,048 stimuli. (From Starr, 1976, with permission.)

terpretations concerning the state of the brain stem pathways must be cautious. Also note that Ferbert et al. (1986) have reported a patient with a posterior fossa hemorrhage who had the clinical features of brain death (including apnea) but preserved EEG and visual EPs.

3.10. Miscellaneous Diseases

3.10.1. Acute Transverse Myelopathy

Ropper et al. (1982) studied 12 consecutive patients with inflammatory acute transverse myelopathy (ATM) and no prior history of neurologic disease (disease evolved over 1 to 10 days, multiple tracts were involved, and there was a discrete sensory level). Brain stem auditory EPs in all were normal; since about one third of patients with MS have abnormal BAEPs, the authors noted that this (along with the normal PSVEPs in these patients) suggested that ATM differs from MS.

3.10.2. Acquired Immunodeficiency Syndrome

Smith et al. (1988) recorded BAEPs in 15 human immunodeficiency virus (HIV)-seropositive but otherwise healthy patients [also without AIDS-related complex (ARC)] and found abnormal wave V absolute latencies in 2 (using 2 SD) and I–V group differences versus controls at the $p < 0.05$ level; Pagano et al. (1992) have also found abnormalities in patients with HIV and AIDS. However, in a large group in a well-performed study Iragui et al. (1994) found only rare BAEP abnormalities in ARC/AIDS patients.

3.10.3. Albinism

Creel et al. (1983a) studied four patients with Chediak-Higashi syndrome and found normal ipsilateral BAEPs. Contralaterally recorded BAEPs were reported as abnormal although replications were not shown and the degree of asymmetry evident in the single figure is probably within normal limits.

3.10.4. Alcoholism

Alcohol in intoxicating doses has small but significant effects on BAEP latencies (Chu et al., 1978; Squires et al., 1978a,b) probably caused by lowered body temperature (Stockard et al., 1978a). Begleiter et al. (1981) studied 17 alcoholic subjects, abstinent for at least 3 weeks, and found marked I–V IPLs prolongations (mean increase 0.95 msec). They suggested demyelination or edema as the mechanism. Chan et al. (1985) reported abnormal BAEPs in 48% of patients with Wernicke-Korsakoff syndrome, 25% of alcoholic patients with cerebellar degeneration, and in 13% of alcoholic patients without the previous two diseases. Hammond et al. (1986) found click polarity-related differences in BAEPs in 24% of patients with Wernicke-Korsakoff syndrome.

3.10.5. Arnold-Chiari Malformation

Lee et al. (1985) found abnormal BAEPs in all 15 patients with type II Arnold-Chiari malformation, I–V prolonged in 9, I–III in 6, and III–V in 4. Some improved postoperatively. However, we have seen a patient with this problem with normal BAEPs, as have Westmoreland et al. (1983).

3.10.6. Basilar Migraine

Serial BAEPs performed in a patient with basilar migraine (Yamada et al., 1986) revealed wave V abnormalities during an attack, only evident with rarefaction clicks.

3.10.7. Cortical Deafness

Ozdamar et al. (1982) and Stockard and Rossiter (1977) have reported patients with bitemporal infarcts and complete cortical deafness who have normal BAEPs bilaterally. This fact underscores the care that must be taken in correlating BAEPs with functional hearing.

3.10.8. Diabetes Mellitus

Donald et al. (1981) studied 20 diabetic patients whose audiometric testing showed no significant hearing loss. They found significant prolongations in I–III and I–V IPLs in group comparisons (normals versus patients), but they did not say how many patients had abnormal IPLs on an individual basis. The mean differences were less than 2 SD. No IPL was correlated with duration of diabetes or with blood glucose measurements. Martini et al. (1985) also found BAEP abnormalities in diabetic patients absolute latencies but not in IPLs.

3.10.9. Epilepsy

Rodin et al. (1980, 1982) studied 80 epileptic patients and found significantly prolonged I–III and I–V IPLs and larger standard deviations compared to their normal subjects. They noted that the prolonged latencies were related more to brain damage (as evidenced on clinical neurologic and EEG examinations) than to the epilepsy alone. The number of different seizure types a given patient had was significantly related to the latency changes, but frequency, type, and duration of seizures were not. Plasma anticonvulsant levels showed a correlation with some IPL parameters (e.g., carbamazepine increased the I–III separation by 0.42 msec, $p < 0.01$) but these findings generally did not follow a consistent pattern. Note that Hirose et al. (1986), Gledhill et al. (1987), and Chan et al. (1990) have commented on effects of phenytoin on BAEPs.

3.10.10. Hemifacial Spasm

Moller et al. (1982) found preoperative absolute wave V latency prolongations on a group statistical basis in 39 patients operated on to relieve hemifacial spasm. Individual data were not available nor IPLs given.

3.10.11. Hysteria-Malingering

Brain stem auditory EPs may be useful in carefully selected patients when the possibility of hysteria-malingering exists (Howard and Dorfman, 1986).

3.10.12. Idiopathic Polyneuritis (Guillain-Barré Syndrome)

Brain stem auditory EP abnormalities were less common in Guillain-Barré syndrome patients (3 of 21) studied by Ropper and Chiappa (1986) than reported by Schiff et al. (1985), whose findings of a shortened or normal I–V IPL, coexisting with the prolonged I–III in some patients, raises the question of proper identification of wave III. Because occasional patients with Guillain-Barré syndrome, usually without significant brain stem symptoms, have abnormal BAEPs, Ropper and Chiappa (1986) urged caution in interpreting abnormal studies in Fisher's syndrome as evidence for CNS lesions since their three patients with Fisher's syndrome had normal BAEPs, except perhaps for one with an abnormal I/V amplitude ratio unilaterally with one click polarity only. Minor accompanying CNS lesions are not excluded by normal EPs, but it is difficult to link electrophysiologic abnormalities to clinical signs. Cases of brain stem encephalitis resembling Fisher's syndrome further confound the relationship between brain stem EP abnormalities and clinical signs (Ropper, 1983; Ropper and Marmarou, 1984).

3.10.13. Meningitis

Since the eighth nerve traverses the subarachnoid space, any inflammatory process may affect conduction in that portion of the nerve. Thus, we have seen abnormal I–III IPLs in patients with bacterial and aseptic (viral) meningitis. The same effect should be expected with other meningitides, for example, carcinomatous, tuberculous, and fungal. See Section 3.11 for a discussion of the utility of BAEPs in detecting sensorineural hearing loss resulting from bacterial meningitis in infants.

3.10.14. Narcolepsy, Primary Insomnia, and Sleep Apnea

Hellekson et al. (1979) studied 10 narcoleptics and 10 primary insomniacs and found no abnormalities in IPLs.

Mosko et al. (1981) found normal IPLs in one child and five adults with obstructive sleep apnea, even when arterial oxygen saturation fell as low as 45% to 70% during the testing period. Stockard et al. (1980a) studied 7 patients with predominantly central and 23 with predominantly obstructive sleep apnea. Three of the seven patients with central sleep apnea had normal BAEPs, the other four had clinical neurologic brain stem dysfunction (infarction and tumor), and all had gross BAEP abnormalities. All but one of the 23 patients with obstructive apnea had normal I–V IPLs.

In another study Stockard (1982) found normal BAEPs in four of eight adults with central sleep apnea, with the other four patients showing central BAEP abnormalities. In 20 adults with mixed/obstructive sleep apnea, BAEPs were normal. Karnaze et al. (1984) and Verma et al. (1987), in 30 patients with sleep apnea, found abnormal BAEPs in only 1 (with a meningeal leukemic infiltrate). Long and Allen (1984) reported abnormal BAEPs in a patient with Odine's Curse of uncertain, perhaps alcoholic toxic, etiology. Snyderman et al. (1982) studied 23 patients with sleep apnea using tone-burst stimuli.

3.10.15. Palatal Myoclonus

Six of 20 patients with palatal myoclonus had abnormal BAEPs, 2 of these with severe head trauma, 1 each with an infarct, tumor, demyelination, and indeterminate inflammatory process (Westmoreland et al., 1983). The 14 patients with normal BAEPs had head trauma (5), infarcts (4), cerebellar tumors (2), and Arnold–Chiari malformation (1).

3.10.16. Postconcussion Syndrome

Rowe and Carlson (1980) studied 27 patients with postconcussion dizziness who had normal neurologic examinations. Three patients had one or more IPLs prolonged beyond the 99% tolerance limit and the group mean I–III, II–III, and I–V IPLs were significantly prolonged. Nineteen of these patients had ENG testing; 11 (58%) had abnormalities of latent or positional nystagmus or caloric-induced nystagmus. However, the ENG abnormality often could not be localized to central or peripheral structures, decreasing its clinical utility. Noseworthy et al. (1981) found normal IPLs both individually and as a group in 11 patients with postconcussion syndrome.

Benna et al. (1982) found a 27% incidence of abnormalities in postconcussion syndrome patients, not correlated with dizziness at the time of recording or with ENG findings. Schoenhuber et al. (1985) studied 165 patients with minor injury within 48 hours and found no group mean differences versus normal controls; using 3 SD as the upper limit of normal they found abnormalities in 11%. The clinical utility of an abnormal BAEP in this area is unclear.

3.10.17. Radiation

Five patients who had had incidental radiation to the rhombencephalon were tested at 11 weeks and 8 months. No BAEP changes were found, nor were there any neurological symptoms (Nightingale et al., 1984).

3.10.18. Renal Disease

Hutchinson and Klodd (1982) found no significant BAEP abnormalities in 15 patients with chronic renal failure on hemodialysis, although in a similar group of patients Rizzo et al. (1982) found 3 of 12 with abnormal BAEPs and related these findings to the action of toxic substances or demyelination. Rossini et al. (1985) found BAEP abnormalities in 24% of patients with chronic renal failure, in close agreement with a 25% abnormality rate given by Pratt et al. (1986a) in 38 patients. Komsuoglu et al. (1985) noted III–IV abnormalities, some of which were reversed by dialysis, and some which were permanent.

3.10.19. Spasmodic Torticollis

Drake (1988) found one of six patients with spasmodic torticollis to have I–III and I–V interpeak latencies at the 99% tolerance limit.

3.10.20. Spastic Dysphonia

Sharbrough et al. (1978) studied 18 patients with spastic dysphonia and found 2 with interpeak latencies prolonged above the 99% confidence limit. They noted that this supports the idea that spastic dysphonia is a symptom due to a disease which, in some cases, incidentally produces asymptomatic slowing of conduction in brain stem auditory pathways. Finitzo-Hieber et al. (1982) have also reported abnormal BAEPs in this disease.

3.10.21. Subacute Sclerosing Panencephalitis

Markand et al. (1980) reported 3 patients with subacute sclerosing panencephalitis (SSPE) who had progressive intellectual deterioration, myoclonic jerks, and periodic complexes in the EEG. All BAEPs were normal. We have seen one patient with SSPE with abnormal BAEPs.

3.10.22. Subacute Spongiform Encephalopathy (Creutzfeldt-Jakob Disease)

We have seen four patients with the typical acute-subacute form of spongiform encephalopathy, usually termed Creutzfeldt-Jakob disease, in whom BAEPs were normal even at an advanced state of the disease. A patient with an atypical form (Case Reports of Massachusetts General Hospital, 1980) also had normal BAEPs. Amantini et al. (1983) reported progressive prolongation of the I–V IPL, indicating brain stem involvement.

3.10.23. Syringobulbia

Kjaer (1980b) mentioned a case of syringobulbia and noted that there were "diffuse" BAEP abnormalities without giving further details on that specific case.

3.10.24. Tourette's Syndrome

Krumholz et al. (1983) reported normal BAEPs in 17 patients with Tourette's syndrome.

3.10.25. Toxic Inhalation

Two patients who had sniffed paint (probable active ingredient was toluene) developed cerebellar dysfunction, optic neuropathy, and dementia; BAEPs had no waves after II (Metrick and Brenner, 1982).

3.10.26. Vitamin Deficiencies

Krumholz et al. (1981) found prolonged I–V IPLs in two B_{12}-deficient patients with clinical evidence of neurologic dysfunction (motor, sensory, and cortical). Neither patient had hearing loss or vestibular dysfunction. After 1 year of therapy, these abnormalities had disappeared. Five other patients with little or no clinical involvement had normal BAEPs. Fine and Hallett (1980, 1981) reported four patients, all with normal BAEPs.

Ten patients with abetalipoproteinemia (vitamin E deficiency) had normal BAEPs (Brin et al., 1986).

3.11. Pediatric Applications

3.11.1. Brain Stem Gliomas

Abnormalities of BAEPs were found in all 21 cases reported in four studies (Starr and Achor, 1975; Jerger et al., 1980; Nodar et al., 1980a; Hecox et al., 1981), with abnormalities most marked ipsilateral to the tumor in most cases (see also Sections 2.4 and 3.7.1). Davis et al. (1985) reported four patients, one with normal BAEPs. Baram et al. (1986) studied 31 children with posterior fossa tumors and found that medulloblastoma was usually associated with normal BAEPs, whereas ependymomas, though they may resemble medulloblastoma on CT, are more likely to have abnormal BAEPs such as are seen in gliomas. Kovnar et al. (1986a) used BAEPs, to follow therapy in brain stem gliomas and noted that the clinical and BAEP findings correlated better with MRI than with contrast-enhanced CT.

3.11.2. Coma Prognosis

Most aspects of this topic have been discussed previously in Section 3.8. Some additional studies are mentioned below.

Hecox and Cone (1981) studied 126 infants who had suffered a significant period of asphyxia. Twenty-one of these had markedly abnormal I:V amplitude ratios (>2.0) and all of these had severe neurologic handicaps, so that it was believed that this was a useful prognostic indicator. Brain stem auditory EPs were more useful than behavioral criteria in this group of patients. However, normal amplitude ratios did not ensure normal neurologic outcome since 10 infants with normal responses were severely handicapped. Lutschg et al. (1983) briefly reported results from 40 asphyxiated infants and concluded that loss of BAEPs or single potentials indicated an unfavorable prognosis concerning survival. Taylor et al. (1983) described a patient with severe hypoxic brain damage after a near drowning whose BAEPs (including wave I) disappeared but subsequently reappeared; they suggested caution in BAEP interpretations in this situation. Karmel et al. (1988) evaluated the use of BAEPs in the assessment of 323 infants at risk for brain injury; detailed statistical analysis indicated that the BAEP helps to establish when the insult occurred, the degree of severity, and the course of recovery.

3.11.3. Giant Axonal Neuropathy

Three patients (14 to 16 years old) all had abnormal I–V IPLs, indicating CNS involvement in giant axonal neuropathy (Majnemer, 1986).

3.11.4. Hydrocephalus

Kraus et al. (1984) studied 38 pediatric patients with hydrocephalus and found some form of BAEP abnormalities in 88%, not correlated with etiology, head circumference, or brain stem symptoms. They suggested that the BAEP can be used to document clinically unsuspected brain stem pathology accompanying hydrocephalus and complicating hearing assessment. McPherson et al. (1985) followed BAEP latencies following shunt insertion in infants 32 to 43 weeks of age and found improvements within 5 days. Cevette (1984) also found BAEP IPLs decreased after shunting in 25 infants.

3.11.5. Hypothyroidism

Laureau et al. (1987) and Hebert et al. (1986) tested children with congenital hypothyroidism at 18 months, 3 years, and 5 to 9 years. No BAEP IPL abnormalities were found on group comparisons with normals, although a few individuals had abnormalities. Correlations between IPLs and serum thyroxine levels were present.

3.11.6. Leigh's Disease

Markand et al. (1980) reported a single patient who had only waves I and II present. Hecox et al. (1981) found BAEP IPL abnormalities in two of three patients with Leigh's disease. Davis et al. (1985) found abnormal BAEPs in all five of their patients, in two prior to the detection of CT abnormalities. However, we have seen one patient who had widespread neuropathologic changes in the brain stem sparing the tegmentum; BAEPs were normal in that patient.

3.11.7. Mental Retardation

Sohmer and Student (1978) studied three groups of children: (1) of 13 autistic children, no responses were found in 4, suggesting a cochlear hearing loss, and the other 9 had a mean I–V IPL about 1 SD above the normal mean; (2) 16 children with minimal brain dysfunction had I–V interpeak latencies about 2.5 SD above the normal mean; and (3) in 2 of 10 children with psychomotor retardation waves IV and V were absent and the other 8 had I–V IPLs about 1 SD above the normal mean. Only one ear was studied in most patients and individual data are not provided. Courchesne et al. (1985) found no BAEP abnormalities in 14 nonretarded autistic patients.

Tanguay et al. (1982) studied BAEPs in 16 autistic children. Three had marked delays of wave I (1 unilateral, 2 bilateral), suggesting a peripheral hearing disorder. Only one had I–V IPLs 3 SD beyond the normal mean at a low stimulus rate and 72 dB HL intensity. With faster rates and lower intensities more differences from normal were found.

Squires et al. (1980) studied 31 retarded adults (16 with Down's syndrome). Thirty-three percent of the ears in the Down's group had I–V IPLs more than 2 SD below the normal mean and only one patient had a value greater than the mean plus 2 SD. In the 15 patients with retardation of unknown etiology, 31% had I–V IPLs greater than the normal mean plus 2 SD. Profound hearing deficits were suggested in one or both ears of four Down's syndrome and two unknown-etiology patients. Lott et al. (1986) reported normal BAEPs in a hydranencephalic infant.

3.11.8. Metabolic Disorders

Markand et al. (1982b) studied four children with nonketotic hyperglycinemia with intractable seizures, multifocal spikes, and slow activity on EEG. Brain stem auditory EPs in all showed well-formed waveforms but were abnormal because of a I–V IPL greater than the normal mean plus 3 SD. Markand et al. thought that this abnormality was correlated with the loss of myelin seen pathologically, especially in those tracts that myelinate after birth. MacDermot et al. (1980) reported absolute latency increases in an infant with hyperglycinemia but IPLs were not given.

Hecox et al. (1981) found I–V IPL abnormalities in maple syrup urine disease and phenylketonuria. Davis et al. (1985) reported normal BAEPs in vitamin E deficiency and citrullinemia, but abnormal BAEPs in pyruvate decarboxylase deficiency and galactosemia.

3.11.9. Precocious Puberty

Normal BAEPs were seen in all 19 patients with precocious puberty of various etiologies (Theodore et al., 1983).

3.11.10. Progressive Myoclonic Epilepsy

Aguglia et al. (1985) reported normal BAEPs in five patients with progressive myoclonic epilepsy with Lafora bodies (Lafora disease).

3.11.11. Screening for Hearing Defects in At-Risk Infants

Normal development of central auditory pathways requires adequate peripheral input. Since conventional, behavioral hearing tests may be difficult to perform reliably in infants and children, the use of BAEPs in this patient population has been the subject of much attention. Sohmer and Feinmesser (1973), Hecox and Galambos (1974), Mokotoff et al. (1977), Starr et al. (1977), Roberts et al. (1982), Smith and Simmons (1982), Picton et al. (1986), and Picton and Durieux-Smith (1988) studied normal and hearing-impaired infants and children, comparing BAEP results with those obtained from conventional audiometric testing; good correlations were found. The importance and utility of testing hearing function in at-risk patients has been shown in several studies.

Schulman-Galambos and Galambos (1979) found on follow-up that 8 (2.1%) of 373 infants treated in a neonatal intensive care unit (NICU) had severe sensorineural hearing deficits, whereas none of 220 normal-term infants had any hearing disability. Brain stem auditory EPs performed in the NICU had revealed the abnormal auditory function in all eight infants (subsequently confirmed on the follow-up conventional audiometric measures) without significant false positives. They recommended routine BAEP testing on all NICU infants prior to discharge. Stein et al. (1981) studied 79 severely developmentally delayed infants and children suspected of being deaf and blind. They concluded that BAEPs were a very useful test of peripheral hearing function in this group and noted that a high percentage of the children were not hearing impaired (as far as brain stem function was concerned). (It must be realized that the BAEP is generated in brain stem structures and it is possible to have behavioral deafness on the basis of supratentorial disease with normal brain stem function and normal BAEPs.)

Kotagal et al. (1981) studied 41 infants and children who had had bacterial meningitis. Twenty-six had normal BAEPs (group 1), 10 had wave I delayed but IPLs normal (group 2), and 5 had no responses (group 3). There was no correlation with age, infective organism, antibiotic therapy, CSF formula, or CSF protein. Five of the infants in group 2 were retested after a mean of 9 months and four had normal responses; all five had normal language development. All five infants in group 3 had the same BAEP abnormality on follow-up.

Salamy et al. (1980) studied 67 normal full-term babies and 67 survivors of the intensive care nursery (ICN). They found no significant I–V IPL differences between these 2 groups (five of the ICN infants had no BAEPs, four had missing waveforms, and all nine of these were excluded from the statistical study). They did find significant absolute latency prolongations in the ICN group, suggesting a peripheral effect.

Kaga et al. (1979) found I–V IPLs normal when measurable in 25 infants with kernicterus, although some had absent waves I and prolonged absolute latencies, and 88% showed elevated thresholds to click, suggesting a peripheral site for the lesion causing the hearing defect. Chisin et al. (1979) found wave I absent in 11 of 13 patients with kernicterus, whereas cochlear microphonics were present in most; they suggested that the hair cells were intact but the eighth nerve damaged.

Picton and Durieux-Smith (1988) have summarized their experience to date and their discussion on this topic is recommended. Note that BAEPs are normal in cortical deafness (Bahls et al., 1988).

3.11.12. Sudden Infant Death Syndrome and Apnea

In sudden infant death syndrome (SIDS), BAEPs were normal in the only reported case where they were performed in an infant who later died a crib death (Stockard and Hecox, 1981; Stockard, 1982).

In near-miss sudden infant death syndrome (NMSIDS), only 3 (11%) of the 28 infants in the study of Stockard and Hecox (1981) had central BAEP abnormalities. In two of these, the abnormalities were thought to be related to anoxic damage incurred in the "near miss," and the third has subsequently displayed delayed development. However, in the study of Stockard (1982), four of the six infants with NMSIDS and normal BAEPs on an individual basis had IPL values that fell 1.2 to 2.2 SD above the normal mean and thus differed significantly from normal as a group. Stockard noted that this was not surprising since these infants have had severe apneic episodes, most with associated bradycardia. Gupta et al. (1981) studied nine infants with NMSIDS and found normal BAEPs in all. The studies of Orlowski et al. (1979) and Nodar et al. (1980a) suffer from methodologic deficiencies detailed by Stockard (1982) which account for the high incidence of BAEP abnormalities that they found in NMSIDS infants. One of the authors from these two articles participated in another study of NMSIDS in the same institution which found normal BAEPs in 14 of 16 infants (Lueders et al., 1984).

In 47 infants with other apnea syndromes unrelated to SIDS, central BAEP abnormalities were found in 15 (32%) and these infants had a higher risk of fatal respiratory arrest (5 of the 15) than those in the group who had normal BAEPs, none of whom died of respiratory arrest during the 6- to 36-month follow-up period (Stockard and Hecox, 1981). Henderson-Smart et al. (1983) found a correlation between presence of apnea and I–V IPL. The number of apneas per day decreased over a period that was similar to the period during which the BAEP IPLs decreased, and ceased when the IPLs equaled those in age-matched, apnea-free infants. Beckerman et al. (1986) reported abnormal BAEPs in four infants with Ondine's Curse.

Evoked Potentials in Clinical Medicine,
3d ed., edited by Keith H. Chiappa.
Lippincott–Raven Publishers, Philadelphia © 1997.

Brain Stem Auditory Evoked Potentials

References

Abbruzzese G, Dall'Agata D, Morena M, Reni L, Favale E (1990): Abnormalities of parietal and prerolandic somatosensory evoked potentials in Huntington's disease. *Electroencephalogr Clin Neurophysiol* 77(5):340–346.

Achor LJ, Starr A (1980a): Auditory brain stem responses in the cat. I. Intracranial and extracranial recordings. *Electroencephalogr Clin Neurophysiol* 48:154–173.

Achor LJ, Starr A (1980b): Auditory brain stem responses in the cat. II. Effects of lesions. *Electroencephalogr Clin Neurophysiol* 48:174–190.

Aguglia U, Farnarier G, Tinuper P, Quattrone A (1985): Brainstem auditory evoked responses in Lafora Disease. *Clin Electroencephalogr* 16:202–207.

Ahmed I (1980): Brainstem auditory evoked potentials in transtentorial herniation. *Clin Electroencephalogr* 11:34–37.

Allen AR, Starr A (1978): Auditory brain stem potentials in monkey (*M. mulatta*) and man. *Electroencephalogr Clin Neurophysiol* 45:53–63.

Allison T, Wood CC, Goff WR (1983): Brainstem auditory, pattern-reversal visual and short-latency somatosensory evoked potentials: Latencies in relation to age, sex, and brain and body size. *Electroencephalogr Clin Neurophysiol* 55:619–636.

Allison T, Hume AL, Wood CC, Goff WR (1984): Development and aging changes in somatosensory, auditory and visual evoked potentials. *Electroencephalogr Clin Neurophysiol* 58:14–24.

Amadeo M, Shagass C (1973): Brief latency click-evoked potentials during waking and sleep in man. *Psychophysiology* 10:244–250.

Amantini A, Ragazzoni A, Zaccara G, Barontini F, Rossi L (1983): SEPs and BAEPs in Creutzfeldt-Jakob disease. *Electroencephalogr Clin Neurophysiol* 55:10P.

Aminoff MJ, Davis SL, Panitch HS (1984): Serial evoked potential studies in patients with definite multiple sclerosis. *Arch Neurol* 41:1197–1202.

Anderson DC, Bundlie S, Rockswold GL (1984): Multimodality EPs in closed head trauma. *Arch Neurol* 41:369–374.

Anderson DC, Slater GE, Sherman R, Ettinger MG (1987): Evoked potentials to test a treatment of chronic multiple sclerosis. *Arch Neurol* 44:1232–1236.

Anderson DC, Bundlie S, Larson DA, Rockswold G, Mastri A (1988): Delayed traumatic midbrain syrinx: Clinical, pathologic, and electrophysiologic features. *Arch Neurol* 45:221–225.

Antoli-Candela F Jr, Kiang NY (1978): Unit activity underlying the N1 potential. In: *Evoked Electrical Activity in the Auditory Nervous System*, edited by RF Naunton and C Fernandez, pp 165–191. Academic Press, New York.

Bahls FH, Chatrian GE, Mesher RA, Sumi SM, Ruff RL (1988): A case of persistent cortical deafness: Clinical, neurophysiologic, and neuropathologic observations. *Neurology* 38:1490–1493.

Baldy-Moulinier M, Rondouin G, Touchon J, DeSaxce B (1984): Brain stem auditory-evoked potentials in the assessment of the transient ischemic attacks of the arterial vertebrobasilar system. *Monogr Neurol Sci* 11:216–221.

Barajas JJ (1982): Evaluation of ipsilateral and contralateral brainstem auditory evoked potentials in multiple sclerosis patients. *J Neurol Sci* 54:69–78.

Baram TZ, Goldie W, van Eys J (1986): Brainstem-evoked potentials in the diagnosis of posterior fossa tumors in children. *Ann Neurol* 20:398.

Barratt H (1980): Investigation of the mastoid electrode contribution to the brain stem auditory evoked response. *Scand Audiol* 9:203–211.

Bastuji H, Larrea LG, Bertrand O, Mauguiere F (1988): BAEP latency changes during nocturnal sleep are not correlated with sleep stages but with body temperature variations. *Electroencephalogr Clin Neurophysiol* 70:9–15.

Bauch CD, Rose DE, Harner SG (1980): Brainstem responses to tone pip and click stimuli. *Ear Hear* 1:181–184.

Beagley HA, Sheldrake JB (1978): Differences in brainstem response latency with age and sex. *Br J Audiol* 12:69–77.

Beckerman R, Meltzer J, Sola A, Dunn D, Wegmann M (1986): Brain-stem auditory response in Ondine's syndrome. *Arch Neurol* 43:698–701.

Begleiter H, Porjesz B, Chou CL (1981): Auditory brainstem potentials in chronic alcoholics. *Science* 211:1064–1066.

Benna P, Bergamasco B, Bianco C, Gilli M, Ferrero P, Pinessi L (1982): Brainstem auditory evoked potentials in postconcussion syndrome. *Ital J Neurol Sci* 4:281–287.

Berry H, Blair RL, Bilbao J, Briant TDR (1976): Click evoked eighth nerve and brain stem responses (electrocochleogram)—experimental observations in the cat. *J Otolaryngol* 5:64–73.

Bhargava VK, McKean CM (1977): Role of 5-hydroxytryptamine in the modulation of acoustic brainstem (far-field) potentials. *Neuropharmacology* 16:447–499.

Bhargava VK, Salamy A, McKean CM (1978): Effect of cholinergic drugs on the auditory evoked responses from brainstem (FFP) and auditory cortex (CER). *Neuroscience* 3:821–826.

Black JA, Fariello RG, Chun RW (1979): Brainstem auditory evoked response in adrenoleukodystrophy. *Ann Neurol* 6:269–270.

Boezeman EHJF, Kapteyn TS, Visser SL, Snel AM (1983a): Effect of contralateral and ipsilateral masking of acoustic stimulation on the latencies of auditory evoked potentials from cochlea and brain stem. *Electroencephalogr Clin Neurophysiol* 55:710–713.

Boezeman EHJF, Kapteyn TS, Visser SL, Snel AM (1983b): Comparison of the latencies between bone and air conduction in the auditory brain stem potential. *Electroencephalogr Clin Neurophysiol* 56:244–247.

Boller F, Jacobson GP (1980): Unilateral gunshot wound of the pons. Clinical, electrophysiologic and neuroradiologic correlates. *Arch Neurol* 37:278–281.

Bolz J and Giedke H (1982): Brain stem auditory evoked responses in psychiatric patients and healthy controls. *J Neural Transm* 54:285–291.

Born J, Schwab R, Pietrowsky R, Pauschinger P, Fegm HL (1989): Glucocorticoid influences on the auditory brain-stem responses in man. *Electroencephalogr Clin Neurophysiol* 74(3):209–216.

Boston JR, Ainslie PJ (1980): Effects of analog and digital filtering on brain stem auditory evoked potentials. *Electroencephalogr Clin Neurophysiol* 48:361–364.

Brin MF, Pedley TA, Lovelace RE, Emerson RG, Gouras P, MacKay C, Kayden HJ, Levy J, Baker H (1986): Electrophysiologic features of abetalipoproteinemia: Functional consequences of vitamin E deficiency. *Neurology* 36:669–673.

Brown FR, Shimizu H, McDonald JM, Moser AB, Marquis P, Chen WW, Moser HW (1981a): Auditory evoked brainstem response and high-performance liquid chromatography sulfatide assay as early indices of metachromatic leukodystrophy. *Neurology* 31:980–985.

Brown RH, Chiappa KH, Brooks EB (1981b): Brainstem auditory evoked responses in 22 patients with intrinsic brainstem lesions: Implications for clinical interpretations. *Electroencephalogr Clin Neurophysiol* 51:38P.

Brunko E, Delecluse F, Herbaut AG, Levivier M, Zegers de Beyl D (1985): Unusual pattern of somatosensory and brain-stem auditory evoked potentials after cardio-respiratory arrest. *Electroencephalogr Clin Neurophysiol* 62:338–342.

Buchwald JS, Huang CM (1975): Far-field acoustic response: Origins in the cat. *Science* 189:382–384.

Buettner UW, Stohr M, Koletzki E (1983): Brainstem auditory evoked potential abnormalities in vascular malformations of the posterior foss. *J Neurol* 229:247–254.

Cacace AT, Shy M, Satya-Murti S (1980): Brainstem auditory evoked potentials: A comparison of two high-frequency filter settings. *Neurology* 30:765–767.

Caird DM, Klinke R (1987): The effect of inferior colliculus lesions on auditory evoked potentials. *Electroencephalogr Clin Neurophysiol* 68:237–240.

Campbell KB, Bartoli EA (1986): Human auditory evoked potentials during natural sleep: The early components. *Electroencephalogr Clin Neurophysiol* 65:142–149.

Cant BR, Hume AL, Judson JA, Shaw NA (1986): The assessment of severe head injury by short-latency somatosensory and brain-stem auditory evoked potentials. *Electroencephalogr Clin Neurophysiol* 65:188–195.

Cascino GD, Adams RD (1986): Brainstem auditory hallucinosis. *Neurology* 36:1042–1047.

Cascino GD, Ring SR, King PJL, Brown RH, Chiappa KH (1988): Evoked potentials in motor system diseases. *Neurology* 38:231–238.

Cazals Y, Aran J-M, Erre J-P, Guilhame A (1980): Acoustic responses after total destruction of the cochlear receptor: Brainstem and auditory cortex. *Science* 210:83–86.

Cevette MJ (1984): Auditory brain-stem response testing in the intensive care unit. *Semin Hear* 5:57–69.

Chakravorty BG (1966): Association of trigeminal neuralgia with multiple sclerosis. *Arch Neurol* 14:95–99.

Chan YW, McLeod JG, Tuck RR, Feary PA (1985): Brain stem auditory evoked responses in chronic alcoholics. *J Neurol Neurosurg Psychiatry* 48:1107–1112.

Chan YW, Woo EKW, Hammond SR, Yiannikas C, McLeod JG (1988): The interaction between sex and click polarity in brain-stem auditory potentials evoked from control subjects of Oriental and Caucasian origin. *Electroencephalogr Clin Neurophysiol* 71:77–80.

Chan YW, Woo E, Yu YL (1990): Chronic effects of phenytoin on brain-stem auditory evoked potentials in man. *Electroencephalogr Clin Neurophysiol* 77:119–126.

Chiappa KH (1980a): Evoked responses. Part 2: Brainstem auditory. In: *Weekly Update: Neurology and Neurosurgery* Vol 2, edited by P Scheinberg, pp 129–135. Continuing Professional Education Center, New Jersey.

Chiappa KH (1980b): Pattern shift visual, brainstem auditory and short-latency somatosensory evoked potentials in multiple sclerosis. *Neurology* 30 (7, part 2):110–123.

Chiappa KH (1982a): Physiologic localization using evoked responses: Pattern shift visual, brainstem auditory and short latency somatosensory. In: *New Perspectives in Cerebral Localization*, edited by RA Thompson and JR Green, pp 63–114. Raven Press, New York.

Chiappa KH (1982b): Utility of lowering click intensity in neurologic applications of brainstem auditory evoked potentials. Presented at Conference on Standards in Clinical BAEP testing, Laguna Beach, California, February, 1982.

Chiappa KH (1983): *Evoked Potentials in Clinical Medicine.* Raven Press, New York.

Chiappa KH (1984): Utility of lowering click intensity in neurologic applications of brainstem auditory evoked potentials. In: *Sensory Evoked Potentials, 1. An International Conference on Standards in Auditory Brainstem Response Testing,* edited by A Starr, C Rosenberg, M Don, and H Davis, pp 131–132. Centro Ricerche e Studi Amplifon, Milan.

Chiappa KH, Parker SW (1984): A simple needle electrode technique for improved registration of wave I in brainstem auditory evoked potentials. In: *Sensory Evoked Potentials, 1. An International Conference on Standards in Auditory Brainstem Response Testing,* edited by A Starr, C Rosenberg, M Don, and H Davis, pp 137–139. Centro Ricerche e Studi Amplifon, Milan.

Chiappa KH, Gladstone KJ, Young RR (1979): Brainstem auditory evoked responses: Studies of waveform variations in 50 normal human subjects. *Arch Neurol* 36:81–87.

Chiappa KH, Harrison JL, Brooks EB, Young RR (1980): Brainstem auditory evoked responses in 200 patients with multiple sclerosis. *Ann Neurol* 7:135–143.

Chisin R, Perlman M, Sohmer H (1979): Cochlear and brain stem responses in hearing loss following neonatal hyperbilirubinemia. *Ann Otol Rhinol Laryngol* 88:352–357.

Chisin R, Gafni M, Sohmer H (1983): Patterns of auditory nerve and brainstem-evoked responses (ABR) in different types of peripheral hearing loss. *Arch Otorhinolaryngol* 237:165–173.

Chu N-S, Squires KC, Starr A (1978): Auditory brain stem potentials in chronic alcohol intoxication and alcohol withdrawal. *Arch Neurol* 35:596–602.

Church MW, Williams HL (1982): Dose- and time-dependent effects of ethanol on brain stem auditory evoked responses in young adult males. *Electroencephalogr Clin Neurophysiol* 54:161–174.

Church MW, Williams HL, Holloway JA (1984): Brain-stem auditory evoked potentials in the rat: Effects of gender, stimulus characteristics and ethanol sedation. *Electroencephalogr Clin Neurophysiol* 59:328–340.

Clemis JD, McGee T (1979): Brainstem electric response audiometry in the differential diagnosis of acoustic tumors. *Laryngoscope* 89:31–42.

Clemis JD, Mitchell C (1977): Electrocochleography and brain stem responses used in the diagnosis of acoustic tumors. *J Otolaryngol* 6:447–459.

Coats AC (1974): On electrocochleographic electrode design. *J Acoust Soc Am* 56:708–711.

Coats AC (1978): Human auditory nerve action potentials and brainstem evoked responses. Latency-intensity function in detection of cochlear and retrocochlear abnormalities. *Arch Otolaryngol* 104:709–717.

Coats AC, Kidder HR (1980): Earspeaker coupling effects on auditory action potential and brainstem responses. *Arch Otolaryngol* 106:339–344.

Coats AC, Martin JL (1977): Human auditory nerve action potentials and brain stem evoked responses. Effects of audiogram shape and lesion location. *Arch Otolaryngol* 103:605–622.

Coats AC, Martin JL, Kidder HR (1979): Normal short-latency electrophysiological filtered click responses recorded from vertex and external auditory meatus. *J Acoust Soc Am* 65:747–758.

Cogan DG, Wray SH (1970): Internuclear ophthalmoplegia as an early sign of brainstem tumors. *Neurology* 20:629–633.

Cohen MS, Britt RH (1982): Effects of sodium pentobarbital, ketamine, halothane, and chloralose on brainstem auditory evoked responses. *Anesth Analg* 61:338–343.

Collet L, Delorme C, Chanal JM, Dubreuil C, Morgon A, Salle B (1987): Effect of stimulus intensity variation on brain-stem auditory evoked potentials: Comparison between neonates and adults. *Electroencephalogr Clin Neurophysiol* 68:231–233.

Corwin JT, Bullock TH, Schweitzer J (1982): The auditory brain stem response in five vertebrate classes. *Electroencephalogr Clin Neurophysiol* 54:629–641.

Courchesne E, Courchesne RY, Hicks G, Lincoln AJ (1985): Functioning of the brain-stem auditory pathway in non-retarded autistic individuals. *Electroencephalogr Clin Neurophysiol* 61:491–501.

Coutin P, Balmaseda A, Miranda J (1987): Further differences between brain-stem auditory potentials evoked by rarefaction and condensation clicks as revealed by vector analysis. *Electroencephalogr Clin Neurophysiol* 66:420–426.

Creel D, Boxer LA, Fauci AS (1983a): Visual and auditory anomalies in Chediak-Higashi syndrome. *Electroencephalogr Clin Neurophysiol* 55:252–257.

Creel D, Conlee JW, Parks TN (1983b): Auditory brainstem anomalies in albino cats. I. Evoked potential studies. *Brain Res* 260:1–9.

Curio G, Oppel F (1988): Intraparenchymatous ponto-mesencephalic field distribution of brain-stem auditory evoked potentials in man. *Electroencephalogr Clin Neurophysiol* 69:259–265.

Daugherty WT, Lederman RJ, Nodar RH, Conomy JP (1983): Hearing loss in multiple sclerosis. *Arch Neurol* 40:33–35.

Davis H (1981): Auditory evoked potentials as a method for assessing hearing impairment. *Trends Neurosci* 4:126–128.

Davis H, Hirsch SK (1979): A slow brain stem response for low-frequency audiometry. *Audiology* 18:445–461.

Davis H, Aminoff MJ, Berg BO (1985): Brain-stem auditory evoked potentials in children with brain-stem or cerebellar dysfunction. *Arch Neurol* 42:156–160.

Decker TN, Howe SW (1981): Auditory tract asymmetry in brainstem electrical responses during binaural stimulation. *J Acoust Soc Am* 69:1084–1090.

Dekaben AS, Sadowsky D (1978): Changes in brain weights during the span of human life: Relation of brain weights to body heights and body weights. *Ann Neurol* 4:345–356.

Deutsch E, Sohmer H, Weidenfeld J, Zelig S, Chowers I (1983): Auditory nerve-brain stem evoked potentials and EEG during severe hypoglycemia. *Electroencephalogr Clin Neurophysiol* 55:714–716.

Dhuna A, Toro C, Torres F, Kennedy WR, Krivit W (1992): Longitudinal neurophysiologic studies in a patient with metachromatic leukodystrophy following bone marrow transplantation. *Arch Neurol* 49:1088–1092.

Dobie RA, Norton SJ (1980): Binaural interaction in human auditory evoked potentials. *Electroencephalogr Clin Neurophysiol* 49:303–313.

Dobie RA, Wilson MJ (1985): Binaural interaction in auditory brain-stem responses: Effects of masking. *Electroencephalogr Clin Neurophysiol* 62:56–64.

Don M, Eggermont JJ (1978): Analysis of the click-evoked brainstem potentials in man using high-pass noise masking. *J Acoust Soc Am* 63:1084–1092.

Don M, Allen AR, Starr A (1977): Effect of click rate on the latency of auditory brain stem responses in humans. *Ann Otol Rhinol Laryngol* 86:186–195.

Donald MW, Bird CE, Lawson JS, Letemendia FJJ, Monga TN, Surridge DHC, Varette-Cerre P, Williams DL, Williams DML, Wilson DL (1981): Delayed auditory brainstem responses in diabetes mellitus. *J Neurol Neurosurg Psychiatry* 44:641–644.

Dorfman LJ, Britt RH, Silverberg GD (1981): Human brainstem auditory evoked potentials during controlled hypothermia and total circulatory arrest. *Neurology* 31 (4, part 2):88–89.

Doyle WJ, Fria TJ (1985): The effects of hypothermia on the latencies of the auditory brain-stem response (ABR) in the rhesus monkey. *Electroencephalogr Clin Neurophysiol* 60:258–266.

Doyle DJ, Hyde ML (1981): Bessel filtering of brainstem auditory evoked potentials. *Electroencephalogr Clin Neurophysiol* 51:446–448.

Doyle DJ, Saad MM, Fria TJ (1983): Maturation of the auditory brain stem response in rhesus monkeys (*Macaca mulatta*). *Electroencephalogr Clin Neurophysiol* 56:210–233.

Drake ME Jr (1988): Brain-stem auditory-evoked potentials in spasmodic torticollis. *Arch Neurol* 45:174–175.

Drummond JC, Todd MM, Sang H (1985): The effect of high dose sodium thiopental on brain stem auditory and median nerve somatosensory evoked responses in humans. *Anesthesiology* 63:249–254.

Durrant JD, Gerich JE, Mitrakou A, Jenssen T, Hyre RJ (1991): Changes in BAEP under hypoglycemia: temperature-related? *Electroencephalogr Clin Neurophysiol* 80(6):547–550.

Ebner A, Dengler R, Meier C (1981): Peripheral and central conduction times in hereditary pressure-sensitive neuropathy. *J Neurol* 226:85–99.

Edwards RM, Buchwald JS, Tanguay PE, Schwafel JA (1982): Sources of variability in auditory brain stem evoked potential measures over time. *Electroencephalogr Clin Neurophysiol* 53:125–132.

Eggermont JJ (1988): On the rate of maturation of sensory evoked potentials. *Electroencephalogr Clin Neurophysiol* 70:293–305.

Eggermont JJ, Don M (1980): Analysis of the click-evoked brainstem potentials in humans using high-pass noise masking. II. Effect of click intensity. *J Acoust Soc Am* 68:1671–1675.

Eggermont JJ, Don M (1986): Mechanisms of central conduction time prolongation in brain-stem auditory evoked potentials. *Arch Neurol* 43:116–120.

Eggermont JJ, Don M, Brackmann DE (1980): Electrocochleography and auditory brainstem electric responses in patients with pontine angle tumors. *Ann Otol Rhinol Laryngol* 89:Suppl 75.

Ehle AL, Stewart RM, Lellelid NA, Leventhal NA (1984): Evoked potentials in Huntington's disease. A comparative and longitudinal study. *Arch Neurol* 41:379–382.

Elberling C (1973): Transitions in cochlear action potentials recorded from the ear canal in man. *Scand Audiol* 2:151–159.

Elberling C (1974): Action potentials along the cochlear partition recorded from the ear canal in man. *Scand Audiol* 3:13–19.

Elberling C (1978): Compound impulse response for the brain stem derived through combinations of cochlear and brainstem recordings. *Scand Audiol* 7:147–157.

Elberling C (1979): Auditory electrophysiology: Spectral analysis of cochlear and brain stem evoked potentials. A comment on: Kevanishvili and Aphonchenko: "Frequency composition of brain stem auditory evoked potentials" (letter). *Scand Audiol* 8:57–64.

Elidan J, Sohmer H, Gafni M, Kahana E (1982): Contribution of changes in click rate and intensity on diagnosis of multiple sclerosis by brainstem auditory evoked potentials. *Acta Neurol Scand* 65:570–585.

Elidan J, Sohmer H, Lev S, Gay I (1984): Short latency vestibular evoked response to acceleration stimuli recorded by skin electrodes. *Ann Otol Rhinol Laryngol* 93:257–261.

Emerson RG, Brooks EB, Parker SW, Chiappa KH (1982): Effects of click polarity on brainstem auditory evoked potentials in normal subjects and patients; unexpected sensitivity of wave V. *Ann NY Acad Sci* 388:710–721.

Epstein CM, Stappenbeck R, Karp HR (1980): Brainstem auditory evoked responses in palatal myoclonus. *Ann Neurol* 7:592.

Fabiani M, Sohmer H, Tait C, Gafni M, Kinarti R (1979): A functional measure of brain activity: Brain stem transmission time. *Electroencephalogr Clin Neurophysiol* 47:483–491.

Facco E, Martini A, Zuccarello M, Agnoletto M, Giron GP (1985): Is the auditory brain-stem response (ABR) effective in the assessment of post-traumatic coma? *Electroencephalogr Clin Neurophysiol* 62:332–227.

Factor SA, Dentinger MP (1987): Early brain-stem auditory evoked responses in vertebrobasilar transient ischemic attacks. *Arch Neurol* 44:544–547.

Ferbert A, Buchner H, Ringelstein EB, Hacke W (1986): Isolated brain-stem death. Case report with demonstration of preserved visual evoked potentials (VEPs). *Electroencephalogr Clin Neurophysiol* 65:157–160.

Ferbert A, Buchner H, Bruckmann H, Zeumer H, Hacke W (1988): Evoked potentials in basilar artery thrombosis: Correlation with clinical and angiographic findings. *Electroencephalogr Clin Neurophysiol* 69:136–147.

Fine EJ, Hallett M (1980): Neurophysiological study of subacute combined degeneration. *J Neurol Sci* 45:331–336.

Fine EJ, Hallett M (1981): Subacute combined degeneration (letter). *Arch Neurol* 38:136.

Finitzo-Hieber T, Freeman FJ, Gerling IJ, Dobson L, Schaefer SD (1982): Auditory brainstem response abnormalities in adductor spasmodic dysphonia. *Am J Otolaryngol* 3:26–30.

Fischer C, Blanc A, Mauguiere F, Courjon J (1981): Apport des potentiels evoques auditifs precoces au diagnostic neurologique. *Rev Neurol* 137:229–240.

Fischer C, Mauguiere F, Echallier JF, Courjon (1982): Contribution of brainstem auditory evoked potentials to diagnosis of tumors and vascular diseases. In: *Clinical Applications of Evoked Potentials in Neurology*, edited by J Courjon, F Mauguiere, and M Revol, pp 177–185. Raven Press, New York.

Fischer C, Joyeux O, Haguenauer JP, Mauguiere F, Schott B (1984): Surdite et acouphenes lors de poussees dans 10 cas de sclerose en plaques. *Rev Neurol* (Paris) 140:117–125.

Fischer C, Bognar L, Turjman F, Lapras C (1995): Auditory evoked potentials in a patient with a unilateral lesion of the inferior colliculus and medial geniculate body. *Electroencephalogr Clin Neurophysiol* 96(3):261–267.

Frank LM, Furgiuele TL, Etheridge JE Jr (1985): Prediction of chronic vegetative state in children using evoked potentials. *Neurology* 35:931–934.

Fujikawa SM, Weber BA (1977): Effects of increased stimulus rate on brainstem electric response (BER) audiometry as a function of age. *J Am Audiol Soc* 3:147–150.

Fujita M, Hosoki M, Miyazaki M (1981): Brainstem auditory evoked responses in spinocerebellar degeneration and Wilson disease. *Ann Neurol* 9:42–47.

Fullerton BC, Levine RA, Hosford-Dunn HL, Kiang NYS (1987): Comparison of cat and human brain-stem auditory evoked potentials. *Electroencephalogr Clin Neurophysiol* 66:547–570.

Furlow TW, Hallenbeck JM, Goodman JC (1980): Adrenergic blocking agents modify the auditory-evoked response in the rat. *Brain Res* 189:269–273.

Gafni M, Sohmer H, Gross S, Weizman Z, Robinson MJ (1980): Analysis of auditory nerve–brainstem responses (ABR) in neonates and very young infants. *Arch Otorhinolaryngol* 229:167–174.

Galambos R, Hecox K (1977): Clinical applications of the brain stem auditory evoked potentials. *Prog Clin Neurophysiol* 2:1–19.

Galbraith GC (1984): Latency compensation analysis of the auditory brain-stem evoked response. *Electroencephalogr Clin Neurophysiol* 58:333–342.

Gandevia SC, Burke D (1990): Projection of thenar muscle afferents to frontal and parietal cortex of human subjects. *Electroencephalogr Clin Neurophysiol* 77(5):353–361.

Ganes T, Lundar T (1988): EEG and evoked potentials in comatose patients with severe brain damage. *Electroencephalogr Clin Neurophysiol* 69:6–13.

Garcia-Larrea L, Betrand O, Artu F, Pernier J, Mauguiere F (1987): Brain-stem monitoring. II. Preterminal BAEP changes observed until brain death in deeply comatose patients. *Electroencephalogr Clin Neurophysiol* 68:446–457.

Garcia-Larrea L, Artru F, Bertrand O, Pernier J, Mauguiere F (1988): Transient drug-induced abolition of BAEPs in coma. *Neurology* 38:1487–1489.

Garcia-Larrea L, Artru F, Bertrand O, Pernier J, Mauguiere F (1992): The combined monitoring of brain stem auditory evoked potentials and intracranial pressure in coma. A study of 57 patients. *J Neurol Neurosurg Psychiatry* 55:792–798.

Garg BP, Markand OM, DeMyer WE (1980): Evoked responses in patients and potential carriers of adrenoleukodystrophy: Implication for carrier detection. *Ann Neurol* 8:219.

Garg BP, Markand ON, Bustion PF (1982): Brainstem auditory evoked responses in hereditary motor-sensory neuropathy: Site of origin of wave II. *Neurology* 32:1017–1019.

Garg BP, Markand ON, DeMyer WE (1983a): Usefulness of BAER studies in the early diagnosis of Pelizaeus-Merzbacher disease. *Neurology* 33:955–956.

Garg BP, Markand OM, DeMyer WE, Warren C Jr (1983b): Evoked response studies in patients with adrenoleukodystrophy and heterozygous relatives. *Arch Neurol* 40:356–359.

Gawel MJ, Das P, Vincent S, Rose FC (1981): Visual and auditory evoked responses in patients with Parkinson's disease. *J Neurol Neurosurg Psychiatry* 44:227–232.

Gerling IJ, Finitzo-Hieber T (1983): Auditory brainstem response with high stimulus rates in normal and patient populations. *Ann Otol Rhinol Laryngol* 92:119–123.

Gilmore RL, Kasarskis EJ, McAllister RG (1985): Verapamil-induced changes in central conduction in patients with multiple sclerosis. *J Neurol Neurosurg Psychiatry* 48:1140–1146.

Gilroy J, Lynn GE (1978): Computerized tomography and auditory-evoked potentials. Use in the diagnosis of olivopontocerebellar degeneration. *Arch Neurol* 35:143–147.

Gilroy J, Lynn GE, Ristow GE, Pellerin RJ (1977): Auditory evoked brain stem potentials in a case of "locked-in" syndrome. *Arch Neurol* 34:492–495.

Glasscock ME, Jackson CG, Josey AF, Dickins JRE, Wiet RJ (1979): Brainstem evoked response audiometry in a clinical practice. *Laryngoscope* 89:1021–1034.

Gledhill RF, DuPont RA, Van der Merwe CA (1987): Phenytoin effect on BAEP. *Neurology* 37:1687–1688.

Goff WR, Allison T, Lyons W, Fisher TC, Conte R (1977): Origins of short latency auditory evoked potentials in man. *Prog Clin Neurophysiol* 2:30–44.

Goitein KJ, Amit Y, Fainmesser P, Sohmer H (1983): Diagnostic and prognostic value of auditory nerve brainstem evoked responses in comatose children. *Crit Care Med* 11:91–94.

Goldie WD, Chiappa KH, Young RR, Brooks EB (1981): Brainstem auditory and short-latency somatosensory evoked responses in brain death. *Neurology* 31:248–256.

Gott PS, Hughes EC (1989): Effect of noise masking on the brain-stem and middle-latency auditory evoked potentials: central and peripheral components. *Electroencephalogr Clin Neurophysiol* 74(2):131–138.

Green JB, McLeod S (1979): Short latency somatosensory evoked potentials in patients with neurological lesions. *Arch Neurol* 36:846–851.

Green JB, Walcoff MR (1982): Evoked potentials in multiple sclerosis. *Arch Neurol* 39:696–697.

Green JB, Price R, Woodbury SG (1980): Short-latency somatosensory evoked potentials in multiple sclerosis. Comparison with auditory and visual evoked potentials. *Arch Neurol* 37:630–633.

Green JB, Walcoff M, Lucke JF (1982): Phenytoin prolongs far-field somatosensory and auditory evoked potentials interpeak latencies. *Neurology* 32:85–88.

Greenberg RP, Becker DP, Miller JD, Mayer DJ (1977): Evaluation of brain function in severe human head trauma with multimodality evoked potentials. Part 2: Localization of brain dysfunction and correlation with posttraumatic neurological conditions. *J Neurosurg* 47:163–177.

Grimes AM, Elks ML, Grunberger G, Pikus AM (1983): Auditory brain-stem responses in adrenomyeloneuropathy. *Arch Neurol* 40:574–576.

Guerit JM, Mahieu P, Houben-Giurgea S, Herbay S (1981): The influence of ototoxic drugs on brainstem auditory evoked potentials in man. *Arch Otorhinolaryngol* 233:189–199.

Gupta PR, Guilleminault C, Dorfman LJ (1981): Brainstem auditory evoked potentials in near-miss sudden infant death syndrome. *J Pediatr* 98:791–794.

Hafner H, Pratt H, Blazer S, Sujov P (1993): Critical ages in brainstem development revealed by neonatal 3-channel Lissajous' trajectory of auditory brainstem evoked potentials. *Hear Res* 66:157–168.

Hafner H, Pratt H, Blazer S, Sujov P (1994): Intra- and extra-uterine development of neonatal 3-channel Lissajous' trajectory of auditory brainstem evoked potentials. *Hear Res* 76:7–15.

Hall JW, Huang-fu M, Gennarelli TA (1982): Auditory function in acute severe head injury. *Laryngoscope* 92:883–890.

Hall JW, Huangfu M, Gennarelli TA, Dolinskas CA, Olson K, Berry GA (1983): Auditory evoked responses, impedance measures, and diagnostic speech audiometry in severe head injury. *Otolaryngol Head Neck Surg* 91: 50–60.

Hammond EJ, Wilder BJ (1982): Short latency auditory and somatosensory evoked potentials in a patient with "locked-in" syndrome. *Clin Electroencephalogr* 13:54–56.

Hammond EJ, Wilder BJ (1983): Evoked potentials in olivopontocerebellar atrophy. *Arch Neurol* 40:366–369.

Hammond SR, Yiannikas C (1987): The relevance of contralateral recordings and patient disability to assessment of brain-stem auditory evoked potential abnormalities in multiple sclerosis. *Arch Neurol* 44:382–387.

Hammond EJ, Wilder BJ, Goodman IJ, Hunter SB (1985): Auditory brain-stem potentials with unilateral pontine hemorrhage. *Arch Neurol* 42:767–768.

Hammond SR, Yiannikas C, Chan YW (1986): A comparison of brainstem auditory evoked responses evoked by rarefaction and condensation stimulation in control subjects and in patients with Wernicke-Korsakoff syndrome and multiple sclerosis. *J Neurol Sci* 74:177–190.

Hansotia PL (1985): Persistent vegetative state. Review and report of electrodiagnostic studies in eight cases. *Arch Neurol* 42:1048–1052.

Hardy RW, Kinney SE, Lueders H, Lesser RP (1982): Preservation of cochlear nerve function with the aid of brain stem auditory evoked potentials. *Neurosurgery* 11:16–19.

Harkins SW, McEvoy TM, Scott ML (1979): Effects of interstimulus interval on latency of the brainstem auditory evoked potential. *Int J Neurosci* 10:7–14.

Hashimoto I (1982): Auditory evoked potentials from the human midbrain: Slow brain stem responses. *Electroencephalogr Clin Neurophysiol* 53:652–657.

Hashimoto I, Ishiyama Y, Tozuka G (1979): Bilaterally recorded brain stem auditory evoked responses. Their asymmetric abnormalities and lesions of the brain stem. *Arch Neurol* 36:161–167.

Hashimoto I, Ishiyama Y, Yoshimoto T, Nemoto S (1981): Brain-stem auditory-evoked potentials recorded directly from human brain-stem and thalamus. *Brain* 104:841–859.

Hausler R, Levine RA (1980): Brain stem auditory evoked potentials are related to interaural time discrimination in patients with multiple sclerosis. *Brain Res* 191:589–594.

Hebert R, Laureau E, Vanasse M, Richard JE, Morissette J, Glorieux J, Desjardins M, Letarte J, Dussault JH (1986): Auditory brainstem response (ABR) audiometry in congenitally hypothyroid children under early replacement therapy. *Pediatr Res* 20:570–573.

Hecox K (1975): Electrophysiological correlates of human auditory development. In: *Infant Perception: From Sensation to Cognition, Vol II: Perception of Space, Speech and Sound,* edited by LB Cohen and P Salapatek, pp 151–191. Academic Press, New York.

Hecox KE, Cone B (1981): Prognostic importance of brainstem auditory evoked responses after asphyxia. *Neurology* 31:1429–1433.

Hecox K, Galambos R (1974): Brain stem auditory evoked responses in human infants and adults. *Arch Otolaryngol* 99:30–33.

Hecox KE, Cone B, Blaw ME (1981): Brainstem auditory evoked response in the diagnosis of pediatric neurologic disease. *Neurology* 31:832–840.

Hellekson C, Allen A, Greeley H, Emery S, Reeves A (1979): Comparison of interwave latencies of brain stem auditory evoked responses in narcoleptics, primary insomniacs and normal controls. *Electroencephalogr Clin Neurophysiol* 47:742–744.

Henderson-Smart DJ, Pettigrew AG, Campbell DJ (1983): Clinical apnea and brain-stem neural function in preterm infants. *N Engl J Med* 308:353–357.

Herskey LA, Gado MH, Trotter JL (1979): Computerized tomography in the diagnostic evaluation of multiple sclerosis. *Ann Neurol* 5:32–39.

Hicks GE (1980): Auditory brainstem response. Sensory assessment by bone conduction masking. *Arch Otolaryngol* 106:392–395.

Hinman CL, Buchwald JS (1983): Depth evoked potential and single unit correlates of vertex midlatency auditory evoked responses. *Brain Res* 264:57–67.

Hirose G, Kitagawa Y, Chujo T, Oda R, Kataoka S, Takado M (1986): Acute effects of phenytoin on brainstem auditory evoked potentials: Clinical and experimental study. *Neurology* 36:1521–1524.

Hopf HC, Maurer K (1983): Wave I of early evoked potentials in multiple sclerosis. *Electroencephalogr Clin Neurophysiol* 56:31–37.

Hosford-Dunn H, Mendelson T, Salamy A (1981): Binaural interactions in the short-latency evoked potentials of neonates. *Audiology* 20:394–408.

House JW, Brackmann DE (1979): Brainstem audiometry in neurotologic diagnosis. *Arch Otolaryngol* 105:305–309.

House JW, Waluch V, Jackler RK (1986): Magnetic resonance imaging in acoustic neuroma diagnosis. *Ann Otol Rhinol Laryngol* 95:16–20.

Howard JE, Dorfman LJ (1986): Evoked potentials in hysteria and malingering. *J Clin Neurophysiol* 3:39–49.

Huang C-M (1980): A comparative study of the brain stem auditory responses in mammals. *Brain Res* 184:215–219.

Huang C-M, Buchwald JS (1977): Interpretation of the vertex short-latency response: A study of single neurons in the brain stem. *Brain Res* 137:291–303.

Huang C-M, Buchwald JS (1978): Factors that affect the amplitudes and latencies of the vertex short latency acoustic responses in the cat. *Electroencephalogr Clin Neurophysiol* 44:179–186.

Hughes JR, Fino J (1980): Usefulness of piezoelectric earphones in recording the brainstem auditory evoked potentials: A new early deflection. *Electroencephalogr Clin Neurophysiol* 48:357–360.

Hutchinson JC, Klodd DA (1982): Electrophysiologic analysis of auditory, vestibular and brain stem function in chronic renal failure. *Laryngoscope* 92:833–843.

Hutchinson M, Blandford S, Glynn D, Martin EA (1984): Clinical correlates of abnormal brain-stem auditory evoked responses in multiple sclerosis. *Acta Neurol Scand* 69:90–95.

Hyde ML, Blair RL (1981): The auditory brainstem response in neuro-otology: Perspectives and problems. *J Otolaryngol* 10:117–125.

Hyde ML, Stephens SDG, Thornton ARD (1976): Stimulus repetition rate and the early brainstem responses. *Br J Audiol* 10:41–50.

Ingram DA, Traub M, Kopelman PG, Summers BA, Swash M (1986): Brain-stem auditory evoked responses in diagnosis of central pontine myelinolysis. *J Neurol* 233:23–24.

Ino T, Mizoi K (1980): Vector analysis of auditory brainstem responses (BSR) in human beings. *Arch Otorhinolaryngol* 226:55–62.

Iragui VJ, Wiederholt WC, Romine JS (1986): Evoked potentials in trigeminal neuralgia associated with multiple sclerosis. *Arch Neurol* 43:444–446.

Iragui VJ, Kalmin J, Thal LJ, Grant I (1994) Neurologic dysfunction in asymptomatic HIV-1 infected man. Evidence from evoked potentials. *Electroenceph Clin Neurophysiol* 92(1):1-10.

Jabbari B, Marsh EE, Gunderson CH (1982a): The site of the lesion in acute deafness of multiple sclerosis—contribution of the brain stem auditory evoked potential test. *Clin Electroencephalogr* 13:241–244.

Jabbari B, Schwartz D, Chikarmane A, Fadden D (1982b): Somatosensory and brainstem evoked response abnormalities in a family with Freidreich's ataxia. *Electroencephalogr Clin Neurophysiol* 53:24P.

Jabbari B, Schwartz DM, Fadden DM (1982c): Far-field brain stem auditory and somatosensory evoked potential findings in palatal myoclonus. *Electroencephalogr Clin Neurophysiol* 53:93P.

Jabbari B, Schwartz DM, MacNeil DM, Coker SB (1983): Early abnormalities of brainstem auditory evoked potentials in Friedreich's ataxia: Evidence of primary brainstem dysfunction. *Neurology (Cleveland)* 33:1071–1074.

Jacobson GP, Newman CW (1989): Absence of rate-dependent BAEP P5 latency changes in patients with definite multiple sclerosis: Possible physiological mechanisms. *Electroencephalogr Clin Neurophysiol* 74:19–23.

Jerger J, Hall J (1980): Effects of age and sex on auditory brainstem response. *Arch Otolaryngol* 106:387–391.

Jerger J, Mauldin L (1978): Prediction of sensorineural hearing level from the brain stem evoked response. *Arch Otolaryngol* 104:456–461.

Jerger J, Neely JG, Jerger S (1980): Speech, impedance and auditory brainstem response audiometry in brainstem tumors. *Arch Otolaryngol* 106:218–233.

Jewett DL (1970): Volume-conducted potentials in response to auditory stimuli as detected by averaging in the cat. *Electroencephalogr Clin Neurophysiol* 28:609–618.

Jewett DL, Romano MN, Williston JS (1970): Human auditory evoked potentials: Possible brain stem components detected on the scalp. *Science* 167:1517–1518.

Kaga K, Kitazumi E, Kodama K (1979): Auditory brainstem responses of kernicterus infants. *Int J Pediatr* 1:255–264.

Kaminer M, Pratt H (1987): Three-channel Lissajous' trajectory of auditory brain-stem potentials evoked by specific frequency bands (derived responses). *Electroencephalogr Clin Neurophysiol* 66:167–174.

Karmel BZ, Gardner JM, Zappulla RA, Magnano CL, Brown EG (1988): Brain-stem auditory evoked responses as indicators of early brain insult. *Electroencephalogr Clin Neurophysiol* 71:429–442.

Karnaze DS, Marshall LF, McCarthy CS, Klauber MR, Bickford RG (1982): Localizing and prognostic value of auditory evoked responses in coma after closed head injury. *Neurology* 32:299–302.

Karnaze DS, Gott P, Mitchell F, Loftin J (1984): Brainstem auditory evoked potentials are normal in idiopathic sleep apnea. *Ann Neurol* 15:406.

Katayama A (1985): Postnatal development of auditory function in the chicken revealed by auditory brain-stem responses (ABRs). *Electroencephalogr Clin Neurophysiol* 62:388–398.

Kayamori R, Dickins S, Yamada T, Kimura J (1984): Brainstem auditory evoked potential and blink reflex in multiple sclerosis. *Neurology* 34:1318–1323.

Ken-Dror A, Pratt H, Zelter M, Sujov P, Katzir J, Benderley A (1987): Auditory brain-stem evoked potentials to clicks at different presentation rates: Estimating maturation of pre-term and full-term neonates. *Electroencephalogr Clin Neurophysiol* 68:209–218.

Kevanishvili ZS (1980): Sources of the human brainstem auditory evoked potential. *Scand Audiol* 9:75–82.

Kevanishvili ZS, Aphonchenko V (1979): Frequency composition of brain-stem auditory evoked potentials. *Scand Audiol* 8:51–55.

Khoshbin S, Hallett M (1981): Multimodality evoked potentials and blink reflex in multiple sclerosis. *Neurology* 31:138–144.

Kiang NY-S (1961): The use of computers in studies of auditory neurophysiology. *Trans Am Acad Ophthalmol Otolaryngol* 65:735–747.

Kiang NY-S, Watanabe T, Thomas EC, Clark LF (1965): *Discharge Patterns of Single Fibers in the Cat's Auditory Nerve*, Research Monograph 35. M.I.T. Press, Cambridge, Massachusetts.

Kinarti R, Sohmer H (1982): Analysis of auditory brain stem response sources along the basilar membrane to low-frequency filtered clicks. *Isr J Med Sci* 18:93–98.

Kjaer M (1980a): Variations of brain stem auditory evoked potentials correlated to duration and severity of multiple sclerosis. *Acta Neurol Scand* 61:157–166.

Kjaer M (1980b): Localizing brain stem lesions with brain stem auditory evoked potentials. *Acta Neurol Scand* 61:265–274.

Kjaer M (1980c): Brain stem auditory and visual evoked potentials in multiple sclerosis. *Acta Neurol Scand* 62:14–19.

Kjaer M (1980d): Recognizability of brain stem auditory evoked potential components. *Acta Neurol Scand* 62:20–33.

Klug N (1982): Brainstem auditory evoked potentials in syndromes of decerebration, the bulbar syndrome and in central death. *J Neurol* 227:219–228.

Klug N, Csecsei G (1985): Brainstem acoustic evoked potentials in the acute midbrain syndrome and in central death. In: *Evoked Potentials. Neurophysiological and Clinical Aspects*, edited by C Morocutti and PA Rizzo, pp 203–210. Elsevier, Amsterdam.

Koffler B, Oberascher G, Pommer B (1984): Brain-stem involvement in multiple sclerosis: A comparison between brain-stem auditory evoked potentials and the acoustic stapedius reflex. *Neurology* 231:145–147.

Komsuoglu SS, Mehta R, Jones LA, Harding GFA (1985): Brainstem auditory evoked potentials in chronic renal failure and maintenance hemodialysis. *Neurology* 35:419–423.

Kotagal S, Rosenberg C, Rudd D, Dunkle LM, Horenstein S (1981): Auditory evoked potentials in bacterial meningitis. *Arch Neurol* 38:693–695.

Kovala T, Tolonen U, Pyhtinen J (1990): Correlation of tibial nerve SEPs with the development of seizures in patients with supratentorial cerebral infarcts. *Electroencephalogr Clin Neurophysiol* 77(5):347–342.

Kovnar EH, Kun LE, Tate J, McHaney VA (1986a): Brainstem auditory evoked responses in children with brainstem glioma. *Ann Neurol* 20:399.

Kovnar EH, Horowitz ME, Tate J, McHaney VA (1986b): Brainstem auditory evoked responses (BAER), audiometry, and ototoxicity in children receiving cisplatin. *Ann Neurol* 20:399.

Kraus N, Ozdam O, Heydemann PT, Stein L, Reed NL (1984): Auditory brain-stem responses in hydrocephalic patients. *Electroencephalogr Clin Neurophysiol* 59:310–317.

Krumholz A, Weiss HD, Goldstein PJ, Harris KC (1981): Evoked responses in vitamin B-12 deficiency. *Ann Neurol* 9:407–409.

Krumholz A, Singer H, Niedermeyer E, Burnite R, Harris K (1983): Electrophysiological studies in Tourette's Syndrome. *Ann Neurol* 14:638–641.

Krumholz A, Felix JK, Goldstein PJ, McKenzie E (1985): Maturation of the brain-stem auditory evoked potential in premature infants. *Electroencephalogr Clin Neurophysiol* 62:124–134.

Kurtzke JF (1970): Clinical manifestations of multiple sclerosis. In: *Handbook of Clinical Neurology, Vol 9: Multiple Sclerosis and Other Demyelinating Diseases,* edited by PJ Vinken and GW Bruyn, pp 161–216. American Elsevier, New York.

Lacey DJ, Terplan K (1984): Correlating auditory evoked and brainstem histologic abnormalities in infantile Gaucher's disease. *Neurology* 34:539–541.

Lacquanti F, Benna P, Gilli M, Troni W, Bergamasco B (1979): Brain stem auditory evoked potentials and blink reflex in quiescent multiple sclerosis. *Electroencephalogr Clin Neurophysiol* 47:607–610.

Lanska DJ, Lanska MJ, Mendez MF (1987): Brainstem auditory halucinosis. *Neurology* 37:1685.

Lasky RE (1984): A developmental study on the effects of stimulus rate on the auditory evoked brain-stem response. *Electroencephalogr Clin Neurophysiol* 59:411–419.

Lasky RE, Rupert A, Waller M (1987): Reproducibility of auditory brain-stem evoked responses as a function of the stimulus, scorer and subject. *Electroencephalogr Clin Neurophysiol* 68:45–57.

Laureau E, Hebert R, Vanasse M, Letarte J, Glorieux J, Desjardins M, Dussault JH (1987): Somatosensory evoked potentials and auditory brain-stem responses in congenital hypothyroidism. II. A cross-sectional study in childhood. Correlations with hormonal levels and developmental quotients. *Electroencephalogr Clin Neurophysiol* 67:521–530.

Lederman RJ, Nodar RH, Conomy JP, Daugherty WT (1978): Hearing loss in multiple sclerosis. *Neurology* 28:406.

Lee JA, Schoener EP, Nielsen DW, Kelly AR, Lin W-N, Berman RG (1990): Alcohol and the auditory brain-stem response, brain temperature, and blood alcohol curves: explanation of a paradox. *Electroencephalogr Clin Neurophysiol* 77(5):362–376.

Lee SI, Park TS, Dalmas AM (1985): Brainstem auditory evoked potentials in Arnold-Chiari malformation. *Electroencephalogr Clin Neurophysiol* 61:20–21P.

Legatt AD, Pedley TA, Emerson RG, Stein BM, Abramson M (1988): Normal brain-stem auditory evoked potentials with abnormal latency-intensity studies in patients with acoustic neuromas. *Arch Neurol* 45:1326–1330.

Lev A, Sohmer H (1972): Sources of averaged neural responses recorded in animal and human subjects during cochlear audiometry (electro-cochleogram). *Arch Klin Exp Ohr-Nas-u Kehlk Heilk* 201:79–90.

Levine RA (1981): Binaural interaction in brain stem potentials of human subjects. *Ann Neurol* 9:384–393.

Levine RA, McGaffigan PM (1983): Right-left asymmetries in the human brain stem auditory evoked potentials. *Electroencephalogr Clin Neurophysiol* 55:532–537.

Levine RA, Gardner JC, Fullerton BC, Stufflebeam SM, Carlisle EW, Furst M, Rosen BR, Kiang NY (1993a): Effects of multiple sclerosis brainstem lesions on sound lateralization and brainstem auditory evoked potentials. *Hear Res.* 68(1):73–88.

Levine RA, Gardner JC, Stufflebeam SM, Fullerton BC, Carlisle EW, Furst M, Rosen BR, Kiang NYS (1993b): Binaural auditory processing in multiple sclerosis subjects. *Hear Res* 68:59–72.

Le Zak RJ, Selhub B (1966): On hearing in multiple sclerosis. *Ann Otol Rhinol Laryngol* 1102–1110.

Long KJ, Allen N (1984): Abnormal brain-stem auditory evoked potentials following Ondine's curse. *Arch Neurol* 41:1109–1110.

Lott IT, McPherson DL, Starr A (1986): Cerebral cortical contributions to sensory evoked potentials: Hydranencephaly. 64:218–223.

Lueders H, Orlowski JP, Dinner DS, Lesser RP, Klem GH (1984): Far-field auditory evoked potentials in near-miss sudden infant death syndrome. *Arch Neurol* 41:615–617.

Lumsden CE (1970): The neuropathology of multiple sclerosis. In: *Handbook of Clinical Neurophysiology, Vol 9,* pp 175–234. North-Holland, Amsterdam.

Lutschg J, Pfenninger J, Ludin HP, Vassella F (1983): BAEPs and early SEPs in neurointensively treated comatose children. *Am J Dis Child* 137:421–426.

Lynn GE, Gilroy J, Taylor PC, Leiser RP (1981): Binaural masking-level differences in neurological disorders. *Arch Otolaryngol* 107:357–362.

MacDermot KD, Nelson W, Reichert CM, Schulman JD (1980): Attempts at use of strychnine sulfate in the treatment of nonketotic hyperglycinemia. *Pediatrics* 65:61–64.

Machado C, Valdes P, Garcia-Tigera J, Virues T, Biscay R, Miranda J, Coutin P, Roman J, Garcia O (1991): Brainstem auditory evoked potentials and brain death. *Electroencephalogr Clin Neurophysiol* 80:392–398.

Majnemer A, Rosenblatt B, Watters G, Andermann F (1986): Giant axonal neuropathy: Central abnormalities demonstrated by evoked potentials. 19:394–396.

Markand ON, Ochs R, Worth RM, DeMyer WE (1980): Brainstem auditory evoked potentials in chronic degenerative central nervous system disorders. In: *Evoked Potentials,* edited by C Barber, pp 367–375. University Park Press, Baltimore.

Markand ON, Garg BP, Brandt IK (1982a): Nonketotic hyperglycinemia: Electroencephalographic and evoked potential abnormalities. *Neurology* 32:151–156.

Markand ON, Garg BP, DeMyer WE, Warren C, Worth RM (1982b): Brain stem auditory, visual and somatosensory evoked potentials in leukodystrophies. *Electroencephalogr Clin Neurophysiol* 54:39–48.

Markand ON, Lee BI, Warren C, Stoelting RK, King RD, Brown JW, Mahomed Y (1987): Effects of hypothermia on brainstem auditory evoked potentials in humans. *Ann Neurol* 22:507–513.

Marsh RR, Yamane H, Potsic WP (1984): Auditory brain-stem response and temperature relationship in the guinea pig. *Electroencephalogr Clin Neurophysiol* 57:289–293.

Marshall NK, Donchin E (1981): Circadian variation in the latency of brainstem responses and its relation to body temperature. *Science* 212:356–358.

Marshall RE, Reichert TJ, Kerley SM, Davis H (1980): Auditory function in newborn intensive care unit patients revealed by auditory brain stem potentials. *J Pediatr* 96:731–735.

Martin MR (1982): Baclofen and the brain stem auditory evoked potential. *Exp Neurol* 76:675–680.

Martin MR, Penix LP (1983): Comparison of the effects of bicuculline and strychnine on brain stem auditory evoked potentials in the cat. *Br J Pharmacol* 78:75–77.

Martin WH, Pratt H, Bleich N (1986): Three-channel Lissajous' trajectory of human auditory brain-stem evoked potentials. II. Effects of click intensity. *Electroencephalogr Clin Neurophysiol* 63:54–61.   •

Martini A, Fedele D, Comacchio F, Cardone C, Bellavere F, Crepaldi G (1985): Auditory brainstem evoked responses in the clinical evaluation of diabetic encephalopathy. In: *Evoked Potentials. Neurophysiological and Clinical Aspects,* edited by C Morocutti and PA Rizzo, pp 231–236. Elsevier, Amsterdam.

Matthews WB, Wattam-Bell JRB, Pountney E (1982): Evoked potentials in the diagnosis of multiple sclerosis. *J Neurol Neurosurg Psychiatry* 45:303–307.

Matheson JK, Harrington H, Hallett M (1983): Abnormalities of somatosensory, visual and brain-stem auditory evoked potentials in amyotrophic lateral sclerosis. *Muscle Nerve* 6:529.

Matheson JK, Harrington HJ, Hallett M (1986): Abnormalities of multimodality evoked potentials in amyotrophic lateral sclerosis. *Arch Neurol* 43:338–340.

Mauldin L, Jerger J (1979): Auditory brain stem evoked responses to bone-conducted signals. *Arch Otolaryngol* 105:656–661.

Maurer K (1985): Uncertainties of topodiagnosis of auditory nerve and brain-stem auditory evoked potentials due to rarefaction and condensation stimuli. *Electroencephalogr Clin Neurophysiol* 62:135–140.

Maurer K, Mika H (1983): Early potentials (EAEPs) in the rabbit. Normative data and effects of lesions in the cerebello-pontine angle. *Electroencephalogr Clin Neurophysiol* 55:586–593.

Maurer K, Marneros A, Schafer E, Leitner H (1979): Early auditory evoked potentials (EAEP) in vertebral basilar insufficiency. *Arch Psychiat Nervenkr* 227:367–376.

Maurer K, Schafer E, Hopf HC, Leitner H (1980a): The location by early auditory evoked potentials (EAEP) of acoustic nerve and brainstem demyelination in multiple sclerosis (MS). *J Neurol* 223:43–58.

Maurer K, Schafer E, Leitner H (1980b): The effect of varying stimulus polarity (rarefaction vs. condensation) on early auditory evoked potentials. *Electroencephalogr Clin Neurophysiol* 50:332–334.

Maurer K, Geyer D, Mika H, Hopf HC (1981): Abnormal wave I of early auditory evoked potentials in multiple sclerosis. *Electroencephalogr Clin Neurophysiol* 52:S15.

Maurer K, Strumpel D, Wende S (1982): Acoustic tumour detection with early auditory evoked potentials and neuroradiological methods. *J Neurol* 227:177–185.

McClelland RJ, McCrea RS (1979): Intersubject variability of the early auditory-evoked brain stem potentials. *Audiologie* 18:462–471.

McGee TJ, Clemis JD (1982): Effects of conductive hearing loss on auditory brainstem response. *Ann Otol Rhinol Laryngol* 91:304–309.

McPherson DL, Amlie R, Foltz E (1985): Auditory brain-stem response in infant hydrocephalus. *Child's Nerv Sys* 1:70–76.

Metrick SA, Brenner RP (1982): Abnormal brainstem auditory evoked potentials in chronic paint sniffers. *Ann Neurol* 12:553–556.

Michalewski HJ, Thompson LW, Patterson JV, Bowman TE, Litzelman D (1980): Sex differences in the amplitudes and latencies of the human auditory brain stem potential. *Electroencephalogr Clin Neurophysiol* 48:351–356.

Mitchell C, Phillips DS, Trune DR (1989): Variables affecting the auditory brainstem response: Audiogram, age, gender and head size. *Hearing Res* 40:75–86.

Mizrahi EM, Maulsby RL, Frost JD (1983): Improved wave V resolution by dual-channel brain stem auditory evoked potential recording. *Electroencephalogr Clin Neurophysiol* 55:105–107.

Mochizuki Y, Go T, Ohkubo H, Tatara T, Motomura T (1982): Developmental changes of brainstem auditory evoked potentials (BAEPs) in normal human subjects from infants to young adults. *Brain Dev* 4:127–136.

Mogensen F, Kristensen O (1979): Auditory double click evoked potentials in multiple sclerosis. *Acta Neurol Scand* 59:96–107.

Mokotoff B, Schulman-Galambos C, Galambos R (1977): Brain stem auditory evoked responses in children. *Arch Otolaryngol* 103:38–43.

Moller AR (1980): A digital filter for brain stem evoked response. *Am J Otolaryngol* 1:372–377.

Moller AR (1988): Use of zero-phase digital filters to enhance brain-stem auditory evoked potentials (BAEPs). *Electroencephalogr Clin Neurophysiol* 71:26–232.

Moller AR, Burgess J (1986): Neural generators of the brain-stem auditory evoked potentials (BAEPs) in the rhesus monkey. *Electroencephalogr Clin Neurophysiol* 65:361–372.

Moller AR, Jannetta PJ (1982a): Evoked potentials from the inferior colliculus in man. *Electroencephalogr Clin Neurophysiol* 53:612–620.

Moller AR, Jannetta PJ (1982b): Auditory evoked potentials recorded intracranially from the brain stem in man. *Exp Neurol* 78:144–157.

Moller AR, Jannetta PJ (1983): Interpretation of brainstem auditory evoked potentials: Results from intracranial recordings in humans. *Scand Audiol* 12:125–133.

Moller AR, Jannetta P, Bennett M, Moller MB (1981a): Intracranially recorded responses from the human auditory nerve: New insights into the origin of brain stem evoked potentials (BSEPs). *Electroencephalogr Clin Neurophysiol* 52:18–27.

Moller AR, Jannetta PJ, Moller MB (1981b): Neural generators of brainstem evoked potentials. Results from human intracranial recordings. *Ann Otol* 90:591–596.

Moller AR, Colletti V, Fiorino FG (1994a): Click-evoked responses from the exposed intracranial portion of the eighth nerve during vestibular nerve section: bipolar and monopolar recordings. *Electroencephalogr Clin Neurophysiol* 92(1):17–29.

Moller AR, Colletti V, Fiorino FG (1994b): Neural conduction velocity of the human auditory nerve: bipolar recordings from the exposed intracranial portion of the eighth nerve during vestibular nerve section. *Electroencephalogr Clin Neurophysiol* 92(4):316–320.

Moller AR, Jannetta PJ, Jho HD (1994c): Click-evoked responses from the cochlear nucleus: a study in human. *Electroencephalogr Clin Neurophysiol* 92(3):215–224.

Moloney JBM, Masterson JG (1982): Detection of adrenoleucodystrophy carriers by means of evoked potentials. *Lancet* October 16:852–853.

Montandon PB (1976): Clinical application of auditory nerve responses recorded from the ear canal. *Acta Otolaryngol* 81:283–290.

Montandon PB, Megill ND, Kahn AR, Peake WT, Kiang NY-S (1975a): Recording auditory-nerve potentials as an office procedure. *Ann Otol* 84:2.

Montandon PB, Shephard NT, Marr EM, Peake WT, Kiang NY-S (1975b): Auditory-nerve potentials from ear canals of patients with otologic problems. *Ann Otol* 84:164.

Morocutti C, Pozzessere G, Floris R, Sancesario G, Argentino C (1985): Brainstem auditory evoked responses in cerebral vascular diseases. In: *Evoked Potentials. Neurophysiological and Clinical Aspects,* edited by C Morocutti and PA Rizzo, pp 211–222. Elsevier, Amsterdam.

Morrison AS, Gibson WPR, Beagley HA (1976): Transtympanic electrocochleography in the diagnosis of retrocochlear tumors. *Clin Otolaryngol* 1:153–157.

Mosko SS, Pierce S, Holowach J, Sassin JF (1981): Normal brain stem auditory evoked potentials recorded in sleep apneics during waking and as a function of arterial oxygen saturation during sleep. *Electroencephalogr Clin Neurophysiol* 51:477–482.

Musiek FE, Geurkink NA (1982): Auditory brain stem response and central auditory test findings for patients with brain stem lesions: A preliminary report. *Laryngoscope* 92:891–900.

Mustafa KY, Aneja IS, Khogali M, Nasreldin A, Arar I (1988): Effect of hyperthermia on brain auditory evoked potentials in the conscious sheep. *Electroencephalogr Clin Neurophysiol* 71:133–141.

Nagao S, Kuyama H, Honma Y, Momma F, Nishiura T, Murota T, Suga M, Tanimoto T, Kawauchi M, Nishimoto A (1987): Prediction and evaluation of brainstem function by auditory brainstem responses in patients with uncal herniation. *Surg Neurol* 27:81–86.

Narayan RK, Greenberg RP, Miller JD, Enas GG, Choi SC, Kishore PRS, Selhorst JB, Lutz HA, Becker DP (1981): Improved confidence of outcome prediction in severe head injury. A comparative analysis of the clinical examination, multimodality evoked potentials, CT scanning, and intracranial pressure. *J Neurosurg* 54:751–762.

Newlon PG, Greenberg RP, Enas GG, Becker DP (1983): Effects of therapeutic pentobarbital coma on multimodality EPs recorded from severely head-injured patients. *Neurosurgery* 12:613–619.

Nightingale S, Schofield IS, Dawes P (1984): Visual, cortical somatosensory and brainstem auditory evoked potentials following incidental irradiation of the rhombencephalon. *J Neurol Neurosurg Psychiatry* 47:91–93.

Nodar RH, Hahn J, Levine HL (1980a): Brain stem auditory evoked potentials in determining site of lesion of brain stem gliomas in children. *Laryngoscope* 90:258–266.

Nodar R, Lonsdale D, Orlowski J (1980b): Abnormal brainstem auditory evoked potentials in infants with threatened sudden infant death syndrome. *Otolaryngol Head Neck Surg* 88:619–621.

Noffsinger D, Olsen W, Carhart R, et al. (1972): Auditory and vestibular aberrations in multiple sclerosis. *Acta Otolaryngol (Stockh)* 303(Suppl):4–63.

Noseworthy JH, Miller J, Murray TJ, Regan D (1981): Auditory brainstem responses in postconcussion syndrome. *Arch Neurol* 38:275–278.

Noseworthy JH, Paty D, Wonnacott T, Feasby T, Ebers G (1983): Multiple sclerosis after age 50. *Neurology* 33:1537–1544.

Nuwer MR, Perlman SL, Packwood JW, Kark RAP (1982): Evoked potential abnormalities in the inherited ataxias: Further results. *Electroencephalogr Clin Neurophysiol* 53:24P.

Nuwer MR, Perlman SL, Packwood JW, Kark RAP (1983): Evoked potential in the various inherited ataxias. *Ann Neurol* 13:20–27.

Nuwer MR, Visscher BR, Packwood JW, Namerow NS (1985): Evoked potential testing in relatives of multiple sclerosis patients. *Ann Neurol* 18:30–34.

Nuwer MR, Packwood JW, Myers LW, Ellison GW (1987): Evoked potentials predict the clinical changes in a multiple sclerosis drug study. *Neurology* 37:1754–1761.

Nuwer MR, Packwood JW, Ellison GW, Myers LW (1988): A parametric scale for BAEP latencies in multiple sclerosis. *Electroencephalogr Clin Neurophysiol* 71:33–39.

Ochs R, Markand OM, DeMyer WE (1979): Brainstem auditory evoked responses in leukodystrophies. *Neurology* 29:1089–1093.

O'Donovan CA, Beagley HA, Shaw M (1980): Latency of brainstem response in children. *Br J Audiol* 14:23–29.

Ogleznev K Ya, Zaretsky AA, Shesterikov SA (1983): Brain stem auditory evoked potentials: Reduction of evaluation errors. *Electroencephalogr Clin Neurophysiol* 55:331–332.

Oh SJ, Kuba T, Soyer A, Choi IS, Bonikowski FP, Vitek J (1981): Lateralization of brainstem lesions by brainstem auditory evoked potentials. *Neurology* 31:14–18.

Orlowski JP, Nodar RH, Lonsdale D (1979): Abnormal brainstem auditory evoked potentials in infants with threatened sudden infant death syndrome. *Cleve Clin Q* 46:77–81.

Ornitz EM, Walter DO (1975): The effect of sound pressure waveform on human brain stem auditory evoked responses. *Brain Res* 92:490–498.

Ornitz EM, Mo A, Olson ST, Walter DO (1980): Influence of click sound pressure direction on brain stem responses in children. *Audiology* 19:245–254.

Osako S, Tokimoto T, Matsuura S (1979): Effects of kanamycin on the auditory evoked responses during postnatal development of the hearing of the rat. *Acta Otolaryngol* 88:359–368.

Ottaviani F, Almadori G, Calderazzo AB, Frenguelli A, Paludetti G (1986): Auditory brain-stem (ABRs) and middle latency auditory responses (MLRs) in the prognosis of severely head-injured patients. *Electroencephalogr Clin Neurophysiol* 65:196–202.

Ozdamar O, Kraus N, Curry F (1982): Auditory brain stem and middle latency responses in a patient with cortical deafness. *Electroencephalogr Clin Neurophysiol* 53:224–230.

Pagano MA, Cahn PE, Garau ML, Mangone CA, Figini HA, Yorio AA, Dellepiane MC, Amores MG, Perez HM, Casiro AD (1992): Brain-stem auditory evoked potentials in human immunodeficiency virus-seropositive patients with and without aquired immunodeficiency syndrome. *Arch Neurol* 49:166–169.

Parker SW, Chiappa KH, Brooks EB (1980): Brainstem auditory evoked responses in patients with acoustic neuromas and cerebello-pontine angle meningiomas. *Neurology* 30:413–414.

Parving A, Elbering C, Smith T (1981): Auditory electrophysiology: Findings in multiple sclerosis. *Audiology* 20:123–142.

Peake WT, Kiang NY-S (1962): Cochlear responses to condensation and rarefaction clicks. *Biophys J* 2:23–34.

Pedersen L, Trojaborg W (1981): Visual, auditory and somatosensory pathway involvement in hereditary cerebellar ataxia, Friedreich's ataxia and familial spastic paraplegia. *Electroencephalogr Clin Neurophysiol* 52:283–297.

Pelosi L, Fels A, Petrillo A, Senatore R, Russo G, Lonegren K, Calace P, Caruso G (1985): Evoked potentials in relation to clinical involvement in Friedreich's ataxia. In: *Evoked Potentials. Neurophysiological and Clinical Aspects,* edited by C Morocutti and PA Rizzo, pp 375–382. Elsevier, Amsterdam.

Phillips KR, Potvin AR, Syndulko K, Cohen SN, Tourtellotte WW, Potvin JH (1983): Multimodality evoked potentials and neurophysiological tests in multiple sclerosis. *Arch Neurol* 40:159–164.

Picton TW, Durieux-Smith A (1988): Auditory evoked potentials in the assessment of hearing. In: *Neurologic Clinics,* Vol 6, No 4, edited by R Gilmore, pp 791–808. W. B. Saunders, Philadelphia.

Picton TW, Hillyard SA (1974): Human auditory evoked potentials. II. Effects of attention. *Electroencephalogr Clin Neurophysiol* 36:191–199.

Picton TW, Hillyard SA, Krausz HI, Galambos R (1974): Human auditory evoked potentials. I. Evaluation of components. *Electroencephalogr Clin Neurophysiol* 36:179–190.

Picton TW, Stapells DR, Campbell KB (1981): Auditory evoked potentials from the human cochlea and brainstem. *J Otolaryngol* 9(Suppl):1–41.

Picton TW, Taylor MJ, Durieux-Smith A, Edwards CG (1986): Brainstem auditory evoked potentials in pediatrics. In: *Electrodiagnosis in Clinical Neurology,* edited by MJ Aminoff, pp 505–534. Churchill Livingstone, New York.

Picton TW, Hunt M, Mowrey R, Rodriguez R, Maru J (1988): Evaluation of brainstem auditory evoked potentials using dynamic time warping. *Electroencephalogr Clin Neurophysiol* 71:212–225.

Pierelli F, Pozzessere G, Bianco F, Floris R, Rizzo PA (1985): Brainstem auditory evoked potentials in neurodegenerative diseases. In: *Evoked Potentials. Neurophysiological and Clinical Aspects,* edited by C Morocutti and PA Rizzo, pp 157–168. Elsevier, Amsterdam.

Plantz RG, Williston JS, Jewett DL (1974): Spatio-temporal distribution of auditory-evoked far field potentials in rat and cat. *Brain Res* 68:55–71.

Pollack MA, Kellaway (1980): Cerebrocortical death vs brain death: Correlation of clinical, EEG and evoked potential studies, abstracted. *Electroencephalogr Clin Neurophysiol* 49:10P.

Polyakov A, Pratt H (1994): Three-channel Lissajous' trajectory of the binaural interaction components in human auditory brain-stem evoked potentials. *Electroencephalogr Clin Neurophysiol* 92(5):396–404.

Prasher DK, Gibson WPR (1980): Brain stem auditory evoked potentials: A comparative study of monaural versus binaural stimulation in the detection of multiple sclerosis. *Electroencephalogr Clin Neurophysiol* 50:247–253.

Prasher DK, Gibson WPR (1981): Phase reversal in brain stem responses: Its use in the detection of asymmetry in the auditory pathways. *Audiology* 20:313–324.

Prasher KD, Sainz M, Gibson WPR, Findley LJ (1982): Binaural voltage summation of brain stem auditory evoked potentials: An adjunct to the diagnostic criteria for multiple sclerosis. *Ann Neurol* 11:86–91.

Pratt H, Bleich N (1982): Auditory brain stem potentials evoked by clicks in notch-filtered masking noise. *Electroencephalogr Clin Neurophysiol* 53:417–426.

Pratt H, Sohmer H (1976): Intensity and rate functions of cochlear and brainstem evoked responses to click stimuli in man. *Arch Otorhinolaryngol* 211:85–92.

Pratt H, Ben-David Y, Peled R, Podoshin L, Scharf B (1981): Auditory brain stem evoked potentials: Clinical promise of increasing stimulus rate. *Electroencephalogr Clin Neurophysiol* 51:80–90.

Pratt H, Bleich N, Martin WH (1985): Three-channel Lissajous' trajectory of human auditory brain-stem evoked potentials. I. Normative measures. *Electroencephalogr Clin Neurophysiol* 61:530–538.

Pratt H, Brodsky G, Goldsher M, Ben-David Y, Harari R, Podoshin L, Eliachar I, Grushka E, Better O, Garty J (1986a): Auditory brain-stem evoked potentials in patients undergoing dialysis. *Electroencephalogr Clin Neurophysiol* 63:18–24.

Pratt H, Bleich N, Martin WH (1986b): Three-channel Lissajous' trajectory of human auditory brain-stem evoked potentials. III. Effects of click rate. *Electroencephalogr Clin Neurophysiol* 63:438–444.

Psatta DM, Matei M (1988): Age-dependent amplitude variation of brain-stem auditory evoked potentials. *Electroencephalogr Clin Neurophysiol* 71:17–26.

Purves SJ, Low MD, Galloway J, Reeves B (1981): A comparison of visual, brainstem auditory, and somatosensory evoked potentials in multiple sclerosis. *Can J Neurol Sci* 8:15–19.

Radtke RA, Erwin A, Erwin CW (1986): Abnormal sensory evoked potentials in amyotrophic lateral sclerosis. *Neurology* 36:796–801.

Ragazzoni A, Amantini A, Rossi L, Pagnini P, Arnetoli G, Marini P, Nencioni C, Versari A, Zappoli R (1982): Brainstem auditory evoked potentials and vertebral-basilar reversible ischemic attacks. In: *Clinical Applications of Evoked Potentials in Neurology,* edited by J Courjon, F Mauguiere, and M Revol, pp 187–194. Raven Press, New York.

Rappaport M, Hall K, Hopkins HK, Belleza T (1981a): Evoked potentials and head injury. 1. Rating of evoked potential abnormality. *Clin Electroencephalogr* 12:154–166.

Rappaport M, Hopkins HK, Hall K, Belleza T (1981b): Evoked potentials and head injury. 2. Clinical Applications. *Clin Electroencephalogr* 12:167–176.

Rappaport M, Maloney JR, Ortega H, et al. (1985): Survival in young children after drowning: Brain evoked potentials as outcome predictors. *Clin Electroencephalogr* 16:183–191.

Richter EA, Norris BA, Fullerton BA, Levine RA, Kiang NY-S (1983): Is there a medial nucleus of the trapezoid body in humans? *Am J Anat* 168:157–166.

Rizzo PA, Pierelli F, Pozzessere G, Verardi S, Casciani CU, Morocutti C (1982): Pattern visual evoked potentials and brainstem auditory evoked responses in uremic patients. *Acta Neurol Belg* 82:72–79.

Roberts JL, Davis H, Phon GL, Reichert TJ, Sturtevant EM, Marshall RE (1982): Auditory brainstem responses in preterm neonates: Maturation and follow-up. *J Pediatr* 101:257–263.

Robinson K, Rudge P (1975): Auditory evoked responses in multiple sclerosis. *Lancet* 1:1164–1166.

Robinson K, Rudge P (1977a): Abnormalities of the auditory evoked potentials in patients with multiple sclerosis. *Brain* 100:19–40.

Robinson K, Rudge P (1977b): The early components of the auditory evoked potential in multiple sclerosis. *Prog Clin Neurophysiol* 2:58–67.

Robinson K, Rudge P (1980): The use of the auditory evoked potential in the diagnosis of multiple sclerosis. *J Neurol Sci* 45:235–244.

Robinson K, Rudge P (1981): Wave form analysis of the brainstem auditory evoked potential. *Electroencephalogr Clin Neurophysiol* 52:583–594.

Robinsin K, Rudge P (1983): The differential diagnosis of cerebello-pontine angle lesions. A multidisciplinary approach with special emphasis on the brainstem auditory evoked potential. *J Neurol Sci* 60:1–21.

Rodin E, Mason K, Perliss R (1980): Investigation of the brainstem auditory evoked potential in patients with severe epilepsy. *Electroencephalogr Clin Neurophysiol* 49:26P.

Rodin E, Chayasirisobhon S, Klutke G (1982): Brainstem auditory evoked potential recordings in patients with severe epilepsy. *Electroencephalogr Clin Neurophysiol* 53:25P.

Ropper AH (1983): The CNS in Guillain-Barré syndrome. *Arch Neurol* 40:397–398.

Ropper AH, Chiappa KH (1986): Evoked potentials in Guillain-Barré syndrome. *Neurology* 36:587–590.

Ropper AH, Marmarou A (1984): Mechanism of pseudotumor in Guillain-Barré syndrome. *Arch Neurol* 41:259–261.

Ropper AH, Miett T, Chiappa KH (1982): Absence of evoked potential abnormalities in acute transverse myelopathy. *Neurology* 32:80–82.

Ropper AH, Miller DC (1985): Acute traumatic midbrain hemorrhage. *Ann Neurol* 18:80–86.

Ropper AH, Shafran B (1984): Brain edema after stroke. Clinical syndrome and intracranial pressure. *Arch Neurol* 41:26–29.

Rosenberg C, Wogensen K, Starr A (1984): Auditory brain-stem and middle- and long-latency evoked potentials in coma. *Arch Neurol* 41:835–838.

Rosenhamer HJ (1977): Observations on electric brain-stem responses in retrocochlear hearing loss. *Scand Audiol* 6:179–196.

Rosenhamer HJ, Lindstrom B, Lundborg T (1980): On the use of click-evoked electric brainstem response in audiologic diagnosis. II. The influence of sex and age upon the normal response. *Scand Audiol* 9:93–100.

Rosenhamer HJ, Lindstrom B, Lundborg T (1981): On the use of click-evoked electric brainstem responses in audiological diagnosis. III. Latencies in cochlear hearing loss. *Scand Audiol* 10:3–11.

Rossi GT, Britt RH (1980): Neural generators of brainstem auditory evoked responses. Part II: Electrode recording studies. *Soc Neurosci Abstr* 6:595.

Rossi GT, Britt RH (1984): Effects of hypothermia on the cat brain-stem auditory evoked response. *Electroencephalogr Clin Neurophysiol* 57:143–155.

Rossi L, Amantini A, Bindi A, Pagnini P, Arnetoli G, Zappoli R (1983): Electrophysiological investigations of the brainstem in the vertebrobasilar reversible attacks. *Eur Neurol* 22:371–379.

Rossini PM, Kula RW, House WJ, Cracco RQ (1982): Alteration of brain stem auditory evoked responses following cardio-respiratory arrest and resuscitation. *Electroencephalogr Clin Neurophysiol* 54:232–234.

Rossini PM, Di Stefano E, Di Paolo B, Albertazzi A (1985): Multimodal evoked potentials in patients with chronic renal failure: Early diagnosis of central nervous system involvement. In: *Evoked Potentials. Neurophysiological and Clinical Aspects,* edited by C Morocutti and PA Rizzo, pp 391–400. Elsevier, Amsterdam.

Rowe MJ III (1978): Normal variability of the brain-stem auditory evoked response in young and old adult subjects. *Electroencephalogr Clin Neurophysiol* 44:459–470.

Rowe MJ III (1981): The brainstem auditory evoked response in neurological disease: A review. *Ear Hear* 2:41–51.

Rowe MJ III, Carlson C (1980): Brainstem auditory evoked potentials in postconcussion dizziness. *Arch Neurol* 37:679–683.

Rumpl E, Prugger M, Battista HJ, Badry F, Gerstenbrand F, Dienstl F (1988): Short latency somatosensory evoked potentials and brain-stem auditory evoked potentials in coma due to CNS depressant drug poisoning. Preliminary observations. *Electroencephalogr Clin Neurophysiol* 70:482–489.

Rushton JG, Olafson RA (1965): Trigeminal neuralgia associated with multiple sclerosis. *Arch Neurol* 13:383–386.

Salamy A (1981): The theoretical distribution of evoked brainstem activity in preterm, high-risk, and healthy infants. *Child Devel* 52:752–754.

Salamy A (1984): Maturation of the auditory brainstem response from birth through early childhood. *J Clin Neurophysiol* 1(3):293–329.

Salamy A, McKean CM (1976): Postnatal development of human brainstem potentials during the first year of life. *Electroencephalogr Clin Neurophysiol* 40:418–426.

Salamy A, McKean CM, Buda FB (1975): Maturational changes in auditory transmission as reflected in human brain stem potentials. *Brain Res* 96:361–366.

Salamy A, McKean CM, Pettett G, Mendelson T (1978): Auditory brainstem recovery processes from birth to adulthood. *Psychophysiology* 15:214–220.

Salamy A, Mendelson T, Tooley WH, Chaplin ER (1980): Differential development of brainstem potentials in healthy and high-risk infants. *Science* 280:553–555.

Salamy A, Mendelson T, Tooley WH (1982): Developmental profiles for the brainstem auditory evoked potential. *Early Human Devel* 6:331–339.

Salamy A, Eldredge L, Wakeley A (1985): Maturation of contralateral brain-stem responses in preterm infants. *Electroencephalogr Clin Neurophysiol* 62:117–123.

Salomon G, Elberling C (1971): Cochlear nerve potentials recorded from the ear canal in man. *Acta Otolaryngol* 71:319–325.

Salomon G, Elberling C, Tos M (1979): Combined use of electrocochleography and brainstem recording in the diagnosis of acoustic neuromas. *Rev Laryngol* 100:697–707.

Sand T (1986): BAEP subcomponents and waveform—relation to click phase and stimulus rate. *Electroencephalogr Clin Neurophysiol* 65:72–80.

Sand T (1991): Clinical correlates of brain-stem auditory evoked potential variables in multiple sclerosis. Relation to click polarity. *Electroencephalogr Clin Neurophysiol* 80(4):292–297.

Sand T, Sulg I (1984): The influence of click phase and rate upon latencies and latency distributions of the normal brain-stem auditory evoked potentials. *Electroencephalogr Clin Neurophysiol* 57:561–570.

Sanders RA, Duncan PG, McCullough DW (1979): Clinical experience with brain stem audiometry performed under general anesthesia. *J Otolaryngol* 8:24–31.

Sanders RA, Smriga DJ, McCullough DW, Duncan PG (1981): Auditory brainstem responses in patients with global cerebral insults. *J Neurosurg* 55:227–236.

Satya-Murti S, Cacace A (1982): Brainstem auditory evoked potentials in disorders of the primary sensory ganglion. In: *Clinical Applications of Evoked Potentials in Neurology,* edited by J Courjon, F Mauguiere, and M Revol, pp 219–225. Raven Press, New York.

Satya-Murti S, Cacace A, Hanson P (1980): Auditory dysfunction in Friedreich ataxia: Result of spiral ganglion degeneration. *Neurology* 30:1047–1053.

Satya-Murti S, Wolpaw JR, Cacace AT, Schaffer CA (1983): Late auditory evoked potentials can occur without brain stem potentials. *Electroencephalogr Clin Neurophysiol* 56:304–308.

Scaioli V, Savoiardo M, Bussone G, Rezzonico M (1988): Brain-stem auditory evoked potentials (BAEPs) and magnetic resonance imaging (MRI) in a case of facial myokymia. *Electroencephalogr Clin Neurophysiol* 71:153–156.

Scherg M, Speulda EW (1982): Brainstem auditory evoked potentials in the neurologic clinic: Improved stimulation and analysis methods. In: *Clinical Applications of Evoked Potentials in Neurology,* edited by J Courjon, F Mauguiere, and M Revol, pp 211–218. Raven Press, New York.

Scherg M, Von Cramon D (1985): A new interpretation of the generators of BAEP waves I-V: Results of a spatio-temporal dipole model. *Electroencephalogr Clin Neurophysiol* 62:277–289.

Schiff JA, Cracco RQ, Cracco JB (1985): Brainstem auditory evoked potentials in Guillain-Barré syndrome. *Neurology* 35:771–773.

Schmidt-Nielsen K (1975): Scaling in biology: The consequences of size. *J Exp Zool* 194:287–307.

Schoenhuber R, Bortolotti P, Malavasi P, DiDonato G, Gentilini M, Nichelli P, Merli GA, Tonelli L (1985): Brainstem acoustic evoked potentials in 165 patients examined within 48 hours of a minor head injury. In: *Evoked Potentials. Neurophysiological and Clinical Aspects*, edited by C Morocutti and PA Rizzo, pp 237–241. Elsevier, Amsterdam.

Schulman-Galambos C, Galambos R (1975): Brain stem auditory-evoked responses in premature infants. *J Speech Hear Res* 18:456–465.

Schulman-Galambos C, Galambos R (1979): Brain stem evoked response audiometry in newborn hearing screening. *Arch Otolaryngol* 105:86–90.

Schwartz DM, Morris MD, Spydell JD, Brink CT, Grim MA, Schwartz JA (1990): Influence of click polarity on the brain-stem auditory evoked response (BAER) revisited. *Electroencephalogr Clin Neurophysiol* 77(6): 445–457.

Schwent VL, Williston JS, Jewett DL (1980): The effects of ototoxicity on the auditory brain stem response and the scalp-recorded cochlear microphonic in guinea pigs. *Laryngoscope* 90:1350–1359.

Seales DM, Rossiter VS, Weinstein ME (1979): Brainstem auditory evoked responses in patients comatose as a result of blunt head trauma. *J Trauma* 19:347–352.

Seales DM, Torkelson RD, Shuman RM, Rossiter VS, Spencer JD (1981): Abnormal brainstem auditory evoked potentials and neuropathology in "locked-in" syndrome. *Neurology* 31:893–896.

Selters WA, Brackmann DE (1977): Acoustic tumor detection with brain stem electric response audiometry. *Arch Otolaryngol* 103:181–187.

Shanon E, Gold S, Himmelfarb MZ (1981a): Assessment of functional integrity of brain stem auditory pathways by stimulus stress. *Audiology* 20:65–71.

Shanon E, Gold S, Himmelfarb MZ (1981b): Auditory brain stem responses in cerebellopontine angle tumors. *Laryngoscope* 91:254–259.

Shanon E, Himmelfarb MZ, Gold S (1981c): Auditory function in Friedreich's ataxia. Electrophysiological study of a family. *Arch Otolaryngol* 107:254–256.

Shanon E, Himmelfarb MZ, Gold S (1981d): Pontomedullary vs pontomesencephalic transmission time. A diagnostic aid in multiple sclerosis. *Arch Otolaryngol* 107:474–475.

Sharbrough FW, Stockard JJ, Aronson AE (1978): Brainstem auditory-evoked responses in spastic dysphonia. *Trans Am Neurol Assoc* 103:198–201.

Smith LE, Simmons FB (1982): Accuracy of auditory brainstem evoked response with hearing level unknown. *Ann Otol Rhinol Laryngol* 94:266–267.

Smith T, Zeeberg I, Sjo O (1986): Evoked potentials in multiple sclerosis before and after high-dose methylprednisolone infusion. *Eur Neurol* 25:67–73.

Smith T, Jakobsen J, Gaub J, Helweg-Larsen S, Trojaborg W (1988): Clinical and electrophysiological studies of human immunodeficiency virus-seropositive men without AIDS. *Ann Neurol* 23:295–297.

Snyderman NL, Moller M, Johnson JT, Thearle PB (1982): Brainstem evoked potentials in adult sleep apnea. *Ann Otol Rhinol Laryngol* 91:597–598.

Sohmer H, Feinmesser M (1973): Routine use of electrocochleography (cochlear audiometry) on human subjects. *Audiology* 12:167–173.

Sohmer H, Student M (1978): Auditory nerve and brainstem evoked responses in normal, autistic, minimal brain dysfunction and psychomotor retarded children. *Electroencephalogr Clin Neurophysiol* 44:380–388.

Sohmer H, Feinmesser M, Szabo G (1974): Sources of electrocochleographic responses as studied in patients with brain damage. *Electroencephalogr Clin Neurophysiol* 37:663–669.

Sohmer H, Feinmesser M, Bauberger-Tell L, Edelstein E (1977): Cochlear, brain stem and cortical evoked responses in nonorganic hearing loss. *Ann Otol* 86:227–234.

Sohmer H, Gafni M, Chisin R (1978): Auditory nerve and brain stem responses. Comparison in awake and unconscious subjects. *Arch Neurol* 35:228–230.

Sohmer H, Kinarti R, Gafni M (1981): The latency of auditory nerve-brainstem responses in sensorineural hearing loss. *Arch Otorhinolaryngol* 230:189–199.

Sohmer H, Gafni M, Chisin R (1982): Auditory nerve-brain stem potentials in man and cat under hypoxic and hypercapnic conditions. *Electroencephalogr Clin Neurophysiol* 53:506–512.

Squires KC, Chu N-S, Starr A (1978a): Acute effects of alcohol on auditory brainstem potentials in humans. *Science* 201:174–176.

Squires KC, Chu N-S, Starr A (1978b): Auditory brainstem potentials with alcohol. *Electroencephalogr Clin Neurophysiol* 45:577–584.

Squires N, Aine C, Buchwald J, Norman R, Galbraith G (1980): Auditory brain stem response abnormalities in severely and profoundly retarded adults. *Electroencephalogr Clin Neurophysiol* 50:172–185.

Starr A (1976): Auditory brainstem responses in brain death. *Brain* 99:543–554.

Starr A, Achor LJ (1975): Auditory brain stem responses in neurological disease. *Arch Neurol* 32:761–768.

Starr A, Achor LJ (1979): Anatomical and physiological origins of auditory brain stem responses (ABR). In: *Human Evoked Potentials: Applications and Problems*, edited by D Lehmann and E Callaway, pp 415–429. Plenum Press, New York.

Starr A, Hamilton AE (1976): Correlation between confirmed sites of neurologic lesions and abnormalities of far-field auditory brainstem responses. *Electroencephalogr Clin Neurophysiol* 41:595–608.

Starr A, Squires K (1982): Distribution of auditory brain stem potentials over the scalp and nasopharynx in humans. *Ann NY Acad Sci* 388:427–442.

Starr A, Amlie RN, Martin WH, Sanders S (1977): Development of auditory function in newborn infants revealed by auditory brainstem potentials. *Pediatrics* 60:831–839.

Stein LK, Ozdamar O, Schnabel M (1981): Auditory brainstem responses (ABR) with suspected deaf-blind children. *Ear Hear* 2:30–40.

Stern BJ, Krumholz A, Weiss H, et al. (1982): Evaluation of brainstem stroke using brainstem auditory evoked responses. *Stroke* 13:705–711.

Stockard JE, Stockard JJ (1982): Brainstem auditory evoked potentials in normal and otoneurologically impaired newborns and infants. In: *Current Clinical Neurophysiology: Update on EEG and Evoked Potentials,* edited by CE Henry. Symposia Specialists, Miami (*in press*).

Stockard JE, Stockard JJ, Westmoreland BF, Corfits JL (1979): Brainstem auditory-evoked responses: Normal variation as a function of stimulus and subject characteristics. *Arch Neurol* 36:823–831.

Stockard JJ (1982): Brainstem auditory evoked potentials in adult and infant sleep apnea syndromes, including sudden infant death syndrome and near-miss for sudden infant death. *Ann NY Acad Sci* 388:443–465.

Stockard JJ, Hecox K (1981): Brainstem auditory evoked potentials in sudden infant death syndrome (SIDS), "near-miss-for-SIDS," and infant apnea syndromes. *Electroencephalogr Clin Neurophysiol* 51:43P.

Stockard JJ, Rossiter VS (1977): Clinical and pathologic correlates of brain stem auditory response abnormalities. *Neurology* 27:316–325.

Stockard JJ, Sharbrough FW (1980): Unique contributions of short-latency somatosensory evoked potentials in patients with neurological lesions. *Prog Clin Neurophysiol* 7:231–263.

Stockard JJ, Rossiter VS, Jones TA (1976a): Effects of focal brainstem cooling on the far-field acoustic response in the cat: Relevance to response abnormalities in CNS demyelinating disease. *Soc Neurosci Abstr* 2:10.

Stockard JJ, Rossiter VS, Wiederholt WC, Kobayashi RM (1976b): Brain stem auditory-evoked responses in suspected central pontine myelinolysis. *Arch Neurol* 33:726–728.

Stockard JJ, Rossiter VS, Jones TA, Sharbrough FW (1977a): Effects of centrally acting drugs on brainstem auditory responses. *Electroencephalogr Clin Neurophysiol* 43:550–551.

Stockard JJ, Stockard JE, Sharbrough FW (1977b): Detection and localization of occult lesions with brainstem auditory responses. *Mayo Clin Proc* 52:761–769.

Stockard JJ, Sharbrough FW, Tinker JA (1978a): Effects of hypothermia on the human brainstem auditory response. *Ann Neurol* 3:368–370.

Stockard JJ, Stockard JE, Sharbrough FW (1978b): Nonpathologic factors influencing brainstem auditory evoked potentials. *Am J EEG Technol* 18:177–209.

Stockard JJ, Hughes JF, Sharbrough FW (1979): Visually evoked potentials to electronic pattern reversal: Latency variations with gender, age and technical factors. *Am J EEG Technol* 19:171–204.

Stockard JJ, Sharbrough FW, Staats BA, Westbrook PR (1980a): Brain stem auditory evoked potentials (BAEPs) in sleep apnea. *Electroencephalogr Clin Neurophysiol* 50:167P.

Stockard JJ, Stockard JE, Sharbrough FW (1980b): Brainstem auditory evoked potentials in neurology: Methodology, interpretation, clinical application. In: *Electrodiagnosis in Clinical Neurology,* edited by MJ Aminoff, pp 370–413. Churchill Livingstone, New York.

Stone JL, Hughes JR, Kumar A, Meyer D, Subramanian KS, Zalkind MS, Fino J (1986): Electrocochleography recorded non-invasively from the external ear. *Electroencephalogr Clin Neurophysiol* 63:494–496.

Stone JL, Ghaly RF, Hughes JR (1988): Evoked potentials in head injury and states of increased intracranial pressure. *J Clin Neurophysiol* 5:135–160.

Strickbine-Van Reet P, Glaze DG, Hrachovy RA (1984): A preliminary prospective neurophysiologic study of coma in children. *Am J Dis Child* 138:492–495.

Sutton LN, Frewen T, Marsh R, Jaggi J, Bruce DA (1982): The effects of deep barbiturate coma on multimodality evoked potentials. *J Neurosurg* 57:178–185.

Suzuki T, Horiuchi K (1977): Effect of high-pass filter on auditory brain stem responses to tone pips. *Scand Audiol* 6:123–126.

Suzuki T, Kobayashi K, Takagi N (1986): Effects of stimulus repetition rate on slow and fast components of auditory brain-stem responses. *Electroencephalogr Clin Neurophysiol* 65:150–156.

Szelenberger W (1983): Brain stem auditory evoked potentials and personality. *Biol Psychiatry* 18:157–174.

Tackmann W, Ettlin T (1982): Blink reflexes elicited by electrical, acoustic and visual stimuli. II. Their relation to visual-evoked potentials and auditory brain stem evoked potentials in the diagnosis of multiple sclerosis. *Eur Neurol* 21:264–269.

Tackmann W, Strenge H, Barth R, Sojka-Raytscheff A (1980): Evaluation of various brain structures in multiple sclerosis with multimodality evoked potentials, blink reflex and nystagmography. *J Neurol* 224:33–46.

Takiguchi T, Myokai K, Shiode A, Ohba O, Ikeda T, Furumoto F, Kaga K (1979): [ABR under deep hypothermia in open heart surgery.] *Nippon Jibiinkoka Gakkai Kaiho* 82:1403–1407.

Tanguay PE, Edwards RM, Buchwald J, Schwafel J, Allen V (1982): Auditory brainstem evoked responses in autistic children. *Arch Gen Psychiatry* 39:174–180.

Taylor MJ, Houston BD, Lowry NJ (1983): Recovery of auditory brain-stem responses after a severe hypoxic ischemic insult. *N Engl J Med* 309:1169–1170.

Terkildsen K, Osterhammel P (1981): The influence of reference electrode position on recordings of the auditory brainstem responses. *Ear Hear* 2:9–14.

Terkildsen K, Osterhammel P, Huis in't Veld F (1973): Electrocochleography with a far-field technique. *Scand Audiol* 2:141–148.

Theodore WH, Comite F, Sato S, Loriaux L, Cutler G (1983): EEG and evoked potentials in precocious puberty. *Electroencephalogr Clin Neurophysiol* 55:69–72.

Thivierge J, Cote R (1987): Brain-stem auditory evoked response (BAER): Normative study in children and adults. *Electroencephalogr Clin Neurophysiol* 68:479–485.

Thomsen J, Terkildsen K, Osterhammel P (1978): Auditory brain stem responses in patients with acoustic neuromas. *Scand Audiol* 7:179–183.

Thornton ARD, Coleman MJ (1975): The adaptation of cochlear and brainstem auditory evoked potentials in humans. *Electroencephalogr Clin Neurophysiol* 39:399–406.

Thornton C, Catley DM, Jordan C, Royston D, Lehane JR, Jones JG (1981): Enflurane increases the latency of early components of the auditory evoked response in man. *Br J Anaesth* 53:1102–1103.

Tobimatsu S, Fukui R, Kato M, Kobayashi T, Kurowa Y (1985): Multimodality evoked potentials in patients and carriers with adrenoleukodystrophy and adrenomyeloneuropathy. *Electroencephalogr Clin Neurophysiol* 62:18–24.

Tolosa ES, Zeese JA (1979): Brainstem auditory evoked responses in progressive supranuclear palsy. *Ann Neurol* 6:369.

Towle VL, Babikian V, Maselli R, Berstein L, Spire J-P (1985): A comparison of multimodality evoked potentials, computed tomography findings and clinical data in brainstem vascular infarcts. In: *Evoked Potentials. Neurophysiological and Clinical Aspects,* edited by C Morocutti and PA Rizzo, pp 383–390. Elsevier, Amsterdam.

Trojaborg W, Jorgensen EO (1973): Evoked cortical potentials in patients with "isoelectric" EEGs. *Electroencephalogr Clin Neurophysiol* 35:301–309.

Tomasulo RA, Peele PB (1988): A new technique for interpreting the BAER in cochlear disease. *Ann Neurol* 23:204–206.

Tsubokawa T, Nishimoto H, Yamamoto T, Kitamura M, Katayama Y, Moriyasu N (1980): Assessment of brainstem damage by the auditory brainstem responses in acute severe head injury. *J Neurol Neurosurg Psychiatry* 43:1005–1011.

Tsuji S, Muraoka S, Kuroiwa Y, Chen KM, Gajdusek CD (1981): [Auditory brainstem evoked response (ABSR) of Parkinson-dementia complex and amyotrophic lateral sclerosis in Guam and Japan.] *Rinsho Shinkeigaku (Clin Neurol Tokyo)* 21:37–41.

Uziel A, Benezech J (1978): Auditory brainstem responses in comatose patients: Relationship with brain-stem reflexes and levels of coma. *Electroencephalogr Clin Neurophysiol* 45:515–524.

van Buggenhout E, Ketelaer P, Carton H (1982): Success and failure of evoked potentials in detecting clinical and subclinical lesions in multiple sclerosis. *Clin Neurol Neurosurg* 84:3–14.

van Olphen AF, Rodenburg M, Verwey C (1978): Distribution of brain stem responses to acoustic stimuli over the human scalp. *Audiology* 17:511–518.

van Olphen AF, Rodenburg M, Verwey C (1979): Influence of the stimulus repetition rate on the brain-stem-evoked responses in man. *Audiology* 18:388–394.

Velasco M, Velasco F, Almanza X, Coats AC (1982): Subcortical correlates of the auditory brain stem potentials in man: Bipolar EEG and multiple unit activity and electrical stimulation. *Electroencephalogr Clin Neurophysiol* 53:133–142.

Verma NP, Kapen S, King SD, Koshorek GJ (1987): Bimodality electrophysiologic evaluation of brainstem in sleep apnea syndrome. *Neurology* 37:1036–1039.

Wada S-I, Starr A (1983a): Generation of auditory brain stem responses (ABRs). I. Effects of injection of a local anesthetic (procaine HCl) into the trapezoid body of guinea pigs and cat. *Electroencephalogr Clin Neurophysiol* 56:326–339.

Wada S-I, Starr A (1983b): Generation of auditory brain stem responses (ABRs). II. Effects of surgical section of the trapezoid body on the ABR in guinea pigs and cat. *Electroencephalogr Clin Neurophysiol* 56:340–351.

Wada S-I, Starr A (1983c): Generation of auditory brain stem responses (ABRs). III. Effects of lesions of the superior olive, lateral lemniscus and inferior colliculus on the ABR in guinea pig. *Electroencephalogr Clin Neurophysiol* 56:352–366.

Wada S-I, Matsuoka S, Urasaki E-I, Yadomi C (1988): Quantitative analysis of reversible dysfunction of brainstem midline structures caused by disturbance of basilar artery blood flow with the auditory brain-stem responses. *Electroencephalogr Clin Neurophysiol* 69:148–159.

Weber BA, Fujikawa SM (1977): Brainstem evoked response (BER) audiometry at various stimulus presentation rates. *J Am Audiol Soc* 3:59–62.

Westmoreland BF, Sharbrough FW, Stockard JJ, Dale AJD (1983): Brainstem auditory evoked potentials in 20 patients with palatal myoclonus. *Arch Neurol* 40:155–158.

Wiederholt WC, Kobayashi RM, Stockard JJ, Rossiter VS (1977): Central pontine myelinolysis. A clinical reappraisal. *Arch Neurol* 34:220–223.

Wielaard R, Kemp B (1979): Auditory brainstem evoked responses in brainstem compression due to posterior fossa tumors. *Clin Neurol Neurosurg* 81:185–193.

Williston JS, Jewett DL, Martin WH (1981): Planar curve analysis of three-channel auditory brain stem response: A preliminary report. *Brain Res* 223:181–184.

Wong PKH, Bickford RG (1980): Brain stem auditory evoked potentials: The use of noise estimate. *Electroencephalogr Clin Neurophysiol* 50:25–34.

Worthington DW, Peters JF (1980): Quantifiable hearing and no ABR: Paradox or error? *Ear Hear* 1:281–285.

Wrege K, Starr A (1981): Binaural interaction in human auditory brainstem evoked potentials. *Arch Neurol* 38:572–580.

Wulff CH (1985): Evoked potentials in acute transverse myelopathy. *Dan Med Bull* 32:282–287.

Yagi T, Baba S (1983): Evaluation of the brain-stem function by the auditory brain-stem response and the caloric vestibular reaction in comatose patient. *Arch Otorhinolaryngol* 238:33–43.

Yamada T, Dickins S, Arensdorf K, Corbett J, Kimura J (1986): Basilar migraine: Polarity-dependent alteration of brainstem auditory evoked potential. *Neurology* 36:1256–1260.

York DH (1986): Correlation between a unilateral midbrain-pontine lesion and abnormalities of brain-stem auditory evoked potential. *Electroencephalogr Clin Neurophysiol* 65:282–288.

Zanette G, Carteri A, Cusumano S (1990): Reappearance of brain-stem auditory evoked potentials after surgical treatment of a brain-stem hemorrhage: contributions to the question of wave generation. *Electroencephalogr Clin Neurophysiol* 77:140–144.

Zappulla RA, Karmel BA, Greenblatt E (1981): Prediction of cerebellopontine angle tumors based on discriminant analysis of brain stem auditory evoked responses. *Neurosurgery* 9:542–547.

Zappulla RA, Greenblatt E, Karmel BZ (1982): The effects of acoustic neuromas on ipsilateral and contralateral brain stem auditory evoked responses during stimulation of the unaffected ear. *J Otolaryngol* 4:118–122.

Zollner Chr, Karnaze Th, Stange G (1976): Input-output function and adaptation behaviour of the five early potentials registered with the earlobe-vertex pick-up. *Arch Otol Rhino Laryngol* 212:23–33.

Evoked Potentials in Clinical Medicine,
3d ed., edited by Keith H. Chiappa.
Lippincott–Raven Publishers, Philadelphia © 1997.

7

Brain Stem Auditory Evoked Potentials in Pediatrics

Susan R. Levy

Departments of Pediatrics, Neurology, and Child Study Center,
Yale University School of Medicine, New Haven, Connecticut 06510

Brain stem auditory evoked potential monitoring (BAEP) is a neurophysiologic technique that is utilized in the pediatric age group to assess hearing and the integrity of the brain stem auditory pathways. The information the BAEP provides is very useful in this group of patients who may not be able to communicate neurologic symptoms. The study can be used as an adjunct to the clinical examination.

1. SPECIAL METHODOLOGY

1.1. Recording Parameters

The BAEP is generally well-tolerated by infants and children. BAEPs are recorded from surface electrodes placed at the vertex and ipsilateral earlobes or mastoids. In young infants, the vertex electrode is placed in the midline anterior to the anterior fontanelle. The ground electrode is placed on the mid-forehead. Electrodes should be applied with nonirritating tape and saline jelly because of skin sensitivity in this age group. In the older child paste and gauze or collodion can be used and is most helpful in the active child. Paste is usually better tolerated as removal of electrodes is faster and collodion application is lengthy, noisy, and malodorous.

The recording sweep time should be longer (15 to 20 msec) in infants because of the slower response seen in this age group. The low-frequency filter cut-off should be 20 to 30 Hz in infants. In children over 18 months of age a low-frequency cut-off of 100 Hz can be used (Picton et al., 1992).

As in adults, two-channel montages are used and consist of vertex to ipsilateral ear and vertex to contralateral ear. When such a two-channel montage is used, wave IV–V differentiation is improved and it is not necessary to switch electrodes if the child rolls over during the study while asleep.

Normative data exist for the technique of broad band clicks presented through earphones (Eggermont and Salamy, 1988; Zimmerman et al., 1987; Gorga et al., 1989; Jiang et al., 1991b; Picton et al., 1992; Brivio et al., 1993). Infants and children are best tested with a single phase click, usually rarefaction. Very young infants may have a high-frequency hearing loss and latency differences between condensation and rarefaction clicks may distort wave I (Stockard et al., 1979; Stockard and Westmoreland, 1981). The intensity of the click is calibrated in relation to normal hearing levels (NHL) for adults. It is reasonable to use 70 to 75 dB initially and observe the resultant waveforms. The stimulus intensity can be increased in 5-dB increments to obtain well-defined waveforms, although 95 dB NHL should not be exceeded. The BAEP can be recorded in newborns with stimulus intensities as low as 30 dB NHL (Durieux-Smith et al., 1985). Earphones should fit snuggly over the ear with care being taken not to occlude the ear canal. It is not necessary to have an airtight seal, but the click generator should be located directly over the ear canal. In infants it is best to lightly hold the earphone over the ear. White-noise masking of the opposite ear may not be possible in premature and small infants because of the large size of the earphones. In the older infant and child, earphones fit comfortably over the ears and white-noise masking should be administered to the nontested ear.

The infant's response is more sensitive to click frequency than that of the older child or adult. Increasing the repetition rate causes a significant increase in the absolute and interpeak latencies and decrease in amplitude of the waveforms (Stockard et al., 1979; Lasky, 1984; Salamy, 1984; Ken-Dorr et al., 1987; Jiang et al., 1991a).

1.2. Sleep

It is best to test infants and young children in sleep because the BAEP waveform amplitudes are smaller than in adults and sleep reduces muscle artifact. Infants are best tested after a feeding and older infants and children should be tested following a short period of sleep deprivation. After application of the electrodes the infant is left in a dark, quiet room with an adult to fall asleep for the test. Children older than 18 to 24 months may tolerate the procedure if they are comfortable with the environment. If they require sedation for the procedure, chloral hydrate is given orally at a dose of 50 to 75 mg/kg.

2. MATURATIONAL CHANGES AND NORMATIVE DATA

The BAEP has been recorded in the fetus during labor (Staly et al., 1990). Waves I, III, and V have been identified utilizing a recording needle scalp electrode and stimulation through a speaker placed on the maternal abdomen. The waveform morphology, absolute latencies, and interpeak latencies (IPLs) are similar to postnatal recordings.

The BAEP waveform morphology changes as a function of maturation. The newborn BAEP differs from that of the adult. The newborn responses are smaller in amplitude, measuring about one-half the adult size. Wave I may be double peaked and waves III and IV are often absent (Starr et al., 1977). There is a prominent negative wave following wave I. Wave II develops between 3 and 4 months of age (Jacobson, 1985) and wave IV begins to separate from wave V. By the end of the first year of life the morphology of the BAEP is similar to that of the adult.

In general the BAEP latencies decrease and amplitudes increase with advancing age. Table 7–1 represents a compilation of normative data adapted from Eggermont and Salamy (1988) and Picton et al. (1992). Brain stem auditory EPs can be recorded in infants as young as 28 to 30 weeks gestation (Schulman-Galambos and Galambos, 1975; Starr et al., 1977; Lary et al., 1985; Picton et al., 1992). In premature infants the response is recorded after stimulation at high intensity and slow rate. The amplitude of all waveforms, especially wave V, is lower than in full-term infants. The latencies of all waveforms decrease with increasing conceptional age, however, there is a greater change in wave V. The I–V IPL, therefore, also decreases with increasing conceptional age. Between 36 and 40 weeks gestational age the latency of wave I decreases by about 0.1 msec and the latency of wave V decreases by 0.4 msec (Picton et al., 1992). There is a rapid change in the BAEP waveforms within the first hours after birth. Wave I latency decreases significantly in the first hours of life (Yamasaki et al., 1991). The latency of wave I in the full-term infant hours after birth has been reported to be 0.48 msec (Adelman et al., 1990) and 0.8 msec (Picton et al., 1992) greater than that of the adult. Wave I latency reaches adult values between 2 weeks (Adelman et al., 1990; Zimmerman et al., 1987) and 2 months (Picton et al., 1992). The latencies of waves III and V decrease rapidly during the first several months of life and reach adult normal values by 2 to 3 years of age (Salamy, 1984; Picton et al., 1992). At term the I–V IPL is about 5 msec and reaches adult values by 2 to 3 years of age (Salamy, 1984; Lauffer and Wenzel, 1990; Picton et al., 1992; Brivio et al., 1993). The amplitude of the waveforms increases with increasing age, with a marked increase after 6 months of age and maximum values by age 4 to 5 years (Salamy, 1984; Jiang et al., 1993). Amplitudes subsequently decrease to adult values. The BAEP matures to adult patterns by about 3 to 4 years of age. The BAEP waveforms and IPLs of the premature infant are similar to those of full-term infants who have reached the same conceptional age (Gorga et al., 1987; Eggermont, 1992). The absolute latency of waveforms is about 0.3 msec longer (Eggermont and Salamy, 1988) and this latency difference persists for the first 2 years of life. The prolonged waveform latencies are possibly caused by a higher incidence of otitis media in infants born prematurely. Gender does cause differences in the BAEP components, however, it is controversial as to when these differences become significant (Stockard et al., 1979; Allison et al., 1984; Thivierge and Cote, 1990; Brivio et al.,

TABLE 7–1. *Pediatric BAEP normative values*

Age	Latency (msec)			
	I	III	V	I–V
33 weeks preterm	2.57 (0.54)	5.68 (0.75)	8.21 (0.79)	5.64 (0.70)
36 weeks preterm	2.41 (0.38)	5.35 (0.49)	7.83 (0.59)	5.43 (0.55)
40 weeks term	2.00 (0.31)	4.82 (0.44)	7.14 (0.43)	5.14 (0.40)
40 weeks preterm	2.34 (0.44)	5.07 (0.60)	7.54 (0.62)	5.20 (0.60)
3 weeks term	1.80 (0.24)	4.50 (0.46)	6.93 (0.37)	5.13 (0.36)
3 weeks preterm	2.01 (0.24)	4.70 (0.37)	7.07 (0.23)	5.07 (0.33)
6 weeks	1.80 (0.20)	4.40 (0.30)	6.60 (0.30)	4.90 (0.30)
12 weeks	1.70 (0.20)	4.30 (0.30)	6.40 (0.30)	4.70 (0.30)
26 weeks	1.70 (0.20)	4.10 (0.30)	6.20 (0.30)	4.60 (0.30)
52 weeks	1.70 (0.20)	4.00 (0.30)	6.0 (0.30)	4.30 (0.20)
2 years	1.70 (0.20)	3.80 (0.20)	5.70 (0.20)	4.00 (0.20)

Brain stem auditory EP normative values adapted from Eggermont and Salamy (1988) for ages 33 weeks preterm to 3 weeks and from Picton et al. (1992) for ages 6 weeks to 2 years of age. Recording techniques for 33 weeks preterm to 3 weeks included clicks 0.1 msec in duration, stimulation at 60 dB NHL, rate of 15/sec, white-noise masking in contralateral ear, band-pass filtered 100 to 3,000 Hz. Recording parameters for ages 6 weeks to 2 years included stimulation with rarefaction clicks at 70 dB NHL, stimulation rate of 11/sec.

1993). Durieux-Smith et al. (1985) did not observe gender differences in neonates. Gender does not affect wave I but the I–V IPL has been found to be shorter in girls (Allison et al., 1984; Thiveierge and Cote, 1990; Fujita et al., 1991). The amplitude of wave V is larger in females (Thiveierge and Cote, 1990; Sand, 1991).

The neonatal BAEP is distributed differently on the scalp compared to the adult. Wave I is larger when recorded ipsilateral to the ear stimulated in a mastoid to mastoid recording compared to a vertex to mastoid recording (Hecox and Burkard, 1982). Waves III and V are small in a recording between the vertex and the contralateral mastoid, making the response difficult to observe at low intensities. These waves may seem to have opposite polarity to those recorded on an ipsilateral montage. Care should be taken to be certain that the recording montage is correct (Hatanaka et al., 1988; Picton et al., 1992).

3. CLINICAL APPLICATIONS

The BAEP is a useful method of evaluating a variety of pathologic conditions that can damage the brain stem auditory pathway. The BAEP may demonstrate a localized lesion but is not specific for etiology.

3.1. Neurodegenerative Disorders

The BAEP can be used as an extension of the clinical examination to uncover otherwise silent lesions in the brain stem auditory pathways. A variety of neurodegenerative disorders that primarily affect white matter or have extensive brain stem involvement are associated with abnormal BAEPs. The BAEP may be abnormal in a child who is neurologically intact and therefore this study can help in the differential diagnosis.

The BAEP is consistently abnormal in the leukodystrophies. Only early BAEP waves are recorded in children with infantile leukodystrophies such as Pelizaeus–Mertzbacher disease or Krabbe's disease. These severe abnormalities are seen as early as 1 month of age (Garg et al., 1983). Older children with demyelinating diseases, including adrenoleukodystrophy and metachromatic leukodystrophy, have abnormalities of BAEPs including IPL increases or, more commonly, absence of waves III and V (Ochs et al., 1979; Markand et al., 1982).

Metabolic disorders that produce a disruption of the central myelin will also cause abnormalities of the BAEP. These disorders include maple syrup urine disease, pyruvate decarboxylase deficiency, and phenylketonuria (Hecox et al., 1981; Cardona et al., 1991). Markand et al. (1982a) studied four children with nonketotic hyperglycinemia and found well-defined waveforms with prologation of the I–V interval in all. Nine of 13 children studied with mucopolysaccharidoses had abnormal BAEPs (Perretti et al., 1990). Abnormalities included delayed absolute latencies of all the waves, absence of waves III and V and increased IPLs.

Brain stem auditory EPs were found to be abnormal in a significant number of patients with neurodegenerative system disorders, including Friedreich's ataxia, olivopontocerebellar atrophy types I and II, hereditary sensorimotor neuropathy type III, and abetalipoproteinemia. None of the patients had hearing impairment (Rossini and Cracco, 1987). In a study involving patients with hereditary motor and sensory neuropathy types I and II (Scaioli et al., 1992), there was a significant prolongation of wave I latency. The BAEP is helpful in differentiating the hereditary ataxias. The BAEP is normal in disorders such as ataxia telangiectasia. Patients with Freidreich's ataxia exhibit a loss of waveforms that begins early in the course of the disease (Pedersen et al., 1981; DePablos et al., 1991). The BAEP abnormalities reflect the rate and progression of disease (Taylor et al., 1985).

Eight children with familial dysautonomia, an autosomal recessive disorder, had abnormal BAEPs (Lahat et al., 1992). The absolute latencies of waves III and V and the I–III and I–V IPLs were prolonged compared to a group of normal controls.

Brain stem auditory EPs have been found to be abnormal in Leigh's syndrome, or subacute necrotizing encephalomyelopathy (Davis et al., 1985; Taylor and Robinson, 1992). This disorder results from a variety of disorders involved in pyruvate metabolism. Included in these disorders are deficiencies of pyruvate dehydrogenase, complex IV or cytochrome oxidase, complex V deficiencies and other mitochondrial disorders. The abnormalities in these disorders vary with the type and age of the patient (Taylor and Robinson, 1992). The BAEPs in children with pyruvate dehydrogenase deficiency had poor morphology and reproducibilty of waveforms. Patients with complex IV or cytochrome oxidase deficiency had increased IPLs and low-amplitude or absent wave IV/V. Six of seven children with complex I deficiency had normal BAEPs and a slowly progressive form of the disease. The other patient with complex I deficiency had only waves I and II and a had a rapidly progressive form of the disease. One patient with complex V deficiency had a normal BAEP at 4 months of age and loss of later waves when retested 10 weeks later.

The BAEP has been found to be abnormal in Niemann–Pick type C disease. Abnormalities have included prolonged IPLs for waves I–V and poor wave morphology (Pikus, 1991). Mondelli et al. (1990) described 11 patients with Leber's hereditary optic atrophy, 7 (64%) of whom had abnormal BAEPs including prolonged IPLs of waves I–II, I–III, III–V and I–V. Abnormal BAEPs have been recorded in children with cerebrohepatorenal (Zellweger's) syndrome, proprionic acidemia, and Menke's kinky hair disease. The III–V IPL has been found to be prolonged in patients with Wilson's disease late in the course of the disease (Fujita et al., 1981; Butnar et al., 1990).

The brain stem auditory pathways have a predilection for bilirubin toxicity, resulting in sensorineural hearing loss. The BAEP is a useful tool to assess early signs of bilirubin encephalopathy in asymptomatic neonates (Perlman and Frank, 1988). The BAEP abnormalities vary: 24 infants with serum bilirubin levels between 15 and 25 µg/dl had BAEPs and in 10 of 24 waves IV/V were absent (Perlman et al., 1983). Increased bilirubin concentrations correlate with prolonged IPLs (Perlman et al., 1983; Vohr et al., 1990; Funato et al., 1994). Abnormalities of the BAEP improve significantly after phototherapy (Tan et al., 1992) and exchange transfusion (Wennberg et al., 1982; Nwaesei et al., 1984; Chin et al., 1985; Bergman et al., 1985; Deliac et al., 1990). Solomon et al., (1990) performed BAEPs in two adolescents with type I Crigler–Najjar syndrome, an autosomal recessive disorder characterized by unconjugated hyperbilirubinemia. Both had normal BAEPs, unlike the neonates with hyperbilirubinemia.

The abnormalities seen in the BAEP increase with progression of degenerative disease and increasing clinical severity. Serial studies help to determine the rate of progression of the diseases.

3.2. Tumors

Posterior fossa tumors are more common in children than in adults and produce abnormalities in the BAEP. The BAEP can therefore complement neuroimaging in the diagnosis and localization of tumors. The BAEP can be serially monitored during treatment to help assess response.

Brain stem gliomas usually produce abnormalities of the BAEP and may do so early in the course of disease. Nodar et al. (1980) described seven children with brain stem gliomas, all of whom had abnormal BAEPs that correctly identified the site of the lesion. Picton et al., (1992) found BAEPs to be abnormal in 23 children with tumors involving the pons or midbrain. In only two patients, the BAEP abnormality did not correctly identify the side of the lesion. There was significant mass effect on the brain stem in these cases. Davis et al. (1985) reported four children with brain stem gliomas diagnosed by computed tomography or biopsy. In three patients the BAEP was abnormal bilaterally and all had signs of brain stem dysfunction at the level of the pons. One child whose tumor involved the thalamus and midbrain had a normal BAEP.

Neurofibromatosis type I (NF1) (von Recklinghausen's disease) is a genetic disorder inherited in an autosomal dominant fashion. There are a wide range of pathologic expressions of this disorder, including brain tumors, heterotopias, and hamartomas. Pensak et al. (1989) studied 44 children and found 32% had significant conduction delay abnormalities of the BAEP. Only one child had an abnormality secondary to an identifiable mass lesion. Picton et al. (1992) found 11 of 25 children with NF1 to have an abnormally delayed I–III or I–V IPL interval. One child had an auditory nerve tumor and another had a brain stem glioma. Duffner et al. (1989) evaluated 47 children with NF1 and found 27% to have abnormal BAEP examinations. Seventy-four percent of children had abnormal magnetic resonance imaging (MRI) studies. The abnormal findings of the BAEP did not consistently correlate with MRI lesions. Therefore, although the BAEP is a useful method of detecting central nervous system (CNS) abnormalities in children with NF1, the clinical impact of these abnormalities is uncertain. A large number of patients must be followed to determine the significance of EP abnormalities and the value of monitoring patients with EP.

3.3. Central Nervous System Malformations

During embryonic development the spinal column may fail to close, leading to myelomeningocele. In addition to spinal anomalies, such children typically have Arnold–Chiari type II malformation, an anomaly of the hindbrain. The cerebellum, brain stem, and fourth venticle are caudally displaced through the foramen magnum into the spinal canal. Patients can develop brain stem dysfunction in infancy or childhood. Symptoms typically include apnea, hypoventilation, and swallowing difficulties. A number of studies have been done to assess whether BAEPs in children with Arnold–Chiari type II malformation can predict the evolution of this syndrome and the need for posterior fossa decompression. Barnet et al. (1993) studied 16 patients one or more times. Waves III and V of the BAEP were typically prolonged in both symptomatic and asymptomatic patients. Lutschg et al. (1984) studied 27 patients with myelomeningocele and found the longest I–V interpeak and wave V latencies in patients with shunted hydrocephalus and cranial nerve deficits. The latencies of myelomeningocele patients were significantly longer than the latencies of the normal population.

Hydrocephalic children usually show abnormalities of the BAEP. Abnormalities of wave V are common (Krause et al., 1984; Edwards et al.,1985) and include reduction of amplitude of wave V and delayed latency. Abnormalities of the BAEP may be transient and improve after a shunting procedure.

Hydranencephaly is a rare condition in which the cerebral hemispheres are absent and are replaced by membranous sacs of cerebrospinal fluid. The BAEP is normal in these patients. The flash visual EP and cortical somatosensory EP are absent (Hanigan and Aldrich, 1988).

3.4. Coma

Multiple diagnostic procedures, including the BAEP, are used to assess the functional status of and prognosis for the head-injured and comatose patient. It has been found in children, as in adults, that a persistently abnormal BAEP is a better predictor of a poor outcome than a normal study is in predicting a good outcome (Rappaport et al., 1985; DeMeirlier and Taylor, 1986; Barelli et al., 1991; Fisher et al., 1992). DeMeileir and Taylor (1986) studied 80 comatose children with various etiologies. Of 15 children with severe neurologic signs, 10 had normal BAEPs, 4 had increased IPLs, and 1 had absent waves. Forty-four patients died and there was a range of BAEP results, with 11 patients having normal BAEPs, 15 having results compatible with brain death, 8 having increased IPLs, and 10 with absent wave V. Seventeen patients had complete absence of waves or only waves I and II recorded and two of these patients survived with minimal neurologic sequelae. Repeat serial testing is necessary, as BAEP abnormalities may be secondary to reversible brain stem dysfunction. Lutschg et al. (1983) examined BAEPs in 43 comatose children who were head-injured or suffered severe hypoxic–ischemic encephalopathy. A bilateral loss of components was observed in all patients who died but one. Prolonged latencies of waves occurred in one third of patients who recovered. Three patients who died had normal BAEPs. Frank et al. (1985) described five infants with nontraumatic coma who had intact BAEPs and absent cortical somatosensory EP responses who persisted in a chronic vegetative state. These studies suggest that BAEPs should not be used alone as criteria for brain death in the pediatric population (Ashwal and Sheider, 1991; Taylor et al., 1983).

3.5. Meningitis

Bacterial meningitis may be associated with long-term neurologic sequelae and hearing impairment. Detection of CNS sequelae is important so that intervention can be started early. The most common abnormalities found in the BAEP are increased IPLs, increased wave V latency, and abnormal latency–intensity functions (Cohen et al., 1988). In a study of 23 children recovered from purulent meningitis, 23% had long-term neurologic sequelae or hearing impairment (Jiang et al., 1990b). Ozdamar and Kraus (1983) studied BAEPs in 60 infants recovering from meningitis and found 10 to have brain stem abnormalities and 25% to have evidence of a hearing loss. Brain stem auditory EP abnormalities have been seen to improve with recovery (Ozdamar et al., 1983; Kotagal et al., 1981).

3.6. Acquired Immunodeficiency Syndrome

It is not currently clear whether serial BAEP studies may provide information about the progression of CNS involvement in children with acquired immunodeficiency syndrome (AIDS). Sixteen infants and children with AIDS had BAEP testing utilizing stimulation rates of 10 and 50/sec. The absolute latencies of waves III, IV, and V were significantly longer unilaterally in the AIDS group with a stimulation rate of 10 Hz. At a stimulation rate of 50 Hz significant differences occurred in the latencies of waves I, III, and V bilaterally (Frank et al., 1992). The differential effect of increasing the stimulus on a group of normals compared to a group of children with AIDS was significant for the absolute latency of wave I and I–III and I–V IPLs. Increased stimulus rates increase these latencies more in the AIDS group. Fourteen children and infants with AIDS had serial BAEPs over a mean follow-up period of 1.95 years. There was a trend toward increasing absolute and IPLs over time and a correlation with the I–V IPL and absolute latency of wave V with a stimulation rate of 50 Hz (Frank and Pahwa, 1993). Schmitt et al. (1992) were unable to document a progression of latencies in pediatric AIDS patients. Improvement in the BAEP IPLs has been reported in response to treatment with AZT (Brivio et al., 1991; Schmitt et al., 1992).

3.7. Neonatal Screening

Fetal and neonatal hypoxic–ischemic events can cause CNS deficits and neurodevelopmental impairments. Evoked potentials have been used to help identify infants at risk for neurologic sequelae so that they may be followed closely and optimally managed (Stockard et al., 1983; Salamy et al., 1989; Majnemer et al., 1988, 1990). Majnemer et al. (1988) performed neonatal and follow-up BAEPs on 34 high-risk neonates and compared findings to a group of age-matched controls. Neonates were identified as at risk if they were asphyxiated, had very low birth weight (<1,501 g), or were small (<3rd%) for gestational age. There was a high incidence of abnormalities in the high-risk group, including increased IPLs, abnormal V/I amplitude ratio, and abnormal waveform morphology. Abnormal brain stem conduction was predictive of gross motor delay and an abnormal neurologic examination at 1 year. Hecox et al. (1981) found a correlation with abnormal V/I amplitude ratios and abnormal neurologic examinations. Stockard et al. (1983) correlated the clinical outcome in 74 children at risk for audiologic or neurologic sequelae with BAEPs. There was no consistent relationship between the BAEP findings and severe brain damage. The BAEP study had greater value when performed several weeks after the perinatal injury. Thirteen of 14 infants with absent waves III–V were severely neurologically impaired at follow-up. Seventeen showed persistent prolonged IPLs and 11 survived with marked neurologic impairment; 4 were normal at follow-up 18 months to 4 years of age and 2 died. Patients with absence of later waves have been reported with only minimal neurologic impairment. The absence of BAEP waveforms does not preclude a favorable outcome. Brain stem auditory EP abnormalities may be transient and therefore serial testing is critical (Stockard et al., 1983; Kitamoto et al., 1990).

Infants ages 32 to 44 weeks postconceptional age exposed to cocaine during pregnancy have been shown to have significant increases in I–V, III–V and I–III IPLs (Salamy et al., 1990). Salamy and Eldredge (1994) evaluated the records of 1,087 full-term and preterm infants and found infants exposed to cocaine in utero with neurologic signs or brain anomalies exhibited abnormal BAEPs four to five times more often than infants without these risk factors. By 3 to 6 months of age cocaine-exposed infants have BAEP latencies similar to normal controls.

Grimmer et al. (1992) performed BAEPs on 39 newborns who were infants of diabetic mothers and found no difference in waveform latencies or amplitudes compared to a control group.

Paccioretti et al. (1992) found normal BAEP absolute and IPLs in a group of neonates treated with extracorporeal membrane oxygenation.

The BAEP is a neurophysiologic technique used to assist in measuring hearing thresholds in infants at risk for hearing loss and in nonverbal children. Hearing impairment early in life leads to abnormal speech and language development. Early identification of hearing impairment can allow for intervention. Those newborn infants considered "at risk" for hearing loss should be tested and include infants with a family history of deafness, congenital infections, prematurity, CNS malformations, perinatal asphyxia, and hyperbilirubinemia.

Approximately 1% to 5% of children leaving a neonatal intensive care unit have bilateral sensorineural hearing loss requiring amplification (Galambos, 1984). Some neonates will have conductive losses that resolve during the first months of life and follow-up studies at 3 months of age should be done. For screening purposes, 30 dB NHL clicks are presented monaurally at a rate of 61/sec and 4,000 responses are average. If recognizable waves are not seen testing is performed at higher intensities until an auditory threshold is identified (Picton et al., 1992). The BAEP is recorded in normal newborns at 30 dB NHL and therefore, if threshold is greater than 30 dB NHL the test should be repeated in several months. Thresholds above 40 dB NHL are predictive of a hearing loss. Care should be taken when assessing auditory thresholds in children with neurologic disorders producing abnormal waveforms. Serial BAEPs should be done to assess whether there is improvement before prescribing amplification (Stockard and Westmoreland, 1981; Bergman et al., 1985; Salamy et al., 1989).

3.8. Apnea and Sudden Infant Death Syndrome

Apnea occurs in some preterm infants and in most cases the etiology is not clear but is thought to be secondary to brain stem immaturity. Fifty-eight infants between 30 and 37 weeks postconceptional age had BAEPs (Henderson-Smart et al., 1983). Apnea was found to occur more frequently at younger postconceptional ages and central brain stem conduction was found to decrease with increasing age. In each postconceptional age group the infants with apnea had brain stem conduction times that were significantly longer than those of the infants without apnea. Brain stem auditory EPs were found not to be helpful in identifying the pathogenesis of cryptogenic infantile apneic episodes or infants at risk for sudden infant death syndrome (Gupta et al., 1981; Stockard, 1982). The BAEP peak latencies and IPLs in infants with near-miss sudden infant death syndrome (prolonged sleep apnea with clinical evidence of hypoxemia requiring resuscitation) were found to be similar to a group of normal controls. Brain stem auditory EPs are not routinely used as a method of screening infants who may be at risk for sudden infant death syndrome.

3.9. Developmental Disorders

Brain stem auditory EPs have been performed in children with autism, learning disabilities, and developmental language disorders. A number of studies have reported significantly longer central brain stem auditory conduction with prolonged I–III, III–V, and I–V IPLs in children with autism compared to normal controls and children with mental retardation (Rosenblum et al., 1980; Wong and Wong, 1991). Courchesne et al. (1985) found BAEPs to normal in a group of nonretarded autistic people aged 14 to 28 years. McClelland et al. (1992) studied 20 children with autism and mental retardation. Children less than 14 years of age had normal central brain stem auditory conduction while 11 of 15 children over 14 years of age had prolonged central conduction compared to a group of normal controls. Brain stem auditory EPs were normal in a group of nonautistic mentally handicapped individuals. The conflicting results of these studies suggest only the possibility of brain stem involvement in autistic individuals. Peripheral thresholds were elevated in some of the patients studied. Hearing should be assessed in this patient population as hearing loss can potentially exacerbate the maladaptive behaviors. No significant differences have been observed in the BAEPs between normal controls and children with learning disorders (Marosi et al., 1990). In children with developmental dysphasia BAEP studies are conflicting with reports of both normal latencies and shorter absolute latencies without a significant difference in brain stem auditory conduction (Roncaglolo et al., 1994).

3.10. Miscellaneous

Santanelli et al. (1990) reported BAEP findings in a case of alternating hemiplegia. The BAEP was normal during and between events.

The I–V IPL was found to be shortened and wave V amplitude smaller in a group of children with Down's syndrome compared to normal controls (Jiang et al., 1990b).

Brain stem auditory EPs were abnormal in 5 of 10 patients with infantile spasms. Abnormalities included low-amplitude wave V in four, prolonged wave V latency and I–V IPL in one patient, and absence of waves IV/V in one patient (Miyazaki et al., 1993).

Sunaga et al. (1992) performed BAEPs in 70 children with congenital heart disease (32 with and 38 without cyanosis) to study the effect of chronic hypoxia on brain stem maturation. The I–V IPLs of cyanotic infants were found to be prolonged compared to controls and patients without cyanosis. The authors postulate that chronic hypoxemia contributes to delayed maturation of the brain stem auditory pathways.

Ten premature infants with low serum thyroxin levels were found to have normal BAEPs (Kohelet et al., 1992) Forty-eight treated early-detected congenitally hypothyroid children, ages 18 months, 3 years, and 5 to 9 years, had BAEPs. In 18-month and 3-year-old congenitally hypothyroid children the most frequent abnormality was an increase in wave I latency. There was no significant difference in IPLs between controls and subjects (Laureau et al., 1987).

CONCLUSION

The BAEP offers a noninvasive, objective method of assessing sensory function in children and can therefore be used as a adjunct to the neurologic examination. Although the study can identify dysfunction in the brain stem auditory pathways, it is not specific as to etiology. Studies should be performed using age-matched normative data and interpreted carefully as there may be hearing impairment or CNS abnormalities affecting the results of the test.

REFERENCES

Adelman C, Levi H, Linder N, Sohmer H (1990): Neonatal auditory brain-stem response threshold and latency: 1 hour to 5 months. *Electroencephalogr Clin Neurophysiol* 77:77–80.

Allison T, Hume AL, Wood CC, Goff WR (1984): Developmental and aging changes in somatosensory, auditory and visual evoked potentials. *Electroencephalogr Clin Neurophysiol* 58:14–24.

Ashwal S, Schneider S (1991): Pediatric brain death: Current perspectives. *Adv Pediatr* 38:181–202.

Barelli A, Valente MR, Clemente A, Bozza P, Proietti R, Corte FD (1991): Serial multimodality-evoked potentials in severely head-injured patients: Diagnostic and prognostic implications. *Crit Care Med* 19:1374–1381.

Barnet AB, Weiss IP, Shaer C (1993): Evoked potentials in infant brain stem syndrome associated with Arnold–Chiari malformation. *Dev Med Child Neurol* 35:42–48.

Bergman I, Hirsch RP, Fria TJ, Shapiro SM, Holzman I, Painter MJ (1985): Cause of hearing loss in the high-risk premature infant. *J Pediatr* 106:95–101.

Brivio L, Tornaghi R, Musetti L, Marschisio P, Principi N (1991): Improvement of auditory brain stem responses after treatment with zidovudine in a child with AIDS. *Pediatr Neurol* 7:53–55.

Brivio L, Grasso R, Salvaggio A, Principi N (1993): Brain-stem auditory evoked potentials (BAEPs): maturation of interpeak latency I–V (IPL I–V) in the first years of life. *Electroencephalogr Clin Neurophysiol* 88:28–31.

Butnar P, Trontelj JV, Khuraibet AJ, Khan RA, Hussein JM, Shakir RA (1990): Brain stem auditory evoked potential in Wilson's disease. *J Neurol Sci* 95:163–169.

Cardona F, Leuzzi V, Antonozzi I, Benedetti P, Loizzo A (1991): The development of auditory and visual evoked potentials in early treated phenylketonuric children. *Electroencephalogr Clin Neurophysiol* 80:3–15.

Chin KC, Taylor MJ, Perlman M (1985): Improvement in auditory and visual evoked potentials in jaundiced preterm infants after exchange transfusion. *Arch Dis Child* 60:714–717.

Cohen BA, Schenk VA, Sweeney DB (1988): Meningitis-related hearing loss evaluated with evoked potentials. *Pediatr Neurol* 4:18–22.

Courchesne E, Courchesne RY, Hicks G, Lincoln AJ (1985): Functioning of the brain-stem auditory pathway in non-retarded autistic individuals. *Electroencephalogr Clin Neurophysiol* 69:491–501.

Davis SL, Aminoff MJ, Berg BO (1985): Brain-stem auditory evoked potentials in children with brain stem or cerebellar dysfunction. *Arch Neurol* 42:156–160.

Deliac P, Demarquez JL, Barberot JP, Sandler B, Paty J (1990): Brain stem auditory evoked potentials in icteric fullterm newborns: alterations after exchange transfusion. *Neuropediatrics* 21:115–118.

DeMeirleir LJ, Taylor MJ (1986): Evoked potentials in comatose children: auditory brain stem responses. *Pediatr Neurol* 2:31–34.

DePablos C, Berciano S, Calleja J (1991): Brain-stem and evoked potentials and blink reflex in Friedreich's ataxia. *J Neurol* 238:212–216.

Duffner PK, Cohen ME, Seidel GF, Shucard DW (1989): The significance of MRI abnormalities in children with neurofibromatosis. *Neurology* 39:373–378.

Durieux-Smith A, Edwards CG, Picton TW, McMurray B (1985): Auditory brain stem response to clicks in neonates. *J Otolaryngol* 14:12–18.

Edwards CG, Durieux-Smith A, Picton TW (1985): Auditory brain stem response audiometry in neonatal hydrocephalus. *J Otolaryngol* 14:40–46.

Eggermont JJ (1992): Development of auditory evoked potentials. *Acta Otolaryngol (Stockh)* 112:197–200.

Eggermont JJ and Salamy A (1988): Maturational time course for the ABR in preterm and full term infants. *Hear Res* 33:35–48.

Frank Y, Pahwa S (1993): Serial brain stem auditory evoked responses in infants and children with AIDS. *Clin Electroencephalogr* 24:160–165.

Frank LM, Furgiuele TL, Etheridge JE (1985): Prediction of chronic vegetative state in children using evoked potentials. *Neurology* 35:931–934.

Frank, Y, Vishnubhakat SM, Pahwa S (1992): Brain stem auditory evoked responses in infants and children with AIDS. *Pediatr Neurol* 8:262–266.

Fujita M, Hosoki M, Miyazaki M (1981): Brain stem auditory evoked responses in spinocerebellar degeneration and Wilson disease. *Ann Neurol* 9:42–47.

Fujita M, Hyde ML, Alberti PW (1991): ABR latency in infants: properties and applications of various measures. *Acta Otolaryngol (Stockh)* 111:53–60.

Funato M, Tamai H, Shimada S, Nakamura H (1994): Vigintiphobia, unbound bilirubin, and auditory brain stem responses. *Pediatrics* 93:50–53.

Galambos R, Hicks GE, Wilson MJ (1984): The auditory brain stem response reliably predicts hearing loss in graduates of an intensive care nursery. *Ear Hear* 5:254–260.

Garg BP, Markand ON, DeMyer WE (1983): Usefulness of BAEP studies in the early diagnosis of Pelizaeus-Merzbacher disease. *Neurology* 33:955–956.

Gorga MP, Reiland JK, Beauchaine KA, Worthington DW, Jesteadt W (1987): Auditory brain stem response form graduates of an intensive care nursery: Normal patterns of response. *J Speech Hear Res* 30:311–318.

Gorga MP, Kaminski JR, Beauchaine KL, Jesteadt W, Neely ST (1989): Auditory brain stem responses from children three months to three years of age: normal patters of response II. *J Speech Hear Res* 32:281–288.

Grimmer I, Trammer RM, Koster K, Kainer F, Obladen M (1992): Normal auditory brain stem evoked responses in infants of diabetic mothers. *Early Hum Dev* 30:221–228.

Gupta PR, Guilleminault C, Dorfman LJ (1981): Brain stem auditory evoked potentials in near-miss sudden infant death syndrome. *J Pediatr* 98:791–794.

Hanigan WC, Aldrich WM (1988): MRI and evoked potentials in a child with hydranencephaly. *Pediatr Neurol* 4:185–187.

Hatanaka T, Shuto H, Yasuhara A, Kobayashi Y (1988): Ipsilateral and contralateral recordings of auditory brain stem response to monaural stimulation. *Pediatr Neurol* 4:354–357.

Hecox K, Burkard R (1982): Developmental dependencies of the human brain stem auditory evoked response. *Ann NY Acad Sci* 388:538–556.

Hecox KE, Cone B, Blaw ME (1981): Brain stem auditory evoked response in the diagnosis of pediatric neurologic diseases. *Neurology* 31:832–840.

Henderson-Smart DJ, Pettigrew AG, Campbell DJ (1983): Clinical apnea and brain-stem neural function in preterm infants. *N Engl J Med* 308:353–357.

Jacobson JT (1985): Normative aspects of the pediatric auditory brain stem response. *J Otolaryngol* 14:7–11.

Jiang ZD, Liu XY, Yun YW, Zheng MS, Liu HC (1990a): Long-term impairments of brain and auditory functions of children recovered from purulent meningitis. *Dev Med Child Neurol* 32:473–480.

Jiang ZD, Wu YY, Liu XY (1990b): Early development of brain stem auditory evoked potentials in Down's syndrome. *Early Hum Dev* 23:41–51.

Jiang ZD, Wu YY, Zheng WS, Sun DK, Feng LY, Liu XY (1991a): The effect of click rate on latency and interpeak interval of the brain-stem auditory evoked potentials in children from birth to 6 years. *Electroencephalogr Clin Neurophysiol* 80:60–64.

Jiang ZD, Zheng MS, Sun DK Liu XY (1991b): Brain stem auditory evoked responses from birth to adulthood: normative data of latency and interval. *Hear Res* 54:67–74.

Jiang ZD, Zhang L, Wu YY, Liu XY (1993): Brain stem auditory evoked responses from birth to adulthood: Development of wave amplitude. *Hear Res* 68:35–41.

Ken-Dorr A, Pratt H, Zeltzer M, Sujov P, Katzir J, Benderley A (1987): Auditory brain-stem evoked potentials to clicks at different presentation rates: estimating maturation of pre-term and full-term neonates. *Electroencephalogr Clin Neurophysiol* 68:209–218.

Kitamoto I, Kukita J, Kurokawa T, Chen YJ, Minami T, Ueda K (1990): Transient neurologic abnormalities and BAEPs in high-risk infants. *Pediatr Neurol* 6:319–325.

Kohelet D, Arbel E, Goldberg M, Arlazzoroff A (1992): Transient neonatal hypothyroxinemia and the auditory brain stem evoked response. *Pediatr Res* 32:530–531.

Kotagal S, Rosenberg C, Rudd D, Dunkle LM, Horenstein S (1981): Auditory evoked potentials in bacterial meningitis. *Arch Neurol* 38:693–695.

Kraus N, Ozdamar O, Heydemann PT, Stein L, Reed NL (1984): Auditory brain-stem responses in hydrocephalic patients. *Electroencephalogr Clin Neurophysiol* 59:310–317.

Lahat E, Aladjem M, Mor A, Azizi E, Arlazarof A (1992): Brain stem auditory evoked potentials in familial dysautonomia. *Dev Med Child Neurol* 34:690–693.

Lary S, Briassoulis G, de Vries L, Dubowitz LMS, Dubowitz V (1985): Hearing threshold in preterm and term infants by auditory brain stem response. *J Pediatr* 107:593–599.

Lasky RE (1984): A developmental study on the effect of stimulus rate on the auditory evoked brain-stem response. *Electroencephalogr Clin Neurophysiol* 59:411–419.

Lauffer H, Wenzel D (1990): Brain stem acoustic evoked responses: maturational aspects from cochlea to midbrain. *Neuropediatrics* 21:57–61.

Laureau E, Hebert R, Vanasse M, Letarte J, Glorieux J, Desjardins M, Dussault JH (1987): Somatosensory evoked potentials in auditory brain-stem responses in congenital hypothyroidism. II. A cross-sectional study in childhood. Correlations with hormonal levels and developmental quotients. *Electroencephalogr Clin Neurophysiol* 67:521–530.

Lutschg J, Pfenninger J, Ludin HP, Vassella F (1983): Brain stem auditory evoked potentials and early somatosensory evoked potentials in neurointensively treated comatose children. *Am J Dis Child* 137:421–426.

Lutschg J, Meyer E, Jeanneret-Iseli C (1984): Brain stem auditory evoked potentials in meningomyelocele. *Neuropediatrics* 16:202–204.

Majnemer A, Rosenblatt B, Riley P (1988): Prognostic significance of the auditory brain stem evoked response in high-risk neonates. *Dev Med Child Neurol* 30:43–52.

Majnemer A, Rosenblatt B, Riley PS (1990): Prognostic significance of multimodality evoked response testing in high-risk newborns. *Pediatr Neurol* 6:367–374.

Markand ON, Garg BP, Brandt IK (1982a): Nonketotic hyperglycinemia: Electroencephalographic and evoked potential abnormalities. *Neurology* 32:151–156.

Markand ON, Garg BP, DeMyer WE, Warren C, Worth RM (1982b): Brain-stem auditory, visual, and somatosensory evoked potential in leukodystrophies. *Electroencephalogr Clin Neurophysiol* 54:39–48.

Marosi E, Harmony T, Becker J (1990): Brain stem evoked potentials in learning disabled children. *Int J Neurosci* 50:233–242.

McClelland RJ, Eyre DG, Watson D, Calvert GJ, Sherrard E (1992): Central conduction time in childhood autism. *Br J Psych* 160:695–763.

Miyazaki M, Hashimoto T, Tayama M, Kuroda Y (1993): Brain stem involvement in infantile spasms: a study employing brain stem evoked potentials and magnetic resonance imaging. *Neuropediatrics* 24:126–130.

Nodar RH, Hahn J, Levine HL (1980): Brainstem auditory evoked potentials in determining site of lesion of brain stem gliomas in children. *Laryngoscope* 90:258–266.

Nwaesei CG, Van Aerde J, Boyden M, Perlman M (1984): Changes in auditory brain stem responses in hyperbilirubinemic infants before and after exchange transfusion. *Pediatrics* 74:800–803.

Ochs R, Markand ON, DeMyer WE (1979): Brain stem auditory evoked responses in leukodystrophies. *Neurology* 29:1089–1093.

Ozdamar O, Kraus N (1983): Auditory brain stem response in infants recovering from bacterial meningitis. *Arch Neurol* 40:499–502.

Ozdamar O, Kraus N, Stein L (1983): Auditory brain stem responses in infants recovering from bacterial meningitis. *Arch Otolaryngol* 109:13–18.

Paccioretti DC, Haluschak MM, Finer NN, Robertson CMT, Pain KS, Hagler M (1992): Auditory brain-stem responses in neonates receiving extracorporeal membrane oxygenation. *J Pediatr* 120:464–467.

Pedersen L, Trojaborg W (1981): Visual, auditory and somatosensory pathway involvement in hereditary cerebellar ataxia, Friedreich's ataxia and familial spastic paraplegia. *Electroencephalogr Clin Neurophysiol* 52:283–297.

Pensak ML, Keith RW, St. John Dignan P, Stowens DW, Towbin RB, Katbamna B (1989): Neuroaudiologic abnormalities in patients with type 1 neurofibromatosis. *Laryngoscope* 99:702–706.

Perlman M, Frank JW (1988): Bilirubin beyond the blood–brain barrier. *Pediatrics* 81:304–315.

Perlman M, Fainmesser P, Sohmer H, Tamari H, Wax Y, Pevsmer B (1983): Auditory nerve-brain stem evoked responses in hyperbilirubimenic neonates. *Pediatrics* 72:658–664.

Perretti A, Petrillo A, Pelosi L, Balbi P, Parenti G, Riemma A, Strisciuglio P (1990): Detection of early abnormalities in the mycopolysaccharidases by the use of visual and brain stem auditory evoked potentials. *Neuropediatrics* 21:83–86.

Picton T, Taylor MJ, Durieux-Smith A (1992): Brain stem auditory evoked potentials in pediatrics. *Electrodiagnosis in Clinical Medicine*, edited by M Aminoff, pp 537–569. Churchill Livingstone, New York.

Pikus A (1991): Audiologic profile in Niemann-Pick C. *Ann NY Acad Sci* 630:313–314.

Rappaport M, Maloney JR, Ortega H, Fetzer D, Hall K (1985): Survival in young children after drowning: brain evoked potentials as outcome predictors. *Clin Electroencephalogr* 16:183–191.

Roncagliolo M, Benitez J, Perez M (1994): Auditory brain stem responses of children with developmental language disorders. *Dev Med Child Neurol* 36:26–33.

Rosenblum SM, Arick JR, Krug A, Stubbs EG, Young NB, Pelson RO (1980): Auditory brain stem evoked responses in autistic children. *J Autism Dev Dis* 10:215–225.

Rossini PM, Cracco JB (1987): Somatosensory and brain stem auditory evoked potentials in neurodegenerative system disorders. *Eur Neurol* 26:176–188.

Salamy A (1984): Maturation of the auditory brain stem response from birth through early childhood. *J Clin Neurophysiol* 1:293–329.

Salamy A, Eldredge L (1994): Risk for ABR abnormalities in the nursery. *Electroencephalogr Clin Neurophysiol* 92:392–395.

Salamy A, Eldredge L, Tooley WH (1989): Neonatal status and hearing loss in high-risk infants. *J Pediatr* 114:847–852.

Salamy A, Eldredge L, Anderson J, Bull D (1990): Clinical and laboratory observations. *J Pediatr* 117:627–629.

Sand T (1991): BAEP amplitudes and amplitude ratios: relation to click polarity, race, age and sex. *Electroencephalogr Clin Neurophysiol* 78:291–296.

Santanelli P, Guerrini R, Dravet C, Genton P, Bureau M, Farnarier G (1990): Brain stem auditory evoked potentials in alternating hemiplegia: ictal vs interictal assessment in one case. *Clin Electroencephalogr* 21:51–54.

Scaioli V, Pareyson D, Avanzini G, Sghirlanzoni A (1992): F response and somatosensory and brain stem auditory evoked potential studies in HMSN type I and II. *J Neurol Neurosurg Psychiatry* 55:1027–1031.

Schmitt B, Seeger J, Jacobi G (1992): EEG and evoked potentials in HIV-infected children. *Clin Electroencephalogr* 23:111–117.

Schulman-Galambos C, Galambos R (1975): Brain-stem auditory-evoked responses in premature infants. *J Speech Hear Res* 18:456–465.

Solomon G, Labar D, Galbraith RA, Schaefer J, Kappas A (1990): Neurophysiological abnormalities in adolescents with type I Crigler-Najjar syndrome. *Electroencephalogr Clin Neurophysiol* 76:473–475.

Staley K, Iragui V, Spitz M (1990): The human fetal auditory evoked potential. *Electroencephalogr Clin Neurophysiol* 77:1–5.

Starr A, Amlie RN, Martin WH, Sanders S (1977): Development of auditory function in newborn infants revealed by auditory brain stem potentials. *Pediatrics* 60:831–839.

Stockard JE, Westmoreland BF (1981): Technical considerations in the recording and interpretation of the brain stem auditory evoked potential for neonatal neurologic diagnosis. *Am J EEG Technol* 21:31–54.

Stockard JE, Stockard JJ, Westmoreland BF, Corfits JL (1979): Brain stem auditory-evoked responses. *Arch Neurol* 36:823–831.

Stockard JE, Stockard JJ, Kleinberg F, Westmoreland BF (1983): Prognostic value of brain stem auditory evoked potentials in neonates. *Arch Neurol* 40:360–365.

Stockard JJ (1982): Brain stem auditory evoked potentials in adult and infant sleep apnea syndromes, including sudden infant death syndrome and near-miss for sudden infant death. *Ann Acad Sci* 388:443–465.

Sunaga Y, Sone K, Nagashima K, Kuroume T (1992): Auditory brain stem responses in congenital heart disease. *Pediatr Neurol* 8:437–440.

Tan KL, Skurr BA, Yip YY (1992): Phototherapy and the brain-stem auditory evoked response in neonatal hyperbilirubinemia. *J Pediatr* 120:306–308.

Taylor MJ, Robinson BH (1992): Evoked potentials in children with oxidative metabolic defects leading to Leigh syndrome. *Pediatr Neurol* 8:25–29.

Taylor MJ, Houston BD, Lowry NJ (1983): Recovery of auditory brain stem responses after a severe hypoxic ischemic insult. *N Engl J Med* 309:1169–1170.

Taylor MJ, Chan-Lui WY, Logan WJ (1985): Longitudinal evoked potential studies in hereditary ataxias. *Can J Neurol Sci* 12:100.

Thivierge J, Cote R (1990): Brain-stem auditory evoked response: normative values in children. *Electroencephalogr Clin Neurophysiol* 77:309–313.

Vohr BR, Karp D, O'Dea C, Darrow D, Coll CG, Lester BM, Brown L, Oh W, Cashore W (1990): Behavioral changes correlated with brain-stem auditory evoked responses in term infants with moderate hyperbilirubinemia. *J Pediatr* 117:288–291.

Wennberg RP, Ahlfors CE, Bickers R, McMurty CA, Shetter JL (1982): Abnormal auditory brain stem response in a newborn infant with hyperbilirubinemia: Improvement with exchange transfusion. *J Pediatr* 100:624–626.

Wong V, Wong SN (1991): Brain stem auditory evoked potential study in children with autistic disorder. *J Autism Dev Dis* 21:329–340.

Yamasaki M, Shono H, Oga M, Ito Y, Shimomura K, Sugimori H (1991): Changes in auditory brain stem responses of normal neonates immediately after birth. *Biol Neonate* 60:92–101.

Zimmerman MC, Morgan DE, Dubno JR (1987): Auditory brain stem evoked response characteristics in developing infants. *Ann Otol Rhinol Laryngol* 96:291–299.

Evoked Potentials in Clinical Medicine,
3d ed., edited by Keith H. Chiappa.
Lippincott–Raven Publishers, Philadelphia © 1997.

8

Short-Latency Somatosensory Evoked Potentials: Methodology

Keith H. Chiappa

*Department of Neurology, Harvard Medical School, and EEG Laboratory,
Massachusetts General Hospital, Boston, Massachusetts 02114*

1. INTRODUCTION

Short-latency somatosensory evoked potentials (SEPs) have been studied and clinically utilized by many different investigators. Unfortunately, there are almost as many different techniques used in the registration of SEPs as there are investigators studying them. Similarly, waveform nomenclature varies markedly among authors. These factors create a methodologic maze capable of discouraging even experienced EP practitioners and make it very difficult to compare and contrast published SEP studies. The publication of guidelines by the American EEG Society [*J Clin Neurophysiol* (1986) 3(Suppl 1):43–92] probably will do little to alleviate this situation. Therefore, taking into account the above problems, the methodologic details will be presented here as SEPs are performed in the EP Unit of the Clinical Neurophysiology Laboratory of the Massachusetts General Hospital. These techniques have been used and developed over the last 5 years in testing more than 200 normal subjects and 8,000 patients with a variety of neurologic diseases. Where appropriate, other methodologies will be discussed to emphasize reasons for or against their use, and to help in comparing studies in the literature. However, in order to minimize confusion, these topics will not be treated exhaustively. Interested readers can confuse themselves to any desired degree by studying the literature.

2. EQUIPMENT

An SEP can be generated by physiologic (e.g., touch and muscle stretch) or electrical stimuli (see Section 9.1.1 for a more detailed discussion). The preferred stimulus for clinical neurologic investigation of the sensory system is electrical since that stimulus (1) is most easily controlled and measured and (2) produces potentials of the greatest amplitude and clarity. Thus, the stimulator should be able to deliver electrical square waves at variable rates (one per several seconds to 100/sec) and durations (10 μsec to 2 msec). The stimulus duration commonly used is 100 to 200 μsec but in patients with peripheral neuropathies it may be necessary to increase this to provide an adequate level of nerve stimulation. The stimulus intensity is varied according to (1) the amount of motor activity (i.e., twitch) produced in muscles controlled by the nerve and/or (2) the patient's appreciation of the stimulus intensity (see Sections 7.3 and 9.1.2). When a peripheral neuropathy is present or when both sides are stimulated simultaneously, it may be necessary for the stimulator to output a current of greater than 20 milliamps (mA), and so an output capability of up to 50 mA is useful. However, it is only rarely necessary to stimulate at greater than 10 to 15 mA and when doing so care must be exercised so that skin damage does not result. The output stage of the stimulator must provide protection so that excessive amounts of current cannot be applied to the patient. Direct current (DC) voltages should not be available through the stimulator or only with special maneuvers. It is very helpful if the stimulus intensity can be controlled close to the patient so that stimulating electrode position and stimulus intensity can be varied simultaneously by one person. A stimulus isolation device is essential to minimize stimulus artifact. This is usually a transformer device which restricts the path of current flow so that little can exit via the amplifiers and thereby produce a stimulus artifact. The number of individual nerve fibers being stimulated is directly related to current flow, which is a product of the voltage divided by the impedance, which is largely (but not entirely) at the stimulating electrode–skin interface. Although this impedance is usually not known and varies widely, a known level of current flow may be obtained using a stimulator that varies the voltage to maintain the current flow at a preset level—this is a constant-current stimulator. Constant voltage stimulators are probably more commonly used, however. Although there is no difference between EP waveforms produced by constant current and constant voltage stimulation (if intensity of nerve stimulation is the same), comparison between laboratories is usually facilitated by the use of the former device because it allows one to speak in terms of milliamps of current used, the factor most closely related to the number and size of nerve fibers stimulated. Note that current flow is measured between the two stimulating electrodes—an unknown fraction of that actually flows across nerve membranes to produce activity there. The possibility of producing extreme patient discomfort or even tissue damage with somatosensory stimulators, especially if long pulse durations and high repetition rates are used, and when recording from comatose or anesthetized patients, dictates that care be exercised with these devices and that they should be operated only by properly trained personnel. Various stimulus electrode types are available on the market. The easiest to use are those that have two metal discs embedded in plastic. A means of holding the stimulating electrodes at the proper stimulus site is necessary; this may be a piece of adhesive tape, or some form of elastic or Velcro band which wraps around the limb. If stimulus artifact is a problem, for example, with trigeminal nerve stimulation, the use of nonpolarizable electrodes (e.g., silver-silver chloride) is just as important for stimulation as for recording purposes. The plastic cup disposable type (pediatric electrocardiography recording electrodes) work quite well in this application. Needle electrodes can be used to stimulate close to the peripheral nerve, thus diminishing the amount of current needed for stimulation and thereby decreasing the stimulus artifact. However, the natural aversion of patients for needles dictates that these should be mainly used when surface stimulation does not produce a sufficient amount of nerve activation. Scalp recording electrodes are of the conventional type used for electroencephalography (EEG) and EP studies; needle electrodes may be used in certain circumstances (see below). With lower-limb stimulation, if lumbar potentials cannot be recorded from the skin surface using similar electrodes, recording at a depth using needle electrodes may be helpful. Monopolar electromyography (EMG) recording needle electrodes are prepared for this purpose by stripping the insulation from 1 cm or so at the tip; normally the only exposed recording surface is the bevel itself and it has insufficient pickup area for SEPs. These needles, after sterilization, are then placed according to techniques described below. The best ground electrodes are flexible metal strips covered with saline-soaked cloth which are wrapped around the limb proximal to the stimulus site and held in place by Velcro strips. Otherwise, large circular plates should be used.

3. PRETEST INSTRUCTIONS

The technician should extract pertinent clinical information from the medical record and/or history from the patient. Information about sensory symptomatology and peripheral nerve injuries are of particular interest. The terminology used to explain the test to the patient should be carefully considered. The use of the word "shock" is best avoided.

4. ELECTRODE APPLICATION

With the patient seated in a chair, electrodes are applied in appropriate positions (see Section 6 for electrode locations used in SEP testing). Any conventional EEG technique may be used for attaching the electrodes to the scalp (see Chapter 2, Section 3, for a discussion of recommended techniques).

4.1. Surface Versus Needle Electrodes

Needle EEG electrodes are completely satisfactory for recording scalp SEPs and are recommended in comatose patients except for long-term monitoring. There is no significant difference in latencies or amplitudes when SEPs are recorded simultaneously with needle and surface electrodes (Siivola and Jarvilehto, 1982) (see also Chapter 1, Section 2.1). Needles are not recommended (1) in monitoring situations, such as the intensive care unit, because of the risk of infection, and (2) in operating room monitoring, unless firmly anchored, because they tend to fall out easily. Needles should be handled very carefully and properly sterilized or discarded. The electrodes are plugged into the proper positions on the electrode board which connects them to the amplifiers and the averager. Impedance must be maintained below 5,000 ohms. Note, however, that needle electrodes may have a slightly higher impedance than this.

4.2. Recording the "Reference" Potentials

In neurologic applications of SEPs, interpeak separations are the only latency parameters used for interpretive purposes, except in special circumstances. These time differences are related to the state of conduction in proximal nerve roots and central nervous system (CNS) pathways. Since the potentials recorded at Erb's point and the lumbar region are generated primarily by activity in nerve trunks and roots close to the spinal cord and root entry zone, they provide a reference point for latency measurements; conduction times between them and later waves accurately represent the state of conduction in central segments of the sensory pathways. This is very similar to the use of wave I in brain stem auditory EPs (BAEPs) (see Chapter 5, Section 3). With good resolution of these reference waves, changes in peripheral nerve conduction velocities produced by peripheral neuropathies and changes in limb temperature can be largely ignored. Thus, clear registration of these waves is integral to reliable clinical neurologic interpretation of SEPs when absolute latencies (stimulus to scalp-recorded cerebral activity) are abnormal. When these reference waveforms cannot be clearly recorded from the skin surface at Erb's point, relocating the electrode will usually allow registration of a good potential. In the most difficult cases it is necessary to stimulate through the recording electrode to find the site where a minimal stimulus elicits a contraction (twitch) in the thumb musculature; this is then the most likely recording site to yield a good brachial plexus potential. Alternatively, a needle electrode may be used (as described below for lumbar point recordings), placed near the brachial plexus. Following lower-limb stimulation, a clear lumbar potential may not be recorded even when several surface recording sites have been used. Inadequate stimulus intensity may be part of the problem; patients may complain that the stimulus is painful, either for psychological reasons or because of dysesthesia from a peripheral neuropathy or other neurologic disease, and may not allow a sufficient stimulus intensity to be used. The only check on the adequacy of posterior tibial nerve stimulation is the technician's observation of a good muscle twitch in the intrinsic foot muscles supplied by the nerve. Registration of the sensory nerve action potential (SNAP) of the posterior tibial nerve from the popliteal fossa (electrodes at the crease and 5 cm proximal, filters 100 to 3,000 Hz) (Figs. 8–1 and 8–11) can be helpful—an amplitude of less than 1 μV may indicate that the stimulus intensity is too low (but note that amplitudes less than 1 μV are often seen with adequate stimulus intensities). (See Section 9.1.2 for a further discussion of this use of posterior tibial SNAP.) Another maneuver that can be tried is to stimulate the tibial nerve in the popliteal fossa. This nerve contains more muscle afferents than either the common peroneal nerve at the knee or the tibial nerve at the ankle, and there is a distinct increase in the amplitudes of the lumbar potentials (Yiannikas, 1983b). If this does not produce good results, yet another technique that can be tried is to use a recording site closer to the spinal cord, thus increasing the amplitude of the waveform (Fig. 8–1). A conventional monopolar EMG electrode with approximately 1 cm of insulation removed from the tip (see Section 2) is inserted in the L1–2 (or L2–3) interspinous space (see Section 6) directed slightly upward (similar to lumbar puncture techniques) to a depth of about 3 or 4 cm, enough to position the tip in or below the interspinous ligament. In adults the subarachnoid space is 5 to 6 cm deep; thus an insertion depth of 3 to 4 cm is nowhere near that which would place the needle tip in spinal fluid. A surface electrode or another similar needle electrode is placed subcutaneously one or two interspinous spaces lower or even further away (e.g., the iliac crest) to provide the reference. (See also Lueders et al., 1981, for an interspinal ligament needle technique.) The usual sterile techniques for needle insertion must be used. Using a second needle electrode rather than a surface electrode as the reference may be helpful because the impedance characteristics of the two types of electrodes are

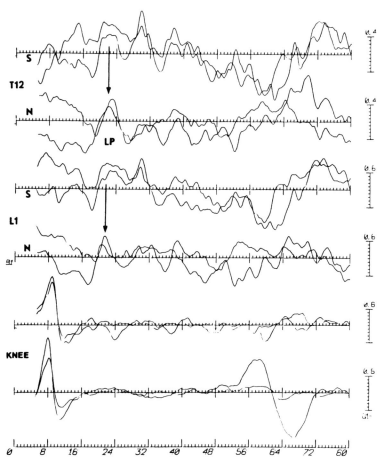

FIG. 8–1. Improvement in cauda equina/spinal cord potentials (LP) gained by use of an interspinal ligament needle electrode. Two channels were recorded at T12 and L1. The upper channel (S) was recorded from a surface disc electrode, and the lower channel (N) from an interspinal ligament electrode (see text for method). Note the improvement in LP resolution at both sites with the needle. Reference was a surface electrode at the iliac crest. Each trace is the average of 512 stimuli. The knee channels were recorded from a pair of electrodes in the popliteal fossa (in the midline at the crease and 5 cm proximal); the posterior tibial nerve was stimulated at the ankle at 5/sec. The surface-recorded channels and the upper-knee channel were acquired simultaneously, at a different time from the needle channels and the lower-knee channel, but the similarity of the knee activity confirms that the improvement in LP is due to the needle recording method. Calibrations are in microvolts.

quite different and may result in the amplifier being so "unbalanced" that excessive amounts of artifact are injected.

5. AMPLIFIER AND AVERAGER CONTROLS

Different makes of equipment require somewhat different setup procedures for a given EP, and some systems need less operator action than others. Also, it is not always possible either to find the same settings as suggested below (use the closest you can find) or even to ascertain at what values a given piece of equipment is operating (e.g., what total amplification the system is producing). The manufacturer's suggested settings usually are reasonably good.

Somatosensory EPs are best recorded by using an amplification of 100,000 to 500,000. The filters used are 1- to 30-Hz low cutoff (high pass) and 3,000 Hz high cutoff (low pass) (see Section 9.1.5 for a further discussion). The averager is set for a total sweep duration of 50 or 100 msec (upper- or lower-limb testing, respectively). Each channel should be sampled with a maximum intersample interval (dwell time) of 0.2 msec (200 µsec). Note that averager and human interpolation between these points allows latency measurements to a greater accuracy than this interval. The automatic sweep repetition control should be set to 1,000. It will be necessary sometimes to continue to 2,000 sweep repetitions if the patient is "noisy" or the responses are unclear for other reasons (e.g., abnormally low amplitude). With a great deal of experience, the waveforms can be examined after 500 stimulus repetitions and, if they are of sufficient clarity, that trial can be deemed complete. Another should always be performed and superimposed (see Section 7.10).

6. CHANNELS TO RECORD

Electrode locations and channel derivations for SEP recordings are based on two principles (Chiappa et al., 1978): (1) the waveforms are best recorded from electrode sites on the body surface closest to the presumed generator sources along the somatosensory pathways, and (2) studies of the potential-field distribution of each waveform of interest dictate the best techniques to be used. A minimum of three channels is required; four is the standard of practice and six or eight is best. Using fewer channels than three necessitates test repetition to obtain complete data and results in a waste of technician and patient time. Schemes which attempt to combine these recording derivations into one or two channels (e.g., Liberson, 1983) are based on insufficient experience with patient testing and with the variety of SEP abnormalities encountered. In clinical practice SEPs cannot be performed with fewer than three channels.

6.1. Upper Limb

6.1.1. Brachial Plexus Potential

For upper-limb testing (median, ulnar, or radial nerves) the reference point for latency measurements is the time when the action potential volley in the mixed peripheral nerve passes through some poorly defined point in the brachial plexus. Use of this reference point allows slowing in nerve conduction due to changes in limb temperature and peripheral neuropathies to be largely ignored, and greatly diminishes the variation due to different body sizes (Chiappa et al., 1980). This activity (labeled EP in Fig. 8–2) is best recorded by an electrode placed at Erb's point in the supraclavicular fossa. Erb's point is at the angle between the clavicle and the posterior border of the sternomastoid, or about 2 cm above the midpoint of the clavicle. There is considerable variation in amplitude of this activity as the recording electrode is moved to different locations in the supraclavicular fossa, so that poor registration of Erb's point is best corrected by relocating the recording electrode, in the most difficult cases, to the site where a minimal stimulus elicits muscular contraction, as discussed above in Section 4.2, or by use of a needle electrode.

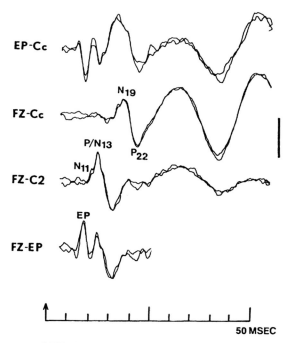

FIG. 8–2. Median nerve SEPs from a normal subject (unilateral stimulation at the wrist at arrow at 5/sec). Each trace is the average of 1,024 stimuli, with two repetitions superimposed. FZ denotes midfrontal, EP, Erb's point, C2, the middle back of the neck over the C2 cervical vertebra, and Cc, the scalp overlying the sensoriparietal cortex (2 cm behind the 10–20 system C3/C4 positions) contralateral to the stimulated limb. Relative negativity at the second electrode caused an upward deflection. Calibration mark is 2 microvolts. (From Chiappa and Ropper, 1982, with permission.)

6.1.2. Cervicomedullary Potentials

With upper-limb stimulation, potentially recordable waveforms are generated in the following structures: (1) brachial plexus, proximal cords, spinal nerves, and dorsal roots; (2) dorsal root entry zone-dorsal horns; (3) posterior columns (primarily cuneate fasciculus); (4) dorsal column nuclei (primarily nucleus cuneatus); and (5) medial lemniscus. The contributions from each of these structures produce a series of waveform peaks. However, they admix with one another in complex ways which vary between normal subjects so that, at the least, there is a good deal of normal variability in amplitude and latency; a given component may even be unrecognizable in a normal subject (see Section 9.1.6, and Emerson and Pedley, 1984, for further discussion). For clinical purposes it is necessary to concentrate attention on components which can be reliably recognized in all normal subjects (Chiappa et al., 1980; Anziska and Cracco, 1980a). A derivation commonly used to record these potentials is FZ–CII (Jones, 1977; Chiappa et al, 1978), where CII is an electrode placed on the nape of the neck in the midline at the level of the second cervical vertebra (an electrode at the level of the eighth cervical vertebra does just about as well). The most consistent and prominent waveforms recorded using this derivation are shown in Fig. 8–2, labeled N11 and P/N13. They are contributed by both electrodes; the FZ electrode primarily contributes positivities at 12 to 15 msec, whereas the neck electrode contributes negativities at slightly earlier latencies (labeled N11 and N12 in Fig. 8–3),

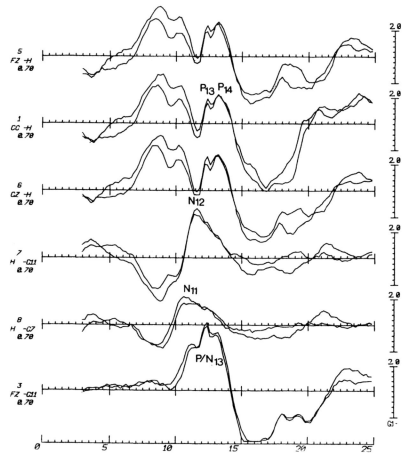

FIG. 8–3. Median nerve SEPs from a normal subject showing the activity present in the two electrodes of the FZ–CII derivation (*bottom channel*) which together generate P/N13. The midfrontal electrode (FZ) is contributing positivity peaking at 13 and 14 msec (*top channel*), whereas the CII electrode is contributing negativity peaking at 12 msec (*fourth channel from the top*); the differential amplifier records the voltage difference between these two electrodes (*bottom channel*). Unilateral stimulation at the wrist at 5/sec. Each trace is the average of 500 stimuli, with two repetitions superimposed. Electrodes as for Fig. 8–2 (CII is the same as C2, C7 is over the spine of the 7th cervical vertebra) and H denotes an electrode on the back of the hand contralateral to the limb being stimulated. Polarity as for Fig. 8–2, so that in the top two channels, relative positivity of G1 (FZ and Cc) causes an upward trace deflection, in the fourth and fifth channels from the top relative negativity of G2 (CII and C7) causes an upward trace deflection. Calibration marks in microvolts and milliseconds.

although these peak latencies are variable. The double label, P/N13, indicates that the first-named electrode (FZ) contributes mainly positivities at 13 msec and the second-named electrode contributes mainly negativities. Thus, the differential amplifier sees a maximum voltage difference between these two electrodes and a large deflection is registered in the FZ–CII channel. These activities are generated in different sources—N11–N12 in root entry zone-dorsal horns and dorsal columns, P13 in dorsal column nuclei, and P14 in medial lemniscus (see Section 9.1.6; Chapter 9, Section 1; and Emerson and Pedley, 1984, for a further discussion). However, it is not possible to register the smaller waveforms and variations reliably in all normal

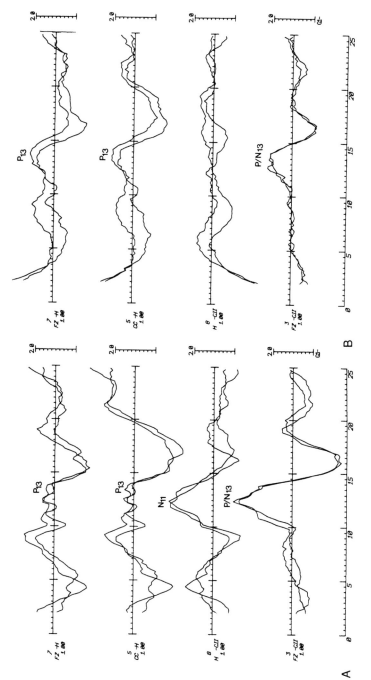

FIG. 8–4. Median nerve SEPs from a patient with nonspecific sensory complaints and examination, **A** following right-sided and **B** following left-sided stimulation. In **A**, note the normal-appearing P/N13 waveform in the bottom (FZ–CII) channel, composed of positivity (P13) from the FZ (top) channel and negativity (N11) from the CII (*third from top*) channel (the latter actually peaks at 12 msec). In **B** (left-sided stimulation) note the normal configuration but low amplitude of P/N13 in the FZ–CII (bottom) channel. The amplitude difference in this waveform between left and right sides is at the upper limit of normal. However, the absence of negativity at the CII electrode (*third channel from top*) in a "quiet" noncephalic reference channel marks the SEP as abnormal, indicating abnormal conduction central to the brachial plexus and caudal to the lower medulla. The FZ positivity is preserved (*top channel*). Each trace is the average of 500 stimuli, with two repetitions superimposed.

subjects. This is especially true with noncephalic references which show the "minor" peaks best in very quiet subjects but unfortunately often inject large amounts of muscle artifact that render the waveforms unrecognizable and uninterpretable. The time and effort needed to record these individual peaks routinely in patients are better spent in other ways, both for the patient and the technologist.

Therefore, rather than using the noncephalic reference derivations shown in Fig. 8–3 (recorded from a very "quiet" normal subject), the FZ–CII "bipolar" channel is used to routinely record and interpret these activities generated in upper cervical and medullary structures, and the composite large deflection labeled P/N13 in Fig. 8–2 is used for clinical interpretation as an indicator for the cervicomedullary junction. If more than four recording channels are available, the noncephalic derivations are sometimes useful in interpreting possible abnormalities seen in the FZ–CII channel, and, in some circumstances, may provide an additional degree of sensitivity and anatomic localization (Larrea and Mauguiere, 1988). For example, Fig. 8–4 shows a patient who demonstrates a dissociation between the potentials recorded in the two locations (neck and scalp) on left-sided stimulation, and here these derivations had clinical utility.

Also, Emerson and Pedley (1984, 1986) have suggested the use of a channel derived from electrodes placed anteriorly and posteriorly on the neck to show dorsal horn activity to best advantage by avoiding picking up persisting scalp P13–14 potentials. Mauguiere and Restuccia (1991) compared cervical SEPs using forehead and anterior cervical reference montages in six patients whose magnetic resonance imaging (MRI) scan showed a cervical syrinx. The N13 potential recorded using the forehead reference was normal in all cases, while the N13 was reduced or absent in 11 out of 12 median nerve SEPs recorded using an anterior cervical reference.

6.1.3. Thalamocortical Potentials

With upper-limb stimulation recordable activity is generated in the thalamus, thalamocortical radiations, and cortex, although the exact relationships between anatomic structures and EP waveforms are still disputed by some (see Chapter 9, Section 1, for a further discussion). The combined contributions from each of these structures produce a series of waveform peaks. However, they also admix with each other in complex ways, producing, here as also in the case of the earlier potentials, a great deal of normal variability and even sometimes "missing" peaks (see Section 9.1.6 for further discussion). Again, for clinical purposes those components which can be reliably recognized in all normal subjects (Chiappa et al., 1980) are most important. A derivation commonly used to record these potentials is FZ–Cc (Halliday and Wakefield, 1963; Giblin, 1964; Namerow, 1968; Desmedt and Noel, 1973; Jones, 1977; Chiappa et al., 1978, 1980). (In the chapters on SEPs, Cc refers to the central scalp area overlying the primary sensory cortex in the parietal lobe contralateral to the limb stimulated, and Ci refers to the same area ipsilateral to the limb stimulated; these electrode locations are 2 cm behind the standard 10–20 system C3/C4 positions.) The waveforms recorded in this channel are shown in Fig. 8–2, labeled N19 and P22. They are contributed by both electrodes; the FZ electrode contributes negativity from 15 to 20 msec, and the Cc electrode contributes negativity over the same latency range but of greater amplitude in the latter part of it (Fig. 8–5). In the early portion of this time span the differential amplifier sees no voltage difference between these two sites and no deflection is registered; then, as the two sites' activities diverge, a voltage difference develops and reaches a maximum at about 19 msec or so when a large deflection is registered (Fig. 8–5). This deflection has been classically labeled N20 (or N19). (See Chapter 9, Section 1, for a further discussion of generator sources of N20

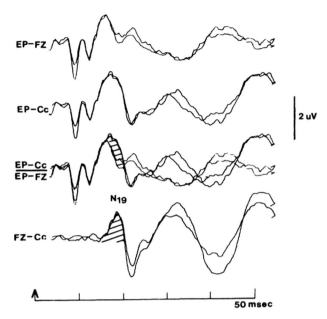

FIG. 8–5. Median nerve SEPs from a normal subject illustrating that N19, as recorded in a FZ–Cc derivation, represents the difference in negativity between those two electrodes. The FZ–Cc channel (*bottom*) shows the actual waveforms registered in that derivation. At the same time, recordings were made from FZ and Cc using a noncephalic reference (Erb's point) in order to register the actual amount of negativity at those two sites (these negativities start earlier (at about 15 msec) than the peak of N19, as can also be seen by comparing the top two channels in Fig. 8–2). The waveforms from the FZ and Cc electrodes were then superimposed, in the third channel, and the difference in negativity between them was crosshatched; this area corresponds to the area under the N19 peak.

and the positivity which follows it.) The actual amount of negativity recordable at Cc is shown in the Cc–hand (or Erb's point) channel in Figs. 8–2 and 8–5. However, the hand reference often injects excessive amounts of artifact, rendering clinical interpretation on that channel difficult in many patients. Therefore, although the FZ–Cc bipolar channel provides an "artificial" view of what is actually going on, it is the most reliable for clinical interpretations. The noncephalic reference channel is recommended as a check on the bipolar channel since an occasional normal subject will have little difference in negativity between these two sites and thus no N19 will be recorded in the bipolar derivation. (See also the comments by Zegers de Beyl and Brunko, 1995, on the use of an earlobe reference.) It may be that it will be possible to demonstrate a dissociation between early and late components of this negativity so that the separate parts will have clinical utility, but this remains to be proved. Raising the low-cutoff filter to 150 or 300 Hz may assist in this endeavor (see Section 9.1.5).

6.1.4. Recommended Montages

The recommended four-channel montage for recording upper limb SEPs is:

Channel 1: FZ to Cc
Channel 2: FZ to CII
Channel 3: FZ to EP
Channel 4: Hand to Cc (optional)

Polarity is arranged so that relative negativity of the second-named electrode causes an upward deflection.

If more than four channels are available, the following derivations may help in interpretation of the above channels:

Channel 5: FZ to Hand
Channel 6: Hand to CII
Channel 7: Hand to CVII
Channel 8: Anterior neck to CV

Cc refers to the central scalp area overlying the primary sensory cortex in the parietal lobe contralateral to the limb stimulated, and Ci refers to the same area ipsilateral to the limb stimulated; EP refers to Erb's point; CII, CV, and CVII refer to the nape of the neck in the midline overlying the level of that cervical vertebra; hand refers to an electrode on the back of the hand (any noncephalic site, such as knee, wrist, or toe, would do just as well); anterior neck refers to the level of the thyroid cartilage in the midline.

6.2. Lower Limb

6.2.1. Cauda Equina—Lower-Cord Potentials

For lower-limb testing (tibial and peroneal nerves) the reference point for latency measurements is the time when the action potential volley in the mixed peripheral nerve passes through the cauda equina and lower spinal cord. Activity in these structures is collectively referred to herein as the lumbar potential, usually labeled LP in the figures. Use of this reference point allows slowing in nerve conduction velocity due to changes in limb temperature and peripheral neuropathies to be largely ignored, and also diminishes the variation due to different body sizes (Wilson et al., 1981). This activity (labeled LP in Figs. 8–6 through 8–9 and 8–11) is best recorded by an electrode placed over the spine at the L1 level, referred to an electrode two or three interspaces away or to a reference electrode on the iliac crest. This is a small potential and reliable recognition of it is greatly assisted by routine use of both of the derivations suggested above. Generator sources of this activity are discussed in Section 9.1.6 and in Chapter 9, Section 1). Emerson (1988) has suggested use of a T12 or T11 recording electrode site since the highest-amplitude LP was seen at that level in 20 of 21 patients studied at eight levels, although our experience at that level has been inconsistent.

Stimulation of the posterior tibial nerve at the ankle usually produces higher-amplitude lumbar and scalp potentials than stimulation of the common peroneal nerve at the knee, as illustrated in Fig. 8–6, both from the same subject. The reason for this amplitude difference is not clear but it may be related to the rich innervation of the sole of the foot; whether or not the posterior tibial nerve at the ankle contains more group Ia muscle afferents than the peroneal nerve at the knee is not known (see also Pelosi et al., 1988). Clinical experience shows that in some patients different results may be seen following stimulation of the two nerves (i.e., one may show normal results and the other abnormal), but this is not in a consistent pattern. In clinically difficult cases testing of both nerves may be helpful (see also Section 9.2.2 below).

If the latencies of the scalp components are abnormal, then it is important to register this lumbar potential reliably since its latency will differentiate delay caused by peripheral sources from delay in conduction rostral to the lower cord. When it is necessary to use the

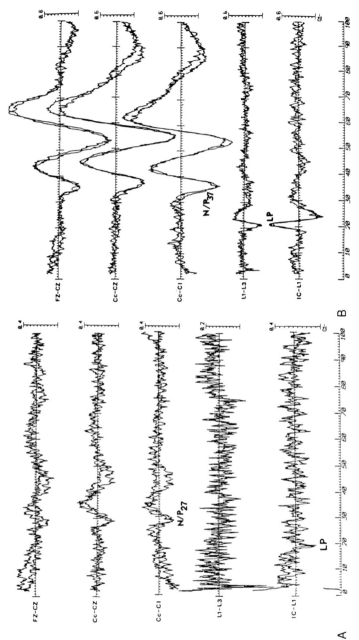

FIG. 8–6. Lower-limb SEPs following unilateral stimulation at 2/sec of the common peroneal nerve at the knee (**A**) and posterior tibial nerve at the ankle (**B**) illustrating the larger-amplitude potentials usually obtained with the latter at both spinal and cerebral levels. With peroneal nerve stimulation the spinal potentials (*lower two channels*) can barely be recognized even at high display magnifications, whereas with tibial nerve stimulation they are very clear. Cerebral potentials (*top three channels*) show similar amplitude differences between **A** and **B**. Each trace is the average of 500 stimuli with two repetitions superimposed. Cc and Ci as for Fig. 8–2, contra- and ipsilateral to the stimulated limb, L1 and L3 are surface electrodes overlying those lumbar spines, and IC is an electrode on the iliac crest contralateral to the stimulated limb. Note that in **A** (peroneal) LP is downgoing since L1 electrode is G2. Also note that in **B** (tibial), fourth channel, electrodes are plugged in opposite to usual fashion, so that LP in this channel also points downward.

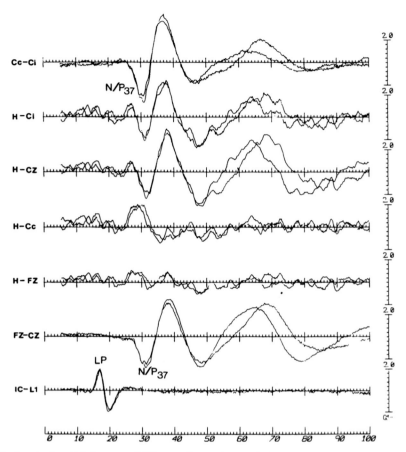

FIG. 8–7. Posterior tibial nerve SEPs (unilateral stimulation at 2/sec) in a normal subject illustrating the most common variation of the scalp potential field distributions from 28 to 40 msec (see text for details). This subject was short—147 cm—so that absolute latencies are earlier than usual. The noncephalic (hand) reference channels all show an initial negativity peaking at 27 to 28 msec, largest in the Cc area. This negativity is replaced by a positivity that appears earliest and has the largest amplitude in central (CZ) and ipsilateral central (Ci) areas. Each trace is the average of 1,000 stimuli, with two repetitions superimposed.

lumbar potential to make this distinction and the surface electrodes do not show an interpretable waveform, then it is important to try both tibial nerve stimulation in the popliteal fossa and the needle electrode recording technique described above in Section 4 to assist in the registration of good waveforms. Also, if the lumbar potential can be recorded from one side and is normal, indicating that the site of the conduction defect is above the cauda equina in the spinal cord or higher, and if the cerebral potential following stimulation of the other side shows the same abnormal absolute latency but no LP can be recorded, then the good LP recording from only the one side is sufficient to localize the conduction defect as rostral to the cauda equina. If LP cannot be recorded despite all maneuvers described above, the H-reflex may be used to assist in the assessment of the peripheral nerves (e.g., De Graaf et al., 1988). However, since stimulation for the H-reflex is delivered at the knee and

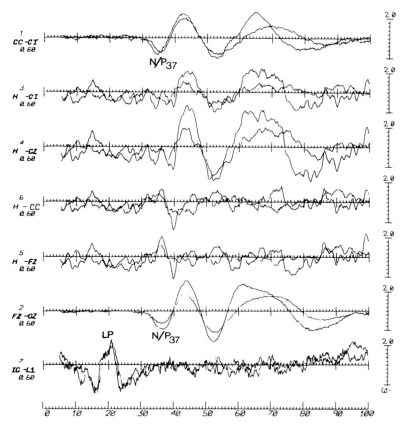

FIG. 8–8. Posterior tibial nerve SEPs (unilateral stimulation at 2/sec) in a normal subject illustrating a variation of the potential field distribution different from that seen in Fig. 8–7. The peak at 36 msec in the FZ–CZ channel (*second from bottom*, labeled N/P37) is usually produced by positivity at CZ (see Fig. 8–7); however, here CZ is inactive at that point and negativity at FZ (*third channel from bottom*) is generating the peak seen in the bipolar channel. Erroneous interpretations result when this peak is small and the second, major downgoing peak in the FZ–CZ channel (here at 52 msec) is assumed to represent the earliest activity, as illustrated in Fig. 8–9. Each trace is the average of 1,000 stimuli, with two repetitions superimposed.

recordings are made over the soleus muscle in the calf, there still remains 20 to 25 cm of peripheral nerve not tested, which could have abnormal conduction. Also, half of the H-reflex latency is contributed by conduction in motor fibers.

Note that these cauda equina and lower-cord potentials are more difficult to record following sural and saphenous nerve stimulation, possibly because those nerves lack muscle Ia afferents which generate a large part of this response.

Registration of the SNAP of the posterior tibial nerve from the popliteal fossa (electrodes at the crease and 5 cm proximal, filters 100 to 3,000 Hz) (Figs. 8–1 and 8–11) may be helpful when LP amplitudes are low. An amplitude of less than 1 μV may indicate that the stimulus intensity is too low (but note that amplitudes less than 1 μV are often seen with adequate stimulus intensities). (See Section 9.1.2 for a further discussion of the use of the knee SNAP in this situation.)

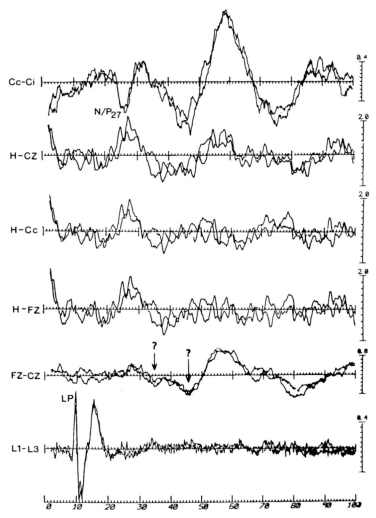

FIG. 8–9. Peroneal nerve SEPs (unilateral stimulation at 2/sec) illustrating a normal variation of the potential field distribution over the scalp which would result in an erroneous interpretation if FZ–CZ (*second channel from bottom*) was the only recording derivation available. The earliest activity at 27 to 28 msec is negative at both FZ (*fourth channel from top*) and CZ (*second channel from top*) so that the FZ–CZ derivation records nothing at this point. The most prominent peaks in the FZ–CZ channel occur later, at the question marks (35 and 45 msec); the Cc–Ci channel shows a clear peak at a normal latency of 26 msec, composed of negative activity from Cc and positive activity from Ci. Each trace is the average of 500 stimuli, with two repetitions superimposed. Note the different display magnification and calibrations on each channel.

6.2.2. Cervicomedullary Potentials

With lower-limb stimulation, waveforms similar to those following upper-limb stimulation thought to be generated in the structures in the spinal canal and brain stem cannot be easily registered from surface electrodes. This may be because the longer distance traveled by the volley results in temporal dispersion, so that its amplitude at any one point in time is not large enough to be seen at the skin surface. Since large numbers of stimuli must be given and the patient must be unusually quiet, definition of these potentials is not routinely useful in clinical practice. An FZ–C5 spine derivation can record the volley at cervical levels (see the third channel from the top in Fig. 8–11). However, this C5 potential is difficult to resolve cleanly and often is not available for analysis when there might be a clinical role for its data, e.g., LP–N/P37 is delayed for height and one would like to localize the conduction delay relative to the neck level.

When clinical circumstances are such that this information would be useful, recordings can be made from needle electrodes (see Section 4.2 and Figs. 8–1 and 8–11). Also, Lueders et al. (1981) have used an interspinal ligament needle electrode technique to reliably record from thoracic and cervical levels, primarily in anesthetized patients.

6.2.3. Thalamocortical Potentials

For various reasons, including temporal dispersion of the afferent volley mentioned above, the thalamocortical potentials generated by lower limb stimulation are smaller than those seen with upper-limb stimulation, and stimulation of sensory nerves lacking muscle afferents generates potentials smaller than those from nerves with muscular connections. Thus, the earliest cerebral potentials with lower-limb stimulation are more difficult to resolve than those from upper-limb stimulation.

To arrive at the best channel derivations for recording the earliest cerebral components, one must consider their timing and scalp potential-field distributions, which are not necessarily what they are commonly assumed to be. For example, the earliest, well-defined cerebral potentials resulting from stimulation of the posterior tibial nerve at the ankle (peaking at 32 to 36 msec after stimulation) are initially negative in all scalp areas, of greatest amplitude and duration in central contralateral and midline anterior regions (Fig. 8–7). This negative activity is preceded by an inconsistent, low-amplitude positivity. At the midline vertex and in ipsilateral central areas this early negativity blends immediately into a well-localized, larger-amplitude positivity which is the activity that has received the greatest attention as registered in the FZ–CZ derivation.

Cruse et al. (1982) have suggested that this positive activity is most consistent and of greatest amplitude at a point midway between CZ and PZ, thus they recommend that recording location. Because the waveform registered at about 37 msec in the FZ–CZ channel is a complex admixture of negative activity at FZ and positive activity at CZ, as described above, the label N/P37 (Figs. 8–6 to 8–8) is most accurate.

However, although this is the most common pattern, there is considerable variation even among normal subjects so that some show negativity at FZ but essentially no activity (positive or negative) at CZ at this time (Fig. 8–8). The apparent positive "downward" deflection seen in the FZ–CZ channel (labeled N/P37 in the second channel from the bottom) is present because CZ is less negative than FZ and thus is relatively more positive as far as the differential amplifier is concerned. Activities in the central areas ipsilateral and contralateral to the limb being stimulated have more consistent polarities than the midline (CZ and FZ) areas, especially following peroneal nerve stimulation; this suggests that the Cc and Ci recording sites be used, in the derivations suggested below, to assist in waveform recognition in the FZ–CZ channel. The differential amplifier sees the opposite polarity activities as a maximum voltage difference between the two points and thus registers a large deflection (Cc–Ci channel in Figs. 8–6 through 8–8 and 8–10). Note that this admixture of activities does not necessarily bear a latency relationship to the activity recorded in the FZ–CZ chan-

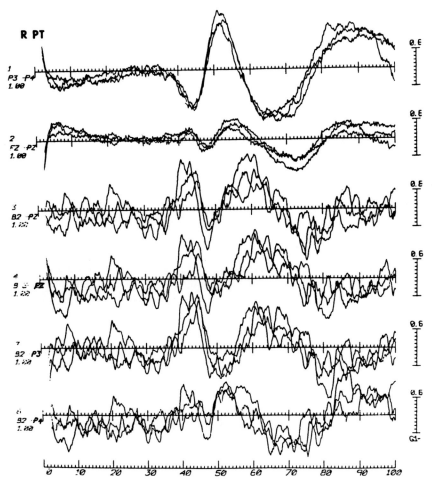

FIG. 8–10. Scalp recordings following stimulation of the right posterior tibial nerve at the ankle. Top channel is the contralateral central area linked to the ipsilateral central area (Cc–Ci), the second channel is FZ–PZ (slightly behind CZ), and the next four channels are PZ, FZ, Cc, and Ci, all referenced to the dorsum of the right hand. Note that N/P37 (in FZ–PZ at *arrow*) occurs about 3.5 msec after the major deflection in Cc–Ci (*small arrow*), so that a different set of normal values is required if the Cc–Ci derivation is used for clinical interpretations. The downward deflection in Cc–Ci is primarily caused by a prominent negativity in the Cc channel (compare bottom two channels). Each trace is the average of 512 stimuli delivered at 5/sec. Relative negativity of the second-named electrode caused an upward trace deflection. Calibration marks are 0.6 μV for all channels.

nel (compare top two channels in Fig. 8–10), so that normal values must be collected specifically for the Cc–Ci channel (peak latency usually about 1 msec shorter).

There are significant differences in scalp topography between peroneal, tibial, and sural nerve EPs, presumably related to their different somatotopic representations and fiber content (sensory nerves lacking muscle afferents). The variability between normal subjects, even with the same nerve being tested, probably relates to normal anatomic variations, as is also the explanation for the great variability in pattern-shift visual EP (PSVEP) P100 potential-field distribution with partial-field stimulation (see Chapter 2, Section 8.1.5, and Fig.

2–15). Differences in subdivisions of the nerve stimulated due to changes in the relative positions of the stimulating electrode and the nerve and nerve fascicles (e.g., superficial versus deep peroneal segments with stimulation of the common peroneal nerve at the fibular head) may also account for some of the intersubject variability. (See also Section 9.1.7 below.)

The potential-field distributions of activities produced by stimulation of the peroneal nerve at the knee show greater variability between normal subjects than those seen with posterior tibial nerve stimulation (hence the greater clinical utility of stimulating the latter nerve)(see also Pelosi et al., 1988). This variability presumably relates to the more lateral somatotopic representation of the leg as compared with the foot, so that a greater change in potential field over the scalp is produced by an anatomic variation. The most marked of these normal peroneal nerve variations may result in incorrect waveform recognition and erroneous interpretations, especially in the midline (FZ–CZ) channel. Figure 8–9 shows such a case, where the question marks indicate the places where one would most likely pick the N/P27 peak (stimulation of peroneal nerve at the knee) in the FZ–CZ derivation. The hand reference channels show that FZ, CZ, and Cc all have a good deal of negativity at the normal latency, but it is not registered in FZ–CZ because the two electrodes are equipotential; the Cc–Ci derivation clearly shows the normal latency peak. Although doubt will always remain in any interpretation of this particular test (i.e., some would say that the lack of positivity at CZ is an abnormality in itself), in conformity with the conservative customs of clinical neurophysiology, it is most properly interpreted as normal, whereas reliance on only the FZ–CZ derivation would result in an abnormal interpretation. Thus, the Cc–Ci derivation is much less susceptible to these variations and, therefore, along with the FZ–CZ derivation, is a recommended derivation for recording following peroneal nerve stimulation (as well as following posterior tibial nerve stimulation).

Even with the relative consistency of the potentials recorded from Cc and Ci (with either posterior tibial or common peroneal nerve stimulation), it is best to record also from Cc, Ci, and CZ using a noncephalic reference so that any anomalies which might cause an erroneous bipolar recording can be recognized. However, the artifact injected by the noncephalic sites is often sufficient to make recognition of the small, early negative potential impossible, thus this derivation is not by itself sufficient for clinical use. (See also Section 9.1.6 for a further discussion.) Certainly the simultaneous use of FZ–CZ and Ci–Cc is highly recommended. The degree of normal variability discussed above, best managed in clinical practice by recording from scalp electrodes using several different derivations, dictates that SEPs from lower limbs be recorded with no less than four channels (see Fig. 8–10).

6.2.4. Recommended Montages

As mentioned above, it is recommended that the posterior tibial nerve be used in routine lower limb testing. A suggested four-channel montage, illustrated in Fig. 8–11 (with an additional channel, L3–L1) for recording SEPs following lower limb stimulation is:

Channel 1: Cc to Ci
Channel 2: FZ to CZ (or mid-CZ/PZ)
Channel 3: Iliac crest to L1 (and/or T12)
Channel 4: Crease of popliteal fossa to 5 cm proximal

Cc refers to the central scalp area overlying the primary sensory cortex in the parietal lobe contralateral to the limb stimulated, and Ci refers to the same area ipsilateral to the

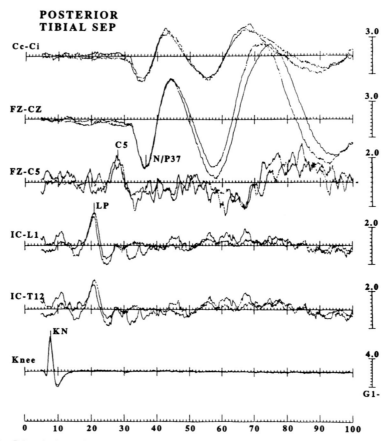

FIG. 8–11. Stimulation of the posterior tibial nerve at the ankle in a normal subject using a recommended recording montage. Each trace is the average of 512 stimuli delivered at 5/sec. The knee channel, recorded from surface disc electrodes in the midline at the popliteal fossa crease and 5 cm proximal, shows the peripheral mixed nerve action potential, useful for judging the adequacy of stimulus intensity and peripheral nerve conduction velocity when LP is absent or poorly defined. Calibrations are in microvolts.

limb stimulated (2 cm behind the 10–20 System C3/C4 locations). Mid-CZ/PZ refers to a point halfway between CZ and PZ. C5, T12, L1, and L3 refer to the midline overlying the level of that vertebra; hand refers to an electrode on the back of the hand (any noncephalic site such as knee, wrist, toe would do just as well). Polarity is assumed to be such that relative negativity of G2 causes an upward trace deflection (positivity is down).

Lower-limb testing is more practically obtained using six-channel recording (Fig. 8–11):

Channel 1: Cc to Ci
Channel 2: FZ to CZ (or mid-CZ/PZ)
Channel 3: FZ to C5
Channel 4: Iliac crest to L1
Channel 5: Iliac crest to T12
Channel 6: Crease of popliteal fossa to 5 cm proximal

Additional channels can be added to record the spinal cord potential at higher levels or to more clearly define the potential-field distributions of activities of interest. Because of the normal variability discussed above, the more information that is available, the easier it is to arrive at a correct interpretation of difficult cases.

7. RUNNING THE TEST

7.1. Subject Relaxation

The test must be performed with the patient supine on a bed with pillows and towels available for head propping to minimize neck muscle tone. The room should be reasonably quiet. The signal-averaging apparatus should be outside the room with a closed door between the averager and the patient. This allows test results to be plotted and discussed without arousing the patient, who, hopefully, has fallen asleep during the test. It is also very helpful if the electrode selection and stimulator controls are outside the room so that no entry is necessary during the test, although the stimulus intensity control is best located close to the patient.

The most common problem encountered with the test is excessive muscle activity. If head propping in various ways does not solve this, other factors must be considered: Is the patient too cold or hot? Does the patient need to go to the bathroom? Is the supine position too uncomfortable (lying on the side may help)? If the problem persists despite consideration of these factors, a mild hypnotic may be given (chloral hydrate and/or diphenhydramine) to induce drowsiness and sleep. Note that the patient should not drive soon after taking a hypnotic. In the most difficult cases it may be necessary to plan the study as for a sleep EEG; the patient is instructed to stay up 2 hours later at night than normal, and take no stimulants with breakfast, and the study is performed in the morning.

7.2. Stimulus Sites

The location of the peripheral nerves and techniques of stimulation can be found in any textbook of EMG. Those most commonly used are the median, ulnar, and radial nerves at the wrist, the posterior tibial nerve at the ankle, the peroneal nerve at the knee, and the sural nerve. The posterior tibial nerve is usually located 2 to 3 cm posterior to the medial malleolus.

Stimulus sites should be prepared by rubbing with fine sandpaper followed by acetone degreasing. The ground site is similarly prepared.

It is the standard of practice in EMG that the cathode of the stimulating pair should be proximal because nerve activation occurs closer to the cathode. However, the difference is slight and over the distance involved (e.g., from wrist to brachial plexus) the latency variation involved (less than 0.5 msec) is not significant when admixed with variations due to limb temperature and length. Furthermore, when the brachial plexus potential is used as the reference point for interpeak latencies (IPLs) and all measurements are taken from that point, the relative positions of the stimulating anode and cathode have no effect.

7.3. Stimulus Intensity

The stimulus intensity is adjusted to produce a minimal movement at the joint involved (e.g., thumb twitch with median nerve stimulation at the wrist). Only a small movement of the toes is required with posterior tibial nerve stimulation. For most peripheral nerves, using

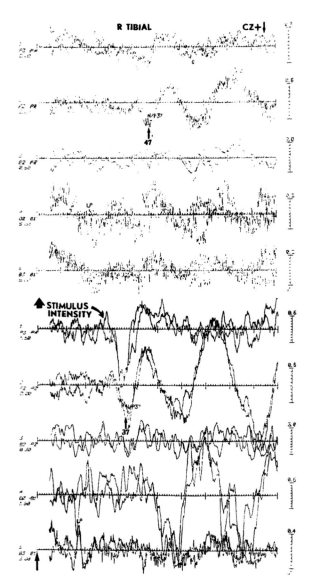

FIG. 8–12. Right posterior tibial nerve stimulation at the ankle in a patient with nonspecific sensory complaints. In the initial test (*upper five channels*) the patient complained about the stimulus and the intensity used was below motor threshold. The apparent N/P37 in the FZ–PZ channel (*second from top*) was at a markedly delayed latency, and LP was poorly defined (*fourth and fifth channels*). The test was repeated with the patient being encouraged and the stimulus intensity slightly above motor threshold (*lower five channels*). N/P37 latency decreased 10 msec into the normal range, and LP was well-defined (*bottom channel*). In each test the channels from the top are Cc–Ci, FZ–PZ, dorsum of hand to PZ, iliac crest to L1, and L3–L1; positivity of the second-named electrode caused a downward trace deflection. Each trace is the average of 512 stimuli delivered at 5/sec. Sweep duration was 100 msec, calibration marks are in microvolts.

surface stimulation, the current required to achieve this will be in the range of 5 to 15 mA (less for needles). If there is a peripheral neuropathy this may be greater and may also require a longer stimulus duration (e.g., 500 μsec). As mentioned above, the possibility of producing extreme patient discomfort or tissue damage, especially if long pulse durations and high repetition rates are used, dictates that care be exercised with these stimulating devices, which

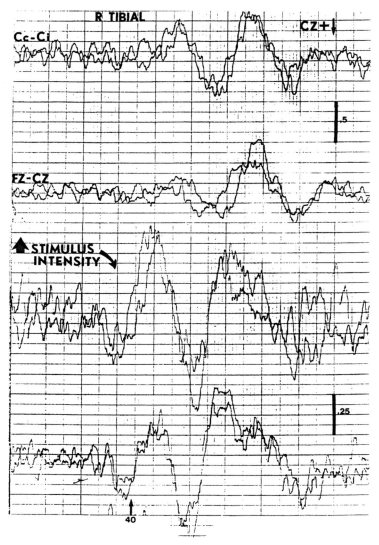

FIG. 8–13. Right posterior tibial nerve stimulation at the ankle in another patient with non-specific sensory complaints. In the initial test (*upper two channels*) the patient complained about the stimulus and the intensity used was below motor threshold. N/P37 may be thought to be absent or markedly delayed (*open arrow in second channel*), although the preceding upward deflection (*thin arrow*) is rarely seen preceding a true N/P37 in the FZ–PZ (or CZ) derivation and suggests that the apparent N/P37 (*open arrow*) is actually the major positivity that follows N/P37 (*open arrow in bottom channel*). With an increase in stimulus intensity (*lower two channels*) N/P37 appeared at a normal latency (*immediately prior to 40 msec label*). Stimulus occurred at arrow at 5/sec and the label shows a 40-msec interval. Calibration marks are in microvolts.

should be operated only by properly trained personnel. (See Section 9.1.2 for a discussion of different types of intensity levels used and their effects on latency and amplitude.)

Inadequate stimulation of the tibial nerve sometimes results in apparently delayed scalp potentials and the latency returns to normal when the stimulus intensity is increased. If the stimulus does not activate group I fibers in the posterior tibial nerve (electrodes improperly placed and/or stimulus intensity too low), only the slower-conducting cutaneous afferents (group II) will generate an apparently delayed potential, with lumbar activity difficult to record. Increasing stimulus intensity will result in latency normalization (Fig. 8–12). Patients may complain that the stimulus is painful, either for psychological reasons or because of dysesthesia from a peripheral neuropathy or other neurologic disease, and may not allow a sufficient stimulus intensity to be used. The only check on the adequacy of posterior tibial nerve stimulation is the technician's observation of a good muscle twitch in the intrinsic foot muscles supplied by the nerve and the presence of good-amplitude lumbar point activity. When recording the sensory nerve action potential from the popliteal fossa (electrodes at the crease and 5 cm proximal, filters 100–3,000 Hz) (see Figs. 8–1 and 8–11) an amplitude of less than 1 μV may indicate that the stimulus intensity is too low (but note that amplitudes less than 1 μV are often seen with adequate stimulus intensities). Another, more subtle indication of the possibility of inadequate stimulus intensity is the waveform configuration of the scalp activities. In the FZ–CZ derivation the initial major deflection is positive (N/P37); with low stimulus intensities this waveform will be of low amplitude or absent and the initial deflection will be the negativity which usually follows N/P37 (Fig. 8–13).

7.4. Unilateral Stimulation

The stimulus is applied to one limb at a time, since many SEP abnormalities are seen following stimulation of only one limb, stimulation of the other limb producing perfectly normal results. For example, in a group of 114 multiple sclerosis (MS) patients (all three diagnostic categories), 48% (29 of 61) of those with abnormal tests had unilateral abnormalities of median SEPs and 22% (16 of 73) had unilateral abnormalities of peroneal SEPs (Brooks et al., 1983). If bilateral stimulation is used, the normal waveforms generated by the "good" side mask the abnormality on the "bad" side. The only possible use for bilateral stimulation in SEP testing may be for obtaining a larger-amplitude response when using the lower-limb SEP to monitor spinal cord functioning during surgery. Here one may be interested only in whether or not the continuity of spinal cord tracts is preserved so that the largest and most visible response is desired. Also, in the latter situation, lateralizing information is less pertinent. (See the discussion of stimulus mode in Section 9.1.4 below.)

7.5. Stimulus Rate

Because SEP waveform amplitudes are so low, it is necessary to use 1,000 or more stimulus repetitions to ensure waveform clarity. The faster the stimulus rate, the less the time taken in performing the test. However, progressive losses in waveform resolution and latency changes occur with rates much above 5/sec, so that that rate is the preferred one. Faster rates only very rarely reveal abnormalities not evident at slower rates. (See Section 9.1.3 for further discussion.)

In lower-limb testing in patients we have found that spinal cord and cerebral potentials may not be recorded well at 5/sec but dramatically improve in appearance at 2/sec. The reason for this is not known and it is not necessarily an indicator of abnormal function in the system, but the frequency of the phenomenon makes it a worthwhile modification of the testing procedure in difficult cases.

7.6. Stimulus Shape

The stimulus is a square wave of 200 μsec duration applied through the isolation transformer. Stimulus polarity has no effect on SEPs.

7.7. Stimulus Artifact

The most difficult technical problem with SEPs, after that of excessive muscle artifact, is stimulus artifact. The approach to this problem should be systematic:

1. Is a stimulus isolation device being used?
2. Has the ground been properly applied? What is the impedance of the ground electrode? It should be less than 7,000 ohms. If it is excessively high the connections of the ground strap may be broken.
3. Is the ground connected to the amplifier input ground terminal (usually on the electrode connector box) or is it connected to the ground post on the stimulator? Switching from one to the other may help.
4. Is the stimulus current excessively high, and, if so, why? Can it be diminished by better application of the stimulating electrodes (i.e., lowering their impedance) or more careful location of the optimum site for nerve stimulation? If neither of these help, then needle electrode stimulation may allow sufficient stimulus current reduction to allow recording.
5. What is the orientation of the stimulating electrode relative to the recording electrodes? Altering this relationship by rotating the stimulating electrode in various directions will change the amount of stimulus artifact recorded.
6. What is the setting of the amplifier low-frequency filters? Sometimes changing this to lower values diminishes stimulus artifact (e.g., 10 Hz to 1 Hz); sometimes the opposite is true. If there is a 60-Hz notch filter being used, switching this off will sometimes help.

The above maneuvers will suffice in the majority of cases. In special circumstances (e.g., trigeminal nerve stimulation) there may still be difficulty. Since most of the problem relates to charge storage at the stimulating electrode interface and in the subject, "fast-recovery" amplifiers are not particularly helpful. Various artifact "suppressor" devices and schemes may or may not help. McGill et al. (1982) have made a systematic theoretical and practical approach to the problem of stimulus artifact. Careful attention to the factors mentioned above will suffice in most cases. Emerson et al. (1988b) have suggested post-hoc removal of stimulus artifact.

7.8. Infant Testing

Special procedures are necessary for infants. Testing must be scheduled for a time when they will be comfortable (fed and dry) and asleep. Small stimulating electrodes must be used. (See Chapter 11 for further details.)

7.9. Artifact Rejection

As discussed, the major factor interfering with registration of good SEPs is ambient muscle artifact, and time spent diminishing this is well-repaid in clarity of results. However, there are transient bursts of artifact that cannot be anticipated and there needs to be a mechanism for excluding these from the average. On the simplest level, the technician watches the ongoing, raw EEG signal (and artifact) on a monitoring oscilloscope set for a sweep speed of 10 msec/cm with automatic triggering. Whenever excessive artifact appears on the screen, the technician manually halts averaging. There is obviously room for error here since there may be a significant lag between artifact appearance and averaging being stopped. Most averaging systems now in use have some form of automatic artifact rejection and this should certainly be used when recording SEPs. (See Chapter 1, Section 2.4, for a discussion of automatic artifact rejection techniques.) Various other on- and offline techniques of artifact suppression and removal are also available (see Chapter 17).

7.10. Trial Repetition

It is *mandatory* in SEP testing to undertake a repeat trial after the first one and superimpose the two to test waveform consistency. It may be necessary to repeat the test two to four times to arrive at a good measure of response variability. Although at least 1,000 stimulus repetitions are usually recommended, with a great deal of experience the waveforms can be examined after 500 stimulus repetitions and, if they are of sufficient clarity, that trial can be deemed complete. At least one other should still be performed and superimposed to verify waveform reliability (see the figures in this chapter and Chapter 9).

7.11. Resolution of Unclear Waveforms

When the SEP waveforms registered using all of the above-recommended procedures are unclear for any reason, operations that can be tried are (1) increasing stimulus repetitions to 2,000, (2) performing multiple trials, (3) increasing stimulus intensity slightly if waveforms have low amplitude and poor definition, and (4) using special stimulating sites or recording electrodes (e.g., with lumbar potentials). These parameter modifications have been discussed in detail in their separate sections above. (See also Chapter 1, Section 5, and Lueders et al., 1985.)

If muscle artifact is a major problem, sedation of the patient should also be considered. Some laboratories use hypnotic or tranquilizing medications to allow the noncephalic references to be used routinely (e.g., 10 mg diazepam PO at the beginning of the test), but this is unacceptable when testing outpatients, who often must drive or otherwise find their own way home.

8. READING THE RESULTS, NORMATIVE DATA, AND VARIATIONS

8.1. Waveform Identification

It is difficult to provide a written method for identification of SEP waveform peaks. The following comments apply reasonably well with normal results but will be increasingly difficult to apply as the degree of abnormality increases.

1. The brachial plexus potential appears as a diphasic, positive–negative waveform in the EP–FZ channel. Although the first deflection, which ends in a positive peak, is used in nerve conduction studies for measurements, it is significantly lower in amplitude than the following negative peak. Since one is looking for a reference point on which to base subsequent latency measurements, the preferred peak is the larger, more consistent negative one, labeled EP in Fig. 8–2.

2. Activity in upper cervical cord and lower brain stem produced by upper-limb stimulation appears as a major deflection in the FZ–CII channel (Fig. 8–2) with superimposed smaller lobulations and peaks. The smaller waveforms cannot be consistently recognized in normal subjects, so the midpoint of the large deflection is estimated (interpolated) and that location used for P/N13 latency measurements (Fig. 8–14).

3. Thalamocortical activity produced by upper-limb stimulation appears as a negative–positive deflection in the FZ–Cc channel (see Fig. 8–2). The initial negative deflection often does not present a well-formed peak, so in those cases a visual interpolation must be performed as with P/N13 (Fig. 8–14). The following positivity (P22) is too variable in shape in normal subjects to use for latency measurements; its amplitude (baseline to peak or N19–P22) is sometimes used in interside comparisons.

4. Thalamocortical activity produced by lower-limb stimulation appears as a major deflection in the Cc–Ci and FZ–CZ channels (labeled N/P37 in Figs. 8–7 and 8–8). Ac-

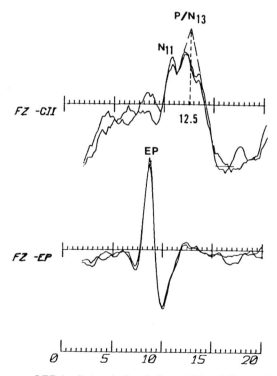

FIG. 8–14. Median nerve SEP (unilateral stimulation at 5/sec) illustrating the interpolation of the P/N13 peak used to arrive at a point of reference for latency measurements in clinical interpretations. This is done because the separate peaks are not recognizable in all normal subjects and patients, often being fused together, and this technique provides a consistent approach. Each trace is the average of 500 stimuli, with two repetitions superimposed.

tivity in either one of these may be less well-formed than in the other; measurements are taken in the channel with the best, that is, clearest, responses. Normal values must be available for whatever derivation is used as the Cc–Ci waveform is usually 1 msec or so earlier than that in FZ–CZ. When a clean peak is not present a visual interpolation must be performed. If there is any doubt about peak location, the Cc, CZ, and other noncephalic reference channels should be examined, if available. If the level of ambient muscle artifact is not excessive, the negative–positive peaks will show clearly there without the admixed contribution from an "active" electrode to confuse the issue.

5. Lumbar activity produced by activity in the cauda equina and root entry zone appears as a positive–negative deflection in the L1 electrode (see Figs. 8–6 to 8–9). The initial major negative deflection in the iliac crest reference derivation is the most reliable and is the best to use in routine clinical interpretations.

8.2. Interpeak Latencies, Interside Differences and Amplitude Ratios

Measurements and calculations performed include (1) absolute latency of N/P37 for lower-limb (posterior tibial nerve at ankle) stimulation, (2) interpeak latencies (IPLs), that is, EP–P/N13, P/N13–N19, EP–N19 for upper limb, and LP–N/P37 for lower limb (if the height-corrected absolute N/P37 latency is abnormal), (3) interpeak, interside differences, and (4) interside amplitude ratios.

The patient's height must be recorded since it is used to correct the lower-limb absolute latencies or lumbar to cerebral conduction times for distance traveled. This correction allows a stricter definition of normality, thus increasing the sensitivity of the test. The patient's height is located on a nomogram which then shows the upper limit (mean plus 3 SD) for that measure (absolute latency of lumbar or scalp potentials or conduction time) (Figs. 8–15 to 8–17).

The distance between the stimulating electrode (midpoint between the anode and cathode) and the electrode recording the lumbar or brachial plexus potentials must be recorded since it is used to compute the mixed nerve conduction velocity over that segment of the peripheral nerve. This datum is sometimes a useful by-product of SEP testing since it may indicate the presence of a previously unsuspected peripheral neuropathy. Nerve conduction velocity in meters per second is the distance in millimeters divided by the latency in milliseconds (or the distance in centimeters divided by the latency in milliseconds multiplied by 10).

→

FIG. 8–15. (A) Plot of the absolute latency of the lumbar point potential using an iliac crest reference (see Figs. 8–6 to 8–8 and 8–11) versus subject height (in centimeters) for posterior tibial nerve stimulation at the ankle using the first negative peak recorded in the iliac crest to L1 derivation. **(B)** is for the knee potential to lumbar point conduction time. (See Table 8–3 for numerical data on these subjects.) This nomogram is used to make allowances for latency differences due to height. In practice this plot would only be used if the absolute latency of the scalp potential (see Fig. 8–16) was abnormal or near the upper limit of normal, so it is necessary to know whether or not the volley is reaching the spinal cord at a normal time (i.e., is there a peripheral conduction delay?). The regression lines were fitted using a least-squares method with a 99% confidence interval (*curved lines*); the dashed straight lines are at 3 SD.

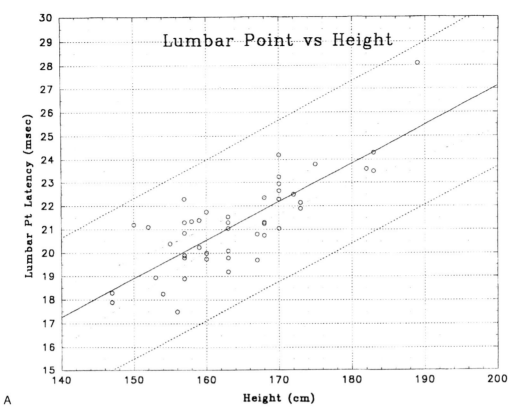

A

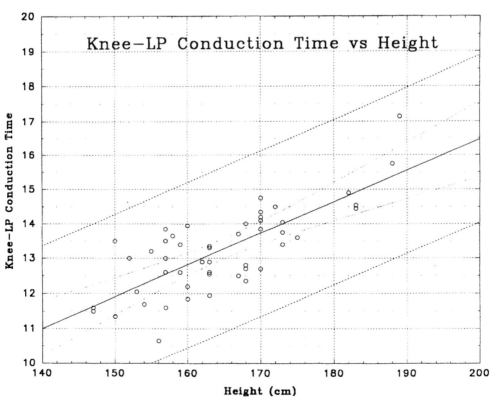

B

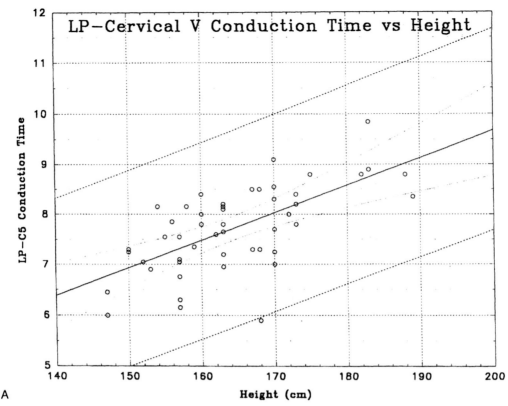

A

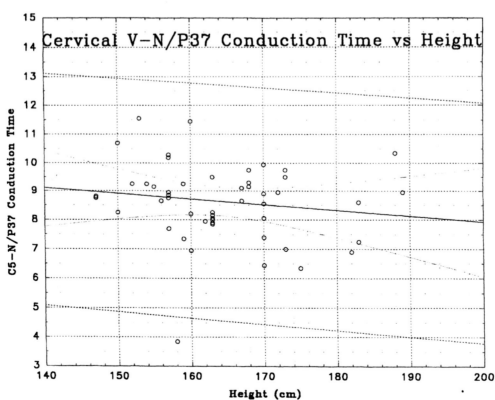

B

TABLE 8–1. *Somatosensory EP median nerve (wrist) normal data*

Parameter	Mean	SD	Mean ± 3 SD	Min	Max
Absolute latency (msec)					
EP	9.7	0.76	12.0	7.9	11.2
P/N13	13.5	0.92	16.3	11.5	15.6
N19	19.0	1.02	22.1	16.7	21.2
P22	22.0	1.29	25.9	19.1	25.2
Intervave latency					
EP–P/N13	3.8	0.45	5.2	2.7	4.5
EP–N19	9.3	0.53	10.9	7.8	10.4
EP–P22	12.3	0.86	14.9	10.0	15.0
P/N13–N19	5.5	0.42	6.8	4.7	6.8
Left–right latency differences					
EP	0.2	0.20	0.8	0.0	0.9
EP–P/N13	0.2	0.17	0.7	0.0	0.6
EP–N19	0.2	0.21	0.8	0.0	0.8
EP–P22	0.3	0.24	1.0	0.0	1.1
P/N13–N19	0.3	0.25	1.1	0.0	1.1
Amplitudes (μV)					
EP	3.0	1.86	8.6	0.5	8.6
P/N13	2.3	0.87	−0.1	0.8	4.4
P/N13 (log transformed)	0.3	0.17	0.7		
N19	1.0	0.56	2.7	0.1	2.7
P22	2.2	1.10	5.5	0.5	5.5
Left–right amplitude difference (%) [(abs(a − b))/((a + b)/2)] × 100					
N19	41.7	33.14	141.1	0.0	144.4
P22	25.7	21.23	89.4	0.0	80.4

Normal data for median nerve SEPs from 50 subjects. Amplitudes were measured from baseline to peak for the Erb's point (EP) potential, P/N13 and N19, and N19 peak to P22 peak for P22 amplitude. Stimulus duration 0.2 msec, rate 5/sec. For P/N13 amplitudes the value given (−0.1) is the mean minus 3 SD; the log transform row was derived by taking the log transform of each data point and finding the mean and standard deviation of that group, with the inverse transform of the log mean minus 3 SD (−0.18) yielding the lower limit of normal of 0.7 μV.

The only difficulties with latency measurements occur when the peaks are poorly defined. In this case, with several trials superimposed, one estimates a point at which to take the measurement. As with other tests in clinical neurophysiology, it is better to err on the side of false negativity (i.e., normality), so that when a visual interpolation is necessary and the peak shape allows some subjective latitude, the preferred technique is to use endpoints that render the result more rather than less normal. When making interside comparisons it is essential to hold the two sheets of paper up to a strong light and optically superimpose the results from the two sides, using the major ascending and descending limbs of the peaks as

FIG. 8–16. Conduction times in the segments below (**A**) and above (**B**) the CV electrode (see Figs. 8–6 to 8–8 and 8–11) versus subject height (in centimeters) for posterior tibial nerve stimulation at the ankle. **A** is for the LP–CV segment and **B** is for the CV–N/P37 segment. (See Table 8-3 for numerical data on these subjects.) This nomogram is used to make allowances for latency differences due to height. The regression line was fitted using a least-squares method with a 99% confidence interval (*curved lines*); the dashed lines are at 3 SD.

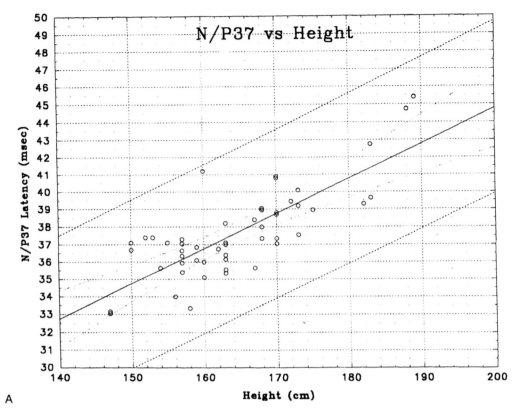

A

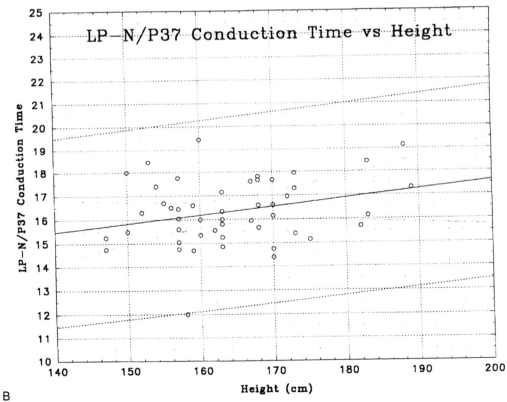

B

FIG. 8–17.

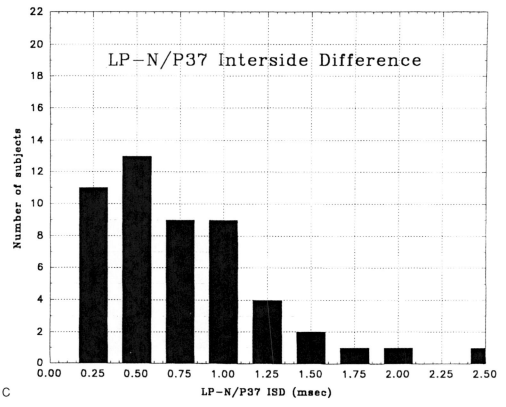

C

FIG. 8–17. (*Continued*) (**A**) Plot of the absolute latency of the scalp potential (N/P37) follow-ing stimulation of the posterior tibial nerve at the ankle. If this result is normal further analysis is usually not necessary. (**B**) Plot of the conduction time between the lumbar (LP) and scalp potentials (N/P37). (**C**) A histogram of the interside difference in this measurement. (See Table 8–3 for numerical data on these subjects.) The nomograms are used to make al-lowances for latency differences due to height. In practice this plot would be used when the lumbar potential is delayed (and thus also absolute latency of N/P37) in order to determine if there is also a conduction delay above lower spinal cord levels. The regression line was fit-ted using a least-squares method with a 99% confidence interval (*curved lines*); the dashed lines are at 3 SD.

guides. This allows a much more reliable comparison than the use of numbers only, or fo-cusing attention solely on a peak.

Complete absence of a wave is a definite abnormality. If the intertrial variability is low, the absolute amplitude of P/N13 can be used in clinical interpretation. However, these am-plitudes in normal subjects do not have a normal (Gaussian) distribution so that nonpara-metric statistics must be used to define the limits of normality. A simple method is to set the lower limit 1 SD below the lowest value seen in a normal subject. Alternatively, the data can be transformed so that they have a normal distribution (Table 8–1). Interside amplitude comparisons must be managed the same way. Amplitude ratios (e.g., EP–P/N13 and P/N13–N19) have too much normal variability to be clinically useful.

TABLE 8–2. *Median, ulnar, and radial nerve normal data*

Peak	Median				Ulnar				Radial	
	Latency (msec) mean ± SD	Amplitude (µV) mean ± SD	Max L–R diff Lat (ms)	Max L–R diff Amp (%)	Latency (msec) mean ± SD	Amplitude (µV) mean ± SD	Max L–R diff Lat (ms)	Max L–R diff Amp (%)	Latency (msec) mean ± SD	Amplitude (µV) mean ± SD
EP	9.6 ± 0.7	5.4 ± 2.5	0.5	49	10.0 ± 0.9	2.9 ± 1.6	0.4	48	9.5 ± 0.8	2.8 ± 1.2
P/N13	13.2 ± 0.8	2.9 ± 1.3	0.6	46	13.9 ± 1.1	1.7 ± 0.8	0.5	56	13.5 ± 1.1	1.4 ± 0.6
N19	18.9 ± 1.0	2.8 ± 1.6	0.9	50	19.3 ± 1.2	1.8 ± 1.1	0.6	55	18.8 ± 1.0	1.5 ± 0.8
EP–P/N13	3.5 ± 0.4		0.8		4.0 ± 0.4		0.5		3.9 ± 0.5	
P/N13–N19	5.8 ± 0.5		0.5		5.3 ± 0.4		0.6		5.3 ± 0.5	

Normal data for median, ulnar, and superficial radial nerves SEPs from 16 subjects. Erb's point (EP) amplitude was negative peak to following positive peak; all others were baseline to peak. Stimulus rate 2/sec. (C. Yiannikas, unpublished data).

TABLE 8–3. *Posterior tibial nerve normal data*

Parameter			
Absolute latencies			
Knee	0.31 ± 0.28	(0–1.1)	39
Lumbar point (LP)	0.42 ± 0.33	(0–1.8)	40
Cervical V (CV)	0.59 ± 0.48	(0–1.8)	41
N/P37	0.81 ± 1.49	(0–10.5)	42
Interpeak latencies			
Knee–LP	0.36 ± 0.42	(0–2.3)	
LP–CV	0.62 ± 0.57	(0–2.5)	
CV–N/P37	0.66 ± 0.53	(0.1–2.3)	
LP–N/P37	0.65 ± 0.48	(0.1–2.3)	
Average amplitudes			
Knee	3.65 ± 1.83	(1.1–8.3)	
LP	1.04 ± 0.40	(0.4–1.95)	
CV	1.06 ± 0.31	(0.5–2.1)	
N/P37	2.52 ± 1.49	(0.4–6.8)	
Amplitude interside differences (abs. L-R/mean)			
Knee	23.6 ± 23.2	(0–88)	
LP	29.1 ± 29.4	(0–150)	
CV	36.9 ± 25.8	(0–92)	
N/P37	31.5 ± 29.9	(0–144)	

Normal data for posterior tibial nerve SEPS from 51 subjects (height 147 to 189 cm, mean 164 cm; age 21 to 65 years, mean 37 years). See Figs. 8–10 through 8–12 for latency–height nomograms on these subjects. N/P37 was measured in the FZ–CZ derivation, lumbar point (LP) as the first negative peak in the IC–L1 derivation (IC, iliac crest). Stimulation was behind the medial malleolus at the ankle, duration 0.2 sec, rate 2 to 5/sec.

8.3. Reproducibility

Tables 8–1 through 8–5 and Figs. 8–15 through 8–17 present data gathered from normal subjects in our laboratory. This is intended to show how such data can be organized to allow comparisons of variability when a laboratory is inexperienced with this test. Since the absolute values are dependent on many variables not likely to be the same in other laboratories,

TABLE 8–4. *Peroneal nerve normal data*

Parameter	Mean	SD	Range
Absolute latency (msec)			
LP	10.8	0.9	8.6–13.1
N/P27	27.3	1.5	24.0–31.3
N/P34	33.5	2.4	30.3–41.3
Conduction time			
(LP–N/P27)	16.5	0.95	15.0–18.8
Left–right latency differences			
LP	0.99	0.14	0.0–0.4
N/P27	0.59	0.55	0.0–2.3
N/P34	1.1	1.62	0.0–7.6
Conduction time	0.6	0.55	0.0–2.3

Normal data for peroneal nerve SEPs from 25 subjects (height 147 to 190 cm, mean 170; age 21 to 51 years, mean 31). See Figs. 8–15 through 8–17 for latency–height nomograms on these subjects. LP was measured as the first positive deflection in the L3–L1 derivation (activity in L3 helped to accentuate this). N/P27 and N/P34 were measured in the CZ–Cc derivation (Cc, central scalp contralateral to limb stimulated). Stimulation was at fibular head at knee, duration 0.2 msec, rate 2 to 5/sec.

TABLE 8–5. *Sural nerve normal data*

Parameter	Mean	SD	Range
Absolute latency (msec)			
LP	20.2	1.6	17.5–22.5
N/P40	38.7	2.9	33.4–42.8
Conduction time			
(LP–N/P40)	18.5	2.0	15.4–21.9
Left–right latency differences			
LP	0.6	0.3	0.3–1.0
N/P40	0.7	0.4	0.1–1.3
Conduction time	0.9	0.6	1.8–0.9

Normal data for sural nerve SEPs from seven subjects. Measurements as in Table 8–3. Stimulation at sural nerve at ankle, duration 0.2 msec, rate 2/sec.

values cannot be used for clinical interpretation except in the laboratory where they were gathered. However, interpeak and interpeak, interside latency measures show only minor differences between laboratories, as does the variability, measured here in standard deviations. In this test, the major purpose of the development of normal standards in each laboratory is to provide experience for the technicians and physicians who will be involved in the clinical application of this highly sophisticated tool. Somatosensory EP results from groups of normal subjects have been published and a study of the methods used and data obtained is useful; for upper-limb results see Giblin (1964), Desmedt and Noel (1973), Cracco and Cracco (1976), Desmedt et al. (1976), Jones (1977), Abbruzzese et al. (1978b), Anziska et al. (1978), Grisolia and Wiederholt (1978), Hume and Cant (1978), Kimura et al. (1978), King and Green (1979), Pratt et al. (1979), Desmedt and Cheron (1980a,b), Eisen and Elleker (1980), Ganes (1980a), Yamada et al. (1980), Leandri et al. (1981), and Jones and Halliday (1982); for lower-limb results see Tsumoto et al. (1972), Perot (1973, 1976), Dorfman (1977), Jones and Small (1978), Kimura et al. (1978), Rowed et al. (1978), Eisen and Nudleman (1979), Eisen and Odusote (1980), Beric and Prevec (1981), Vas et al. (1981), and Pelosi et al. (1987). [See Section 9.2.6 for a discussion of the consistency of SEPs over long periods of recording and when recording at repeated intervals for several months. Refer to Chapter 1, Section 4.3, for a discussion of the concepts relating values obtained from normal subjects and those obtained from patients (whose results are possibly abnormal).]

9. NONPATHOLOGIC FACTORS AFFECTING RESULTS

9.1. Technical Factors

9.1.1. Stimulus Mode—Electrical Versus Others

It may be that closer approximation to natural stimuli will improve the sensitivity and specificity and SEPs can be elicited by stimuli other than electrical. Ishiko et al. (1980), Larsson and Prevec (1970), Pratt and Starr (1981), Pratt et al. (1979, 1980), and Kakigi and Shibasaki (1984) have studied mechanical taps to various parts of the body, including the face, tongue, trunk, and fingers. Pratt and Starr (1981) compared mechanical stimulation of the fingernail with electrical stimulation at the wrist. The waveforms produced by the former were similar to those produced by the latter but of lower amplitude, as is also the case with electrical stimulation of digital nerves. Since good SEPs could be registered with the mechanical stimulation it was suggested that results using this technique when compared with those following electrical stimulation could provide a means of defining receptor and nerve-ending impairments in peripheral neuropathies. Zarola and Rossini (1991) found no difference in central SEP components with peripheral magnetic stimulation.

Starr et al. (1981) and Cohen and Starr (1985) studied SEPs following plantar flexion movements of the ankle and percussion of the tibialis anterior tendon. The earliest component was a biphasic positive wave at 45 and 65 msec, of greatest amplitude at the vertex. Ischemia, cooling and nerve block experiments, and the effects of vibration and muscle stretch suggested that the afferent nerves involved arose from primary muscle spindles. Passive joint position alteration (Grunewald et al., 1984; Desmedt and Ozaki, 1991), tactile air-jet stimulation (Schieppati and Ducati, 1984), voluntary foot and finger movements (Shibasaki et al., 1980, 1981), biceps muscle loading or unloading during voluntary contraction (Angel et al., 1984), air-puff (Hashimoto 1988; Forss et al., 1994), high-frequency vibration (Hamano et al., 1993), mechanical tapping (Onofrj et al., 1990), magnetic (Kunesch et al., 1993) and chemical stimuli (Kobal and Hummel, 1988) have also been used as EP stimuli. However, none of these stimulus modes has yet proven to have the reliability necessary for clinical applications. Jones (1981), Cheron and Borenstein (1991) and Weerasinghe and Sedgwick (1994) have studied the interference with conventional electrical SEPs caused by various natural stimuli and Dietz et al. (1985) and El-Abd and Ibrahim (1994) have used SEPs to study the blocking of group I afferents during gait. Okajima et al. (1991) studied the interactions resulting from simultaneous stimulation of two nerves. Rossini et al. (1990) found that SEPs had maximum amplitude during complete muscle relaxation, whereas contraction depressed all components following the N20. Seyal et al. (1993) used transcranial magnetic stimulation prior to an electrical stimulation of the median nerve at the wrist and discovered that this enhanced the SEP components after N20 when the SEP volley was timed to arrive at the cortex between 50 and 120 msec after the cortical stimulation, presumably related to intracortical phasing mechanisms, either inhibitory or excitatory.

Since pain is such a common and difficult clinical problem, an objective means for study of the pain system would be very useful. The correlation between SEPs obtained using current techniques and clinical sensory symptoms is well-established. Patients whose deficit lies in pain and temperature modalities have normal SEPs, whereas disorders of joint position, touch, vibration, and stereognosis are usually associated with SEP abnormalities (see Chapter 9, Section 1.1.2, for a detailed discussion). However, the intensity of the electrical stimulus used for SEPs excites only the largest myelinated fibers in the peripheral nerves (cutaneous and subcutaneous somaesthetic and proprioceptive fibers, and alpha motor axons), and thus does not directly test the pain system. Stimulation strong enough to produce activity in pain fibers is too painful for clinical use. It is even difficult to stimulate these fibers with needles placed intradermally (Hallin and Torebjork, 1973). Although Chatrian et al. (1975) and Jacobson et al. (1985) studied EPs to pain in humans by stimulation of tooth pulp, this is obviously not a technique that will be useful for most investigators. Thus, a new approach is needed to allow investigation of this system. Morgan et al. (1984) investigated event-related EPs to warm and painful thermal stimuli and Dowman and Goshko (1992) evaluated reference sites for painful sural nerve stimulation. Although long-latency EPs have a greater intrasubject and intersubject variability than the short-latency EPs currently most clinically useful, this may be the only means of investigating this system on a routine clinical basis. Kakigi et al. (1989) used laser stimulation and recorded a P320 which they considered to be transmitted in A-delta fibers and generated in the thalamus. Kakigi and Shibasaki (1991) used a similar technique and estimated the conduction velocity in spinothalamic tracts at 8 to 10 m/sec. Bromm et al. (1991) used laser stimulation to study patients with dissociated sensory deficits (mechanosensibility versus pain and temperature). Beydoun et al. (1993) have contributed a study of normal variability using the laser technique. Cole and Katifi (1991) recorded SEPs at a latency of 84 msec in a patient with a complete large myelinated fiber sensory neuropathy below the neck, presumably conducted along A-delta fibers. See Chudler and Dong (1983) for a good review of EPs in the assessment of pain.

9.1.2. Stimulus Intensity

Changes in stimulus intensity have little effect on peripheral nerve conduction velocities. Practical aspects of the effects of decreased stimulus intensity in patients prone to find the stimulus uncomfortable have been discussed above (see Section 7.3).

Hume and Cant (1978) studied median nerve SEPs in a few normal subjects at different intensities (sensory threshold, just below motor threshold, thumb twitch, and maximal tolerated level). They found no significant effect on the absolute latency of any SEP component in the 14- to 30-msec range. The amplitude of all components increased significantly when the stimulus intensity was increased from just above sensory threshold to a level which was just below that producing a thumb twitch, but further increases in intensity produced only slight increases in amplitude.

Lesser et al. (1979) in a similar study found no changes in the absolute latencies of the brachial plexus potential or N18 at various intensities but noted that P/N13 absolute latency had a tendency to decrease slightly with increasing intensity. The brachial plexus potential to N18 IPL remained unchanged, whereas there was a slight decrease in brachial plexus to P/N13 and a slight increase in P/N13 to N18 with increasing stimulus intensity. Whether or not these IPL changes were due to a change in the shape of the P/N13 complex was not noted. They found that motor threshold stimulation gave submaximal amplitude responses, whereas a level equal to the sum of motor plus sensory thresholds produced maximal or nearly maximal amplitude. Since this was a comfortable level of stimulation they suggested this for routine clinical use. With increasing stimulus intensities the brachial plexus component showed a greater rise in amplitude than did the central potentials.

Kritchevsky and Wiederholt (1978) found that SEPs became more well-defined and of larger amplitude as stimulus intensity was increased. They found the greatest difference when the stimulus intensity was increased from a level producing no twitch of the thumb to one producing a slight twitch.

TABLE 8–6. *Effect of stimulus intensity for stimulation of the posterior tibial nerve at the ankle in normal subjects*

A. Mean latencies (msec) Stimulus strength	N/P37	LP	LP–N/P37	Knee	Knee amplitude (range) μV
Minimal	39.8 (3.8)*	21.7 (2.4)	18.0 (2.0)*	8.0 (1.0)*	1.5 (0–4.7)
Intermediate	38.5 (3.1)	21.4 (2.3)	17.2 (1.4)	8.3 (1.2)	3.0 (1.0–6.3)
Strong	38.6 (3.2)	21.4 (2.3)	17.1 (1.4)	8.3 (1.2)	3.5 (1.5–7.3)
B. Group comparisons: p values on paired t-test					
Minimal vs intermediate	.0002*	.0008	.0019*	.0007*	<.0001
Minimal vs strong	.0012*	.0128	.0064*	.0105*	<.0001
Intermediate vs strong	.8981	.5070	.9333	.5490	<.0001

*N = 16 (NP37 was absent in one subject and the knee potential was absent in another at minimal intensity). N = 17 for all other values. Numbers in parentheses are 1 SD except for knee amplitude.

Minimal intensity was a barely perceptible twitch in the intrinsic foot muscles; strong was the maximum intensity that felt comfortable to the subject; and intermediate was midway between these two (probably closest to the intensity used in routine clinical practice). (King and Chiappa, unpublished data.)

Eisen et al. (1982) for the median nerve studied the relationship between the amplitudes of peripheral nerve sensory action potentials and cerebral SEPs as intensity was increased, using this as a measure of CNS amplification. They compared results obtained in normals with those recorded in patients with MS and postulated that central amplification is attenuated in MS and that this may be a sensitive indicator of early disease. Whether or not this measure as computed in their study was related more to the recording geometry of the peripheral versus central situations than to CNS amplification is not clear. Also, amplitude was taken peak to peak, whereas an area measure might be more physiologic.

Phillips and Daube (1980) studied the lumbar potential produced by peroneal and tibial nerve stimulation and found that latency was not affected by increasing stimulus intensity

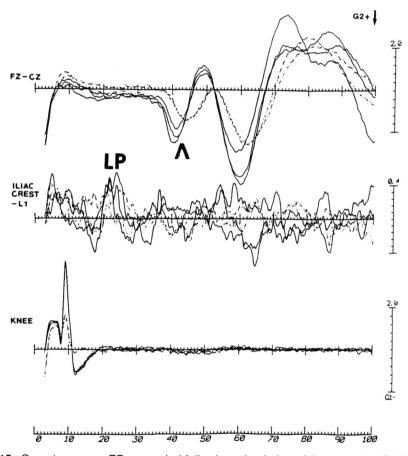

FIG. 8–18. Somatosensory EPs recorded following stimulation of the posterior tibial nerve at the ankle with strong (*solid traces*) and minimal (*dashed traces*) stimulus intensities in one of four normal subjects in whom the difference in latency of N/P37 (*open arrow*) for the two intensities (3.6 msec) exceeded the upper limit of normal for side-to-side differences (mean plus 3 SD = 1.7 msec). Thus, erroneous interpretation might occur if the stimulus intensity was too low on one side. At minimal intensity LP–N/P37 was at the upper limit of normal for height (mean plus 3 SD = 21.8 msec). Note the marked reduction in knee amplitude and small reduction in knee latency with minimal compared to strong stimulus intensity. Minimal intensity was a barely perceptible twitch in the intrinsic foot muscles, strong was the maximum intensity that felt comfortable to the subject. Each trace is the average of 512 stimuli delivered at 5/sec. The knee channel is recorded as in Fig. 8–11. Calibration marks are in microvolts.

but that, under those circumstances, amplitude was increased until a vigorous muscle twitch was being evoked, after which no further change was seen.

King and Chiappa (1988) studied the effects of changes in stimulus intensity in 17 normal subjects. Intensities used were based on the twitch in intrinsic foot muscles: "minimal," "intermediate," and "strong." The LP, N/P37, and LP–N/P37 latencies were significantly increased for minimal compared with intermediate and strong, but not for intermediate compared with strong (Table 8–6 and Figs. 8–18 and 8–19). At minimal intensity, in four subjects the latency shift in N/P37 exceeded 3 SD for interside differences, in one N/P37 absolute latency was greater than 3 SD, and in another the LP–N/P37 was at 3 SD. Most N/P37 prolongation was due to increased LP–N/P37 latency. Amplitude of the sensory nerve action potential at the knee was greater than or equal to 1 μV for intermediate and strong but was less than 1 μV in 8 of 17 subjects at minimal intensities. In two patients, submotor threshold stimuli produced markedly delayed and low-amplitude EPs (see Figs. 8–12

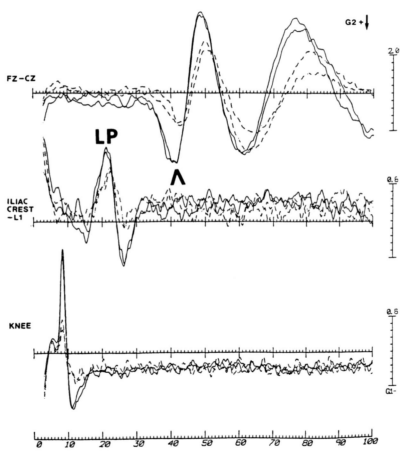

FIG. 8–19. Somatosensory EPs recorded following stimulation of the posterior tibial nerve at the ankle with strong (*solid traces*) and minimal (*dashed traces*) stimulus intensities in another normal subject in whom the difference in latency of N/P37 (*open arrow*) for the two intensities (2.0 msec) and the N/P37 latency at minimal intensity (1.2 msec over the upper limit of normal for height) might lead to an erroneous interpretation. (See Fig. 8–18 for stimulus and recording parameters.)

and 8–13), presumably mediated via cutaneous rather than posterior tibial nerve activation, which normalized at intermediate intensities.

Tsuji et al. (1984) studied the effects of stimulus intensity on posterior tibial nerve SEPs and recommended a level of at least three times sensory threshold for clinical studies. If greater reproducibility is required, Kukulka et al. (1991) have recommended an objective technique for assessing graded electrically evoked afferent activity in humans.

9.1.3. Stimulus Rate

Since SEP amplitudes and signal-to-noise ratios are quite low, a large number of responses (500 to 1,000) must be averaged to produce clear components. Thus, the fastest stimulus rate allowing good registration of SEPs is the most practical. Animal studies (Wiederholt, 1978) suggested that a rate of 5/sec would have little detrimental effect on SEPs while allowing a large series of stimuli to be delivered in a reasonable period of time.

Pratt et al. (1980) studied the effects of stimulus rates of 2, 4, 8, 16, and 32/sec on median nerve SEPs (mechanical and electrical stimulation). They concluded that in normal subjects a stimulus rate of 8/sec could be used without significant sacrifice in definition of the early components of the SEP (up to P/N13) but that 4/sec was optimal for N20 amplitude.

Kritchevsky and Wiederholt (1978) compared 4 and 10/sec for the median nerve and found amplitude loss but no significant latency changes at the higher rate. Recovery curves of peripheral and central median nerve SEP components were reported by Reisin et al. (1988) and Meyer-Hardting et al. (1983), and common peroneal, posterior tibial, and sural nerve recovery functions were described by Saito et al. (1992).

Phillips and Daube (1980) studied lumbar potentials following stimulation of the peroneal and tibial nerves and found that amplitude remained constant at rates from 0.5 to 5/sec. Jones et al. (1982) recorded spinal potentials epidurally and, even at 50/sec, found only a slight amplitude decrement.

Onishi et al. (1991) examined the effect of increasing the stimulus rate from 2.3 to 5.1/sec following stimulation of the common peroneal, posterior tibial, and sural nerves and found a significant reduction in amplitude of later cortical components (P40–N50, N50–P60), following common peroneal and posterior tibial nerve stimulation only. Following median nerve and digital nerve stimulation at 1.6 to 5.7/sec, Delberghe et al. (1990) found the amplitude of the N13 potential decreased, whereas the P14 and N20 remained stable. Delberghe et al. (1990) noted a dissociation of the amplitudes of the N13 versus P14 and N20 versus P22 components with increasing stimulus rate. See also Larrea et al. (1992), Manzano et al. (1995), and Fujii et al. (1994b).

9.1.4. Stimulus Mode—Unilateral Versus Bilateral

Bilateral stimulation approximately doubles SEP component amplitudes (Kritchevsky and Wiederholt, 1978). However, when there is a long distance between the stimulus site and the anatomic structure whose activity is to be recorded, there may be difficulty in synchronizing the volleys from the two sides. Peripheral neuropathies, pressure palsies, and other factors may defeat the purpose of the bilateral stimulation. In addition, unilateral stimulation provides more specific anatomic information and is more sensitive in revealing abnormalities. For example, in MS, 48% of patients with abnormal tests had unilateral abnormalities of median SEPs; the proportion was 22% for peroneal SEPs (see Section 7.4 above). If bilateral stimulation is used, the normal waveforms generated by the "good" side mask the abnormality in the "bad" side. The only possible reason to use bilateral stimulation in SEP testing is to obtain a larger-amplitude response when using the lower-limb SEP to monitor spinal cord functioning during surgery. Here one may be interested only in whether or not the spinal cord has any continuity, so that the largest and most visible response is desired. Also, lateralizing information is not pertinent.

9.1.5. Recording Band-Pass

The SEP components discussed here contain significant activity in the 25- to 2,500-Hz frequency range; thus, they are usually recorded using a filter band-pass exceeding that window. When the high-cutoff filter is lowered much below the value stated above, distortion of components results (Desmedt et al., 1974).

When the low-cutoff filter is raised from 1 or 5 Hz to 100 or 150 Hz, multiple small subcomponents appear in the SEP (King and Green, 1979; Rossini et al., 1981; Maccabee et al., 1983, 1986; Eisen et al., 1984, 1985). These authors found that these subcomponents were well-defined and stable within and across normal subjects. McKay and Galloway (1979) and Rossini et al. (1981) reported similar results, that is, appearance of multiple, small subcomponents, when studying spinal EPs. The clinical utility of these subcomponents is presently uncertain, especially since they cannot be clearly recorded in all normal subjects.

9.1.6. Potential-Field Distribution

Synaptic activity in gray matter and propagating action potentials in fiber tracts generate electrical activity potentially recordable at skin and scalp surfaces. In the cortex, current flow produced by inhibitory and excitatory postsynaptic potentials in the dendrites of cortical neurons produces scalp-recorded activity. Subcortical gray matter may or may not have an electrical geometry ("open," "open-closed," or "closed" fields) that results in surface-recordable activity (see Emerson and Pedley, 1984, for a review of these considerations), predictions based on anatomy are unreliable, and extrapolations from animal work are problematic. Solving the reverse problem via dipole theories (i.e., predicting the anatomic generator sources from the surface potential-field distribution) is equally difficult. Conclusions are often based on the assumption that the generators are very small sources, whereas, in fact, they occupy a significant volume within the bounds of the recording surface (skin and scalp), have an irregular and asymmetric shape, and may be only partially affected (i.e., inactivated) by lesions. Furthermore, some surface-recorded potentials are generated when the tissue surrounding a propagating volley suddenly changes its geometry or conductive properties (Nakanishi, 1982, 1983; Kimura et al., 1983, 1984, 1986; Deupree and Jewett, 1988; Eisen et al., 1986; Yamada et al., 1985; Lueders et al., 1983a,c; Sonoo et al., 1992). Thus, considerations of potential-field distributions of SEP activity and their relationship to generator sources are complex (and sometimes controversial) issues. Although a detailed discussion is beyond the scope of this book, a summary of current ideas will be presented; references can be consulted for more detailed treatment.

A large number of SEP potentials can be differentiated in most normal subjects but many of these are rather small and inconsistent between normal subjects; therefore, this discussion will focus on those potentials that appear to be of large enough amplitude to be reliably recorded.

Note that these potentials usually follow one another quite closely and often merge (e.g., N11–N13, P15–N19, and N19–P23), so it is difficult, if not impossible, to say where one ends and the other starts. More important is the fact that activity generated in a single source is often recorded as a negativity in one head or neck area, and as a positivity elsewhere (or vice versa). For example, the afferent volley in the cervical dorsal columns following median nerve stimulation produces negative activity over the back of the neck and simultaneous positive activity on the scalp. This "duplication" can be confusing, especially if one author focuses on one part of the field and the next author on another, and the two may use slightly different latency labeling. However, if this "duplication" effect is kept in mind, less confusion will result as the section below is traversed.

9.1.6.1. Upper Limb

The scalp potential-field distributions of upper-limb SEPs are similar for the nerves usually studied (median, ulnar, radial, and digital).

Brachial Plexus Potentials. Activity in the brachial plexus has a maximum amplitude in the supraclavicular fossa. Its potential field has a wide distribution and it is seen routinely as a small positive potential at scalp electrodes (when they are referred to a distant, noncephalic reference, e.g., knee or toe) (Cracco and Cracco, 1976; Desmedt and Cheron, 1980a; Grisolia and Wiederholt, 1978; King and Green, 1979; Kritchevsky and Wiederholt, 1978; Pratt and Starr, 1981; Desmedt et al., 1983; Lueders et al., 1983a,c; Desmedt, 1984; Desmedt and Cheron, 1983; Emerson and Pedley, 1984; Emerson et al., 1984; Frith et al., 1986). This scalp positivity is nearly simultaneous with the peripherally recorded brachial plexus activity, at 9 to 10 msec. Desmedt et al. (1983) have shown that supporting the shoulder in a high position significantly increases the latency of the scalp-recorded potential P9, and Kameyama et al. (1988) and Yasuhara et al. (1990) also noted changes in components with different arm positions.

Electrodes arrayed vertically along the anterior border of the ipsilateral sternocleidomastoid muscle record a traveling wave similar in waveform and polarity to that seen at Erb's point (Emerson et al., 1984). This is delayed slightly from the latter activity and presumably is generated by activity in the trunks of the brachial plexus and/or cervical roots (Emerson et al., 1984). This activity may be recorded from scalp electrodes as a negativity.

Cervical Spinal Cord Potentials. Activity from structures in the cervical cord and medulla can be recorded at all head and neck locations 11 to 15 msec after a stimulus at the wrist. The waveforms consist of negative potentials recorded from the posterior neck and low back of the head, and positive potentials recorded from the anterior scalp. Although ear reference recordings have been used to study the distribution of these potentials (Cracco, 1972, 1980), a good deal of activity is present at the ears themselves and results using this technique can be expected to differ from those using noncephalic references (Pratt and Starr, 1981; Kritchevsky and Wiederholt, 1978; Grisolia and Wiederholt, 1978; King and Green, 1979; Desmedt and Cheron, 1981a; Anziska and Cracco, 1981; Favale et al., 1982; Lueders et al., 1983a,c; Nakanishi, 1983; Desmedt, 1984; Emerson et al., 1984; Iragui, 1984). Various "bipolar" studies have also been performed (Hume and Cant, 1978; Favale et al., 1982; Ganes, 1982; Kaji and Sumner, 1987). Caccia et al. (1976) and Beric et al. (1986) have compared surface and epidural recordings in humans.

The negative potentials appearing over the posterior neck and low back of the head tend to peak earlier in the 11- to 13-msec period than the positive potentials recorded from the scalp, as can be seen in Fig. 8–3 (compare the peaks labeled N11 and N12 in the second and third channels from the bottom with the peaks labeled P13 and P14). Desmedt and Cheron (1981a) recorded this early negative activity using esophageal electrodes and noted a latency shift with recording at progressively higher levels corresponding to a conduction velocity of 58 m/sec. Taking this with the potential-field distribution, they concluded that N11 is generated by the ascending volley in the dorsal columns. Lesser et al. (1981) recorded directly from the cervical cord during intraoperative monitoring and found that the maximum amplitude of activity occurring at 11 msec was seen at CVI, with a progressive latency increase in more rostral segments. Other studies with direct recordings have confirmed these results (Hallstrom et al., 1989; Jeanmond et al., 1989). Emerson et al. (1984) recorded similar activity at the neck and also over the scalp.

In addition to this traveling wave, another negativity may be recorded over the posterior neck which has a constant latency at different levels but maximum amplitude in low- to middle-cervical regions (Desmedt and Cheron, 1981a; Lueders et al., 1983a,c; Desmedt, 1984; Desmedt and Nguyen, 1984; Emerson et al., 1984), and has a positive reflection anteriorly at the neck level. There is general agreement that this activity is generated postsynaptically in the gray matter of the cervical cord (dorsal horns) from axon collateral input up to two levels above and below the root entry level. Scalp electrodes record a positive reflection of the dorsal column traveling negativity (N11) but the dorsal horn activity, whose equivalent dipole is oriented horizontally, does not appear at the scalp (Desmedt, 1984; Desmedt and Nguyen, 1984; Hallstrom et al., 1989; Jeanmond et al., 1989). Beall et al. (1977) have shown similar activity in medullary recordings in monkeys, as have Urasaki et al. (1990a) and Morioka et al. (1991a) in humans.

These possible sources (root entry zone/dorsal horn, dorsal column, dorsal column nucleus, and medial lemniscus) include the localizations and potential-field distributions suggested by most other studies (Pratt and Starr, 1981; Jones, 1977; Hume and Cant, 1978; Anziska and Cracco, 1981; El-Negamy and Sedgwick, 1978; Desmedt and Cheron, 1980a; Ganes, 1982; Shimoji et al., 1978; Kritchevsky and Wiederholt, 1978; Ertekin, 1976; Allison et al., 1980; Tsuji and Murai, 1986; Yamada et al., 1984; Sances et al., 1978). They also are in general agreement with studies of recovery curves of the various components (Ganes, 1982; Iragui, 1984; Favale et al., 1982; Kaji and Sumner, 1987). (See Chapter 9, Section 1.1, for a further discussion of the generator sources of these activities.)

Brain Stem–Cerebral Potentials. Potentials generated in medullary and cerebral structures have wide scalp distributions. Their potential-field distributions are difficult to study with bipolar or ear reference derivations (as was done by Cracco, 1980, and Goff et al., 1977) because of the activity present at both electrodes. For example, Fig. 8–20 shows the median nerve SEP from a normal subject with hand reference recordings from both earlobes as well as Cc and FZ (relative negativity of second electrode produces an upward deflection). Note that both earlobes contain as much negativity at 15 to 18.5 msec as FZ. Tomberg et al. (1991a) have confirmed this earlobe activity and have also noted an asymmetry according to side of stimulation.

Widespread positive activity is recorded over the scalp at 13 to 14 msec using a noncephalic reference; in the best recordings this activity presents two distinct peaks (see Fig. 8–3) although this distinction can be made in a minority of subjects (Chiappa, 1983; Desmedt and Cheron, 1980a; Anziska and Cracco, 1981; Hume and Cant, 1978). Although there is some uncertainty about the first of these positivities, it is considered to be generated postsynaptically in nucleus cuneatus. Based on considerations of conduction times P14 is generally agreed to be generated in the medial lemniscus (Desmedt and Cheron, 1980a, 1981a; Desmedt, 1984; Desmedt and Nguyen, 1984). Human data affirm this localization and are discussed in Chapter 9, Section 1.1.3. Moller et al. (1986) recorded from the surface of the cuneate nucleus in humans and monkeys and concluded that P14 is generated by the termination of the dorsal column fibers and that the cuneate nucleus itself contributes little to the far-field potentials.

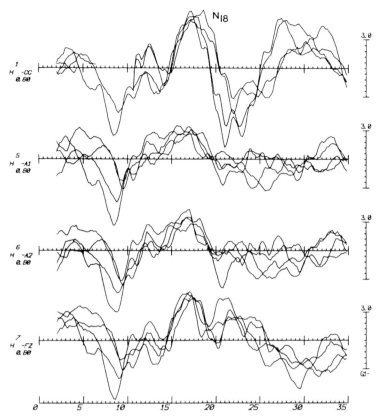

FIG. 8–20. Left and right median nerve SEPs (two traces from each side are superimposed) in a normal subject demonstrating the large amount of activity present at earlobe recording sites (A1 is left and A2 is right). The earlobes (*middle two traces*) show nearly as much negativity at 15 to 18 msec as is present at FZ (*bottom channel*) and a significant proportion of that seen at Cc (*top channel*), using a noncephalic reference electrode on the right hand; unilateral stimulation at 5/sec. Each trace is the average of 1,000 stimuli.

Shortly after the widespread positivity with a peak at 13 to 14 msec, a widespread negativity appears at all scalp locations and the earlobes (see Figs. 8–2 through 8–5 and 8–20), including scalp and earlobe ipsilateral to the limb stimulated, with a peak at about 18 msec. Although this activity was noted by some (Abbruzzese et al., 1978b; Kritchevsky and Wiederholt, 1978; Chiappa et al., 1979), and much of it was considered to have a thalamic origin (Abbruzzese et al., 1978b; Chiappa et al., 1978, 1979, 1980), it was ignored by others (Desmedt and Cheron, 1980a) who focused attention on the more restricted negativity (which has a slightly later peak) seen in parietal scalp regions contralateral to the limb stimulated. Most authors now recognize this earlier, widespread, negative activity (Desmedt and Cheron, 1981b; Pratt and Starr, 1981; Lueders et al., 1983c; Yamada et al., 1984; Kakigi and Shibasaki, 1984; Desmedt and Bourguet, 1985; Desmedt et al., 1987; Rossini et al., 1987) and there is agreement on its thalamic origin (see Chapter 9, Section 1.1.3, for further discussion). Note also that brain-dead patients may show an apparent N18, which is actually "uncovered" negativity from the region of the cervicomedullary junction, its appearance facilitated by the absence of P14, N18, N19, and P22 generators, also seen in extensive lesions of the pons (Raroque et al., 1993) and in a patient with a lesion at the pontomedullary junction but absent with a dorsal column lesion at C1–2 (Sonoo et al., 1992b). Much of the confusion about this topic is related to nomenclature, because the labels N2, N19, and N20 were used in different ways by different authors without the significance of the difference in usage being understood by some.

The widespread negativity has a longer duration in parietal scalp areas contralateral to the limb stimulated than in frontal and ipsilateral areas. Thus, when electrodes in this area are linked in a bipolar fashion with electrodes elsewhere on the head, only the difference in negativity, that is, the localized activity, is registered (see also Chapter 6, Section 5.1, and Fig. 8–5). This localized activity may have this distribution for either of two reasons: (1) It may be generated by distant, deep structures (e.g., thalamus or radiations) and yet have an asymmetrical spread over the scalp. This would not be surprising since there is precedent for this; for example, BAEP wave III (see Chapter 6, Section 8.1.8), known to be generated in the lower pons, has a very asymmetrical scalp distribution, indicating that "far-field" potentials can be asymmetrically distributed. (2) It may be generated locally in primary sensory parietal cortex. This seems less likely because of its preservation in patients with cortical lesions (see Chapter 9, Section 1.1.3, for a further discussion of this controversy). Rossini et al. (1987) used 12- to 36-channel recordings to study the scalp topography of SEPs to mixed and pure sensory stimulation of the median nerve, and evaluated the influence of stimulus rate and intensity changes.

The positivity (P22 in Fig. 8–2) that follows these negative activities is generally agreed to be a cortical component. Its variability renders it less useful in clinical applications and its potential-field distribution has been well-described (Pratt and Starr, 1981; Kritchevsky and Wiederholt, 1978; Desmedt and Cheron, 1980b, 1981b; Yamada et al., 1984; Desmedt and Bourguet, 1985; Kakigi and Shibasaki, 1984; Rossini et al., 1987; Lueders et al., 1983c; Desmedt et al., 1987; Deiber et al., 1986; Tsuji et al., 1988; Dinner et al., 1987). These authors usually have also considered in detail the frontal negative activity appearing at about the same time as P22, and have debated whether or not it represents a separate, frontal generator or is merely the other side of the dipole generating P22. (See also the dipole modeling study of Franssen et al., 1992, in normal subjects and patients with small subcortical infarcts.)

9.1.6.2. Lower Limb

Cauda Equina—Spinal Cord Potentials. The potential-field distributions of cauda equina and spinal cord potentials are difficult to study using bipolar derivations (as done by Cracco, 1973; Cracco et al., 1980; Rossini et al., 1981; Jones and Small, 1978). Stimulating the posterior tibial nerve in the popliteal fossa, using distant reference sites (iliac crest, thigh, hand), and recording from the skin surface at the S1 level, two large negative peaks are seen at about 9 and 13.5 msec (Yiannikas, 1983b; Yiannikas and Shahani, 1988) (Fig. 8–21). As can be seen in the figure, as one records from progressively higher levels (L5, L3, L1, and T12) these two potentials converge in time and fuse into a single peak. Recording at even higher levels shows primarily only this single peak, its latency increasing as the volley ascends in the spinal cord. The first peak is the afferent volley ascending to the cord which it enters at about the T12–L1 vertebral level. The second potential is efferent activity in motor axons activated in the H-reflex; the top trace shows the H-reflex as recorded from the muscle itself. Vibration of the muscle or increased intensity of the stimulus causes this sec-

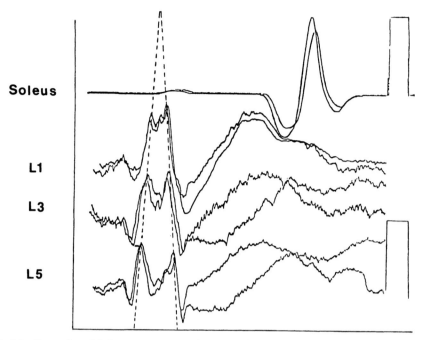

FIG. 8–21. Posterior tibial nerve (popliteal fossa) SEPs (unilateral stimulation at 1/2 sec) recorded from L5 up to L1 levels, showing the earlier afferent volley and the later efferent volley (which will generate an H-reflex recordable from soleus muscle) gradually converging in time at progressively higher levels (they eventually fuse completely at the T10 level). The top trace shows the H-reflex recorded from the soleus muscle. Any maneuvers which abolish the H-reflex (vibration of the muscle, increased stimulus intensity and increased stimulus rate) also abolish the later, efferent component. Recordings were at the L5, L3, and L1 levels, referenced to the iliac crest. Relative negativity of the lumbar electrodes caused an upward trace deflection. Sweep duration was 50 msec. Each trace is the average of 500 stimuli, with two repetitions superimposed. Calibration marks are 5 μV for spinal channels and 2 mV for the compound muscle action potential. (From Yiannikas C, unpublished data.)

ond potential to be greatly attenuated in amplitude (Yiannikas, 1983b; Yiannikas and Shahani, 1988).

When a nerve which does not subserve an H-reflex (sural, peroneal, tibial at the ankle) is stimulated these two traveling potentials are not present in this form (Yiannikas, 1983b). Rather, the afferent negative peak is visible with a second peak which does not change latency up to T12–L1 (Fig. 8–22). This second, standing, waveform is postsynaptic activity in the dorsal gray matter of the root entry zone of the spinal cord, being recorded as a far-field potential both above and below its site of generation. A relatively long refractory period (Seyal and Gabor, 1985) is consistent with this localization. Above the T12–L1 level, the traveling wave is seen as usual as the volley continues to ascend in the spinal cord gracile tract (Seyal et al., 1983; Seyal and Gabor, 1985, 1987; Desmedt and Cheron, 1983; Emerson, 1988).

As the volley ascends in the cord above the entry level, gradual dispersion secondary to slightly different conduction velocities causes the duration of the peak to gradually increase and the amplitude to decrease so that it is usually not recordable (unless special care is taken) above mid- to upper-thoracic levels (see below).

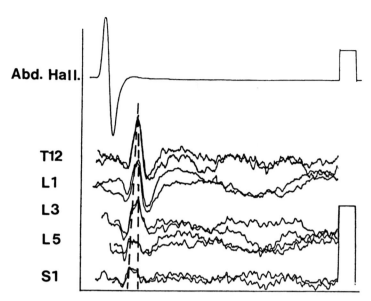

Abd. Hall.

T12

L1

L3

L5

S1

FIG. 8–22. Posterior tibial nerve (ankle) SEPs (unilateral at 1/2 sec) recorded from S1 up to T12 levels, showing the earlier afferent volley and a later standing potential. The latency of the afferent volley increases at progressively higher levels so that it converges on the standing potential whose latency remains constant. Since this nerve does not usually subserve an H-reflex no efferent volley is registered. The top trace shows the direct M-response only, recorded from the abductor hallucis muscle. Recordings, techniques, and calibrations same as for Fig. 8–21. (From Yiannikas C, unpublished data.)

Findings similar in part to those described above have been reported by Dimitrijevic et al. (1978), Phillips and Daube (1980), Delbeke et al. (1978), El-Negamy and Sedgwick (1978), Yamada et al. (1982a), Kakigi et al. (1982), and Sonoo et al. (1992b).

Recordings from intrathecal electrodes in normal subjects and patients (Magladery et al., 1951; Ertekin, 1973, 1976; Ertekin et al., 1980, 1984; Maruyama et al., 1982) and epidural (Jones et al., 1982; Caccia et al., 1976; Shimizu et al., 1979, 1982; Jeanmond et al., 1989, 1991; Halonen et al., 1989) or intraspinal ligament (Lueders et al., 1981) recordings during scoliosis surgery have allowed correlations with the surface recordings. Jones et al. (1982) showed that the volley at thoracic levels has segregated into at least three distinct peaks, corresponding to activity in different axonal populations. Snyder and Holliday (1984) and Feldman et al. (1980) have made similar recordings in animals.

Cervicomedullary Potentials. Because of dispersion of the volley over the relatively long distance traveled from the leg, the potentials which follow upper-limb stimulation and are generated in the medulla and possibly lower pons usually cannot be seen following lower-limb stimulation. Special techniques such as averaging the responses to large numbers of stimuli (2,000–4,000) in well-relaxed, normal subjects (Cracco, 1973; Cracco et al., 1980), or the use of intraspinal ligament needle electrodes (see Section 4 above and Lueders et al., 1981) are necessary. Thus, the registration of these potentials is not routinely attempted in patients, although Tinazzi and Mauguiere (1995) have reported good clinical utilization of Fpz–Cv6 recorded P30 in 70 patients with cervical cord, brain stem, or hemispheric lesions.

Seyal et al. (1987) recorded a localized, synapse-dependent negativity at 29 msec over the upper cervical spine after bilateral stimulation of the posterior tibial nerve at the ankle. Its amplitude was maximal at the C2 level and its latency was constant at different levels. Its long refractory period indicated that the nucleus gracilis was the most likely generator source.

Lueders et al. (1981), Kakigi et al. (1982), Jones and Small (1978), Vas et al. (1981), Rossini et al. (1981), Seyal et al. (1983, 1987), Lueders et al. (1983a), and Desmedt and Cheron (1983) have also studied the potential-field distribution of these early activities seen with lower limb stimulation.

Thalamocortical Potentials. Potentials generated in the thalamus are the first that can be routinely recorded from the scalp following lower-limb stimulation. The discussion of their potential-field distribution has already been covered in detail above in Section 6.2.3, because it is necessary to understand the potential-field distribution to determine the best recording derivations. An important aspect is the difference between posterior tibial, sural,

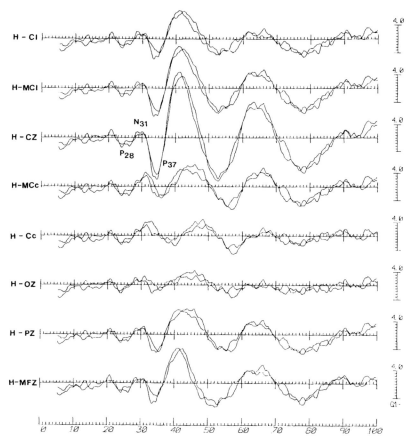

FIG. 8–23. Posterior tibial nerve (ankle) SEPs (unilateral stimulation at 2/sec) in a normal subject demonstrating in detail the potential field distribution over the scalp of early (and middle) latency components. The early negativity at 30 msec is seen in all head regions; this is replaced by positive activity appearing earliest and with largest amplitude at ipsilateral and central locations, peaking at 34 to 35 msec. Its amplitude at PZ is lower than at CZ. Each trace is the average of 500 stimuli, with a repetition superimposed. The "M" label in a derivation denotes an electrode placed halfway between two conventional positions (e.g., mCi is halfway between Ci and CZ). (From Yiannikas C, unpublished data.)

and peroneal nerves with respect to intersubject variability, especially at the midline FZ and CZ sites, the latter two nerves showing more variability than the first. The typical patterns of distribution are shown in Figs. 8–6 to 8–8, and Fig. 8–9 demonstrates how the increased variability of the midline activity can lead to problems in waveform recognition and interpretation, especially with peroneal nerve stimulation (see discussion in Section 6.2.3). Figure 8–23 shows in more detail than available in the earlier figures the typical development and distribution of activity over the scalp of a normal subject following stimulation of the posterior tibial nerve at the ankle, using noncephalic (hand) reference recordings (Yiannikas, 1983b). These data have also been presented previously for the common peroneal nerve by Wilson et al. (1981).

This distribution of activity has been referred to as "paradoxical" by Cruse et al. (1982) and Lesser et al. (1987) but it is only "paradoxical" if one assumes that the positivity at 36 msec has some specific anatomic generator (which is not known at the present time), and/or that for some reason it is "logical" for it to be recorded with maximum amplitude contralateral to the limb stimulated (there seems to be no reason to suspect that that should be so—see the case with half-field PSVEPs).

These potentials have also been studied by others with similar results (Kakigi et al., 1982; Desmedt and Bourguet, 1985; Emerson, 1988), or with magnetoencephalography (Rogers et al., 1994), often, however, with an emphasis on bipolar or ear reference derivations (Vas et al., 1981; Rossini et al., 1981; Burke et al., 1981; Beric and Prevec, 1981; Jones and Small, 1978; Tsumoto et al., 1972; Kimura et al., 1978; Eisen and Elleker, 1980; Vera et al., 1983; Wang et al., 1989), which are subject to the problems of activity in the "reference" electrode mentioned above. Nagamine et al. (1992) have used current source density mapping to study the localization of generator sources of both median and tibial SEPs.

9.1.7. Nerve Location and Fiber Composition

The integrity of somatosensory pathways is usually tested by stimulation of a mixed nerve, for example, median nerve at the wrist or the tibial or peroneal nerves in the lower limbs. However, the localization of plexus or root pathology using SEPs may be dependent on stimulation of peripheral nerves containing fibers contributing to the clinical suspect cords, trunks, or spinal segments (Table 8–7), and the correlation of cutaneous sensory loss with SEP abnormalities may be improved by the stimulation of sensory nerves subserving those dermatomes. Somatosensory EPs obtained with cutaneous nerve stimulation have configurations similar to those obtained with mixed-nerve stimulation; however, the responses have smaller amplitudes, particularly the cervical and lumbar spinal responses, which may not be registered from some normal subjects when the digits, musculocutaneous, saphenous, or sural nerves are stimulated. Strong electrical stimuli (about three times sensory threshold) to these cutaneous nerves elicit scalp SEPs about half the size of SEPs seen following stimulation of mixed nerves. In the upper limbs, all SEP components show appropriate latency shifts when stimulating proximal (musculocutaneous) or distal (digit) to the wrist. Superficial radial nerve stimulation at the wrist produces responses with latencies similar to the mixed median nerve but with lower amplitudes (see Table 8–2). In the lower limbs, sural nerve stimulation produces low-amplitude EPs at the scalp with prolonged latencies relative to those produced by stimulation of the posterior tibial nerve at the ankle (mean difference in scalp latency is 2–3 msec—see Tables 8–3 and 8–5), even though the distance between stimulus site and spinal cord is approximately the same (Chiappa,

TABLE 8–7. *Plexus and root relationships for the peripheral nerves commonly used in SEP testing*

| Nerve | Plexus | | Root afferents |
	Cords	Trunks	
Median	Lateral	Upper	C6-7—Cutaneous
	Medial	Middle	
		Lower	C8-T1—Muscle
Ulnar	Medial	Lower	C8—Cutaneous
			C8-T1—Muscle
Superficial radial	Posterior	Upper	C6—Cutaneous
Musculocutaneous	Lateral	Upper	C5-6—Cutaneous
Posterior tibial (popliteal fossa)			L4-S2—Cutaneous
			L4-S2—Muscle
Posterior tibial (ankle)			L4-S2—Cutaneous
			S1-2—Muscle
Common peroneal			L4-5—Cutaneous
			L4-S1—Muscle
Sural			S1-2—Cutaneous
Saphenous			L3-4—Cutaneous
Superficial peroneal			L4-5—Cutaneous

1983; Burke et al., 1981, 1982; Vogel et al., 1986). This may be related to the contribution of the more rapidly conducting muscle afferents to the potentials produced by mixed nerve (posterior tibial) stimulation; it is believed that muscle afferents from the lower limbs travel in dorsolateral (spinocerebellar) pathways rather than in the posterior columns, whereas cutaneous afferents (e.g., from sural and posterior tibial nerves) travel predominantly in the posterior columns. Since the average diameter of posterior column axons (Ohnishi et al., 1976) is less than the diameter of axons in the spinocerebellar tracts, the conduction velocity is faster in the muscle afferent (posterior tibial nerve) than in the cutaneous (sural nerve) paths. In the upper limbs, both cutaneous and muscle afferents are believed to travel in the posterior columns, consistent with the equal conduction times in cutaneous (superficial radial and digital nerves) and mixed (median) nerves (when distances are normalized) (see Webster, 1977, for a more detailed discussion of somasthetic pathways).

The effect of cutaneous stimulation concurrent with electrical elicitation of SEPs has been studied with both upper (Jones, 1981; Kakigi and Jones, 1985; Jones and Power, 1984; Kakigi, 1986) and lower limbs (Burke et al., 1982; Kakigi and Jones, 1986; Burke and Gandevia, 1988; Greenwood and Goff, 1987). The effects of vibration, joint movement, and muscle contractions have also been investigated (Abbruzzese et al., 1980, 1981b; Cohen and Starr, 1985; Angel et al., 1984, 1986; Seyal et al., 1987; Cheron and Borenstein, 1987; Desmedt and Ozaki, 1991), and concurrent electrical stimulation of the same and nearby nerves (Nardone and Schieppati, 1989). These findings and results obtained from microneuronography experiments have led Burke and Gandevia (1986) to suggest that the dominant afferent input for lower-limb mixed-nerve SEPs are group I muscle afferents. A similar conclusion was reached by Gandevia et al. (1984) for the median nerve SEP, and for intercostal nerves (Gandevia and Macefield, 1989), although controversy exists (Halonen et al., 1988; Jones et al., 1989). Further microneuronography experiments by Gandevia and Burke (1990) using noncephalic references to record scalp potentials after stimulation of muscle afferents from the upper limb have revealed (1) the cortical projection produces both a focal negativity over the contralateral parietal cortex and a focal positivity over the frontal cortex; (2) using the amplitude of the N20–P25 component, the projection from the cutaneous nerves is about three times greater than that from the thenar muscle afferents; and (3) the conduction velocity along the entire pathway (peripheral and central) was similar for the fastest cutaneous and muscle afferents. Other forms of concurrent limb activity have also been shown to affect cortical but not brain stem components (Huttunen and Homberg, 1991).

When stimulating the various mixed nerves, differences in latency and amplitude can partially be accounted for by different stimulus site to spinal cord distances (e.g., peroneal nerve at the knee versus posterior tibial nerve at the ankle), and the number of sensory afferents in each nerve. For example, stimulation of the ulnar nerve (wrist), which contains only C8–T1 sensory afferents, produces SEPs of lower amplitude than those registered following stimulation of the median nerve (wrist), which contains C6–T1 sensory afferents (C8–T1 muscle and C6–C8 cutaneous afferents). In addition, the latencies of the Erb's point potential (EP) and the EP–P/N13 IPL are usually longer for the ulnar nerve; presumably, this is related to a longer anatomic course and entry into the cord at a lower level for the ulnar nerve. In the lower limbs, posterior tibial nerve EPs, besides being of appropriately increased latency because of the more distal stimulus site, are of greater amplitude than peroneal EPs; the reason for this amplitude difference is not clear but it may be related to the rich innervation of the sole of the foot, and the posterior tibial nerve at the knee may contain more group Ia muscle afferents than the peroneal nerve.

Pelosi et al. (1987) studied afferent conduction characteristics of the peroneal, tibial, and sural nerves over peripheral nerve, spinal cord, and from spine to cerebral cortex; they also noted changes in conduction times and apparent velocities in different segments of the pathways. They confirmed previous suggestions (Chiappa, 1983) that the posterior tibial nerve is the most useful for routine clinical use because of the larger amplitude of its SEPs and less intersubject variability when compared with the other lower-limb nerves.

Goodridge et al. (1987) have suggested the use of paraspinal stimulation for localization of spinal lesions.

9.2. Subject/Patient Factors

9.2.1. Age

Normal premature infants, neonates, and children are discussed in Chapter 11.

Age changes in adults have received much less attention in SEPs than in PSVEPs and BAEPs. Lueders (1970) studied median nerve SEPs in 40 male subjects 19 to 70 years old, dividing them into four groups: 19 to 29, 30 to 45, 46 to 58, and 59 to 70 years old. Absolute latencies of N19 and P23 showed no differences between the groups (earlier potentials were not measured). The N19 to P23 amplitude showed a significant decline in the 30- to 45-year-old group and then increased above that age. Hume et al. (1982) found no changes in P/N13 to N19 IPL from 10 to 49 years but noted an abrupt increase of about 0.3 msec between the fifth and sixth decades, with little change thereafter. Allison et al. (1983, 1984) studied median nerve SEPs in 286 subjects from 4 to 95 years of age and have provided detailed data on latency changes in the 4- to 17- and 18- to 95-year-old age groups (Figs. 8–24 and 8–25). Kakigi (1987) studied age effects in posterior tibial nerve SEPs in 20 normal young subjects and 45 subjects divided into 61- to 74-year-old and 75- to 88-year-old groups.

Dorfman and Bosley (1979) studied 15 young adults (mean age 31.6 years) and 15 elderly subjects (mean age 74.1 years). They concluded that (1) median nerve conduction velocities slowed with advancing age at about 0.16 msec/year for sensory fibers; (2) SEP on-

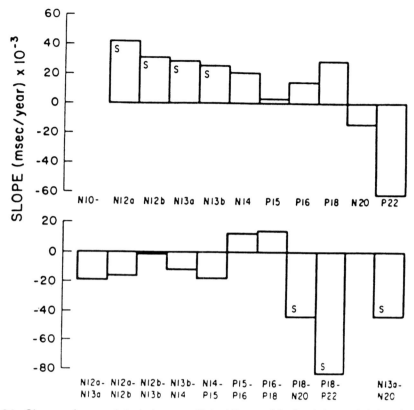

FIG. 8–24. Slopes of age-related changes (4 to 17 years) in the interpeak latencies (IPLs) of SEP components (there were no gender differences and pooled data are shown), e.g., the 40 level on the vertical axis is a change in latency of 40 msec/year. Significant slopes ($p < 0.01$) have an S in the upper left of the bar. The *upper graph* shows IPLs relative to brachial plexus activity, and the *lower graph* shows sequential IPLs. Approximate waveform nomenclature correlations are N10 with EP, N13a with P/N13, and N13a–N20 with P/N13–N19. Total subjects for 4 to 95 years = 130 males, 156 females. (Adapted from Allison et al., 1984.)

set latencies increased with age at 0.015 msec/year for median and 0.08 msec/year for tibial (ankle) stimulation—these increases were thought to be produced in both the peripheral and central segments of the pathway; (3) spinal sensory conduction velocity (indirectly estimated) was stable over 18 to 60 years, then declined at 0.78 msec/year.

Desmedt and Cheron (1980b) studied digital nerve SEPs in 25 normal subjects 20 to 30 years old and 19 normal subjects 80 to 90 years old. Normalizing for distance, they found a significant difference in N14 onset latency (12.6 versus 14.8 msec; $p < 0.001$) for the two groups, and also a decrease in peripheral sensory conduction velocity (71.1 versus 61.2 m/sec). The onset of N22 (equivalent of N19) normalized for distance was 18.4 versus 20.7 msec ($p < 0.001$). The latency difference between the N14 equivalent and N22 was shorter in the older subjects (6.1 versus 5.5 msec; $p < 0.005$) unless normalized for distance, when the latency difference was not significant. They commented that the primary afferent neurons appeared to age faster than the second- or third-order neurons.

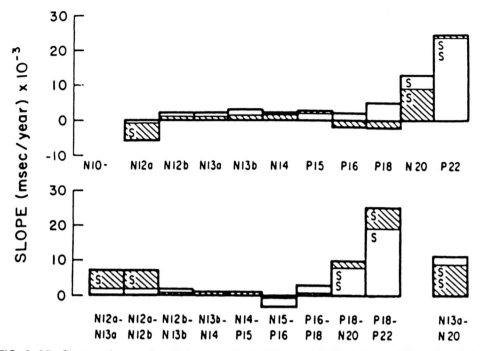

FIG. 8–25. Slopes of age-related changes (18 to 95 years) in the interpeak latencies (IPLs) of SEP components (cross-hatched = male, clear = female), e.g., the 40 level on the vertical axis is a change in latency of 40 msec/year. Significant slopes ($p < 0.01$) have an S in the *upper left* of the bar, and slopes with a significant gender difference have an S at the border between the areas. Upper and lower graphs and nomenclature correlations same as for Figure 8–24. Total subjects for 4 to 95 years = 130 males, 156 females. (Adapted from Allison et al., 1984.)

Cracco et al. (1975) and Cracco and Cracco (1979) studied spinal EPs in 95 infants, children, and adults who had no evidence of peripheral nerve or spinal cord pathology, including 10 premature and term infants. They found that in all age groups the speed of conduction was nonlinear, being slower over caudal cord segments than over peripheral nerves or rostral cord segments. Newborns had both spinal cord and peripheral nerve conduction velocities that were about one half of adult values and progressively increased with age. They found that peripheral nerve values reached adult levels by about 3 years of age, whereas spinal cord values did not reach adult levels until about 5 years of age.

Mervaala et al. (1988) and Zegers de Beyl et al. (1988) found no height or age correlation for interpeak latency (N13–N19) (see also Tsuji et al., 1984).

Eggermont (1988), using a simple developmental model, has defined three exponential functions with time constants of 4 weeks, 40 weeks, and 4 years which describe maturational latency changes.

9.2.2. Gender

Green et al. (1982a) found that in a group of 31 normal subjects the females (21) had shorter central conduction times than the males (10) by about 1 msec (12.1 versus 13.1

msec, $p < 0.00001$). The reason for this difference (e.g., head and brain size, body temperature) is not known. Note that Mervaala et al. (1988) found no such correlation.

9.2.3. Body Size

The absolute latency of SEPs is obviously related to the distance between stimulus site and waveform generator (see also Kritchevsky and Wiederholt, 1978; Sauer and Schenck, 1977; Desmedt and Brunko, 1980; Small et al., 1978, 1980; Mervaala et al., 1988; Chu, 1986; Tsuji et al., 1984; Chu and Hong, 1985). With upper-limb testing, the standard deviations of absolute latencies (around 0.8 msec) are twice that of IPLs (around 0.4 msec) and most of the extra variability in the absolute latencies is due to differences in body size. Thus, if absolute latencies are used for interpretations, the normal range will be twice that for IPLs, with a resulting loss of interpretation accuracy, unless a correction for body size is applied. When latencies are taken relative to the brachial plexus (Erb's point) potential, the recommended procedure, the effect of differences in body size on the IPLs is small enough that it can be disregarded.

As expected, the effect of body size is much more prominent with lower-limb testing and a correction for height must be applied to both absolute latencies and the conduction time from lower cord to cerebrum, as discussed above in Section 8 and Figs. 8–15 to 8–17 (see also Dorfman, 1977; Phillips and Daube, 1980; Wilson et al., 1981; Small and Matthews, 1984; and Lastimosa et al. 1982).

9.2.4. Body/Limb Temperature

Peripheral nerve conduction velocities are significantly affected by changes in limb temperature so that the accepted practice in EMG laboratories is to measure and control it (e.g., Bolton et al., 1981; Denys, 1991).

Matthews et al. (1979) raised the body temperature of normal subjects 1°C and found that P/N13 and N19 decreased in absolute latency by 0.7 and 1.0 msec, respectively, while the brachial plexus to N19 conduction time was shortened by only 0.18 msec. Kazis et al. (1982) found no significant changes in SEP latencies in 17 control subjects studied during fever (38.0°C to 39.7°C due to viral infection, etc.) and 2 to 3 days later. Markand et al. (1990a,b) and Guerit et al. (1990) reported the effects of controlled hypothermia down to 19.0°C and noted more marked changes for later components.

9.2.5. Drugs

The short-latency SEPs discussed here are remarkably unaffected by drugs. For example, when barbiturates are given in doses sufficient to render the EEG isoelectric, little change is seen in the SEPs. Hume et al. (1979) studied comatose patients and found no relationship between blood levels of phenobarbital (0 to 146 µg/ml, median 56 µg/ml) and upper-limb SEP central conduction times. In another study of head-injured patients they did find some correlation with serum phenobarbital levels (none with blood gases and pH) but the combined effects of drug and body temperature contributed to only 4% of the variance in conduction times (Hume and Cant, 1981). Sutton et al. (1982) found no short-latency SEP changes in cats at therapeutic coma levels induced by pentobarbital. Rumpl et al. (1988a) observed prolonged P/N13–N19 IPL in patients in coma due to severe CNS depressant drug overdose (amitryptyline, barbiturates, meprobamate, and nitrazepam), with a return to normal at therapeutic levels. Although we have not systematically studied this question, we have consistently noted normal SEP IPLs in patients in intensive care units who are being treated with high-dose barbiturates as a therapy for increased intracranial pressure and who have burst-suppression or isoelectric EEGs (as long as the primary intracerebral lesion does not involve the sensory structures).

Green et al. (1982a,b) studied the effects of phenytoin on SEPs in 163 epileptic patients. Using analysis of variance, they found no effect of seizure type, duration of epilepsy, frequency of seizures, or abnormal EEG on SEP central conduction times. Age ($p < 0.001$), sex ($p < 0.00001$) and serum levels of phenytoin ($p < 0.012$) were related to SEP central conduction time; levels of phenytoin in the toxic range had an even greater effect ($p < 0.005$). Mean values for central conduction (corrected for age and body size) were 13.02 msec for normal subjects, and for patients taking only phenytoin with blood levels 0, 1 to 9, 10 to 20, and greater than 20 µg/ml 13.24, 13.09, 13.53, and 14.15, respectively. In another study of 108 patients, Green et al. (1982a,b) found that phenytoin, but not phenobarbital, was associated with prolonged IPLs at concentrations over 20 µg/ml, but that neither carbamazepine nor primidone produced changes.

Mavroudakis et al. (1991) reported that a phenytoin infusion increased the latency of the spinal N13 potential and increased central conduction time.

Prevec (1980) studied four children before and after intravenous administration of 10 mg diazepam. Although he did not measure N19, inspection of the available traces shows no apparent changes in latency or amplitude of that wave. He noted a slightly shorter peak latency of P25 after diazepam (mean 1.8 msec), perhaps due more to an amplitude and shape change than to an actual latency shift.

9.2.6. Peripheral Neuropathies

Peripheral neuropathies obviously will affect absolute latencies. However, those of the purely axonal type will have much less effect on latency than demyelinating types. Thus, patients with Friedreich's ataxia may show absent Erb's point potentials and low-amplitude but normal latency cerebral potentials. In this case the few axons remaining conduct at normal velocities.

Demyelinating lesions produce large delays in absolute latencies, hence the importance of measuring central latencies relative to a point as close to the CNS as possible. It is important to note that with upper-limb stimulation there is still 8 to 12 cm of nerve with peripheral-type myelin interposed between the reference point and the point in the spinal canal where the myelin changes to central type so that a peripheral neuropathy (e.g., in Guillain-Barré disease) can still cause apparent increases in central conduction times. With lower-limb stimulation the potentials recorded over the lower spine are generated in the spinal canal in cauda equina very close to the root entry zone and in the root entry zone itself so that the same problem cannot occur even though most of the cauda equina has peripheral-type myelin. (For further discussion, see sections on appropriate diseases in Chapter 9.)

9.2.7. Radiation of Brain Stem

Nightingale et al. (1984) saw no median nerve SEP changes in five patients studied up to 8 months following a mean brain stem dose of radiation of about 2,000 rads over 22 to 35 days for tumor therapy. Lecky et al. (1980) saw no changes in six patients studied up to 6 months after incidental spinal cord irradiation.

9.2.8. Reproducibility—Reliability

There are no systematic studies of the consistency of SEPs over long periods of time and with repeat studies. Matthews and Small (1979) recorded SEPs from 27 patients with MS on two or more occasions, the interval between the first and last recordings varying from 1 to 40 months (mean 14 months). In seven of these patients testing was performed every 1 to 3 months and in these patients the SEP waveforms did not change significantly in the four in whom no relapse occurred; there were SEP changes in the three who had clinical relapses. Vogel and Vogel (1982) studied lower-limb SEPs in 10 normal subjects over 2 to 8 weeks and found up to a 4-msec variability in N/P37 absolute latency.

9.2.9. State

Desmedt and Manil (1970) and Desmedt et al. (1980) studied the differences in SEPs in newborn infants in rapid eye movement (REM) sleep, slow-wave sleep, and waking (see Section 9.2.1). Cracco (1980) tested five normal subjects awake and asleep and noted no change in P13 but commented that peak latencies of subsequent components often increased during sleep. Yamada et al. (1988) compared median nerve SEPs in waking and stages II, IV, REM, and non-REM sleep and found amplitude and absolute latency changes significant at the $p < 0.01$ level (for N20 the latency change was 0.36 msec—$p < 0.02$). Interpeak latency changes were not described. Addy et al. (1989) found prolonged cortical latencies during stage II sleep. Noguchi et al. (1995) found that the amplitudes of frontal components, particularly P22, were increased in sleep, whereas the amplitudes of parietal components were decreased in sleep. Santamaria et al. (1994) described a significant increase in central conduction time with median nerve SEPs during stage II sleep in young and old healthy subjects. Emerson et al. (1988) noted sleep versus waking alterations of N20 latency and morphology on a minute-by-minute basis using special analysis techniques. Their observed shifts of up to 0.9 msec for the EP–N20 IPL might be significant in interside comparisons since the two sides are tested at different times (the upper limit of normal being 0.8 msec).

Yamauchi et al. (1976) found no latency changes but decreased amplitude of N19 during electrical acupuncture to two points on the hand. The acupuncture stimulus consisted of 1.3 to 3 pulses/sec of 1 msec duration at "maximum tolerable stimulation without undue discomfort." De-Xuan et al. (1983) and Kang et al. (1983) also have found no SEP changes during acupuncture.

Evoked Potentials in Clinical Medicine,
3d ed., edited by Keith H. Chiappa.
Lippincott–Raven Publishers, Philadelphia © 1997.

9

Short-Latency Somatosensory Evoked Potentials: Interpretation

Keith H. Chiappa, and °Rosamund A. Hill

*Department of Neurology, Harvard Medical School, and EEG Laboratory,
Massachusetts General Hospital, Boston, Massachusetts 02114; and
°Neuroservices Unit, Auckland Hospital, Auckland, New Zealand*

1. ANATOMIC AND PHYSIOLOGIC BASIS OF SOMATOSENSORY EVOKED POTENTIALS

1.1. Human Data

1.1.1. Anatomy

The stimulus intensity used for somatosensory evoked potentials (SEPs) excites only the largest myelinated fibers in the peripheral nerve (cutaneous and subcutaneous somaesthetic and proprioceptive fibers, and alpha motor axons). Stimulation strong enough to produce activity in smaller fibers is too painful for clinical use. It may not be possible to stimulate the smallest (pain—C) fibers electrically without producing skin damage [it is even difficult to stimulate them with needles placed intradermally but outside the nerve itself (Hallin and Torebjork, 1973)].

Cell bodies of the large-fiber dorsal column sensory system lie in the dorsal root ganglia; their central processes travel rostrally in ipsilateral posterior columns of the spinal cord and synapse in the dorsal column nuclei at the cervicomedullary junction. Second-order fibers cross to the opposite side shortly after origination and travel to the primary receiving nucleus (ventroposterolateral, VPL) of the thalamus via the medial lemniscus. Third-order fibers continue from thalamus to frontoparietal sensorimotor cortex. Whether or not any of the activity generating SEPs in humans travels in ascending paths other than the posterior columns is not known (also see below).

1.1.2. Sensory Tracts Involved

Note that there is some uncertainty about the localization of vibration, joint position, and tactile sensation in the dorsal columns (Greenberg et al., 1987; Wall and Noordenbos, 1977).

Clinical studies have consistently found that SEP abnormalities are associated with disorders of joint position, touch, vibration, and stereognosis but are not seen in disorders affecting only pain and temperature sensations (see Section 2.1 for a more complete presentation of these data). However, there is little direct human evidence relating to whether or not the posterior columns of the spinal cord and medial lemnisci are the only structures involved in the transmission of the volleys responsible for the generation of these SEPs. Namerow (1969) studied three patients who had unilateral percutaneous cordotomies for intractable pain; the interruption of the lateral spinothalamic tract produced hypalgesia and hypesthesia below the lesion but no changes in N19–P23 on either side. Domino et al. (1965) tested SEPs during cryothalamectomy, performed, without premedication, to relieve incapacitating motor symptoms. They found that lesions in VPL nucleus produced the most marked changes in the SEP. Blair et al. (1975) studied tibial SEPs during direct electrical stimulation of the dorsal columns and found attenuation of late components but little effect on early ones. If stimulus intensities greater than those necessary to relieve pain were used, the amplitudes of all components were diminished. Jones et al. (1982) recorded in humans directly from the epidural space at various levels of the spinal cord. They found a complex set of waveforms which they were able to resolve into at least three components with different activation thresholds and conduction velocities. They suggested that the faster activity was conducted in the dorsal spinocerebellar tracts and the slower waves in the posterior columns since they could not record activity of the fastest fibers with stimulation of any intensity at the ankle and the posterior tibial nerve contains many fewer Ia and Ib afferents at that location than at the knee. Macon et al. (1982) recorded epidural SEPs in a patient who had a surgically induced lesion of one dorsal column and noted that the cord potentials rostral to the lesion were abolished, whereas a patient with a complete anterior quadrant lesion did not have a significant SEP change. A case of autopsy-proven anterior spinal artery infarction showed no abnormality of the posterior tibial SEPs (Zornow et al., 1990). Yamada et al. (1981) studied the effect of tourniquet-induced ischemia on median nerve SEPs and found that the components up to and including N18 were abolished before later components. They believed that this suggests that SEP components are not transmitted through a single pathway but are mediated through independent routes, probably involving different first-order fibers. In summary, the last study aside, these human findings suggest that the large-fiber sensory system (posterior columns of the spinal cord and lemniscal system) carries the impulses responsible for these SEPs.

Cusick et al. (1978) studied 10 macaque monkeys by surgically isolating or sparing the posterior columns and recording EPs from epidural and subdural spaces anterior and posterior to the spinal cord. Segmental resection of the dorsal columns both at thoracic and cervical levels resulted in total obliteration of the responses recorded rostral to this lesion, whereas isolated segmental dorsal column preservation did not significantly alter response latency or waveforms recorded at the rostral electrodes. Zornow et al. (1990) recorded normal lower-limb SEPs in a patient with an anterior spinal artery syndrome who was later shown to have an infarction of the anterior portion of the thoracolumbar spinal cord with preservation of the posterior columns.

Until further evidence is forthcoming, these short-latency SEPs can reasonably be considered to be generated by volleys traversing the posterior columns and medial lemnisci. Note that Ia afferents produce no conscious sensation so that conduction defects in them might produce SEP abnormalities without abnormal sensation. There is also considerable evidence (although controversial) indicating that muscle afferents are involved in SEP generation (see Chapter 8, Section 9.1.7).

1.1.3. Clinicopathologic Correlations

Clinical interpretation of SEP data is based on knowledge of the anatomic sites generating the waveforms. This information in humans is provided by potential-field distribution studies, physiologic behavior (e.g., refractory period, response to interfering stimuli), microneuronography, and clinicopathologic correlations in patients with appropriately located, well-defined (clinical, radiologic, and, best if all, pathologic) lesions. Although computed tomography (CT) or magnetic resonance imaging (MRI) scans are often taken as the final word on anatomic involvement, they are not completely reliable for these purposes and should be used very carefully, certainly more carefully than in many published studies. Another confounding factor is the retrograde degeneration that occurs in many central nervous systems (CNS) after tract or nuclear lesions. For example, VPL neurons show degenerative changes within days to weeks after a purely cortical lesion and presumably are functionally inactive even earlier. Thus, the SEP studies that correlate waveforms with lesions present more than a few days are subject to ever-increasing errors (e.g., Sonoo et al., 1991a,b). Many of these studies do not even give the time interval between lesion and SEP testing.

Sections 6, 9.1.6, and 9.1.7 in Chapter 8 should be read carefully before proceeding here. Their conclusions are initially summarized in the sections below, followed by a discussion of the human clinicopathologic correlations available for the same area.

1.1.3.1. Brachial Plexus and Cauda Equina/Spinal Cord

The diphasic, positive–negative waveform recorded at the Erb's point electrode (labeled EP in Fig. 8–2) following stimulation of a peripheral nerve of the upper limb is generated by the ascending volley in motor and sensory fibers as it approaches and passes through the brachial plexus. Most of this negativity is generated in sensory fibers (rather than in the few antidromically stimulated alpha motor fibers) since it remains prominent in patients who have longstanding, flaccid paralysis of a limb following ventral root avulsions. Note that it is also unchanged in patients with dorsal root avulsions (if the brachial plexus is uninjured) since the nerve cell body remains in continuity with its axons (Fig. 9–1). If this continuity is broken in a plexus injury, after 5 to 10 days Wallerian degeneration proceeds peripherally and EP will be lost, as well as any mixed-nerve action potentials at the elbow or wrist.

The initial component of the waveform recorded from the lower lumbar region (labeled LP in Figs. 8–6 to 8–8) following stimulation of a peripheral nerve in the lower limb is generated by the afferent volley in the cauda equina. There are no good human clinicopathologic correlations of this activity. The second component of LP is generated in the root entry zone/dorsal horns of the lower spinal cord (like N13/P13 with upper-limb stimulation). This activity is unchanged in spinal shock (Sedgwick et al., 1980) but abnormal in lesions in-

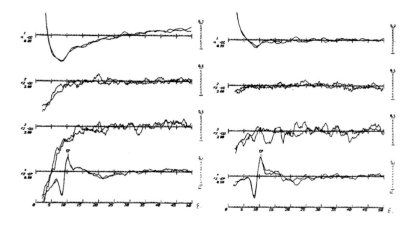

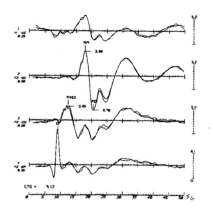

FIG. 9–1. Upper-limb SEPs in a 22-year-old man 1 month after a traumatic injury to the right arm. The arm was flaccid and all sensation was absent distal to a line 5 cm above the elbow. The left median nerve SEPs were normal (*lower panel*), but right median (*upper left*) and ulnar (*upper right*) nerve SEPs showed only EP (brachial plexus) activity and no subsequent waveforms. There was no muscle response to the stimulation, nor could the patient feel the stimulus. The preservation of EP at this time interval from the injury indicates that the peripheral sensory axons are still in continuity with their cell bodies in the sensory ganglia, suggesting relative sparing of the brachial plexus; the lack of central SEPs indicates interruption of the sensory paths central to the ganglia, presumably root avulsion. Recording montages same as for Fig. 8–2. Stimulation of median and ulnar nerves at the wrist at 5/sec. Each trace is the average of 512 stimuli. Calibrations marks from the top are 6.0, 0.6, 0.6, and 3.0 for the upper panels, and 6.0, 3.0, 3.0, and 6.0 for the bottom panel. Stimulus artifact is visible in the upper panels because a higher stimulus intensity was used.

volving that level (Ertekin et al., 1980; Restuccia et al., 1993) or with chronic lesions at higher levels (Lehmkuhl et al., 1984). Children with tethered-cord malfunctions have a caudal displacement of this activity (Rossini et al., 1981; Roy et al., 1986a,b; Emerson, 1986).

The volley can be followed as it ascends in the posterior columns of the spinal cord but it becomes more dispersed rostrally because of slightly different conduction velocities in the involved axons and is difficult to record above midthoracic levels.

Latencies of central components are measured relative to the components recorded at Erb's point and cauda equina because this diminishes the effects of peripheral nerve conduction velocity alterations resulting from changes in limb temperature and neuropathies. For upper limb testing, this also negates the effect of subject height.

1.1.3.2. Cervical Cord

With lower-limb testing, activity in the cervical cord and medulla cannot be routinely recorded in human subjects unless large numbers of stimulus repetitions or special needle electrodes are used (see Chapter 8, Section 4, and Lueders et al., 1981).

With upper-limb stimulation, the potentials appearing at 11 to 12 msec over the neck and low back of the head after a stimulus at the wrist are negative, as recorded and illustrated in Figs. 8–2 and 8–3 at the N11 label. This activity is generated by the ascending volley in the posterior columns (cuneate tract).

Dissociation between N11 and later waves is occasionally seen. Almost three quarters of brain-dead patients have preservation of P/N13 (Goldie et al., 1981), but some of those lacking this wave had preservation of N11 (also noted by Anziska and Cracco, 1980b). Stohr et al. (1982) presented clinical, radiologic, and SEP data in 17 patients with cervical cord lesions. They found some cases where P/N13 was exclusively abolished; these were restricted lesions in the lower cervical segments. Larger cervical cord lesions which seemed likely to involve the root entry zone also produced attenuation or loss of N11, as also noted for traumatic dorsal root avulsion (Jones, 1979). Patients with cervical cord lesions (Fig. 9–2; see *N Engl J Med* 316:150–157, 1987, for a full report of this case, and Fig. 9–20) or lower medullary lesions (Fig. 9–3) often show relative sparing of N11 in the face of abnormalities of N13, P13, and P14. Emerson and Pedley (1986), Urasaki et al. (1988) and Sonoo et al. (1990) have also described patients with cervical cord lesions (syrinxes, ependymomas, compressions) with N11 (their DCV) and N13 (their CERV N13/P13) abnormalities consistent with the suggested localizations. Taylor et al. (1985) studied the effects of profound hypothermia and noted dissociations between some of these components.

For purposes of clinical interpretation it can reasonably be assumed that N11 is generated in the dorsal columns. The posterior neck negative activity (with its dipolar positive reflection anteriorly on the neck) is generated in the upper cervical cord by postsynaptic activity in the central gray matter (dorsal horns).

1.1.3.3. Dorsal Column Nucleus, Medial Lemniscus

With lower-limb testing, activity in the cervical cord and medulla cannot be routinely recorded in human subjects unless large numbers of stimulus repetitions or special needle electrodes are used (see Chapter 8, Sections 4, and 9.1.6).

Following upper-limb stimulation, positive potentials are registered at 13 to 15 msec over the scalp, as illustrated in Fig. 8–3 in the FZ–hand and Cc–hand channels at the P13 label (FZ and Cc relative positivity causes an upward deflection in these channels). As discussed

text continued on p. 352

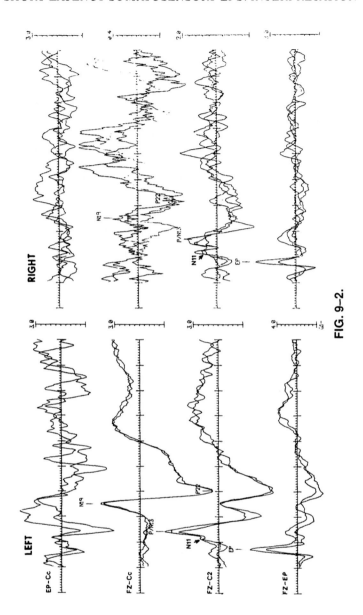

FIG. 9–2.

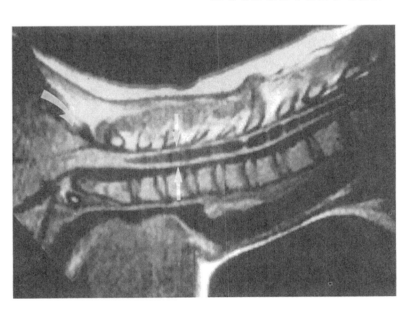

FIG. 9–2. (*Continued*) Median nerve SEPs and MRI scan in a 17-year-old woman with symptoms and signs indicative of a lesion in the left brain stem. Left-sided stimulation produced normal results; right-sided stimulation showed P/N13 and N19/P22 of abnormally low amplitude but normal N11, suggesting a conduction defect in the upper cervical cord on the right. The MRI scan shows an Arnold–Chiari type I malformation with the cerebellar tonsils below the plane of the foramen magnum (*curved arrow*). Syringomyelia was also present, with the syrinx extending from C2 downward to just above the conus medullaris. The arrows indicate the anterior and posterior borders of the spinal cord, somewhat expanded by the syrinx visible in the middle. Despite the prominent clinical signs pointing to a lesion in the medulla, syringobulbia was seen in the MRI scan; presumably the cavity was too narrow to be detected. Lower-limb SEPs were normal. Recording montage same as for Fig. 8–2. Each trace is the average of 512 stimuli delivered at 5/sec. Calibrations are 3.0 μV (4.0 for bottom channel) for left panel, and 3.0, 0.4, 2.0, and 3.0 for right panel (from the top). (From Case Records of the Massachusetts General Hospital, *N Engl J Med* 316:150–157, 1987, with permission; see that text for case details.)

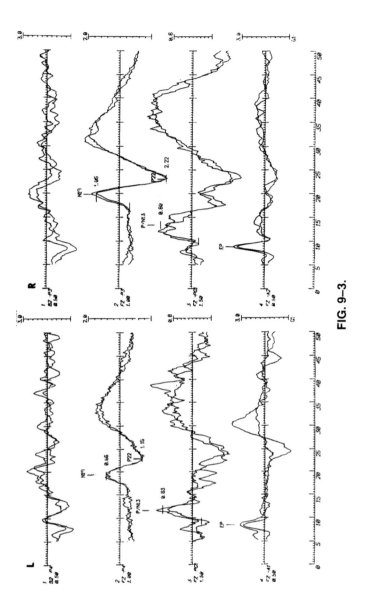

FIG. 9–3.

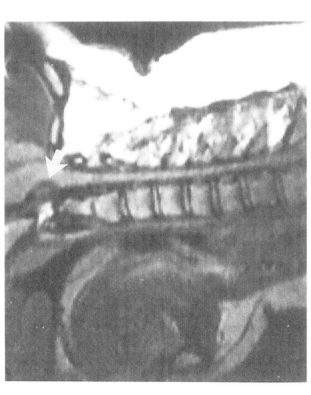

FIG. 9–3. (*Continued*) Median nerve SEPs and MRI scan in a 20-year-old man with increased leg stiffness for 3 months, and a long previous history of hydrocephalus (shunted at 19 months of age) secondary to posterior fossa arachnoid cysts. The SEP bilaterally shows an abnormal P/N13 with a best baseline to peak amplitude of 0.6 μV, below the lower limit of normal. As in the previous figure the early cervical component (N11) is relatively preserved, indicating bilateral conduction defects in the upper cervical cord. N19/P22 amplitude is abnormally low following left-sided stimulation (compared with right). The MRI scan shows large posterior fossa arachnoid cysts (*visible to the right and above the arrow*) displacing the brain stem anteriorly and compressing the anterior medulla around a soft tissue mass at the craniocervical junction (*arrow*) that presumably is a blood vessel. Recording montage and parameters same as for Fig. 9–2. Calibration marks from the top are 3.0, 2.0, 0.8, and 3.0 μV.

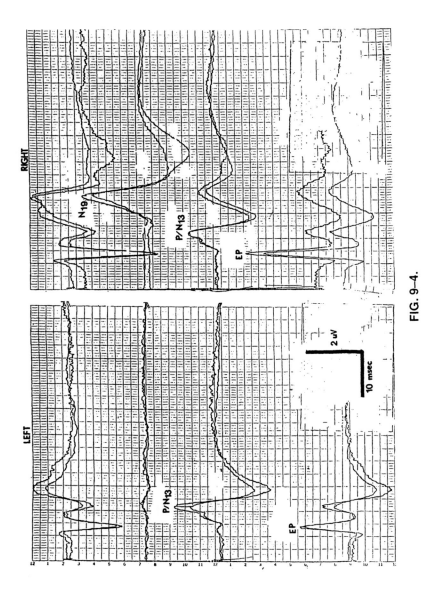

FIG. 9-4.

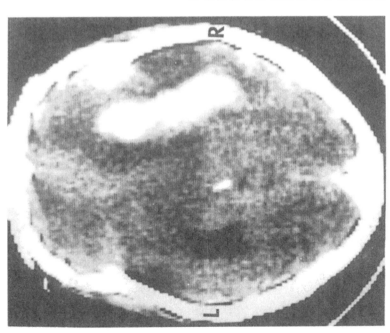

FIG. 9–4. (*Continued*) Median nerve SEPs and CT scan from a 42-year-old hypertensive man with an intracerebral hemorrhage involving the putamen and frontal and temporal lobes, with compression of the lateral ventricle, subfalcial herniation, and intraventricular blood. Computed tomography scan at other levels showed that the hemorrhage had not extended downward into the pons. Somatosensory EPs were done with the patient in barbiturate coma for control of intracranial pressure. Stimulation of the clinically affected side (*left*) had a normal P/N13 (*third channel from top*), whereas N19 and P22 were absent (*top two channels*). Right-sided stimulation was normal. Brain stem auditory EPs from the left ear were normal; the right ear showed a peripheral hearing deficit. Intracranial pressure could not be controlled and brain death ensued 2 days after the SEPs were done. Each trace is the average of 512 stimuli delivered at 5/sec. Recording montage and parameters same as for Fig. 9–2. Stimulation occurred 3.2 msec prior to sweep onset.

in Chapter 8, Sections 6 and 9.1.6, these are most likely generated postsynaptically in the dorsal column nuclei and medial lemniscus.

On the basis of latency and potential-field distribution, it was initially thought that P13 and P14 were generated in the caudal brain stem (Jones, 1977; Liberson et al., 1966) or more rostrally in the thalamus (Cracco and Cracco, 1976; Kritchevsky and Wiederholt, 1978). Others had either mentioned this activity only briefly (Goff et al., 1977) or not at all (Noel and Desmedt, 1975, 1976; Desmedt et al., 1976; Desmedt and Noel, 1973, 1975; Giblin, 1964; Halliday and Wakefield, 1963; Namerow, 1968, 1970).

Human clinicopathologic correlations have been very helpful in indicating the possible generator sites of these potentials. Chiappa et al. (1978, 1979, 1980) and Chiappa (1982) studied patients with CNS disease at a variety of levels and found P/N13 preserved in patients with thalamic hemorrhages (Fig. 9–4), midbrain hemorrhages, pontine infarcts and brain death, indicating a low medullary or cerebellar, or both, origin. Of these, the brain-dead patients provide the data which best define the rostral limit of the generator sources since, if appropriate criteria are used (especially including the lack of spontaneous respirations when off a respirator long enough for carbon dioxide tension to exceed 50 mmHg), the neuropathologic examination always reveals complete necrosis of brain stem structures down to at least the middle part of the medulla. About two thirds of patients who meet these criteria have some of P/N13 (usually mostly P13) present (Figs. 9–5 and 9–6) (Goldie et al., 1981); Wagner (1991) used nasopharyngeal electrodes to study this differentiation. The noncephalic reference channels (Fig. 9–5) usually show that the later positivity appearing in normal subjects at about 14 msec is absent, as also seen by Buchner et al. (1988); this activity is a contribution from the medial lemniscus in the medulla and low pons. Note that these patients, when P13 is present, also may show at the scalp a considerable amount of negativity at 13 to 14 msec which presumably is generated at the level of the cervicomedullary junction and normally leads into and is obscured by the higher-amplitude negativity generated in the thalamus. In brain-dead patients this "uncovered" negative activity may erroneously be considered to have a thalamic origin.

In patients with neurologic diseases where the extent of the lesion can be defined clinically and/or radiologically [this usually excludes multiple sclerosis (MS)], it is possible to find a dissociation between the negativity over the neck and low back of the head and the positive potentials seen over the scalp (Figs. 9–2 and 9–3) (Stohr et al., 1982; Emerson and Pedley, 1986). A particularly good example of this was presented by Mauguiere et al. (1983c), who tested a patient with a unilateral, low medullary lemniscal transection from a bone fragment. When stimulating the median nerve on the side clinically affected with a dense sensory loss, N13 recorded from the neck was normal, whereas P14 was absent. The fact that a perfectly normal side was available for comparison in the case of Mauguiere et al. makes it especially valuable. Mavroudakis et al. (1993) have presented a case of a focal lesion at the spinomedullary junction with similar results. The clear preservation of P13 in the brain-dead patients (with only the lowest parts of the medulla intact) (Fig. 9–5) does not fit completely with the latter case but the patient of Mauguiere et al. probably had a normal variation in which P13 was poorly developed bilaterally since it is not registered well even on the unaffected side. Although this dissociation is frequently seen as an abnormality in MS (see Fig. 8–4) the lack of definite anatomic localization renders these cases less useful for generator source considerations.

Suzuki et al. (1982) recorded directly from the ventral surface of the brain stem in humans and recorded peaks of positive activity at the same latencies as those recorded from the scalp. Lesser et al. (1981), recording from the spinal cord surface, registered high-amplitude potentials at the level of the foramen magnum, with latencies approximating or

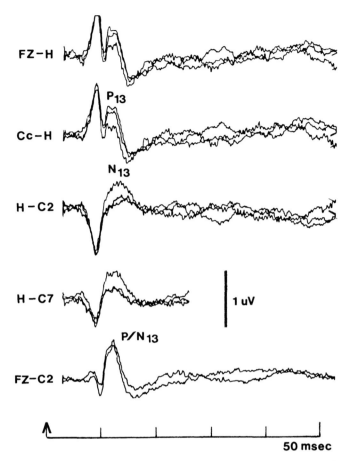

FZ–H

Cc–H

P_{13}

N_{13}

H–C2

H–C7

1 uV

P/N_{13}

FZ–C2

50 msec

FIG. 9–5. Median nerve SEPs from a patient who met all clinical criteria of brain death, including no spontaneous respirations at a carbon dioxide tension of 50 mmHg. In the FZ–C2 channel (*bottom trace*) P/N13 has a normal appearance except that the P14 peak usually seen on the downslope in many normal subjects is absent. Hand reference recordings show that the neck negativity (N11–N13) is preserved, as is P13, but P14 from the scalp is absent. Each trace is the average of 500 responses, with three repetitions superimposed (two for bottom channel). In upper two channels, relative positivity of the scalp electrode causes an upward deflection; in the neck channels, relative negativity of the neck causes an upward trace deflection (i.e., in all channels relative negativity of G2 causes an upward trace deflection).

following the major positivity recorded at the scalp at about 13 to 14 msec. They suggested that this potential is generated in ipsilateral dorsal column pathways at the level of the cervicomedullary junction. Hashimoto (1984) recorded from the fourth and third ventricles in a patient who was undergoing ventriculography for delineation of an arteriovenous malformation (AVM). He concluded that P13 and P14 reflected synchronized volleys of the medial lemniscus and its branches to various pontine and mesencephalic nuclei. Jacobson and Tew (1988) recorded intraoperatively from the cervicomedullary junction in two patients and concluded that P14 was generated rostral to that point. Katayama and Tsubokawa (1987) recorded from VPL and concluded that P13 and P14 reflected activity in the medial lemniscus (Morioka et al., 1991a,b).

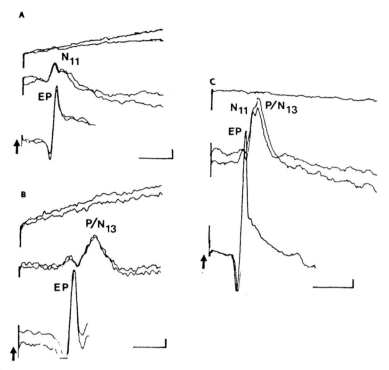

FIG. 9–6. Median nerve SEPs from brain-dead patients. N19–P22 complexes are absent from each—they would normally appear in the top channel (FZ–Cc). **A** shows a complete lack of N13, P13, and P14, with some of N11 preserved (*middle trace*—FZ–CII). **B** shows a small P/N13 preserved but delayed and distorted, possibly because of hypothermia (<92°F). **C** shows normal N11 and N13 and probably P13, but the lack of noncephalic reference recording does not allow definite statements about the presence or absence of P13 and P14. Microscopic neuropathologic examination in **C** showed complete necrosis in all areas examined, including upper medulla and pons; thus, any EPs present could not have been generated in those structures. Each trace is the average of 1,024 stimuli, with a repetition superimposed. Calibration marks are 10 msec and 0.25 μV. (From Goldie et al., 1981, with permission.)

Other studies of patients with brain stem lesions have confirmed these findings (Anziska and Cracco, 1980a, Greenberg et al., 1977; Small et al., 1980; Marra, 1982; Mauguiere and Courjon, 1981; Green and McLeod, 1979; Hume and Cant, 1978; Emerson and Pedley, 1986; Yamada et al., 1986; Delestre et al., 1986; Suzuki and Mayanagi, 1984).

Tomberg et al. (1991b) recorded a large N18 from nasopharyngeal electrodes and suggested that this was being generated in the medulla.

In summary, it can reasonably be assumed that the scalp positive activity at about 13 msec after a stimulus at the wrist is generated postsynaptically in the dorsal column nucleus (cuneatus), and that at 14 msec or so is generated in the medial lemniscus in the medulla and low pons. As was discussed above and in Chapter 8, the use of noncephalic reference derivations may allow dissociations between dorsal column (neck N11), dorsal horn (neck posterior/anterior N13/P13), dorsal column nuclei (scalp P13), and medial lemniscus (scalp P14) activities. However, the subjects/patients need to be especially quiet for these recordings to be interpretable at a confidence level appropriate for clinical work. Although we have routinely registered these derivations in several thousand patients, I do not find that they can routinely be well-defined without special effort, and even then the extra informa-tion is usually not clinically significant. Use of the FZ–CII deriviation and the "P/N13" waveform as described in Chapter 8 localizes the site of the lesion to the region of the cervi-comedullary junction (upper cervical cord and lower medulla), which is usually enough to direct clinical and/or radiologic attention to the proper area. Further anatomic delineation by electrophysiologic techniques would, in any case, require radiologic confirmation before any clinical decisions were made.

1.1.3.4. Thalamus, Cortex

Major lesions of the thalamus abolish all waves after the lower medullary components (i.e., after 15 msec following upper-limb stimulation). The most common examples of this are provided by thalamic hemorrhages (see Fig. 9–4). Thalamic infarcts (e.g., lacunes) and tumors may or may not affect these SEP components, the SEP results usually paralleling clinical symptomatology. Specific anatomic structures (VPL) must be involved for the SEP to be abnormal. For example, patients with thalamic lacunar infarcts may have normal SEPs even if there are sensory symptoms and/or signs. Usually the SEP parallels the clinical ex-amination and the SEP is abnormal when there are significant clinical deficits (Hammond et al., 1982; see also Section 2.1 below).

The wide scalp potential-field distribution of much of the negative activity after 15 msec led to suggestions that it had a subcortical, that is, thalamic, origin (Abbruzzese et al., 1978b; Chiappa et al., 1978, 1979, 1980; Chiappa, 1982). Note that there is a polarity rever-sal across the central sulcus with pial recordings and across the cortex with depth record-ings in epileptic patients undergoing surgery (Wood et al., 1988). However, intrathalamic recordings (Ervin and Mark, 1964; Pagni, 1967; Larson and Sances, 1968; Fukushima et al., 1976; Celesia, 1979; Chiappa, 1982; Tsuji et al., 1984; Albe-Fessard et al., 1986; Katayama and Tsubokawa, 1987; Morioka et al., 1989; Urasaki et al., 1990b) showed a great deal of ac-tivity in the primary receiving nucleus of the thalamus (VPL) at about the same time that the peak of widespread negativity was seen on the scalp (Fig. 9–7). This does not prove that the activity recorded at the scalp is the same as that seen at the surface, but suggests a relation-ship. Urasaki et al. (1990a,b, 1993b) also made direct recordings in the medulla and pons and found no latency shift of the negative activity above the upper pons, suggesting that N18 originates from between the upper pons and the mid-brain rather than from the thalamus. Sonoo et al. (1991a) found the widespread N18 preserved in a patient with a lesion of the pontine medial lemniscus and a profound unilateral disturbance of deep sensation, suggest-ing an even lower origin of some of this activity. Tomberg et al. (1991a) used nasopharyn-geal electrodes which are situated approximately at the level of the cervicomedullary junc-tion to record a large N18, also suggesting a medullary origin for the widespread component of the negativity. Sonoo et al. (1992b) showed a patient with a lesion at the pontomedullary junction with a normal N18, whereas a lesion in the dorsal columns at C1–2 abolished N18.

Again, human clinicopathologic correlations are very helpful. Chiappa et al. (1978, 1979, 1980) and Goldie et al. (1981) published a series of patients with specific lesions indicating that much of the scalp negativity after 15 msec was being generated in the thalamus. A pa-tient with an acute centrum semiovale leukoencephalopathy with marked sensory loss had preservation of the negativity on the appropriate side with complete absence of subsequent positivity (Fig. 9–8), a dissociation that would be difficult to produce if the generators of

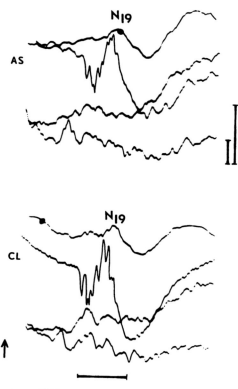

FIG. 9–7. Right median nerve SEPs (at 5/sec) from a patient with a left intrathalamic (VPL) depth electrode placed for investigation and treatment of a pain syndrome. Channel derivations (*top to bottom*) were FZ–Cc, AS (left ear) or CL (left clavicle) to VPL, FZ–CII, and FZ–EP; relative negativity at G2 and in the thalamus produced an upward trace deflection. Note the large peak of negative activity in VPL that precedes N19 (*top channel*) by a millisecond or so (maximum at same time as scalp Cc negativity when it is recorded with a noncephalic reference). Calibration marks are 10 msec and 2 μV (the smaller mark refers to the VPL channel). (From Chiappa, 1982, with permission.)

both activities were in the cortex. Also, the CT scan in that patient (Fig. 9–8) showed significant lesions in the white matter surrounding the thalamus (the centrum semiovale), indicating that as the site of the functional transection (Chiappa et al., 1980). The most convincing cases are those patients with apallic syndrome (persistent vegetative state) following anoxic insults. The patient whose SEPs are shown in Fig. 9–9 suffered a cardiac arrest and was tested about 3 days later (a period of time sufficient for neuropathologic changes to become manifest) when he was clinically in an apallic state. The median SEPs showed a normal-appearing N19 and subsequent positivity was absent or very poorly seen (Fig. 9–9). He died a few hours later, so the correlation between neuropathology and SEP results should be good; detailed examination of both sensory and motor cortex showed widespread and complete necrosis with a normal-appearing thalamus (Fig. 9–9). Even when recorded in bipolar fashion (FZ–Cc) N19 appeared normal, suggesting that even the localized component of the scalp negativity was not affected by the cortical necrosis. Patients with advanced Creutzfeldt–Jakob disease, a cortical degenerative disease, also show essentially the same pattern at advanced stages of the disease (Chiappa, 1982). More severe cases of anoxic dam-

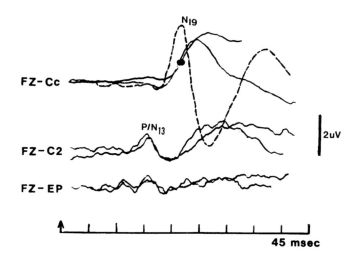

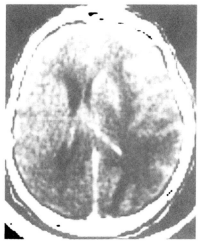

FIG. 9–8. Median nerve SEPs (unilateral stimulation at 5/sec) and CT scan from a patient with a centrum semiovale leukoencephalopathy, primarily affecting right cerebral structures (note lucent area in CT scan). Stimulating the clinically less affected side (*right*), the N19–P22 complex has a normal configuration (*dashed line in top channel*). Stimulating the clinically severely affected side (*left*), the N19 negativity is present, although slightly delayed, but the P22 positivity is entirely absent with the trace either remaining negative for 10 msec or more (*one trace*) or returning to baseline over 20 msec (*second trace*). This dissociation between N19 and P22, with the lesion location, suggests that N19 is generated caudal to the centrum semiovale, that is, in the thalamus. Each trace is the average of 1,024 stimuli, with a repetition superimposed from left-sided stimulation. (From Chiappa et al., 1980, with permission.)

age will not show N19 (Wytrzes et al., 1989). Note also that brain-dead patients may show an apparent N18 which is actually "uncovered" negativity from the region of the cervicomedullary junction, its appearance facilitated by the absence of P14, N18, N19, and P22 generators, also seen in extensive lesions of the pons (Raroque et al., 1994). Urasaki et al. (1992) have studied N18 amplitude abnormalities in patients with midbrain–pontine lesions and concluded that much of this activity (far-field components) is generated in this region. Although clinicopathologic correlations had been attempted previously (Desmedt and Noel, 1973, 1975; Anziska and Cracco, 1980; Williamson et al., 1970; Tsumoto et al., 1973; Mauguiere et al., 1983a,b; Obeso et al., 1980), all of these studies ignored the complete retrograde degeneration of the primary thalamic nuclei which occurs within 6 to 12 weeks after a cortical insult (Powell, 1952; Russell, 1958; Peacock and Combs, 1965). None of the SEP studies mentioned above indicated the time interval between the lesion and SEP testing, although in some it was obvious that months to years had elapsed (e.g., in Figs. 11–13 of Noel and Desmedt, 1980). In one study (Obeso et al., 1980) it was stated that at least 2 weeks had elapsed, and in another (Mauguiere et al., 1982) it was stated that at least 3 months had

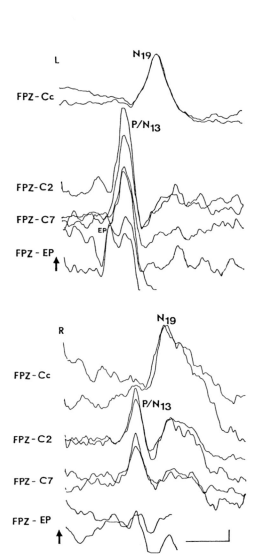

FIG. 9–9. Median nerve SEPs (unilateral stimulation at 5/sec) from a patient 4 days after cardiac arrest, clinically in an apallic (persistent vegetative) state. Upper set obtained following left and lower set following right-sided stimulation. Note the preservation of P/N13 and N19, with P22 absent. The microscopic picture of the parietal primary sensory cortex shows that the entire depth of the cortex was necrotic; this appearance was consistent over the entire cerebral cortex of both hemispheres, whereas the thalamus had a normal appearance. The patient died only a few hours after the SEP tests were performed, so this neuropathology was present at the time of SEP testing. Thus, the N19 negativity could not have been generated in the cortex. Each trace is the average of 1,024 stimuli, with two repetitions superimposed. Calibration marks are 10 msec and 0.25 μV. (From Goldie et al., 1981, with permission.)

elapsed. The time interval between the cortical damage and the SEP is critical and should be no greater than a few days if these correlations are to be reliable. Regli and Despland (1982) and Despland and Regli (1985) studied 70 patients with acute infarctions and found N19 preserved in small lesions confined to the postcentral gyrus, but absent in large lesions involving the underlying white matter and thalamus. When one of these patients was retested after several months, an N19 that had been previously present had disappeared, a correlation that is in agreement with the results of retrograde degeneration. Nakanishi et al. (1983), Spudis (1983), and Molaie (1987) had similar results. Macdonell et al. (1991) followed patients with strokes for 6 months and concluded that the major effect of stroke on SEPs occurs acutely and is little affected by secondary degenerative processes. However, inspection of their data shows that five of their cases had no joint position sense loss at outset, in two more it had returned to normal at 6 weeks, and in another two it eventually returned to normal. Of the remaining three, two showed a progressive amplitude loss and one never had N19/P22 potentials. There was a substantial loss of negativity at 20 msec in two of the five cases shown; these were two of the four who had cortical involvement, and they had the most severe sensory loss in that group. Thus, these data suggest that in patients with a persistent dysfunction in large-fiber sensory systems from lesions rostral to the thalamus, there will be a progressive decline in N19/P22 amplitude. In the cases presented by Tsuji et al. (1988) the lesions involved subcortical as well as cortical structures, so they did not bear directly on this question. The case of Slimp et al. (1986), in which the primary sensory cortex was removed, is not particularly helpful since there was no preoperative SEP and the cortex removed was pathologically abnormal. Since this was a longstanding cortical lesion, any thalamic retrograde degeneration would have occurred and presumably altered the SEP. Intraoperative recordings in epileptic patients (Wood et al., 1988) show a polarity reversal at 18 to 19 msec across the central sulcus (negative posteriorly and positive anteriorly) and across the cortex vertically, but it is not clear from comparative amplitudes and potential-field distributions whether or not this is the activity being registered at the scalp.

Furthermore, lesions of the sensory cortex that are epileptogenic often produce augmentation of P23 but not N19 (measured from baseline to peak). This has been seen in epilepsia partialis continua (Giblin, 1964; Chiappa et al., 1980), focal lesions (Furlong et al., 1993) and many myoclonic disorders (Halliday, 1967a,b,c; Dorfman et al., 1978b; Shibasaki et al., 1977, 1978, 1985, 1990), and can have diagnostic utility.

The cases in which marked abnormalities of P23 are present but N19 is normal (even recorded in a bipolar, frontal to parietal derivation) are particularly difficult to reconcile with a cortical generator of the N19 activity. Since the cortex is only a few millimeters thick this differential involvement would have to be selective for one neuronal population (or site) while sparing another which is admixed anatomically (see Shibasaki et al., 1990, for a further discussion of this topic, and Peterson et al., 1995, for a detailed microelectrode study in monkeys confirming parallel activation of different cellular and anatomic elements in sensorimotor cortices). This might be reasonable for the myoclonic and degenerative conditions but how this would be possible in infarcts and apallia (persistent vegetative state) is problematic. It seems unlikely that these lesions affect certain areas of sensory cortex and not others. Along similar lines, Seyal et al. (1993) used transcranial magnetic stimulation prior to an electrical stimulation of the median nerve at the wrist and discovered that this enhanced the SEP components after N20 when the SEP volley was timed to arrive at the cortex between 50 and 120 msec after the cortical stimulation, presumably related to intracortical phasing mechanisms, either inhibitory or excitatory. The discrepancies among the data and the clinicopathologic correlations described above are rarely discussed and need to be resolved before we can consider this case closed. In summary, it can presently be reasonably assumed that the negative activity appearing in scalp electrodes between 16 and 19 msec after stimulating the median nerve at the wrist is being generated in the thalamus. Some slightly later negative activity localized to the parietal scalp is generated from thalamocortical radiations or primary cortex. It is generally agreed that the subsequent positivity (P22) is generated in the parietal sensory cortex (see Dinner et al., 1987, for recordings from chronically implanted subdural electrodes).

With lower-limb stimulation, there is only a small amount of clinicopathologic confirmation of the generator sites which have been hypothesized on the basis of parallels with upper-limb SEPs. The suggested correlations are (1) the negative activity seen at 30 to 34 msec following stimulation of the posterior tibial nerve at the ankle and at 25 to 28 msec following stimulation of the peroneal nerve at the knee (the initial widespread negativity) is presumably generated in the brain stem and thalamus (the equivalent of N18 seen with upper-limb stimulation); (2) the subsequent positive activity at 36 to 38 msec following stimulation of the posterior tibial nerve at the ankle (N/P37) and 31 to 34 msec (N/P34) following stimulation of the peroneal nerve at the knee is generated in the parietal sensory cortex (the equivalent of P22 seen with upper-limb stimulation). Molaie (1987) showed loss of N/P34 in patients with restricted cortical lesions, and Lesser et al. (1987) recorded from subdural electrodes within the interhemispheric fissure. Ebner et al. (1982) saw no changes in five patients with parasagittal tumors. Urasaki et al. (1993b) made recordings from the floor of the fourth ventricle during surgery for mengiomas and hydrocephalus and found these results to be in substantial agreement with these localizations. (See also Chapter 8, Section 9.1.7, for a more detailed discussion of the possible fiber types involved in lower-limb SEP generation.)

1.2. Animal Data

A great deal of animal work has been done but adds little to the conclusions stated above (Cracco and Evans, 1978; Dong, 1982; Dong et al., 1982; Greenberg et al., 1981; Wiederholt and Iragui-Madoz, 1977; Zhuravin et al., 1981; Gardner et al., 1984; McCarthy et al., 1991).

1.3. Summary

For purposes of clinical interpretation, until further evidence is forthcoming, it can reasonably be assumed for upper-limb stimulation that (1) SEPs are generated by volleys traversing the posterior columns and medial lemnisci, and, presumably, the spinocerebellar tracts; (2) N11 is generated in the posterior columns; (3) the negative activity recorded from the neck and low back of the head (positive when recorded from the anterior neck) at 13 msec is generated by postsynaptic activity in the central cord gray matter (dorsal horns); (4) the scalp positive activity at about 13 msec after a stimulus at the wrist is generated postsynaptically in the dorsal column nucleus cuneatus; (5) the scalp positive activity at 14 msec or so is generated in the medial lemniscus in the medulla and low pons; (6) the negative activity appearing between 16 and 19 msec after stimulating the median nerve at the wrist is being generated in the thalamus (some slightly later negative activity localized to the parietal scalp may be generated from thalamocortical radiations or primary cortex); (7) the subsequent positivity (P22) is generated in the parietal sensory cortex.

For a summary of lower-limb stimulation generator sites, see the paragraph preceding Section 1.2 above.

2. PATHOPHYSIOLOGY AND CLINICAL INTERPRETATIONS

2.1. Clinical Sensation and SEP Abnormalities

See Chapter 8, Section 9.1.7, for a discussion of the relative contributions of muscle versus cutaneous afferents in different nerves; also see Section 1.1.2 in this chapter.

Giblin (1964) and Halliday and Wakefield (1963) found a good correlation in patients with lesions of the spinal cord and brain stem between changes in the SEP and the type of sensory loss. The correlation was best with position sense and passive joint movement: if that modality was more than minimally impaired, the SEP was abnormal. Somatosensory EPs were unchanged in patients with lesions affecting only pain and temperature sensation.

In patients with cerebral lesions, the correlation is less precise. Giblin (1964) found SEP amplitude abnormalities in 34 of 42 patients with lesions in the sensory cortex; of the remaining 8 patients, 1 had absent SEPs but no clinical deficit and 7 had normal SEPs but definite sensory loss (impairment of two-point discrimination, stereognosis, and joint position sense). He believed that the lesions in these patients spared the primary somatosensory receiving areas. Williamson et al. (1970) found a good correlation between degree of loss of joint position sense and SEP abnormality. No patients with mild clinical sensory loss had marked changes in the SEPs. Mauguiere et al. (1982) tested patients with lesions of the thalamocortical pathways and found (1) normal SEPs in five patients who had no clinical sensory loss (although two of these exhibited extinction to double simultaneous tactile stimulation), (2) asymmetrical but present SEP N19–P23 waveforms in six patients who had normal "tactile exploration," and (3) absent N19–P23 waveforms in patients with sensory loss. Noel and Desmedt (1975) found normal SEPs in three patients with brain stem lesions (two with Wallenberg syndrome and one with Weber's syndrome) causing loss of pain and temperature sensation, whereas patients with loss of sensation in all modalities had absent SEPs. Patients with congenital indifference to pain have been reported to have normal SEPs (Halliday, 1967b), as do patients with hysterical and hypnotically induced sensory loss (Halliday, 1967b). Anziska and Cracco (1980a) found normal SEPs in six of seven patients with impaired pain and temperature sensation but normal proprioception, and abnormal SEPs in all three patients with impaired joint position and vibration but normal pain and temperature sensation. They also found normal SEPs in two patients with impairment of all modalities. Shibasaki et al. (1977) in a group of 62 patients with cerebral lesions found SEP N19 abnormalities in 80% of patients with a "deep or cortical" sensory deficit, in 44% of patients with a pain-temperature sensory deficit, in 100% of patients with both modalities involved, and in 35% of patients with no sensory deficit. Mauguiere and Desmedt (1991) used median SEPs to evaluate four patients with a subcortical lesion due to a focal vascular accident in the internal capsule. They reported selective involvement of cortical SEP components with three patients with hemiparesis and normal somatic sensation showing loss of the precentral P22 and N30 and preserved parietal components, and one patient with sensory loss only, showing preservation of the precentral components and loss of the parietal components.

There have been many studies on the relationship between clinical sensory findings and SEPs in patients with MS (see Section 3.2, below). Since the site of the lesions is not definitely known, these are of less interest in the context of this discussion. Suffice it to say that a significant proportion of MS patients have abnormal SEPs despite no clinical sensory symptoms or signs, with a lesser proportion having normal SEPs despite abnormal sensation.

The relationship between lower-limb SEPs and myelograms is of clinical importance. In a consecutive series of more than 500 patients tested with lower-limb SEPs, 68 also had a myelogram. Twenty-four of these patients had both the myelogram and SEP normal, 23 had a normal myelogram and abnormal SEP, 16 had both tests abnormal, and 5 had a normal SEP and an abnormal myelogram (Wilson and Brooks, unpublished data). Also, median and ulnar SEPs have been reported to be differentially involved in focal cortical infarcts (Youl et al., 1991).

2.2. Latency Abnormalities

Because exact generator sources of SEP waveforms are not known (synaptic versus tract potentials or both), the pathophysiology of abnormalities is also speculative. The variety of diseases in which SEP abnormalities are found suggests that multiple factors can be involved, presumably including segmental demyelination and axonal and neuronal loss. McDonald (1977) measured the length of 20 optic nerve plaques in 14 patients who died from MS; the length of the individual plaques varied from 3 to 30 mm, with a mean of 10.5 mm. Using this information, Noel and Desmedt (1980) have speculated that if the largest CNS somatosensory axons have an internode length of about 0.5 mm, then about 20 internodes would be involved in an average MS plaque; with a 20 times slowing of the internode conduction time the extra delay from roots to the cortex would be about 10 msec. Most latency prolongations in MS are roughly within this range at medullary and thalamic points. Noel and Desmedt also pointed out that longer delays could be attributed to (1) more than

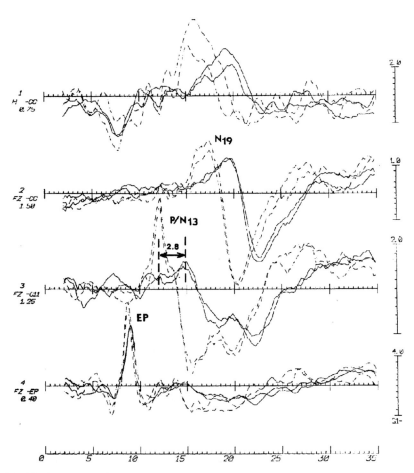

FIG. 9–10. Median nerve SEPs (unilateral stimulation at 5/sec) from a patient with possible MS, illustrating an abnormal EP–P/N13 separation (2.8 msec interside difference versus upper limit of normal of 0.7 msec—see Table 8–1) and somewhat decreased amplitude of P/N13. Left- and right-sided SEPs were superimposed, the normal (*left*) SEPs are dashed. These abnormalities, with the normal Erb's point potential, suggest a conduction defect central to the brachial plexus and at or below the lower medulla (i.e., in the cervical cord). The P/N13–N19 conduction time was normal bilaterally. Noncephalic reference recordings (*not shown*) revealed a normal N13 and P13 bilaterally, with apparent delay of P14 only on the abnormal side. Each trace is the average of 1,000 stimuli, with two repetitions superimposed.

one plaque, (2) larger plaques, and (3) the necessity for the low amplitude and desynchronized afferent volley to rely on temporal summation of synaptic potentials for eliciting a response from the next element in the pathway.

Axonal loss (e.g., following ischemic lesions) would be expected to produce amplitude changes without latency shifts since the remaining axons will be conducting at normal velocities. Therefore, compressive lesions that produce a mixture of segmental demyelination and axonal loss result in a combination of latency delays and amplitude changes.

See Chapter 8, Section 8, for a discussion of the measurements that should be taken for interpretation. If waves are clearly seen following upper-limb stimulation, the final part of the interpretation might read:

1. When there is an abnormal interpeak latency (IPL) between the brachial plexus potential (Erb's point, EP) and P/N13 (P/N13 amplitude and configuration normal) (Fig. 9–10)—"This abnormality suggests a conduction defect in the large-fiber sensory system central to the brachial plexus and below the lower medulla (or cervicomedullary junction) on the right/left."

2. When P/N13 is absent or of abnormally low amplitude (Fig. 9–11) (with or without an abnormal EP–N19 IPL)—"This abnormality suggests a conduction defect in the large-fiber sensory system central to the brachial plexus and at or below the lower medulla (or cervicomedullary junction) following left/right limb stimulation. The absence of the medullary potentials renders it impossible to determine the state of tract conduction above the lower medulla." Since the lesion would be ipsilateral (to the side of stimula-

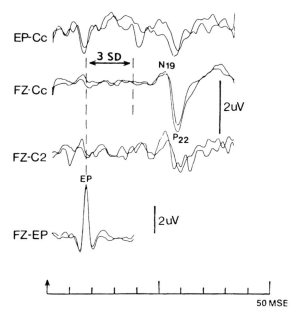

FIG. 9–11. Median nerve SEPs (unilateral stimulation at 5/sec) from a patient with MS, illustrating a complete lack of P/N13 with preservation of N19–P22; the EP–N19 separation is markedly abnormal. These abnormalities suggest conduction defects central to the brachial plexus and at or below the lower medulla. The lack of the lower medullary waveforms makes it impossible to comment on conduction above that level. (From Chiappa and Ropper, 1982, with permission.)

tion) if below the medulla, ipsilateral or contralateral or both if at the level of the medulla, and contralateral if above the medulla, the lateralization is best stated in terms of the side stimulated.

3. When there is an abnormal IPL between P/N13 and N19 (wave amplitudes and configurations normal)—"This abnormality suggests a conduction defect in the large-fiber sensory system above the lower medulla and below the thalamus on the right/left" (contralateral to the side stimulated).

4. When P/N13 is normal and N19–P22 are absent (see Fig. 9–4, right-sided stimulation)—"This abnormality suggests a conduction defect in the large-fiber sensory system above the lower medulla on the right/left" (contralateral to the side stimulated). If the lesion is recent, that is, within a few days, and if the disease process is supratentorial, the absence of N19 suggests that the thalamus is involved; with new, purely cortical or centrum semiovale (white matter) lesions initially only P22 is lost (e.g., Figs. 9–8 and 9–9). Within days to weeks after such a lesion, retrograde thalamic degeneration occurs, resulting in loss of N19, so this anatomic distinction cannot be made.

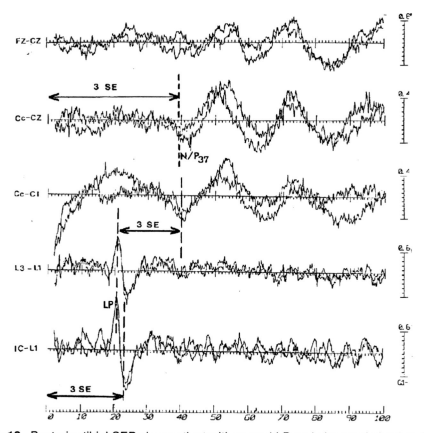

FIG. 9–12. Posterior tibial SEPs in a patient with normal LP and abnormal absolute latency of LP–N/P37 IPL. The first dashed line (in FZ–CZ channel) indicates the normal mean plus 3 SD for the N/P37 absolute latency for this patient's height (158 cm). The other dashed lines show the upper limits of normal for the LP–N/P37 interval and for LP absolute latency. This pattern suggests a conduction defect above the level of the cauda equina/lower spinal cord.

5. When both the EP–P/N13 and P/N13–N19 IPLs are abnormal—"This abnormality suggests conduction defects in the large-fiber sensory system central to the brachial plexus both below and above the medulla (but caudal to the thalamus) following right/left-sided stimulation."

6. When the brachial plexus potential cannot be recorded, if the absolute latencies for P/N13 and N19 are normal for body size, then the test can be interpreted as normal. If the absolute latencies are abnormal, then the test cannot be interpreted as normal but the interpretation must reflect the fact that the latency delay could be due to slowing in the peripheral nerve. Of course, abnormalities of the P/N13–N19 segment can be interpreted as usual.

7. Note that there is a length of peripheral nerve and myelin interposed between the generator site of the brachial plexus potential and the CNS, so that an abnormal EP–P/N13 IPL does not definitely indicate a CNS lesion; there could be a radiculopathy, for example.

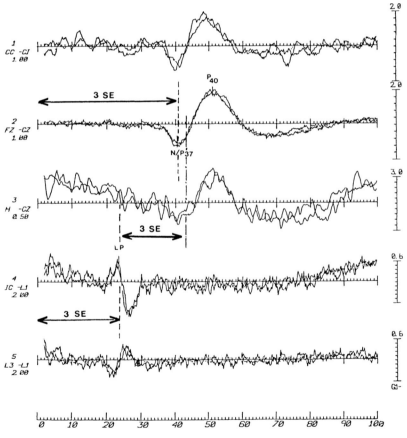

FIG. 9–13. Posterior tibial SEPs in a patient with LP absolute latency borderline abnormal but LP–N/P37 IPL normal. The first dashed line (in FZ–CZ channel) indicates the normal mean plus 3 SD for the absolute latency of N/P37 for this patient's height (164 cm). The others show the upper limits of normal for the LP–N/P37 IPL, the patient being well within normal limits, and the upper limit of normal for absolute LP latency. This pattern suggests a conduction defect in the peripheral nervous system, caudal to the cauda equina and lower spinal cord.

With lower-limb stimulation (e.g., posterior tibial nerve at the ankle), the final part of the interpretation might read:

1. When LP is not seen but the absolute latency of N/P37 is normal (corrected for height), the test can be interpreted as normal and extra time need not be taken in registering LP.
2. When LP absolute latency is normal and LP–N/P37 IPL is abnormal (Fig. 9–12) (corrected for height) (N/P37 absolute latency will then also usually be abnormal)—"This abnormality suggests a conduction defect in the large-fiber sensory system above the cauda equina and below the sensory cortex following right/left-sided stimulation." Since the tracts cross in the medulla and there is no way of knowing whether the lesion is caudal or rostral to that point, one cannot be more specific as to the vertical location of the lesion. Where this information might be clinically very useful, additional recordings from the neck using sedation, large numbers of stimuli, and needle recording techniques may reveal the afferent volley at this level (see Chapter 8, Sections 4 and 6). If N/P37 is absent or its amplitude and configuration are grossly abnormal, the relationship of the conduction defect to the cortex cannot be determined since the lesion might involve the cortex.
3. When LP is present but delayed (corrected for height) and the LP–N/P37 IPL is normal (Fig. 9–13), the conduction defect must be peripheral to the cauda equina. The absolute latency of P/N37 will usually be abnormal in these cases.
4. When LP is present but delayed and the LP–N/P37 IPL is abnormal, this usually indicates both peripheral and central conduction delays, although a single lesion at the cauda equina/lower cord is a less-likely possibility.
5. When LP is absent and N/P37 absolute latency is delayed (corrected for height), since the conduction defect could be in peripheral nerve, the interpretation must reflect this possibility.

Since LP is generated very close to the place where peripheral myelin meets central myelin, a situation where LP is normal and yet there is still a lesion in peripheral myelin is very unlikely. This contrasts with upper-limb testing in which the EP potential (brachial plexus) can be normal, the EP–N/P13 IPL be abnormal, and the lesion involve peripheral myelin (e.g., in the proximal roots).

2.3. Amplitude Abnormalities

As discussed in Chapter 8, Section 8, the most reliable abnormality in this sphere is complete absence of a wave. Low amplitude is only reliable when the intertrial variability is low and the amplitude is less than the minimum amplitude seen in a group of normals minus one standard deviation (SD) (or the mean minus 3 SD for transformed data or some nonparametric statistical measure). The interpretations of these abnormalities have been discussed above.

The interside comparison is helpful when the absolute amplitude is near the limits of normal. An amplitude difference between the two sides of more than 2.5 times can be considered abnormal if there is no significant difference in the amplitude of the Erb's point potential. However, one must be conservative in the interpretation when the only abnormality is an interside amplitude comparison.

There are occasions when P22 and N/P37 amplitudes are abnormally large (usually epileptic and myoclonic states). The same conservative approach to these interpretations must be taken as when the amplitudes are too low; amplitudes more than twice the maximum seen in a group of normal subjects can be considered abnormal.

2.4. Laterality of Abnormalities

This is a straightforward matter with SEPs compared to the complexity of this topic in brain stem auditory EPs (BAEPs). The sensory tract involved, crossing to the opposite side in the lower medulla just above the dorsal column nuclei, is well-defined.

The lower- and upper-limb fibers are usually involved equally if the lesion is at an anatomic level at which both tracts are present. However, differential involvement can be present, e.g., in MS (see Table 9–4), where the lesion size presumably is small enough to involve the fibers from only one limb (since they remain largely segregated in the medial lemniscus). The same differential involvement of upper- (abnormal) and lower- (normal) limb SEPs may be seen in patients with pontine gliomas. This is caused by the central pontine location of the tumor, which, as it expands, first encounters the medial aspects of the medial lemniscus. In the dorsal columns of the spinal cord the lower-limb sensory fibers lie medially, but as the medial lemniscus is formed and ascends through the medulla and pons the upper-limb fibers come to lie medially and hence are first affected by the tumor.

3. CLINICAL CORRELATIONS

3.1. Introduction

Clinical utility of SEPs stems from the close relationship between the EP waveforms and specific anatomic structures. This specificity allows localization of conduction defects in the brain stem to within a few centimeters or so. In addition, SEPs are very resistant to alteration by anything other than structural pathology in the somatosensory pathways. For example, barbiturate doses sufficient to render the electroencephalogram (EEG) "flat" (isoelectric) and general anesthesia do not significantly affect SEPs. These factors of anatomic specificity and physiologic and metabolic immutability are the basis of the clinical utility of SEPs.

Somatosensory EPs offer a look at "physiologic anatomy." They provide a sensitive tool for assessment of spinal cord and brain stem posterior columns and medial lemniscal tracts and nearby structures. Abnormalities demonstrated by SEPs are etiologically nonspecific and must be carefully integrated into the clinical situation by a physician familiar with the clinical use of this test. He or she must decide if other procedures [e.g., electromyography (EMG), radiologic studies, subspecialty consultation] are indicated to differentiate the possible causes of the conduction delay.

Somatosensory EPs are used to test (1) the peripheral nervous system (nerves and roots) and (2) the large-fiber sensory tracts in the central nervous system. The knowledge of neuroanatomy and neurologic diseases required to guide the performance of the test and provide a clinical correlation dictates that only physicians with special training in these matters be responsible for it.

3.2. Multiple Sclerosis

Multiple sclerosis is a demyelinating disease of the CNS characterized by foci of myelin destruction with relative preservation of axons and nerve cell bodies. Central myelin is formed by extensions of the cytoplasmic membrane of oligodendrocytes which wrap around the axon, resulting in concentric layers of lipid and protein. The acute MS plaque shows myelin breakdown and inflammation with perivenous infiltrates of mononuclear cells and lymphocytes; older lesions contain microglial phagocytes and reactive astrocytes. Inactive lesions (sclerotic plaques) contain relatively acellular fibroglial tissue (gliosis) and show loss of axis cylinders (see Ludwin, 1981, for a review of the pathology of demyelination and remyelination). The pathogenesis of MS is unknown but this is a very active research area (see Matthews et al., 1985, for a review of related infectious and immunologic data).

The biochemistry and electrophysiology of nerve conduction with normal and abnormal myelination has been well-studied, and Waxman (1981), Waxman and Ritchie (1981), Rasminsky (1981), Sears and Bostock (1981), and Sedgwick (1983) provide excellent reviews of pertinent topics. Although these principles provide a starting point for understanding EP abnormalities seen in patients with demyelinating diseases the generation of EPs often involves complex physiologic mechanisms whose response to partial anatomic and physiologic lesions is difficult, if not impossible, to predict or understand.

The clinical utility of EPs in MS is based on their ability (1) to demonstrate abnormal sensory system function when the history and/or neurologic examination are equivocal, (2) to reveal the presence of clinically unsuspected malfunction in a sensory system when demyelinating disease is suspected because of symptoms and/or signs in another area of the CNS, (3) to help define the anatomic distribution of a disease process, and (4) to monitor objective changes in a patient's status. Although some of the information they provide is similar to that elicitable at the bedside by an experienced clinician, these tests are very helpful in the evaluation of patients with suspected demyelinating disease because (1) they provide data unobtainable without the use of amplifiers and oscilloscopes, (2) they quantify and objectify data which the clinician may only sense, and (3) they can localize lesions within a pathway, whereas clinicians often cannot.

3.2.1. Incidence of Abnormalities

There have been a large number of studies of SEPs in patients with MS (Abbruzzesse et al., 1981a; Anziska et al., 1978; Chiappa, 1980; Chiappa et al., 1980; Dau et al., 1980; Dorfman et al., 1978a; Eisen and Nudleman, 1979; Eisen and Odusote, 1980; Eisen et al., 1979, 1981, 1982; Ganes, 1980c; Green et al., 1980; Kazis et al., 1982; Khoshbin and Hallett, 1981; Kjaer, 1980a,b; Mastaglia et al., 1978; Matthews and Esiri, 1979; Matthews et al., 1979; Matthews and Small, 1979; Namerow, 1968, 1970; Noel and Desmedt, 1980; Purves et al., 1981; Small et al., 1978; Tackmann et al., 1980; Trojaborg and Petersen, 1979; Trojaborg et al., 1981; van Buggenhout et al., 1982; Walsh et al., 1982; Weiner and Dawson, 1980; Larrea and Mauguiere, 1988). Of 1,006 patients with varying classifications of MS in some of the above studies, 58% (500 of 855) had abnormal median/digital SEPs, and 76%

TABLE 9–1. *Incidence of median nerve SEP abnormalities in patients with MS, with and without clinical sensory system symptoms and/or signs*

Clinical status	Definite	Probable	Possible	Total
With sensory symptoms and/or signs	12/14 (86%)	12/16 (75%)	3/9 (33%)	27/39 (69%)
Without sensory symptoms and/or signs	7/14 (50%)	10/17 (59%)	4/10 (40%)	21/41 (51%)
All patients	19/28 (68%)	22/33 (67%)	7/19 (37%)	48/80 (60%)

From Chiappa, 1980, with permission.

TABLE 9–2. *Laterality of median nerve SEP abnormalities in patients with MS*

Laterality	Definite	Probable	Possible	Total
Unilateral abnormality	5/18 (28%)	6/22 (27%)	3/7 (43%)	14/47 (30%)
Bilateral, same abnormality	8/18 (44%)	15/22 (68%)	4/7 (57%)	27/47 (57%)
Bilateral, different abnormalities	5/18 (28%)	1/22 (5%)	0	6/40 (15%)
Total bilateral abnormalities	13/18 (72%)	16/22 (73%)	4/7 (57%)	33/47 (70%)

(90 of 118) had abnormal peroneal/tibial SEPs. In 270, 112, and 98 patients classified as definite, probable, or possible MS, the average abnormality rates were 77%, 67%, and 49%, respectively. Grouping the probable and possible patients from this collection together, the abnormality rate was 59%. The data presented in Tables 9–1 through 9–5 for patients seen in our laboratory are representative of findings in this patient population.

3.2.2. Importance of Unilateral Stimulation

Thirty-four percent (81 of 239) of patients with abnormal tests for whom the data were available had unilateral abnormalities (see also Table 9–2). This dictates that unilateral testing be used since one third of patients with abnormal tests would show normal SEPs with the bilateral testing (the potentials from the normal side mask the abnormal response).

3.2.3. Influence of Stimulus Rate

Although the effect of stimulus rate has been studied in normals, there has been no study of rate effects in patients with MS. Smith et al. (1986) saw no change in median and tibial SEPs with infusion of high-dose methylprednisolone. Gilmore et al. (1985b) noted minor SEP improvement in one of eight MS patients infused with the calcium-antagonist drug verapamil. Nuwer et al. (1985) studied first-degree relatives of MS patients and found some abnormal interarm EP–N18 latency differences, although all other SEP parameters were normal.

3.2.4. Clinical Findings and SEP

The relationship between clinical symptomatology and SEP findings has been discussed above in Section 2.1. There have been many studies of the relationship between clinical sensory findings and SEPs in patients with MS (Small et al., 1978; Spudis et al., 1980;

TABLE 9–3. *Incidence of median and peroneal nerve SEP abnormalities in patients with MS (two patients did not have both sides tested)*

	Definite	Probable	Possible	All patients
Median(s) abnormal (one or both sides)	71% (25/35)	58% (25/43)	31% (11/36)	54% (61/114)
Peroneal(s) abnormal (one or both sides)	83% (29/35)	72% (31/43)	36% (13/36)	64% (73/114)
Either or both tests abnormal (one or both sides)	91% (32/35)	79% (34/43)	42% (15/36)	71% (81/114)

From Brooks et al., 1983, with permission.

TABLE 9–4. *Combined SEP results (median and peroneal) in 114 MS patients*

	Definite	Probable	Possible	All patients
Group i Both tests normal	9% (3/35)	21% (9/43)	58% (21/36)	29% (33/114)
Group ii Medians normal, peroneal(s) abnormal	20% (7/35)	21% (9/43)	11% (4/36)	18% (21/114)
Group iii Peroneals normal, median(s) abnormal	9% (3/35)	7% (3/43)	6% (2/36)	7% (8/114)
Group iv Median(s) and peroneal(s) abnormal	63% (22/35)	52% (22/43)	25% (9/36)	46% (53/114)

From Brooks et al., 1983, with permission.

Mastaglia et al., 1978; Namerow, 1968; Khoshbin and Hallett, 1981; Kjaer, 1980a,b; Ganes, 1980a; Green et al., 1980; Eisen et al., 1979; Anziska et al., 1978; van Buggenhout et al., 1982; Chiappa, 1980; Davis et al., 1985). Forty-two percent (249 of 598) of patients reported to have no symptoms or signs referrable to the sensory system had abnormal SEPs, whereas 75% (250 of 335) of patients with sensory system symptoms and/or signs had abnormal SEPs (both upper and lower limbs included) (see also Tables 9–1, 9–3, and 9–4). The data presented below will show that there is a higher incidence of clinically silent SEP abnormalities found on testing the lower limbs (as compared with the upper limbs).

3.2.5. Types of SEP Abnormalities

Data shown in Tables 9–3 and 9–4 from a group of 114 MS patients seen in our laboratory exemplify the findings that can be expected when using SEPs to test patients with (or suspected of having) MS. Twenty-nine percent of the patients had completely normal tests (both upper and lower limb). Upper-limb SEPs were abnormal in 54% of patients, lower-limb SEPs in 64%. In 18% of the patients, upper-limb SEPs were normal when lower-limb SEPs were abnormal, whereas the converse was true in 7%. Only 2% of patients had bilat-

TABLE 9–5. *Incidence of types of median nerve SEP abnormalities seen in MS patients*

Type of abnormality	Definite	Probable	Possible	Total
Only EP	6	2	0	8
Only EP and P/N13	2	2	1	5
↓ P/N13 amp	1	0	0	1
No P/N13	1	3	0	4
No P/N13, delayed N19	4	3	2	9
Delayed P/N13, N19, P/N13 to N19	0	2	1	3
Delayed P/N13	0	1	0	1
Delayed N19, P/N13 to N19	3	7	3	13
Delayed N19, normal P/N13–N19	0	2	0	2
No N19, delayed P22	1	0	0	1
P/N13 duration prolonged	1	0	0	1
Total	19	22	7	48

EP, Erb's point.
From Chiappa, 1980, with permission.

erally abnormal upper-limb and bilaterally normal lower-limb SEPs, but the reverse was found in 11% of the patients. Thirty-seven percent of normal upper-limb SEPs were associated with abnormal lower-limb SEPs on the same side, whereas only 12% of normal lower-limb SEPs were associated with abnormal upper-limb SEPs ipsilaterally. Some of the conclusions that may be drawn from these results are (1) when lower-limb testing is normal, upper-limb testing will reveal abnormalities in an additional, although small, group of patients, (2) SEP abnormalities in one limb (upper or lower) are not necessarily associated with SEP abnormalities in the other limb on the same side, although lower-limb abnormali-

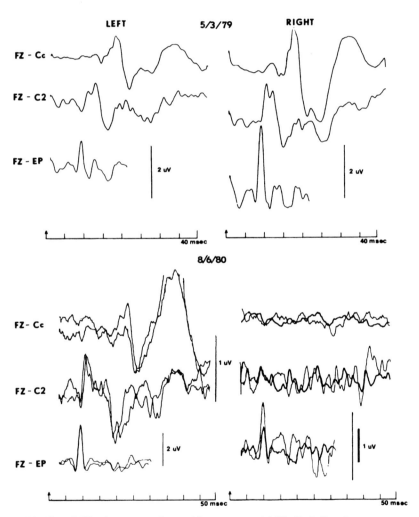

FIG. 9–14. Median SEPs from a patient with suspected MS. Ill-defined sensory complaints were the initial clinical presentation, with neurologic examination not revealing a definite abnormality. Initial median SEPs (5/3/79) were normal bilaterally. Fifteen months later (8/6/80) there had been no change in the clinical features but the SEP had become markedly abnormal following right-sided stimulation, with P/N13 and later waves absent. This suggested a lesion central to the brachial plexus on the right, at or below the level of the lower medulla, presumably in the cervical spinal cord. A myelogram was normal. In the lower right panel the thicker amplitude calibration mark refers to the thicker trace in the bottom channel.

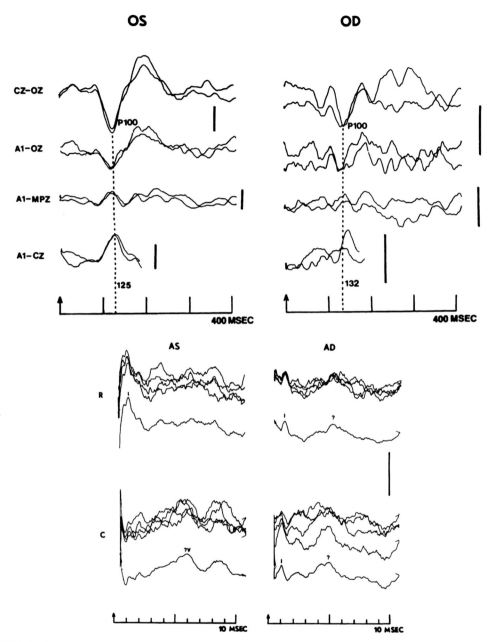

FIG. 9–15. Pattern-shift visual, brain stem auditory, and peroneal somatosensory EPs from a 59-year-old patient with multiple symptoms and signs, demonstrating the etiologic non-specificity of EPs. The patient was being evaluated for left-ear tinnitus and 1-year progressive unsteadiness of gait; neurologic examination revealed decreased hearing bilaterally, normal visual function, normal corneal reflexes, dysarthria, multiple cerebellar abnormalities, and bilateral extensor plantar reflexes. The PSVEPs show markedly abnormal absolute latencies bilaterally (upper limit of normal = 117 msec), suggesting bilateral conduction defects in the visual system. Brain stem auditory EPs show only wave I bilaterally with either click polarity (R, rarefaction, C, condensation), with perhaps a low-amplitude wave V visible, suggesting bilateral low pontine or proximal eighth nerve conduction defects. Median nerve SEPs (*not shown*) were normal, but peroneal nerve SEPs showed an abnormal N/P27

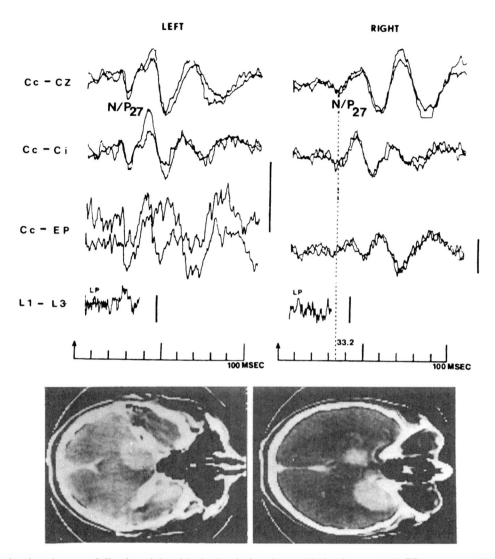

absolute latency following right-sided stimulation (upper limit of normal (3 SD) corrected for this patient's height was 31.4 msec—note dashed line at N/P27 = 33.2 msec). LP was not well-defined. Despite these multiple, separate conduction defects, all of which could be seen in MS, the disease process was not MS but multiple meningiomas, demonstrated on CT scan. Calibration marks: PSVEP 5 μV; BAEP 0.5 μV; peroneal SEP 1 μV for upper three channels and 0.1 μV for bottom channel in each panel. (From Chiappa, 1983, with permission.)

ties will be more commonly associated with upper-limb abnormalities than vice versa. Others have had similar results, the yield of abnormalities being greater with lower-limb stimulation (Eisen and Odusote, 1980; Khoshbin and Hallett, 1981; Shibasaki et al., 1982; Trojaborg and Petersen, 1979; Riffel et al., 1984).

Figure 9–14 shows median SEPs in a patient with sensory symptoms but no definite abnormalities on neurologic examination. Initial testing (May 1979) showed no abnormalities, but 15 months later, without change in clinical features, marked SEP abnormalities appeared (lower-limb SEPs at this time were also abnormal but had not been previously tested). Because pattern-shift visual EPs (PSVEPs) and BAEPs were normal a focal process at the level of the upper cervical cord was suspected but a myelogram was normal; MS remains the most likely diagnosis. Similarly, other patients with suspected MS have been tested and a similar pattern (all EPs normal except for SEPs pointing to the upper cervical cord) has prompted a myelogram that revealed significant cervical cord compression from spondylotic bars; some of these patients have improved with surgical decompression. Conversely, of course, multiple EP abnormalities do not necessarily indicate MS. Figure 9–15 shows abnormal PSVEPs, BAEPs, and lower-limb SEPs (median SEPs were normal) in a patient who had multiple meningiomas (CT scan).

Tables 9–1, 9–3, and 9–4 show the incidence of abnormal SEPs in patients with MS. Table 9–5 shows the incidence of types of abnormalities seen in the median SEP for 48 patients. Although every conceivable abnormality was seen, the most interesting is the absence of P/N13 with preservation of N19–P23 and a normal brachial plexus to N19 separation. The pathophysiology of such a finding and how it relates to the generation of the SEP waveforms are matters of pure speculation. In this group of patients, 30% of the abnormalities were unilateral and 70% were bilateral, an incidence quite similar to the grand average given above. Of the bilateral abnormalities, 79% were identical and 21% were different on the two sides.

Roberts et al. (1983) have used the dispersion of the thalamocortical waveforms, as determined by Fourier analysis, as an additional analysis parameter. Rossini et al. (1981) registered SEP short-latency wavelets using restricted band-pass digital filtering and thereby increased the yield of abnormalities. Yamada et al. (1982b) studied long-latency in addition to short-latency SEP components and found additional abnormalities; they also believed that the long-latency components helped to resolve interpretive difficulties encountered with short-latency testing, especially when bilateral stimulation was used. Delwaide et al. (1985) studied lumbosacral spinal SEPs in MS patients and noted a correlation between intensity of spasticity and some elements of the EP waveform.

3.2.6. Comparison with PSVEP and BAEP

The relative utility of PSVEPs, BAEPs, and median SEPs was compared in patients (combined definite, probable, and possible groups) who had had each of the three tests (see Tables 3–3 and 3–4). Note that not all patients in Table 3–3 had all three tests. Only two patients had a clinically unsuspected lesion revealed by all three tests, as might be expected since it would be unlikely for a diagnosis of MS to be made clinically if at least one of the systems involved in the EP tests had not already shown clinical evidence of dysfunction. Thus, as was postulated on the basis of length of white matter tracts involved, the order of relative utility of the tests in revealing evidence of clinically unsuspected lesions was SEP, PSVEP, and BAEP. This is in agreement with similar studies of Trojaborg and Petersen (1979), Khoshbin and Hallett (1981), Green et al. (1980), Matthews et al. (1979), and Purves et al. (1981). These data, and the overall abnormality rates found with the three tests irrespective of clinical findings (60%, 56%, and 32% in the SEP, PSVEP, and BAEP, respectively), suggest that there is not a specific differential susceptibility to demyelination in the systems involved in the tests. Rather, it is the length and amount of white matter tracts being tested which determines the likelihood of detection of a lesion in a given system.

Matthews et al. (1982) followed for 38 months after SEP testing 84 patients in whom the diagnosis of MS was under consideration. In only three of these patients an abnormal SEP at initial presentation subsequently proved to be of diagnostic value in that it revealed a separate, clinically silent lesion, indicating multifocal disease (and the patient on follow-up proved to have MS). Aminoff et al. (1984) and Davis et al. (1985) found that clinical motor and sensory findings in MS patients in the corresponding limb frequently correlated with abnormalities of the median-nerve SEP cervical response. When new clinical features appeared, the SEP deteriorated in some patients but improved in others, and overall disability sometimes increased despite improved SEPs. Most SEP changes were not accompanied by clinical changes.

3.2.7. Indirect Measurements of Spinal Cord Conduction

H-reflex and F-wave latencies have been used in conjunction with SEPs for "indirect" measurement of spinal cord conduction velocities in patients with MS (Eisen and Nudleman, 1979; Dorfman et al., 1978a). Objections to this technique are (1) the central delay (synaptic or other) used in calculation of F or H conduction velocities can only be estimated and may vary by different amounts in different diseases, (2) the efferent limb of the H-reflex and both limbs of the F-wave are mediated via motor axons that have diameters and responses to diseases different from the sensory axons involved in SEP testing—thus the factors used to correct for the conduction velocity differences between sensory and motor fibers will be inconsistent, and (3) H-reflexes are reliably obtainable only from the soleus muscle (unless abnormally enhanced reflexes are present) and so may not be mediated via the same roots involved in SEP testing.

3.2.8. Spinal Cord Syndromes

Ropper et al. (1982) studied EP abnormalities in 12 consecutive patients with inflammatory acute transverse myelopathy (ATM) as their first neurologic illness. All nine patients tested with median SEPs had normal findings, the lesions being below cervical levels mediating that response. Five of six patients tested with peroneal SEPs had abnormal findings (the sixth was tested 8 months after onset when there was no residual neurologic deficit). All of these patients had normal PSVEPs and BAEPs and none developed new neurologic signs during 18 months mean follow-up. The authors believed that the lack of other lesions by EP testing and the failure to develop new clinical lesions indicates that ATM, when defined as a virtually or totally complete transverse inflammatory lesion of the cord, is a different process from MS.

Attempts have been made to use SEPs—and other EPs—to gauge the effectiveness of plasmapheresis therapy in MS but only a few patients have been studied so far and it is not yet possible to draw conclusions (Dau et al., 1980; Weiner and Dawson, 1980).

3.2.9. Repeat Testing

Effects on SEPs of raising body temperature in patients with MS have been studied by Matthews et al. (1979) and Kazis et al. (1982). The former authors used intercurrent extra-CNS infection (viral or bacterial) as the hyperthermic agent and the effect of toxins cannot be discounted as the cause of the observed SEP changes. Matthews et al. (1979) used external heat to raise the body temperature of their subjects and found that P/N13 amplitude was markedly diminished by the temperature increase. Phillips et al. (1983) found that hyperthermia increased the yield of peroneal SEP abnormalities in MS patients.

3.2.10. Combined Evoked Potential Studies

The comparative utility of PSVEPs, BAEPs, and SEPs has been studied in several groups of patients (Chiappa et al., 1980; Green et al., 1980; Khoshbin and Hallett, 1981; Kjaer, 1980b; Mastaglia et al., 1976; Matthews et al., 1982; Phillips et al., 1983; Purves et al., 1981; Tackmann et al., 1982; Trojaborg and Petersen, 1979). As might be postulated on the basis of length of white matter tracts involved, the order of relative utility of the tests in revealing evidence of clinically unsuspected lesions was SEP, PSVEP, and BAEP. These data suggest that there is not a specific differential susceptibility to demyelination in the systems involved in the tests. Rather, it is the length and amount of white matter tracts being tested which determine the likelihood of detection of a lesion in a given system. Phillips et al. (1983) found increased abnormality rates in all EPs during hyperthermia.

Bottcher et al. (1982) followed patients for 2 to 4 years after PSVEP, SEP, and CSF immunoglobulin G (IgG) testing and found that 81% of those in whom both the EPs and the IgG index was abnormal initially had entered a higher MS diagnostic class at the later evaluation. Those patients in whom either the EPs or IgG index were normal initially remained in the same diagnostic class. Walsh et al. (1982) followed 56 patients for 2.5 years and found an increased number of abnormalities in multimodality EPs which was paralleled by an increase in overall clinical disability. However, Aminoff et al. (1984) have noted that the correlation between changes in specific clinical features and EPs may be poor.

Noseworthy et al. (1983) have studied PSVEP, BAEP, and blink reflexes in patients presenting after age 50 with suspected MS. They found both the EPs and cerebrospinal fluid (CSF) electrophoresis to have high diagnostic yield in this difficult diagnostic group.

Nuwer et al. (1987) performed EPs annually during a 3-year, double-blind, placebo-controlled study of azathioprine with or without steroids in chronic progressive MS. Treatment-related visual and somatosensory EP changes became statistically different 1 year before corresponding differences were seen in the Standard Neurological Examination scores, and the statistical significance of the EP changes was substantially greater than seen for changes in other clinical scales. The degree of significance was increased by using EP latency values, rather than simple criteria for change. Anderson et al. (1987) were less impressed with EP utility in clinical MS trials.

3.2.11. Magnetic Resonance Imaging and Evoked Potentials

Magnetic resonance imaging is proving to be an invaluable tool in the investigation of patients with suspected demyelinating disease, especially the T_2-weighted images (see Drayer and Barrett, 1984, for a review). Immediate postmortem studies have shown that demyelinated lesions 3 mm in diameter are seen, and that the apparent lesion size on MRI is accurate (Stewart et al., 1986). Where signal intensity varied, so did the degree of inflammation, demyelination, and gliosis, and it was thought that MRI could distinguish gliotic and nongliotic demyelinated lesions. Serial MRI scans show the appearance and evolution of asymptomatic lesions (Paty et al., 1986) and enhancement may afford a measure of activity (Gonzalez-Scarano et al., 1986). Magnetic resonance imaging has been shown to be better than EPs and CT in revealing multiple lesions in the CNS (Cutler et al., 1986; Kirshner et al., 1985; Gebarski et al., 1985; Ormerod et al., 1986; Guerit et al., 1988; Farlow et al., 1986; Giesser et al., 1987; Paty et al., 1988; Eisen et al., 1987; Gilmore et al., 1989; Lee et al., 1991), including the spinal cord (Maravilla et al., 1985; Turano et al., 1991), but, of course, MRI is no more specific than EPs with respect to etiology. However, in the brain stem EPs reveal a significant number of conduction defects not seen by MRI (Kirshner et al., 1985; Baumhefner et al., 1986; Giesser et al., 1986; Cutler et al., 1986; Ross et al., 1992). Similarly, it can be expected that optic nerve lesions will be detected more reliably by EPs than MRI (Farlow et al., 1986), although Miller et al. (1986) recently suggested an improved MRI technique for searching for demyelinating lesions in the optic nerve. Thus, although as a general statement it can be said that the overall neurologic workup of the patient suspected of having demyelinating disease is better served by MRI (and most patients with MS will eventually have an MRI scan), in selected cases specific questions are better answered by EPs, and some anatomic areas are better tested by EPs.

3.3. Other Demyelinating Diseases

Markand et al. (1982a,b) have studied SEPs in patients with leukodystrophies. In five patients with Pelizaeus–Merzbacher disease (PMD) there were no P/N13 components recordable despite good brachial plexus potentials, whereas their three patients with adrenoleukodystrophy (ALD) had normal P/N13 components. In nine patients (eight with PMD, one with metachromatic leukodystrophy, MLD) N19 and P23 components were missing, whereas in four (one with PMD, three with ALD) although N19 and P23 were present, one or both were prolonged in latency, as were the IPLs. Posterior tibial nerve SEPs were abnormal in all six patients tested. In three (two with PMD, one with ALD) no cerebral components could be recorded and in two others the earliest positive components had prolonged latencies. Garg et al. (1980, 1983) reported abnormal tibial SEPs in three patients and in four of seven ALD carriers studied, including both of the obligate heterozygotes, and Tobimatsu et al. (1985) found SEP abnormalities in patients and carriers with ALD and adrenomyeloneuropathy. Wulff and Trojaborg (1985) found abnormal SEPs in two adult patients with MLD. Aubourg et al. (1992) described SEP abnormalities in 17 patients with clinical adrenomyeloneuropathy.

3.4. OTHER DEGENERATIVE DISEASES

3.4.1. Alzheimer's Disease

Abbruzzese et al. (1984) found only 1 of 30 patients with Alzheimer's disease with an abnormal P/N13–N19 IPL and 3 with abnormal N19–P22 peak-to-peak amplitude, contrasted with abnormal P/N13–N19 IPL in 7 and low-amplitude N19–P22 in 3 of 18 patients with multi-infarct dementia.

3.4.2. Charcot–Marie–Tooth Disease

Jones and Halliday (1982) studied 13 cases of Charcot–Marie–Tooth disease and found N19–P23 generally present but of low amplitude at normal or markedly delayed absolute latencies. They found forearm sensory conduction velocities normal in two patients but slowed in the remainder. The lower medullary (P/N13) to thalamic (N19) conduction was essentially normal, although in two cases there was some indication of a central delay. Noel and Desmedt (1980) studied eight patients with markedly reduced conduction velocities in the median nerve in both motor and sensory systems. Although the P/N13 potential was delayed, the IPL between it and N19 was normal, indicating that conduction rostral to the lower medulla was preserved.

3.4.3. Friedreich's Ataxia

Large-diameter afferent fibers gradually degenerate in this condition. Pain and temperature sensation in Friedreich's ataxia is usually normal, whereas vibration and joint position sense are eventually always abnormal. Peripheral motor nerve conduction velocities are normal, as are peripheral sensory conduction velocities when measurable, but the sensory nerve action potentials have progressively lower amplitudes and eventually cannot be registered. Desmedt and Noel (1973) and Noel and Desmedt (1976, 1980) have studied six patients with disease duration of 6 to 21 years, all with normal median nerve motor conduction studies. They found a dispersed initial scalp negativity with the first element appearing at latencies normal for N19. The separate peaks do not change relationships when the stimulus point in the limb is changed, thus the authors suggested that the effect is a central rather than peripheral one, produced by collateral reinnervation.

Jones et al. (1980) studied 22 patients with Friedreich's ataxia. They found marked attenuation of the brachial plexus potential but no latency delay of that component or the lower medullary potentials (P/N13). The latter potentials also were attenuated to varying degrees. N19 was delayed in all patients but two, in whom it could not be recognized. Stimulation at different limb sites showed that the N19 peak was mediated by peripheral nerve fibers with normal conduction velocities. Thus, this study also provided evidence of a central conduction disturbance in the pathways mediating these SEPs. Patients with Friedreich's ataxia were also tested by Mastaglia et al. (1978) (8 patients, all with abnormal P/N13 and N19 components), Pedersen and Trojaborg (1981) (10 patients, at least 5 with abnormal P/N13 to N19 IPL), Sauer and Schenck (1977), Chiappa et al. (1980), and Pelosi et al. (1985).

3.4.4. Huntington's Disease

Oepen et al. (1981) studied 13 patients with Huntington's disease (HD) and 9 clinically unaffected offspring. Of the SEP components discussed in this book, only N19 and P23 were recorded by their techniques. They found prolonged latencies (mean was at the upper limit of normal) and decreased amplitudes on a group statistical basis, but individual data were not presented. Three of the nine offspring had normal N19–P23 components but later waves were sometimes abnormal.

Takahashi et al. (1972) tested four patients and found that three of them had an abnormal N19 latency. Ehle et al. (1984) studied 12 patients with HD and repeated the test in 8 at 1 and 2 years. Somatosensory EP latencies were normal but the peak-to-peak N19–P22 amplitude showed a progressive decline. This was also observed by Noth et al. (1984), who studied 37 patients with HD and 43 children of HD patients and found marked amplitude reduction of N19–P22 for the median nerve and N33–P40 for the tibial nerve. Almost half of those at risk showed significant amplitude reduction of these components.

Bollen et al. (1985) had similar results in 21 patients with HD. Abbruzzese et al. (1990) found that the prerolandic P22/N30 components were consistently affected and were unrecognizable in two thirds of the patients, whereas the parietal N20/P27 were always present although the N20 latency and central conduction time were increased. Yamada et al. (1991) also saw similar abnormalities.

3.4.5. Motor System Disease

The motor system disorders are a group of degenerative disorders with variable expression of involvement of motor neurons and their axons in cortex, brain stem, and spinal cord. The major clinical syndromes include amyotrophic lateral sclerosis (ALS), primary lateral sclerosis (PLS), progressive spinal muscular atrophy (PSMA), pseudobulbar palsy (PBP), and bulbar palsy (BP). Usually there is preservation of mental, sensory, and autonomic function despite progressive motor deficits. Sensory symptoms, predominantly pain (due to muscle cramping) and paresthesiae, have been reported in MSD (Dyck et al., 1975; Lawyer and Netsky, 1953; Mulder, 1982), although computerized sensory examinations have detected abnormal vibratory sensation in 14 out of 80 patients with MSD (Mulder et al., 1983). Quantitative measurements of cutaneous touch-pressure sensation have also indicated abnormalities in two out of four ALS patients (Dyck et al., 1975). Consistent with the usual clinical abnormalities, the pathologic findings in MSD have been predominantly restricted to the motor system (Tandan and Bradley, 1985). However, morphometric examination of the sural and superficial peroneal nerves have noted a reduction in the total number of myelinated fibers in MSD patients (Dyck et al., 1975; Bradley et al., 1983). Significant degeneration in the neurons of Clarke's nucleus and the spinocerebellar tracts in patients with sporadic ALS has been recognized, but the posterior columns have been generally spared (Lawyer and Netsky, 1953; Averback and Crocker, 1982). In familial ALS there is evidence for posterior column, spinocerebellar tract, and Clarke's nucleus involvement in over 50% of patients (Emery and Holloway, 1982). However, pathologic evidence for sensory involvement does not necessarily correlate with clinical sensory abnormalities (Lawyer and Netsky, 1953; Mulder, 1982). A review of previous reports on upper-limb SEPs in MSD shows conflicting and problematic results. Our study (Cascino et al., 1988) showed normal results in 29 of 30 cases and no statistical trend toward abnormality in the EP–N19 IPL of patients with MSD compared with controls. This is in agreement with Oh et al. (1985), who reported normal median nerve cervical and cortical SEPs in 21 out of 22 ALS patients. Their lone abnormal patient had a unilaterally prolonged IPL between Erb's point and the cervical potential associated with C6/C7 discs. In our study we were careful to eliminate the possibility that disc or other compressive lesions might cause abnormalities in SEPs because we, along with others, recognize that the incidence of SEP abnormalities is high in these disorders (Oh et al., 1985; Yiannikas et al., 1986) and that they may coexist in patients with MSD. Thus four patients with ALS were excluded from our study because they had evidence of spinal cord compression on myelography. The only median SEP abnormality found in our MSD patients (prolonged P/N13–N19 IPL) (Fig. 9–16) is not one usually associated with spinal cord compression. A further 16 patients had myelograms, all of which were normal. Median SEP abnormalities (mainly EP–P/N13 prolongation) have been found in 70% to 100% of patients with cervical spondylotic myelopathy (Oh et al., 1985; Bosch et al., 1985). It has been suggested that SEPs may be a useful test in the differentiation of MSD from cervical spondylotic myelopathy (Oh et al., 1985; Bosch et al., 1985) because of the high incidence of abnormalities in cervical spondylotic myelopathy

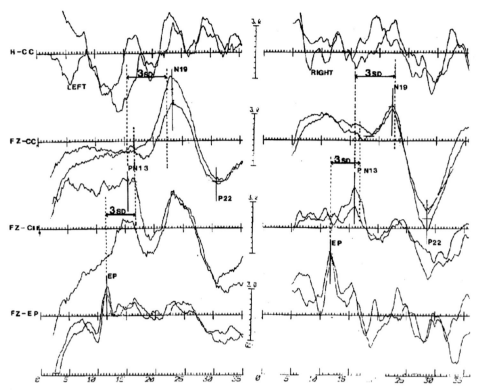

FIG. 9–16. Median nerve SEPs in a 57-year-old patient with familial ALS. There is a prolonged P/N13–N19 IPL following left-sided stimulation (normal mean ± 3 SD = 6.8 msec), indicating a conduction defect rostral to the lower medulla (the dotted lines show the upper limit of normal for the IPLs). This was the only central conduction abnormality in 20 patients with ALS and 30 with all varieties of motor system diseases. Recording montage and parameters same as for Fig. 9–2. Calibration marks are 3.0 μV in all channels. (From Cascino et al., 1988, with permission.)

and the relatively low incidence of abnormalities in MSD. We would agree with this and add that they may help differentiate MSD from other causes of cord compression as well. We attempted to differentiate peripheral from central causes of median SEP abnormalities by utilizing interpeak rather than absolute latencies and by examining the EP–P/N13 (peripheral and/or central segment) and the P/N13–N19 (central segment) IPLs separately. Other studies which have found a high incidence of abnormal median SEPs in MSD have either not addressed the possibility of coincidental cord compression or have used EP methods which have not best allowed central and peripheral causes for abnormalities to be differentiated. Matheson et al. (1986) reported 11 of 32 patients with abnormal median SEPs. In 8 of 11 the abnormality was in N13 only (N19 was normal, the Erb's point potential was not measured). No patient had N19 abnormal with N13 normal. Thus all abnormalities could have been caused by peripheral lesions. It was not stated whether myelography was performed on the patients with abnormalities. Cosi et al. (1984) found abnormalities in 11% to 26% (various parameters studied) of their 45 patients, 32 of whom had documented cervical spondylosis. No separate analysis was carried out on the group with MSD alone.

Radke et al. (1986) found 2 of 16 patients with abnormalities and, although they were careful to exclude cord compression (all patients had myelograms), the use of EP–N19 only as a criterion for abnormality did not best allow separation of central from peripheral lesions. Anziska and Cracco (1983) found prolonged EP–N19 and P/N13–N19 IPLs in one of three ALS patients (only one side was examined). Dasheiff et al. (1985) reported one ALS patient who had sequential EP studies over a period of 10 months. Initial median SEP studies were normal but 10 months later there was an increased P25 latency bilaterally with normal EP–N20 interwave latencies. Sensory examination was normal. This patient was similar to one of our patients who had poorly formed and apparently delayed P22 waves bilaterally (Fig. 9–17). Our patient had sporadic PLS and elevated serum aluminum levels. However, many laboratories, including our own, do not make clinical interpretations based solely on P22–25 because of the high intersubject variability of this waveform in normal controls. Nevertheless, this observation is interesting. Bosch et al. (1985), using simultaneous bilateral stimulation of the median nerve, found an abnormality in 11 of 30 patients with MSD in absolute latency of long-latency SEPs (components greater than 30 msec), and unilateral stimulation revealed short-latency abnormalities (N19 absolute latency only) in 6 of 30 pa-

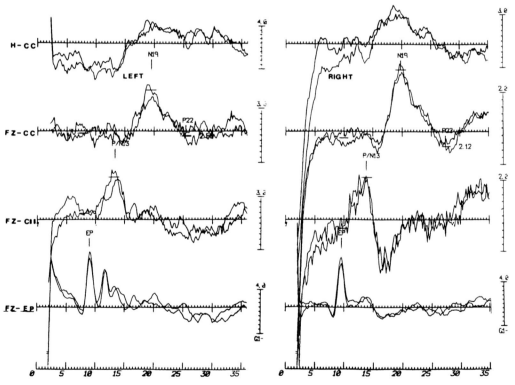

FIG. 9–17. Normal median nerve SEPs in a 38-year-old patient with sporadic primary lateral sclerosis (and markedly elevated serum aluminum level). The EP, P/N13, and N19 components are at normal latencies. P22 has an abnormal configuration; however, this component is not used in clinical interpretation because of large latency and amplitude variability in normal subjects. Recording montage and parameters same as for Fig. 9–2. Calibration marks from top are 4, 3, 3, and 4 μV on left, and 3, 2, 2, and 4 on right. (From Cascino et al., 1988, with permission.)

tients. They concluded that the median SEPs suggested somatosensory involvement at the cortical or subcortical level in patients with MSD. We have not used long-latency SEPs because of the variability found in normal subjects and their dependency on mental state. Assessment of the N19 absolute latency alone does not take into account limb length, limb temperature and possible neuropathic effects. We found no statistical group tendency toward abnormalities in the EP–P/N13, P/N13–N19, and EP–N19 IPLs in the patients with normal studies when compared with controls. It is apparent, therefore, that many of the abnormalities reported in median SEP studies may be accounted for by peripheral lesions. Our data suggest that rarely a patient may have abnormal IPLs due to MSD alone. The finding of abnormal IPLs should prompt a search for other diseases more commonly associated with these SEP abnormalities such as cervical spondylotic myelopathy.

Similarly with lower-limb SEPs there have been various reports of abnormalities found in patients with MSD. However, often a distinction has not been made between central and peripheral abnormalities, the role of inadequate stimulation as a cause for delayed latency of scalp components has not been considered, and possible coexisting cervical spondylosis or other compressive lesions have not been adequately excluded in those patients in whom abnormalities have been found. Matheson et al. (1986) noted that 20 out of 32 patients had abnormalities in lower-extremity SEPs, and they attributed 13 of these to defects in central conduction. The LP was not measured but H-reflexes were utilized to attempt to differentiate peripheral from central conduction defects; if the H-reflex was normal the defect was assumed to be central. However, the posterior tibial nerve studies were performed by stimulation at the ankle while the H-reflexes were obtained with stimulation at the popliteal fossa (Matheson et al., 1986). Therefore 30 to 40 cm of peripheral sensory nerve which was not being evaluated by the H-reflex may have contributed to the SEP latency. In addition, two patients in our study with ALS had delayed scalp EPs (corrected for height) and normal H-reflexes, but the lumbar recording showed that the delay was peripheral and that central conduction was normal. This suggests that it may not be correct to attribute delayed scalp potentials to defects in central conduction by utilizing H-reflexes with stimulation at the knee. In addition, it is possible that some of their patients may have had coexisting cervical spondylosis, as details of how this was excluded were not given.

Cosi et al. (1984) noted that 19 of 33 MSD patients had delayed cortical (N34–P45) waves, but LPs were not reported, so it is not possible to ascertain whether the conduction defects were central or peripheral. Also, 32 of 45 of their patients had cervical spondylosis. There is an even higher incidence of abnormal SEPs in myelopathy associated with cervical spondylosis when lower rather than upper limbs are studied (Bosch et al., 1985). Dasheiff et al. (1985) reported tibial studies that revealed a prolonged lower cord to sensory cortex conduction (LIII–P1 interwave latency) bilaterally in a patient with ALS who had a normal myelogram. Radtke et al. (1986) reported abnormal lower-limb SEPs in 7 of 16 patients with MSD, but central conduction was abnormal in only four of these. No patient had a significant abnormality on myelography. Our study identified only 1 of 18 MSD patients with definite central conduction abnormalities following tibial stimulation. Eight others had delayed or absent scalp potentials on one or both sides, but in only three of these the LPs were bilaterally delayed, suggesting definite peripheral pathology alone. Sural conduction velocity was normal in all four cases in which it was studied (a low-amplitude response was seen on one side of one study). However, as with H-reflexes, normal sural sensory conduction does not preclude a peripheral conduction abnormality in tibial SEPs. In normal subjects the scalp latency following stimulation of the posterior tibial nerve at the ankle is 4 to 11 msec shorter than that following stimulation of the sural nerve at the ankle (at the same distance from the spinal cord) (Burke et al., 1981), and so a different axon population is being tested during tibial compared with sural stimulation. This may be due to the exclusive cutaneous content (group II) of sural fibers compared with the muscle afferent (group I), motor, and cutaneous fibers in the tibial nerve and/or to their central connections in the spinal cord. In addition, at least theoretically, patients may be subject to mononeuropathy of the tibial nerve which spares the sural nerve. Inadequate stimulation of the tibial nerve sometimes results in apparently delayed scalp potentials and the latency returns to normal when the stimulus intensity is increased (see Chapter 8, Section 9.1.2, and Figs. 8–12 and 8–13). If the stimulus does not activate group I fibers in the posterior tibial nerve (electrodes improperly placed and/or stimulus intensity too low), only the slower conducting cutaneous afferents (group II) will generate an apparently delayed scalp EP, with lumbar activity difficult to record. The only check on the adequacy of posterior tibial nerve stimulation is the technician's observation of a good muscle twitch in the intrinsic foot muscles supplied by the posterior tibial nerve and the presence of good lumbar activity. In our patients with normal central conduction (all but one with good lumbar activity), there was no statistical group tendency toward abnormality in central conduction when patients were compared with normal controls. These data suggest that when other coexisting disease and technical factors are carefully excluded, abnormal central conduction is rarely seen in patients with MSD. However, abnormal central conduction in lower-limb SEPs is very common in patients with cervical spondylotic myelopathy (Bosch et al., 1985). When delayed central conduction is found in a patient in whom the diagnosis of MSD is being considered, it would be wise, therefore, to exclude other lesions, such as cervical myelopathy, which much more commonly produce central conduction abnormalities, before attributing the abnormalities to MSD.

This is illustrated by four of our patients with MSD who were excluded from this study because of myelographic evidence of spinal cord compression. Two had normal median SEPs and did not benefit from surgery for cervical spondylosis, suggesting that MSD may have been the etiology for their symptoms. In a contrasting case, EPs were of diagnostic use because they detected abnormalities which our data show are unusual in MSD. This patient with a painless progressive spastic quadriparesis had normal joint position sensation, light touch and pain perception, and bilateral extensor plantar responses. Tibial SEP studies revealed bilateral central conduction abnormalities with prolonged LP–N/P37 IPLs. Myelography demonstrated an incomplete block at C6–7 and significant spinal stenosis at C4–5 and C5–6. The patient refused surgery, but remained entirely unchanged 2 years later.

A curious finding in our study was that the patient with the unusually formed N19/P22 on median nerve stimulation and the patient with the central conduction prolongation on tibial stimulation both had elevated serum aluminum levels (Fig. 9–17). The former patient had sporadic PLS and the latter had sporadic PSMA. None of our patients exhibited raised serum or urine lead levels. Yanagihara (1982) demonstrated raised aluminum levels in the spinal cords of ALS patients from regions of the Guam Islands with endemic MSD. However, we are not aware of previous reports of EP abnormalities and raised aluminum levels in MSD.

In summary, in our laboratory we have found no consistent or reproducible abnormalities of PSVEPs and BAEPs in the 38 patients we have examined, and only rare abnormalities in SEP central conduction. After exclusion of technical factors, the finding of abnormal EPs in patients with a diagnosis of MSD should prompt a search for coexisting, often treatable disease or an alternative diagnosis. Most reported sensory conduction defects have involved lower-extremity studies, which may be difficult to interpret.

3.4.6. Parkinson's Disease

Upper-limb SEPs have been normal in this laboratory in patients with Parkinson's disease. Rossini et al. (1989) found normal N20 but abnormal later components. Rossini et al. (1995) saw enhancement of frontal but no change in parietal SEP components with subcutaneous injection of apomorphine chloride.

3.4.7. Progressive Supranuclear Palsy

Mastaglia et al. (1978) found "enhanced cortical" SEPs in two of six patients with progressive supranuclear palsy, but no other descriptions were given.

3.4.8. Spinocerebellar Brain Stem Ataxias/Degenerations

There are several reports of SEPs in spinocerebellar brain stem ataxias/degenerations. The diversity of these syndromes and the quality of the work are such that the reports themselves must be read for details before meaningful conclusions or comparisons can be made on clinical and technical grounds.

Mastaglia et al. (1978) reported low-amplitude or absent P/N13 in two patients with peroneal muscular atrophy and two others with mixed sensorimotor polyneuropathies. Of seven patients with hereditary spastic paraparesis, three had abnormal P/N13 components and in two of these, N19 was also delayed and reduced in amplitude. Of 10 patients with cerebellar degenerations, the P/N13 components were abnormal in 3; N19 could be recorded only in 6, in one of whom it was abnormal. Of five patients with mixed spinocerebellar degenerations, four had abnormal SEPs.

Pedersen and Trojaborg (1981) studied 11 patients with hereditary cerebellar ataxia and 13 with hereditary spastic paraplegia. Eight of the 11 with cerebellar ataxia and 4 of the 13 with spastic paraplegia had abnormal SEPs (all but one had normal central conduction times from the upper limb). Noel and Desmedt (1980) tested six patients with a "late spinocerebellar degeneration," with ataxia, minimal or absent disorders of sensation, and hyperactive reflexes. The SEP results were similar to those seen in patients with Friedreich's ataxia, with low-amplitude, dispersed N19 components, the first of which was at a normal latency.

Thomas et al. (1981) studied median SEPs in 18 patients with hereditary spastic paraplegia and normal peripheral nerve conduction velocities. In one third of the patients the lower medullary potentials were absent and they were reduced in amplitude in the remainder.

See also Uncini et al. (1987)—Strumpell's familial spastic paraplegia, Chokroverty et al. (1985) and Hammond and Wilder (1983)—olivopontocerebellar atrophy, Majnemer et al. (1986)—giant axonal neuropathy, Imai et al. (1991)—xeroderma pigmentosum, and Anziska and Cracco (1983), Yamada et al. (1986), Nousiainen et al. (1987), and Nuwer et al. (1983)—a variety of ataxias and degenerative diseases.

3.5. INTRINSIC BRAIN STEM LESIONS

3.5.1. Tumors

There are only a few reports of patients with intrinsic brain stem tumors tested with SEPs. Anziska and Cracco (1980) reported two patients, one with a brain stem glioma and the other with a thalamic glioma; both were only confirmed radiographically, both had normal sensation, and both had normal median SEPs (patients 10 and 23 in that study). Green and McLeod (1979) reported three patients with cerebellar tumors who had normal SEPs and one patient with a bithalamic tumor in whom N19 was absent. Niazy and Lundervold (1982) reported median nerve SEPs in a group of patients with thalamic and other supratentorial tumors. One patient with a thalamic tumor, hemianesthesia, and hemiataxia had normal SEPs. Four patients with frontal lobe tumors had normal SEPs. One patient with a parietal lobe tumor (and normal sensation) had normal SEPs but five others with sensory deficits all had abnormal SEPs. Kaplan et al. (1988a) studied SEPs in a patient with a cervical cord glioma extending from C3 to C7; tibial SEPs were normal and median SEPs were markedly abnormal, and they related the differential involvement to the distribution of upper- and lower-limb tracts in the spinal cord.

The same differential involvement of upper- (abnormal) and lower- (normal) limb SEPs may be seen in patients with pontine gliomas. This is caused by the central pontine location of the tumor, which, as it expands, first encounters the medial aspects of the medial lemniscus. In the dorsal columns of the spinal cord the lower-limb sensory fibers lie medially, but as the medial lemniscus is formed and ascends through the medulla and pons the upper-limb fibers come to lie medially and hence are first affected by the tumor.

We have seen a patient who had a thalamic glioma but normal clinical examination and median SEPs. The patient came to medical attention because of an incidental, minor head injury and the tumor was found on a CT scan performed for evaluation of the head injury. This is in agreement with the experience reported above; the nature of gliomas, which is to infiltrate initially instead of destroying parenchyma, allows normal functioning of a sufficient number of thalamic neurons so that the SEPs are normal.

3.5.2. Hemorrhages, Infarctions, and Ischemia

Most of the case reports of patients with brain stem vascular disease have been discussed above in Section 1.1.3 since they usually have been presented as data relating to the generator sources of SEP potentials. Other case reports have been discussed above in Section 2.1. As these discussions together present the data in their most useful contexts, they will not be repeated here.

One clinical utility of SEPs in this area is illustrated by Fig. 9–18, which shows median SEPs from a patient who began to complain of left hand pain several months following a subarachnoid hemorrhage and spasm-induced infarction. Clinically it was not clear whether the "pain" was thalamic or psychiatric in origin. Median SEPs revealed a clear abnormality (absence of N19–P22) on left-sided stimulation, thus providing an objective indication of CNS disease. Here, the reliability of the SEPs made them useful purely in an objective demonstration of an abnormality in sensory system function.

There has been considerable interest in the use of SEPs for stroke prognosis (La Joie et al., 1982; Zeman and Yiannikas, 1989; Chester and McLaren, 1989; Gott et al., 1990; Kovala, 1991; Macdonell et al., 1991), and a majority of these patients with substantial deficits have SEP abnormalities. For example, La Joie et al. (1982) studied median nerve SEPs on admission in 68 patients with right hemiplegia following a stroke. Forty-two patients had absent N19–P23 potentials and only one of these showed some functional improvement before discharge. Of eight having a normal SEP, three had some functional gain. Although the SEPs offer the advantages of objectivity and quantification via numeric data (Zeman and Yiannikas, 1989) and may be complementary to the clinical examination, especially the tibial SEPs (Kovala, 1991), they probably are no better prognostically than pertinent elements of the neurologic examination (e.g., Chester and McLaren, 1989 and Gott et al., 1990) since

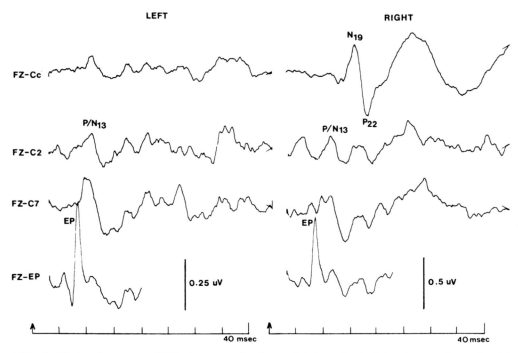

FIG. 9–18. Median nerve SEPs from a patient complaining of pain following a subarachnoid hemorrhage with cerebral infarction secondary to arterial spasm. Clinically it was not clear whether or not the pain had an "organic" basis. The SEP demonstrates an absent N19–P22 following left-sided stimulation, providing objective evidence of somatosensory system malfunction. Each trace is the average of 1,000 stimuli.

motor function is of prime importance clinically and the SEP does not assess this area. Kovala et al. (1990) have suggested that tibial SEPs have predictive value for the development of seizures in the first year following a cerebral infarction. Kovala et al. (1991) followed posterior tibial SEPs for 1 year after cerebral infarction and noted no significant changes in latency or amplitude values.

Macdonell et al. (1991) followed patients with strokes for 6 months and concluded that the major effect of stroke on SEPs occurs acutely and is little affected by secondary degenerative processes. However, inspection of their data shows a substantial loss of negativity at 20 msec in two of the five cases shown; these were two of the four who had cortical involvement and they had the most severe sensory loss in that group.

Mori et al. (1984) studied three patients with ataxic hemiparesis from capsular lesions, all with abnormal N19 and/or P22 components; they postulated that patients with an ataxic hemiparesis from a pontine lesion would have normal SEPs. Hammond and Wilder (1982) recorded absent N19–P22 on one side in a patient with locked-in syndrome secondary to a basilar infarction. Ferbert et al. (1988) reported similar findings in 7 of 28 patients with basilar thrombosis, and in another 6 the N19–P22 amplitude was abnormally low; 7 patients had absent N19–P22 components bilaterally. SEP results in thalamic infarction syndromes have been reported by Graff-Radford et al. (1985) and Mauguiere and Desmedt (1988), and the possible utility of the SEPs in differentiating the subtypes of Dejerine–Roussy syndrome was discussed by the latter authors. A variety of cases with infarctions have been reported by Mauguiere et al. (1983a,b), Nakashima et al. (1985), Stejskal and Sobota (1985), de Weerd et al. (1985), and Reisecker et al. (1986), some with transient syndromes. Kovala et al. (1990) found a high correlation between the side-to-side amplitude difference of tibial nerve SEPs and the development of seizures in patients following nonhemorrhagic cerebral infarction.

3.6. Coma

Goldie et al. (1979, 1981) studied median SEPs in 36 patients who were in coma (clinically poorly responsive but with some preservation of brain stem function) from various etiologies. All had identifiable Erb's point and P/N13 waves. Twelve patients (33%) had no identifiable N19–23 waves bilaterally; six of them died and six remained in a vegetative state.

Eight patients (22%) had identifiable N19–P23 waveforms only unilaterally; three died, three remained in a vegetative state, and two became functional. Sixteen (44%) had N19–P23 waves present bilaterally (normal or abnormal); 3 died, 4 remained in a vegetative state, and 9 became functional. In many of these patients the N19–P23 waves were distorted or delayed in latency relative to normal standards. Follow-up of some of these patients showed improvement in configuration and latency of these waveforms, usually paralleling clinical improvement. Six of the 12 patients with no identifiable N19–P23 waveforms died. Two of them had autopsies; one autopsy did not demonstrate a cerebral abnormality because the patient died only a few hours after a cardiac arrest and the other showed widespread necrosis of the cerebral hemispheres. The other patients survived and left the hospital with varying degrees of disability. Of the 24 patients (67%) who had at least unilateral N19–P23 responses, 6 died and none had autopsies. Patients who initially had well-preserved N19–P23 components survived if no new complications ensued, but the precise level of subsequent disability varied.

One comatose but not brain-dead patient had suffered cardiac arrest and at the time of SEP testing was clinically apallic (see Ingvar et al., 1978). He died less than 8 hours after the test and neuropathologic examination documented complete necrosis of the cortex. His SEP (Fig. 9–9) showed normal P/N13 and N19, but absent or distorted P23 waves. Biniek et al. (1989) found absent SEPs in four patients with the complete apallic syndrome with isoelectric EEGs who lived 6 weeks to 13 months following the hypoxic event.

Thirty-three comatose but not brain-dead patients had both BAEP and SEP tests. Combinations of the results including differences between sides were many and complex. Using criteria requiring both sides to have a normal response for the test to be judged normal, three patients had both tests normal and all three remained in a vegetative state. Thirteen patients had normal BAEPs and abnormal SEPs; four of these had functional recovery, six remained in a vegetative state, and three died. Two patients had normal SEPs and abnormal BAEPs; both had functional recovery. Using the best result obtained (irrespective of side) 10 patients had both tests normal; 5 of them remained in a vegetative state and 5 had functional recovery. Five patients had normal BAEPs but only SEP waves P/N13; two of them died and three remained in a vegetative state. Six patients had abnormal BAEP waves and only SEP waves P/N13; three of them died, two remained in a vegetative state, and one had functional recovery. Thus the SEP results were much more accurate in prognosis for no or poor recovery since no patient with absent N19–P23 waveforms bilaterally had a good outcome.

Hume et al. (1979) studied median SEPs in 24 comatose patients (various etiologies) and found that the lower medullary to N19 IPL (termed central conduction time by them) (1) was increased in 11 of the patients, (2) showed no relationship with serum phenobarbital levels (0 to 146 μg/ml, mean 56 μg/ml) or body temperature (35.0°C to 38.5°C), and (3) had a correlation with clinical outcome when obtained within 10 to 35 days of the onset of coma. They also noted short-term central conduction delays during temporary metabolic disorders and sustained delays with gradual recovery over many months, particularly after head injury. All 11 of their patients who made a good recovery had normal conduction times at or before the end of the 35-day period, whereas the conduction time remained abnormal or N19–P23 could not be recorded in 11 of the 13 who did not make a good recovery.

Hume et al. (1982) studied 94 patients in coma secondary to head injury. Of 49 patients tested within 3.5 days of the injury, the SEP was normal in 14 of the 20 patients who made a good recovery and abnormal in 24 of 29 who died or were left disabled. All eight patients who had absent N19–P23 waveforms died. The outcome was not correlated with SEP results at all times; for example, they found that 10 patients among the 44 who did not make a good recovery had normal SEPs at some point in time. Three patients who had normal SEPs on all occasions remained disabled and two who died had normal results early but not later. Fifteen of the group of 31 patients who made a good recovery had abnormal SEPs at some point.

Another study from the same group (Cant et al., 1986) in 35 patients with posttraumatic coma also resulted in the conclusion that the SEPs reliably predicted both good and bad outcomes, whereas the BAEP did not. All 17 patients in whom SEPs were normal had a favorable outcome and 15 of 18 with abnormal SEPs had an unfavorable outcome, whereas only 19 of 28 with normal BAEPs had a favorable outcome. Of 14 patients with absent N19–P22 (unilateral or bilateral not differentiated in this study), 12 died, 1 was severely disabled, and 1 was moderately disabled.

Walser et al. (1986) studied 63 comatose patients, classified the SEPs into five grades of severity, and showed a good correlation with outcome and degree of post mortem pathologic change. Judson et al. (1990) in a study of 100 intensive care unit patients claimed that SEPs recorded within 24 hrs of head injury are a reliable predictor of outcome and that predictive accuracy was not influenced by the time of recording or cumulative recordings over the first 4 days after injury.

Lindsay et al. (1981) tested median SEPs using a vertex to Cc derivation in 32 patients in coma secondary to head injury. They counted the number of waves present on the worst side in the first 200 msec (N19 was not identified) and found a positive correlation with outcome. De la Torre et al. (1978) used a similar method of counting peaks present and reported good correlations in 17 patients. Rappaport et al. (1981a,b) studied SEPs in head-injured patients using a nine-point rating scale and found significant correlations between admission and 1-year outcome disabilities and the EPs. Gutling et al. (1994) followed 50 patients for 18 months after severe head injury and found that a combined analysis of frontal and parietal SEP components improved the outcome prediction and that the predictive power of the parietal component alone decreased with time. Narayan et al. (1981) studied 133 severely head-injured patients and found that "multimodality" EPs were the most accurate single prognostic indicator (with a 91% accuracy rate) when compared with clinical examination, CT scan, and intracranial pressure. In a series of 255 comatose patients studied by Haupt (1988), all 57 with absent N19–P22 bilaterally did not recover.

Hansotia (1985) has noted increased central conduction times and decreased P22 amplitudes in patients with persistent vegetative state. Patients with severe anoxic damage will have flat or near-flat EEGs and absent thalamocortical components (N19–P23) (Wytrzes et al., 1989).

Serial EPs may be of prognostic significance and play an important role in decision-making in patients who are unable to be examined neurologically due to barbiturate coma or neuromuscular blockade as the configuration and latencies of these potentials do not change (de Weerd et al., 1985). However, in patients in coma due to severe CNS depressant drug overdose the central somatosensory conduction time after median nerve stimulation is prolonged and N20 is dispersed and BAEP IPLs are delayed (Rumpl et al., 1988a).

In summary, the absence of N19–P22 bilaterally remains one of the best prognostic rules in these patients, that is, if a comatose patient is missing N19–P22 bilaterally, then that patient's outcome will be a persistent vegetative state at best. All studies in adults (Anderson et al., 1984; Goldie et al., 1981; Hume and Cant, 1981; Cant et al., 1986; Ropper and Miller, 1985; Brunko and Zegers de Beyl, 1987; Ganes and Lundar, 1988; Haupt 1988; Rumpl et al., 1988a,b; Rothstein et al., 1991; Facco et al., 1990, 1991; Guerit, 1992) and children (see Chapter 11) have revealed no good exceptions to this rule. Table 9–6 presents a summary of data encompassing 629 comatose patients from centers around the world; of the 258 who had bilaterally absent N19–P22 83% died, 11% were left in a persistent vegetative state, and 6% were left with a disability. The articles usually did not define "disability" well enough for a further analysis or discussion; the patient listed as having made a good recovery had no further clinical description and a child tested on day 3 following a lightning strike made a normal recovery. Our experience indicates that patients in coma

TABLE 9–6. *Somatosensory EPs in coma*

Authors	Age	Year	Country	Total	Bilat. absent N20/P22	Died	PVS	Disability	SEP time	Follow-up
Anderson et al.	A	84	U.S.A.	23	8	2	4	2 dependent	<5 days	5 months
Biniek et al.	A/C	89	Germany	4	4	3	1	0	?	6 months
Brunko & Zegers de Beyl	A	87	Belgium	50	30	30	0	0	<8 hrs	week
Cant et al.	A	86	New Zealand	40	7	6	0	1 dependent	<4 days	2 months
DeMeirleir	C	87	Canada	33	13	4	0	9 severe	1 week	?
DeWeerd & Groeneveld	A	85	Netherlands	18	8	6	2	0	<1 week	6 months
Facco et al.	A	90	Italy	49	19	19[a]	0	0	<4 days	days
Frank et al.	C	85	U.S.A.	5	5	0	5	0	<1 day	months
Goldie et al.	A	81	U.S.A.	65	41	35	6	0	<3 weeks	hospital discharge
Goodwin et al.	A/C	91	U.S.A.	41	27	23	4	0	<3 days	?
Judson et al.	A	90	New Zealand	100	30	27	2	1 severe	<5 days	6 months
Lindsay et al.	A	90	Scotland	101	24	22	1	1[b] good recovery	<13 days	6 months
Taylor & Farrell	C	89	Canada	37	19	15	3	1[c] normal	?	weeks
Walser et al.	A	86	Switzerland	63	23	22	1	0	<3 weeks	3 months
Total				629	258	214 (83%)	29 (11%)	15 (6%)		

Outcome of coma related to bilateral absence of SEP N19/P22 components. Disability as stated without further description available in report. (A/C, adults or children; PVS, persistent vegetative state).
[a]Outcome either dead or PVS not separated in report.
[b]Not further described in report.
[c]Child tested on day 3 following a lightning strike, SEPs normal on day 10.

with absent N19–P22 bilaterally will uniformly have a persistent vegetative state as the best possible outcome.

Obviously, the clinical utility of SEPs in comatose patients is related to whether or not the patient is brain-dead, that is, if a patient is brain-dead, then the finding of bilateral absence of the hemispheral/cortical SEP components (N19/P22) is clinically less helpful since the prognosis from the clinical examination is completely reliable. If these patients are removed from consideration, the overall numbers are smaller but the conclusion remains the same.

This bilateral absence of N19–P22 needs to be clearly distinguished from unilateral absence since these patients may have a good outcome (although the absent EP waveforms on that side indicate that the functional recovery of the involved limbs will be poor).

Also see the appropriate sections in Chapter 11 for a discussion of these considerations in the pediatric age group.

3.7. Brain Death

Goldie et al. (1981) studied median SEPs in 29 brain-dead patients. All patients had identifiable Erb's point waves; they were at latencies representing normal peripheral conduction velocities in 27 and in the other two, prolonged Erb's point latencies implied slowed peripheral conduction due to subnormal body temperature (< 92°F). One patient had too much ambient muscle artifact to exclude identifiable CNS responses. None of these patients had identifiable N19–P23 waveforms despite increased amplifier sensitivity during two separate trials.

Of the 29 brain-dead patients, 69% showed preservation of the P/N13 waves. Two patients with preserved P/N13 waves were autopsied and extensive necrosis of the pons was demonstrated. Three additional patients with preserved P/N13 waves showed severe cerebral and brain stem autolysis and so formal neuropathologic evaluation could not be done. All of these patients were autopsied within 36 hours and often within 12 hours of the evoked potential studies. These findings support the postulate that the P/N13 wave originates in structures caudal to the pons which can be preserved even with clinical evidence of brain stem disruption.

Nine patients showed loss of the P/N13 wave despite preserved Erb's point responses. Two of these cases were shown pathologically to have transections of the cervical spinal cord at C2–3 and C5–6, respectively. (The other seven cases did not have autopsies.) These results again support the postulated location of the P/N13 wave somewhere between the cervical roots and pons. Preservation of the P/N13 wave in 69% of brain-dead patients indicates that the stimulus-generated signal has reached the spinal cord. Failure of further rostral conduction, indicated by lack of subsequent waves, is then an indicator of brain stem dysfunction. This situation contrasts with the BAEP where 77% of brain-dead patients did not have a wave (wave I) that proved the input signal had activated the eighth nerve.

The variable preservation of P/N13 in brain-dead patients is probably the result of an interaction between cessation of intracranial circulation (due to increased intracranial pressure following cerebral necrosis) and the pattern of blood supply to the lower medulla. The site of P/N13 generation, in the region of the cervicomedullary junction, is where an interface between intracranial and extracranial blood supply exists. Since the dorsal column nuclei are the most likely candidates for the P/N13 generator, this suggests that these nuclei were functionally preserved in 69% of brain-dead patients. In a multicenter study, 57% of 127 brain-dead patients had neuropathologically intact cervicomedullary junctions (Walker et al., 1975), although the state of the dorsal column nuclei themselves was not systematically defined. Preservation of the lower medulla and P/N13 might also parallel preservation of some cerebral respiratory function in patients who meet al.l other criteria of brain death. Among previous reports of SEPs in the assessment of brain death (Trojaborg and Jorgensen,

1973; Hume et al., 1979; Anziska and Cracco, 1980b), only Hume et al. recorded short-latency responses with simultaneous pickup of the signal at optimum locations along the somatosensory pathways, as we did. None of their patients met clinical criteria of brain death.

Twenty-seven brain-dead patients (Goldie et al., 1981) had both BAEP and SEP tests. Sixteen had no BAEP waves and only P/N13 in the SEP, two had only BAEP wave I and SEP P/N13 waves, one had only BAEP waves I and II and SEP P/N13 wave, and eight had no waves in either test.

Anziska and Cracco (1980b) studied median SEPs in 11 patients in deep coma using central scalp electrodes and ear or noncephalic references. Although their patients met most accepted brain-death criteria, the apnea test was "the absence of spontaneous respiration manifested by the need for controlled ventilation (that is, the patient makes no effort to override the respirator) for at least 15 minutes." An EEG was obtained in 7 of the 11 patients, arteriography in 4, CT scan in 1, and an autopsy in 1. They found N17–18 present in one of these patients who had had a right-hemisphere infarction; brain death was confirmed by arteriography but there was no EEG or autopsy. On the basis of our experience, the finding of a preserved N18 indicates that the thalamus was at least partially intact and probably suggests that the patient was not brain-dead as currently defined. Note also that brain-dead patients may show an apparent N18 which is actually "uncovered" negativity from the region of the cervicomedullary junction, its appearance facilitated by the absence of P14, N18, N19, and P22 generators, also seen in extensive lesions of the pons (Raroque et al., 1994). Myogenic sources may also confuse the issue (Guerit, 1986). Buchner et al. (1988) followed the evolution of the brain-dead state in 35 patients and noted loss of P14 within 3 hours of onset of brain death, followed by N13 alterations; N11 was preserved until severe systemic effects (hypotension, hypoxia) were present. Belsh and Chokroverty (1987) reported N19 and later waves lost in 10 adult brain-dead patients.

3.8. Miscellaneous Diseases

3.8.1. Acquired Immune Deficiency Syndrome

Abnormal SEPs have been found in patients with acquired immune deficiency syndrome (AIDS) (Arimura et al., 1987; Smith et al., 1988). Kakigi et al. (1992) found decreased conduction velocities in spinothalamic and posterior column tracts in patients with human T-cell lymphotropic virus type 1-associated myelopathy, more than half of whom had no clinical impairment of sensation. Iragui et al. (1994) studied 159 human immune deficiency virus-infected subjects who had no neurologic symptoms or signs [129 asymptomatic, 30 with AIDS-related complex (ARC)/AIDS] and found central conduction delays in both groups, whereas peripheral abnormalities were seen only in the ARC/AIDS group. They found only rare abnormalities in BAEPs and PSVEPs.

3.8.2. Arnold–Chiari Malformation

Although patients with Arnold–Chiari malformation have been reported to have both abnormal and normal BAEPs, our patients have usually had normal BAEPs. There are no reports in the literature on SEPs in this condition; one of our patients had abnormal SEPs, not in the cervicomedullary region but with an abnormal P/N13 to N19 IPL and an abnormal configuration of N19–P22, with absent cortical potentials from posterior tibial stimulation (Fig. 9–19).

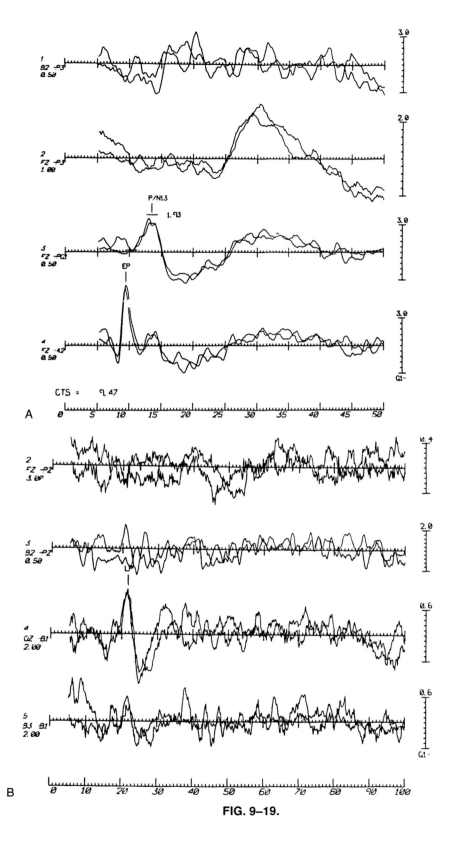

FIG. 9–19.

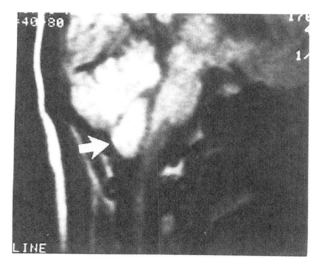

FIG. 9–19. (*Continued*) Upper- and lower-limb SEPs in a 30-year-old woman with a 1-year history of balance problems and several months of upper-limb symptoms suggestive of carpal tunnel syndrome. Tendon reflexes in the legs were brisk but plantar responses were flexor; cerebellar testing was normal. The upper limbs had findings on examination consistent with carpal tunnel syndrome. Initial CT was normal. Brain stem auditory and pattern-shift visual EPs were normal. Median and peroneal nerve SEPs were similar to the median and posterior tibial nerve SEPs recorded 3 years later (*shown above*). The right median nerve SEP (*panel* **A**) was similar to the left and shows normal EP and P/N13 but absent N19; the nature of the upgoing peak in FZ–Cc (*second channel from top*) is unknown. The left posterior tibial SEP (*panel* **B**) was similar to the right and had a normal LP but no cortical components. Multiple sclerosis was considered a likely possibility. Three years later an MRI scan (*above*) showed an Arnold–Chiari type I malformation (*arrow*). Recording montage and parameters for median SEPs same as for Fig. 9–2. Tibial SEP montage from top was FZ–CZ, dorsum of hand to CZ, iliac crest to L1 spinous process, and L3–L1; each trace is the average of 1,000 stimuli delivered at 2/sec (tibial) and 5/sec (median). Calibrations are in microvolts.

3.8.3. Diabetes

Cracco et al. (1980b), using the mean value plus 2 SD to define abnormality, and measuring conduction velocities for segments of the spinal cord, found abnormalities over rostral cord (T6–C7) in 20% (6 of 30) of their diabetic patients (aged 5 to 24 years), whereas caudal segments were normal.

Gupta and Dorfman (1980, 1981) used "indirect" measurements and found delays in the spinal cord but not in central conduction. Comi et al. (1985) found abnormal central conduction in 31% (lower limbs) and 20% (upper limbs) of 30 patients with diabetes.

3.8.4. Creutzfeldt–Jakob Disease

Two patients with advanced Creutzfeldt–Jakob disease have shown normal median SEPs up to and including N19 (Chiappa, 1982). However, the P23 potential was essentially absent in these patients.

3.8.5. Hepatic Disease

Chu et al. (1985) followed a patient with Wilson's disease and hepatic failure. The P/N13–N19 IPL was within normal limits, but decreased slightly following liver transplantation. Selwa et al. (1993) studied 20 patients and showed abnormal median SEPs, usually bilaterally prolonged N/P13–N20 latencies, in 65% of patients. Grimm et al. (1992) showed significantly abnormal EPs in the group of 28 neurologically symptomatic patients as compared to controls.

3.8.6. Hysteria–Malingering

Somatosensory EPs cannot be affected significantly voluntarily, so an abnormal SEP as defined in Chapter 8 and above in Section 2 is a definite indicator of CNS dysfunction, although the presenting problems and the SEP may not necessarily be related. On the other hand, although lesions in the sensory system usually produce abnormal SEPs (see above Section 2.1), this is not always so (e.g., with thalamic lacunar disease). A normal SEP does not necessarily indicate the complete absence of lesions in the sensory system (see also Howard and Dorfman, 1986).

3.8.7. Multi-Infarct Dementia

Abbruzzese et al. (1984) found increased P/N13–N19 IPL in 7 of 18 patients with multi-infarct dementia, and abnormally low N19–P22 peak-to-peak amplitude in three. They contrasted this with 30 patients who had Alzheimer's disease, only one of whom had an abnormal P/N13–N19 IPL and 3 of whom had abnormal N19–P22 amplitudes.

3.8.8. Myoclonic Epilepsy

Halliday (1967a,c) looked at P33 in 26 patients with myoclonic epilepsy of various etiologies (amaurotic family idiocy, Lafora body disease, Unverricht–Lundborg disease, idiopathic) and found it abnormally large in about one third of them, the largest responses usually being found in the most incapacitated patients. Shibasaki et al. (1978, 1985, 1990) found normal N19 amplitudes but abnormally large later potentials in 17 of 19 patients with progressive myoclonic epilepsy, and also in diseases with similar clinical features (lipidoses, neuronal ceroid lipofuscinosis, posthypoxic myoclonus, Creutzfeldt–Jakob disease), but no SEP abnormalities in patients with a variety of other diseases associated with myoclonus (midbrain infarction, epilepsy with myoclonus, essential myoclonus, and others). They also have investigated the scalp topography of these giant SEPs in myoclonic epilepsies (Shibasaki et al., 1990, 1991). Ugawa et al. (1991) studied recovery functions by paired stimuli in patients with myoclonus. Mastaglia et al. (1978) found enhanced SEPs, presumably after N19, in four patients with familial myoclonic epilepsy. Dorfman et al. (1978b) studied two brothers with a progressive myoclonus epilepsy and found abnormally large potentials after N19.

3.8.9. Myotonic Dystrophy

Bartel et al. (1984) reported abnormal median nerve SEPs in almost one third of 21 patients with myotonic dystrophy.

3.8.10. Renal Disease

All of 10 chronic hemodialysis patients, studied with nerve conduction tests as well as both electrically and mechanically evoked SEPs (upper limb), showed delays of sensory conduction in at least some portion of the peripheral nerve (none of the patients had symptoms of neuropathy) (Vaziri et al., 1981). Electrical stimulation of the ulnar nerve at the wrist showed abnormal conduction between the brachial plexus and the spinal cord–lower medulla in eight patients (two of whom had only brachial plexus components). Four patients showed an abnormal conduction time between lower medulla and thalamus–cortex. Although spinal cord to thalamus–cortex conduction times were normal in 8 of 10 patients using electrical stimulation of the digital nerves, all 8 patients tested with mechanical stimulation of the finger had abnormalities of the same segment. Another study, using both upper- and lower-limb stimulation, found central delays and, also, increased amplitudes in their 16 chronic uremia patients (Serra et al., 1981). Ganji and Mahajan (1983) found normal central conduction times in eight patients undergoing hemodialysis. Rossini et al. (1985b) reported both upper- and lower-limb SEP abnormalities in patients with chronic renal failure.

3.8.11. Subarachnoid Hemorrhage

Symon et al. (1979) measured central conduction time from P/N13 to N19–P23 in 16 patients with subarachnoid hemorrhage. Central conduction was normal on the unaffected side and prolonged during the development of ischemic complications. In one patient central conduction showed a close relationship to cerebral blood flow and degree of arm weakness.

3.8.12. Syringomyelia

Patients with cervical cord syrinxes may show abnormalities in median nerve SEPs, indicating a lesion in the upper cervical cord, with relative sparing of lower-limb SEPs (see Fig. 9–2) (see *N Engl J Med* 316:150–157, 1987 for a full report of this case, and Fig. 9–20). In our experience, normal tibial SEPs accompanying abnormal median SEPs indicating a lesion in the upper cervical cord (Fig. 9–20) should strongly raise the question of syringomyelia. The differential involvement presumably results from the lesion involving the root entry zone (collateral) portions of the spinal cord rather than the dorsal columns.

Veilleux and Stevens (1987) studied 44 patients with syringomyelia and noted that median and ulnar SEPs were usually normal in the presence of a dissociated sensory loss, and were usually abnormal (ulnar more frequently than median) when all sensory modalities were impaired; abnormalities of tibial SEPs were frequent and were related to impaired proprioceptive sensation in the lower extremities. Emerson and Pedley (1986) and Urasaki et al. (1988) have also described patients with cervical cord lesions (syrinxes, ependymomas, compressions) with N11 (their DCV) and N13 (their CERV N13/P13) abnormalities consistent with the suggested localizations. Jabbari et al. (1990) found abnormal tibial and/or median SEPs in 16 of 22 patients with syringomyelia. Prestor et al. (1991) made subpial cervical spinal cord recordings in patients with syringomyelia. Morioka et al. (1993) also made direct recordings from the dorsal columns and found in two patients that median nerve SEPs were normal, whereas posterior tibial SEPs were abnormal, suggesting that the gracile dorsal column, lying more medially, is more vulnerable when a cervical syrinx is present.

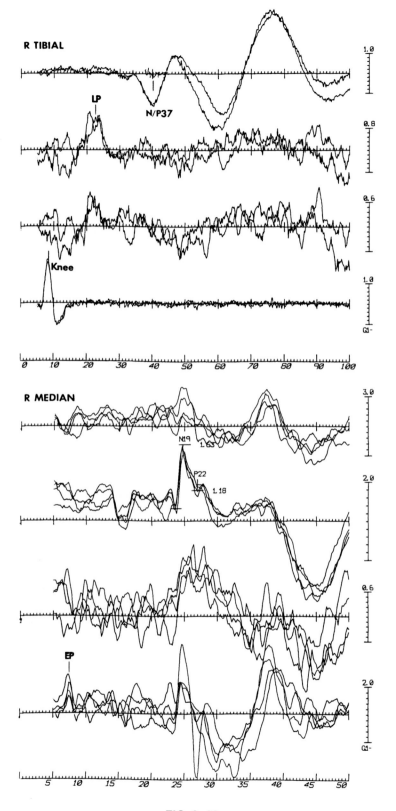

FIG. 9–20.

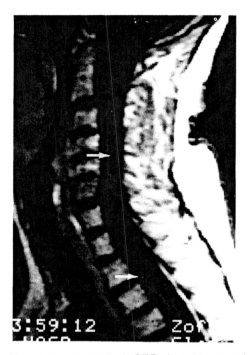

FIG. 9–20. (*Continued*) Upper- and lower-limb SEPs in a 68-year-old woman with left neck pain radiating to the shoulder, progressive numbness of the left forearm, and painless "burning" of the left hand. Pain sensation was decreased over the left shoulder and upper arm with absent reflexes on that side. The right median SEP (similar to left) showed a normal Erb's point potential, absent P/N13, and N19 at an abnormal latency from EP, suggesting bilateral conduction defects in the upper cervical cord. The right posterior tibial SEP (similar to left) was normal. The MRI scan showed syringomyelia, with a cavity extending from C3 to T3, distending the cord (*arrows*). Median nerve recording montage and parameters same as for Fig. 9–2. Posterior tibial SEP channels from top are FZ–CZ, iliac crest to T12 and L1 spinous processes, and a bipolar recording in the popliteal fossa (see Fig. 8–11); each trace is the average of 500 stimuli delivered at 5/sec.

Mauguiere and Restuccia (1991) concluded that the anterior neck reference is significantly superior to the forehead reference in detecting a cervical centromedullary lesion after comparing the N13 potential in six patients with cervical syringomyelia using both montages. In a study of median nerve SEPs in 24 patients with syringomyelia using an anterior cervical montage and measuring the N13/P9 amplitude ratio, Restuccia and Mauguiere (1991) found an absent or reduced N13 in 83% of median nerve SEPs studied. This was significantly correlated with loss of pain and temperature sensation. Masur et al. (1992) used posterior tibial nerve SEPs and found that IPLs were increased in 52% of the limbs.

3.8.13. Thyroid Disease

Takahashi and Fujitani (1970) studied median SEPs in 14 hyperthyroid patients (using an Fz–Cc derivation). They found the N19–P23 amplitude was significantly higher in the patients (mean 30.0 μV) than in the normal controls (mean 8.9 μV). All but one of the patients' N19–P23 amplitudes exceeded the normal mean plus 3 SD. All patients with amplitudes greater than 30 μV had had the disease for more than 6 months. There were no significant differences in latency, or correlation with I-131 uptake, BMR, or resin-sponge uptake.

Straumanis and Shagass (1976) tested the effects of triiodothyronine (T3) and T3 and propanolol on six normal subjects. T3 increased the amplitude of the early SEP components and this effect was eliminated by propanolol.

3.8.14. Tourette's Syndrome

Krumholz et al. (1983) found no SEP abnormalities in 17 patients with Tourette's syndrome.

3.8.15. Vitamin Deficiencies

Both upper- and lower-limb SEPs have been found abnormal in patients with vitamin B_{12} deficiency, often showing no components or only the peripheral EP peak. Fine and Hallett (1980) performed sural and median SEPs in three patients with subacute combined degeneration (SCD) and found bilateral abnormalities in all tests. Krumholz et al. (1981) tested median and peroneal SEPs (using a single scalp channel) in seven patients with SCD; all median SEPs were normal, and five peroneal SEPs were normal. In the two patients in whom the peroneal responses were absent initially, they were present when tested 1 year later. Ludvigsson et al. (1980) studied a 9-year-old boy with SCD. They found normal lumbar and thoracic SEPs but absent cerebral potentials. These were normal after 3 months of therapy. Di Lazzaro et al. (1992) reported on four patients with B_{12} deficiency.

Central SEP conduction abnormalities have been described in abetalipoproteinemia (Harding et al., 1982; Johnson, 1985; Brin et al., 1986) and in vitamin E deficiency (Harding et al., 1982; Kaplan et al., 1988b).

3.9. Trigeminal Nerve Testing

Trigeminal SEPs have been investigated as another area where EP techniques can provide useful clinical data. The different techniques that have been used have produced results that are not easily reconciled, given the present level of knowledge and experience in this field.

Macon et al. (1981) recorded intraoperative trigeminal root EPs in 42 patients during differential radiofrequency thermal rhizotomies and were able to record activities at latencies corresponding to conduction velocities of 64, 3, and 1 m/sec. The amount of heat used in producing the lesion and loss of these EP components correlated well with the clinical outcome.

Larsson and Prevec (1970) used mechanical stimulation of the face and registered an initial positive peak at about 20 msec (F3–C3 derivation). Drechsler et al. (1977) and Drechsler (1980) stimulated at slightly above sensory threshold via a pair of discs placed over the foramen mentale and middle of the chin, recording from bipolar derivations (frontal to central and central to occipital). These recordings showed negative peaks at 5, 14, and 34 msec, positive peaks at 9 and 23 msec, with standard deviations increasing from 1.5 to 2.0 msec for N5 to 3.0 to 3.6 msec for P23 msec in 20 normal subjects. Amplitudes ranged from 1.4 to 2.6 μV for N5–P9, 1.0 to 1.6 for P9–N14, and 1.9 to 2.3 for N14–P23. N5 and P9 were missing after thermocoagulation of the Gausserian ganglion in patients with intractable trigeminal neuralgia and a negativity with a peak at 5 msec was recorded from the ganglion during surgery, suggesting that structure as the origin of N5. Later waves were postulated as being cortical in origin.

Stohr and Petruch (1979), Stohr et al. (1981), and Buettner et al. (1982) stimulated at 3 times sensory threshold via electrodes on the upper and lower lips at the corner of the mouth, recording from FZ to C5 or C6. They found a negative peak at 12 msec (SD 0.87) and a positive peak at 18.5 msec (SD 1.5), with a left–right difference of 0.55 msec (SD 0.55). N12 was not reliably recognized and the N12–P19 amplitude also varied greatly (0.5–6.5 μV, mean 2.7) and so was not thought to be of clinical utility. Using the normal mean plus 2.5 SD as the upper limit of normal, they found that 41% of 17 patients with trigeminal neuralgia had abnormal SEPs (using 3 SD this drops to 35%). Interside latency differences were the most sensitive parameter. Of 46 patients with MS, 61% had abnormal SEPs and 60% of these were asymptomatic. Of seven patients with Wallenberg's syndrome, three had absent waveforms and three had P19 delayed or low in amplitude. Of 11 patients with cerebellopontine angle tumors and trigeminal nerve compression, six had abnormal SEPs.

Bennett and Jannetta (1980) stimulated at 3 to 4 times sensory threshold via electrodes 1 cm apart on the gums over the maxillary first bicuspid, recording from Cc to an earlobe reference. They found consistent N20 (SD 1.8), P34 (SD 4.0), and N51 (SD 6.6) peaks, with considerable variation as stimulus and recording sites were altered. The N20 and P35 components had shorter latencies in females. When the inside of the lip was stimulated, producing a visible lip twitch but less sensation, the amplitude of the potentials was significantly reduced, indicating that muscle potentials were not a major part of the observed activity.

Salar et al. (1982) stimulated at sensory threshold via a coaxial subcutaneous needle placed near the point of emergence of the branch of the trigeminal nerve being tested, recording from CZ to Cc and Ci. They registered P20 and N30 components but thought that P50 was the most reliable. The SEPs were found to be normal in branches affected by trigeminal neuralgia. The SEP was repeated after percutaneous trigeminal thermocoagulation and the SEPs were altered when tactile sensation was disturbed, but not when pain sensation was the only modality affected. Singh et al. (1982) stimulated at 3 times sensory threshold via subcutaneous needles placed near the mentalis nerve at its exit point from the mandibular foramen, recording from bipolar derivations. They registered N3 (mean 3.2 msec, SD 0.47), P9 (mean 9.8 msec, SD 0.29), N14 (mean 14.1 msec, SD 1.05), P23 (mean 24.6 msec, SD 1.9), and N34 (mean 33.7 msec, SD 2.49). N3, P9, N14, P23, and N34 were recognized in 100%, 56%, 56%, 44%, and 36% of normal faces, respectively. The early negative potential disappeared when stimulus polarity was reversed halfway through the test. Amplitudes were too variable for clinical use. In 25 patients with trigeminal neuralgia, atypical facial pain, facial hemispasm, and myokymia the SEPs were within normal limits. In two patients with acoustic neuromas who had unilateral facial anesthesia to pin and loss of the corneal response, no potentials could be recorded on that side although those on the opposite side were normal. Delayed SEPs were seen on the affected side of a patient with recurrent facial paralysis due to meningeal sarcoidosis.

Findler and Feinsod (1982) stimulated the upper and lower lips with 20-mA stimuli via disc electrodes, recording from FpZ to Cc. Lower lip latencies were slightly longer (by about 0.5 msec) than upper-lip latencies, and polarities were reversed. Potentials recorded from upper lip were N8 (mean 7.6 msec, SD 0.7), P14 (mean 14.5 msec, SD 1.1), N19 (mean 19.0 msec, SD 1.73), N23 (mean 23.26 msec, SD 2.76), P37 (mean 37.2 msec, SD 3.9), with P33 from lower lip (mean 33.0 msec, SD 4.55). These peaks and polarities are similar to those obtained by Bennett and Jannetta (1980) with upper-gum stimulation, and by Drechsler (1980) with stimulation over the foramen mentale (compared with lower-lip stimulation here).

Eisen et al. (1981) stimulated at 2.5 times threshold at the corner of the mouth, recording from FpZ to Cc. Peaks recorded were N13 (mean 12.8 msec, SD 0.9), P19 (mean 19.3 msec, SD 1.4), and N30 (mean 28.6 msec, SD 1.7). Abnormalities were found in 41% of 29 patients with MS, none of whom had clinical symptoms or signs of fifth nerve involvement. Four of seven patients with progressive spinal MS and both of two patients who had only optic neuritis had abnormal SEPs.

Leandri et al. (1985, 1988a,b) and Leandri and Campbell (1986) recorded simultaneously from the scalp and the trigeminal pathway following stimulation of the infraorbital nerve in patients undergoing thermocoagulation rhizotomy. They correlated successive scalp components with the entry point of the maxillary nerve into the Gausserian ganglion, the point of entry of the trigeminal root into the pons, and the presynaptic portion of the trigeminal spinal tract. Chapman et al. (1986) stimulated the tooth pulp and maxillary gingiva in 16 volunteers but could not record consistent EPs from the teeth. Leandri et al. (1988a) have reported results of infraorbital nerve stimulation in patients with tumors at the base of the skull and trigeminal neuralgia. They have also reported that blink reflex components may mimic trigeminal EPs (Leandri et al., 1994). See also Seyal and Browne (1989), Altenmuller et al. (1990), Soustiel et al. (1991), Hummel and Kobal (1992), Aziz et al. (1995), and Fujii et al. (1994a) for a variety of studies on SEPs from facial, oral, and esophageal sites.

3.10. Neurourologic Evoked Potentials

Haldeman et al. (1982) stimulated with comfortable intensities via ring electrodes around the base of the penis (1 cm apart) in males and adjacent to the clitoris in females, recording over the lumbar spine and from FpZ to 2 cm behind CZ on the scalp. Somatosensory EPs to stimulation of the posterior tibial nerve were also tested. The responses recorded from over the scalp were quite similar in all three cases (dorsal nerve of the penis, dorsal nerve of the clitoris, and posterior tibial nerve at the ankle), with an initial peak positivity at 39 to 42 msec, followed by a negative peak at 49 to 52 msec. The maximum amplitude was in the midline, 0.2 to 1 μV for clitoral stimulation, 0.5 to 2 μV for penile stimulation, and 1 to 5 μV for posterior tibial nerve stimulation at the ankle. Penile stimulation gave a spinal response at a mean of 12.9 msec (SD 0.8), whereas posterior tibial stimulation had a mean latency of 24.6 msec (SD 2.3). Consistent spinal responses could not be recorded following clitoral stimulation. The spinal conduction time for penile stimulation had a mean of 30.0 msec (SD 3.2); for posterior tibial stimulation this was 16.5 msec (SD 1.6). The difference in peripheral conduction time (stimulus to spinal response) was suggested as being caused by the different distance involved, the nerves having been shown to have similar conduction velocities (Chautraine et al., 1973). The slower central conduction of the penile afferents is presumably related to axon diameter since the pudendal nerve contains only cutaneous afferents, whereas the posterior tibial nerve contains muscle afferents.

Goldstein (1983a,b) and Goldstein et al. (1982a,b) also have used SEPs in the investigation of neurourologic disorders. In their pudendal EP studies, unilateral stimulation via block electrodes placed on either side of the penis was employed, providing localizing data not available with the ring electrode technique. Potential-field distribution studies showed significant amounts of negative activity frontally and contralaterally similar to that seen with lower-limb stimulation. Maximum activity was seen contralaterally with little seen ipsilaterally. They stressed the use of the pudendal EP in patients with erectile dysfunction and suspected suprasacral neurologic pathology [e.g., in MS patients (Goldstein et al., 1982a,b)].

Fernandez-Gonzalez and Suarez (1985) studied pudendal EPs in normals and in 12 patients with MS and 14 patients with peripheral neuropathies. Badr et al. (1982) reported on EPs produced by bladder stimulation, some in patients with neurologic disorders; patients with complete transverse spinal cord lesions had absent EPs. Sarica and Karacan (1986) reported EPs evoked by stimulation of the vesicourethral junction. See also Opsomer et al. (1989), Hansen et al. (1990), Fitzpatrick et al. (1989), Vodusek (1990), Guerit and Opsomer (1991), Loening-Baucke et al. (1991), and Loening-Baucke and Yamada (1993).

Evoked Potentials in Clinical Medicine,
3d ed., edited by Keith H. Chiappa.
Lippincott–Raven Publishers, Philadelphia © 1997.

Somatosensory Evoked Potentials

References

Abbruzzese M, Favale E, Leandri M, Ratto S (1978a): Spinal components of the cerebral somatosensory evoked response in normal man: The "S wave." *Acta Neurol Scand* 58:221–229.

Abbruzzese M, Favale E, Leandri M, Ratto S (1978b): New subcortical components of the cerebral somatosensory evoked potential in man. *Acta Neurol Scand* 58:325–332.

Abbruzzese G, Abbruzzese M, Favale E, Ivaldi M, Leandri M, Ratto S (1980): The effect of hand muscle vibration on the somatosensory evoked potential in man: An interaction between lemniscal and spinocerebellar inputs? *J Neurol Neurosurg Psychiatry* 43:433–437.

Abbruzzese G, Cocito L, Ratto S, Abbruzzese M, Leandri M, Favale E (1981a): A reassessment of sensory evoked potential parameters in multiple sclerosis: A discriminant analysis approach. *J Neurol Neurosurg Psychiatry* 44:133–139.

Abbruzzese G, Ratto S, Favale E, Abbruzzese (1981b): Proprioceptive modulation of somatosensory evoked potentials during active or passive finger movements in man. *J Neurol Neurosurg Psychiatry* 44:942–949.

Abbruzzese G, Reni L, Cocito L, Ratto S, Abbruzzese M, Favale E (1984): Short-latency somatosensory evoked potentials in degenerative and vascular dementia. *J Neurol Neurosurg Psychiatry* 47:1034–1037.

Abbruzzese G, Dall'Agata D, Morena M, Reni L, Favale E (1990): Abnormalities of parietal and prerolandic somatosensory evoked potentials in Huntington's disease. *Electroencephalogr Clin Neurophysiol* 77:340–346.

Abe Y, Kuroiwa Y (1990): Amplitude asymmetry of hemifield pattern reversal VEPs in healthy subjects. *Electroencephalogr Clin Neurophysiol* 77:81–85.

Addy RO, Dinner DS, Luders H, Lesser RP, Norris HH, Wyllie E (1989): The effects of sleep on median nerve short latency somatosensory evoked potentials. *Electroencephalogr Clin Neurophysiol* 74(2):105–111.

Albe-Fessard D, Tasker R, Yamashiro K, Chodakiewitz J, Dostrovsky J (1986): Comparison in man of short latency averaged evoked potentials recorded in thalamic and scalp hand zones of representation. *Electroencephalogr Clin Neurophysiol* 65:405–415.

Allison T, Goff WR, Williamson PD, VanGilder JC (1980): On the neural origin of early components of the human somatosensory evoked potential. *Prog Clin Neurophysiol* 7:51–68.

Allison T, Wood CC, Goff WR (1983): Brain stem auditory, pattern-reversal visual, and short-latency somatosensory evoked potentials: Latencies in relation to age, sex, and brain and body size. *Electroencephalogr Clin Neurophysiol* 55:619–636.

Allison T, Hume AL, Wood CC, Goff WR (1984): Developmental and aging changes in somatosensory, auditory and visual evoked potentials. *Electroencephalogr Clin Neurophysiol* 58:14–24.

Allison T, Wood CC, McCarthy G, Spencer DD (1991): Cortical somatosensory evoked potentials. II. Effects of excision of somatosensory or motor cortex in humans and monkeys. *Journal of Neurophysiology* 66(1):64–82.

Altenmuller E, Cornelius CP, Buettner UW (1990): Somatosensory evoked potentials following tongue stimulation in normal subjects and patients with lesions of the afferent trigeminal system. *Electroencephalogr Clin Neurophysiol* 77(6):403–415.

Aminoff MJ, Davis SL, Panitch HS (1984): Serial evoked potential studies in patients with definite multiple sclerosis. *Arch Neurol* 41:1197–1202.

Anderson DC, Bundlie S, Rockswold GL (1984): Multimodality evoked potentials in closed head trauma. *Arch Neurol* 41:369–374.

Anderson DC, Slater GE, Sherman R, Ettinger MG (1987): Evoked potentials to test a treatment of chronic multiple sclerosis. *Arch Neurol* 44:1232–1236.

Angel RW, Boylls CC, Weinrich M (1984): Cerebral evoked potentials and somatosensory perception. *Neurology* 34:123–126.

Angel RW, Weinrich M, Rodnitzky R (1986): Recovery of somatosensory evoked potential amplitude after movement. *Ann Neurol* 19:344–348.

Anziska B, Cracco RQ (1980a): Short latency somatosensory evoked potentials: Studies in patients with focal neurological disease. *Electroencephalogr Clin Neurophysiol* 49:227–239.

Anziska B, Cracco RQ (1980b): Short latency somatosensory evoked potentials in brain dead patients. *Arch Neurol* 37:222–225.

Anziska BJ, Cracco RQ (1981): Short latency SEPs to median nerve stimulation: Comparison of recording methods and origin of components. *Electroencephalogr Clin Neurophysiol* 52:531–539.

Anziska BJ, Cracco RQ (1983): Short-latency somatosensory evoked potentials to median nerve stimulation in patients with diffuse neurologic disease. *Neurology* 33:989–993.

Anziska B, Cracco RQ, Cook AW, Feld EW (1978): Somatosensory far field potentials: Studies in normal subjects and patients with multiple sclerosis. *Electroencephalogr Clin Neurophysiol* 45:602–610.

Arimura K, Rosales R, Osame M, Igata A (1987): Clinical electrophysiologic studies of HTLV-I-associated myelopathy. *Arch Neurol* 44:609–612.

Aubourg P, Adamsbaum C, Lavallard-Rousseau MC, Lemaitre A, Boureau F, Mayer M, Kalifa G (1992): Brain MRI and electrophysiologic abnormalities in preclinical and clinical adrenomyeloneuropathy. *Neurology* 42:85–91.

Averback P, Crocker P (1982): Regular involvement of Clarke's nucleus in sporadic amyotrophic lateral sclerosis. *Arch Neurol* 39:155–156.

Aziz Q, Furlong PL, Barlow J, Hobson A, Alani S, Bancewicz J, Ribbands M, Harding FGA, Thompson DG (1995): Topographic mapping of cortical potentials evoked by distension of the human proximal and distal oesophagus. *Electroencephalogr Clin Neurophysiol* 96(3):219–228.

Badr G, Carlsson CA, Fall M, Friberg S, Lindstrom L, Ohlsson B (1982): Cortical evoked potentials following stimulation of the urinary bladder in man. *Electroencephalogr Clin Neurophysiol* 54:494–498.

Bartel P, Conradie J, Robinson E, Prinsloo J, Becker P (1988): The relationship between median nerve somatosensory evoked potential latencies and age and growth factors in young children. *Electroencephalogr Clin Neurophysiol* 68:180–186.

Bartel PR, Lotz BP, Van Der Meyden CH (1984): Short-latency somatosensory evoked potentials in dystrophia myotonica. *J Neurol Neurosurg Psychiatry* 47:524–529.

Baumhefner RW, Tourtellotte WW, Ellison G, et al (1986): Multiple sclerosis: Correlation of magnetic resonance imaging with clinical disability. Quantitative evaluation of neurologic function, evoked potentials and intrablood-brain-barrier IgG synthesis. *Neurology* 36(1):283.

Beall JE, Foremann RD, Willis WD (1977): Spinal cord potentials evoked by cutaneous afferents in the monkey. *J Neurophysiol* 40:199–211.

Bell HJ, Dykstra DD (1985): Somatosensory evoked potentials as an adjunct to diagnosis of neonatal spinal cord injury. *J Pediatr* 106:298–301.

Belsh JM, Chokroverty S (1987): Short-latency somatosensory evoked potentials in brain-dead patients. *Electroencephalogr Clin Neurophysiol* 68:75–78.

Bennett MH, Jannetta PJ (1980): Trigeminal evoked potentials in humans. *Electroencephalogr Clin Neurophysiol* 48:517–526.

Beric A, Prevec TS (1981): The early negative potential evoked by stimulation of the tibial nerve in man. *J Neurol Sci* 50:299–306.

Beric A, Dimitrijevic MR, Prevec TS, Sherwood AM (1986): Epidurally recorded cervical somatosensory evoked potentials in humans. *Electroencephalogr Clin Neurophysiol* 65:94–101.

Beydoun A, Morrow TJ, Shen JF, Casey KL (1993): Variability of laser-evoked potentials: attention, arousal and lateralized differences. *Electroencephalogr Clin Neurophysiol* 88(3):173–181.

Biniek R, Ferbert A, Rimpel J, Paepke U, Berns TH, Schuchardt V, Heitmann R (1989): The complete apallic syndrome—a case report. *Intensive Care Med* 15:212–215.

Blair RDG, Lee RG, Vanderlinden G (1975): Dorsal column stimulation. Its effect on the somatosensory evoked response. *Arch Neurol* 32:826–829.

Bollen EL, Arts RJ, Roos RA, Van der Velde EA, Buruma OJ (1985): Somatosensory evoked potentials in Huntington's chorea. *Electroencephalogr Clin Neurophysiol* 62:235–240.

Bolton CF, Sawa GM, Carter K (1981): The effects of temperature on human compound action potentials. *J Neurol Neurosurg Psychiatry* 44:407–413.

Bosch EP, Yamada T, Kimura J (1985): Somatosensory evoked potentials in motor neuron disease. *Muscle Nerve* 8:556–562.

Bottcher J, Trojaborg W (1982): Follow-up of patients with suspected multiple sclerosis: A clinical and electrophysiological study. *J Neurol Neurosurg Psychiatry* 45:809–814.

Bradley WG, Good P, Rasool CG, Adelman LS (1983): Morphometric and biochemical studies of peripheral nerves in amyotrophic lateral sclerosis. *Ann Neurol* 14:267–277.

Brin MF, Pedley TA, Lovelace RE, Emerson RG, Gouras P, MacKay C, Kayden HJ, Levy J, Baker H (1986): Electrophysiologic features of abetalipoproteinemia: Functional consequences of vitamin E deficiency. *Neurology* 36:669–673.

Bromm B, Frieling A, Lankers J (1991): Laser-evoked brain potentials in patients with dissociated loss of pain and temperature sensibility. *Electroencephalogr Clin Neurophysiol* 80(4):284–291.

Brooks EB, Wilson SL, Lentz KE, Chiappa KH, Young RR (1983): A comparison of upper and lower limb somatosensory evoked potentials in multiple sclerosis. In: *Actual Problems in Multiple Sclerosis Research*, edited by E Pederson, J Clausen, and L Oades, pp 38–44. FADL's Forlag, Copenhagen.

Brunko E, Zegers de Beyl D (1987): Prognostic value of early cortical somatosensory evoked potentials after resuscitation from cardiac arrest. *Electroencephalogr Clin Neurophysiol* 66(1):15–24.

Buchner H, Ferbert A, Hacke W (1988): Serial recording of median nerve stimulated subcortical somatosensory evoked potentials (SEPs) in developing brain death. *Electroencephalogr Clin Neurophysiol* 69:14–23.

Buettner UW, Petruch JF, Schlegmann K, Stohr M (1982): Diagnostic significance of cortical somatosensory evoked potentials following trigeminal nerve stimulation. In: *Clinical Applications of Evoked Potentials in Neurology*, edited by J Courjon, F Mauguiere, M Revol, pp 339–345. Raven Press, New York.

Burke D, Gandevia SC (1986): Muscle afferent contribution to the cerebral potentials of human subjects. In: *Frontiers of Clinical Neuroscience*, Vol 3, *Evoked Potentials*, edited by RQ Cracco and I Bodis-Wollner, pp 262–268. A R Liss, New York.

Burke D, Gandevia SC (1988): Interfering cutaneous stimulation and the muscle afferent contribution to cortical potentials. *Electroencephalogr Clin Neurophysiol* 70:118–125.

Burke D, Skuse NF, Lethlean AK (1981): Cutaneous and muscle afferent components of the cerebral potential evoked by electrical stimulation of human peripheral nerves. *Electroencephalogr Clin Neurophysiol* 51:579–588.

Burke D, Gandevia SC, McKeon B, Skuse NF (1982): Interactions between cutaneous and muscle afferent projections to cerebral cortex in man. *Electroencephalogr Clin Neurophysiol* 53:349–360.

Caccia MR, Ubiali E, Andreussi L (1976): Spinal evoked responses recorded from the epidural space in normal and diseased humans. *J Neurol Neurosurg Psychiatry* 39:962–972.

Cadhilac J, Zhu Y, Georgesco M (1986): Somatosensory evoked potentials during maturation in normal children. A comparative study of SEPs to median and to posterior tibial nerve stimulations. In: *Maturation of the CNS and Evoked Potentials*, edited by V Gallai, pp 107–111. Excerpta Medica, Amsterdam.

Cant BR, Hume HL, Judson JA, Shaw NA (1986): The assessment of severe head injury by short-latency somatosensory and brain-stem auditory evoked potentials. *Electroencephalogr Clin Neurophysiol* 65:188–195.

Cascino GD, Ring SR, King PJL, Brown RH, Chiappa KH (1988): Evoked potentials in motor system diseases. *Neurology* 38:231–238.

Celesia GG (1979): Somatosensory evoked potentials recorded directly from human thalamus and Sm I cortical area. *Arch Neurol* 36:399–405.

Chapman CR, Gerlach R, Jacobson R, Buffington V, Kaufmann E (1986): Comparison of short-latency trigeminal evoked potentials elicited by painful dental and gingival stimulation. *Electroencephalogr Clin Neurophysiol* 65:20–26.

Chatrian GE, Canfield RC, Knauss TA, Lettich E (1975): Cerebral responses to electrical tooth pulp stimulation in man. *Neurology* 25:745–757.

Chautraine A, de Leval J, Onkelinx A (1973): Motor conduction velocity in the internal pudendal nerves. In: *New Developments in EMG and Clinical Neurophysiology*, edited by JE Desmedt, pp 433–438. Karger, Basel.

Cheron G, Borenstein S (1987): Specific gating of the early somatosensory evoked potentials during active movement. *Electroencephalogr Clin Neurophysiol* 67:537–548.

Cheron G, Borenstein S (1991): Gating of the early components of the grontal and parietal somatosensory evoked potentials in different sensory-motor interference modalities. *Electroencephalogr Clin Neurophysiol* 80(6):522–530.

Chester CS, McLaren CE (1989): Somatosensory evoked response and recovery from stroke. *Arch Phys Med Rehabil* 70:520–525.

Chiappa KH (1980): Pattern shift visual, brainstem auditory, and short latency somatosensory evoked potentials in multiple sclerosis. *Neurology* 30 (7, part 2):110–123.

Chiappa KH (1982): Physiologic localization using evoked responses: Pattern shift visual, brainstem auditory and short latency somatosensory. In: *New Perspectives in Cerebral Localization*, edited by RA Thompson and JR Green, pp 63–114. Raven Press, New York.

Chiappa KH (1983): Evoked potentials in clinical medicine. In: *Clinical Neurology*, edited by AB Baker and LH Baker, Chapter 7. JB Lippincott, Philadelphia.

Chiappa KH, Ropper AH (1982): Evoked potentials in clinical medicine. *N Engl J Med* 306:1140–1150, 1205–1211.

Chiappa KH, Choi S, Young RR (1978): The results of a new method for the registration of human short latency somatosensory evoked responses. *Neurology* 28:385.

Chiappa KH, Young RR, Goldie WD (1979): Origins of the components of human short-latency somatosensory evoked responses (SER). *Neurology* 29:598.

Chiappa KH, Choi S, Young RR (1980): Short latency somatosensory evoked potentials following median nerve stimulation in patients with neurological lesions. In: *Progress in Clinical Neurophysiology*, Vol 7, edited by JE Desmedt, pp 264–281. Karger, Basel.

Chokroverty S, Duvoisin RC, Sachedeo R, Sage J, Lepore F, Nicklas W (1985): Neurophysiologic study of olivopontocerebellar atrophy with or without glutamate dehydrogenase deficiency. *Neurology* 35:652–659.

Chu NS (1986): Somatosensory evoked potentials: Correlations with height. *Electroencephalogr Clin Neurophysiol* 65(3):169–176.

Chu NS, Hong CT (1985): Erb's and cervical somatosensory evoked potentials: Correlations with body size. *Electroencephalogr Clin Neurophysiol* 62(5):319–322.

Chu NS, Yang SS, Cheng CL (1985): Somatosensory evoked potentials: Monitoring cerebral functions following liver transplantation. *Clin Electroencephalogr* 16:192–194.

Chudler EH, Dong WK (1983): The assessment of pain by cerebral evoked potentials. *Pain* 16:221–244.

Cohen LG, Starr AS (1985): Vibration and muscle contraction affect somatosensory evoked potentials. *Neurology* 35:691–698.

Cole JD, Katifi HA (1991): Evoked potentials in a man with a complete large myelinated fibre sensory neuropathy below the neck. *Electroencephalogr Clin Neurophysiol* 80(2):103–107.

Comi GC, Locatelli T, Ghilardi MF, Medaglini S, Martinelli V, Mandelli A (1985): Median and tibial somatosensory evoked potentials in diabetes mellitus. In: *Evoked Potentials, Neurophysiological and Clinical Aspects*, edited by C Morocutti and PA Rizzo, pp 89–96. Elsevier, New York.

Cosi V, Poloni M, Mazzini L, Callieco R (1984): Somatosensory evoked potentials in amyotrophic lateral sclerosis. *J Neurol Neurosurg Psychiatry* 47:857–861.

Cracco RQ (1972): The initial positive potential of the human scalp-recorded somatosensory evoked response. *Electroencephalogr Clin Neurophysiol* 32:623–629.

Cracco RQ (1973): Spinal evoked responses: Peripheral nerve stimulation in man. *Electroencephalogr Clin Neurophysiol* 35:379–386.

Cracco RQ (1980): Scalp-recorded potentials evoked by median nerve stimulation: Subcortical potentials, travelling waves and somatomotor potentials. *Prog Clin Neurophysiol* 7:1–14.

Cracco RQ, Cracco JB (1976): Somatosensory evoked potentials in man: Far field potentials. *Electroencephalogr Clin Neurophysiol* 46:58–64.

Cracco JB, Cracco RQ (1979): Somatosensory spinal and cerebral evoked potentials in children with occult spinal dysraphism. *Neurology* 29:543.

Cracco JB, Cracco RQ (1982): Spinal somatosensory evoked potentials: Maturational and clinical studies. *Ann NY Acad Sci* 388:526–537.

Cracco JB, Cracco RQ (1986): Spinal, brainstem and cerebral SEP in the pediatric age group. In: *Evoked Potentials,* edited by RQ Cracco and I Bodis-Wollner, pp 471–482. A R Liss, New York.

Cracco RQ, Evans B (1978): Spinal evoked potential in the cat: Effects of asphyxia, strychnine, cord section and compression. *Electroencephalogr Clin Neurophysiol* 44:187–201.

Cracco JB, Cracco RQ, Graziani L (1974): Spinal evoked responses in infants with myelodysplasia. *Neurology* 24:359–360.

Cracco JB, Cracco RQ, Graziani LJ (1975): The spinal evoked response in infants and children. *Neurology* 25:31–36.Cracco JB, Cracco RQ, Stolove R (1979): Spinal evoked potentials in man: A maturational study. *Electroencephalogr Clin Neurophysiol* 46:58–64.

Cracco JB, Bosch VV, Cracco RQ (1980): Cerebral and spinal somatosensory evoked potentials in children with CNS degenerative disease. *Electroencephalogr Clin Neurophysiol* 49:437–455.

Cracco JB, Castells S, Mark E (1984): Spinal somatosensory evoked potentials in juvenile diabetes. *Ann Neurol* 15:55–58.

Cracco JB, Udani V, Cracco RQ (1988): MN-SSEPs in infants. *Electroencephalogr Clin Neurophysiol* 69:79P.

Cruse R, Lem G, Lesser RP, Lueders H (1982): Paradoxical lateralization of cortical potentials evoked by stimulation of posterior tibial nerve. *Arch Neurol* 39:222–225.

Cullity P, Franks CI, Duckworth T, Brown BH (1976): Somatosensory evoked cortical responses: Detection in normal infants. *Dev Med Child Neurol* 18:11–18.

Cusick JF, Myklebust J, Larson SJ, Sances JA (1978): Spinal evoked potentials in the primate: Neural substrate. *J Neurosurg* 49:551–557.

Cutler JR, MJ, Brant-Zawadzki M (1986): Evaluation of patients with multiple sclerosis by evoked potentials and magnetic resonance imaging: A comparative study. *Ann Neurol* 20:645–648.

Dasheiff RM, Drake ME, Brendle A, Erwin CW (1985): Abnormal somatosensory evoked potentials in amyotrophic lateral sclerosis. *Electroencephalogr Clin Neurophysiol* 60:306–311.

Dau PC, Petajan JH, Johnson KP, Panitch HS, Bornstein MB (1980): Plasmapheresis in multiple sclerosis: Preliminary findings. *Neurology* 30:1023–1028.

Davis SL, Aminoff MJ, Panitch HS (1985): Clinical correlations of serial somatosensory evoked potentials in multiple sclerosis. *Neurology* 35:359–365.

De Graaf RJ, Visser SL, De Rijke (1988): H reflex latency as an adequate predictor of the spinal evoked potential latency. *Electroencephalogr Clin Neurophysiol* 70:62–67.

Deiber MP, Giard MH, Mauguiere F (1986): Separate generators with distinct orientations for N20 and P22 somatosensory evoked potentials to finger stimulation. *Electroencephalogr Clin Neurophysiol* 65:321–334.

de la Torre JC, Trimble JL, Beard RT, Hanlon K, Surgeon JW (1978): Somatosensory evoked potentials for the prognosis of coma in humans. *Exp Neurol* 60:304–317.

Delbeke J, McComas AJ, Kopec SJ (1978): Analysis of evoked lumbosacral potentials in man. *J Neurol Neurosurg Psychiatry* 41:293–302.

Delberghe X, Mavroudakis N, Zegers de Beyl D, Brunko E (1990): The effect of stimulus frequency on post- and precentral short-latency somatosensory evoked potentials (SEPs). *Electroencephalogr Clin Neurophysiol* 77:86–92.

Delestre F, Lonchampt P, Dubas F (1986): Neural generator of P14 far-field somatosensory evoked potential studied in a patient with a pontine lesion. *Electroencephalogr Clin Neurophysiol* 65(3):227–230.

Delwaide PJ, Schoenen J, De Pasqua V (1985): Lumbosacral spinal evoked potentials in patients with multiple sclerosis. *Neurology* 35:174–179.

DeMeirleir LJ, Taylor MJ (1987): Prognostic utility of SEPs in comatose children. *Pediatr Neurol* 3:78–82.

DeMeirleir LJ, Taylor MJ, Logan WJ (1988): Multimodal evoked potential studies in leukodystrophies of children. *Can J Neurol Sci* 15:26–31.

Denys EH (1991): AAEM minimonograph #14: The influence of temperature in clinical neurophysiology. *Muscle Nerve* 14:795–811.

Desmedt JE (1984): Non-invasive analysis of the spinal cord generators activated by somatosensory input in man: Near field and far field potentials. *Exp Brain Res* Suppl 9:45–62.

Desmedt JE, Bourguet M (1985): Color imaging of parietal and frontal somatosensory potential fields evoked by stimulation of median or posterior tibial nerve in man. *Electroencephalogr Clin Neurophysiol* 62:1–17.

Desmedt JE, Brunko E (1980): Functional organization of far-fields and cortical components of somatosensory evoked potentials in normal adults. In: *Progress in Clinical Neurophysiology*, Vol 7, edited by JE Desmedt, pp 27–50. Karger, Basel.

Desmedt JE, Cheron G (1980a): Central somatosensory conduction in man: Neural generators and interpeak latencies of the far-field components recorded from neck and right or left scalp and earlobes. *Electroencephalogr Clin Neurophysiol* 50:382–403.

Desmedt JE, Cheron G (1980b): Somatosensory evoked potentials to finger stimulation in healthy octogenarians and in young adults: Wave forms, scalp topography and transit times of parietal and frontal components. *Electroencephalogr Clin Neurophysiol* 50:404–425.

Desmedt JE, Cheron G (1981a): Prevertebral (oesophageal) recording of subcortical somatosensory evoked potentials in man: The spinal P13 component and the dual nature of the spinal generators. *Electroencephalogr Clin Neurophysiol* 52:257–275.

Desmedt JE, Cheron G (1981b): Non-cephalic reference recording of early somatosensory potentials to finger stimulation in adult or aging normal man: Differentiation of widespread N18 and contralateral N20 from the prerolandic P22 and N30 components. *Electroencephalogr Clin Neurophysiol* 52:553–570.

Desmedt JE, Cheron G (1983): Spinal and far-field components of human somatosensory evoked potentials to posterior tibial nerve stimulation analysed with oesophageal derivations and non-cephalic reference recording. *Electroencephalogr Clin Neurophysiol* 56:635–651.

Desmedt JE, Manil J (1970): Somatosensory evoked potentials of the normal human neonate in REM sleep, in slow wave sleep and in waking. *Electroencephalogr Clin Neurophysiol* 29:113–126.

Desmedt JE, Nguyen TH (1984): Bit-mapped colour imaging of the potential fields of propagated and segmental subcortical components of somatosensory evoked potentials in man. *Electroencephalogr Clin Neurophysiol* 58:481–497.

Desmedt JE, Noel P (1973): Average cerebral evoked potentials in the evaluation of lesions of the sensory nerves and of the central somatosensory pathway. In: *New Developments in Electromyography and Clinical Neurophysiology*, Vol 2, edited by JE Desmedt, pp 352–371. Karger, Basel.

Desmedt JE, Noel P (1975): Cerebral evoked potentials. In: *Peripheral Neuropathy*, edited by PJ Dyck, PK Thomas, and EH Lambert, pp 480–491. WB Saunders, Philadelphia.

Desmedt JE, Ozaki I (1991): SEPs to finger joint input lack the N20-P20 response that is evoked by tactile inputs: contrast between cortical generators in areas 3b and 2 in humans. *Electroencephalogr Clin Neurophysiol* 80:513–521.

Desmedt JE, Brunko E, Debecker J, Carmelit J (1974): The system bandpass required to avoid distortion of early components when averaging somatosensory evoked potentials. *Electroencephalogr Clin Neurophysiol* 37:407–410.

Desmedt JE, Brunko E, Debecker J (1976): Maturation of the somatosensory evoked potentials in normal infants and children, with special reference to the early N1 component. *Electroencephalogr Clin Neurophysiol* 40:43–58.

Desmedt JE, Brunko E, Debecker J (1980): Maturation and sleep correlates of the SEP. *Prog Clin Neurophysiol* 7:146–161.

Desmedt JE, Nguyen TH, Carmelit J (1983): Unexpected latency shifts of stationary P9 somatosensory evoked potential far field with changes in shoulder position. *Electroencephalogr Clin Neurophysiol* 56:628–634.

Desmedt JE, Nguyen TH, Bourguet M (1987): Bit-mapped color imaging of human evoked potentials with reference to N20, P22, P27 and N30 somatosensory responses. *Electroencephalogr Clin Neurophysiol* 68:1–19.

Despland PA, Regli F (1985): Somatosensory evoked response changes in patients with unilateral vascular lesions. In: *Evoked Potentials, Neurophysiological and Clinical Aspects*, edited by C Morocutti and PA Rizzo, pp 57–67. Elsevier, New York.

Deupree DL, Jewett DL (1988): Far-field potentials due to action potentials traversing curved nerves, reaching curt nerve ends, and crossing boundaries between cylindrical volumes. *Electroencephalogr Clin Neurophysiol* 70:355–362.

De Weerd AW, Groeneveld C (1985): The use of evoked potentials in the management of patients with severe cerebral trauma. *Acta Neurol Scand* 72:489–494.

De Weerd AW, Looijenga A, Veldhuizen RJ, Van Huffelen AC (1985): Somatosensory evoked potentials in minor cerebral ischaemia: Diagnostic significance and changes in serial records. *Electroencephalogr Clin Neurophysiol* 62:45–55.

De-Xuan K, Bin-rong M, Lundervold A (1983): The effect of acupuncture on somatosensory evoked potentials. *Clin Electroencephalogr* 14:53–56.

Dietz V, Quintern J, Berger W (1985): Afferent control of human stance and gait: evidence for blocking of group I afferents during gait. *Exp Brain Res* 61:153–163.

Di Lazzaro V, Restuccia D, Fogli D, Nardone R, Mazza S, Tonali P (1992): Central sensory and motor conduction in vitamin B12 deficiency. *Electroencephalogr Clin Neurophysiol* 84(5):433–439.

Dimitrijevic MR, Larsson LE, Lehmkuhl D, Sherwood A (1978): Evoked spinal cord and nerve root potentials in humans using a non-invasive recording technique. *Electroencephalogr Clin Neurophysiol* 45:331–340.

Dinner DS, Luders H, Lesser RP, Morris HH (1987): Cortical generators of somatosensory evoked potentials to median nerve stimulation. *Neurology* 37:1141–1145.

Domino EF, Matsuoka S, Waltz J, Cooper IS (1965): Effects of cryogenic thalamic lesions in the somesthetic evoked response in man. *Electroencephalogr Clin Neurophysiol* 19:127–138.

Dong WK (1982): Trigeminal evoked potentials: Origins in the cat. *Brain Res* 233:205–210.

Dong WK, Harkins SW, Ashleman BT (1982): Origins of cat somatosensory far-field and early near-field evoked potentials. *Electroencephalogr Clin Neurophysiol* 53:143–165.

Dorfman LJ (1977): Indirect estimate of spinal cord conduction velocity in man. *Electroencephalogr Clin Neurophysiol* 42:26–34.

Dorfman LJ, Bosley TM (1979): Age-related changes in peripheral and central nerve conduction in man. *Neurology* 29:38–44.

Dorfman LJ, Bosley TM, Cummins KL (1978a): Electrophysiological localization of central somatosensory lesions in patients with multiple sclerosis. *Electroencephalogr Clin Neurophysiol* 44:742–753.

Dorfman LJ, Pedley TA, Tharp BR, Scheithauer BW (1978b): Juvenile neuroaxonal dystrophy: Clinical, electrophysiological and neuropathological features. *Ann Neurol* 3:419–428.

Dorfman LJ, Donaldson SS, Gupta PR, Bosley TM (1980a): Subclinical radiation myelopathy in humans. *Neurology* 31:67.

Dorfman LJ, Perkash I, Bosley TM, Cummins KL (1980b): Use of cerebral evoked potentials to evaluate spinal somatosensory function in patients with traumatic and surgical myelopathies. *J Neurosurg* 52:654–660.

Dowman R, Goshko L (1992): Evaluation of reference sites for scalp potentials evoked by painful and non-painful sural nerve stimulation. *Electroencephalogr Clin Neurophysiol* 84:477–485.

Drayer BP, Barrett L (1984): Magnetic resonance imaging and CT scanning in multiple sclerosis. *Ann NY Acad Sci* 436:294–314.

Drechsler F (1980): Short and long latency cortical potentials following trigeminal nerve stimulation in man. In: *Evoked Potentials*, edited by C Barber, pp 415–422. University Park Press, Baltimore.

Drechsler F, Wickboldt J, Neuhauser B, Miltner F (1977): Somatosensory trigeminal evoked potentials in normal subjects and in patients with trigeminal neuralgia before and after thermocoagulation of the ganglion Gasseri. *Electroencephalogr Clin Neurophysiol* 43:496.

Dyck PJ, Stevens JC, Mulder DW, Espinosa RE (1975): Frequency of nerve fiber degeneration of peripheral motor and sensory neurons in amyotrophic lateral sclerosis. *Neurology* 25:781–785.

Ebner A, Einsiedel-Lechtape H, Lucking CH (1982): Somatosensory tibial nerve evoked potentials with parasagittal tumours: A contribution to the problem of generators. *Electroencephalogr Clin Neurophysiol* 54:508–515.

Eggermont JJ (1988): On the rate of maturation of sensory evoked potentials. *Electroencephalogr Clin Neurophysiol* 70:293–305.

Ehle AL, Stewart RM, Lellelid NA, Leventhal NA (1984): Evoked potentials in Huntington's Disease. *Arch Neurol* 41:379–382.

Eisen A, Elleker G (1980): Sensory nerve stimulation and evoked cerebral potentials. *Neurology* 30:1097–1105.

Eisen A, Nudleman K (1979): Cord to cortex conduction in multiple sclerosis. *Neurology* 29:189–193.

Eisen A, Odusote K (1980): Central and peripheral conduction times in multiple sclerosis. *Electroencephalogr Clin Neurophysiol* 48:253–265.

Eisen A, Stewart J, Nudleman K, Cosgrove JBR (1979): Short-latency somatosensory responses in multiple sclerosis. *Neurology* 29:827–834.

Eisen A, Paty D, Purves S, Hoirch M (1981): Occult fifth nerve dysfunction in multiple sclerosis. *Can J Neurol Sci* 8:221–225.

Eisen A, Purves S, Hoirch M (1982): Central nervous system amplification: Its potential in the diagnosis of early multiple sclerosis. *Neurology* 32:359–364.

Eisen A, Hoirch M, Moll A (1983): Evaluation of radiculopathies by segmental stimulation and somatosensory evoked potentials. *Can J Neurol Sci* 10:178–182.

Eisen A, Roberts K, Low M, Hoirch M, Lawrence P (1984): Questions regarding the sequential neural generator theory of the somatosensory evoked potential raised by digital filtering. *Electroencephalogr Clin Neurophysiol* 59:388–395.

Eisen A, Hoirch M, Fink M, Goya T, Calne D (1985): Noninvasive measurement of central sensory and motor conduction. *Neurology* 35:503–509.

Eisen A, Odusote K, Bozek C, Hoirch M (1986): Far-field potentials from peripheral nerve: Generated at sites of muscle mass change. *Neurology* 36:815–818.

Eisen A, Odusote K, Li D, Robertson W, Purvis S, Eisen K, Paty D (1987): Comparison of magnetic resonance imaging with somatosensory testing in MS suspects. *Muscle Nerve* 10:385–390.

El-Abd MAR, Ibrahim IK (1994): Impaired afferent control in patients with spastic hemiplegia at different recovery stages: Contribution to gait disorder. *Arch Phys Med Rehabil* 75:312–317.

El-Negamy E, Sedgwick EM (1978): Properties of a spinal somatosensory evoked potential recorded in man. *J Neurol Neurosurg Psychiatry* 41:762–768.

Emerson RG (1988): Anatomic and physiologic bases of tibial nerve somatosensory evoked potentials. In: *Neurologic Clinics*, Vol 6, edited by R Gilmore, pp 735–749. WB Saunders, Philadelphia.

Emerson RG, Pedley TA (1984): Generator sources of median somatosensory evoked potentials. *J Clin Neurophysiol* 1:159–202.

Emerson RG, Pedley TA (1986): Effect of cervical spinal cord lesions on early components of the median nerve somatosensory evoked potential. *Neurology* 36:20–26.

Emerson RG, Seyal M, Pedley TA (1984): Somatosensory evoked potentials following median nerve stimulation. *Brain* 107:169–182.

Emerson RG, Pavlakis SG, Carmel PC, DeVino DC (1986): Use of spinal somatosensory evoked potentials in the diagnosis of tethered cord. *Ann Neurol* 20:443.

Emerson RG, Sgro JA, Pedley TA, Hauser WA (1988a): State-dependent changes in the N20 component of the median nerve somatosensory evoked potential. *Neurology* 38:64–68.

Emerson RG, Sgro JA, Stanton PC (1988b): Post-hoc removal of stimulus artifact in evoked potential recordings. *J Clin Neurophysiol* 5:363.

Emery AEH, Holloway S (1982): Familial motor neuron diseases. In: *Human Motor Neuron Diseases. Advances in Neurology*, Vol 36, edited by LP Rowland, pp 139–147. Raven Press, New York.

Ertekin C (1973): Human evoked electrospinogram. In: *New Developments in Electromyography and Clinical Neurophysiology*, Vol 2, edited by JE Desmedt, pp 344–351. Karger, Basel.

Ertekin C (1976): Studies on the human evoked electrospinogram. I and II. *Acta Neurol Scand* 53:3–37.

Ertekin C, Mutlu R, Sarica Y, Uckardesler L (1980): Electrophysiological evaluation of the afferent spinal roots and nerves in patients with conus medullaris and cauda equina lesions. *J Neurol Sci* 48:419–433.

Ertekin C, Sarica Y, Uckardesler L (1984): Somatosensory cerebral potentials evoked by stimulation of the lumbosacral spinal cord in normal subjects and in patients with conus medullaris and cauda equina lesions. *Electroencephalogr Clin Neurophysiol* 59:57–66.

Ervin FR, Mark VH (1964): Studies of the human thalamus: IV. Evoked responses. *Ann NY Acad Sci* 112:81–92.

Erwim CW, Erwin AC, Hartwell JW, Wilson WH (1991): P100 latency as a function of head size. *Am J EEG Technol* 31:279–288.

Facco E, Munari M, Baratto F, Dona B, Giron GP (1990): Somatosensory evoked potentials in severe head trama. *New Trends Adv Tech Clin Neurophysiol* Suppl.41:330–341.

Facco E, Baratto F, Munari M, Dona B, Casartelli Liviero M, Behr AU, Giron GP (1991): Sensorimotor central conduction time in comatose patients. *Electroencephalogr Clin Neurophysiol* 80(6):469–476.

Fagan ER, Taylor MJ, Logan WJ (1987a): Somatosensory evoked potentials. Part 1: A review of neural generators and special considerations in pediatrics. *Neurology* 3:189–196.

Fagan ER, Taylor MJ, Logan WJ (1987b): Somatosensory evoked potentials. Part II: A review of clinical applications in pediatric neurology. *Pediatr Neurol* 3:249–255.

Farlow MR, Markand ON, Edwards MK, Stevens JC, Kolar OL (1986): Multiple sclerosis: Magnetic resonance imaging, evoked responses, and spinal fluid electrophoresis. *Neurology* 36:828–831.

Favale E, Ratto S, Leandri M, Abbruzzese M (1982): Investigations on the nervous mechanisms underlying the somatosensory cervical response in man. *J Neurol Neurosurg Psychiatry* 45:796–801.

Feldman MH, Cracco RQ, Farmer P, Mount F (1980): Spinal evoked potential in the monkey. *Ann Neurol* 7:238–244.

Ferbert A, Buchner H, Bruckmann H, Zeumer H, Hacke W (1988): Evoked potentials in basilar artery thrombosis: Correlation with clinical and angiographic findings. *Electroencephalogr Clin Neurophysiol* 69:136–147.

Fernandez-Gonzalez F, Suarez T (1985): Pudendal nerve evoked potentials: Neurophysiological and clinical applications. In: *Evoked Potentials, Neurophysiological and Clinical Aspects*, edited by C Morocutti and PA Rizzo, pp 97–106. Elsevier, New York.

Findler G, Feinsod M (1982): Sensory evoked response to electrical stimulation of the trigeminal nerve in humans. *J Neurosurg* 56:545–549.

Fine EJ, Hallett M (1980): Neurophysiological study of subacute combined degeneration. *J Neurol Sci* 45:331–336.

Fitzpatrick DF, Hendricks SE, Graber B, Balogh SE, Wetzel M (1989): Somatosensory evoked potentials elicited by dorsal penile and posterior tibial nerve stimulation. *Electroencephalogr Clin Neurophysiol* 74(2):95–104.

Forss N, Salmelin R, Hari R (1994): Comparison of somatosensory evoked fields to airpuff and electric stimuli. *Electroencephalogr Clin Neurophysiol* 92(6):510–517.

Frank LM, Furgiuele TL, Etheridge JE (1985): Prediction of chronic vegetative state in children using evoked potentials. *Neurology* 35:931–934.

Franssen H, Stegeman DF, Moleman J, Schoobaar RP (1992): Dipole modelling of median nerve SEPs in normal subjects and patients with small subcortical infarcts. *Electroencephalogr Clin Neurophysiol* 84(5):401–417.

Frith RW, Benstead TJ, Daube JR (1986): Stationary waves recorded at the shoulder after median nerve stimulation. *Neurology* 36:1458–1464.

Froehlich J, Kaufman DI (1992): Improving the reliability of pattern electroretinogram recording. *Electroencephalogr Clin Neurophysiol* 84:394–399.

Fujii M, Toleikis JR, Logemann JA, Larson CR (1994a): Glossopharyngeal evoked potentials in normal subjects following mechanical stimulation of the anterior faucial pillar. *Electroencephalogr Clin Neurophysiol* 92(3):183–195.

Fujii M, Yamada T, Aihara M, Kokubun Y, Noguchi Y, Matsubara, Yeh MH (1994b): The effects of stimulus rates upon median, ulnar and radial nerve somatosensory evoked potentials. *Electroencephalogr Clin Neurophysiol* 92(6):518–526.

Fukushima T, Mayanagi Y, Bouchard G (1976): Thalamic evoked potentials to somatosensory stimulation in man. *Electroencephalogr Clin Neurophysiol* 40:481–490.

Furlong PL, Wimalaratna S, Harding GFA (1993): Augmented P22-N31 SEP component in a patient with a unilateral space occupying lesion. *Electroencephalogr Clin Neurophysiol* 88(1):72–76.

Gallai V, Mazzotta G, Cagini L, DelGatto F, Agnelotti F (1986): Maturation of SEPs in preterm and full-term neonates. In: *Maturation of the CNS and Evoked Potentials*, edited by V Gallai, pp 95–106. Excerpta Medica, Amsterdam.

Gandevia SC, Burke D (1990): Projection of thenar muscle afferents to frontal and parietal cortex of human subjects. *Electroencephalogr Clin Neurophysiol* 77:353–361.

Gandevia SC, Macefield G (1989): Projection of low-threshold afferents from human intercostal muscles to the cerebral cortex. *Respiration Pysiology* 77:203–214.

Gandevia SC, Burke D, McKeon B (1984): The projection of muscle afferents from the hand to cerebral cortex in man. *Brain* 107:1–13.

Ganes T (1980a): A study of peripheral, cervical and cortical evoked potentials and afferent conduction times in the somatosensory pathway. *Electroencephalogr Clin Neurophysiol* 49:446–451.

Ganes T (1980b): Somatosensory conduction times and peripheral, cervical and cortical evoked potentials in patients with cervical spondylosis. *J Neurol Neurosurg Psychiatry* 43:683–689.

Ganes T (1980c): Somatosensory evoked responses and central afferent conduction times in patients with multiple sclerosis. *J Neurol Neurosurg Psychiatry* 43:948–953.

Ganes T (1982): Synaptic and non-synaptic components of the human cervical evoked response. *J Neurol Sci* 55:313–326.

Ganes T, Lundar T (1988): EEG and evoked potentials in comatose patients with severe brain damage. *Electroencephalogr Clin Neurophysiol* 69:6–13.

Ganji S, Mahajan S (1983): Changes in short-latency somatosensory evoked potentials during hemodialysis in chronic renal failure. *Clin Electroencephalogr* 14:202–206.

Gardner EP, Hamalainen HA, Warren S, Davis J, Young W (1984): Somatosensory evoked potentials (SEPs) and cortical single unit responses elicited by mechanical tactile stimuli in awake monkeys. *Electroencephalogr Clin Neurophysiol* 58:537–552.

Garg BP, Markand ON, DeMyer WE (1980): Evoked responses in patients and potential carriers of adrenoleukodystrophy: Implications for carrier detection. *Ann Neurol* 8:219.

Garg BP, Markand ON, DeMyer WE, Warren Jr C (1983): Evoked response studies in patients with adrenoleukodystrophy and heterozygous relatives. *Arch Neurol* 40:356–359.

Gebarski SS, Gabrielsen TO, Gilman S, et al (1985): The initial diagnosis of multiple sclerosis: Clinical impact of magnetic resonance imaging. *Ann Neurol* 17:469–474.

Giblin DR (1964): Somatosensory evoked potentials in healthy subjects and in patients with lesions of the nervous system. *Ann NY Acad Sci* 112:93–142.

Giesser BS, Kurtzberg D, Arezzo JC, et al (1986): Trimodal evoked potentials compared with magnetic resonance imaging in the diagnosis of multiple sclerosis. *Neurology* 36:158.

Giesser BS, Kurtzberg D, Vaughan HG, Arezzo JC, Aisen ML, Smith CR, LaRocca NG, Scheinberg LC (1987): Trimodal evoked potentials compared with magnetic resonance imaging in the diagnosis of multiple sclerosis. *Arch Neurol* 44:281–284.

Gilles FH, Shankle EC, Dooling EC (1983): Myelinated tracts: Growth patterns. In: *The Developing Human Brain,* edited by FH Gilles, A Leviton, and EC Dooling, pp 117–183. John Wright, Boston.

Gilmore R (1986): Developmental profile of lumbar spinal cord and early cortical evoked potentials after tibial nerve stimulation during the neonatal period and childhood: Assessment of age and stature. In: *Maturation of the CNS and Evoked Potentials,* edited by V Gallai, pp 112–118. Excerpta Medica, Amsterdam.

Gilmore RL, Bass NH, Wright EA, Greathouse D, Stanback K, Norvell E (1985a): Developmental assessment of spinal cord and cortical evoked potentials after tibial nerve stimulation: Effects of age and stature on normative data during childhood. *Electroencephalogr Clin Neurophysiol* 62:241–251.

Gilmore RL, Kasarskis EJ, McAllister RG (1985b): Verapamil-induced changes in central conduction in patients with multiple sclerosis. *J Neurol Neurosurg Psychiatry* 48:1140–1146.

Gilmore RL, Brock J, Hermansen MC, Baumann R (1987): Development of lumbar spinal cord and cortical evoked potentials after tibial nerve stimulation in the pre-term newborns: Effects of gestational age and other factors. *Electroencephalogr Clin Neurophysiol* 68:28–39.

Gilmore RL, Kasarskis EJ, Carr WA, Norvell E (1989): Comparative impact of paraclinical studies in establishing the diagnosis of multiple sclerosis. *Electroencephalogr Clin Neurophysiol* 73:433–442.

Goff GD, Matsumiya Y, Allison T, Goff WR (1977): The scalp topography of human somatosensory and auditory evoked potentials. *Electroencephalogr Clin Neurophysiol* 42:57–76.

Goldie WD, Chiappa KH, Young RR (1979): Brainstem auditory evoked responses and short-latency somatosensory evoked responses in the evaluation of deeply comatose patients. *Neurology* 29:551.

Goldie WD, Chiappa KH, Young RR, Brooks EB (1981): Brainstem auditory and short-latency somatosensory evoked responses in brain death. *Neurology* 31:248–256.

Goldstein I (1983a): Controversies in evoked response evaluations. In: *Controversies in Neuro-Urology,* edited by DB Barrett and AJ Wein. Churchill Livingstone, NY.

Goldstein I (1983b): Neurologic impotence. In: *Male Sexual Dysfunction,* edited by RJ Krane and MB Siroky. Little Brown, Boston.

Goldstein I, Siroky MB, Davidson MM, Pavlakis AP, Krane RJ (1982a): Studies of the central afferent pathway of the pudendal nerve. Proceedings of the International Incontinence Society, Leiden, pp 149–150.

Goldstein I, Siroky MB, Sax DS, Krane RJ (1982b): Neurourologic abnormalities in multiple sclerosis. *J Urol* 128:541–545.

Gonzalez-Scarano F, Grossman RI, Galetta SL, et al (1986): Enhanced magnetic images in multiple sclerosis. *Neurology* 36:285.

Goodridge A, Eisen A, Hoirch M (1987): Paraspinal stimulation to elicit somatosensory evoked potentials: An - approach to physiological localization of spinal lesions. *Electroencephalogr Clin Neurophysiol* 68:268–276.

Goodwin SR, Friedman WA, Bellefleur M (1991): Is it time to use evoked potentials to predict outcome in comatose children and adults? *Critical Care Med* 19:518–524.

Gorke W (1986): Somatosensory evoked cortical potentials indicating impaired motor development in infancy. *Dev Med Child Neurol* 28:633–641.

Gorke W (1987): Diagnostic value of somatosensory evoked potentials as compared to neurologic score, EEG and CT in infancy—a prospective study. *Neuropediatrics* 18:205–209.

Gott PS, Karnaze DS, Fisher M (1990): Assessment of median nerve somatosensory evoked potentials in cerebral ischemia. *Stroke* 21:1167–1171.

Graff-Radford NR, Damasio H, Yamada T, Eslinger PJ, Damasio AR (1985): Nonhaemorrhagic thalamic infarction. *Brain* 108:485–516.

Green JB, McLeod S (1979): Short latency somatosensory evoked potentials in patients with neurological lesions. *Arch Neurol* 36:846–851.

Green JB, Price R, Woodbury SG (1980): Short-latency somatosensory evoked potentials in multiple sclerosis. Comparison with auditory and visual evoked potentials. *Arch Neurol* 37:630–633.

Green JB, Walcoff MR, Lucke JF (1982a): Comparison of phenytoin and phenobarbital effects on far-field auditory and somatosensory evoked potential interpeak latencies. *Epilepsia* 23:417–421.

Green JB, Walcoff M, Lucke JF (1982b): Phenytoin prolongs far-field somatosensory and auditory evoked potential interpeak latencies. *Neurology* 32:85–88.

Greenberg JA, Kaplan PW, Erwin CW (1987): Somatosensory evoked potentials and the dorsal column myth. *J Clin Neurophysiol* 4:189–196.

Greenberg RP, Mayer DJ, Becker DP, Miller JD (1977): Evaluation of brain function in severe human head trauma with multimodality evoked potentials. *J Neurosurg* 47:150–177.

Greenberg RP, Stablein DM, Becker DP (1981): Noninvasive localization of brain-stem lesions in the cat with multimodality evoked potentials. Correlation with human head-injury data. *J Neurosurg* 54:740–750.

Greenwood PM, Goff WR (1987): Modification of median nerve somatic evoked potentials by prior median nerve, peroneal nerve, and auditory stimulation. *Electroencephalogr Clin Neurophysiol* 68:295–302.

Grimm G, Madl C, Katzenschlager R, Oder W, Ferenci P, Gangl A (1992): Detailed evaluation of evoked potentials in Wilson's disease. *Electroencephalogr Clin Neurolphysiol* 82:119–124.

Grisolia JS, Wiederholt WC (1978): Short latency somatosensory evoked potentials from radial, median and ulnar nerve stimulation in man. *Electroencephalogr Clin Neurophysiol* 50:375–381.

Grunewald G, Grunewald-Zuberbier E, Schuhmacher H, Mewald J, Noth J (1984): Somatosensory evoked potentials to mechanical disturbances of positioning movements in man: Gating of middle-range components. *Electroencephalogr Clin Neurophysiol* 58:525–536.

Guerit JM (1986): Unexpected myogenic contaminants observed in the somatosensory evoked potentials recorded in one brain-dead patient. *Electroencephalogr Clin Neurophysiol* 64:21–26.

Guerit JM (1992): Evoked potentials: A safe brain-death confirmatory tool? *Europ J Medicine* 1(4):233–243.

Guerit JM, Argiles AM (1988): The sensitivity of multimodal evoked potentials in multiple sclerosis. A comparison with magnetic resonance imaging and cerebrospinal fluid analysis. *Electroencephalogr Clin Neurophysiol* 70:230–238.

Guerit JM, Opsomer RJ (1991): Bit-mapped imaging of somatosensory evoked potentials after stimulation of the posterior tibial nerves and dorsal nerve of the penis/clitoris. *Electroencephalogr Clin Neurophysiol* 80(3):228–237.

Guerit JM, Soveges L, Baele P, Dion R (1990): Median nerve somatosensory evoked potentials in profound hypothermia for ascending aorta repair. *Electroencephalogr Clin Neurophysiol* 77(3):163–173.

Gupta PR, Dorfman LJ (1980): Spinal somatosensory conduction in diabetes. *Neurology* 30:414–415.

Gupta PR, Dorfman LJ (1981): Spinal somatosensory conduction in diabetes. *Neurology* 31:841–845.

Gutling E, Gonser A, Imhof H-G, Landis T (1994): Prognostic value of frontal and parietal somatosensory evoked potentials in severe head injury: a long-term follow-up study. *Electroencephalogr Clin Neurophysiol* 92(6):568–570.

Haldeman S, Bradley WE, Bhatia NN, Johnson BK (1982): Pudendal evoked responses. *Arch Neurol* 39:280–283.

Halliday AM (1967a): Cerebral evoked potentials in familial progressive myoclonic epilepsy. *J R Coll Phys Lond* I:123–134.

Halliday AM (1967b): Changes in the form of cerebral evoked responses in man associated with various lesions of the nervous system. *Electroencephalogr Clin Neurophysiol* Suppl 25:178–192.

Halliday AM (1967c): The electrophysiological study of myoclonus in man. *Brain* 90:241–284.

Halliday AM, Wakefield GS (1963): Cerebral evoked potentials in patients with dissociated sensory loss. *J Neurol Neurosurg Psychiatry* 26:211–219.

Hallin RG, Torebjork HE (1973): Electrically induced A and C fibre responses in intact human skin nerves. *Exp Brain Res* 16:309–320.

Hallstrom YT, Lindblom U, Meyerson BA, Prevec TS (1989): Epidurally recorded cervical spinal activity evoked by electrical and mechanical stimulation in pain patients. *Electroencephalogr Clin Neurophysiol* 74(3): 175–185.

Halonen JP, Jones S, Shawkat F (1988): Contribution of cutaneous and muscle afferent fibres to cortical SEPs following median and radial nerve stimulation in man. *Electroencephalogr Clin Neurophysiol* 71:331–335.

Halonen JP, Jones SJ, Edgar MA, Ransford AO (1989): Conduction properties of epidurally recorded spinal cord potentials following lower limb stimulation in man. *Electroencephalogr Clin Neurophysiol* 74(3):161–174.

Hamano T, Kaji R, Diaz AF, Kohara N, Takamatsu N, Uchiyama T, Shibasaki H, Kimura J (1993): Vibration-evoked sensory nerve action potentials derived from Pacinian corpuscles. *Electroencephalogr Clin Neurophysiol* 89:278–286.

Hammond EJ, Wilder BJ (1982): Short latency auditory and somatosensory evoked potentials in a patient with "Locked-In" syndrome. *Clin Electroencephalogr* 13:54–56.

Hammond EJ, Wilder BJ (1983): Evoked potentials in olivopontocerebellar atrophy. *Arch Neurol* 40:366–369.

Hammond EJ, Wilder BJ, Ballinger WE (1982): Electrophysiologic recordings in a patient with a discrete unilateral thalamic infarction. *J Neurol Neurosurg Psychiatry* 45:640–643.

Hansen MV, Ertekin C, Larsson L-E (1990): Cerebral evoked potentials after stimulation of the posterior urethra in man. *Electroencephalogr Clin Neurophysiol* 77(1):52–58.

Hansotia PL (1985): Persistent vegetative state. *Arch Neurol* 42:1048–1052.

Harding AE, Muller DPR, Thomas PK, Willison HJ (1982): Spinocerebellar degeneration secondary to chronic intestinal malabsorption: A vitamin E deficiency syndrome. *Ann Neurol* 12:419–424.

Hashimoto I (1984): Somatosensory evoked potentials from the human brain-stem: Origins of short latency potentials. *Electroencephalogr Clin Neurol* 57:221–227.

Hashimoto I (1988): Trigeminal evoked potentials following brief air puff: Enhanced signal-to-noise ratio. *Ann Neurol* 23:332–338.

Haupt WF (1988): Prognostischer Wert multimodaler evozierter Potentiale bei neurologischen Intensivpatienten. *Klin Wochenschr* 66:53–61.

Hornabrook RSL, Miller DH, Newton MR, MacManus DG, du Boulay GH, Halliday AM, McDonald WI (1992): Frequent involvement of the optic radiation in patients with acute isolated optic neuritis. *Neurology* 42:77–79.

Howard JE, Dorfman LJ (1986): Evoked potentials in hysteria and malingering. *J Clin Neurophysiol* 3:39–49.

Hrbek A, Karlberg P, Olsson T (1973): Development of visual and somatosensory evoked responses in pre-term newborn infants. *Electroencephalogr Clin Neurophysiol* 34:225–232.

Hrbek A, Karlberg P, Kjellmer I, Olsson T, Riha M (1977): Clinical application of evoked electroencephalographic responses in newborn infants. I. Perinatal asphyxia. *Dev Med Child Neurol* 19:34–44.

Hume AL, Cant BR (1978): Conduction time in central somatosensory pathways in man. *Electroencephalogr Clin Neurophysiol* 45:361–375.

Hume AL, Cant BR (1981): Central somatosensory conduction after head injury. *Ann Neurol* 10:411–419.

Hume AL, Cant BR, Shaw NA (1979): Central somatosensory conduction time in comatose patients. *Ann Neurol* 5:379–384.

Hume AL, Cant BR, Shaw NA, Cowan JC (1982): Central somatosensory conduction time from 10 to 79 years. *Electroencephalogr Clin Neurophysiol* 54:49–54.

Hummel T, Kobal G (1992): Differences in human evoked potentials related to olfactory of trigeminal chemosensory activation. *Electroencephalogr Clin Neurophysiol* 84(1):84–89.

Huttunen J, Homberg V (1991): Modification of cortical somatosensory evoked potentials during tactile exploration and simple active and passive movements. *Electroencephalogr Clin Neurophysiol* 81:216–223.

Imai T, Ishikawa Y, Minami R, Nagaoka M, Okabe M, Kameda K, Tachi N, Matsumoto H (1991): Delayed central conduction of somatosensory evoked potentials in xeroderma pigmentosum. *Neurology* 41:933–935.

Ingvar DH, Brun A, Johansson L (1978): Survival after severe cerebral anoxia. *Ann NY Acad Sci* 315:184–214.

Iragui VJ (1984): The cervical somatosensory evoked potential in man: Far-field, conducted and segmental components. *Electroencephalogr Clin Neurol* 57:228–235.

Iragui VJ, Kalmijn J, Thal LJ, Grant I, The HNRC Group (1994): Neurological dysfunction in asymptomatic HIV-1 infected men: evidence from evoked potentials. *Electroencephalogr Clin Neurophysiol* 92(1):1–10.

Ishiko N, Hanamori T, Murayama N (1980): Spatial distribution of somatosensory responses evoked by tapping the tongue and finger in man. *Electroencephalogr Clin Neurophysiol* 50:1–10.

Jabbari B, Geyer C, Gunderson C, Chu A, Brophy J, McBurney JW, Jonas B (1990): Somatosensory evoked potentials and magnetic resonance imaging in syringomyelia. *Electroencephalogr Clin Neurophysiol* 77:277–285.

Jacobson GP, Tew JM (1988): The origin of the scalp recorded P14 following electrical stimulation of the median nerve: Intraoperative observations. *Electroencephalogr Clin Neurophysiol* 71:73–76.

Jacobson RC, Chapman CR, Gerlach R (1985): Stimulus intensity and inter-stimulus interval effects on pain-related cerebral potentials. *Electroencephalogr Clin Neurophysiol* 62:352–363.

Jeanmonod D, Sindou M, Mauguiere F (1989): Three transverse dipolar generators in the human cervical and lumbo-sacral dorsal horn: evidence from direct intraoperative recordings on the spinal cord surface. *Electroencephalogr Clin Neurophysiol* 74(3):236–240.

Jeanmonod D, Sindou M, Mauguiere F (1991): The human cervical and lumbo-sacral evoked electrospinogram. Data from intra-operative spinal cord surface recordings. *Electroencephalogr Clin Neurophysiol* 80(6):477–489.

Johnson S (1985): Somatosensory evoked potentials in abetalipoproteinemia. *Electroencephalogr Clin Neurophysiol* 60:27–29.

Jones SJ (1977): Short latency potentials recorded from the neck and scalp following median nerve stimulation in man. *Electroencephalogr Clin Neurophysiol* 43:853–863.

Jones SJ (1979): Investigation of brachial plexus traction lesions by peripheral and spinal somatosensory evoked potentials. *J Neurol Neurosurg Psychiatry* 42:107–116.

Jones SJ (1981): An "interference" approach to the study of somatosensory evoked potentials in man. *Electroencephalogr Clin Neurophysiol* 52:517–530.

Jones SJ, Halliday AM (1982): Subcortical and cortical somatosensory evoked potentials: Characteristic waveform changes associated with disorders of the peripheral and central nervous system. In: *Clinical Applications of Evoked Potentials in Neurology,* edited by J Courjon, F Mauguiere, and M Revol, pp 313–320. Raven Press, New York.

Jones SJ, Power CN (1984): Scalp topography of human somatosensory evoked potentials: The effect of interfering tactile stimulation applied to the hand. *Electroencephalogr Clin Neurophysiol* 58:25–36.

Jones SJ, Small DG (1978): Spinal and sub-cortical evoked potentials following stimulation of the posterior tibial nerve in man. *Electroencephalogr Clin Neurophysiol* 44:299–306.

Jones SJ, Baraitser M, Halliday AM (1980): Peripheral and central somatosensory nerve conduction defects in Friedreich's ataxia. *J Neurol Neurosurg Psychiatry* 43:495–503.

Jones SJ, Edgar MA, Ransford AO (1982): Sensory nerve conduction in the human spinal cord: Epidural recordings made during scoliosis surgery. *J Neurol Neurosurg Psychiatry* 45:446–451.

Jones SJ, Halonen J-P, Shawkat (1989): Centrifugal and centripetal mechanisms involved in the "gating" of cortical SEPs during movement. *Electroencephalogr Clin Neurophysiol* 74:36–45.

Judson JA, Cant BR, Shaw NA (1990): Early prediction of outcome from cerebral trauma by somatosensory evoked potentials. *Crit Care Med* 18:363–368.

Kaji R, Sumner AJ (1987): Bipolar recording of short-latency somatosensory evoked potentials after median nerve stimulation. *Neurology* 37:410–418.

Kakigi R (1986): Ipsilateral and contralateral SEP components following median nerve stimulation: Effects of interfering stimuli applied to the contralateral hand. *Electroencephalogr Clin Neurophysiol* 64:246–259.

Kakigi R (1987): The effect of aging on somatosensory evoked potentials following stimulation of the posterior tibial nerve in man. *Electroencephalogr Clin Neurophysiol* 68:277–286.

Kakigi R, Jones SJ (1985): Effects on median nerve SEPs of tactile stimulation applied to adjacent and remote areas of the body surface. *Electroencephalogr Clin Neurophysiol* 62:252–265.

Kakigi R, Jones SJ (1986): Influence of concurrent tactile stimulation on somatosensory evoked potentials following posterior tibial nerve stimulation in man. *Electroencephalogr Clin Neurophysiol* 65:118–129.

Kakigi R, Shibasaki H (1984): Scalp topography of mechanically and electrically evoked somatosensory potentials in man. *Electroencephalogr Clin Neurophysiol* 59:44–56.

Kakigi R, Shibasaki H (1991): Estimation of conduction belocity of the spino-thalamic tract in man. *Electroencephalogr Clin Neurophysiol* 80(1):39–45.

Kakigi R, Shibasaki H, Hashizume A, Kuroiwa Y (1982): Short latency somatosensory evoked spinal and scalp-recorded potentials following posterior tibial nerve stimulation in man. *Electroencephalogr Clin Neurophysiol* 53:602–611.

Kakigi R, Shibasaki H, Ikeda A (1989): Pain related somatosensory evoked potentials following CO2 laser stimulation in man. *Electroencephalogr Clin Neurophysiol* 74(2):139–146.

Kakigi R, Kuroda Y, Takashima H, Endo C, Neshige R, Shibasaki H (1992): Physiological functions of the ascending spinal tracts in HTLV-1-associated myelopathy. *Electroencephalogr Clin Neurophysiol* 84(2):110–114.

Kameyama S, Yamada T, Matsuoka H, Fuchigama Y, Nakazumi Y, Suh C-k, Kimura J (1988): Stationary potentials after median nerve stimulation: Changes with arm positions. *Electroencephalogr Clin Neurophysiol* 71:348–356.

Kang DX, Ma BR, Lundervold A (1983): The effect of acupuncture on somatosensory evoked potentials. *Clin Electroencephalogr* 14(1):53–56.

Kaplan PW, Hosford DA, Werner MH, Erwin CW (1988a): Somatosensory evoked potentials in a patient with a cervical glioma and syrinx. *Electroencephalogr Clin Neurophysiol* 70:563–565.

Kaplan PW, Rawal K, Erwin CW, D'Souza BJ, Spock A (1988b): Visual and somatosensory evoked potentials in vitamin E deficiency with cystic fibrosis. *Electroencephalogr Clin Neurophysiol* 71:266–272.

Katayama Y, Tsubokawa T (1987): Somatosensory evoked potentials from the thalamic sensory relay nucleus (VPL) in humans: Correlations with short latency somatosensory evoked potentials recorded at the scalp. *Electroencephalogr Clin Neurophysiol* 68:187–201.

Kazis A, Vlaikidis N, Xafenias D, Papanastasiou J, Pappa P (1982): Fever and evoked potentials in multiple sclerosis. *J Neurol* 227:1–10.

Khoshbin S, Hallett M (1981): Multimodality evoked potentials and blink reflex in multiple sclerosis. *Neurology* 31:138–144.

Kimura J, Yamada T, Kawamura H (1978): Central latencies of somatosensory cerebral evoked potentials. *Arch Neurol* 35:683–688.

Kimura J, Mitsudome A, Beck DO, Yamada T, Dickens QS (1983): Field distribution of antidomically activated digital nerve potentials. Model for far field recording. *Neurology* 33:1164–1169.

Kimura J, Mitsudome A, Yamada T, Dickens QS (1984): Stationary peaks from a moving source in far-field recording. *Electroencephalogr Clin Neurophysiol* 58:351–361.

Kimura J, Ishida T, Suzuki S, Kudo Y, Matsuoka H, Yamada T (1986a): Far field recording of the junctional potential generated by median nerve volleys at the wrist. *Neurology* 36:1451–1457.

Kimura J, Kimura A, Ishida T, Kudo Y, Suzuki S, Machida M, Yamada T, Matsuoka H (1986b): What determines the latency and amplitude of stationary peaks in far-field recordings? *Ann Neurol* 19:479–486.

Kimura J, Kimura A, Machida M, Yamada T, Mitsudome A (1986c): Model for far-field recordings of sep. In: *Evoked Potentials,* edited by RQ Cracco and I Bodis-Wollner, pp 246–261. A R Liss, New York.

King DW, Green JB (1979): Short latency somatosensory potentials in humans. *Electroencephalogr Clin Neurophysiol* 46:702–708.

King PJL, Chiappa KH (1988): Effect of stimulus intensity on latency of tibial evoked potentials. *J Clin Neurophysiol* 5:203.

Kirshner HS, Tsai SI, Runge VM, et al (1985): Magnetic resonance imaging and other techniques in the diagnosis of multiple sclerosis. *Arch Neurol* 42:859–863.

Kjaer M (1980a): Variations of brain stem auditory evoked potentials correlated to duration and severity of multiple sclerosis. *Acta Neurol Scand* 61:157–166.

Kjaer M (1980b): The value of brain stem auditory, visual and somatosensory evoked potentials and blink reflexes in the diagnosis of multiple sclerosis. *Acta Neurol Scand* 62:220–236.

Klimach VJ, Cooke RW (1988): Short-latency cortical evoked somatosensory evoked responses of preterm infants with ultrasound abnormality of the brain. *Dev Med Child Neurol* 30:215–221.

Kobal G, Hummel C (1988): Cerebral chemosensory evoked potentials elicited by chemical stimulation of the human olfactory and respiratory nasal mucosa. *Electroencephalogr Clin Neurophysiol* 71:241–250.

Kovala T (1991): Prognostic significance of somatosensory potentials evoked by stimulation of the median and posterior tibial nerves: A prospectice 1-year follow-up study in patients with supratentorial cerebral infarction. *Eur Neurol* 31:141–148.

Kovala T, Tolonen U, Pyhtinen J (1990): Correlation of tibial nerve SEPs with the development of seizures in patients with supratentorial cerebral infarcts. *Electroencephalogr Clin Neurophysiol* 77:347–352.

Kovala T, Tolonen U, Pyhtinen J (1991): A prospective 1 year follow-up study with somatosensory potentials evoked by stimulation of the posterial tibial nerve in patients with supratentorial cerebral infarction. *Electroencephalogr Clin Neurophysiol* 80(4):262–275.

Kritchevsky M, Wiederholt WC (1978): Short latency somatosensory evoked potentials. *Arch Neurol* 35:706–711.

Krumholz A, Weiss HD, Goldstein PJ, Harris KC (1981): Evoked responses in vitamin B12 deficiency. *Ann Neurol* 9:407–409.

Krumholz A, Singer HS, Niedermeyer E, Burnite R, Harris K (1983): Electrophysiological studies in Tourette's Syndrome. *Ann Neurol* 14:638–641.

Kukulka CG, Brown DA, Weightman MM (1991): An objective method for assessing graded electrically evoked afferent activity in humans. *Electroencephalogr Clin Neurophysiol* 81:312–318.

Kunesch E, Knecht S, Classen J, Roick H, Tyercha C, Benecke R (1993): Somatosensory evoked potentials (SEPs) elicited by magnetic nerve stimulation. *Electroencephalogr Clin Neurophysiol* 88(6):459–467.

Laget P, Salbreux R, Raimbault J, d'Allest AM, Mariani J (1976): Relationship between changes in somesthetic evoked responses and electroencephalographic findings in the child with hemiplegia. *Dev Med Child Neurol* 18:620–631.

LaJoie WJ, Reddy NM, Melvin JL (1982): Somatosensory evoked potentials: Their predictive value in right hemiplegia. *Arch Phys Med Rehab* 63:223–226.

Larrea LG, Mauguiere F (1988): Latency and amplitude abnormalities of the scale far-field P14 to median nerve stimulation in multiple sclerosis. A SEP study of 122 patients recorded with a non-cephalic reference montage. *Electroencephalogr Clin Neurophysiol* 71:180–186.

Larrea LG, Bastuji H, Mauguiere F (1992): Unmasking of cortical SEP components by changes in stimulus rate: a topographic study. *Electroencephalogr Clin Neurophysiol* 84(1):71–83.

Larson SJ, Sances A (1968): Averaged evoked potentials in stereotaxic surgery. *J Neurosurg* 28:227–232.

Larson SJ, Holst RA, Hemmy DC, Sances A (1976): Lateral extracavitary approach to traumatic lesions of the thoracic and lumbar spine. *J Neurosurg* 45:628–637.

Larsson LE, Prevec TS (1970): Somato-sensory response to mechanical stimulation as recorded in the human EEG. *Electroencephalogr Clin Neurophysiol* 28:162–172.

Lastimosa ACB, Bass NH, Stanback K, Norvell EE (1982): Lumbar spinal cord and early cortical evoked potentials after tibial nerve stimulation: Effects of stature on normative data. *Electroencephalogr Clin Neurophysiol* 54:499–507.

Lauffer H, Wenzel D (1986): Maturation of central somatosensory conduction time in infancy and childhood. *Neuropediatrics* 17:72–74.

Laureau E, Hebert R, Vanasse M, Letarte J, Glorieux J, Desjardins M, Dussault JH (1987): Somatosensory evoked potentials and auditory brain-stem responses in congenital hypothyroidism. II. A cross-sectional study in childhood. Correlation with hormonal levels and developmental quotients. *Electroencephalogr Clin Neurophysiol* 67:521–530.

Laureau E, Majnemer A, Rosenblatt B, Riley P (1988): A longitudinal study of short latency evoked responses in healthy newborns and infants. *Electroencephalogr Clin Neurophysiol* 71:100–108.

Lawyer T, Netsky MG (1953): Amyotrophic lateral sclerosis: A clinico-anatomical study of 53 cases. *Arch Neurol Psychiatry* 69:171–192.

Leandri M, Campbell JA (1986): Origin of early waves evoked by infraorbital nerve stimulation in man. *Electroencephalogr Clin Neurophysiol* 65:13–19.

Leandri M, Favale E, Ratto S, Abbruzzese M (1981): Conducted and segmental components of the somatosensory cervical response. *J Neurol Neurosurg Psychiatry* 44:718–722.

Leandri M, Parodi CI, Favale E (1985): Early evoked potentials detected from the scalp of man following infraorbital nerve stimulation. *Electroencephalogr Clin Neurophysiol* 62:99–107.

Leandri M, Parodi CI, Favale E (1988a): Early trigeminal evoked potentials in tumours of the base of the skull and trigeminal neuralgia. *Electroencephalogr Clin Neurophysiol* 71:114–124.

Leandri M, Parodi CI, Favale E (1988b): Normative data on scalp responses evoked by infraorbital nerve stimulation. *Electroencephalogr Clin Neurophysiol* 71:415–421.

Leandri M, Schizzi R, Favale E (1994): Blink reflex far fields mimicking putative cortical trideminal evoked potentials. *Electroencephalogr Clin Neurophysiol* 93:240–242.

Lecky BRF, Murray NMF, Barry RJ (1980): Transient radiation myelopathy: Spinal somatosensory evoked responses following incidental cord exposure during radiotherapy. *J Neurol Neurosurg Psychiatry* 43:747–750.

Lee KH, Hashimoto SA, Hooge JP, Kastrukoff LF, Oger JJF, Li DKB, Paty DW (1991): Magnetic resonance imaging of the head in the diagnosis of multiple sclerosis: A prospective 2-year follow-up with comparison of clinical evaluation, evoked potentials, oligoclonal banding, and CT. *Neurology* 41:657–660.

Lehmkuhl LD, Dimitrijevic MR, Renouf F (1984): Electrophysiological characteristics of lumbosacral evoked potentials in patients with established spinal cord injury. *Electroencephalogr Clin Neurophysiol* 59(2):142–155.

Lesser RP, Koehle R, Lueders H (1979): Effect of stimulus intensity on short latency somatosensory evoked potentials. *Electroencephalogr Clin Neurophysiol* 47:377–382.

Lesser RP, Lueders H, Hahn J, Klem G (1981): Early somatosensory potentials evoked by median nerve stimulation: Intraoperative monitoring. *Neurology* 31:1519–1523.

Lesser RP, Lueders H, Hahn J, Morris H, Wyllie E, Resor S (1987): The source of "paradoxical lateralization" of cortical evoked potentials to posterior tibial nerve stimulation. *Neurology* 37:82–88.

Liberson WT (1983): More on one-channel recording of somato-sensory evoked potentials (SEP) of multiple origin. *Electroencephalogr Clin Neurophysiol* 23:607–611.

Liberson WT, Gratzer M, Zalis A, Grabinski B (1966): Comparison of conduction velocities of motor and sensory fibers determined by different methods. *Arch Phys Med* 47:17–23.

Light JK, Beric A, Wise PG (1987): Predictive criteria for failed sphincterotomy in spinal cord injury patients. *J Urol* 138:1201–1204.

Lindsay K, Pasaoglu A, Hirst D, Allardyce G, Kennedy I, Teasdale G (1990): Somatosensory and auditory brain stem conduction after head injury: a comparison with clinical features in prediction of outcome. *Neurosurgery* 26:278–285.

Lindsay KW, Carlin J, Kennedy I, Fry J, McInnes A, Teasdale GM (1981): Evoked potentials in severe head injury—analysis and relation to outcome. *J Neurol Neurosurg Psychiatry* 44:796–802.

Loening-Baucke V, Yamada T (1993): Cerebral potentials evoked by rectal distention in humans. *Electroencephalogr Clin Neurophysiol* 88(6):447–452.

Loening-Baucke V, Read NW, Yamada T (1991): Cerebral evoked potentials after rectal stimulation. *Electroencephalogr Clin Neurophysiol* 80(6):490–495.

Ludvigsson P, Hassink SE, Bernstein M, Widzer S, Grover WD (1980): Ataxia, cerebral atrophy, and abnormal somatosensory evoked potentials in a 9-year-old boy with vitamin B12 deficiency. *Ann Neurol* 8:234.

Ludwin SK (1981): Pathology of demyelination and remyelination. In: *Demyelinating Disease: Basic and Clinical Electrophysiology,* edited by SG Waxman and JM Ritchie, pp 123–168. Raven Press, New York.

Lueders H (1970): The effects of aging on the wave form of the somatosensory cortical evoked potential. *Electroencephalogr Clin Neurophysiol* 29:450–460.

Lueders H, Andrish J, Gurd A, Weiker G, Klem G (1981): Origin of far-field subcortical potentials evoked by stimulation of the posterior tibial nerve. *Electroencephalogr Clin Neurophysiol* 52:336–344.

Lueders H, Dinner DS, Lesser RP, Klem G (1983a): Origin of far-field subcortical evoked potentials to posterior tibial and median nerve stimulation. *Arch Neurol* 40:93–97.

Lueders H, Lesser RP, Hahn J, Dinner DS, Klem G (1983b): Cortical somatosensory evoked potentials in response to hand stimulation. *J Neurosurg* 58:885–894.

Lueders H, Lesser R, Hahn J, Little J, Klem G (1983c): Subcortical somatosensory evoked potentials to median nerve stimulation. *Brain* 106:341–372.

Lueders H, Lesser RP, Dinner DS, Morris HM (1985): Optimizing stimulating and recording parameters in somatosensory evoked potential studies. *J Clin Neurophysiol* 2:383–396.

Lutschg J, Pfenninger J, Ludin HP, Vassella F (1983): Brain stem auditory evoked potentials and early somatosensory evoked potentials in neurointensively treated comatose children. *Am J Dis Child* 137:421–426.

Maccabee PJ, Pinkhasov EI, Cracco RQ (1983): Short latency somatosensory evoked potentials to median nerve stimulation: Effect of low frequency filter. *Electroencephalogr Clin Neurophysiol* 55:34–44.

Maccabee PJ, Hassan NF, Cracco RQ, Schiff JA (1986): Short latency somatosensory and spinal evoked potentials: Power spectra and comparison between high pass analog and digital filter. *Electroencephalogr Clin Neurophysiol* 65:177–187.

Macdonell RAL, Donnan GA, Bladin PF (1991): Serial changes in somatosensory evoked potentials following cerebral infarction. *Electroencephalogr Clin Neurophysiol* 80:276–283.

Macon JB, Poletti CE, Sweet WH (1981): Human trigeminal root evoked potentials during differential thermal and chemical trigeminal rhizotomy. *Surg Forum* 32:486–488.

Macon JB, Poletti CE, Sweet WH, Ojemann RG, Zervas NT (1982): Conducted somatosensory evoked potentials during spinal surgery. Part 1: Clinical applications. *J Neurosurg* 57:354–359.

Magladery JW, Porter WE, Park AM, Teasdale RD (1951): Electrophysiological studies of nerve and reflex activity in normal man; (IV) the two-neurone reflex and identification of certain action potentials from spinal roots and cords. *Bull Johns Hopkins Hosp* 88:499–519.

Majnemer A, Rosenblatt B, Watters G, Andermann F (1986): Giant axonal neuropathy: Central abnormalities demonstrated by evoked potentials. *Ann Neurol* 19:394–396.

Majnemer A, Rosenblatt B, Riley P, Laureau E, O'Gorman AM (1987): Somatosensory evoked response abnormalities in high risk newborns. *Pediatr Neurol* 3:350–355.

Manzano GM, De Navarro JM, Nobrega JAM, Novo NF, Juliano Y (1995): Short latency median nerve somatosensory evoked potential (SEP): increase in stimulation frequency from 3 to 30 Hz. *Electroencephalogr Clin Neurophysiol* 96(3):229–235.

Maravilla KR, Weinreb JC, Suss R, et al (1985): Magnetic resonance demonstration of multiple sclerosis plaques in the cervical cord. *Am J Rad* 144:381–385.

Markand ON, DeMyer WE, Worth RM, Warren C (1982a): Multimodality evoked responses in leukodystrophies. In: *Clinical Applications of Evoked Potentials in Neurology*, edited by J Courjon, F Mauguiere, and M Revol, pp 409–416. Raven Press, New York.

Markand ON, Garg BP, DeMeyer WE, Warren C, Worth RM (1982b): Brain stem auditory, visual and somatosensory evoked potentials in the leukodystrophies. *Electroencephalogr Clin Neurophysiol* 54:39–48.

Markand ON, Warren C, Mallik GS, King RD, Brown JW, Mahomed Y (1990a): Effects of hypothermia on short latency somatosensory evoked potentials in humans. *Electroencephalogr Clin Neurophysiol* 77(6):416–424.

Markand ON, Warren C, Mallik GS, Williams CJ (1990b): Temperature-dependent hysteresis in somatosensory and auditory evoked potentials. *Electroencephalogr Clin Neurophysiol* 77(6):425–435.

Marra TR (1982): The origins of the subcortical component of the median nerve somatosensory evoked potentials. *Clin Electroencephalogr* 13:116–121.

Maruyama Y, Shimoji K, Shimizu H, Kuribayashi H, Fujioka H (1982): Human spinal cord potentials evoked by different sources of stimulation and conduction velocities along the cord. *J Neurophysiol* 48:1098–1107.

Mastaglia FL, Black JL, Collins DWK (1976): Visual and spinal evoked potentials in the diagnosis of multiple sclerosis. *Br Med J* 2:732.

Mastaglia FL, Black JL, Edis R, Collins DWK (1978): The contribution of evoked potentials in the functional assessment of the somatosensory pathway. *Clin Exp Neurol* 15:279–298.

Masur H, Oberwittler C, Fahrendorf G, Heyen P, Reuther G, Nedjat S, Ludolph AC, Brune GG (1992): The relation between functional deficits, motor and sensory conduction times and MRI findings in syringomyelia. *Electroencephalogr Clin Neurophysiol* 83:321–330.

Matheson JK, Harrington HJ, Hallett M (1986): Abnormalities of multimodality evoked potentials in amyotrophic lateral sclerosis. *Arch Neurol* 43:338–340.

Matthews WB, Esiri M (1979): Multiple sclerosis plaque related to abnormal somatosensory evoked potentials. *J Neurol Neurosurg Psychiatry* 42:940–942.

Matthews WB, Small DG (1979): Serial recording of visual and somatosensory evoked potentials in multiple sclerosis. *J Neurol Sci* 40:11–21.

Matthews WB, Read DJ, Pountney E (1979): Effect of raising body temperature on visual and somatosensory evoked potentials in patients with multiple sclerosis. *J Neurol Neurosurg Psychiatry* 42:250–255.

Matthews WB, Wattam-Bell JRB, Pountney E (1982): Evoked potentials in the diagnosis of multiple sclerosis: A follow up study. *J Neurol Neurosurg Psychiatry* 45:303–307.

Matthews WB, Acheson ED, Batchelor JR, et al (eds) (1985): *McAlpine's Multiple Sclerosis.* Churchill Livingstone, London.

Mauguiere F, Courjon J (1981): The origins of short-latency somatosensory evoked potentials in humans. *Ann Neurol* 9:607–611.

Mauguiere F, Desmedt JE (1988): Thalamic pain syndrome of Dejerine-Roussy. *Arch Neurol* 45:1312–1320.

Mauguiere F, Desmedt JE (1991): Focal capsular vascular lesions can selectively deafferent the prerolandic or the parietal cortex: Somatosensory evoked potentials evidence. *Ann Neurol* 30:71–75.

Mauguiere F, Restuccia D (1991): Inadequacy of the forehead reference montage for detecting abnormalities of the spinal N13 SEP in cervical cord lesions. *Electroencephalogr Clin Neurophysiol* 79:448–456.

Mauguiere F, Brunon AM, Echallier JF, Courjon J (1982): Early somatosensory evoked potentials in lesions of the lemniscal pathway in humans. In: *Clinical Applications of Evoked Potentials in Neurology*, edited by J Courjon, F Mauguiere, and M Revol, pp 321–338. Raven Press, New York.

Mauguiere F, Desmedt JE, Courjon J (1983a): Neural generators of N18 and P14 far-field somatosensory evoked potentials studied in patients with lesion of thalamus or thalamo-cortical radiations. *Electroencephalogr Clin Neurophysiol* 56:283–292.

Mauguiere F, Desmedt JE, Courjon J (1983b): Astereognosis and dissociated loss of frontal or parietal components of somatosensory evoked potentials in hemispheric lesions. *Brain* 106:271–311.

Mauguiere F, Courjon J, Schott B (1983c): Dissociation of early SEP components in unilateral traumatic section of the lower medulla. *Ann Neurol* 13:309–313.

Mavroudakis N, Brunko E, Nogueira MC, Zegers de Beyl D (1991): Acute effects of diphenylhydantoin on peripheral and central somatosensory conduction. *Electroencephalogr Clin Neurophysiol* 78:263–266.

Mavroudakis N, Brunko E, Delberghe X, Zegers de Beyl D (1993): Dissociation of P13-P14 far-field potentials: clinical and MRI correlation. *Electroencephalogr Clin Neurophysiol* 240–242.

McCarthy G, Wood CC, Allison T (1991): Cortical somatosensory evoked potentials I. Recordings in the monkey Macaca fascicularis. *J Neurophysiol* 66(1):53–63.

McDonald WI (1977): Pathophysiology of conduction in central nerve fibers. In: *Visual Evoked Potentials in Man: New Developments*, edited by JE Desmedt, pp 427–437. Clarendon Press, Oxford.

McGill KC, Cummins KL, Dorfman LJ, Berlizot BB, Luetkemeyer K, Nishimura DG, Widrow B (1982): On the nature and elimination of stimulus artifact in nerve signals evoked and recorded using surface electrodes. *IEEE Trans Biomed Eng* 29:129–136.

McKay WB, Galloway BL (1979): Technological aspects of recording evoked potentials from the cauda equina and lumbosacral spinal cord in man. *Am J EEG Technol* 19:83–96.

Meredith JT, Celesia GG (1982): Pattern-reversal visual evoked potentials and retinal eccentricity. *Electroencephalogr Clin Neurophysiol* 53:243–253.

Mervaala E, Paakkonen A, Partanen JV (1988): The influence of height, age and gender on the interpretation of median nerve SEPs. *Electroencephalogr Clin Neurophysiol* 71:109–113.

Meyer-Hardting E, Wiederholt WC, Budnick B (1983): Recovery function of short-latency components of the human somatosensory evoked potential. *Arch Neurol* 40:290–293.

Miller DH, Johnson G, McDonald WI, et al (1986): Detection of optic nerve lesions in optic neuritis with magnetic resonance imaging. *Lancet* 1490–1491.

Molaie M (1987): Scalp-recorded short and middle latency peroneal somatosensory evoked potentials in normals: Comparison with peroneal and median nerve SEPs in patients with unilateral hemispheric lesions. *Electroencephalogr Clin Neurophysiol* 68:107–118.

Moller AR, Jannetta PJ, Burgess JE (1986): Neural generators of the somatosensory evoked potentials: Recording from the cuneate nucleus in man and monkeys. *Electroencephalogr Clin Neurophysiol* 65:241–248.

Morgan JM, Van Hees J, Gybels J (1984): ERPs associated with decisions based on slowly increasing warm and painful stimuli. *Electroencephalogr Clin Neurophysiol* 58:343–350.

Mori E, Yamadori A, Kudo Y, Tabuchi M (1984): Ataxic hemiparesis from small capsular hemorrhage. *Arch Neurol* 41:1050–1053.

Morioka T, Shima F, Kato M, Fukui M (1989): Origin and distribution of thalamic somatosensory evoked potentials in humans. *Electroencephalogr Clin Neurophysiol* 74(3):186–193.

Morioka T, Shima F, Kato M, Fukui M (1991a): Direct recording of somatosensory evoked potentials in the vicinity of the dorsal column nuclei in man: their fenerator mechanisms and contribution to the scalp far-field potentials. *Electroencephalogr Clin Neurophysiol* 80(3):215–220.

Morioka T, Tobimatsu S, Fujii K, Fukui M, Kato M, Matsubara T (1991b): Origin and distribution of brain-stem somatosensory evoked potentials in humans. *Electroencephalogr Clin Neurophysiol* 80(3):221–227.

Morioka T, Katsura T, Fujii K, Kato M, Fukui M (1993): Discrepancy between SEPs directly recorded from the dorsal column nucleio following upper and lower limb stimulation in patients with syringomyelia. *Electroencephalogr Clin Neurophysiol* 88(6):453–458.

Mulder DW (1982): Clinical limits of amyotrophic lateral sclerosis. In: *Human Motor Neuron Diseases. Advances in Neurology*, Vol 36, edited by LP Rowland, pp 15–22. Raven Press, New York.

Mulder DW, Bushek W, Spring E, Karnes J, Dyck PJ (1983): Motor neuron disease (ALS): Evaluation of detection thresholds of cutaneous sensation. *Neurology* 33:1625–1627.

Mutoh K, Okuno T, Mikawa H, Hojo H (1988): Maturation of somatosensory evoked potentials upon posterior tibial nerve stimulation. *Pediatr Neurol* 4:342–349.

Nagamine T, Kaji R, Suqazono S, Hamano T, Shibasaki H, Kimura J (1992): Current source density mapping of somatosensory evoked responses following median and tibial nerve stimulation. *Electroencephalogr Clin Neurophysiol* 84:248–256.

Nakanishi T (1982): Action potentials recorded by fluid electrodes. *Electroencephalogr Clin Neurophysiol* 53:343–346.

Nakanishi T (1983): Origin of action potentials recorded by fluid electrodes. *Electroencephalogr Clin Neurophysiol* 55:114–155.

Nakanishi T, Tamaki M, Ozaki Y, Arasaki K (1983): Origins of short latency somatosensory evoked potentials to median nerve stimulation. *Electroencephalogr Clin Neurophysiol* 56:74–85.

Nakashima K, Kanba M, Fujimoto K, Sato T, Takahashi K (1985): Somatosensory evoked potentials over the non-affected hemisphere in patients with unilateral cerebrovascular lesions. *J Neurol Sci* 70:117–127.

Namerow NS (1968): Somatosensory evoked responses in multiple sclerosis patients with varying sensory loss. *Neurology* 18:1197–1204.

Namerow NS (1969): Somatosensory evoked responses following cervical cordotomy. *Bull LA Neurol Soc* 34:184–189.

Namerow NS (1970): Somatosensory recovery functions in multiple sclerosis patients. *Neurology* 20:813–817.

Narayan RK, Greenberg RP, Miller JD, Enas GG, Choi SC, Kishore PS, Selhorst JB, Lutz HA, Becker DP (1981): Improved confidence of outcome prediction in severe head injury. A comparative analysis of the clinical examination, multimodality evoked potentials, CT scanning, and intracranial pressure. *J Neurosurg* 54:751–762.

Nardone A, Schieppati M (1989): Influences of transcutaneous electrical stimulation of cutaneous and mixed nerves on subcortical and cortical somatosensory evoked potentials. *Electroencephalogr Clin Neurophysiol* 74:24–35.

Nash CL, Schatzinger LH, Brown RH, Brodkey J (1977): The unstable thoracic compression fracture. Its problems and the use of spinal cord monitoring in the evaluation of treatment. *Spine* 2:261–265.

Nelson FW, Goldie WD, Hecht JT, Butler IJ, Scott CI (1984): Short latency somatosensory evoked potentials in the management of patients with achondroplasia. *Neurology* 34:1053–1058.

Nelson FW, Hecht JT, Horton WA, Butler IJ, Goldie WD, Miner M (1988): Neurological basis of respiratory complications in achondroplasia. *Ann Neurol* 24:89–93.

Niazy HMA, Lundervold A (1982): Correlation of evoked potentials (SEP and VEP), EEG and CT in the diagnosis of brain tumors and cerebrovascular disease. *Clin Electroencephalogr* 13:71–81.

Nightingale S, Schofield IS, Dawes PJDK (1984): Visual, cortical somatosensory and brainstem auditory evoked potentials following incidental irradiation of the rhombencephalon. *J Neuro Neurosurg Psychiatry* 47:91–93.

Noel P, Desmedt JE (1975): Somatosensory cerebral evoked potentials after vascular lesions of the brain stem and diencephalon. *Brain* 98:113–128.

Noel P, Desmedt JE (1976): The somatosensory pathway in Friedreich's ataxia. *Acta Neurol Belg* 76:271.

Noel P, Desmedt JE (1980): Cerebral and far-field somatosensory evoked potentials in neurological disorders involving the cervical spinal cord, brainstem, thalamus and cortex. *Prog Clin Neurophysiol* 7:205–230.

Noguchi Y, Yamada T, Yeh M, Matsubara M, Kokubun Y, Kawada J, Shiraishi G, Kajimoto S (1995): Dissociated changes of frontal and parietal somatosensory evoked potentials in sleep. *Neurology* 45:154–160.

Noseworthy J, Paty D, Wonnacott T, Feasby T, Ebers G (1983): Multiple sclerosis after age 50. *Neurology* 33:1537–1544.

Noth J, Engel L, Friedemann HH, Lange HW (1984): Evoked potentials in patients with Huntington's Disease and their offspring. I. Somatosensory evoked potentials. *Electroencephalogr Clin Neurophysiol* 59:134–141.

Nousiainen U, Partanen J, Laulumaa V, Paakkonen A (1987): Involvement of somatosensory and visual pathways in late onset ataxia. *Electroencephalogr Clin Neurophysiol* 67:514–520.

Nuwer MR, Perlman SL, Packwood JW, Pieter Kark RA (1983): Evoked potential abnormalities in the various inherited ataxias. *Ann Neurol* 13:20–27.

Nuwer MR, Visscher BR, Packwood JW, Namerow NS (1985): Evoked potential testing in relatives of multiple sclerosis patients. *Ann Neurol* 18:30–34.

Nuwer MR, Packwood JW, Myers LW, Ellison GW (1987): Evoked potentials predict the clinical changes in a multiple sclerosis drug study. *Neurology* 37:1754–1761.

Obeso JA, Marti-Masso JF, Carrerra N (1980): Somatosensory evoked potentials: Abnormalities with focal brain lesions remote from the primary sensorimotor area. *Electroencephalogr Clin Neurophysiol* 49:59–65.

Oepen G, Doerr M, Thoden U (1981): Visual (VEP) and somatosensory (SSEP) evoked potentials in Huntington's Chorea. *Electroencephalogr Clin Neurophysiol* 51:666–670.

Oh SJ, Sunwoo IN, Kim HS, Faught E (1985): Cervical and cortical somatosensory evoked potentials differentiate cervical spondylotic myelopathy from amyotrophic lateral sclerosis. (Abstract) *Neurology* 35(Suppl 1):147–148.

Ohnishi A, O'Brien PC, Okazaki H, Dyck PJ (1976): Morphometry of myelinated fibers of fasciculus gracilis of man. *J Neurol Sci* 27:163–172.

Onishi H, Yamada T, Saito T, Emori T, Fuchigami T, Hassegawa A, Nagaoka T, Ross M (1991): The effect of stimulus rate upon common peroneal, posterior tibial, and sural nerve somatosensory evoked potentials. *Neurology* 41:1972–1977.

Okajima Y, Chino N, Saitoh E, Kimura A (1991): Interactions of somatosensory evoked potentials: simultaneous stimulation of two nerves. *Electroencephalogr Clin Neurophysiol* 80(1):26–31.

Onofrj M, Basciani M, Fulgente T, Bazzano S, Malatesta G, Curatola L (1990): Maps of somatosensory evoked potentials (SEPs) to mechanical (tapping) stimuli: comparison with P14, N20, P22, N30 of electrically elicited SEPs. *Electroencephalogr Clin Neurophysiol* 77(4):314–319.

Opsomer RJ, Caramia MD, Zarola F, Pesce F, Rossini PM (1989): Neurophysiological evaluation of central-peripheral sensory and motor pudendal fibres. *Electroencephalogr Clin Neurophysiol* 74(4):260–270.

Ormerod IEC, McDonald WI, du Boulay GH, et al (1986): Disseminated lesions at presentation in patients with optic neuritis. *J Neurol Neurosurg Psychiatry* 49:124–127.

Pagni CA (1967): Somatosensory evoked potentials in thalamus and cortex of man. *Electroencephalogr Clin Neurophysiol Suppl* 26:147–155.

Parry GJ, Aminoff MJ (1987): Somatosensory evoked potentials in chronic acquired demyelinating peripheral neuropathy. *Neurology* 37:313–316.

Paty DW, Isaac CD, Grochowski E, et al (1986): Magnetic resonance imaging in multiple sclerosis: A serial study in relapsing and remitting patients with quantitative measurements of lesion size. *Neurology* 36:177.

Paty DW, Oger JJF, Kastrukoff LF, Hashimoto SA, Hooge JP, Eisen AA, Eisen KA, Purves SJ, Low MD, Brandejs V, Robertson WD, Li DKB (1988): MRI in the diagnosis of MS: A prospective study with comparison of clinical evaluation, evoked potentials, oligoclonal banding, and CT. *Neurology* 38:180–185.

Peacock JH, Combs CM (1965): Retrograde cell degeneration in diencephalic and other structures after hemidecortication of rhesus monkeys. *Exp Neurol* 11:367–399.

Pedersen L, Trojaborg W (1981): Visual, auditory and somatosensory pathway involvement in hereditary cerebellar ataxia, Friedreich's ataxia and familial spastic paraplegia. *Electroencephalogr Clin Neurophysiol* 52:283–297.

Pelosi L, Fels A, Petrillo A, Senatore R, Russo G, Lonegren K, Calace P, Caruso G (1985): Evoked potentials in relation to clinical involvement in Friedreich's ataxia. In: *Evoked Potentials, Neurophysiological and Clinical Aspects*, edited by C Morocutti and PA Rizzo, pp 375–381. Elsevier, New York.

Pelosi L, Cracco JB, Cracco RQ (1987): Conduction characteristics of somatosensory evoked potentials to peroneal, tibial and sural nerve stimulation in man. *Electroencephalogr Clin Neurophysiol* 68:287–294.

Pelosi L, Cracco JB, Cracco RQ, Hassan NF (1988): Comparison of scalp distribution of short latency somatosensory evoked potentials (SSEPs) to stimulation of different nerves in the lower extremity. *Electroencephalogr Clin Neurophysiol* 71:422–428.

Perot PL (1973): The clinical use of somatosensory evoked potentials in spinal cord injury. *Clin Neurosurg* 20:367–381.

Perot PL (1976): Somatosensory evoked potentials in the evaluation of patients with spinal cord injury. In: *Current Controversies in Neurosurgery,* edited by TP Marley, pp 160–167. Saunders, Philadelphia.

Perot PL, Vera CL (1982): Scalp-recorded somatosensory evoked potentials to stimulation of nerves in the lower extremities and evaluation of patients with spinal cord trauma. *Ann NY Acad Sci* 388:359–368.

Peterson NN, Schroeder CE, Arezzo JC (1995): Neural generators of early cortical somatosensory evoked potentials in the awake monkey. *Electroencephalogr Clin Neurophysiol* 96(3):248–260.

Phillips LH, Daube JR (1980): Lumbosacral spinal evoked potentials in humans. *Neurology* 30:1175–1183.

Phillips KR, Potvin AR, Syndulko K, Cohen SN, Tourtellotte WW, Potvin JH (1983): Multimodality evoked potentials and neurophysiological tests in multiple sclerosis. *Arch Neurol* 40:159–164.

Powell TPS (1952): Residual neurons in the human thalamus following decortication. *Brain* 75:571–584.

Pratt H, Starr A (1981): Mechanically and electrically evoked somatosensory potentials in humans: Scalp and neck distributions of short latency components. *Electroencephalogr Clin Neurophysiol* 51:138–147.

Pratt H, Starr A, Amlie RN, Politoske D (1979): Mechanically and electrically evoked somatosensory potentials in normal humans. *Neurology* 29:1236–1244.

Pratt H, Politoske D, Starr A (1980): Mechanically and electrically evoked somatosensory potentials in humans: Effects of stimulus presentation rate. *Electroencephalogr Clin Neurophysiol* 49:240–249.

Prestor B, Zgur T, Dolenc VV (1991): Subpially recorded cervical spinal cord evoked potentials in syringomyelia. *Electroencephalogr Clin Neurophysiol* 80(2):155–158.

Prevec TS (1980): Effect of valium on the somatosensory evoked potentials. *Prog Clin Neurophysiol* 7:311–318.

Purves SJ, Low MD, Galloway J, Reeves B (1981): A comparison of visual, brainstem auditory and somatosensory evoked potentials in multiple sclerosis. *Can J Neurol Sci* 8:15–19.

Radtke RA, Erwin A, Erwin CW (1986): Abnormal sensory evoked potentials in amyotrophic lateral sclerosis. *Neurology* 36:796–801.

Rappaport M, Hall K, Hopkins HK, Belleza T (1981a): Evoked potentials and head injury. 1. Rating of evoked potential abnormality. *Clin Electroencephalogr* 12:154–166.

Rappaport M, Hopkins HK, Hall K, Belleza T (1981b): Evoked potentials and head injury. 2. Clinical applications. *Clin Electroencephalogr* 12:167–176.

Raroque HG, Batjer H, White C, Bell WL, Bowman G, Greenlee R (1994): Lower brain-stem origin of the median nerve N18 potential. *Electroencephalogr Clin Neurophysiol* 90:170–172.

Rasminsky M (1981): Hyperexcitability of pathologically myelinated axons and positive symptoms in multiple sclerosis. In: *Demyelinating Disease: Basic and Clinical Electrophysiology,* edited by SG Waxman and JM Ritchie, pp 289–298. Raven Press, New York.

Regli F, Despland PA (1982): Usefulness of short-latency SEPs in 50 cases with cerebrovascular lesions. *Neurology* 32 (4, part 2):A116.

Reid CS, Pyeritz RE, Kopits SE, Maria BL, Wang W, McPherson RW, Hurko O, Phillips JA, Rosenbaum AE (1987): Cervicomedullary compression in young patients with achondroplasia: Value of comprehensive neurologic and respiratory evaluation. *J Pediatr* 110:522–530.

Reisecker F, Witzmann A, Deisenhammer E (1986): Somatosensory evoked potentials (SEPs) in various groups of cerebro-vascular ischaemic disease. *Electroencephalogr Clin Neurophysiol* 65:260–268.

Reisin RC, Goodin DS, Aminoff MJ, Mantle MM (1988): Recovery of peripheral and central responses to median nerve stimulation. *Electroencephalogr Clin Neurophysiol* 69:585–588.

Restuccia D, Mauguiere F (1991): The contribution of median nerve SEPs in the functional assessment of the cervical spinal cord in syringomyelia. *Brain* 114:361–379.

Restuccia D, Di Lazzaro V, Valeriani M, Colosimo C, Tonali P (1993): N24 spinal response to tibial nerve stimulation and magnetic resonance imaging in lesions of the lumbosacral spinal cord. *Neurology* 43:2269–2275.

Riffel B, Stohr M, Korner S (1984): Spinal and cortical evoked potentials following stimulation of the posterior tibial nerve in the diagnosis and localization of spinal cord diseases. *Electroencephalogr Clin Neurophysiol* 58:400–407.

Roberts KB, Lawrence PD, Eisen A (1983): Dispersion of the somatosensory evoked potential in multiple sclerosis. *IEEE Trans Biomed Eng* 30:360–364.

Rogers RL, Basile LFH, Taylor S, Sutherling WW, Papanicolaou AC (1994): Somatosensory evoked fields and potentials following tibial nerve stimulation. *Neurology* 44:1283–1286.

Ropper AH, Chiappa KH (1986): Evoked potentials in Guillain-Barré Syndrome. *Neurology* 36:587–590.

Ropper AH, Miller DC (1985): Acute traumatic midbrain hemorrhage. *Ann Neurol* 18:80–86.

Ropper AH, Miett T, Chiappa KH (1982): Absence of evoked potential abnormalities in acute transverse myelopathy. *Neurology* 32:80–82.

Ross MA, Leis AA, Krain L, Mitchell G (1992): Normal conduction in pathways traversing an asymptomatic multiple sclerosis plaque. *Electroencephalogr Clin Neurophysiol* 85:42–45.

Rossini PM, Cracco JB (1987): Somatosensory and brainstem auditory evoked potentials in neurodegenerative disorders. *Eur Neurol* 26:176–188.

Rossini PM, Cracco RQ, Cracco JB, House WJ (1981): Short latency somatosensory evoked potentials to peroneal nerve stimulation: Scalp topography and the effect of different frequency filters. *Electroencephalogr Clin Neurophysiol* 52:540–552.

Rossini PM, Basciani M, Di Stefano E, Febbo A, Mercuri N (1985a): Short-latency scalp somatosensory evoked potentials and central spine to scalp propagation characteristics during peroneal and median nerve stimulation in multiple sclerosis. *Electroencephalogr Clin Neurophysiol* 60:197–206.

Rossini PM, Di Stefano E, Di Paolo B, Albertazzi A (1985b): Multimodal evoked potentials in patients with chronic renal failure: Early diagnosis of central nervous system involvement. In: *Evoked Potentials, Neurophysiological and Clinical Aspects,* edited by C Morocutti and PA Rizzo, pp 391–399. Elsevier, New York.

Rossini PM, Zarola F, di Capua M, Cracco JB (1986): Somatosensory evoked potential studies in neurodegenerative system disorders. In: *Maturation of the CNS and Evoked Potentials,* edited by V Gallai, pp 125–134. Excerpta Medica, Amsterdam.   •

Rossini PM, Gigli GL, Marciani MG, Zarola F, Caramia M (1987): Non-invasive evaluation of input-output characteristics of sensorimotor cerebral areas in healthy humans. *Electroencephalogr Clin Neurophysiol* 68:88–100.

Rossini PM, Babiloni F, Bernardi G, Cecchi L, Johnson PB, Malentacca A, Stanzione P, Urbano A (1989): Abnormalities of short-latency somatosensory evoked potentials in parkinsonian patients. *Electroencephalogr Clin Neurophysiol* 74(4):277–289.

Rossini PM, Paradiso C, Zarola F, Mariorenzi R, Traversa R, Martino G, Caramia MD (1990): Bit-mapped somatosensory evoked potentials and muscular reflex responses in man: comparative analysis in different experimental protocols. *Electroencephalogr Clin Neurophysiol* 77(4):266–276.

Rossini PM, Bassetti MA, Pasqualetti P (1995): Median nerve somatosensory evoked potentials. Apomorphine-induced transient potentiation of frontal components in Parkinson's disease and in parkinsonism. *Electroencephalogr Clin Neurophysiol* 96(3):236–247.

Rothstein TL, Thomas EM, Sumi SM (1991): Predicting outcome in hypoxic-ischemic coma. A prospective clinical and electrophysiologic study. *Electroencephalogr Clin Neurophysiol* 79:101–107.

Rowed DW, McLean JAG, Tator Ch (1978): Somatosensory evoked potentials in acute spinal cord injury: Prognostic value. *Surg Neurol* 9:203–210.

Roy MW, Gilmore R, Walsh JW (1986a): Evaluation of children and young adults with tethered cord syndrome. Utility of spinal and scalp recorded somatosensory evoked potentials. *Surg Neurol* 26:241–248.

Roy MW, Gilmore R, Walsh JW (1986b): Somatosensory evoked potentials in tethered cord syndrome. *Electroencephalogr Clin Neurophysiol* 64:42P.

Rumpl E, Prugger M, Battista HJ, Badry F, Gerstenbrand F, Dienstl F (1988a): Short latency somatosensory evoked potentials and brain-stem auditory evoked potentials in coma due to CNS depressant drug poisoning. Preliminary observations. *Electroencephalogr Clin Neurophysiol* 70:482–489.

Rumpl E, Prugger M, Gerstenbrand F, Brunhuber W, Badry F, Hackl JM (1988b): Central somatosensory conduction time and acoustic brainstem transmission time in post-traumatic coma. *J Clin Neurophysiol* 5:237–260.

Russell GV (1958): Histologic alterations in thalamic nuclei of man following cortical lesions. *Texas Rep Biol Med* 16:483–492.

Saito T, Yamada T, Hasegawa A, Matsue Y, Emori T, Onishi H, Fuchigami T (1992): Recovery functions of common peroneal, posterior tibial and sural nerve somatosensory evoked potentials. *Electroencephalogr Clin Neurophysiol* 85:337–344.

Salar G, Iob I, Mingrino S (1982): Somatosensory evoked potentials before and after percutaneous thermocoagulation of the Gasserian ganglion for trigeminal neuralgia. In: *Clinical Applications of Evoked Potentials in Neurology,* edited by J Courjon, F Mauguiere, and M Revol, pp 359–365. Raven Press, New York.

Sances A, Larson SJ, Cusick JF, Myklebust J, Ewing CL, Jodat R, Ackmann JJ, Walsh P (1978): Early somatosensory evoked potentials. *Electroencephalogr Clin Neurophysiol* 45:505–514.

Santamaria J, Orteu N, Pujol M, Reolid A, Chimeno E, Solanas A (1994): Changes in median nerve short latency somatosensory evoked potentials during sleep in healthy adults. *Electroencephalogr Clin Neurophysiol* 91:63P.

Sarica Y, Karacan I (1986): Cerebral responses evoked by stimulation of the vesico-urethral junction in normal subjects. *Electroencephalogr Clin Neurophysiol* 65:440–446.

Sauer M, Schenck E (1977): Electrophysiologic investigations in Friedreich's heredoataxia and in hereditary motor and sensory neuropathy. *Electroencephalogr Clin Neurophysiol* 43:623.

Schieppati M, Ducati A (1984): Short-latency cortical potentials evoked by tactile air-jet stimulation of body and face in man. *Electroencephalogr Clin Neurophysiol* 58:418–424.

Sears TA, Bostock H (1981): Conduction failure in demyelination: Is it inevitable? In: *Demyelinating Disease: Basic and Clinical Electrophysiology,* edited by SG Waxman and JM Ritchie, pp 357–376. Raven Press, New York.

Sedgwick EM (1983): Pathophysiology and evoked potentials in multiple sclerosis. In: *Multiple Sclerosis: Pathology, Diagnosis and Management,* edited by JF Hallpike, et al. Williams and Wilkins, Baltimore.

Sedgwick EM, El-Negamy E, Frankel H (1980): Spinal cord potentials in traumatic paraplegia and quadriplegia. *J Neurol Neurosurg Psychiatry* 43:823–830.

Selwa LM, Vanderzant CW, Brunberg JA, Brewer GJ, Drury I, Beydoun A (1993): Correlation of evoked potential and MRI findings in Wilson's disease. *Neurology* 43:2059–2064.

Serra C, Rossi A, Palma V, Fusaro A, d'Angelillo A, Romano A (1981): Visual, auditory and somatosensory evoked potentials in uremic patients. *Electroencephalogr Clin Neurophysiol* 52:S14.

Seyal M, Browne JK (1989): Short latency somatosensory evoked potentials following mechanical taps to the face. Scalp recordings with a non-cephalic reference. *Electroencephalogr Clin Neurophysiol* 74(4):271–276.

Seyal M, Gabor AJ (1985): The human posterior tibial somatosensory evoked potential: Synapse dependent and synapse independent spinal components. *Electroencephalogr Clin Neurophysiol* 62:323–331.

Seyal M, Gabor AJ (1987): Generators of human spinal somatosensory evoked potentials. *J Clin Neurophysiol* 4(2):177–187.

Seyal M, Emerson RG, Pedley TA (1983): Spinal and early scalp-recorded components of the somatosensory evoked potential following stimulation of the posterior tibial nerve. *Electroencephalogr Clin Neurophysiol* 55:320–330.

Seyal M, Kraft LW, Gabor AJ (1987): Cervical synapse-dependent somatosensory evoked potential following posterior tibial nerve stimulation. *Neurology* 37:1417–1421.

Seyal M, Browne JK, Masuoka LK, Gabor AJ (1993): Enhancement of the amplitude of somatosensory evoked potentials following magnetic pulse stimulation of the human brain. *Electroencephalogr Clin Neurophysiol* 88(1):20–27.

Shibasaki H, Yamashita Y, Tsuji S (1977): Somatosensory evoked potentials. Diagnostic criteria and abnormalities in cerebral lesions. *J Neurol Sci* 34:427–439.

Shibasaki H, Yamashita Y, Kuroiwa Y (1978): Electroencephalographic studies of myoclonus. Myoclonus-related cortical spikes and high amplitude somatosensory evoked potentials. *Brain* 101:447–460.

Shibasaki H, Barrett G, Halliday E, Halliday AM (1980): Cortical potentials following voluntary and passive finger movements. *Electroencephalogr Clin Neurophysiol* 50:201–213.

Shibasaki H, Barrett G, Halliday E, Halliday AM (1981): Cortical potentials associated with voluntary foot movement in man. *Electroencephalogr Clin Neurophysiol* 52:507–516.

Shibasaki H, Kakigi R, Tsuji S, Kimura S (1982): Spinal and cortical somatosensory evoked potentials in Japanese patients with multiple sclerosis. *J Neurol Sci* 57:441–453.

Shibasaki H, Yamashita Y, Neshige R, Tobimatsu S, Fukui R (1985): Pathogenesis of giant somatosensory evoked potentials in progressive myoclonic epilepsy. *Brain* 108:225–240.

Shibasaki H, Nakamura M, Nishida S, Kakigi R, Ikeda A (1990): Wave form decomposition of 'giant SEP' and its computer model for scalp topography. *Electroencephalogr Clin Neurophysiol* 77(4):286–294.

Shibasaki H, Kakaigi R, Ikeda A (1991): Scalp topography of giant SEP and pre-myoclonus spike in cortical reflex myoclonus. *Electroencephalogr Clin Neurophysiol* 81:31–37.

Shimizu H, Shimoji K, Maruyama Y, Sato Y, Harayama H, Tsubaki T (1979): Slow cord dorsum potentials elicited by descending volleys in man. *J Neurol Neurosurg Psychiatry* 42:242–246.

Shimizu H, Shimoji K, Maruyama Y, Matsuki M, Kuribayashi H, Fujioka H (1982): Human spinal cord potentials produced in lumbosacral enlargement by descending volleys. *J Neurol* 48:1108–1120.

Shimoji K, Shimizu H, Maruyama Y (1978): Origin of somatosensory evoked responses recorded from the cervical skin surface. *J Neurosurg* 48:980–984.

Siivola J, Jarvilehto M (1982): Spinal evoked potentials evaluated with two relevant electrode types. *Acta Physiol Scand* 115:103–107.

Singh N, Sachdev KK, Brisman R (1982): Trigeminal nerve stimulation: Short latency somatosensory evoked potentials. *Neurology* 32:97–101.

Sitzoglou C, Fotiou F (1985): A study of the maturation of the somatosensory pathway by evoked potentials. *Neuropediatrics* 16:205–208.

Slimp JC, Tamas LB, Stolov WC, Wyler AR (1986): Somatosensory evoked potentials after removal of somatosensory cortex in man. *Electroencephalogr Clin Neurophysiol* 65:111–117.

Small M, Matthews WB (1984): A method of calculating spinal cord transit time from potentials evoked by tibial nerve stimulation in normal subjects and in patients with spinal cord disease. *Electroencephalogr Clin Neurophysiol* 59:156–164.

Small DG, Matthews WB, Small M (1978): The cervical somatosensory evoked potential (SEP) in the diagnosis of multiple sclerosis. *J Neurol Sci* 35:211–224.

Small DG, Beauchamp M, Matthews WB (1980): Subcortical SEPs in normal man and in patients with CNS lesions. *Prog Clin Neurophysiol* 7:190–204.

Smith T, Zeeberg I, Sjo O (1986): Evoked potentials in multiple sclerosis before and after high-dose methylprednisolone infusion. *Eur Neurol* 25:67–73.

Smith T, Jakobsen J, Gaub J, Helweg-Larsen S, Trojaborg W (1988): Clinical electrophysiological studies of human immunodeficiency virus-seropositive men without AIDS. *Ann Neurol* 23:295–297.

Snowden ML, Haselkorn JK, Kraft GH, Bronstein AD, Bigos SJ, Slimp JC, Stolov WC (1992): Dermatomal somatosensory evoked potentials in the diagnosis of lumbosacral spinal stenosis: Comparison with imaging studies. *Muscle Nerve* 15:1036–1044.

Snyder BGE, Holliday TA (1984): Pathways of ascending evoked spinal cord potentials of dogs. *Electroencephalogr Clin Neurophysiol* 58:140–154.

Sonoo M, Shimpo T, Genba K, Kunimoto M, Mannen T (1990): Posterior cervical N13 in median nerve SEP has two components. *Electroencephalogr Clin Neurophysiol* 77(1):28–38.

Sonoo M, Sakuta M, Shimpo T, Genba K, Mannen T (1991a): Widespread N18 in median nerve SEP is preserved in a pontine lesion. *Electroencephalogr Clin Neurophysiol* 80(3):238–240.

Sonoo M, Shimpo T, Takeda K, Genba K, Nakano I, Mannen T (1991b): SEPs in two patients with localized lesions of the poscentral gyrus. *Electroencephalogr Clin Neurophysiol* 80(6): 536–546.

Sonoo M, Genba K, Iwatsubo T, Mannen T (1992a): P15 in tibial nerve SEPs as an example of the junctional potential. *Electroencephalogr Clin Neurophysiol* 84:486–491.

Sonoo M, Genba K, Zai W, Iwata M, Mannen T, Kanazawa I (1992b): Origin of the widespread N18 in median nerve SEP. *Electroencephalogr Clin Neurophysiol* 84(5):418–425.

Soustiel JF, Feinsod M, Hafner H (1991): Short latency trigeminal evoked potentials: normative data and clinical correlations. *Electroencephalogr Clin Neurophysiol* 80(2):119–125.

Spielholz NI, Benjamin MV, Engler G, Ransohoff J (1979): Somatosensory evoked potentials and clinical outcome in spinal cord injury. In: *Neural Trauma*, edited by AJ Popp, pp 217–222. Raven Press, New York.

Spudis EV (1983): Value of N20 evoked response in acute sensory stroke. *Stroke* 14:634–635.

Spudis EV, Fullerton W, Fernandez H, Green P, Tatum T, Howard G (1980): Somatosensory central latencies and disc discrimination in multiple sclerosis. *Clin Electroencephalogr* 11:48–56.

Starr A, McKeon B, Skuse N, Burke D (1981): Cerebral potentials evoked by muscle stretch in man. *Brain* 104:149–166.

Stejskal L, Sobota J (1985): Somatosensory evoked potentials in patients with occlusions of cerebral arteries. *Electroencephalogr Clin Neurophysiol* 61:482–490.

Stewart WA, Hall LD, Berry K, et al (1986): Magnetic resonance imaging (MRI) in multiple sclerosis (MS): Pathological correlation studies in eight cases. *Neurology* 36:320.

Stohr M, Petruch F (1979): Somatosensory evoked potentials following stimulation of the trigeminal nerve in man. *J Neurol* 220:95–98.

Stohr M, Petruch F, Schleglmann K (1981): Somatosensory evoked potentials following trigeminal nerve stimulation in trigeminal neuralgia. *Ann Neurol* 9:63–66.

Stohr M, Buettner UW, Riffel B, Koletzki E (1982): Spinal somatosensory evoked potentials in cervical cord lesions. *Electroencephalogr Clin Neurophysiol* (in press).

Straumanis JJ, Shagass C (1976): Electrophysiological effects of triiodothyronine and propranolol. *Psychopharmacologia (Berlin)* 46:283–288.

Sutton LN, Frewen JT, Marsh R, Jaggi J, Bruce DA (1982): The effects of deep barbiturate coma on multimodality evoked potentials. *J Neurosurg* 57:178–185.

Suzuki I, Mayanagi Y (1984): Intracranial recording of short latency somatosensory evoked potentials in man: Identification of origin of each component. *Electroencephalogr Clin Neurophysiol* 59:286–296.

Suzuki I, Mayanagi Y, Sano S (1982): Intracranial recordings of short-latency somatosensory evoked potentials. *Appl Neurophysiol* 45:410–412.

Symon L, Hargadine J, Zawirski M, Branston N (1979): Central conduction time as an index of ischaemia in subarachnoid haemorrhage. *J Neurol Sci* 44:95–103.

Synek VM (1986): Diagnostic importance of somatosensory evoked potentials in the diagnosis of thoracic outlet syndrome. *Clin Electroencephalogr* 17:112–116.

Synek VM (1986c): Validity of median nerve somatosensory evoked potentials in the diagnosis of supraclavicular plexus lesions. *Electroencephalogr Clin Neurophysiol* 65:27–35.

Tackmann W, Strenge H, Barth R, Sojka-Raytscheff A (1980): Evaluation of various brain structures in multiple sclerosis with multimodality evoked potentials, blink reflex and nystagmography. *J Neurol* 224:33–46.

Tackmann W, Ettlin T, Strenge H (1982): Multimodality evoked potentials and electrically elicited blink reflex in optic neuritis. *J Neurol* 227:157–163.

Takahashi K, Fujitani Y (1970): Somatosensory and visual evoked potentials in hyperthyroidism. *Electroencephalogr Clin Neurophysiol* 29:551–556.

Takahashi K, Okada E, Fujitani Y (1972): [Somatosensory and visual evoked potentials in Huntington's Chorea.] *Rinsho Shinkeigakku* 12(8):381–385.

Tandan R, Bradley WG (1985): Amyotrophic lateral sclerosis. I. Clinical features, pathology and ethical issues in management. II. Etiopathogenesis. *Ann Neurol* 18:271–280, 419–431.

Taylor MJ, Chan-Lui WY (1985): Longitudinal evoked potential studies in hereditary ataxias. *Can J Neurol Sci* 12:100–105.

Taylor MJ, Fagan ER (1988): SEPs to median nerve stimulation: Normative data for paediatrics. *Electroencephalogr Clin Neurophysiol* 71:323–330.

Taylor MJ, Farrell EJ (1989): Comparison of the prognostic utility of VEPs and SEPs in comatose children. *Pediatr Neurol* 5:145–150.

Taylor MJ, Borrett DS, Coles JC (1985): The effects of profound hypothermia on the cervical SEP in humans: Evidence of dual generators. *Electroencephalogr Clin Neurophysiol* 62:184–192.

Thomas PK, Jeffreys JGR, Smith IS, Loulakis D (1981): Spinal somatosensory evoked potentials in hereditary spastic paraplegia. *J Neurol Neurosurg Psychiatry* 44:243–246.

Tinazzi M, Mauguiere F (1995): Assessment of intraspinal and intracranial conduction by P30 and P39 tibial nerve somatosensory evoked potentials in cervical cord, brainstem, and hemispheric lesions. *J Clin Neurophysiol* 12(3):237–253.

Tobimatsu S, Fukui R, Kato M, Kobayashi T, Kuroiwa Y (1985): Multimodality evoked potentials in patients and carriers with adrenoleukodystrophy and adrenomyeloneuropathy. *Electroencephalogr Clin Neurophysiol* 62: 18–24.

Tomberg C, Desmedt JE, Ozaki I (1991a): Right or left ear reference changes the boltage of frontal and parietal somatosensory evoked potentials. *Electroencephalogr Clin Neurophysiol* 80(6)504–512.

Tomberg C, Desmedt JE, Ozaki I, Noel P (1991b): Nasopharyngeal recordings of somatosensory evoked potentials document the medullary origin of the N18 far-field. *Electroencephalogr Clin Neurophysiol* 80:496–503.

Tomita Y, Nishimura S, Tanaka T (1986): Short latency SEPs in infants and children: Developmental changes and maturational index of SEPs. *Electroencephalogr Clin Neurophysiol* 65:335–343.

Tomita Y, Tanaka T, Kamimura N, Shimozawa N, Takashima S, Takeshita K (1988): Origin and clinical significance of subcortical components in short-latency somatosensory evoked potentials in children. *Electroencephalogr Clin Neurophysiol* 69:199–208.

Torok B, Meyer M, Wildberger H (1992): The influence of pattern size on amplitude, latency and wave form of retinal and cortical potentials elicited by checkerboard pattern reversal and stimulus onset-offset. *Electroencephalogr Clin Neurophysiol* 84:13–19.

Trojaborg W, Jorgensen EO (1973): Evoked cortical potentials in patients with "isoelectric" EEGs. *Electroencephalogr Clin Neurophysiol* 35:301–309.

Trojaborg W, Peterson E (1979): Visual and somatosensory evoked cortical potentials in multiple sclerosis. *J Neurol Neurosurg Psychiatry* 42:323–330.

Trojaborg W, Bottcher J, Saxtrup O (1981): Evoked potentials and immunoglobulin abnormalities in multiple sclerosis. *Neurology* 31:866–871.

Tsuji S, Murai Y (1986): Scalp topography and distribution of cortical somatosensory evoked potentials to median nerve stimulation. *Electroencephalogr Clin Neurophysiol* 65(6):429–439.

Tsuji S, Shibasaki H, Kato M, Kuroiwa Y, Shima F (1984): Subcortical, thalamic and cortical somatosensory evoked potentials to median nerve stimulation. *Electroencephalogr Clin Neurophysiol* 59:465–476.

Tsuji S, Murai Y, Kadoya C (1988): Topography of somatosensory evoked potentials to median nerve stimulation in patients with cerebral lesions. *Electroencephalogr Clin Neurophysiol* 71:280–288.

Tsumoto T, Hirose N, Nonaka S, Takahashi M (1972): Analysis of somatosensory evoked potentials to lateral popliteal nerve stimulation in man. *Electroencephalogr Clin Neurophysiol* 33:379–388.

Tsumoto T, Hirose N, Nonaka S, Takahashi M (1973): Cerebrovascular disease: Changes in somatosensory evoked potentials associated with unilateral lesions. *Electroencephalogr Clin Neurophysiol* 35:463–473.

Turano G, Jones SJ, Miller DH, Du Boulay GH, Kakigi R, McDonald WI (1991): Correlation of SEP abnormalities with brain and cervical cord MRI in multiple sclerosis. *Brain* 114:663–681.

Udani V, Cracco JB, Hittelman J, Hotson G, Fikrig S (1988): Clinical and developmental evaluation, evoked potentials and MRI in pediatric AIDS. *Electroencephalogr Clin Neurophysiol* 69:87P.

Ugawa Y, Genba K, Shimpo T, Mannen T (1991): Somatosensory evoked potential recovery (SEP-R) in myoclonic patients. *Electroencephalogr Clin Neurophysiol* 80(1):21–25.

Uncini A, Treviso M, Basciani M, Gambi D (1987): Strumpell's familial spastic paraplegia: An electrophysiological demonstration of selective central distal axonpathy. *Electroencephalogr Clin Neurophysiol* 66:132–136.

Urasaki E, Wada S, Kadoya C, Matsuzaki H, Yokota A, Matsuoka S (1988): Absence of spinal N13-P13 and normal scalp far-field P14 in a patient with syringomyelia. *Electroencephalogr Clin Neurophysiol* 71:400–404.

Urasaki E, Wada S, Kadoya C, Yokata A, Matsuoka S (1990a): Spinal intramedullary recording of human somatosensory evoked potentials. *Electroencephalogr Clin Neurophysiol* 77(3):233–236.

Urasaki E, Wada S, Kadoya C, Yokota A, Matsuoka S, Shima F (1990b): Origin of scalp far-field N18 of SSEPs in response to median nerve stimulation. *Electroencephalogr Clin Neurophysiol* 77(1):39–51.

Urasaki E, Wada S, Kadoya C, Tokimura T, Yokota A, Yamamoto S, Fukumura A, Hamada S (1992): Amplitude abnormalities in the scalp far-field N18 of SSEPs to median nerve stimulation in patients with midbrain-pontine lesion. *Electroencephalogr Clin Neurophysiol* 84:232–242.

Urasaki E, Tokimura T, Yasukouchi H, Wada S-i, Yokota A (1993a): P30 and N33 of posterior tibial nerve SSEPs are analogous to P14 and N18 of median nerve SSEPs. *Electroencephalogr Clin Neurophysiol* 88(6): 525–529.

Urasaki E, Uematsu S, Lesser RP (1993b): Short latency somatosensory evoked potentials recorded around the human upper brain-stem. *Electroencephalogr Clin Neurophysiol* 88(2):92–104.

van Buggenhout E, Ketelaer P, Carton H (1982): Success and failure of evoked potentials in detecting clinical and subclinical lesions in multiple sclerosis patients. *Clin Neurol Neurosurg* 84:3–14.

Vas GA, Cracco JB, Cracco RQ (1981): Scalp-recorded short latency cortical and subcortical somatosensory evoked potentials to peroneal nerve stimulation. *Electroencephalogr Clin Neurophysiol* 52:1–8.

Vaziri D, Pratt H, Saiki JK, Starr A (1981): Evaluation of somatosensory pathway by short latency evoked potentials in patients with end-stage renal disease maintained on hemodialysis. *Int J Artif Organs* 4:17–22.

Veale JL, Mark RF, Rees S (1973): Differential sensitivity of motor and sensory fibres in human ulnar nerve. *J Neurol Neurosurg Psychiatry* 36:75–86.

Vera CL, Perot PL, Fountain EL (1983): Scalp recorded somatosensory evoked potentials to posterior tibial nerve stimulation in humans. *Electroencephalogr Clin Neurophysiol* 56:159–168.

Veilleux M, Stevens JC (1987): Syringomyelia: Electrophysiological aspects. *Muscle and Nerve* 10:449–458.

Vodusek DB (1990): Pudendal SEP and bulbocavernsosus reflex in women. *Electroencephalogr Clin Neurophysiol* 77(2):134–136.

Vogel P, Vogel H (1982): Somatosensory cortical potentials evoked by stimulation of leg nerves: Analysis of normal values and variability; diagnostic significance. *J Neurol* 228:97–111.

Vogel P, Ruber P, Klein R (1986): The latency difference of the tibial and sural nerve SEP: Peripheral versus central factors. *Electroencephalogr Clin Neurophysiol* 65:269–275.

Wagner W (1991): SEP testing in deeply comatose and brain dead patients: the role of nasopharyngeal, scalp and earlobe erivations in recording the P14 potential. *Electroencephalogr Clin Neurophysiol* 80:352–363.

Walk D, Fisher MA, Doundoulakis SH, Hemmati M (1992): Somatosensory evoked potentials in the evaluation of lumbosacral radiculopathy. *Neurology* 42:1197–1202.

Walker AE, Diamond EL, Moseley J (1975): The neuropathological findings in irreversible coma. *J Neuropathol Exp Neurol* 34:295–323.

Wall PD, Noordenbos W (1977): Sensory functions which remain in man after complete transection of dorsal columns. *Brain* 100:641–653.

Walser H, Emre M, Janzer R (1986): Somatosensory evoked potentials in comatose patients: correlation with outcome and neuropathological findings. *J Neurol* 233:34–40.

Walsh JC, Garrick R, Cameron J, McLeod JG (1982): Evoked potential changes in clinically definite multiple sclerosis: A two year follow up study. *J Neurol Neurosurg Psychiatry* 45:494–500.

Wang L, Cohen LG, Hallett M (1989): Scalp topography of somatosensory evoked potentials following electrical stimulation of femoral nerve. *Electroencephalogr Clin Neurophysiol* 74(2):112–123.

Waxman SG (1981): Clinicopathological correlations in multiple sclerosis and related diseases. In: *Demyelinating Disease: Basic and Clinical Electrophysiology*, edited by SG Waxman and JM Ritchie, pp 169–182. Raven Press, New York.

Waxman SG, Ritchie JM (1981): Electrophysiology of demyelinating diseases: Future directions and questions. In: *Demyelinating Disease: Basic and Clinical Electrophysiology*, edited by SG Waxman and JM Ritchie, pp 511–514. Raven Press, New York.

Webster KE (1977): Somaesthetic pathways. *Br Med Bull* 33:113–120.

Weerasinghe V, Sedgwick M (1994): Effect of manipulation and fractionated finger movements on subcortical sensory activity in man. *Electroencephalogr Clin Neurophysiol* 92(6):527–535.

Weiner HL, Dawson DM (1980): Plasmapheresis in multiple sclerosis: A preliminary study. *Neurology* 30:1029–1033.

White LE, Frank LM, Furgiuele TL, Montes JE, Etheridge JE (1985): Childhood coma: Improved prediction of outcome with somatosensory and brainstem auditory evoked potentials. *Ann Neurol* 18:417.

Wiederholt WC (1978): Recovery function of short latency components of surface and depth recorded somatosensory evoked potentials in the cat. *Electroencephalogr Clin Neurophysiol* 45:259–267.

Wiederholt WC, Iragui-Madoz VJ (1977): Far field somatosensory potentials in the rat. *Electroencephalogr Clin Neurophysiol* 42:456–465.

Williamson PD, Goff WR, Allison T (1970): Somatosensory evoked responses in patients with unilateral cerebral lesions. *Electroencephalogr Clin Neurophysiol* 28:566–575.

Willis J (1986): Effects of state and stimulus rate on short latency somatosensory evoked potentials in infants. *Ann Neurol* 20:411.

Willis J, Seales D, Frazier E (1984): Short latency somatosensory evoked potentials in infants. *Electroencephalogr Clin Neurophysiol* 59:366–373.

Willis J, Duncan C, Bell R (1987): Short latency somatosensory evoked potentials in perinatal asphyxia. *Pediatr Neurol* 3:203–207.

Wilson SL, Brooks EB, Chiappa KH (1981): Scalp and spinal short-latency somatosensory evoked potentials following lower extremity stimulation in normal subjects. *Electroencephalogr Clin Neurophysiol* 51:40P.

Wood CC, Spencer DD, Allison T, McCarthy G, Williamson PD, Goff WR (1988): Localization of human sensorimotor cortex during surgery by cortical surface recording of somatosensory evoked potentials. *J Neurosurg* 68:99–111.

Wulff CH, Trojaborg W (1985): Adult metachromatic leukodystrophy: Neurophysiologic findings. *Neurology* 35:1776–1778.

Wyrtzes LM, Chatrian G-E, Shaw C-M, Wirch AL (1989): Acute failure of forebrain with sparing of brain-stem function. Electroencephalographic, multimodality evoked potential, and pathologic findings. *Arch Neurol* 46:93–97.

Yakovlev P, Lecours A (1967): The myelogenetic cycle of regional maturation of the brain. In: *Regional Development of the Brain in Early Life*, edited by A Minkowski, pp 3–69. F. A. Davis, Philadelphia.

Yamada T, Kimura J, Nitz DM (1980): Short latency somatosensory evoked potentials following median nerve stimulation in man. *Electroencephalogr Clin Neurophysiol* 48:367–376.

Yamada T, Muroga T, Kimura J (1981): Tourniquet-induced ischemia and somatosensory evoked potentials. *Neurology* 31:1524–1529.

Yamada T, Machida M, Kimura J (1982a): Far-field somatosensory evoked potentials after stimulation of the tibial nerve. *Neurology* 32:1151–1158.

Yamada T, Shivapour E, Wilkinson JT, Kimura J (1982b): Short- and long-latency somatosensory evoked potentials in multiple sclerosis. *Arch Neurol* 39:88–94.

Yamada T, Kayamori R, Kimura J, Beck DO (1984): Topography of somatosensory evoked potentials after stimulation of the median nerve. *Electroencephalogr Clin Neurophysiol* 59:29–43.

Yamada T, Machida M, Oishi M, Kimura A, Kimura J, Rodritzky RL (1985): Stationary negative potentials near the source vs. positive far-field potentials at a distance. *Electroencephalogr Clin Neurophysiol* 60:509–524.

Yamada T, Ishida T, Kudo Y, Rodnitzky RL, Kimura J (1986): Clinical correlates of abnormal P14 in median SEPs. *Neurology* 36:765–771.

Yamada T, Kameyama S, Fuchigami Y, Nakazumi Y, Dickins QS, Kimura J (1988): Changes of short latency somatosensory evoked potential in sleep. *Electroencephalogr Clin Neurophysiol* 70:126–136.

Yamada T, Rodnitzky RL, Kameyama S, Matsuoka H, Kimura J (1991): Alteration of SEP topography in Huntington's patients and their relatives at risk. *Electroencephalogr Clin Neurophysiol* 80(4):251–261.

Yamauchi N, Okazari N, Sato T et al (1976): The effects of electrical acupuncture on human somatosensory evoked potentials and spontaneous brain waves. *Yonago Acta Med* 20:88–100.

Yanagihara R (1982): Heavy metals and essential minerals in motor neuron diseases. In: *Human Motor Neuron Diseases. Advances in Neurology,* Vol 36, edited by LP Rowland, pp 233–247. Raven Press, New York.

Yasuhara A, Yamada T, Seki Y, Emori T, Vachatimanont P, Andoh K, Ando M, Ross M, Kimura J (1990): Presence of two subcomponents in P9 far-field potential following stimulation of the median nerve. *Electroencephalogr Clin Neurophysiol* 77:93–100.

Yiannikas C (1983a): Cervical radiculopathies. In: *Evoked Potentials in Clinical Medicine,* edited by KH Chiappa, pp 281–285. Raven Press, New York.

Yiannikas C (1983b): Spinal components of tibial somatosensory evoked potentials. In: *Evoked Potentials in Clinical Medicine,* edited by KH Chiappa, pp 240–241 and Fig. 6–14. Raven Press, New York.

Yiannikas C, Shahani BT (1988): The origins of lumbosacral spinal evoked potentials in humans using a surface electrode recording technique. *J Neurol* 51:499–508.

Yiannikas C, Shahani BT, Young RR (1986): Short-latency somatosensory-evoked potentials from radial, median, ulnar and peroneal nerve stimulation in the assessment of cervical spondylosis. *Arch Neurol* 43:1264–1271.

Youl BD, Adams RW, Lance JW (1991): Parietal sensory loss simulating a peripheral lesion, documented by somatosensory evoked potentials. *Neurology* 41:152–154.

Young W (1982): Correlation of somatosensory evoked potentials and neurological findings in spinal cord injury. In: *Early Management of Acute Spinal Cord Injury,* edited by CH Tator, pp 153–165. Raven Press, New York.

Zarola F, Rossini PM (1991): Nerve, spinal cord and brain somatosensory evoked responses: a comparative study during electrical and magnetic peripheral nerve stimulation. *Electroencephalogr Clin Neurophysiol* 80:372–377.

Zegers de Beyl D, Brunko E (1995): Thoughts about the IFCN recommendations for the recording of short latency somatosensory evoked potentials. *Electroencephalogr Clin Neurophysiol* 94:151–152.

Zegers de Beyl D, Borenstein S, Dufaye P (1984): Irreversible cortical damage in acute postanoxic coma: Predictive value of somatosensory-evoked potentials. *Transplant Proc* 26(1):98–101.

Zegers de Beyl D, Delberghe X, Herbaut AG, Brunko E (1988): The somatosensory central conduction time: Physiological considerations and normative data. *Electroencephalogr Clin Neurophysiol* 71:17–26.

Zeman BD, Yiannikas C (1989): Functional prognosis in stroke: use of somatosensory evoked potentials. *J Neurol Neurosurg Psychiatry* 52:242–247.

Zhu Y, Georgesco M, Cadilhac J (1987): Normal latency values of early cortical somatosensory evoked potentials in children. *Electroencephalogr Clin Neurophysiol* 68:471–474.

Zhuravin IA, Dobrylko AK, Kadantseva AG, Tolkunov BF (1981): Effect of local cooling of the cortex on evoked potentials in the reticular formation in response to somatosensory stimulation. *Neurophysiology* 13:25–30.

Ziganow S, Rowed DW (1980): The cortical somatosensory evoked potential in acute spinal cord injuries. Presented at the International Symposium on Clinical Applications of Evoked Potentials in Neurology. Lyon (France), October 16 and 17, 1980.

Zornow MH, Grafe MR, Tybor C, Swenson MR (1990): Preservation of evoked potentials in a case of anterior spinal artery syndrome. *Electroencephalogr Clin Neurophysiol* 77:137–139.

Evoked Potentials in Clinical Medicine,
3d ed., edited by Keith H. Chiappa.
Lippincott–Raven Publishers, Philadelphia © 1997.

10

Short-Latency Somatosensory Evoked Potentials in Peripheral Nerve Lesions, Plexopathies, and Radiculopathies

Con Yiannikas

Department of Neurology, Concord Hospital, Concord NSW 2137, Sydney, Australia

1. INTRODUCTION

The assessment of pathology affecting the proximal segment of nerves at a root or plexus level can be difficult. Electrophysiologic assessment is important in determining the site of the lesion, the level (pre- or postganglionic), and the presence of functional continuity. Conventional electromyography (EMG) may be of use particularly when assessing muscles that receive their supply directly from the roots (paraspinals, serratus anterior) or plexus (trunks, e.g., supraspinatus, rhomboids) or by determining the pattern of involvement which may reflect pathology of a particular part of the plexus and differentiate it from peripheral nerve pathology (e.g., tibialis anterior, tibialis posterior, and gluteus medius in an L5 lesion). However, EMG cannot differentiate between pre-and postganglionic involvement and active denervation may be absent in the presence of conduction block or in the first 4 or 5 days after injury.

Sensory nerve action potentials (SNAPs) may be useful in localizing root or plexus pathology. Ferrante and Wilbourn (1995) reviewed the localizing value of the medial antebrachial, lateral antebrachial, radial, median D1, D2, and D3, and ulnar D5 SNAPs and were able to predict with some accuracy pathology affecting the C6–T1 roots and the various components of the plexus. Despite these findings the method is indirect and the absence of a SNAP does not necessarily mean loss of axonal continuity. Furthermore, the SNAP may be preserved early on and is normal in the presence of conduction block.

Somatosensory evoked potentials (SEPs) have the advantage of assessing conduction across the lesion, therefore providing more accurate information regarding axonal continuity, conduction block, and the ganglionic level. In addition the amplification effect of the central nervous system (CNS) allows the recording of an SEP when the SNAPs may be unobtainable. This confers greater sensitivity in detecting axonal continuity and early nerve regeneration.

2. PERIPHERAL NERVE LESIONS

The SEP may be used to document sensory nerve continuity when SNAPS are unrecordable because they are too small or too desynchronized or both. The ability to elicit an SEP in the absence of a SNAP implies that incoming peripheral volleys have been amplified within the central nervous system (Eisen et al., 1982). Stimulation of the sensory nerve at two sites allows the estimation of conduction velocity by subtracting the latencies of the N19 peaks.

The neuropathies most extensively studied have been Charcot–Marie–Tooth and Friedreich's ataxia (see Chapter 9, Section 3.4, for further discussion). This technique has also been used in the assessment of spinal cord sensory involvement in nutritional neuropathy such as B_{12} deficiency (Jones et al., 1987) and in diabetes (Cracco et al., 1980; Nakumara et al., 1992; Ziegler et al., 1993; Palma et al., 1994). Pozzessere et al. (1988) suggested SEPs were useful in detecting early involvement of the peripheral nervous system of patients with diabetes prior to the clinical appearance. In severe traumatic lesions of peripheral nerves SNAPS may not be recordable for many months. The presence of SEPs would provide clear evidence for axonal continuity and, by using different stimulation sites, the rate of regeneration can be determined (Desmedt and Noel, 1973).

In Guillain–Barré syndrome (GBS) SEPs can detect slowing in proximal segments of peripheral nerves in the presence of normal conduction distally. Walsh et al. (1984) and Brown and Feasby (1984) found an increase in Erb's point (EP)–P/N13 conduction time and/or reduction in amplitude and dispersion of P/N13 in 12 of 17 (71%) and 10 of 11 (99%) of their cases, respectively, In both studies this was abnormal at times when motor and sensory velocities over more distal segments were normal. Furthermore, it was suggested by Walsh et al. (1984) that the yield from SEPs were higher than measuring F-wave latencies. Ropper and Chiappa (1986) found abnormalities in 10 of 21 median SEPs (47%) but noted a higher yield from lower-limb nerve studies (75%). Significantly, all patients with abnormal SEPs had abnormal F-waves and some patients with normal SEPs had abnormal F-waves. This difference in the relative sensitivity of SEPs versus F-waves may be related to the method of analysis of the F-waves; Walsh et al. looked only at minimal latencies, whereas Ropper and Chiappa measured other parameters, such as persistence and chronodispersion, that may have increased the abnormality rate, particularly in the first 2 weeks when conduction block is the major finding. Our further experience has shown that occasional patients may have normal F-wave studies (using all parameters) and still have abnormal SEPs, particularly early in their course. This finding has been supported by Vasjar et al. (1992), who studied 23 children with GBS and found that SEPs, particularly from the lower limbs, were more sensitive in detecting abnormality early in the disease than nerve conduction studies and F-wave analysis. Similarly Gilmore and Nelson (1989) found greater abnormalities in tibial nerve SEPs than from F-waves from the same nerve.

The most common finding suggestive of proximal nerve demyelination is an increase in EP–P/N13 conduction time and less frequently the P/N13 may be absent with a delayed EP–P/N19 conduction time. The central conduction time is usually normal. Figure 10–1 illustrates the SEP from a 47-year-old female who developed acute, progressive weakness 2 weeks after an acute viral illness. Physical examination revealed generalized weakness of upper and lower limbs with a mild distal sensory loss. Electromyography and peripheral

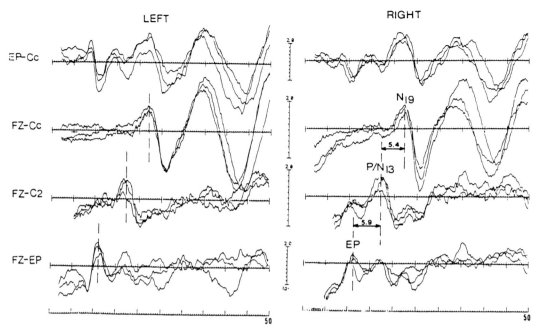

FIG. 10–1. Median SEPs from a patient with GBS demonstrating bilateral prolongation of EP–P/N13 IPLs (L = 6.0 msec; R = 5.9 msec versus an upper limit of normal of 5.2 msec—see Table 10–1) with normal P/N13–N19 IPLs (5.1 and 5.4 msec on left and right sides, respectively). In the presence of normal sensory conduction distally these findings suggest sensory conduction abnormalities at the root or proximal plexus level. Each trace is an average of 500 stimuli. Calibrations are in microvolts.

nerve conduction studies were consistent with a generalized motor neuropathy; SNAPs were normal. On median nerve stimulation SEPs demonstrated bilateral prolongation of EP–P/N13 conduction time with normal central conduction. In the presence of normal forearm conduction in the median nerve, the SEPs suggested a proximal conduction defect. Subsequent clinical course confirmed the diagnosis of GBS. Figure 10–2 illustrates the median and tibial SEPs from a 63-year-old male with progressive weakness and minor patchy sensory loss. The nerve conduction studies for the median nerve showed velocities at the lower limits of normal, but the F-waves were markedly delayed. The median SEPs show normal conduction to Erb's point but absent spinal potentials and delayed responses from the scalp suggesting demyelination at a radicular level.

It is clear that SEPs can demonstrate proximal conduction defects, even in the presence of normal distal conduction. Although F-wave studies demonstrate abnormal proximal conduction in the large majority of GBS patients, occasionally SEPs may reveal proximal abnormalities despite normal F-waves; in selected patients they should be performed in addition to F-waves. Presumably this differential involvement is because the SEPs assess a different fiber population.

Somatosensory EPs have also been used to investigate peripheral and central conduction in hereditary pressure-sensitive neuropathies (Ebner et al., 1981; Strenge et al., 1982) and chronic acquired demyelinating neuropathy (Parry and Aminoff, 1987).

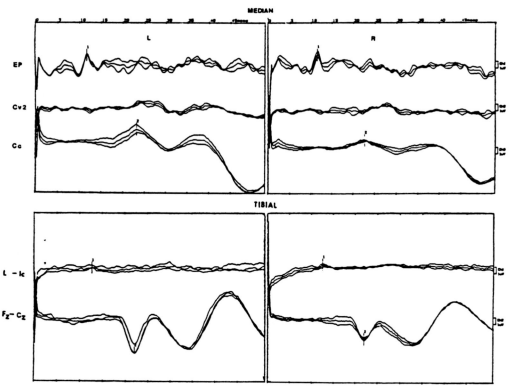

FIG. 10–2. Median and tibial SEPs from a patient with GBS. The median studies demonstrate normal conduction up to Erb's point (1 = EP) but absent P/N13 potentials bilaterally and prolonged EP–N19 (2 = N19) conduction time (11.4, 11.3 msec). These features are consistent with demyelination at a dorsal root level. The tibial SEPs show delayed, poorly formed spinal potentials (1 = N20 or LP) (25.6, 25.2 msec) but normal central conduction time (2 = P37) (N20–P37 was 18.8, 18.4 msec), consistent with pathology at or distal to the dorsal roots. Each trace is an average of 512 stimuli, with two superimposed and a mean trace. Median nerve channels referred to FZ. *L*, L1; *Ic*, iliac crest. Sweep duration of tibial EP was 100 msec. Calibration bars are 1μV.

3. BRACHIAL PLEXUS AND CERVICAL ROOT TRAUMA

The brachial plexus and associated spinal roots (C8–T1) are particularly prone to traction injury. The extent of location of the lesion is an important factor in assessing the prognosis of these cases (Table 10–1). A rupture proximal to the dorsal root ganglion carries a poor prognosis in comparison to postganglionic lesion, which may recover spontaneously when the nerves remain in continuity or are surgically repaired. It is thus important to establish the location of the lesion and to attempt to document the presence of functional continuity as accurately as possible. Conventional EMG may be of help in this assessment. The presence of SNAPs on peripheral nerve stimulation suggests continuity between sensory axons and their cell bodies in the dorsal nerve root ganglia (Bonney and Gilliatt, 1958), and, in association with anesthesia in the appropriate segments, suggests preganglionic pathology. In addition, the lack of motor units under voluntary control and the presence of features consistent with active denervation, particularly in muscles that receive their nerve supply di-

TABLE 10–1. *Plexus and root relationships for the peripheral nerves commonly used in SEP testing*

Nerve	Plexus		Root afferents
	Cords	Trunks	
Median	Lateral	Upper	C6–7—Cutaneous
	Medial	Middle	
		Lower	C8–T1—Muscle
Ulnar	Medial	Lower	C8—Cutaneous
			C8–T1—Muscle
Superficial radial	Posterior	Upper	C6—Cutaneous
Musculocutaneous	Lateral	Upper	C5–6—Cutaneous
Posterior tibial (popliteal fossa)			L4–S2—Cutaneous
			L4–S2—Muscle
Posterior tibial (ankle)			L4–S2—Cutaneous
			S1–2—Muscle
Common peroneal			L4–5—Cutaneous
			L4–S1—Muscle
Sural			S1–2—Cutaneous
Saphenous			L3–4—Cutaneous
Superficial peroneal			L4–5—Cutaneous

rectly from spinal roots (paraspinals, serratus anterior), may also help in the assessment of functional continuity of the ventral roots and in the localization of the lesion.

Despite the usefulness of peripheral nerve sensory potentials in the localization of dorsal root plexus pathology, the method is indirect and the absence of SNAPs does not necessarily mean loss of continuity in all axons. Furthermore, at an early stage of Wallerian degeneration the inevitable preservation of peripheral sensory potentials and the absence of denervation on EMG may be misleading as to the site of the lesion (i.e., preganglionic or postganglionic) and as to the presence of functional continuity. Gilliatt and Hjorth (1972) showed that motor fibers continued to conduct for 4 or 5 days after peroneal nerve section (baboon), and sensory fibers for an additional 2 to 3 days. Other workers (Salafsky and Jasinski, 1967; Harris and Thesleff, 1972) have demonstrated that these changes are related to the length of the isolated section of nerve. In this situation, recording the potentials at Erb's point (closer to the site of the lesion) or the cervical spine and somatosensory cortex (proximal to the site of the lesion) would provide early information on the characteristics of the lesion, that is, distal or proximal to the spinal ganglion, and whether or not there is functional continuity of sensory axons.

A number of early workers (Zalis et al., 1970; Zverina and Kredba, 1977) effectively combined somatosensory cerebral evoked potentials (SCEPs) and SNAPs in the assessment of brachial plexus injuries, but their numbers of patients were small and failure to record a cervical potential made the exclusion of an additional central lesion difficult. Rosen et al. (1977) described two cases where they recorded SNAPs and cervical spinal potentials and confirmed the presence of root avulsion.

Jones (1979) and Jones et al. (1981) have studied a large series of cases with brachial plexus trauma. Recording at three levels (Erbs's point, cervical spine, and somatosensory cortex) following stimulation of the median and/or ulnar nerve at the wrist, they were able to determine conduction in the central segments of the peripheral nerve and in the CNS. The patients fell into four groups: (1) total lesion in the distribution of C5–T1; (2) C5–7 root distribution with minimal involvement of C8–T1; (3) C5–6; and (4) C8–T1. Complete lesions were by far the most common and lesions of the lower part of the plexus (C8–T1) the least common. They considered the Erb's point potential to reflect the propagation of the mixed-nerve action potential through the brachial plexus; the P/N13 potential was thought to arise from the cervical spinal cord or the lower brain stem, and the N19 from the cortex.

The criteria for abnormality were differences in amplitude of the P/N13 and the Erb's point responses of greater than 40% when compared to the unaffected limb. If the P/N13 was absent or was reduced to a greater extent than the Erb's point response, then the lesion was considered preganglionic. If the Erb's point response was reduced to an equal or greater degree than the P/N13, the lesion was considered postganglionic. In the situation where the P/N13 was absent and the Erb's point potential was of low amplitude, a combined lesion was suspected. No attention was paid to changes that may have occurred in conduction times. Using this yardstick they accurately predicted the site of the lesions in 10 of the 16 cases that went to surgery. The major difficulty was in the prediction of combined lesions, particularly if some roots had preganglionic and others postganglionic lesions. The presence of a severe lesion at the postganglionic level precluded the diagnosis of an additional root avulsion lesion (unless the root was stimulated during surgery). Furthermore, the reduction in the amplitude of the response at Erb's point did not necessarily mean a postganglionic lesion but may have been related to other factors, such as loss of motor axons or the recoil of the avulsed root (in which case the surface electrode may have been inappropriately placed). In this situation the additional recording of peripheral SNAPS and EMG analysis of relevant muscles would assist in the accuracy of the diagnosis.

Some inaccuracy in these studies may be related to the nerves studied. The exclusive stimulation of the median nerve trunk reduced the precision of the study since the sensory fibers which constitute the afferent volley are contributed to not only by the cutaneous fibers innervating the C6–7 segments but also by the muscle afferents which arise from C8–T1 innervated muscles (see Table 10–1). Thus on some occasions clinical cutaneous deficits may not be associated with abnormal SEPs if the muscle spindle afferents are intact. The importance of the contribution of muscle afferents to the SEP has been recently established (Burke et al., 1981; Starr et al., 1981). Another potential problem in the use of mixed-nerve stimulation is related to the contribution of antidromic motor activity to the response at Erb's point. Dawson and Scott (1949) in their early studies suggested that with supramaximal stimulation 70% of the amplitude of the action potential in a mixed nerve was due to large-diameter sensory afferents and the remaining 30% was predominantly due to antidromic motor activity. In this situation the comparison of the amplitudes of the P/N13 and the Erb's point potential may lead to errors if there is a significant loss of motor fibers. As SEPs are performed here (with minimal motor axon activation), the proportion of the Erb's point potential due to antidromic activity in motor fibers is much less (10%–20% perhaps).

Some authors (Eisen et al., 1983; Desmedt, and Noel, 1973) have used segmental sensory stimulation to accurately assess root lesions, but the recording of adequate cervical responses on single-digit or dermatomal stimulation is often difficult, even in normal subjects. In a series of cases with brachial plexus trauma studied with conventional EMG, nerve conduction studies (including late responses), and SEPs (from the median, ulnar, and superficial radial nerves), Yiannikas et al. (1983) found that those with lesions of the upper trunk of the brachial plexus or C5–6 roots were more accurately assessed using the superficial radial and musculocutaneous nerves, whereas those affecting the lower trunk or medial cord were more accurately assessed by using the ulnar nerve. The median nerve gave less specific information about the location of the pathology. These findings have been confirmed subsequently in a larger series of 35 patients with brachial plexus trauma (Yiannikas, unpublished data).

Figure 10–3 illustrates the case of a 25-year-old man with an occupational blunt injury to the right shoulder who had on clinical examination weakness predominantly affecting C5–7 muscles (biceps, triceps, deltoid, and forearm extensors) with minimal weakness of the small muscles of the hand. Sensory loss was in the C5–7 dermatomes with relative sparing of C8–T1. The EP, P/N13, and N19 responses on stimulating the radial nerve were absent. On median nerve stimulation the Erb's point response was absent but low amplitude, delayed P/N13 and N19 potentials were seen. In contrast, the potentials on ulnar nerve stimu-

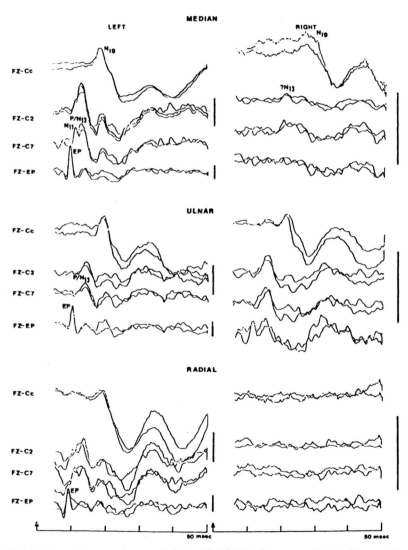

FIG. 10–3. Median, ulnar, and superficial radial SEPs from a patient with an injury to the right shoulder. The radial SEPs are absent at all levels; median studies show an absent EP and delayed P/N13 and N19, and ulnar SEPs have only a slight increase in latencies of all components. These findings suggest C6–T1 pathology at the level of the brachial plexus on the right with no apparent functional continuity of C6 sensory fibers. Calibration bars are 5 μV. Each trace is the average of 1,000 stimuli on the right, 500 on the left.

lation were preserved although the latency of all components was a little longer, suggesting loss of some of the larger-diameter fibers. The median and radial SNAPs were absent but a normal ulnar SNAP was present. These features suggest postganglionic pathology affecting the lateral posterior cords of the brachial plexus with only minor involvement of the medial cords. Here the radial SEPs have helped to localize the lesion more precisely. Conversely, another patient with a similar lesion also had absent radial nerve SNAPs and complete denervation with no voluntary units seen on EMG in C5 and C6 muscles. The superficial radial SEP (stimulating at the wrist), however, showed a scalp (cerebral) response, even though EP and P/N13 responses were absent, indicating continuity of some sensory axons (and thus the gross nerve itself). This suggested that surgical exploration was not necessary.

The importance in these patients of combining EMG and SEP was demonstrated in the case of a 36-year-old woman who sustained an injury from a sharp object to the neck following a motor vehicle accident (Fig. 10–4). Clinical examination revealed an anesthetic

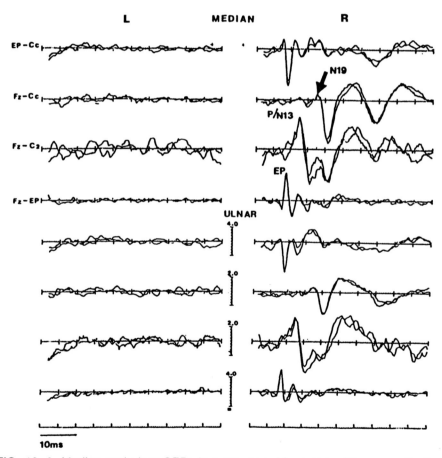

FIG. 10–4. Median and ulnar SEPs in a 36-year-old woman with an anesthetic limb with movement only in small hand and some forearm muscles, subsequent to trauma. There were no SEPs recorded with left median or ulnar nerve stimulation at any level. These features suggest extensive (C5–T1) postganglionic pathology. The presence of denervation in the paraspinal muscles suggest additional root pathology. Each trace is the average of 512 stimuli. Calibrations are in microvolts.

limb with movement only in the small muscles of the hand and some of the forearm muscles. There were no SEPs recorded at any level on stimulating the median, ulnar, or radial nerves. The radial and median SNAPs were absent and the ulnar SNAP was of abnormally low amplitude. Compound muscle action potentials could be evoked from the median, radial, and ulnar nerves but were of low amplitude. Electromyography showed no voluntary activity in C5–7 muscles and reduced activity in C8–T1 muscles. Paraspinal EMG demonstrated fibrillation potentials from C5–8. The most severe damage was at the C5–7 level, with no apparent functional continuity, whereas in the C8–T1 segments there was some preservation of motor fibers. The presence of active denervation in the paraspinal muscles localized the lesions to the root level but the absence of SNAPs placed it distal to the dorsal ganglion. These conclusions correlated well with operative findings, where the C5–6 roots were apparently still in continuity but on stimulation of the roots (still distal to the lesion) no SEPs could be recorded, indicating a lack of functional continuity centrally.

The patient whose SEPs are shown in Fig. 10–5 is a 22-year-old woman who was involved in an industrial accident and developed weakness of the C8–T1 muscles of the right hand and forearm. In addition there was decreased appreciation of light touch and pinprick in C8–T1 dermatomes. The EPs on right median nerve stimulation were of low amplitude at all levels and an increase in the EP–P/N13 interpeak latency (IPL). Ulnar nerve studies showed absent EP and P/N13 potentials and delayed low-amplitude N19. The radial nerve studies were normal. The nerve conduction studies showed an absent ulnar SNAP and denervation in C8–T1 muscles on the appropriate side. These features were typical of medial cord or upper trunk pathology with preservation of continuity.

The findings in our experience and by other authors (Synek and Cowan, 1982; Synek, 1987; Aminoff, 1987) would suggest that in the majority of situations the necessary information is obtainable from conventional EMG and nerve conduction studies. For lesions involving the upper segments only, SEPs are useful because late responses and SNAPs from these segments are less accessible. Furthermore, by recording proximal to the lesion, preganglionic pathology is easily determined and, taking advantage of the amplifying characteristics of the CNS, SEPs provide the most accurate method of assessing axonal continuity, which is integral to determining the need for surgical intervention.

The patient whose SEPs are shown in Fig. 10–6 is a 25-year-old woman who was involved in a motor vehicle accident and developed weakness of the C8–T1 muscles of the right hand and forearm with extreme wasting. In addition, there was decreased appreciation of light touch and pinprick in C8–T1 dermatomes. The EPs on median, ulnar, and radial nerve stimulation were normal (although the response at Erb's point was slightly smaller on the right than on the left). A compound muscle action potential could not be evoked on either median or ulnar nerve stimulation and the sensory nerve action potentials (median, ulnar, radial) were normal in the presence of sensory loss. These features suggest a preganglionic lesion of C8–T1 roots most severely affecting the motor fibers and sparing the large-diameter sensory fibers. The complete loss of motor axons has produced very little change in the SEPs (either at Erb's point or more centrally) and it must be the preservation of muscle afferents that has produced normal EPs in the presence of some clinical cutaneous deficit, suggesting that (1) on mixed-nerve stimulation SEPs are generated more by muscle than by cutaneous afferents, and (2) the Erb's point potential primarily reflects activity in sensory rather than motor axons with this level of submaximal stimulation (minimal twitch).

The use of intraoperative stimulation of specific roots with recording over the cervical epidural space, contralateral scalp, and relevant peripheral nerves (Landi et al., 1980; Sugioka et al., 1982; Murase et al., 1993) may add valuable information to the preoperative

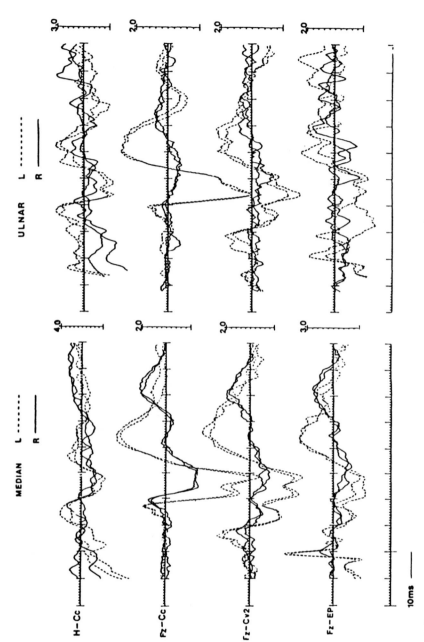

FIG. 10–5. Median and ulnar SEPs from a 22-year-old woman with brachial plexus trauma. Left-sided stimulation (*dotted trace*) was normal. Right ulnar nerve stimulation showed absent EP and P/N13 potentials, and a delayed, low-amplitude N19. Right median SEPs showed low-amplitude potentials at all levels and an increase in the EP–P/N13 IPL. Radial nerve studies were normal. These features suggest a lesion affecting the lower trunk or medial cord of the brachial plexus with preserved axonal continuity. The normal side (*dotted line*) is superimposed on the affected side (*filled line*). Each trace is the average of 512 stimuli. Calibrations are microvolts.

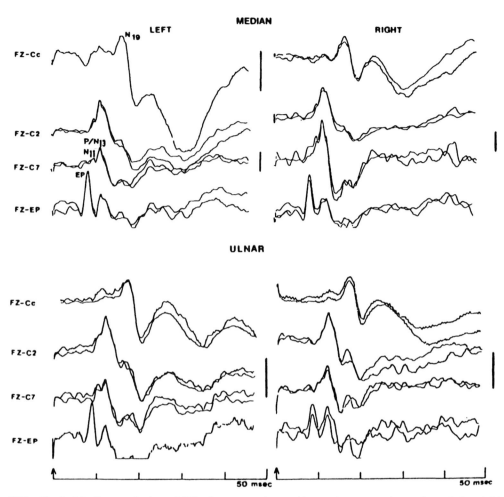

FIG. 10–6. Median and ulnar SEPs from a patient with weakness and wasting of the right C8–T1 muscles subsequent to trauma. The SEPs were normal (minor differences only in the amplitude at Erb's point) from both nerves bilaterally. These features suggest that at this intensity of stimulation (minimal twitch) the contribution of the antidromic motor activity to the Erb's point (*EP*) potential is small; see discussion of the contribution of muscle afferents to the SEP in the text. Each trace is the average of 500 stimuli. Calibration marks are 2.5 µV.

studies. The presence of lesions at multiple levels may be determined and a comparison of functional and anatomic continuity may be assessed. This is of importance when considering the prognosis and the suitability of ruptured roots for grafting. The authors of these studies suggested that the anatomic appearance of the plexus at operation may be misleading since the presence of intact epineurium did not mean continuityof the nerve fascicles. These findings would explain the disappointing results of operations based on anatomic morphology alone.

Somatosensory EPs also have a place in trauma cases at early stages of regeneration when no compound-nerve action potentials are evokable by stimulating the peripheral nerve. The rate of advance of regenerating sensory axons can be worked out by stimulating the nerve at various distances from the cord and determining the most distal level from which cerebral potentials can be evoked (Desmedt and Noel, 1973).

4. PLEXOPATHIES AND RADICULOPATHIES

4.1. Thoracic Outlet Syndrome

The thoracic outlet syndrome (TOS) is a broad term which includes patients who have symptoms due to compression of the neurovascular structures at the base of the neck by muscular (scalenus anticus syndrome), fibrous band, or bony (cervical rib, enlarged C7 transverse process) abnormalities. It may be characterized by a combination of pain in the arm provoked by traction, vascular changes characterized by color changes in the hand (vasculogenic), and a C8–T1 radicular pattern of sensory loss, weakness, and wasting with intact tendon reflexes (neurogenic). In the absence of significant neurologic deficit, the diagnosis may be difficult to make on clinical grounds. Electrophysiologic abnormalities in motor and sensory conduction in the peripheral segments of the median and ulnar nerve in patients with cervical ribs or bands have been described by Gilliatt et al. (1978), Wulff and Gilliatt (1979), and Eisen et al. (1977) and include a reduction in the amplitude of the ulnar SNAP, chronic partial denervation in the small muscles of the hand and prolongation of the F-wave latencies from these muscles. In some patients with wasted hands the nerve conduction studies were normal, and, in the group of patients in whom there were symptoms of TOS but no objective signs, the diagnostic yield from EMG, nerve conduction, and late-response studies was low. Difficulties that arise in electrophysiologic diagnosis of this condition are related to the problem of assessing nerve conduction across the brachial plexus and the results of transclavicular nerve conduction studies have been conflicting. This is particularly a problem if the symptoms are predominantly due to vascular compression.

There have been relatively few studies of SEP in patients with thoracic outlet syndrome. Siivola et al. (1979) studied one case and found an absent response from Erb's point on ulnar nerve stimulation below and above the elbow with normal responses on median nerve stimulation. Glover et al. (1981) studied 21 cases of suggested TOS with median and ulnar nerve stimulation and found a high incidence of abnormalities (13 of 19 new patients). Of the nine cases that had surgical treatment, eight showed reversal of the EP abnormalities. In their cases, however, the clinical criteria for the diagnosis of TOS and the EP abnormalities were not discussed. Inouye and Buchthal (1977) used root recording techniques in a small group of patients with cervical ribs and found abnormalities in only one case when stimulating digit V. This case had wasting of the hand and classical features on EMG of TOS.

Yiannikas and Walsh (1983) studied 12 cases with radiologically proven cervical ribs and symptoms suggestive of TOS. Conventional nerve conduction studies (without F-waves) and EMG were performed and SEPs were recorded while stimulating the median and ulnar nerves at the wrist. The patients were divided into two groups depending on the presence or absence of neurologic signs. In the first group, with no objective neurologic signs, the SEP amplitude, latencies, and conduction times were normal, as was the EMG. The second group, with both symptoms and objective neurologic disturbances, demonstrated two distinct types of abnormalities on stimulating the ulnar nerve. In two patients the Erb's point component was present and of normal latency, with P/N13 abnormal or absent. This could result from a proximal lesion on either side of the dorsal ganglion leading to conduction block. In the other three cases the SEP showed an attenuation and prolongation of the latency of the Erb's point component with the P/N13 affected to an equal or lesser extent, and an increase in the EP–P/N13 conduction time. This suggested a lesion distal to the dorsal ganglion involving the medial cord of the brachial plexus affecting large diameter motor and sensory fibers. In one of the cases in group 2 with abnormal ulnar SEP the EMG and nerve conduction studies were normal. Therefore, it was thought that SEPs were potentially of use in addition to conventional nerve conduction studies and EMG.

Subsequently there have been a number of studies confirming these findings (Siivola et al., 1983; Jerrett et al., 1984; Chodoroff et al., 1985; Newmark et al., 1985; Synek, 1986). Siivola et al. (1983) studied 13 patients, 9 of whom had abnormal studies, and of these 3 showed normalization of results postoperatively. Chodoroff et al. (1985) suggested an increased yield in ulnar nerve SEP abnormalities in patients with TOS if these are recorded in a "dynamic" position, that is, with the arm abducted and externally rotated. Veilleux et al. (1988) have some reservations regarding this technique as the maneuver produced amplitude reduction of greater than 50% in four of their normal subjects (this has also been observed in our laboratory). They studied 20 patients with TOS and found abnormal ulnar SEPs in 3 patients (15%), whereas the nerve conduction studies and F-waves were abnormal in only 1 case. Electromyography of the hand muscles showed chronic neurogenic changes in five patients. Therefore, it was thought that eh routine use of SEPs was not worthwhile. This belief was also expressed by Aminoff et al. (1987), who found that in 10 patients with non-neurogenic TOS there were no SEP abnormalities.

The discrepancy between these studies and earlier studies is difficult to reconcile and may be related to patient selection. One of the main problems in comparing the diagnostic utility of various tests in different studies is the lack of uniformity in the clinical diagnosis of TOS and the absence of an investigative benchmark with which to compare electrodiagnostic studies.

We have reappraised our experience over the last 7 years assessing 65 patients with the diagnosis of TOS. These patients were classified as neurogenic (objective signs of neurogenic dysfunction)—15 patients; vasculogenic (objective signs of vascular occlusion, obliteration of pulse, venous thrombosis, radiographic evidence of vascular compression)— 17 patients; symptomatic (no objective abnormalities)—33 patients. Thirty-eight of the patients (58%) had cervical ribs and 23 of the 33 (70%) patients with symptomatic TOS had cervical ribs or enlarged transverse processes. Consistent with our earlier study (Yiannikas and Walsh, 1983) and subsequent studies the patients with neurogenic TOS, all had abnormal ulnar SEPs, with normal median studies. The most common finding was low-amplitude N9 and/or increased N9/N13 IPL, but absent N9 and P/N13 potentials were seen in four patients. Interestingly, three patients had abnormal SEPs but normal EMG and nerve conduction studies; these patients had sensory deficit only. Figure 10–7 shows the SEPs from a 48-year-old man with a history of numbness in the ulnar aspects of the left hand and forearm, with some loss of appreciation to light touch and pinprick in this distribution. There was no evidence of weakness or wasting. Somatosensory EPs on left radial and median nerve stimulation were within normal limits, although there was an asymmetry in the amplitude of the responses on median nerve stimulation. On stimulation of the left ulnar nerve there was mild reduction in the amplitude of the Erb's response, an essentially absent spinal response (P/N13) and an increased EP–N19 conduction time with a low-amplitude N19 potential. The EMG, late responses, and nerve conduction studies were normal. These features suggested conduction block at the level of the medial cord of the brachial plexus affecting C8–T1 sensory fibers predominantly.

Of the 17 patients with vasculogenic TOS, 6 (35%) had abnormalities in the ulnar SEPs. These abnormalities were predominantly low-amplitude responses at Erb's point and, occasionally, an increase in the N9–N/P13 IPL. Only two patients had abnormal EMG and nerve

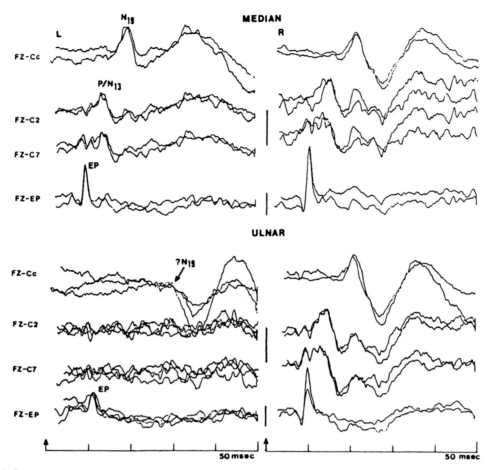

FIG. 10–7. Median and ulnar SEPs from a patient with left-sided sensory loss in a C8–T1 distribution. The responses on median nerve stimulation were normal. The left ulnar SEPs show a mild reduction in the amplitude of the Erb's point (*EP*) potential, an absent P/N13, and a prolonged EP–N19 IPL. In the presence of a normal ulnar sensory nerve action potential, this suggests a conduction defect at the level of the left medial cord or lower trunk of the brachial plexus. Each trace is the average of 1,000 stimuli on the left, 500 on the right. Calibration marks are 1 μV.

conduction studies, one of whom had normal SEPs. Figure 10–8 is from a 28-year-old woman who presented with paresthesia in her left hand, discoloration and obliteration of her pulse with the arm abducted, and an episode of subclavian vein thrombosis. Neurologic examination was normal. The median SEPs were normal, but the ulnar studies showed low-amplitude responses at all levels and marginally increased EP–P/N13. At operation she was found to have a band constricting the brachial plexus. The nerve conduction studies and EMG were normal.

In the symptomatic group of patients 7 of 33 (21%) had abnormal ulnar SEPs. They all had reduced-amplitude Erb's point potentials and/or increased EP–P/N13 IPLs. The nerve conduction studies were abnormal in two patients, one of whom had normal SEPs. Figure 10–9 illustrates the EPs from a 45-year-old woman with a left cervical rib and paresthesia

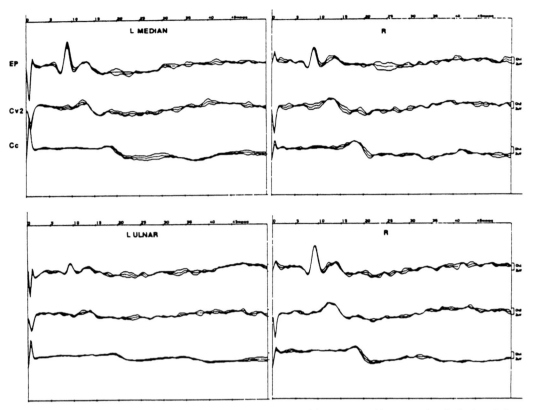

FIG. 10–8. Median and ulnar SEPs from a 28-year-old woman with paresthesia in her left hand and obliteration of her pulse and discoloration of her hand with abduction of her arm. The median SEPs are normal. The ulnar SEPs show a low-amplitude Erb's point potential and an increase in the EP–P/N13 IPL on the left. Each trace is the average of 512 stimuli, with two superimposed and a mean trace. Reference was FZ for all channels. Calibration marks are 2 μV.

and numbness and some intermittent discoloration of the left hand. The median SEPs are normal but the ulnar studies show a smaller response, on the left, particularly the P/N13 response, and an increase in the EP–N/13 IPL on that side compared to the right (0.8 msec). The nerve conduction studies and EMG were normal.

On the basis of these results it may be concluded that in patients with typical neurogenic TOS and neurologic signs there is a high incidence of ulnar SEP abnormalities. The incidence is lower in the vasculogenic and symptomatic group (20% to 30%). This is less than that reported in some studies (Jerrett 79%, Chodoroff 43%, Siivola 69%, Glover 68%), similar to that of Veilleux (15%), and more than that of Aminoff (0%). In our laboratory the SEPs were more sensitive than conventional EMG and nerve conduction studies (18% had abnormal SEPs and normal EMG), particularly in the non-neurogenic group, although there were three cases (5%) with abnormal nerve conduction/EMG and normal SEPs.

These findings suggest that SEPs to ulnar nerve stimulation are useful in the diagnosis of TOS. More importantly, in the group who do not have neurologic signs there is still a significant yield. Furthermore, in combination with nerve conduction studies and EMG, the sen-

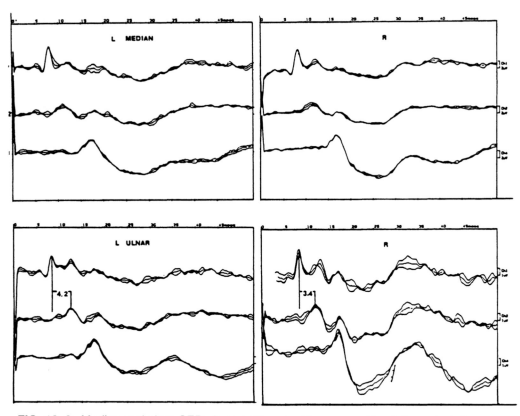

FIG. 10–9. Median and ulnar SEPs from a 45-year-old woman with a left cervical rib, paresthesias, and episodes of discoloration of her left hand. The median SEPs are normal. The left ulnar studies show a normal EP potential but a 48% drop in P/N13 amplitude (L = 1.4 μV, R = 2.6 μV) and an increased EP–P/N13 IPL (the interside difference was 0.8 msec, upper limit of normal is 0.5 msec; see Table 8–2). Each trace is the average of 512 stimuli, with two superimposed and a mean trace. Reference was FZ in all channels. Calibration marks are 2 μV.

sitivity may be increased. Although it has been recently suggested that the routine use of SEPs in TOS is not helpful (Veilleux et al., 1988, Passero et al., 1994). Machleder et al. (1987) found that SEPs were abnormal on the affected side in 74% of patients and 85% of those with abnormal studies showing improvement in the SEPs postoperatively. Excellent clinical correlation was evident in 92% of patients who had pre- and postoperative tests. Walsh et al. (1995) assessed the correlation of preoperative SEP abnormalities and surgical outcome and found that patients with abnormal SEP had a good outcome in 93% of cases as compared to 60% of those with normal preoperative SEPs.

In the study by Veilleaux EMG was more sensitive but the patients in that study did not have neurogenic TOS. Furthermore, they demonstrated a 15% incidence of SEP abnormalities compared to only one patient with abnormalities in nerve conduction studies or F-waves (5%). The major increase in sensitivity was with EMG and then only one subject showed active denervation with the majority of changes consistent with chronic denervation. This assessment of subtle chronic denervation on EMG is subjective and, therefore, more open to differences in interpretation and less useful than SEPs in follow-up assessment of the effectiveness of surgery.

4.2. Cervical Radiculopathies

The objective diagnosis of cervical radiculopathy is problematic in clinical neurology. Electrophysiologic evaluation in the past has been limited to EMG and nerve conduction studies. Conventional nerve conduction studies are usually normal unless compression is severe enough to cause significant Wallerian degeneration and consequently a drop in amplitude of the compound muscle action potential and possible slowing of motor conduction. Although Eisen et al. (1977) have found significant prolongation of F-wave latencies in some of his patients with abnormal cervical myelograms secondary to spondylosis, the general experience is that F-wave studies from muscles innervated by the median and ulnar nerve are unrewarding (this is related to the fact that they test only the C8–T1 segments that are generally not affected by cervical spondylosis). The most useful studies are the EMG analysis of muscles innervated by the appropriate roots and the analysis of F-waves from those muscles, but these only take account of motor root dysfunction, whereas the most common clinical deficit is sensory (pain or numbness). In the lower limbs, this problem is overcome by the use of H-reflexes, but these are usually not present in the upper limbs.

Somatosensory EPs should be useful because such recordings monitor afferent sensory impulses passing through the roots. In a series of patients studied in this laboratory (Yiannikas, 1983; Yiannikas et al., 1986) with clinical and radiologic diagnosis of cervical radiculopathy, the sensitivity of EMG, nerve conduction, and late responses was compared to SEPs recorded by stimulating the median, ulnar, and superficial radial nerves. It was suggested that SEPs were of limited use in patients with only symptoms of root compression. In patients with signs of root compression, EMG was the most sensitive procedure, although additional information was obtained from superficial radial nerve SEPs. Median nerve SEPs were usually normal in this group, whereas in patients with clinical features of a myelopathy there was a high incidence of SEP abnormality, particularly when SEPs from the lower limbs were studied.

These findings have been confirmed and extended in a recent review of our findings in 68 patients with cervical radiculopathy and/or myelopathy. This included 20 patients with radicular symptoms only, 26 with objective neurologic signs of root compression, and 22 with clinical and radiologic features of spinal cord compression. In the patients with radicular symptoms, only two (10%) had abnormal EMG and one (5%) had abnormal radial SEPs. In patients with signs of root compression (sensory changes, weakness, or reflex changes), eight (39%) had abnormal radial SEPs, whereas only two (8%) had abnormal median SEPs. These changes included a low-amplitude or absent P/N13, with increase in the EP–P/N13 conduction time occurring less frequently. The EMG was abnormal in 16 (61%) of patients and included features consistent with active denervation in the appropriate muscles. The nerve conduction studies and late responses were normal in all. In only 2 was the SEP abnormal with a normal EMG, but in 10 the EMG was abnormal with normal SEPs.

The EPs were very useful in confirming the presence of a myelopathy, with 15 (68%) having abnormal median SEPs and 21 of 22 (95%) patients having abnormal tibial or peroneal studies. The abnormalities seen were a low amplitude or absent P/N13 and N19 and a prolonged EP– P/N13 conduction time and increase in the central conduction time and low-amplitude scalp responses from the lower limbs. Nine (41%) of these patients had abnormalities in EMG suggesting a radiculomyelopathy. Figure 10–10 is from a 42-year-old man who presented with pain in the neck radiating down the left arm. There was an area of sensory loss over the C6 dermatome and weakness of biceps with depressed biceps and triceps jerks. Electromyography showed features of denervation in biceps and triceps. The SEPs on median and ulnar nerve stimulation were normal. On radial nerve stimulation there was a significant reduction in amplitude of the P/N13 and N19 components on the appropriate

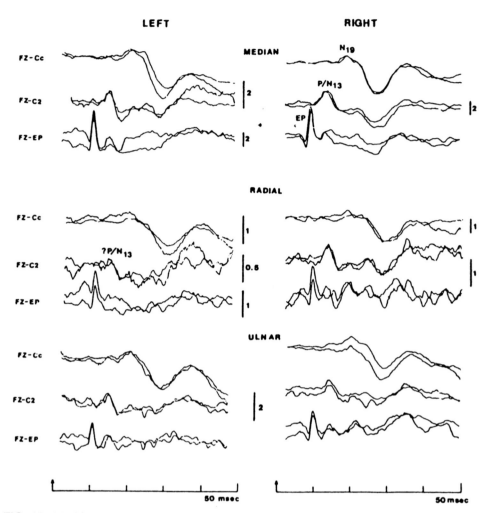

FIG. 10–10. Median, radial, and ulnar SEPs in a patient with clinical features suggesting a left cervical radiculopathy. The median and ulnar SEPs were normal but left radial studies showed abnormally low-amplitude P/N13 and N19 potentials, with normal IPLs. The left median SEP P/N13 amplitude was reduced but still within normal limits. These features were consistent with a left C6 root compression. Each trace is the average of 1,000 stimuli. Calibration marks are in microvolts.

side with normal conduction times. These features were consistent with the diagnosis of C6–7 cervical root compression on the left. Figure 10–11 illustrates a case of a 42-year-old woman with history of acute pain and dysesthesia in the left upper extremity with paraesthesia in digits 1 to 3 and decreased appreciation to pinprick and light touch over digit 3. There was weakness of triceps and finger extensors with depression of the triceps reflex. Median nerve SEPs were within normal limits. Radial studies showed increase in the EP–P/N13 IPL on the left and a poorly formed N19 on that side. The nerve conduction studies were normal. Electromyography showed chronic partial denervation in triceps and extensor digitorum communis. These features were conistent with cervical radiculopathy af-

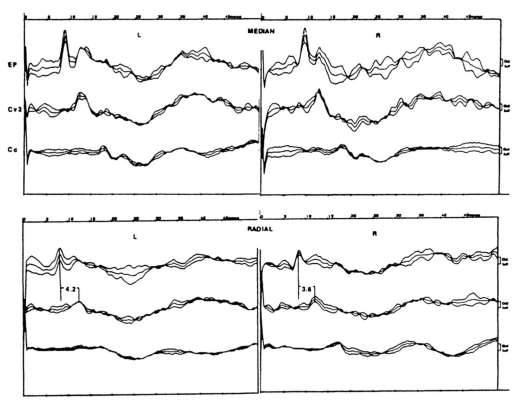

FIG. 10–11. Median and radial SEPs from a 42-year-old woman with clinical features suggesting C6–7 root compression on the left. The median SEPs are normal. The left radial SEPs show an increased EP–P/N13 IPL compared to the right and an absent N19 on that side. These features are consistent with a left C6 radiculopathy. Each trace is the average of 512 stimuli, with 2 superimposed and a mean trace. The calibration bars are 1 μV.

fecting the C6–7 roots on the left. This was confirmed by myelography showing amputation of the C7 roots on the left (Fig. 10–12). The EPs in Fig. 10–13 are from a 57-year-old man with weakness of his right arm greater than left and C5–7 muscle and bilateral lower-limb weakness in a pyramidal distribution, brisk reflexes in his legs, and extensor plantar responses. The right biceps and triceps jerks were absent. Myelography revealed canal stenosis at C4–6 and some root compression of the right. Median SEPs were abnormal bilaterally with P/N13 absent on the left with an increased EP–N19 conduction time; on the right there was an increased EP–P/N13 IPL. The tibial SEPs showed an abnormal absolute latency of P37 bilaterally.

Earlier workers (Mastaglia et al., 1978; El-Negamy and Sedgwick, 1979; Ganes, 1980; Siivola et al., 1981) have studied patients with a clinical and radiologic diagnosis of cervical spondylosis using SEPs performed by stimulating the median nerve at the wrist. These authors found changes similar to those described in the patients presented above, although the changes in the EP–P/N13 conduction time in patients with signs of root compression noted by Ganes (1980) and Siivola et al. (1981) were not seen by the others. Matsukado et al. (1976) and Caccia et al. (1976) attempted to increase the sensitivity of the study by the

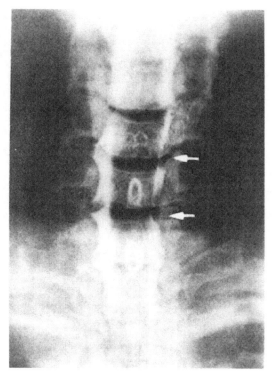

FIG. 10–12. Cervical myelogram from the patient whose SEPs are shown in Fig. 10–11. There is a C7 root amputation on the left (*arrow*).

use of epidural recording electrode (electrospinogram). They found significant reduction in the amplitude of the spinal response on the impaired side with normal latencies. The invasive nature of this procedure precludes its routine clinical use.

More recently Yu and Jones (1985), using median, ulnar, and tibial nerve stimulation in 34 patients with cervical spondylosis, found similar high correlation of SEP abnormalities with myelopathy (particularly with lower-limb stimulation) but not with radiculopathy, although 3 of 13 patients with radiculopathy had abnormal SEPs. Significantly, 6 of 21 patients with clinical myelopathy had abnormal tibial SEPs but no evidence of cord compression, suggesting that blood supply may be a significant factor in the development of myelopathy and confirming the diagnostic importance of the SEPs versus radiology. Interestingly, Veilleux and Daube (1987) and Perlik and Fisher (1987) have confirmed the high sensitivity of tibial SEPs compared to median SEPs but the former authors suggested that ulnar SEPs were the most sensitive, which is not our experience nor that of Yu and Jones (1985). This may be related to the fact that only 24 of their patients had tibial N20–P37 IPLs calculated and 30 of the 37 pateints had bilateral tibial nerve stimulation, which would prevent the detection of interside differences.

There have been attempts to improve sensitivity of the technique in patients with radiculopathy only, with either more specific stimulation of the digits or dermatomal stimulation (Eisen et al., 1983; Synek, 1986; Leblhuber et al., 1988; Schimsheimer et al., 1988; Schmid et al., 1988). The results were not consistent with those of Schimsheimer et al. reporting a high yield (68%), whereas Schmid et al. had a low yield (28%) but 22% false positive re-

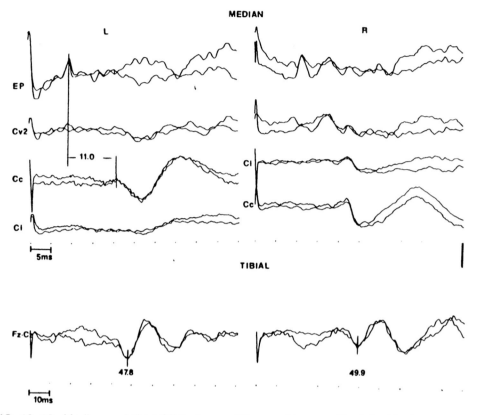

FIG. 10–13. Median and tibial SEPs from a 57-year-old man with clinical features sugges-tive of a cervical myelopathy, worse on the left. The median SEPs are bilaterally abnormal with absent left P/N13 and an abnormal EP–N19 conduction time; the EP– P/N13 conduction time on the right was also increased. The tibial SEPs have an abnormal absolute latency of P37 bilaterally. Each trace is the average of 1,024 stimuli. Reference for all median channels was FZ. The calibration bar is 2 μV for all channels.

sults on the asymptomatic side. Although theoretically the technique should have a higher sensitivity than when using a multisegmental nerve such as the median nerve, the reliability is questionable because of the small amplitude of the responses and the frequent inability to obtain reproducible EP and P/N13 potentials in normals. Most studies have shown improve-ment in the EPs after surgery, particularly in the radiculopathy group (Heiskari et al., 1986, Yu and Jones 1985; Kubota et al., 1984).

From these studies it is apparent that in patients with cervical myelopathy, SEPs (particu-larly from the tibial nerve) are useful, but in patients with radiculopathy without features of myelopathy SEPs evoked by median or ulnar nerve stimulation have limited diagnostic suc-cess. This is due to stimulation of a mixed-nerve trunk that has multisegmental composition (median—C6–T1) and thus is unlikely to show significant changes when a single root is compressed. Some improvement in specificity may result from the use of the superficial ra-dial nerve (C6), especially when there is cutaneous sensory loss in a C6 distribution, or from stimulation using the digits, but the frequency of abnormalities is low and certainly less than with the conventional EMG. The use of multiple-nerve testing increases the sensitivity and accuracy of the SEP but greatly increases testing time. In selected cases the additional information gained may be of diganostic utility, but often the same information is available with less effort via conventional EMG techniques.

4.3. Lumbar Radiculopathies

The results from the application of SEPs to pathology of the lumbosacral roots has been conflicting. Ertekin et al. (1980, 1984) studied 52 patients with various lesions of the cauda equina and the conus medullaris with electrospinograms and cortical evoked responses (CEPs). In nine classified as grade I (no weakness, no sacral sensory loss, and normal EMG), the EPs were normal. In the presence of monoparesis, absent knee or ankle jerks, and EMG features of denervation, the EPs always showed significant abnormalities, which included a delayed low-amplitude spinal response and a low-amplitude response from the scalp. Some early works attempted to increase the specificity of their studies by stimulating cutaneous nerves, such as the saphenous, superficial peroneal, and sural nerves (Eisen and Elleker, 1980), or by stimulating cutaneous dermatomes (Scarff et al., 1981; Sedgwick et al., 1985; Katifi and Sedgwick, 1986; Tans and Vredeveld, 1992) and recording over the scalp. These authors found SEPs useful with good correlation between physiologic, myelographic, and operative findings. Scarff et al. (1981) found abnormalities in SEPs in 90 of their cases as compared to EMG, where fewer than 50 of the patients had abnormalities, and the SEP was thought to be more sensitive than myelography. In a later dermatomal study Dvonch et al. (1986) found an accuracy of 85.7% for dermatomal SEPs when using myelography as the gold standard, and 87.7% when using surgical outcome as the gold standard. These results have not been confirmed by others. Aminoff et al. (1985a,b) and Aminoff (1987) compared the diagnostic utility of dermatomal SEPs with EMG and late responses and found that in 25% of patients the dermatomal SEP was abnormal, in two cases with all other electrophysiology normal, but that the single most useful technique was EMG. Peroneal derived SEPs were always normal. More recently Rodriguez et al. (1987) found that dermatomal SEPs were less sensitive and accurate than conventional EMG or in anatomic studies. In addition, a significant incidence of false positive localization to the asymptomatic side has been described (Aminoff et al., 1985a,b; Rodriguez et al., 1987).

These studies had some limitations in that recordings were not done over the lumbar spine, so the presence of a coexisting central lesion, particularly at a cervical level, could not be detected. Furthermore, the amplitude of scalp potentials to dermatomal stimulation is small when compared to mixed-nerve or cutaneous nerve stimulation and may provide technical difficulties in interpretation. In addition, a more theoretical objection may be raised that it is difficult to be certain that only cutaneous fibers are being stimulated in the dermatome and not muscle afferents from the underlying muscle, which may subserve different segmental innervation.

There may be significant advantages gained in stimulating cutaneous nerve trunks such as the superficial peroneal, sural, and saphenous nerves in that scalp responses are larger and spinal potentials more readily available than those obtained from dermatomal stimulation. Furthermore, greater specificity is obtained when compared to results from a multisegmental mixed nerve such as the tibial nerve. In a series of 20 patients with lumbosacral radiculopathies, confirmed by computed tomography scan or myelography, studied in this laboratory (Yiannikas, unpublished data) with EMG, late responses including the H-reflex, nerve conduction studies, and SEPs (tibial, peroneal and sural with stimulation at the ankle), it was found that in 9 with symptoms but no objective neurologic signs the EMG was abnormal in 3 (33%), whereas the SEP was abnormal in 2 (22%). In the other 11 patients with signs of root compression there was evidence of denervation in the appropriate muscles on EMG in all patients and the SEP was abnormal in 10 of 11 (91%) when the relevant nerve was stimulated. Significantly, of the 12 patients who had abnormal SEPs only 6 had abnormal posterior tibial studies.

Figure 10–14 illustrates SEPs from a 44-year-old man who complained of sudden onset of back pain radiating down the right leg with weakness and paresthesias and numbness over the dorsum of the right foot. Physical examination revealed an area of sensory loss in the L4–5 dermatome, weakness of dorsiflexion of the ankle, and normal reflexes. Nerve conduction studies were normal but F-waves from tibialis anterior were abnormal and the EMG showed denervation in L4–5 innervated muscles including gluteus medius. The tibial EPs were normal, whereas on right peroneal nerve stimulation the lumbar spinal response

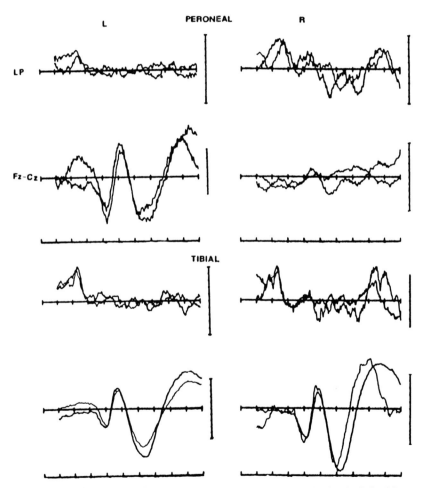

FIG. 10–14. Peroneal and tibial SEPs from a 44-year-old man who had clinical features consistent with a right L4–5 radiculopathy. Tibial SEPs were normal. Right peroneal SEPs showed no reproducible spinal potential and a dispersed and low-amplitude scalp response. The sweep duration was 100 msec; the calibration bar is 1 μV. The LP channel derivation is L1 to iliac crest.

was absent and the scalp responses were dispersed. These features suggested compression of L4–5 roots, which was confirmed at myelography and at operation.

Figure 10–15 is from a 26-year-old woman who presented with pain and weakness. There was some minor weakness of the gastrocnemius, sensory loss in an S1 distribution, and a depressed left ankle jerk. Electromyography showed chronic denervation in the

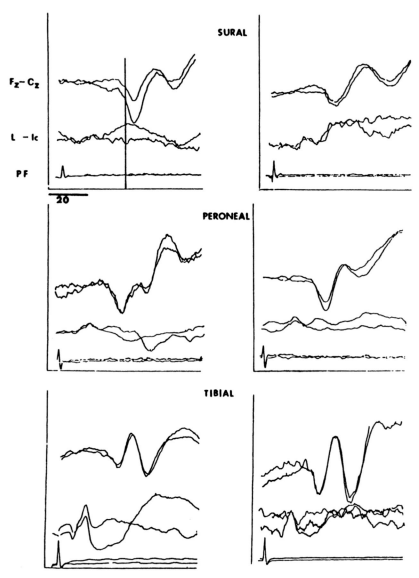

FIG. 10–15. Sural, peroneal , and tibial SEPs from a 26-year-old woman with a history suggestive of a left radiculopathy. The peroneal and tibial SEPs were normal. The left sural SEPs (*left panel*) show a low-amplitude, dispersed spinal potential and a delayed P37 (the vertical cursor in the left sural nerve panel marks the right sural nerve P37 latency). These features are consistent with an S1 root lesion on the left side. (*L*, L1 lumbar spine; *Ic*, iliac crest; *PF*, popliteal fossa). Each trace is the average of 1,024 stimuli. The stimulus occurred at the left vertical line (e.g., at the beginning of the 20-msec calibration mark). The calibration bar is 2 μV for the cortical and knee channels and 1 μV for spinal channels.

gastrocnemius and there was a delay in the tibial F-waves. Somatosensory EPs on tibial and peroneal nerve stimulation were normal. In comparison, the sural studies showed absent spinal potentials and a major difference in the latency of the scalp potential, suggesting pathology affecting predominantly the S1 root. This was confirmed by myelogram and operatively.

On the basis of these findings it appears that the use of SEPs in lumbosacral root disease suffers from limitations similar to those in the cervical area and may be used in conjunction with conventional EMG in patients with objective findings to provide support in the selection of those to undergo disc surgery, but they do not confer a major advantage to conventional EMG in the majority of patients (see also Synek, 1987). Intraoperative application of SEPs is of some interest, and Gepstein and Brown (1989), in a study of 41 patients, found that good outcome correlated with intraoperative improvement of SEPs and thus may be useful in assessing the adequacy of decompression.

REFERENCES

Aminoff MJ (1987): Use of somatosensory evoked potentials to evaluate the peripheral nervous system. *J Clin Neurophysiol* 4:135–144.

Aminoff MJ, Goodin DS, Barbaro NM, Weinstein PR, Rosenblum ML (1985a): Dermatomal somatosensory evoked potentials in unilateral lumbosacral radiculopathy. *Ann Neurol* 17:171–176.

Aminoff MJ, Goodin DS, Barbaro NM, Weinstein PR, Rosenblum ML (1985b): Electrophysiologic evaluation of lumbosacral radiculopathies: Electromyography, late responses, and somatosensory evoked potentials. *Neurology* 35:1514–1518.

Aminoff MJ, Olney RK, Parry GJ, Raskin NH (1987): Electrophysiological evaluation of brachial plexopathy: Clinical relevance. *Ann Neurol* 22:165.

Bonney G, Gilliatt RW (1958): Sensory nerve conduction after traction lesions of the brachial plexus. *Proc R Soc Med* 51:365–367.

Brown WF, Feasby FE (1984): Sensory evoked potentials in Guillain–Barré polyneuropathy. *J Neurol Neurosurg Psychiatry* 47:288–291.

Burke D, Skuse NF, Lethlean AK (1981): Cutaneous and muscle afferent components of the cerebral potential evoked by electrical stimulation of human peripheral nerves. *Electroencephalogr Clin Neurophysiol* 51:579–588.

Caccia MR, Ubiali E, Andreussi L (1976): Spinal evoked responses recorded from the epidural space in normal and diseased humans. *J Neurol Neurosurg Psychiatry* 39:962–972.

Chodoroff G, Lee DW, Honet JC (1985): Dynamic approach in the diagnosis of thoracic outlet syndrome using somatosensory evoked responses. *Arch Phys Med Rehabil* 66:3–6.

Cracco JB, Castells S, Mark E (1980): Conduction velocity in peripheral nerve and spinal afferent pathways in juvenile diabetics. *Neurology* 30:370–371.

Dawson GD, Scott JW (1949): Recording of nerve action potentials through the skin in man. *J Neurol Neurosurg Psychiatry* 12:259–267.

Desmedt JE, Noel P (1973): Average cerebral evoked potentials in the evaluation of lesions of the sensory nerves and of the central somatosensory pathway. In: *New Developments in Electromyography and Clinical Neurophysiology*, Vol 2, edited by JE Desmedt, pp 352–371. Karger, Basel.

Dvonch V, Scarff T, Buch WH, Smith D, Boscardin J, Lebarge H, Ibrahim K (1986): Dermatomal somatosensory evoked potentials: Their use in lumbar radiculopathy. *Spine* 9:291–293.

Ebner A, Dengler R, Meier C (1981): Peripheral and central conduction times in hereditary pressure-sensitive neuropathy. *J Neurol* 226:85–99.

Eisen A, Elleker G (1980): Sensory nerve stimulation and evoked cerebral potentials. *Neurology* 30:1097–1105.

Eisen A, Schomer D, Melamed C (1977): The application of F-wave measurements in the differentiation of proximal and distal upper limb entrapments. *Neurology* 27:662–668.

Eisen A, Purves S, Hoirch M (1982): Central nervous system amplification: Its potential in the diagnosis of early multiple sclerosis. *Neurology* 32:359–364.

Eisen A, Hoirch M, Moll A (1983): Evaluation of radiculopathies by segmental stimulation and somatosensory evoked potentials. *Can J Neurol Sci* 10:178–182.

El-Negamy E, Sedgwick EM (1979): Delayed cervical somatosensory evoked potentials in cervical spondylosis. *J Neurol Neurosurg Psychiatry* 42:238–241.

Ertekin C, Mutlu R, Sarica Y, Uckardesler L (1980): Electrophysiological evaluation of the afferent spinal roots and nerves in patients with conus medullaris and cauda equina lesions. *J Neurol Sci* 48:419–433.

Ertekin C, Sarica Y, Uckardesler L (1984): Somatosensory cerebral potentials evoked by stimulation of the lumbosacral spinal cord in normal subjects and in patients with conus medullaris and cauda equina lesions. *Electroencephalogr Clin Neurophysiol* 59:57–66.

Ferrante A, Wilbourn AJ (1995): The utility of various sensory nerve conduction responses in assessing brachial plexopathies. *Muscle Nerve* 18:879–889.

Ganes T (1980): Somatosensory conduction times and peripheral, cervical and cortical evoked potentials in patients with cervical spondylosis. *J Neurol Neurosurg Psychiatry* 43:683–689.

Gepstein R, Brown MD (1989): Somatosensory evoked potentials in lumbar nerve root decompression. *Clin Orthop* 245:69–71.

Gilliatt RW, Hjorth RJ (1972): Nerve conduction during Wallerian degeneration in the baboon. *J Neurol Neurosurg Psychiatry* 35:335–441.

Gilliatt RW, Willison RG, Dietz V, Williams IR (1978): Peripheral nerve conduction in patients with cervical rib and band. *Ann Neurol* 4:124–129.

Gilmore RL, Nelson KR (1989): SSEP and F-wave studies in acute inflammatory demyelinating neuropathy. *Muscle Nerve* 12(7):538–543.

Glover JL, Worth RM, Bendick PJ, Hall PV, Markand OM (1981): Evoked responses in the diagnosis of thoracic outlet syndrome. *Surgery* 89:86–92.

Harris JB, Thesleff S (1972): Nerve stump length and membrane changes in denervated skeletal muscle. *Nature* (NB) 276:60–61.

Heiskari M, Siivola J, Heikkinen ER (1986): Somatosensory evoked potentials in evaluation of decompressive surgery of cervical spondylosis and herniated disc. *Ann Clin Res* 47:107–113.

Inouye Y, Buchthal F (1977): Segmental sensory innervation determined by potentials recorded from cervical spinal nerves. *Brain* 100:731–748.

Jerrett SA, Cuzzone LJ, Pasternalk BM (1984): Thoracic outlet syndrome: Electrophysiological reappraisal. *Arch Neurol* 41:960–963.

Jones SJ (1979): Investigation of brachial plexus traction lesions by peripheral and spinal somatosensory evoked potentials. *J Neurol Neurosurg Psychiatry* 42:107–116.

Jones SJ, Wynn Parry CB, Landi A (1981): Diagnosis of brachial plexus traction lesions by sensory nerve action potentials and somatosensory evoked potentials. *Injury* 12:376–382.

Jones SJ, Yu YL, Rudge P, Kriss A, Gilois C, Hirani N, Nijhawan R, Norman P, Will R (1987): Central and peripheral SEP defects in neurologically symptomatic and asymptomatic subjects with low vitamin B12 levels. *J Neurol Sci* 82:55–65.

Katifi HA, Sedgwick EM (1986): Somatosensory evoked potentials from posterior tibial nerve and lumbosacral dermatomes. *Electroencephalogr Clin Neurophysiol* 65:249–259.

Kubota S, Masuda T, Ohmori S, Nagashima C (1984): Evaluation of cord functions in patients with cervical radiculomyelopathy using cortical and spinal somatosensory evoked potentials. *No To Shinkei* 36:339–348.

Landi A, Copeland SA, Wynn Parry CB, Jones SJ (1980): The role of somatosensory evoked potentials and nerve conduction studies in the surgical management of brachial plexus injuries. *J Bone Joint Surg* 62-B:492–496.

Lai DT, Walsh J, Harris JP, May J (1995): Predicting outcomes in thoracic outlet syndrome. *Med J Aust* 162(7):345–347.

Leblhuber MD, Reisecker F, Boehm-Jurkovic H, Witzmann A, Deisenhammer E (1988): Diagnostic value of different electrophysiologic tests in cervical disk prolapse. *Neurology* 38:1879–1881.

Machleder HI, Moll F, Nuwer M, Jordan S (1987): Somatosensory evoked potentials in the assessment of thoracic outlet compression syndrome. *J Vasc Surg* 6(2):177–184.

Mastaglia FL, Black JL, Edis R, Collins DWK (1978): The contribution of evoked potentials in the functional assessment of the somatosensory pathway. *Clin Exp Neurol* 15:279–298.

Matsukado Y, Yoshida M, Goya T, Shimoji K (1976): Classification of cervical spondylosis or disc protrusion by preoperative evoked spinal electrogram. *J Neurosurg* 44:435–441.

Murase T, Kawai H, Masatomi T, et al (1993): Evoked spinal cord potentials for diagnosis during brachial plexus surgery. *J Bone Joint Surg* 75(5):775–781.

Nakumara R, Noritake M, Hosoda Y, et al (1992): Somatosensory conduction delay in central and peripheral nervous system of diabetic patients. *Diabetes Care* 15(4):532–535.

Nelson JI, Seiple WH (1992): Human VEP contrast modulation sensitivity: separation of magno- and parvocellular components. *Electroencephalogr Clin Neurophysiol* 84:1–12.

Newmark J, Levy SR, Hochberg FH (1985): Somatosensory evoked potentials in thoracic outlet syndrome. *Arch Neurol* 42:1036.

Palma V, Serra LL, Armentano V, et al (1994): Somatosensory evoked potentials in non-insulin diabetics with different degrees of neuropathy. *Diabetes Res Clin Pract* 1994;25(2):91–96.

Parry GJ, Aminoff MJ (1987): Somatosensory evoked potentials in chronic acquired demyelinating peripheral neuropathy. *Neurology* 37:313–316.

Passero S, Paradiso C, Giannini F, et al (1994): Diagnosis of thoracic outlet syndrome. Relative value of electrophysiological studies. *Acta Neurol Scand* 90(3):179–185.

Perlik SJ, Fisher MA (1987): Somatosensory evoked response evaluation of cervical spondylitic myelopathy. *Muscle Nerve* 10(6):481–489.

Pozzessere G, Rizzo PA, Valle E, et al (1988): Early detection of neurological involvement in IDDM and NIDDM. Multimodal evoked potential versus metabolic control. *Diabetes Care* 11(6):473–480.

Rodriguez AA, Kanis L, Lane D (1987): Somatosensory evoked potentials from dermatomal stimulation as an indicator of L5 and S1 radiculopathy. *Arch Phys Med Rehabil* 68:266–368.

Ropper AH, Chiappa KH (1986): Evoked potentials in Guillain-Barré Syndrome. *Neurology* 36:587–590.

Rosen I, Sornas R, Elmqvist D (1977): Cervical root avulsion–electrophysiological analysis with electrospino-gram. *Scand J Plast Reconstr Surg* 11:247–250.

Salafsky B, Jasinski D (1967): Early electrophysiological changes after denervation of fast skeletal muscle. *Exp Neurol* 19:375–387.

Scarff TB, Dallmann DE, Bunch WH (1981): Dermatomal somatosensory evoked potentials in the diagnosis of lumbar root entrapment. *Surg Forum* 32:489–491.

Schimsheimer RJ, Ongerboer de Visser BW, Bour J, Kropveld D, Van Ammers VCPJ (1988): Digital nerve so-matosensory evoked potentials and flexor carpi radialis H reflexes in cervical disc protrusion and involvement of the sixth and seventh root: Relations to clinical and myelographic findings. *Electroencephalogr Clin Neuro-physiol* 70:313–324.

Schmid UD, Hess CW, Ludin HP (1988): Somatosensory evoked potentials following nerve and segmental stimu-lation do not confirm cervical radiculopathy with sensory deficit. *J Neurol Neurosurg Psychiatry* 51:182–187.

Sedgwick EM, Katifi HA, Docherty TB, Nicpon K (1985): Dermatomal somatosensory evoked potentials in lum-bar disc disease. In: *Evoked Potentials: Neurophysiological and Clinical Aspects*, edited by C Morocutti and PA Rizzo, pp 77–88. Elsevier, New York.

Siivola J, Myllylla VV, Sulg I, Hokkanen E (1979): Brachial plexus and radicular neurography in relation to corti-cal evoked responses. *J Neurol Neurosurg Psychiatry* 42:1151–1158.

Siivola J, Sulg I, Heiskari M (1981): Somatosensory evoked potentials in diagnostics of cervical spondylosis and herniated disc. *Electroencephalogr Clin Neurophysiol* 52:276–282.

Siivola J, Pokela R, Sulg I (1983): Somatosensory evoked responses as a diagnostic aid in thoracic outlet syn-drome: A post-operative study. *Acta Chir Scand* 149:147–150.

Starr A, McKeon B, Skuse N, Burke D (1981): Cerebral potentials evoked by muscle stretch in man. *Brain* 104:149–166.

Strenge H, Soyka D, Tackmann W (1982): Visual and somatosensory evoked potentials and F-wave latency mea-surements in hereditary neuropathy with liability to pressure palsies. *J Neurol* 226:269–273.

Sugioka H, Tsuyama N, Hara T, Nagao A, Tachibona S, Acheai N (1982): Investigation of brachial plexus injuries by intraoperative cortical somatosensory evoked potentials. *Arch Orthop Traumat Surg* 99:143–151.

Synek VM (1986): Somatosensory evoked potentials after stimulation of digital nerves in upper limbs: Normative data. *Electroencephalogr Clin Neurophysiol* 65:460–463.

Synek VM (1987): Role of somatosensory evoked potentials in the diagnosis of peripheral nerve lesions: Recent advances. *J Clin Neurophysiol* 4:55–73.

Synek VM, Cowan JC (1982): Somatosensory evoked potentials in patients with supraclavicular brachial plexus injury. *Neurology* 32:1347–1352.

Tans RJ, Vredeveld JW (1992): Somatosensory evoked potentials (cutaneous nerve stimulation) and electromyog-raphy in lumbosacral radiculopathy. *Clin Neurol Neurosurg* 94(1):15–17.

Vasjar J, Taylor MJ, MacMillan LJ, et al. (1992): Somatosensory evoked potentials and nerve conduction studies in patients with Guillain- Barré Syndrome. *Brain Dev* 14(5):315–318.

Veilleux M, Daube JR (1987): The value of ulnar somatosensory evoked potentials (SEPs) in cervical myelopathy. *Electroencephalogr Clin Neurophysiol* 68:415–423.

Veilleux M, Stevens JC, Campbell JK (1988): Somatosensory evoked potentials: Lack of value for diagnosis of thoracic outlet syndrome. *Muscle Nerve* 11:571–575.

Walsh JC, Yiannikas C, Mcleod JG (1984): Abnormalities of proximal conduction in acute idiopathic polyneuritis: Comparison of short latency somatosensory evoked potentials and F-waves. *J Neurol Neurosurg Psychiatry* 47:197–200.

Wulff CH, Gilliatt RW (1979): F-waves in patients with hand wasting caused by a cervical rib and band. *Muscle Nerve* 2:452–457.

Yiannikas C (1983): Cervical radiculopathies. In: *Evoked Potentials in Clincial Medicine*, edited by KH Chiappa, pp 281–285. Raven Press, New York.

Yiannikas C, Walsh JC (1983): Somatosensory evoked potentials in thoracic outlet syndrome. *J Neurol Neurosurg Psychiatry* 46:234–240.

Yiannikas C, Shahani BT, Young RR (1983): The investigation of traumatic lesions of the brachial plexus by elec-tromyography and short latency somatosensory potentials evoked by stimulation of multiple peripheral nerves: *J Neurol Neurosurg Psychiatry* 46:1014–1022.

Yiannikas C, Shahani BT, Young RR (1986): Short-latency somatosensory- evoked potentials from radial, median, ulnar and peroneal nerve stimulation in the assessment of cervical spondylosis. *Arch Neurol* 43:1264–1271.

Yu YL, Jones SJ (1985): Somatosensory evoked potentials in cervical spondylosis: Correlation of median, ulnar and posterior tibial nerve responses with clinical and radiological findings. *Brain* 108:273–300.

Zalis AW, Oester YT, Rodriquez AA (1970): Electrophysiological diagnosis of cervical nerve root avulsion. *Arch Phys Med* 51:708–710.

Zeigler D, Muhlen H, Dannehl K, Gries FA (1993). Tibial nerve somatosensory evoked potentials at various stages of peripheral neuropathy in insulin dependent diabetic patients. *J Neurol Neurosurg Psychiatry* 56(1):58–64.

Zverina E, Kredba J (1977): Somatosensory cerebral evoked potentials in diagnosing brachial plexus injuries. *Scand J Rehab Med* 9:47–54.

Evoked Potentials in Clinical Medicine,
3d ed., edited by Keith H. Chiappa.
Lippincott–Raven Publishers, Philadelphia © 1997.

11

Somatosensory Evoked Potentials in Pediatrics

Susan R. Levy

*Departments of Pediatrics, Neurology, and Child Study Center,
Yale University School of Medicine, New Haven, Connecticut 06510*

Somatosensory evoked potential (SEP) testing can provide a noninvasive objective method of evaluating the central and peripheral nervous systems and can also generate information about the maturation of the human afferent sensory system. This testing is particularly useful because the clinical sensory neurologic examination is often difficult and unreliable in infants and young children. Although in childhood the clinical applications of SEPs are less well-established than those in the adult population, abnormalities have been described in children with diffuse and focal neurologic disorders. The utility of these tests as diagnostic aids depends upon the ability to generate reproducible data and to compare the data to normative values. Accurate and age-specific normative data are critical if SEP testing is used in the pediatric population as a prognostic tool to determine the functional integrity of the somatosensory pathways. There are changes in response patterns during normal growth and development. These changes must not be mistaken for alterations occurring in various disease states.

1. SPECIAL METHODOLOGY

1.1. Recording and Stimulating Parameters

Somatosensory EP testing is generally well-tolerated by infants and young children. Data are easily collected because children are more relaxed in the testing situation and thus have less muscle artifact than adults. Somatosensory EPs have been recorded after electrical stimulation of the median (Cullity et al., 1976; Willis et al., 1984; Cracco and Cracco, 1986;

Cracco et al., 1988; Lafreniere et al., 1990; Laureau and Marlot, 1990; George and Taylor, 1991; Gibson et al., 1992), posterior tibial (Gilmore et al., 1985, 1987; Gilmore, 1986; Laureau and Marlot, 1990), and peroneal nerves (Cracco et al., 1975, 1979; Cracco and Cracco, 1982) in infants and children. The responses are recorded from surface electrodes. In premature or term newborns the electrodes should be applied with electrode paste and nonirritating tape after gentle abrasion of the skin. Collodion should not be used in this age group because of skin sensitivity. In older children electrodes can be applied with paste and tape or collodion.

Somatosensory EPs to median nerve stimulation are recorded from a midclavicular site (Erb's point, ipsilateral to stimulation) cervical spine (C2, C5, or C7) and the contralateral sensory cortex (C3' or C4', 2 cm behind the C3 or C4 site in the standard 10–20 system)

TABLE 11–1. *Median nerve normative data*

Age	Arm Length (cm)		Latency (msec)			
			N13	P14	N20	N13–N20
0–2 wks	—	Mean	9.7	—	26.7	17.2
		SD	0.9	—	5.7	6.4
3–6 wks	—	Mean	—	16	21.79	—
		SD	—	2.14	3.05	—
7–13 wks	—	Mean	—	14.54	20.71	—
		SD	—	1.85	2.54	—
4–8 mos	26	Mean	8.27	10.6	17.74	9.63
		SD	0.53	1.11	0.85	0.94
		U limit	9.6	13.37	19.86	11.98
9–15 mos	30	Mean	8.01	9.45	15.71	7.89
		SD	0.5	0.95	0.94	0.97
		U limit	9.26	11.83	18.06	10.31
16–22 mos	33	Mean	7.82	10.13	15.41	7.76
		SD	0.32	0.52	0.63	0.44
		U limit	8.62	11.43	16.98	8.86
2–3 yrs	37	Mean	7.77	—	14.88	7.1
		SD	0.3	—	0.93	1.04
		U limit	8.52	—	17.2	9.7
3–5 yrs	44	Mean	8.62	10.82	15.28	6.69
		SD	0.45	0.51	0.58	0.49
		U limit	9.74	12.09	16.73	7.91
6–8 yrs	54	Mean	9.63	11.56	15.52	5.71
		SD	0.43	0.45	0.54	0.47
		U limit	10.71	12.69	16.87	6.89
9–11 yrs	60	Mean	10.7	12.63	16.53	5.84
		SD	0.37	0.5	0.6	0.43
		U limit	11.63	13.88	18.03	6.92
12–16 yrs	66	Mean	11.6	13.36	17.24	5.64
		SD	0.68	0.61	0.69	0.4
		U limit	13.3	14.88	18.97	6.64
14–18 yrs	73	Mean	12.21	13.94	17.73	5.6
		SD	0.89	0.83	0.79	0.48
		U limit	14.43	16.01	19.7	6.8

Normative data for median nerve SEPs from Laureau and Marlot (1990) for age 0 to 2 weeks, George and Taylor (1991) for ages 3 to 13 weeks and Taylor and Fagan (1988) for ages 4 months to 18 years. Recording techniques for 0 to 2 weeks include unilateral stimulation, stimulation rate of 2 to 5 Hz, bandpass of 20 to 2,000 Hz. Recording techniques for 3 to 13 weeks include unilateral stimulation, stimulation rate of 1.1 Hz, band-pass of 30 to 3,000 Hz with a 100K gain, sweep of 200 msec, 64 trials recorded. Recording parameters for older children differed with a sweep of 50 msec, stimulation rate of 4.1 Hz, and 256 trials recorded. Potentials were recorded over the cervical spine at C2 for the 1 to 2 week age group and at C7 for the other ages, and contralateral somatosensory cortex (C3', C4') referenced to FpZ.

TABLE 11–2. *Posterior tibial nerve normative data*

Age		Latency (msec)					
1–8 yrs		N14 (LP)	N20	P28	N14–N20	N20–P28	N14–P28
	Mean	13.7	19.96	27.74	6.27	6.79	13.28
	SD	1.33	1.63	3.17	0.64	1.27	1.54
	U limit	16.56	24.24	33.12	7.68	8.88	18.6
Preterm newborn		N16 (LP)	N27	P55	N16–N27	N27–P55	N16–P55
	Mean	16.07	27.37	54.97	11.08	25.35	37.81
	SD	2.5	4.36	8.9	4.24	8.63	7.85
	U limit	22.4	34.56	72.32	18.88	39.36	44.8
Term newborn		N8 (LP)		P32			N8–P32
	Mean	7.8		32.5			24.6
	SD	1.2		3.1			3.1
	U limit	10.4		38.4			31.2

Normative data for posterior tibial nerve SEPs from Gilmore (1985, 1987) for the preterm newborn (post conceptional age of 26 to 38.2 weeks, with a mean of 32.3 weeks) and children ages 1 to 8 years and from Laureau and Marlot (1990) for term newborns (post conceptional age 37 to 43 weeks, mean 41 weeks). The recording techniques used in Gilmore's studies included stimulation at the ankle at a rate or 5 Hz, band-pass of 30 to 1500 Hz with a 40K gain, sweep of 81.92 to 102.4 msec, 1,000 to 3,000 trials averaged. The following montages were used: N16 and N14 (spL1–spT6), N27 (spC7–FpZ), P55 (CZ'–FpZ), N20 (spC7–FZ), P28 (CZ'–FZ). In term newborns the tibial nerve was stimulated at the popliteal fossa at a rate of 2 to 5 Hz. N8 was recorded from L2 to L4 and P32 from FpZ to CZ. Five hundred to 1,000 responses were averaged.

referenced to FZ (Chiappa, 1983), FpZ, or a noncephalic reference (Chiappa, 1983). The potentials are designated, as in adults, according to their peak latency and polarity. In newborns, the Erb's point potential is best recorded 1 cm above the axilla (Cracco et al., 1988) and the cervical potential at the C7 vertebral prominence. In older infants and children the placement of the stimulating electrode is similar to that in adults. In very young infants the stimulator can be placed with the anode in the palm and the cathode at the wrist. Stimulating electrodes have also been placed on opposite sides of the wrist with the cathode ventral and the anode dorsal (Hrbek et al., 1973; Willis et al., 1984). This method can eliminate the possibility of a salt bridge between stimulating electrodes on these small wrists. Lower stimulus rates (1.1 Hz) produce higher-amplitude SEPs in neonates and older infants (George and Taylor, 1991; Willis, 1986). The optimal band-pass in children and infants older than 4 months is 30 to 3,000 Hz, with a sweep of 50 msec (Taylor and Fagan, 1988). The cortical EP may be difficult to record in the first 3 months of life. George and Taylor (1991) have suggested using two recording techniques: (1) 30 to 3,000 Hz band-pass and a 80- to 100-msec sweep, and (2) 5 to 1,500 Hz and a 200-msec sweep. Fifty to 60 trials are averaged with each technique. If the first set of parameters provides reproducible results, then the other settings are not needed.

Lower-extremity SEPs are generated by stimulation of the posterior tibial nerve at the ankle or the peroneal nerve at the knee. The recording sites for peroneal and tibial nerve stimulation are similar to those in adults. Spinal recordings utilize the spinous processes of the first or third lumbar vertebrae referenced to the contralateral iliac crest (Chiappa, 1983) or a rostral spinous process such as T6 (Cracco et al., 1975; Gilmore et al., 1985). Scalp potentials are recorded at CZ referenced to FZ (Chiappa, 1983), CZ' (2 cm behind CZ) referenced to FZ (Gilmore et al., 1985), or CZ' to FpZ'(midway between FpZ and FZ) (Cracco and Cracco, 1986). Additionally, potentials over the C7, T6, and T12 vertebral processes are of greater amplitude than in the adult and thus bipolar spine recordings are more easily elicited than in the adult. Each limb can be stimulated separately in older infants and children. In premature and newborn infants bilateral nerve stimulation is necessary to obtain reproducible results (Cracco et al., 1979; Gilmore et al., 1987). Recording techniques are similar to those for the median nerve. The sweep time should be 80 to 100 msec.

Results are compared to normative data based upon height and age for peak latencies. (Tables 11–1 and 11–2) Criteria for abnormalities include absence of waveforms normally recorded and peripheral conduction velocities and interpeak latencies (IPLs) which are 2.5 to 3.0 standard deviations (SD) from the mean of age-matched controls (see American EEG Society Guidelines for Clinical Evoked Potential Studies, *J Clin Neurophysiol* 1:3–54, 1984, and 3 (Suppl. 1):43–92, 1986).

1.2. Sedation

Although many children can cooperate for SEP testing, children less than 3 years of age or those with developmental delay may require sedation to eliminate movement and muscle artifact. Oral chloral hydrate (50 to 75 mg/kg) is most often administered. The scalp-recorded responses in children sedated in this manner may change unpredictably. Changes have consisted of amplitude reduction and latency shifts in the cortical potential after upper-limb stimulation (Fagan et al., 1987a). Similar changes have not been observed in the peripheral and spinal components. If cortical potentials are abnormal after the child has been sedated, the study must be repeated without sedation.

1.3. Sleep

Sleep may also induce changes in the SEP waveform. In preterm infants, Gilmore et al. (1987) recorded a cortical potential after posterior tibial nerve stimulation more often during rapid eye movement (REM) sleep and slow-wave sleep than during waking. Desmedt and Manil (1970) measured a difference in peak latency and duration of the cortical waveforms between the waking state and quiet sleep (mean increase of peak latency of 2.5 msec, $p < 0.01$) but no significant difference between waking and REM sleep among 34 normal term neonates. Willis (1986) examined 15 normal infants 1 year of age or younger and found similar cerebral potentials during REM sleep and quiet sleep in neonates. In older infants, the amplitude of SEP cerebral components was higher in the waking state than in stage 2 sleep. Sleep could also induce latency shifts. Fagan et al. (1987a) found little effect of natural sleep on the SEP components in children older than 4 months of age, although rarely changes in amplitude and latency were observed. These studies provide evidence that when latency shifts or loss of cortical components are observed during sleep the study should be repeated with the infant awake to determine whether the responses are abnormal or are sleep induced.

2. MATURATIONAL CHANGES AND NORMATIVE DATA

Somatosensory EPs can be recorded from premature and term infants and children. There are maturational changes which occur during normal growth and development. The changes seen in waveform latency and morphology are secondary to the combined effects of synaptic expansion and myelination of the peripheral and central somatosensory pathways and the increase in length of these pathways with body growth. The peripheral and central segments of the somatosensory pathways mature asynchronously with earlier maturation in the periphery (Yakovlev et al., 1967). Myelination of the peripheral fibers progresses earlier and more rapidly than that of the central pathways (Gilles et al., 1983). Electrophysiological data reflect these trends.

The mean latency of the Erb's point potential remains constant over time, whereas latencies of cervical and cortical potentials decrease with maturation in normal infants from birth to 12 months (Willis et al., 1984). Cracco et al. (1988) found latencies over Erb's point and cervical cord to be stable in newborns and older infants. The conduction velocity over the peroneal nerve is about one half the adult value in the newborn and increases rapidly during the first year of life, reaching the adult value by 3 to 4 years of age (Cracco et al., 1979). Gilmore et al. (1985) studied 32 healthy children ages 1 to 8 years and found that all had an electronegative potential recorded over the first lumbar vertebra after tibial nerve stimulation (13.70 msec ± 1.33). The latency of the potential was correlated positively with height and age. These data reflect the early maturation in the peripheral nervous system.

Cracco et al. (1979) recorded sequentially over lumbar, thoracic and cervical spinal cord levels in 95 normal infants, children, and adults. The conduction velocity was nonlinear and slower over the lower thoracic spine than over the cauda equina and more rostral portions of the spinal cord. The conduction velocities in these central afferent pathways were one half the adult values at birth and increased to adult values by 5 to 7 years of age.

The latency of potentials recorded over the cervical cord remain relatively constant until 2 to 3 years of age and then increase to adult values by 14 to 18 years (Taylor et al., 1988). Fagan et al. (1987a,b) demonstrated that the IPL between the potentials recorded over the cervical cord and cortex decreases from a mean of 11.6 msec at 4 to 8 months of age to a mean of 7 msec at 6 to 8 years of age and remains constant into adulthood. Allison et al. (1984) studied IPLs in patients 4 to 17 years of age. The most striking developmental change was a decrease in latency of the cortical components as compared to the spinal cord and brainstem portions of the somatosensory pathway.

Desmedt et al. (1976) studied the maturational changes in the cortical component after mechanical stimulation of the median nerve. The latency of the initial negative component decreased in early childhood until 8 years of age and then increased to adult values as body size increased and conduction velocity remained unchanged. The latency of the cortical wave after median nerve stimulation decreases from 18 msec at 4 to 8 months of age to 15 msec at 2 to 3 years of age and then gradually increases to adult values (Taylor and Fagan, 1988). A cortical potential was recorded in all subjects ages 1 to 8 years after tibial nerve stimulation at 27.74 msec ± 3.17 (Gilmore et al., 1985). The latency of this potential is more variable in children than in adults and is not as highly correlated with height as in adults. Conduction times in the central somatosensory pathways are the greatest in the infant and young child and decrease with age (Fig 11–1) (Hume et al., 1982; Chiappa, 1983; Cadilhac et al., 1986; Cracco and Cracco, 1986; Lauffer and Wenzel, 1986; Tomita and Tanaka, 1986; Fagan et al., 1987a,b; Zhu et al., 1987; Bartel et al., 1988; Gilmore, 1988; Taylor and Fagan, 1988; Mutoh et al., 1988; Tomita et al., 1988).

Hrbek et al. (1973) stimulated the median nerve and recorded a long-latency (>200 msec), long-duration negative potential in infants 25 to 28 weeks gestation. After 29 weeks gestation an initial negative component was recorded which progressively decreased in am-

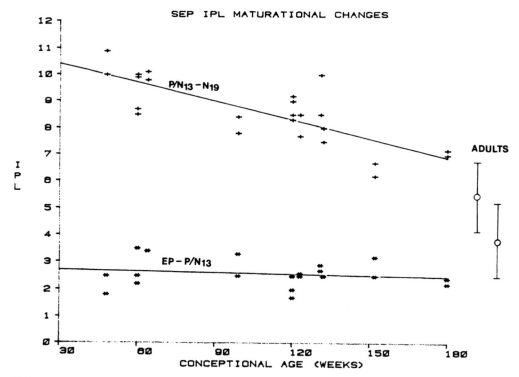

FIG. 11–1. Median nerve SEP maturational changes in IPLs. Conceptual age is gestational age plus chronologic age. Interpeak latency is in milliseconds.

plitude and duration, reaching a mature newborn response at 37 to 38 weeks gestational age. Gallai et al. (1986) studied 40 preterm (32 to 37 weeks) and 42 full-term infants and found a cortical component in all with the latency significantly decreasing with advancing age. Majnemer et al. (1990b) compared normative data obtained from term infants with data from low-risk premature infants tested at term utilizing median nerve stimulation. The study demonstrated that there are no significant differences in absolute or interwave latencies at similar conceptional ages.

Gilmore (1986) studied preterm newborns (26 to 36 weeks) utilizing bilateral tibial nerve stimulation and found an electronegative potential over the first lumbar vertebral prominence in all subjects. The latency of this potential varied widely (16.07 msec ± 2.50) and decreased with increasing postconceptual age and length. This inverse relationship suggests that the increased conduction velocity exceeds linear growth in this age group.

There is a gradual change in the form of the evoked responses with increasing age. The cortical components generated by upper- and lower-extremity stimulation are broader in children than in adults and there is a decrease in the duration of the cerebral components with maturation (Desmedt et al., 1976; Willis et al., 1984; Sitzouglou and Fotiou, 1985; Cracco and Cracco, 1986). Bifid patterns of the scalp recorded component of the median nerve SEP begin to develop at 1 year of age and are well-developed in childhood by 3 to 5 years of age (Fig. 11–2). The bifid appearance of the cervical component of the median nerve SEP disappears in early childhood, with the typical adult pattern recorded consistently in teenage years (Taylor and Fagan, 1988). Components arising from the peripheral nerve, spinal cord, and brainstem are of greater amplitude and complexity in children compared to those of adults (Cracco and Cracco 1979, 1986). Overall, waveform morphology becomes similar to adults between 5 and 8 years of age.

Although complex maturational changes in the brainstem and cerebral portions of the somatosensory system begin in the fetus, they continue during the first 2 years of life. As a consequence of incomplete maturation at term, some components of the SEP may not be recorded consistently in infancy. Therefore it is necessary to define the time when SEP components should be reliably recorded. Gilmore et al. (1987) found the scalp-recorded component of the

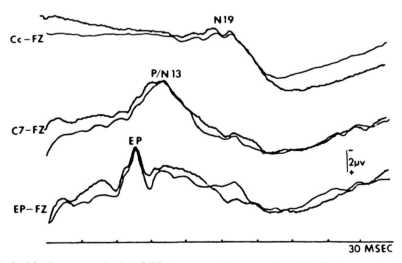

FIG. 11–2. Median nerve (wrist) SEP in a normal 6-year-old child. Each trace is the average of 1,024 stimuli, delivered at 5/sec. System band-pass was 30 to 3,000 Hz.

tibial nerve SEP to be present in approximately 50% of newborns and absent in infants younger than 31 weeks postconceptual age. Among full-term newborns, cortical EPs to median nerve stimulation have been reportedly present in 66% (Willis et al., 1984) and in 85% (Laureau et al., 1988) of cases. Cracco et al. (1988) found the cortical component of the median nerve SEP to be present consistently in infants 6 weeks of age post-term and Willis et al. (1984) recorded this potential after 8 weeks post-term. These data underscore the necessity of performing serial follow-up SEP studies in newborns who initially demonstrate abnormalities.

3. CLINICAL APPLICATIONS

The clinical usefulness of SEP in the pediatric population is increasing as the availability of normative data has improved. The conduction times within the peripheral and central somatosensory pathways have been seen to be altered by a variety of disease states.

3.1. Neurodegenerative Disorders

Several SEP studies of children with neurodegenerative disorders affecting gray and white matter describe abnormal responses to both upper- and lower-extremity stimulation. (Cracco et al., 1980; Markand et al., 1982; Tobimatsu et al., 1985; Rossini et al., 1986 and 1987; De Meirleir et al., 1988.) Cracco et al. (1980) studied the EPs to median nerve and peroneal stimulation in 17 children with neurodegenerative disorders. Within this group of patients, there were 10 with Tay-Sachs disease, 2 with Canavans' disease, 1 with Sandhoff's disease, 1 with Hunter's disease, 1 with neuroaxonal dystrophy, 1 with GM3 gangliosidosis, and 1 with juvenile-onset neuronal ceroid lipofuscinosis. In all patients the cauda equina and peripheral nerve conduction velocities were normal. The responses over the caudal and rostral spinal cord segments, brainstem, and cortex were abnormal. Alterations in waveform morphology, delay in latency, or absence of components were seen in degrees proportional to severity of disease.

Markand et al. (1982) studied 18 patients with leukodystrophy [Pelizaeus–Merzbacher disease (PMD), 12; adrenoleukodystrophy (ALD), 3; metachromatic leukodystrophy (MLD), 3]. Median nerve SEPs showed abnormalities of central components and in the patients with metachromatic leukodystrophy an absence of Erb's point potential reflecting peripheral nerve involvement. In 15 patients with a consistent Erb's point potential, normal cervical and scalp potentials were seen in only one patient with ALD in an early stage. Two other ALD patients showed a delay between cervical and scalp potentials. Scalp components were absent in 12 patients (11 PMD, 1 MLD). Ten of 11 patients had abnormal tibial SEPs. In five (four PMD, one ALD), no cortical responses could be recorded. Two patients with PMD had unilateral absence of cortical potentials and in three (one PMD, one ALD, one MLD) cortical responses were prolonged.

DeMeirleir et al. (1988) studied 22 children with leukodystrophy (10 MLD, 2 ALD, 4 PMD, 3 Krabbe's disease, 1 Canavan's disease, 1 Alexander's disease, 1 multiple sulfatase deficiency) and in all but four mild cases cortical SEPs were absent. Peripheral and/or central conduction delays were seen in the four mildly affected children and reflected the areas of demyelination early in the course of their disease. No SEPs were normal.

Tobimatsu et al. (1985) performed SEPs on five patients, including two with ALD, one with adrenomyeloneuropathy (AMN), one female carrier of AMN, and one female carrier of ALD. The two cases of ALD had a prolonged central conduction time between cervical cord and cortex. The patient and carrier with AMN had delayed Erb's point potential in addition to a similar central conduction delay. These findings differentiated AMN from ALD and reflect the peripheral nerve involvement in AMN.

Rossini et al. (1986) and Rossini and Cracco (1987) studied SEPs in patients with other neurodegenerative disorders, including Friedreich's ataxia (FA), hereditary motor sensory neuropathy, late-onset cerebellar atrophy, familial spastic paraplegia, olivopontocerebellar atrophy, and ataxia telangiectasia. Abnormalities only of peroneal SEPs were seen in patients with hereditary motor sensory neuropathy II, ataxia telangiectasia, and in two with olivopontocerebellar atrophy. Somatosensory EPs to upper- and lower-limb stimulation were abnormal in 25 of 33 patients, including all patients with FA and hereditary motor sensory neuropathy I and III, and one with olivopontocerebellar atrophy. As in other studies, patients with FA had impaired central conduction and normal or slightly prolonged peripheral nerve potential latencies (Taylor and Chan-Lui, 1985). Upper- and lower-limb SEPs were normal in patients with familial spastic paraplegia and late-onset cerebellar atrophy. Somatosensory EPs have been found to be more severely altered than brain stem auditory EPs and serial testing parallels the clinical progression of disease (Rossini and Cracco, 1987). Johnson (1985) described prolonged central conduction and normal peripheral nerve conduction of median nerve SEPs in a patient with abetalipoproteinemia. Somatosensory EPs are generally normal in acute cerebellar ataxia and in chronic ataxias of unknown etiology (Fagan et al., 1987b).

3.2. Coma

Somatosensory EPs can be useful in the assessment of the comatose child. Somatosensory EP studies of comatose children may have prognostic value (Lutschg et al., 1983; Frank et al., 1985; White et al., 1985; DeMeirleir and Taylor, 1987; Taylor and Farrell, 1989; Goodwin et al., 1991; Beca et al., 1995). DeMeirleir et al. (1987) recorded SEPs in 73 comatose children with multiple etiologies admitted to an intensive care unit. Fourteen children who recovered normally had increased IPLs or normal SEPs; the IPL prolongations normalized on serial examinations in patients with normal outcomes. The persistence of a unilaterally absent cortical SEP in five patients was predictive of a hemiparesis. Children with bilaterally absent cortical responses either died (19) or developed severe neurologic sequelae (12). None of the patients who died had normal initial SEPs. Lutschg et al. (1983) studied 43 comatose children with median nerve SEP. Coma was due to head trauma in 26 and hypoxic-ischemic encephalopathy in 17. Of the 15 fatal cases, initial SEP studies showed bilateral absence of the cortical potential in 12, unilateral absence in 1, and delayed latency of the cortical potential in 1; 1 patient had a normal study. The cause of death of these latter three cases was not given. Follow-up SEP studies of patients who eventually died were described as severely abnormal. All five patients with brain death confirmed by arch aortogram had bilaterally absent cortical components. Patients surviving with neurologic sequelae had either unilateral loss or a latency prolongation of the cortical potential. Patients who experienced normal outcomes had initially normal or mildly delayed cortical SEPs. Of the 13 patients with bilateral absence of N19–P22, 12 died and 1 was left with neurologic deficits (not further defined). Frank et al. (1985) found bilateral absence of the cortical potentials after median nerve stimulation in five children with nontraumatic coma. Brainstem auditory EPs were preserved. Serial EP testing remained unchanged and all five children are in a chronic vegetative state. In this study, EP testing proved more reliable than the clinical examination or electroencephalography (EEG) for prediction of outcome. Similar findings were described in a study of 62 children with traumatic and nontraumatic coma (White et al.,

1985). Of 31 patients with absent cortical responses (unilateral or bilateral), 13 died, 16 survived in a chronic vegetative state, and 2 others (under 2 months of age) recovered. Of nine patients who had absent N19–P22 bilateral), four died and five developed a chronic vegetative state. Taylor and Farrell (1989) studied 37 children ages 7 months to 15 years in coma with multiple etiologies with serial median nerve SEPs. Of the 19 patients with bilateral absence of N19–P22, 15 died, 3 had severe sequelae, and 1 had a normal outcome. The one child who recovered had been struck by lightning. Goodwin et al. (1991) performed SEPs in 41 comatose children (ages 6 weeks to 18 years). Of 27 children who had bilaterally absent cortical responses, 23 died and 4 survived in a chronic vegetative state. Beca et al. (1995) prospectively evaluated SEPs as a predictor of outcome in 109 brain-injured children ages 0.1 to 16.8 years. Normal SEPs predicted a favorable outcome in 93% of patients. Abnormal SEPs predicted an unfavorable outcome, defined as severe disabilty or persistent vegetative state in 92% of cases. There were four cases in which SEPs were absent and a favorable outcome occurred. Two of these patients had meningitis and bilateral subdural hematomas, one had a midbrain hemorrhage, and one had a craniectomy for uncontrolled increased intracranial pressure. If these cases producing a physical barrier to the recording of the SEP were excluded, absent SEPs predicted an unfavorable outcome in 100% of the patients.

In summary, in the above seven studies, of 213 children in coma following a variety of insults, when N19–P22 was absent bilaterally, 110 died and 42 had severe disabilities [described as severe sequelae (28), neurologic deficits (1), and chronic vegetative state (23)]. Thus, as in adults, the bilateral absence of N19–P22 in coma is highly predictive of a very poor outcome in traumatic and atraumatic coma. The SEP can be used to help determine the level of support in the comatose child.

3.3. Encephalopathies

There has been no prospective study addressing the role of SEPs in the assessment of children with developmental delay. In infants and young children with mild nonspecific findings on examination, SEPs may be abnormal and suggest the need for further evaluations. In the older child with a nonprogressive or static encephalopathy, SEPs are generally normal (Fagan, 1987a,b).

Children with acquired immune deficiency syndrome (AIDS) often experience neurologic dysfunction and developmental regression. Udani et al. (1988) studied 18 HIV positive children with AIDS or AIDS-related complex using clinical and developmental assessments, BAEPs, SEPs, and magnetic resonance imaging (MRI). The mean age at disease onset was 19 months; 33% were microcephalic and 56% had motor abnormalities. All children were developmentally delayed. Twelve of fourteen median nerve and 4 of 16 peroneal nerve SEPs were abnormal centrally. Three of sixteen BAEPs had prolonged central conduction times and 4 of 16 had peripheral abnormalities. Only 3 of 14 MRI scans showed specific abnormalities, whereas all showed some degree of atrophy. The high frequency of abnormal SEPs early in pediatric AIDS suggests they may provide a method for monitoring the clinical course of these children.

3.4. Perinatal Asphyxia

Somatosensory EP testing has proven to be a useful adjunct to the clinical examination in high-risk neonates. Somatosensory EP abnormalities have been observed in term infants with perinatal asphyxia (Laget et al., 1976; Hrbek et al., 1977; Gorke, 1986, 1987; Majnemer et al., 1987, 1990a; Willis et al., 1984, 1987; Klimach and Cooke, 1988; de Vries et al., 1991; Taylor et al., 1992; de Vries, 1993). Willis et al. (1987) studied 10 asphyxiated term infants ages 2 to 6 months with subsequent follow-up evaluations to a mean age of 20 months to determine if SEP findings were predictive of future clinical findings. All children with prolonged latency or unilateral or bilateral absence of the cortical response after median nerve stimulation experienced subsequent neurologic sequelae. Results of the median nerve SEP testing correlated positively with outcome in all patients. Although SEP findings helped to distinguish normal from abnormal infants, they were not predictive of the degree of disability. Majnemer et al. (1987) found 10 of 34 neonates at risk for neurodevelopmental sequelae to have abnormal SEPs to median nerve stimulation. Abnormalities included increased latency of cortical potentials, increased interwave latency between cervical spinal cord and cortex and unilateral or bilateral absence of cortical potentials. Somatosensory EP findings correlated positively with clinical outcome. All three children with bilaterally absent cortical potentials which persisted on serial tests developed spastic quadriparesis. One patient with a unilaterally absent cortical potential had greater motor impairments on the side corresponding to this abnormality. One patient with a unilaterally absent response and a prolonged latency on the other side, had a spastic diplegia greatest on the side with the flat response. Serial SEPs in four patients showing increased absolute and interwave latencies normalized. Clinically these children have mild developmental delay and abnormalities of muscle tone. One patient in this series with an initially normal SEP suffered a hemispheric infarction. Follow-up SEP studies at 2 and 6 months of age demonstrated a unilateral absence of the cortical potential. At 6 months a hemiparesis was apparent clinically. The clinical status of the other 14 neonates with normal SEP responses was not provided. Laget et al. (1976) studied 43 children with focal motor deficits and found SEPs to be superior to EEG for localization of the responsible lesion. Taylor et al. (1992) performed serial median nerve EP studies on asphyxiated neonates and found that SEPs performed at the end of the first week provided the highest predictive ability regarding outcome.

Somatosensory EPs may also prove useful in the assessment of premature infants with intraventricular hemorrhage. Willis et al. (1984) demonstrated abnormal SEPs to median nerve stimulation in two premature infants with intraventricular hemorrhage. Somatosensory EP abnormalities correlated with the side of hemorrhage and subsequent neurologic sequelae. Pierrat et al. (1993) studied a group of infants with extensive cystic leukomalacia. Somatosensory EPs were performed between 31 and 49 weeks postmenstrual age in 27 infants. Fourteen of these infants had normal N19 latencies but developed neurologic sequelae. A large percentage of these infants had cysts restricted to the occipital periventricular white matter, posterior to the somatosensory tracts. Keenan et al. (1992) performed visual evoked potentials (VEPs) and SEPs in premature infants to establish whether these studies are predictive of neurodevelopmental outcome. Both SEPs and VEPs were reliably obtained but the results have as yet to be correlated with long-term follow-up studies.

Klimach and Cooke (1988) compared findings on cranial ultrasound with bilateral median nerve SEPs. Thirty patients had abnormal ultrasounds of varying severity and 14 of them had normal SEPs. These 14 infants had normal neurologic examinations at 6 months of age. Only those infants with bilateral abnormalities of the cortical SEP (prolonged peak latency or absence) manifested developmental delay in addition to motor deficits. No children with bilateral SEP abnormalities were normal. Among six infants with normal computed tomography scans and abnormal development, four had abnormal SEPs (Gorke, 1987). These studies suggest that SEP testing may have more predictive value for neurologic function than imaging studies. Somatosensory EPs can help to identify children at risk for impairments of motor development. The number of infants studied to date is small and therefore serial SEP examinations are currently necessary for correlation with clinical findings over time.

3.5. Compressive Lesions

Compressive lesions of the brainstem and spinal cord can produce abnormalities of SEPs. Neurologic complications occur in achondroplasia as a result of cervical or brainstem compression. Nelson et al. (1984) evaluated 23 patients with achondroplasia with median and peroneal nerve SEPs. Sixteen patients were asymptomatic and seven had neurologic signs. All symptomatic patients had normal SEPs with the level of abnormality correlating with the patient's clinical signs or radiographic findings. Forty-four percent of asymptomatic patients had abnormal SEPs and several were found subsequently to have foramen magnum stenosis. Abnormalities included prolonged interwave latencies or absence of responses over cervical cord and scalp. Although abnormal SEPs identify individuals with cervicomedullary stenosis (Nelson et al., 1984; Reid et al., 1987), SEPs have not been predictive of respiratory dysfunction or apnea in these patients (Nelson et al., 1988).

3.6. Structural Lesions

There is often a good correlation between clinical deficits and spinal SEP abnormalities in children with myelodysplasia (Cracco et al., 1974, 1979; Cracco and Cracco, 1982). In some

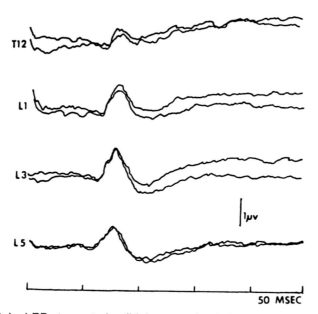

FIG. 11–3. Spinal EPs to posterior tibial nerve stimulation (ankle) in a 10-year-old boy with bladder dysfunction and lower-extremity weakness. The spinal potential is displaced caudally with maximal amplitude over L3 (normally this would be at 11 or 12). A sacral lipoma and tethered spinal cord were documented with MRI and surgery. Each trace is the average of 1,024 stimuli, delivered at 2/sec. The reference electrode was on the iliac crest. Relative negativity of the back electrodes caused an upward trace deflection. The system band-pass was 20 to 2,000 Hz.

patients with myelodysplasia, occult spinal dysraphism, or sacral lipomas, the spinal cord is caudally displaced or tethered. In these circumstances, the spinal potential normally recorded over the lower thoracic or upper lumbar levels is recorded over lower lumbar processes (Fig. 11–3) or is absent. Emerson et al. (1986) described three such patients in whom myelography confirmed a tethered cord. Roy et al. (1986a,b) found that posterior tibial nerve SEPs were predictive of the level of the lesion in patients with radiographically or surgically confirmed tethered cord. Somatosensory EPs may be a useful screening test for this disorder. In some instances, if the traction on the spinal cord is relieved surgically, the SEP may improve.

Patients with myelomeningocele also have structural anomalies involving the brainstem. Barnet et al. (1993) studied EPs in infants with myelomeningocele and Arnold–Chiari malformation to determine their usefulness in the assessment of brainstem dysfunction. All patients with symptomatic brainstem dysfunction and a small number of asymptomatic patients had abnormal central SEPs. A normal central median SEP is reassuring in an infant with Arnold–Chiari malformation.

Posterior tibial nerve somatosensory EP studies have been shown to be valuable in the diagnosis of spinal cord disorders in young children who are unable to cooperate with sensory testing. They are especially helpful when MRI studies are normal (Mutoh et al., 1991).

3.7. Peripheral Nerve Lesions

A number of children with birth-related brachial plexus injuries (Erb's palsy) evaluated with SEPs have been reported (Cracco and Cracco, 1986; Fagan et al., 1987b). With a root avulsion, the dorsal root ganglion is intact and a sensory potential can be recorded over Erb's point but more rostral potentials are absent. A lesion of the brachial plexus produces absence of the Erb's point potential and rostral components.

3.8. Miscellaneous

Cracco et al. (1984) documented slowed spinal conduction velocities over rostral spinal cord (T6–C7) in 25% of patients with juvenile-onset diabetes mellitus without clinical evidence of neurologic involvement. Conduction velocity over the caudal spinal cord (T12–T6) was normal.

Bell and Dykstra (1985) described an infant with a birth-related traumatic spinal cord injury in whom median nerve SEPs were normal and tibial nerve SEPs were abnormal. Spinal EPs were recorded over lumbar and mid-thoracic regions and there was an absence of cortical potentials. At autopsy, the spinal cord was atrophic in the lower cervical and upper thoracic regions.

Laureau et al. (1987) studied SEPs in 48 congenitally hypothyroid, early-detected, treated children, aged 18 months, 3 years, and 5 to 9 years of age, and in 9 three-year-old congenitally hypothyroid children before and after 1 month of therapy. Bongers-Schokking et al. (1993) used SEPs to assess the influence of treatment on the development of the somesthetic pathway in infants with hypothyroidism. They found that for normal central nervous system (CNS) development euthyroidism should be achieved as quickly as possible and later overtreatment should be avoided.

Bongers-Schokking et al. (1990) studied SEPs in jaundiced neonates and found it a helpful technique to monitor the effect of bilirubin on the CNS.

The effect of prenatal treatment with betamethasone and thyrotropin releasing hormone (TRH) on neural maturation was studied by performing serial SEPs in preterm infants (gestational ages 29 to 36 weeks) (deZegher et al., 1992). The cortical latencies were found to be shorter in the infants exposed to betamethasone/TRH on the first postnatal day compared to a group of controls. This difference did not persist at the age of 1 week, suggesting that this therapy accelerates SEP-assessed neural maturation.

Kaufmann et al. (1995) performed SEPs in patients ages 6 months to 44 years with classic galactosemia and undetectable erythrocyte galactose-1-phosphate uridyltransferase activity to assess the integrity of the myelinated pathways. Median nerve SEPs were abnormal in 17 of 60 patients (28%), showing central slowing in 14. Posterior tibial SEPs were abnormal in 26 of 34 patients (77%), showing central slowing in 12. The EPs correlated with the severity of presenting symptoms, age at the time of testing, and presence of focal white matter lesions on MRI. There was no relationship between age at diagnosis of galactosemia, cognitive outcome, or presence of tremor, dysmetria, ataxia, and EP abnormalities.

Majnemer and Rosenblatt (1992) performed SEPs in nine healthy full-term infants to determine whether there were functional asymmetries and whether electrophysiologic measures might be early indicators of hand dominance. Three of the nine children were left-handed and all of them had a clear N19 over the right hemisphere. Two of the three had absent N19 after right median nerve stimulation and the response was questionable in the third. Asymmetries were not present in the right handers and interhemispheric differences were not evident in follow-up studies at two months of age. This study suggests that hemispheric asymmetry occurs early in development.

4. CONCLUSION

The neurologic examination of the pediatric patient is, at times, difficult and unreliable. Somatosensory EPs provide a noninvasive, reproducible, objective method of evaluating the somatosensory system in infants and children. Pediatric SEPs must be interpreted with an understanding of the maturational changes that affect normative data. Somatosensory EPs provide useful, reliable information for prognostication in comatose children and asphyxiated neonates and contribute data for diagnosis of static and progressive disorders of the nervous system.

REFERENCES

Allison T, Hume AL, Wood CC, Goff WR (1984): Developmental and aging changes in somatosensory, auditory and visual evoked potentials. *Electroencephalogr Clin Neurophysiol* 58:14–24.

American EEG Society (1984): Guidelines for clinical evoked potential studies. *J Clin Neurophysiol* 1:3–35.

Barnet AB, Weiss IP, Shaer C (1993): Evoked potentials in infant brainstem syndrome associated with Arnold–Chiari malformation. *Dev Med Child Neurol* 35:42–48.

Bartel P, Conradie J, Robinson E, Prinsloo J, Becker P (1988): The relationship between median nerve somatosensory evoked potential latencies and age and growth factors in young children. *Electroencephalogr Clin Neurophysiol* 68:180–186.

Beca J, Cox PN, Taylor MJ, Bohn D, Butt W, Logan WJ, Rutka JT, Barker G (1995): Somatosensory evoked potentials for prediction of outcome in acute severe brain injury. *J Pediatr* 126:44–49.

Bell HJ, Dykstra DD (1985): Somatosensory evoked potentials as an adjunct to diagnosis of neonatal spinal cord injury. *J Pediatr* 106:298–301.

Bongers-Schokking JJ, Colon EJ, Hoogland RA, Van Den Brande JLV, DeGroot CJ (1990): Somatosensory evoked potentials in neonatal jaundice. *Acta Paediatr Scand* 79:148–155.

Bongers-Schokking JJ, Colon EJ, Mulder PGH, Hoogland RA, deGroot CJ, Van den Brande JL (1993): Influence of treatment on the maturation of the somesthetic pathway in infants with primary congenital hypothyroidism during the first year of life. *Pediatr Res* 34:73–78.

Cadilhac J, Zhu Y, Georgesco M (1986): Somatosensory evoked potentials during maturation in normal children. A comparative study of SEPs to median and to posterior tibial nerve stimulations. In: *Maturation of the CNS and Evoked Potentials,* edited by V Gallai, pp 107–111. Excerpta Medica, Amsterdam.

Chiappa KH (1983): *Evoked Potentials in Clinical Medicine.* Raven Press, New York.

Cracco JB, Cracco RQ (1979): Somatosensory spinal and cerebral evoked potentials in children with occult spinal dysraphism. *Neurology* 29:543.

Cracco JB, Cracco RQ (1982): Spinal somatosensory evoked potentials: maturational and clinical studies. *Ann NY Acad Sci* 388:526–537.

Cracco JB, Cracco RQ (1986): Spinal, brainstem and cerebral SEP in the pediatric age group. In: *Evoked Potentials,* edited by RQ Cracco and I Bodis-Wollner, pp 471–482. Alan R Liss, New York.

Cracco JB, Cracco RQ, Graziani L (1974): Spinal evoked responses in infants with myelodysplasia. *Neurology* 24:359–360.

Cracco JB, Cracco RQ, Graziani LJ (1975): The spinal evoked response in infants and children. *Neurology* 25:31–36.

Cracco JB, Cracco RQ, Stolove R (1979): Spinal evoked potentials in man: a maturational study. *Electroencephalogr Clin Neurophysiol* 46:58–64.

Cracco JB, Bosch VV, Cracco RQ (1980): Cerebral and spinal somatosensory evoked potentials in children with CNS degenerative disease. *Electroencephalogr Clin Neurophysiol* 49:437–455.

Cracco J, Castells S, Mark E (1984): Spinal somatosensory evoked potentials in juvenile diabetes. *Ann Neurol* 15:55–58.

Cracco JB, Udani V, Cracco RQ (1988): MN-SSEPs in infants. *Electroencephalogr Clin Neurophysiol* 69:79P.

Cullity P, Franks CI, Duckworth T Brown BH (1976): Somatosensory evoked cortical responses: detection in normal infants. *Dev Med Child Neurol* 18:11–18.

DeMeirleir LJ, Taylor MJ (1987): Prognostic utility of SEPs in comatose children. *Pediatr Neurol* 3:78–82.

DeMeirleir LJ, Taylor MJ, Logan WJ (1988): Multimodal evoked potential studies in leukodystrophies of children. *Can J Neurol Sci* 15:26–31.

Desmedt JE, Manil J (1970): Somatosensory evoked potentials of the normal human neonate in REM sleep, in slow wave sleep and in waking. *Electroencephalogr Clin Neurophysiol* 29:113–126.

Desmedt JE, Brunko E, Debecker J (1976): Maturation of the somatosensory evoked potentials in normal infants and children, with special reference to the early N1 component. *Electroencephalogr Clin Neurophysiol* 40:43–58.

de Vries LS (1993): Somatosensory-evoked potentials in term neonates with postasphyxial encephalopathy. *Clin Perinatol* 20:463–482.

de Vries LS, Pierrat V, Eken P, Minami T, Daniels H, Casaer P (1991): Prognostic value of early somatosensory evoked potentials for adverse outcome in full-term infants with brain asphyxia. *Brain Dev* 13:320–325.

deZegher F, de Vries L, Pierrat V, Daniels H, Spitz B, Casaer P, Devlieger H, Eggermont E (1992): Effect of prenatal betamethasone/thyrotropin releasing hormone treatment on somatosensory evoked potentials in preterm newborns. *Pediatr Res* 32:212–214.

Emerson RG, Pavlakis SG, Carmel PC, DeVino DC (1986): Use of spinal somatosensory evoked potentials in the diagnosis of tethered cord. *Ann Neurol* 20:443.

Fagan ER, Taylor MJ, Logan WJ (1987a): Somatosensory evoked potentials, Part 1: A review of neural generators and special considerations in pediatrics. *Pediatr Neurol* 3:189–196.

Fagan ER, Taylor MJ, Logan WJ (1987b): Somatosensory evoked potentials Part II: a review of clinical applications in pediatric neurology. *Pediatr Neurol* 3:249–255.

Frank LM, Furgiuele TL, Etheridge JE (1985): Prediction of chronic vegetative state in children using evoked potentials. *Neurology* 35:931–934.

Gallai V, Mazzotta G, Cagini L, DelGatto F, Agnelotti F (1986): Maturation of SEPs in preterm and full-term neonates. In: *Maturation of the CNS and Evoked Potentials.* Edited by V Gallai, pp 95–106. Excerpta Medica, Amsterdam.

George SR, Taylor MJ (1991): Somatosensory evoked potentials in neonates and infants: developmental and normative data. *Electroencephalogr Clin Neurophysiol* 80:94–102.

Gibson NA, Brezinova V, Levene MI (1992): Somatosensory evoked potentials in the term newborn. *Electroencephalogr Clin Neurophysiol* 84:26–31.

Gilles FH, Shankle EC, Dooling EC (1983): Myelinated tracts: growth patterns. In: *The Developing Human Brain.* Edited by FH Gilles, A Leviton, and EC Dooling, pp 117–183. John Wright, Boston.

Gilmore R (1986): Developmental profile of lumbar spinal cord and early cortical evoked potentials after tibial nerve stimulation during the neonatal period and childhood: assessment of age and stature. In: *Maturation of the CNS and Evoked Potentials.* Edited by V Gallai, pp 112–118. Excerpta Medica, Amsterdam.

Gilmore R (1988): Somatosensory evoked potentials in infants and children. *Neurol Clin* 6:839–859.

Gilmore R, Bass NH, Wright EA, Greathouse D, Stanback K, Norvell E (1985): Developmental assessment of spinal cord and cortical evoked potentials after tibial nerve stimulation: effects of age and stature on normative data during childhood. *Electroencephalogr Clin Neurophysiol* 62:241–251.

Gilmore RL, Broch J, Hermansen MC, Baumann R (1987): Development of lumbar spinal cord and cortical evoked potentials after tibial nerve stimulation the pre-term newborns: effect of age and other factors. *Electroencephalogr Clin Neurophysiol* 68:28–39.

Goodwin SR, Friedman WA, Bellefleur M (1991): Is it time to use evoked potentials to predict outcome in comatose children and adults? *Crit Care Med* 19:518–524.

Gorke W (1986): Somatosensory evoked cortical potentials indicating impaired motor development in infancy. *Dev Med Child Neurol* 28:633–641.

Gorke W (1987): Diagnostic value of somatosensory evoked potentials as compared to neurologic score, EEG and CT in infancy—a prospective study. *Neuropediatrics* 18:205–209.

Hrbek A, Karlberg P, Olsson T (1973): Development of visual and somatosensory evoked responses in pre-term newborn infants. *Electroencephalogr Clin Neurophysiol* 34:225–232.

Hrbek A, Karlberg P, Kjellmer I, Olsson T, Riha M (1977): Clinical application of evoked electroencephalographic responses in newborn infants. I. Perinatal asphyxia. *Dev Med Child Neurol* 19:34–44.

Hume AL, Cant BR, Shaw NA, Cowan JC (1982): Cerebral somatosensory conduction time from 10–19 years. *Electroencephalogr Clin Neurophysiol* 54:49–54.

Johnson S (1985): Somatosensory evoked potentials in abetalipoproteinemia. *Electroencephalogr Clin Neurophysiol* 60:27–29.

Kaufman FR, Horton EJ, Gott P, Wolff JA, Nelson MD, Azen C, Manis FR (1995): Abnormal somatosensory evoked potentials in patients with classic galactosemia: correlation with neurologic outcome. *J Child Neurol* 10:32–36.

Keenan NK, Taylor MJ, Whyte HEA (1992): Somatosensory evoked potentials and visual evoked potentials in premature babies. *Ann Neurol* 32:481.

Klimach VJ, Cooke RW (1988): Short-latency cortical evoked somatosensory evoked responses of preterm infants with ultrasound abnormality of the brain. *Dev Med Child Neurol* 30:215–221.

Lafreniere L, Laureau E, Vanasse M, Forest L, Ptito M (1990): Maturation of a short latency somatosensory evoked potentials by median nerve stimulation: a cross-sectional study in a large group of children. *Electroenceph Clin Neurophysiol* Suppl 41:236–242.

Laget P, Salbreux R, Raimbault J, d'Allest AM, Mariani J (1976): Relationship between changes in somesthetic evoked responses and electroencephalographic findings in the child with hemiplegia. *Dev Med Child Neurol* 18:620–631.

Lauffer H, Wenzel D (1986): Maturation of central somatosensory conduction time in infancy and childhood. *Neuropediatrics* 17:72–74.

Laureau E, Marlot D (1990): Somatosensory evoked potentials after median and tibial nerve stimulation in healthy newborns. *Electroencephalogr Clin Neurophysiol* 76:453–458.

Laureau E, Majnemer A, Rosenblatt B, Riley P (1988): A longitudinal study of short latency evoked responses in healthy newborns and infants. *Electroencephalogr Clin Neurophysiol* 71:100–108.

Laureau E, Hebert R, Vanasse M, Letark J, Glorieux J, Desjardinio M, Dussault JH (1987): Somatosensory evoked potentials and auditory brain stem responses in congenital hypothyroidism. II. A cross-sectional study in childhood. Correlation with hormonal levels and developmental quotients. *Electroencephalogr Clin Neurophysiol* 67:521–530.

Lutschg J, Pfenninger J, Ludin HP, Vassella F (1983): Brain stem auditory evoked potentials and early somatosensory evoked potentials in neurointensively treated comatose children. *Am J Dis Child* 137:421–426

Majnemer A, Rosenblatt B (1992): Functional Interhemispheric asymmetries at birth as demonstrated by somatosensory evoked potentials. *J Child Neurol* 7:408–412.

Majnemer A, Rosenblatt B, Riley P, Laureau E, O'Gorman AM (1987): Somatosensory evoked response abnormalities in high risk newborns. *Pediatr Neurol* 3:350–355.

Majnemer A, Rosenblatt B. Riley PS (1990a): Prognostic significance of multimodality evoked response testing in high risk newborns. *Pediatr Neurol* 6:367–374.

Majnemer A, Rosenblatt B, Willis D, Lavallee J (1990b): The effect of gestational age at birth on somatosensory evoked potentials performed at term. *J Child Neurol* 5:329–335.

Markand ON, Garg BP, DeMeyer WE, Warren C, Worth RM (1982): Brain stem auditory, visual and somatosensory evoked potentials in the leukodystrophies. *Electroencephalogr Clin Neurophysiol* 54:39–48.

Mutoh K, Okuno T, Mikawa H, Hojo H (1988): Maturation of somatosensory evoked potentials upon posterior tibial nerve stimulation. *Pediatr Neurol* 4:342–349.

Mutoh K, Okuno T, Ito M, Fujii T, Mikawa H, Asata R (1991): Somatosensory evoked potentials after posterior nerve stimulation in focal spinal cord diseases. *Pediatr Neurol* 7:326–333.

Nelson FW, Goldie WD, Hecht JT, Butler IJ, Scott CI (1984): Short latency somatosensory evoked potentials in the management of patients with achondroplasia. *Neurology* 34:1053–1058.

Nelson FW, Hecht JT, Horton WA, Bulter IJ, Goldie WD, Miner M (1988): Neurological basis of respiratory complications in achondroplasia. *Ann Neurol* 24:89–93.

Pierrat V, Eken P, Duquennoy C, Rousseau S, de Vries LS (1993): Prognostic value of early somatosensory evoked potentials in neonates with cystic leukomalacia. *Dev Med Child Neurol* 35:683–690.

Reid CS, Pyeritz RE, Kopits SE, Marla BL, Wang W, McPherson RW, Hurko O, Phillips JA, Rosenbaum AE (1987): Cervicomedullary compression in young patients with achondroplasia: value of comprehensive neurologic and respiratory evaluation. *J Pediatr* 110:522–530.

Rossini PM, Cracco JB (1987): Somatosensory and brainstem auditory evoked potentials in neurodegenerative disorders. *Eur Neurol* 26:176–188.

Rossini PM, Zarola F, di Capua M, Cracco JB (1986): Somatosensory evoked potential studies in neurodegenerative system disorders. In: *Maturation of the CNS and Evoked Potentials*. Edited by V Gallai, pp 125–134. Excerpta Medica, Amsterdam.

Roy MW, Gilmore R, Walsh JW (1986a): Evaluation of children and young adults with tethered cord syndrome. Utility of spinal and scalp recorded somatosensory evoked potentials. *Surg Neurol* 26:241–248.

Roy MW, Gilmore R, Walsh JW (1986b): Somatosensory evoked potentials in tethered cord syndrome. *Electroencephalogr Clin Neurophysiol* 64:42P.

Sitzoglou C, Fotiou F (1985): A study of the maturation of the somatosensory pathway by evoked potentials. *Neuropediatrics* 16:205–208.

Taylor MJ, Chan-Lui WY (1985): Longitudinal evoked potential studies in hereditary ataxias. *Can J Neurol Sci* 12:100–105.

Taylor MJ, Fagan ER (1988): SEPs to median nerve stimulation: normative data for paediatrics. *Electroencephalogr Clin Neurophysiol* 71:323–330.

Taylor MJ, Farrell EJ (1989): Comparison of the prognostic utility of VEPs and SEPs in comatose children. *Pediatr Neurol* 5:145–150.

Taylor MJ, Murphy WJ, Whyte HE (1992): Prognostic reliability of somatosensory and visual evoked potentials of asphyxiated term infants. *Dev Med Child Neurol* 34:507–515.

Tobimatsu S, Fukui R, Motohiro K, Kobayashi T, Kuroiw (1985): Multimodality evoked potentials in patients and carriers with adrenoleukodystrophy and adrenomyeloneuropathy. *Electroencephalogr Clin Neurophysiol* 62:18–24.

Tomita Y, Tanaka T (1986): Short latency SEPs in infants and children: developmental changes and maturational index of SEPs. *Electroencephalogr Clin Neurophysiol* 65:335–343.

Tomita Y, Tanaka T, Kamimura N, Shimozawa N, Takashima S, Takeshita K (1988): Origin and clinical significance of subcortical components in short-latency somatosensory evoked potentials in children. *Electroencephalogr Clin Neurophysiol* 69:199–208.

Udani A, Cracco JB, Hittleman J, Hotson G, Fikrig S (1988): Clinical and developmental evaluation, evoked potentials and MRI in pediatric AIDS. *Electroencephalogr Clin Neurophysiol* 69:87P.

White LE, Frank LM, Furgluele TL, Montes JE, Etheridge JE (1985): Childhood coma: improved prediction of outcome with somatosensory and brainstem auditory evoked potentials. *Ann Neurol* 18:417.

Willis J (1986): Effects of state and stimulus rate on short latency somatosensory evoked potentials in infants. *Ann Neurol* 20:411.

Willis J, Duncan C, Bell R (1987): Short latency somatosensory evoked potentials in perinatal asphyxia. *Pediatr Neurol* 3:203–207.

Willis J, Seales D, Frazier E (1984): Short latency somatosensory evoked potentials in infants. *Electroencephalogr Clin Neurophysiol* 59:366–373.

Yakovlev P, Lecours A (1967): The myelogenetic cycle of regional maturation of the brain. In: *Regional Development of the Brain in Early Life*. Edited by A Minkowski, pp 3–69. F.A. Davis, Philadelphia.

Zhu Y, Georgesco M, Cadilhac J (1987): Normal latency values of early cortical somatosensory evoked potentials in children. *Electroencephalogr Clin Neurophysiol* 68:471–474.

Evoked Potentials in Clinical Medicine,
3d ed., edited by Keith H. Chiappa.
Lippincott–Raven Publishers, Philadelphia © 1997.

12

Dermatomal Somatosensory Evoked Potentials

°Keith H. Chiappa and †Didier Cros

*Department of Neurology, Harvard Medical School, and °EEG Laboratory; and
†EMG Unit–Bigelow 12; Massachusetts General Hospital, Boston, Massachusetts 02114*

1. INTRODUCTION

The integrity of somatosensory pathways is usually tested by stimulation of a large mixed nerve, such as the median nerve at the wrist or the tibial nerve of the ankle. However, the localization of plexus or root pathology using somatosensory evoked potentials (SEPs) may be improved by stimulation of peripheral nerves containing fibers contributing to the clinically suspect cords, trunks, or spinal segments, and the correlation of cutaneous sensory changes or loss with SEP abnormalities may be improved by the stimulation of sensory nerves subserving those dermatomes. "Dermatomal" SEPs (DSEPs) obtained with cutaneous nerve or skin patch stimulation have waveform configurations similar to those obtained with mixed nerve stimulation. However, the responses have smaller amplitudes, particularly the cervical and lumbar spinal responses, which may not be registered from some normal subjects when the digital, musculocutaneous, saphenous, or sural nerves or dermatomes are stimulated. Even strong electrical stimuli (about three times sensory threshold) to these cutaneous nerves elicit scalp DSEPs less than half the size of SEPs seen following stimulation of mixed nerves. This presents greater difficulties with waveform identification and reliable latency and amplitude measurements than is the case for the mixed nerve results. This results in a wider range of normal values [see the excellent study of Slimp et al. (1992) for examples of gross asymmetries in normal subjects which required special recording derivations for elucidation], a need for larger numbers of normal control subjects with representation from more subpopulations (height, gender) and a consequent greater difficulty in the definition of abnormality.

In addition to the difficulties presented by the above nonpathologic factors, DSEPs give the initial impression, largely unwarranted, of being suitable for the investigation of a wide range of nonspecific neurologic complaints in the limbs. Together, these elements of DSEPs have resulted in an overestimation of their clinical utility. They have also been overprescribed by some practitioners (for obvious reasons), which has not helped the reputation of either party. The determination of the appropriate clinical application of DSEPs requires a careful review of the available data on normal, control subjects, and clinical trials in which the DSEP results are compared with a suitable "gold standard," and the best of these reveal poor sensitivity and specificity in most clinical areas.

In the upper limbs, all SEP components show appropriate latency shifts when stimulating proximal (musculocutaneous) or distal (digit) to the wrist. Superficial radial nerve stimulation at the wrist produces responses with latencies similar to the mixed median nerve but with lower amplitudes (see Table 8–2). In the lower limbs, sural nerve stimulation produces low-amplitude EPs at the scalp with prolonged latencies relative to those produced by stimulation of the posterior tibial nerve at the ankle (mean difference in scalp latency is 2 to 3 msec—see Tables 8–3 and 8–5), even though the distance between stimulus site and spinal cord is approximately the same (Burke et al., 1981, 1982; Chiappa, 1983; Vogel et al., 1986). This may be related to the contribution of the more rapidly conducting muscle afferents to the potentials produced by mixed nerve (posterior tibial) stimulation. It is believed that muscle afferents from the lower limbs travel in dorsolateral (spinocerebellar) pathways rather than in the posterior columns, whereas cutaneous afferents (e.g., from sural and posterior tibial nerves) travel predominantly in the posterior columns. Since the average diameter of posterior column axons (Ohnishi et al., 1976) is less than the diameter of axons in the spinocerebellar tracts, the conduction velocity is faster in the muscle afferent (posterior tibial nerve) than in the cutaneous (sural nerve) paths. The muscle afferents may also follow a shorter path and have fewer interposed synapses (Gandevia et al., 1984; Vogel et al., 1986). In the upper limbs, both cutaneous and muscle afferents are believed to travel in the posterior columns, consistent with the equal conduction times in cutaneous (superficial radial and digital nerves) and mixed (median) nerves (when distances are normalized) [see Webster (1977) for a more detailed discussion of somasthetic pathways].

2. METHODS

It is reasonable to use the methods of the group with the largest published experience in normal subjects. This allows direct comparison of results obtained in one's own laboratory. Thus, the methods used in the study of Slimp et al. (1992) are recommended.

3. NORMAL SUBJECTS AND VARIABILITY

Techniques and normal values for DEPs have been described for the L5 and S1 dermatomes in 54 subjects (Katifi and Sedgwick, 1986), for C4–8, the even-numbered thoracic segments, L2–5, and S1 in 41 subjects (Slimp et al., 1992), for the superficial peroneal and sural nerves and L5 and S1 dermatomes (Dumitru et al., 1993), and for the C6–8 and L5 and S1 in 15 to 20 subjects (Liguori et al., 1991). Root specificity has been studied experimentally in 32 monkeys (Owen et al., 1993) and hogs (Terada et al., 1993), as well as occasional intraoperative correlations made in humans. Articles on clinical correlations of DEPs also often contained results from normal subjects, although this is certainly not universal.

The pitfalls awaiting the unwary are well-demonstrated in Figs. 5 and 6 of Slimp et al. (1992), the best study of normal variability in DSEPs. In Fig. 5 the CZ'–FZ derivation, second from the top on the left, shows the left and right tibial DSEPs superimposed, with a dramatic amplitude asymmetry evident between the two sides. Their Fig. 6 shows a similar amplitude asymmetry in the L5 and S1 DSEPs. Without prior knowledge of this degree of normal asymmetry this result would certainly be interpreted as abnormal since many practitioners use only the midline recording derivations. Slimp et al. (1992) note that it would be advisable to record DSEPs using at least four recording channels, three devoted to FZ to parietal derivations and the fourth to a FZ–mastoid derivation. In addition, they note that occasionally additional derivations may contribute to interpretations, that is, help to identify an anomalous set of waveforms as a normal variant. Most practitioners performing DSEPs do not have the EP machine channel capacity, the inclination, or the knowledge to incorporate these complexities into their clinical practice, so that false positives will result. Thus, DSEP results cannot be readily taken by themselves to provide confirmatory evidence for lesions only hinted at by vague clinical complaints. Slimp et al. (1992), Katifi and Sedgwick (1986), and Dumitru et al. (1993) all found that the amplitude asymmetry in normal subjects could be more than a factor of four.

Furthermore, although the paper by Slimp et al. (1992) is a superb presentation of normal data, is the best on DSEPs and is a model for such studies in any EP modality, they excluded from their numerical summaries the results obtained from their most atypical normal subject. Absent a valid reason, this is an incorrect maneuver according to statistical practices and is potentially misleading since few practitioners will read the paper carefully enough beyond the summary tables to uncover this omission. If this normal finding is included, the normal range becomes so large that the measurement is of limited use clinically and must be employed very carefully.

Replication of EP waveforms (i.e., repeating a test using exactly the same parameters for stimulation and recording, and superimposing the results so that an immediate visual estimation of component variability can be achieved) is standard practice. Given the low amplitude of many DSEP components, this guideline is even more important but it is frequently ignored in the performance of DSEPs. Slimp et al. (1992) used this practice but showed only grand averages for simplicity. In their study of normal subjects Dumitru et al. (1993) found that the single trial maximum interside latency differences were up to 10.4 msec for the S1 dermatome, and the percent amplitude interside differences were up to 83%, so that the use of a 3-standard-deviation (SD) measure here would "essentially render amplitude of minimal diagnostic relevance." Thus, Dumitru et al. (1993) have recommended using the arithmetic mean of at least two trials for both latency and amplitude measurements. Dermatomal SEPs performed with single trials are unacceptable for clinical utilization in any manner, and articles on clinical studies of DSEPs should show such replicated waveforms or else they should be routinely rejected for publication.

Finally, the definition of abnormality (e.g., the use of 2 versus 3 SDs as the upper limit of normal), the population of patients, and the "gold standard" all have major influences upon study results and need to be given careful attention (see Aminoff and Goodin, 1988; Katifi and Sedgwick, 1988; Dumitru and Dreyfuss, 1996).

There are few recent studies on the specificity and reliability of DSEPs relative to their correlation with a given nerve root. Owen et al. (1993) used 32 macaque monkeys and recorded DSEPs from C5 to C8 and L4 to L6, then randomly sectioned dorsal nerve rootlets and observed the changes in the DSEPs. They concluded that DSEPs should be recorded at multiple levels proximal and distal to a level of decompression to help to take into account the variations in peripheral innervation patterns of the dorsal roots. Terada et al. (1993) studied DSEPS in eight hogs and found considerable interindividual and side-to-side variability similar to that described above in humans. They then proceeded to investigate the sensitivity of DSEPs to S1 nerve root function in these hogs. They obtained baseline DSEPs and then on one side sectioned only the S1 root, whereas on the other side they sectioned the L5, L6, and S2 nerve roots, leaving the S1 root intact. Abnormal postsectioning results were found in only half of the S1-sectioned limbs. When only the S1 root was preserved the results were always normal. There are also sensitivity and specificity results reported in humans, which will be presented below in the section on clinical studies. Evaluation of these human results must be performed critically with a clear understanding of the reliability of the "gold standard" being applied, that is, the method by which it was decided that nerve compression was or was not present.

4. CLINICAL STUDIES

This topic has already been covered from one point of view in Chapter 10 of this book, with a discussion of the use of SEPs in peripheral nerve lesions, brachial plexus and cervical root trauma, thoracic outlet syndrome, and cervical and lumbar radiculopathies. In Chapter 14, Kiers and Chiappa discuss the use of SEPs in spinal cord disease. Aminoff (1995) has presented a useful review.

Studies available in the literature concerning lumbosacral radiculopathies include those of Tullberg et al. (1993), Walk et al. (1992), Owen et al. (1991), Tokuhashi et al. (1991), Seyal et al. (1988), Rodriquez et al. (1987), Katifi and Sedgwick (1987), Perlik et al. (1986), Aminoff et al. (1985a,b), Eisen et al. (1983) and Scarff et al. (1981). Dumitru and Dreyfuss (1996) applied strict criteria for a "gold standard" to define a group of 20 patients with a unilateral/unilevel L5/S1 radiculopathy (1 to 6 months of pain and/or paresthesia in a clearly defined L5 or S1 dermatomal distribution radiating into a single lower limb, limb pain greater than back pain, no history of surgery, examination showing a partial loss of sensation unilaterally in the dermatome, an absent or reduced ankle jerk with S1, motor weakness not necessary but if present consistent with the sensory features, positive straight-leg raising, computed tomography or magnetic resonance imaging scan clearly consistent with unilateral/unilevel nerve root encroachment, positive sharp waves or fibrillation potentials in at least two muscles per myotome, absent or unilaterally prolonged H-reflex with S1, and normal sural nerves). Superficial peroneal and sural nerve as well as L5 and S1 dermatomal SEPs were performed and compared with appropriate statistical rigor with the results from 43 normal controls. Regression analyses for cortical P1 latencies revealed segmental and dematomal sensitivities for L5 radiculopathies to be 70% and 50% at 90% confidence intervals, and the side-to-side comparison showed sensitivities of 40% and 40% at 2 SDs. Similar values for S1 radiculopathies were 30% and 20%, and 50% and 10%. They concluded that the clinical utility of both segmental and dermatomal SEPs is questionable in patients with known unilateral/unilevel L5 and S1 nerve root compromise. Since these SEP results were obtained in patients with very clear evidence of nerve compression, only lower sensitivity rates could be expected with lesser degrees of nerve involvement. This is the best study to date on this topic and, pending further studies to the contrary, this must remain as the final word.

Lumbar stenosis may present a special case, perhaps because of the number of nerve roots involved and the length of the compression. Snowden et al. (1992) have shown sensitivities of 78% and 93% for dermatomal SEPs in this disease, depending on the number of roots involved.

REFERENCES

Aminoff MJ (1995): Segmentally specific somatosensory evoked potentials. In: *Diagnosis and Management of Disorders of the Spinal Cord,* edited by RR Young and RM Woolsey, pp 170–176. WB Saunders, Philadelphia.
Aminoff MJ, Goodin DS (1988): Dermatomal somatosensory evoked potentials in lumbosacral root compression. *J Neurol Neurosurg Psychiatry* 51:740–741.

Aminoff MJ, Goodin DS, Barbaro NM, Weinstein PR, Rosenblum ML (1985a): Dermatomal somatosensory evoked potentials in unilateral lumbosacral radiculopathy. *Ann Neurol* 17:171–176.

Aminoff MJ, Goodin DS, Parry GJ, Barbaro NM, Weinstein PR, Rosenblum ML (1985b): Electrophysiologic evaluation of lumbosacral radiculopathies: electromyography, late responses, and somatosensory evoked potentials. *Neurology* 35:1514–1518.

Burke D, Skuse NF, Lethlean AK (1981): Cutaneous and muscle afferent components of the cerebral potential evoked by electrical stimulation of human peripheral nerves. *Electroencephalogr Clin Neurophysiol* 51:579–588.

Burke D, Gandevia SC, McKeon B, Skuse NF (1982): Interactions between cutaneous and muscle afferent contributions to cerebral cortex in man. *Electroencephalogr Clin Neurophysiol* 53:349–360.

Dumitru D, Dreyfuss P (1996): Dermatomal/segmental somatosensory evoked potential evaluation of L5/S1 unilateral/unilevel radiculopathies. *Muscle Nerve* 19:442–449.

Dumitru D, Newton BY, Dreyfuss P (1993): Segmental v dermatomal somatosensory evoked potentials: Normal intertrial variation and side-to-side comparison. *Am J Phys Med Rehabil* 72:75–83.

Eisen A, Hoirch M, Moll A (1983): Evaluation of radiculopathies by segmental stimulation and somatosensory evoked potentials. *Can J Neurol Sci* 10:178–182.

Gandevia SC, Burke D, McKeon B (1984): The projection of muscle afferents from the hand to cerebral cortex in man. *Brain* 107:1–13.

Katifi HA, Sedgwick EM (1986): Somatosensory evoked potentials from posterior tibial nerve and lumbosacral dermatomes. *Electroencephalogr Clin Neurophysiol* 65:249–259.

Katifi HA, Sedgwick EM (1987): Evaluation of the dermatomal somatosensory evoked potential in the diagnosis of lumbo-sacral root compression. *J Neurol Neurosurg Psychiatry* 50:1204–1210.

Katifi HA, Sedgwick EM (1988): Dermatomal somatosensory evoked potentials in lumbosacral root compression. *J Neurol Neurosurg Psychiatry* 51:741–742.

Liguori R, Taher G, Trojaborg W (1991): Somatosensory evoked potentials from cervical and lumbosacral dermatomes. *Acta Neurol Scand* 84:161–166.

Ohnishi A, O'Brien PC, Okazaki H, Dyck PJ (1976): Morphometry of myelinated fibers of fasciculus gracilis of man. *J Neurol Sci* 27:163–172.

Owen JH, Padberg AM, Spahr-Holland L, Bridwell KH, Keppler L, Steffee AD (1991): Clinical correlation between degenerative spine disease and dermatomal somatosensory-evoked potentials in humans. *Spine* 16:S201–S205.

Owen JH, Bridwell KH, Lenke LG (1993): Innervation pattern of dorsal roots and their effects on the specificity of dermatomal somatosensory evoked potentials. *Spine* 18:748–754.

Perlik S, Fisher MA, Patel DV, Slack C (1986): On the usefulness of somatosensory evoked responses for the evaluation of lower back pain. *Arch Neurol* 43:907–913.

Rodriquez AA, Kanis L, Rodriquez AA, Lane D (1987): Somatosensory evoked potentials from dermatomal stimulation as an indicator of L5 and S1 radiculopathy. *Arch Phys Med Rehabil* 68:366–368.

Scarff TB, Dallman DE, Toleikis R, Bunch WH (1981): Dermatomal somatosensory evoked potentials in the diagnosis of lumbar root entrapment. *Surg Forum (Neurol Surg)* 32:489–491.

Seyal M, Palma GA, Sandhu LS, Mack YP, Hannam JM (1981): Spinal somatosensory evoked potentials following segmental sensory stimulation. A direct measure of dorsal root function. *Electroencephalogr Clin Neurophysiol* 69:390–393.

Slimp JC, Rubner DE, Snowden ML, Stolov WC (1992): Dermatomal somatosensory evoked potentials: cervical, thoracic, and lumbosacral levels. *Electroencephalogr Clin Neurophysiol* 84(1):55–70.

Snowden ML, Haselkorn JK, Kraft GH, Bronstein AD, Bigos SJ, Slimp JC, Stolov WC (1992): Dermatomal somatosensory evoked potentials in the diagnosis of lumbosacral spinal stenosis: comparison with imaging studies. *Muscle Nerve* 15:1036–1044.

Terada K, Larson BJ, Owen JH, Sugioka Y (1993): The effect of nerve root lesioning on various somatosensory evoked potentials in the hog. *Spine* 18:1090–1095.

Tokuhashi Y, Satoh K, Funami S (1991): A quantitative evaluation of sensory dysfunction in lumbosacral radiculopathy. *Spine* 16:1321–1328.

Tullberg T, Svanborg E, Isacsson J, Grane P (1993): A preoperative and postoperative study of the accuracy and value of electrodiagnosis in patients with lumbosacral disc herniation. *Spine* 18:837–842.

Vogel P, Ruber P, Klein R (1986): The latency difference of the tibial and sural nerve SEP: peripheral versus central factors. *Electroencephalogr Clin Neurophysiol* 65:269–275.

Walk D, Fisher MA, Doundoulakis SH, Hemmati M (1992): Somatosensory evoked potentials in the evaluation of lumbosacral radiculopathy. *Neurology* 42:1197–1202.

Webster KE (1977): Somaesthetic pathways. *Br Med Bull* 33:113–120.

Evoked Potentials in Clinical Medicine,
3d ed., edited by Keith H. Chiappa.
Lippincott–Raven Publishers, Philadelphia © 1997.

13

Motor Evoked Potentials

°Didier Cros and †Keith H. Chiappa

*Department of Neurology, Harvard Medical School, and °EMG Unit–Bigelow 12; and
†EEG Laboratory; Massachusetts General Hospital, Boston, Massachusetts 02114*

1. INTRODUCTION

Conventional neurophysiologic assessment of the motor system is limited to motor nerve conduction studies and electromyography (EMG). Whereas these techniques are very useful in disorders affecting the peripheral nervous system, they yield little information in disease affecting the central motor pathways. In such cases, only indirect evidence of disease can be deduced from abnormal motor unit firing and recruitment patterns.

The development of transcranial *electrical* stimulation by Merton and Morton (1980) marked the beginning of a new era in clinical neurophysiology. For the first time it became possible to excite the central motor pathways noninvasively in intact human subjects and quantitatively assess central motor conduction. However, transcranial electrical stimulation is quite uncomfortable, a limitation to its widespread use in patients and normal subjects alike.

Barker and colleagues (1985) described a transcranial magnetic stimulation (TMS) technique which has the advantages of being painless and safe. In the past decade, the availability of this approach has triggered a flurry of clinical and physiologic studies and this test appears ready to take a major place as a clinical and research method of investigation of the human motor system. In this chapter, essential physiologic data pertinent to transcranial stimulation and magnetic stimulation with special reference to the motor system are reviewed, along with relevant information in disease states.

2. PHYSIOLOGY OF TRANSCRANIAL STIMULATION

Magnetic or electrical transcranial stimulation activates the cortical motor neuronal (CM) pathways, resulting in descending excitation reaching the spinal motor neurons and generating a compound muscle action potential (CMAP) easily recorded via surface electrodes. This muscle response has a high amplitude on the order of a millivolt and does not require the signal averaging necessary to record sensory evoked potentials (EPs) [e.g., somatosensory (SEPs), pattern-shift visual (PSVEPs), and brain stem auditory evoked potentials (BAEPs)]. The global motor conduction time so determined corresponds to conduction from cortex to muscle. It can be conveniently subdivided into a central conduction time (CCT) and a peripheral conduction time (PCT), the latter one obtained using the same equipment to stimulate the spinal roots over the cervical enlargement and the cauda equina (see Section 4).

In experimental animals a single stimulus to the surface of the motor cortex produces multiple descending waves which may be recorded at the medullary pyramids or from the contralateral pyramidal tract in the spinal cord (Kitagawa and Moller, 1994). The earliest D-wave (D for direct) occurs at a latency too short for any interposed synapse. It can also be elicited by direct stimulation of subcortical white matter after ablation of the cortex. This D-wave is thought to result from direct excitation of the proximal segment of the axon of fast-conducting CM cells (Amassian et al., 1987). The subsequent I-waves (I for indirect) are thought to result from the excitation of cortical elements presynaptic relative to the CM cell. There is no dispersion of the I-waves relative to the D-wave in successively lower parts of the pyramidal tracts, suggesting that both use the same fast-conducting descending pathway.

The actual depth of stimulation using TMS is at present uncertain. Comparison of onset latency of motor evoked potentials (MEPs) elicited electrically and magnetically suggests that, at least at lower intensities of TMS, the white matter may not be involved. Thus, transcranial electrical stimulation in humans triggers a descending volley consisting of D- and I-waves, whereas TMS induces only I-waves (Amassian et al., 1987; Day et al., 1987). These descending excitatory inputs reach the spinal alpha motor neuron presumably through a monosynaptic pathway. They cause a series of excitatory postsynaptic potentials (EPSPs) which summate and cause the motor neuron to fire.

The magnitude and time course of descending excitation is such that some motor neurons fire repeatedly, which has been shown using collision experiments (Hess et al., 1987a; Kiers et al., 1993) (Figs. 13–1 and 13–2). It is known that the motor neurons excited by reflex activation in the spinal cord of the cat are recruited in an orderly manner determined by physical characteristics of the cell bodies. This property is known as *Henneman's size principle* (Henneman et al., 1965). It had been assumed though not demonstrated that the size principle also applies to the recruitment of spinal motor neurons by the corticospinal excitatory command. Experiments comparing the motor unit potentials recruited using threshold TMS and low-grade voluntary contraction identified the same motor unit, which provides further support to that assumption (Hess et al., 1987a).

Cortical magnetic stimulation is an ill-chosen term, as the magnetic pulse does not stimulate the neural structures but rather induces current flow in the volume conductor subjected to the magnetic pulse. This current in turn excites nerve cells and/or their processes by a mechanism identical to that of transcranial electrical stimulation. From correlations between the direction of coil current flow and the size of MEPs it has been established that a posterior to anterior induced current is most effective in evoking activation of CMs. With a large circular coil positioned symmetrically over the head (centered at the vertex), both hemispheres can be stimulated. However, based on direction of coil current flow, the hemi-

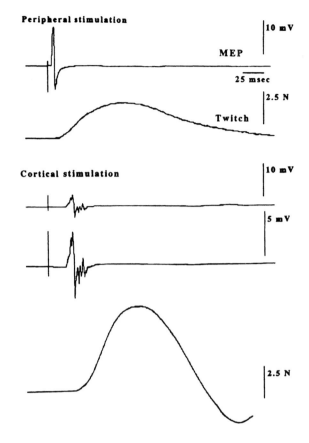

FIG. 13–1. Compound muscle action potential (CMAP) and twitch recordings produced by supramaximal ulnar nerve electrical stimulation at the wrist (peripheral) and magnetic cortical stimulation. Stimulus intensity was at 40% of maximum stimulator output above resting motor threshold; 5% of maximum background voluntary contraction. The twitch amplitude evoked by cortical magnetic stimulation is much larger than that evoked by peripheral stimulation, despite the reverse finding for the CMAP amplitude. Note the long-duration polyphasic waveform produced by cortical stimulation. (From Kiers et al., 1995, with permission.)

sphere subjected to induction of a posterior to anterior current is stimulated at lower magnetic stimulation intensities. By using a carefully defined methodology, it is possible to determine the excitation threshold of both hemispheres at rest. Interestingly, in right-handed normal subjects, the motor cortex of the left hemisphere is more excitable, which is possibly related to the asymmetry of organization of the brain in humans (Triggs et al., 1994).

The amplitude and latency of MEPs vary over time as consecutive stimuli of the same intensity are delivered to relaxed target muscles. This variability is most likely due to some yet unidentified mechanism intrinsic to the nervous system as it persists with optimal control of stimulus parameters, which guarantees consistency of excitatory input to the neural elements (Kiers et al., 1993) (Fig. 13–3). Presumably this is a random fluctuation of the resting threshold. Interestingly, the amplitude of MEPs recorded from two resting muscles in the same subject in response to the same stimulus over time does not covary, suggesting that there is no central "tone" setting the gain of the response to TMS (Kiers et al., 1993).

The MEP amplitude and latency evoked by stimuli of the same intensity also vary depending on the state (relaxation or contraction) of the target muscle. Motor EP latency shortens and amplitude augments with tonic contraction of the target muscle, a phenomenon known as *facilitation of MEPs*. The changes in MEP latency and amplitude are maximum for tonic contraction of 5% to 15% of maximum voluntary contraction (Hess et al., 1987; Figs. 13–4 and 13–5). These changes can be explained in part by tonic excitation of the motor neuron pool causing subliminally excited motor neurons to fire more easily when

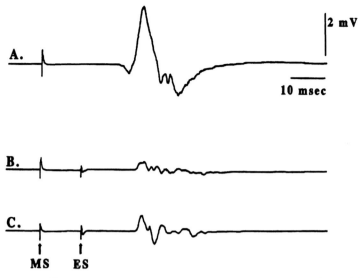

FIG. 13–2. Surface CMAP recordings from first dorsal interosseus (relaxed) following **(A)** cortical magnetic stimulation at a stimulus intensity of 30% above resting motor threshold; **(B)** cortical magnetic stimulation followed 12 msec later by supramaximal electrical ulnar nerve stimulation (ES); cortical stimulation was at 20% above resting motor threshold. The contribution of the ulnar CMAP resulting from ES has been subtracted by collision from the cortically evoked CMAP but some CMAP remains. **(C)** As in **B** but the cortical stimulation was at 30% above threshold. (From Kiers et al., 1995, with permission.)

the phasic excitation induced by TMS reaches them. Participation of cortical mechanisms to facilitation has not yet been clearly elucidated. This property can be used in clinical studies to maximize the size of a pathologically low MEP amplitude. In pathologic situations in which the cortical excitation threshold is abnormally increased, MEPs are occasionally obtainable only with background contraction of the target muscles.

Cervical root stimulation can easily be achieved using magnetic or transcutaneous electrical stimulation with a high-voltage stimulator (Cros et al., 1990; Mills and Murray, 1986) (see Section 4 for the technical aspects). Comparison of the latency of the compound muscle responses evoked by cervical stimulation and F-response latencies suggests that the site of excitation using cervical magnetic stimulation is within a few millimeters of the cell body of the lower motor neuron (Cros et al., 1990; Siao et al., 1992). This finding is of importance as it establishes that the peripheral conduction time obtained with cervical magnetic stimulation includes conduction along the entire length of the peripheral motor pathway. Consequently, this method is valid to accurately calculate a PCT, and, by subtraction, a CCT. The locus of excitation using transcutaneous cervical electrical stimulation and cervical root needle stimulation is similarly very close to the emergence of the motor axon from the cell body and, consequently, these methods are valid alternatives for PCT determination (Cros et al., 1990; Mills and Murray, 1986.)

Lumbosacral root stimulation has been attempted by several authors but has met with greater difficulty than cervical root stimulation (Macdonell et al., 1992; Chokroverty et al., 1993; Maccabee et al., 1996). Magnetic coil stimulation does not consistently elicit a motor

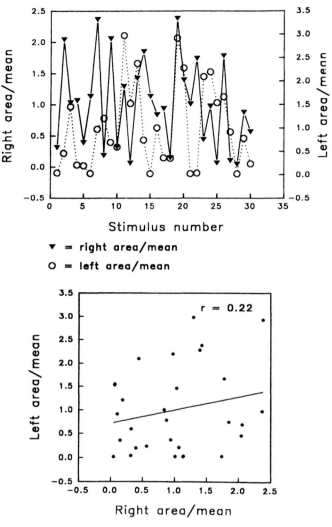

FIG. 13–3. The relationship between variability in mean normalized MEP area in right and left first dorsal interosseus, showing lack of covariance. Linear regression analysis; correlation coefficient (r) - 0.22, not significant. The minimum interstimulus interval was 5 sec, thus the 35 stimuli (x-axis) encompass about 3 minutes. (From Kiers et al., 1993, with permission.)

response when applied over the lumbosacral spinal column. A more reliable technique to calculate a peripheral conduction time consists of needle electrical stimulation.

There is no reason or evidence to suggest that there is any significant risk attached to the use of the magnetic stimulator for central motor stimulation. Electroencephalograms (EEGs) have showed no change related to magnetic stimulation (Boyd and Dasilva, 1986; Cohen and Hallett, 1987; Bridgers and Delaney, 1989). Serum prolactin and cognitive studies have shown no changes (Bridgers and Delaney, 1989; Chokroverty et al., 1995), and single photon emission computed tomography studies have shown no changes in regional cerebral blood flow (Dressler et al., 1990). Considerations of charge density and tissue heating

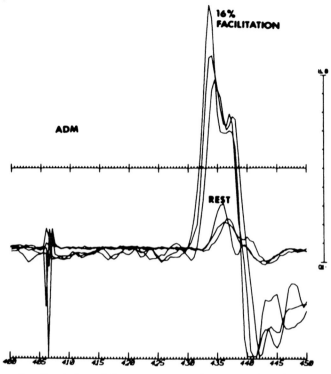

FIG. 13–4. Magnetic stimulation of the motor cortex in a normal subject at rest and during a small contraction of the target muscle (facilitation). Facilitation has caused the CMAP latency to decrease by about 2 msec and the amplitude to increase fivefold. Stimulation was at 80% of the maximum output (1.5 tesla) of a 9-cm mean-diameter coil centered at the vertex (stimulus intensity 20% above the threshold at rest). Recordings are from the abductor digiti minimi. The root-mean-square of the EMG activity prior to stimulation, when compared with that of a maximum voluntary contraction, showed that the facilitation was 16% of maximum. Three single stimuli are superimposed in each condition. Calibrations are in milliseconds and 6 mV.

are insignificant (Barker et al., 1987). The intensity and pattern of stimulation used (single stimuli, several seconds apart, limited number of stimuli in one setting) radically differ from the parameters necessary to induce kindling in experimental animals (Cain, 1979). Many investigators have stimulated themselves thousands of times, and hundreds of patients have been tested without serious side effects. Patients with recent strokes have been tested and had no untoward effects, and the results were highly significant prognostically (Heald et al., 1993a,b). Two such patients have been reported to have had a clinical seizure temporally related to the stimulation. Epileptic patients have been stimulated without adverse effects or exacerbation or initiation of seizures; CMAPs were unchanged during petit mal discharges but were attenuated or absent during polyspike bursts. However, large numbers of stimuli given to patients with known epileptic foci have initiated seizures.

Counter et al. (1991) found morphologic damage to the cochlea and functional hearing abnormalities in young rabbits 3 or more weeks after exposure to repeated magnetic stimulation. However, Counter (personal communication) found no audiogram abnormalities in six members of our group who had received thousands of suprathreshold magnetic stimuli.

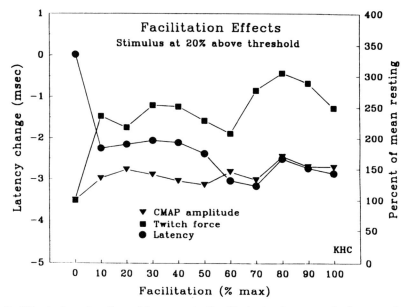

FIG. 13–5. Effect of contraction of the muscle (facilitation) prior to cortical magnetic stimulation. Both the amplitude of the CMAP and the twitch force are markedly increased by the prior activation of the muscle, and the latency is decreased by 2 to 3 msec, most of this effect occurring in the first 10% of facilitation, the latter expressed as percentage of a maximum voluntary contraction. The CMAP amplitude was expressed as the percentage of the mean CMAP obtained with the muscle at rest. The data are the mean of a group of normal subjects.

Similar results were reported by the National Institutes of Health group (Pascual-Leone et al., 1992).

Rapid-rate stimulation is now used by some centers and exciting prospects such as therapeutic use in neurologic disease are being explored (see Sections 5.5 and 5.8). With this method, there is a risk of inducing focal seizures in healthy subjects depending on intensity and number of stimuli in a train. Safety guidelines have therefore been suggested (Pascual-Leone et al., 1993). Recent observations by the same group (Wasserman et al., 1996) suggest that these guidelines need revision.

Even if seizures are, on very rare occasions, caused by the stimulation, this is not an absolute contraindication to the test; other tests in routine use in clinical neurophysiology may cause the patient to have a grand mal convulsion. For example, photic strobe stimulation is routinely used in every EEG test and about 1% of patients have a paroxysmal (epileptiform) response to strobe stimulation. When this paroxysmal response appears, the technologist stops the stimulation immediately. However, in rare instances (about 0.03% of all patients) the paroxysmal activity continues to build despite cessation of stimulation, and the patient has a grand mal convulsion. The occurrence rate of clinical seizures with magnetic stimulation must be much smaller even than the 0.03% rate given above for seizures during routine EEGs because transcranial stimulation has been used in Europe for 10 years in large numbers of patients without a single seizure being reported. Corroborating this, the Food and Drug Administration has declared magnetic stimulation a nonsignificant-risk device in 1994, requiring only approval of clinical or research projects using magnetic stimulation by institutional review boards in each institution.

It should be noted that electrical brain stimulation has been used in neurosurgery for many years without side effects. Electroconvulsive therapy (ECT), in which cortical stimulation is intentionally given in sufficient strength, duration, and pattern to cause a seizure, has been rarely reported to initiate or worsen pre-existing epilepsy. The electrical charge delivered to the brain following magnetic stimulation is relatively very small, less than 0.05% of that used for ECT.

Metal objects in the magnetic field may intensify the induced currents or be subject to significant forces and these effects need to be considered when drawing up guidelines for clinical use of the test. Presently our guidelines are that the magnetic stimulator will not be used on, near, or by persons wearing pacemakers or other implanted mechanical or electrical devices, or any metal in the brain or head (e.g., vascular clips, bullet fragments, metal intracranial pressure measurement devices, cochlear implants, bone plates), or on any person with a skull defect; the test will not be performed on patients who have any indications of increased intracranial pressure or on any person who has a history of epilepsy or any clinical indications of lowered seizure threshold (e.g., photoconvulsive response on EEG, myoclonic jerks). Normal children 2 weeks and older have been tested in some laboratories (Muller et al., 1991) without problems, although most investigators do not study this age group.

There are also hazards for the personnel adjacent to the magnetic stimulator. Magnetically encoded information on computer disks and credit and other cards may be corrupted if these are placed too close to the magnet (within a meter or so).

3. EQUIPMENT AND SETUP

3.1. Magnetic Stimulation

Transcranial magnetic stimulation is now the method of choice for scalp stimulation, primarily because it is much better tolerated than electrical stimulation (see below). The magnetic field is not attenuated by the scalp and skull and induces an electric field in the brain, primarily the cortex, which results in excitation of descending motor pathways. Because there is no attenuation of the magnetic field by the tissues interposed between the brain and the coil, its intensity at the scalp does not need to be as great as an electrical field, which is attenuated by the resistivity of the scalp, skull, and meninges up to 30-fold before reaching the cortex. Thus, the induced current at the scalp is much smaller than the electric current required for transcranial electrical stimulation, which results in activation of many fewer pain receptors in the scalp. Also, the intensity of magnetically induced current is inversely proportional to the resistance of a given tissue so that the current induced in the high-resistance skin remains of low intensity, minimizing the number of high-threshold unmyelinated pain fibers being stimulated. There are differences in the physiologic results obtained with electrical and magnetic stimulation, which, at moderate intensity, excite different elements in the cortex (see Section 2).

The stimulator consists of a capacitor bank which is charged and subsequently discharged rapidly though a coil. The peak magnetic field in the center of a circular coil is 1.5 to 2.5 tesla depending on coil size and current flow. The field intensity generated by a given stimulator is directly related to the coil size and shape, a factor which should be taken into account when comparing different devices. For example, a commercial stimulator which develops a 1.5-tesla peak field at the center of its standard 9-cm-diameter coil produces 2.1- and 5-tesla fields at the center of a 7- and 4-cm-diameter coil, respectively.

A smaller coil has a stronger field at its center than a larger coil for the same current pulse. However, a smaller coil provides less stimulation at a distance because the magnetic field strength falls off more rapidly with distance than with a larger coil. The field strength of a coil falls off as the inverse square of the distance until the "dipole distance" (about three times the coil radius) is reached, after which it falls off as the inverse cube of the distance. Since the dipole distance is reached earlier with a smaller coil, the more rapid decrement begins earlier.

The shape of the magnetic pulse produced by a magnetic stimulator is important to consider as different physiologic effects are obtained with a largely monophasic-current pulse as compared with a biphasic-decaying sine-wave pulse. Using monophasic pulses and large circular coils centered on the vertex, it has been shown that posterior to anterior induced currents activate preferentially the motor cortex (Hess et al., 1987a; Santamaria et al., 1988). Because its effect is simpler to understand, use of a monophasic-current pulse is probably preferable. The rise time of the magnetic pulse is of the order of 200 msec.

3.2. Transcranial Electrical Stimulation

The main technical feature of transcranial electrical stimulation is use of a high-voltage electrical stimulator. Commercially available instruments deliver a pulse of up to 750 volts with a very short rise and decay time of 50 to 100 msec. A bipolar stimulating electrode is most commonly used, consisting of 15-mm-diameter stainless steel bolts covered with gauze and dipped in saline before use (King et al., 1988). Others have used cup electrodes attached to the skin with collodion and filled with conductive jelly (Rothwell et al., 1987). The anode is positioned over the central area and the cathode anterior to the anode (upper- and lower-limb studies) or at the vertex (upper-limb studies). An alternative method of transcranial electrical stimulation allows the use of a conventional peripheral nerve stimulator (Rossini et al., 1985a,b). In this method, the anode consists of a disc electrode positioned as described above and the cathode of a flexible stainless steel belt or a series of interconnected electrodes placed in a crownlike fashion around the head just above the inion–nasion plane. In another method used intraoperatively in anesthetized patients by Levy et al. (1984), the cathode was positioned in the mouth against the hard palate, the motor cortex being stimulated using a conventional stimulator.

3.3. Amplifiers and Recording Parameters

Standard, preferably multichannel EMG equipment is optimal for transcranial motor stimulation. The band-pass used is similar to that of EMG motor studies (including 10 to 5,000 Hz). Appropriate sweep durations are 50 and 100 msec for upper- and lower-extremity studies. Of note is that marked delay of MEPs has occasionally been noted, for instance, in progressive lateral sclerosis and in demyelinating polyneuropathies, which requires adjustment of the sweep duration. The amplitude of the MEPs varies greatly and the gain setting is best determined by trials. Monitoring of the state of relaxation of the target muscle should best be conducted using a free-running, high-gain EMG display using the same pick-up electrodes in all cases. As the phenomenon of facilitation is seen at very low degrees of contraction of the target muscles (0% to 5% of maximum voluntary contraction), it is essential to ensure that complete relaxation be achieved prior to the recording of resting MEPs.

4. RUNNING THE TEST

4.1. Electrical Cortical Stimulation

Magnetic stimulation has supplanted electrical stimulation for clinical purposes at this time, therefore, this technique will not be discussed in detail further. The reader is referred to the reviews of Rossini et al. (1985a,b); Rothwell et al. (1987); and Macdonnell et al. (1989) if detailed information is needed.

4.2. Cortical Magnetic Stimulation

Several types of coil have been developed, including circular and figure-of-eight coils. The relative advantage of circular coils is accurate and easily reproducible positioning, particularly when hand-held and centered over the vertex. A relative disadvantage in certain types of study (e.g., mapping; see below) stems from the fact that large coils induce current in a large cortical areas, for instance, vertex stimulation beyond a certain intensity routinely stimulates the primary motor cortex bilaterally. Attempts to reduce the diameter of circular coils for more focal stimulation have been made (Cohen D. and Kazumoto Y., personal communication). Drawbacks were threefold: The energy required for each current pulse was maximized, therefore the battery of accumulators needed became extremely heavy and cumbersome, and the passage of each current pulse dissipated enough energy to rapidly lead to overheating of the coil, limiting its routine use for more than a few stimuli in a row. Finally, the high current intensity used generated mechanical constraints in the coil, necessitating use of special casing because of safety requirements. Researchers and clinicians have therefore turned to a different tool, the figure-of-eight coil. In this device, the turns of copper wire are arranged in an "8" shape so that the coil seems formed of two tangent circles. There are twice as many copper wires at the point of overlap of the circles, resulting in a high magnetic field density underneath this region which decreases rapidly with distance. This magnetic coil is therefore more focal. The size of the available figure-of-eight coils varies and technical limitations toward smaller sizes are similar to those described above for small circular coils.

Coils must be kept in the same position relative to the head during the study. This is best achieved by marking the scalp using the EEG anatomic landmarks. If the coil is hand-held, great care must be taken to maintain the position of the coil from one stimulation to the next as slight changes in position may result in a significantly different physiologic effect, particularly obvious with smaller, more focal coils and stimulation intensity close to threshold. To address this potential pitfall, we attach the coil to a gooseneck-type device which is rigidly clamped to the subject's chair. This chair is comfortable, reclinable, and equipped with a headrest, which helps the subject to remain still, although uncomfortable stiffness develops in the neck after a moment. These considerations apply more often to research studies, which are lengthier than clinical ones.

Single transcranial magnetic stimuli are sufficient for most clinical applications to date. At least two or three repetitions of MEP recordings at the desired intensity of stimulation are obtained to demonstrate consistency of the results. It should be noted that there is some variability from trial to trial (see Fig. 13–3). Use of multiple stimuli may be required for certain applications which remain in the domain of research so far. Double stimulation may be obtained by time-locking the output of two magnetic stimulators firing though the same coil, the interstimulus interval being adjusted by the experimentor. Another approach to repetitive TMS consists of using especially designed repetitive stimulators capable of delivering long trains of stimuli at set frequencies. Useful references on these techniques are by Pascual-Leone et al. (1994a,b,c) and Nielsen (1996). Repetitive TMS has caused seizures in several normal subjects (see above).

4.3. Stimulation of the Cervical Spinal Roots

Cervical root stimulation is easily performed using a large (9 cm) circular coil (Cros et al., 1990). In our laboratory, we record simultaneously from three or four muscles in each upper extremity (abductor pollicis brevis, abductor digiti minimi, biceps, and triceps). The coil is applied over the midline of the cervical region in a subject in the sitting position with a slight degree of neck flexion to reduce the cervical lordosis. The coil is discharged twice at maximum output while centered over the spinous process of the third, fourth, and fifth cervical vertebrae. The coil current is clockwise for right-sided recordings and counter-clockwise for left-sided recordings. The largest CMAP amplitude for each target muscle irrespective of the level of stimulation is selected and the corresponding latency measured. This technique is generally well tolerated. We consider the following situations as contraindications to cervical magnetic stimulation: Tight cervical stenosis, cervical cord compression, cervical spine instability, and multiple (more than two) cervical fusions. Magnetic cervical root stimulation does not always elicit a supramaximal response and is therefore not the "gold standard" technique to assess for proximal conduction block of the motor fibers. It does provide an accurate assessment of the peripheral conduction time as demonstrated by magnetic stimulations at different intensity levels.

4.4. Lumbosacral Root Stimulation

We use needle electrical stimulation at L1 to stimulate the lumbosacral roots at or near their emergence from the conus medullaris, as magnetic stimulation fails to elicit a compound response in 50% of subjects at this location (Menkes et al., 1994). Using this method, the PCT reflects conduction along most of the peripheral conduction pathway, whereas stimulation at the lumbosacral level (L5) bypasses the proximal intraspinal segment of this pathway (Maccabee et al., 1996). The target muscles most often used are the tibialis anterior and flexor hallucis brevis muscles. The motor cortex is stimulated by positioning a large circular coil on the midline centered on a point 2 to 3 cm anterior to the vertex. The CCT calculated includes conduction from cortex to the lumbosacral spinal motor neurons.

4.5. Motor Evoked Potentials

Determination of a motor conduction time from cortex to target muscle and of a PCT to the same muscle allows easy calculation of the CCT (motor conduction time minus PCT) (Fig. 13–6). This latency includes conduction along the fast-conducting axons of the corticospinal pathway as well as the time to bring to excitation the CM cells on the one hand and the spinal motor neurons on the other hand. It is therefore advisable not to calculate a conduction velocity as the physiologic phenomena underlying the CCT are considerably more complex than those underlying motor conduction studies in the peripheral nervous system.

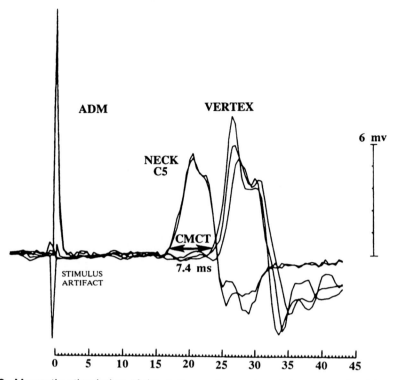

FIG. 13–6. Magnetic stimulation of the motor cortex and neck in a normal subject, with the results from the two levels superimposed. The latency difference between the CMAPs recorded in the target muscle is the central motor conduction time (CMCT). This includes the time required to depolarize corticocortical neurons activated by the induced current, one or two interposed synapses to the corticospinal neuron, depolarization of the corticospinal neuron, conduction time in the pyramidal tract, depolarization of the spinal alpha motor neuron, and conduction time in its axon to the site of its activation by the neck magnetic stimulation (at the foramen). The magnetic coil was centered at the vertex, and the stimulus (at artifact) was delivered during a small voluntary contraction (facilitation) of the target muscle (abductor digiti minimi). Three single stimuli are superimposed for the cortical stimulation, two for the neck. Calibrations are in millivolts and milliseconds. The calibration bar is 3.1 mV for neck stimulation.

The CCTs vary in the upper and lower extremity, and in each extremity with the target muscle considered. In the field of MEPs as well as other areas of neurophysiology, it is essential for each laboratory to determine its own clinical procedure, and to obtain the corresponding normal values in a sufficient number of control subjects prior to engaging in the study of patients. Examples of procedural details to decide upon is the intensity of cortical magnetic stimulation (in percentage of maximum output above resting threshold) at which the resting and facilitated MEPs will be evoked.

4.6. Cortical Mapping

Many investigators have used this technique in investigations of the motor system. The usual method consists of measuring the MEP evoked from a given muscle while moving a figure-of-eight shaped coil systematically over the scalp. The map generated generally includes an optimal position in its center where the MEP is of maximum amplitude, whereas smaller MEPs are obtained toward the edges (Brasil-Neto et al., 1992b). A good correlation between the hemodynamically based functional magnetic resonance imaging (fMRI) maps and TMS maps of the primary sensorimotor hand representation was documented recently (Krings et al., 1997).

Mapping techniques or their variants have been useful to document reorganization of the cortex following amputation (Cohen et al., 1991a; Hall et al., 1990), immobilization (Liepert et al., 1995), and spinal cord injury (Levy et al., 1990; Cohen et al., 1991a,b). Similar tech-

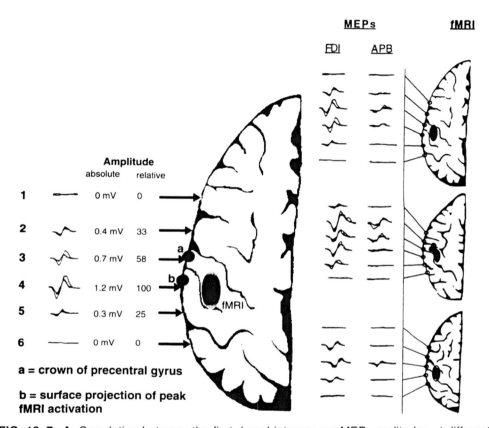

FIG. 13–7. **A.** Correlation between the first dorsal interosseus MEP amplitudes at different scalp sites of transcranial magnetic stimulation (TMS), cortical surface anatomy, and motor cortical activation for a fist-clenching task as revealed by functional magnetic resonance imaging (fMRI). The radially projected surface location of the peak fMRI activation (*gray-black oval on the genu of the central sulcus*) corresponded well to the cortical area from which TMS could elicit the peak response (site 4), although the center of the TMS coil actually was situated directly over the postcentral gyrus. Functional MRI was performed using a multislice, asymmetric, spin-echo, echo-planar pulse sequence. Transcranial magnetic stimulation stimulus sites were coregistered with the MRI images in real time during TMS stimulation by a frameless stereotaxy system, which used a jointed mechanical arm with position sensors in each joint, the tip of the arm attached to the center of the TMS coil, and the location of this point displayed in the MRI slices on a work-station screen. MEP amplitudes are peak-to-peak. **B.** Same data for two other MRI slices in the same subject, same task, with MEP data for abductor pollicis brevis also shown. (From Krings et al., 1997, *Neurology*, in press.)

niques have revealed rapid and reversible modulation of motor cortex organization in response to transient deafferentation of the forearm using local anesthetics (Brasil-Neto et al., 1992a).

4.7. Poststimulus Time Histogram

Single motor unit firing recorded during a weak tonic contraction reflects the activity of a single spinal motor neuron. This activity reflects the convergence of many inputs on the motor neuron, many of which are corticospinal. It is possible to study these connections by assessing the modulation of the tonic voluntary discharge of a motor unit by defined inputs elicited in the cortex by TMS (Mills, 1991). This is conducted by plotting the times of occurrence of spikes relative to stimulation on multiple consecutive trials. An example of the resulting poststimulus time histogram (PSTH) is shown in Fig. 13–8.

Small deviations from the prestimulus firing level are detected by cusum analysis of the PSTH. A sorted raster plot is useful to assess the effect of the stimulus relative to the firing history of the motor unit.

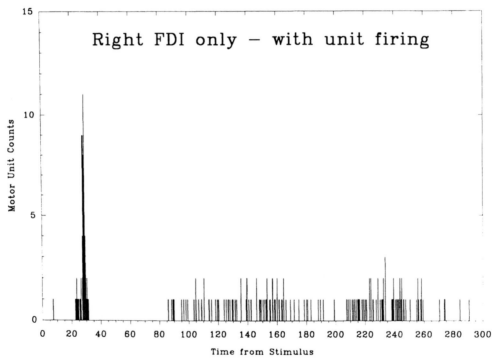

FIG. 13–8. Poststimulus time histogram in a normal subject from a single motor unit in the right first dorsal interosseus for sorted trials in which the unit fired in direct relationship to a cortical magnetic stimulation at time 0. This unit has a high probability of firing at latencies 23 to 32 msec and a silent period from 32 to 86 msec after the stimulus. The recordings were made from concentric needle electrodes positioned so that the earliest voluntarily recruited units had a large amplitude relative to the other one or two units that were usually visible. With the unit being voluntarily fired at about 10/sec the magnetic stimuli were delivered at random intervals of 4 to 5 secs, and the latency data from about 100 stimuli were plotted in this figure as a histogram. (From Chiappa et al., 1991, with permission.)

At a low intensity of stimulation, the motor unit firing probability decreases in the small muscles of the hand (Boniface et al., 1994). At a higher stimulus intensity, the slowing of discharge turns into an increase in firing probability, consisting of a narrow primary peak at 25 to 30 msec in a hand muscle followed by a secondary peak at about 70 msec. In multiple sclerosis the primary peak is often delayed and dispersed as expected from the demyelination of the central motor pathway (Boniface et al., 1994).

4.8. Cortical Stimulation Silent Period

In addition to MEPs, which are readily elicited from relaxed (resting MEPs) or contracting target muscles (facilitated MEPs), a silent period can be induced in a tonically active muscle (Fuhr et al., 1991; Cantello et al., 1992; Triggs et al., 1992). This silent period follows the MEP and is generally followed by a rebound of EMG activity. The cortically stim-

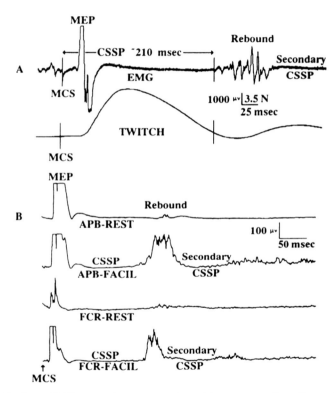

FIG. 13–9. **A.** Surface EMG trace (*upper trace*) and force recording (*lower trace*) following TMS at 25% of stimulator output above resting motor threshold (magnetic coil stimulation, MCS) during voluntary contraction of abductor pollicis brevis (APB) at 10% of maximum force, showing the cortically stimulated silent period (CSSP) and muscle twitch force accompanying the MEP. The MEP is clipped at the gain used in this illustration. Note that the falling phase of the cortically evoked muscle twitch occurs well in advance of the rebound phase of excitation terminating the CSSP. **B.** Rectified averaged (n=10) surface EMG recorded at REST (*first and third traces*) and during mild voluntary contraction (FACIL; *second and fourth traces*) of the APB (*first and second traces*) and flexor carpi radialis (FCR; *third and fourth traces*) muscles showing silent periods and "rebound" late responses following MCS. (From Triggs et al., 1993, with permission.)

ulated magnetic silent period (CSSP) (Triggs et al., 1993) is characterized by its duration, which should be assessed at a given stimulation intensity relative to excitation threshold, and with a given type of magnetic coil, as it changes with the magnitude of stimulator output (Fig. 13–9). The CSSP can be obtained using vertex stimulation with a circular coil or a butterfly coil positioned over the central region contralateral to the active target muscle, and also using ipsilateral stimulation of the motor cortex with a focal coil (Wasserman et al., 1991; Ferbert et al., 1992, Chiappa et al., 1995), in which case it is not preceded by an MEP and is thought to be generated though activation of a transcallosal pathway. The peripheral silent period induced by stimulation of the mixed nerve supplying a contracting target muscle is mostly thought to be due to spinal mechanisms secondary to changes in peripheral input (Merton, 1951; Shahani and Young, 1973) and is of shorter duration than the CSSP. The physiologic mechanisms underlying the CSSP have been studied by Triggs et al. (1993) and Inghilleri et al. (1993). It is generally agreed that the first 50 msec of the CSSP are due to peripheral factors, whereas the later part (from 50 msec onward) involves cortical inhibitory mechanisms.

5. CLINICAL CORRELATIONS

5.1. Stroke

Reports of abnormal MEPs in ischemic disorders affecting the corticospinal pathways rapidly followed the development of clinically applicable techniques for transcranial stimulation. Berardelli et al. (1987) described the MEP abnormalities noted in stroke patients using transcranial electrical stimulation. They found that MEPs evoked by stimulation of the damaged hemisphere were often absent and occasionally delayed.

An important question was to determine whether cortical stimulation performed early in the course of a stroke has any value in predicting outcome. As SEPs have already proved useful for this purpose (LaJoie et al., 1982), Macdonell and colleagues (1989) compared electrically evoked MEPs and SEPs as predictors of outcome in 19 stroke patients in the acute phase. The functional disability caused by the stroke was assessed at the time of neurophysiologic testing and 1 to 6 months later. Macdonell et al. found that the presence or absence of MEPs or SEPs was closely linked to the degree of functional recovery, the MEPs having a slightly better predictive value than the SEPs. These findings were subsequently confirmed by Kandler et al. (1991) in a study of 22 stroke patients in the acute phase. Other authors stressed that the sensitivity of TMS in stroke was lower than that of transcranial electrical stimulation based on a series study of 27 patients examined with both techniques (Berardelli et al., 1991).

A most informative study of stroke outcome as a function of initial TMS studies was conducted in Newcastle, UK, and included 118 patients with a first stroke evaluated within 72 hours of clinical onset (Heald et al., 1993a,b). Clinical assessment included a neurologic examination, the Motricity Index for muscle strength, the Nine-Hole Peg Test for manual dexterity, the Barthel Score for activities of daily living, and the modified Rankin Scale for functional outcome. Initial assesment was in the first 72 hours just preceding the initial neurophysiologic evaluation. Serial studies were repeated over 12 months or until death. The patients were divided into three groups based on the results of the initial neurophysiologic examination: normal MEP, delayed MEP, and absent MEP groups. Patients with normal MEPs achieved better functional recovery at 12 months. Patients with absent MEPs did poorly on neurologic and functional tests during the 12-month study period. Patients with obtainable but delayed MEPs were intermediate in terms of neurologic and functional testing during the follow-up period but their outcome at 12 months was similar to that of patients with initially normal MEPs. When the threshold to TMS was abnormally high the functional outcome was generally poor. Patients with absent MEPs have a high risk of poor functional recovery at 12 months and a greater risk of death during the first year after stroke. This study establishes the prognostic value of TMS in stroke, which was subsequently confirmed by others (Catano et al., 1995). Cortical magnetic stimulation can thus be used as a predictor of stroke outcome so that rehabilitative resources can be focused on those patients with a greater potential for recovery.

Early cortical stimulation studies in stroke patients showed either absent or delayed MEPs or, in a minority of cases, normal MEPs on stimulation of the affected hemisphere (Berardelli et al., 1987). The question of correlation of the type of stroke and type of MEP abnormality was later addressed by Macdonell and colleagues (1989), who found that only subcortical lesions delayed the MEPs, which is consistent with normal generation of the descending volley in the cortical layers and conduction delay due to functional or anatomic alterations in the descending pathways. If the corticospinal pathways are severely damaged, the MEPs are unobtainable in subcortical lesions. Interestingly, stimulation of the affected hemisphere in patients with a capsular stroke and MRI evidence of degeneration of the pyramidal tract elicited bilateral responses in the thenar muscles, whereas stimulation of the intact hemisphere at the same intensity caused only contralateral MEPs (Fries et al., 1991). These findings suggest unmasking of bilateral corticospinal projections, possibly corticoreticulospinal, after pyramidal tract lesions. Such a mechanism could explain functional recovery after a capsular stroke, and would also provide a pathophysiologic basis for the mirror movements occasionally seen after recovery from stroke (Fries et al., 1991). In cortical strokes using electrical and transcranial magnetic stimulation, the MEP is absent if the number of surviving corticospinal connections is too small to generate EPSPs in the anterior horn cells. The same patterns of MEP abnormalities are noted in stroke patients examined using TMS, with three patient groups characterized by absent, delayed, or normal responses (Heald et al., 1993a).

Other TMS parameters have been assessed in stroke patients. Heald et al. (1993a) and Catano et al. (1995) found that TMS excitation thresholds measured at rest were pathologically elevated in the affected hemisphere in stroke patients when the MEPs were initially obtainable. The threshold values decreased in subsequent studies during the first year to reach, somewhat surprisingly, values inferior to the contralateral intact hemisphere on the average. In some patients with initially unobtainable MEPs, motor responses reappeared in serial studies and initially were obtainable only at 100% of output of the magnetic stimulator (Heald et al., 1993a). Several groups emphasize the importance of testing patients during a facilitating voluntary contraction. Facilitation decreases the excitation threshold of the stimulated hemisphere and therefore may result in elicitation of MEPs which were not obtainable at rest. This was the case in 18% of the 118 patients examined by Heald and colleagues (1993a,b), who performed all the studies used in their correlations with outcome with facilitation when possible (e.g., except in paralyzed muscles, where they had the patient contract the contralateral muscles). Catano et al. (1995), who confirmed the predictive value of TMS in ischemic stroke, stress the importance of TMS testing with facilitation as patients with facilitated TMS responses only (and absent MEPs at rest) should be considered as subjects with obtainable MEPs for the purpose of prognosis.

Braune and Fritz (1995) found that the TMS silent period (SP) is prolonged in patients with ischemic stroke on stimulation of the affected hemisphere relative to contralateral values. The degree of SP abnormality tended to correlate with the severity of stroke deficits, and remained the sole neurophysiologic abnormality after complete clinical recovery in some cases (see Section 5.3 for further details on pathologic SP).

An unresolved question is that of the optimal number and choice of target muscles. Some investigators only examined one or two intrinsic hand muscles with useful outome correlations (Macdonell et al., 1989; Kandler et al., 1991; Catano et al., 1995). Heald et al. (1993 a,b) examined four upper-extremity muscles (pectoralis major, biceps, triceps, and thenar group) and found that the best correlations with outcome were obtained with the thenar recordings. Arac et al. (1994) recorded from hand and lower-leg muscles in 27 patients and found no correlations with outcome, arguing that differences from previous studies may stem from inclusion of lower-extremity MEP data.

5.2. Multiple Sclerosis

Unlike computed tomography and MRI techniques, which provide information on anatomic changes in the brain, central motor conduction studies provide functional information on the central motor pathways. Central motor conduction time complements the battery of neurophysiologic tests already available, such as sensory EPs and EEG, for the investigation of disorders of the brain and spinal cord.

Many patients with multiple sclerosis (MS) have already been studied using TMS. In these patients, several types of CMCT abnormalities have been demonstrated, including low-amplitude MEP, MEP of prolonged latency, delayed *and* low-amplitude MEP, and un-

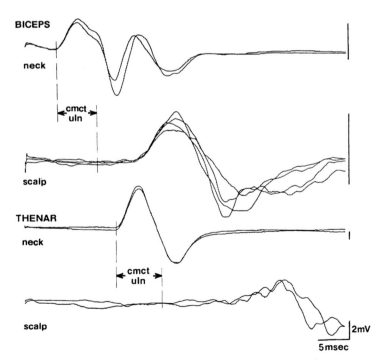

FIG. 13–10. Electrical scalp and neck stimulation in a 29-year-old woman with MS. Central motor conduction time (cmct) is about twice the upper limit of normal (uln) for both biceps and thenar muscles.

obtainable motor responses on transcranial stimulation (Fig. 13–10). In a study of 83 MS patients, Hess et al. (1987b) found abnormal CMCT to abductor digiti minimi in 60 individuals (72%). There were 62 patients with definite MS, 11 patients with probable MS, and 10 patients with possible MS; the CMCT was *normal* in 21, 46, and 50% of the subjects in each of these three groups, respectively. The delay noted in CMCT relative to normal mean value was considerable in many cases (the CMCT was more than twice the mean normal value in one third of the abnormal recordings, and more than three times this value in 10% of the abnormal recordings). A low-amplitude MEP was also a common finding usually found in association with prolonged CMCT. In one patient only, no MEP could be evoked by cortical magnetic stimulation on one side in the abductor digiti minimi. Motor EP CMAPs could be evoked by cortical magnetic stimulation on one side. Motor EP abnormalities limited to low amplitude without concomitant delay in CMCT was noted in 7 of 161 upper extremities tested in 83 patients, all having definite MS. All results summarized above were obtained with facilitation (sustained tonic contraction) of the target muscle. Hess and colleagues compared the result of TMS performed with and without facilitation in 39 MS patients, and found no advantage in testing the abductor digiti minimi at rest.

The neurologic signs which correlated best with abnormal CMCT abnormalities were ipsilateral hyperreflexia (including brisk finger flexor jerks) and increased tone. It is clear from this study that the presence of physical signs correlates with a high frequency of CMCT abnormalities. However, in 7 of 32 upper extremities which were neurologically normal, CMCTs were abnormal and thus demonstrated the presence of subclinical lesion(s).

Comparison of CMCT abnormalities with EP data revealed significant correlation between abnormal median sensory EP and abnormal central motor conduction (Table 13–1). There was no correlation between abnormal VEPs or BAEPs and abnormal CMCT. Finally, comparison of MRI data and central conduction indicated that abnormal CMCT is occasionally found in patients with questionable or no MRI changes. The diagnostic yield of CMCT in MS is comparable to that of established neurophysiologic tests such as PSVEPs.

In other studies, a close agreement was found between MEPs and the MRI, with a concordance of 85% (Ravnborg et al., 1992). Pyramidal tract conduction times did not differ in MS patients between rested and fatigued conditions (Sandroni et al., 1992). Masur et al. (1992) used a visual suppression paradigm to demonstrate slowing of conduction in the visual system and found a close relationship with delayed VEPs.

TABLE 13–1. *Comparison of central motor conduction (CMC) and EPs results in 83 patients with MS*

Evoked potential	CMC abnormal	CMC normal
VEP abnormal	43	11
VEP normal	17	10
SEP abnormal	35	1
SEP normal	8	17
BAEP abnormal	21	3
BAEP normal	24	13

VEP, pattern reversal check stimulation (81 patients); SEP, median nerve stimulation (61 patients); BAEP, brain stem auditory testing (61 patients); the EP numbers refer to patients rather than sides. CMC was determined with cortical and cervical (C7-T1 interspace) magnetic stimulation with CMAP recorded from the surface over abductor digiti minimi during a slight tonic contraction using the shortest latency and largest amplitude produced by three stimuli. The upper limit of normal for latency values was the normal mean plus 2.5 standard deviations. MEP amplitudes of less than 15% of the peripheral wrist amplitude were considered to be abnormal. (Hess et al, 1987b)

5.3. Motor Neuron Disease

Ingram and Swash (1987) reported a study of 12 patients with motor neuron disease using transcranial electrical stimulation, and Schriefer and colleagues (1989) evaluated 22 patients with TMS. The MEPs were abnormal in the majority of patients with both techniques, the abnormalities consisting of unobtainable or low-amplitude motor responses on cortical stimulation with preserved responses on root stimulation, and less often prolongation of CMCT. Pathologic decrease in cortical excitability, demonstrable by measuring excitation thresholds, is commonly noted and often corresponds with the low-amplitude MEPs (Schriefer et al., 1989; Cros and Chiappa, 1993; Eisen and Shtybel, 1990). As lower motor neuron loss and pathology of the CM pathway may both play a role in the genesis of low-amplitude MEPs, cortical threshold determination is a simple physiologic indicator of dysfunction of the upper motor neuron pathway which can be easily determined even if the corresponding peripheral response is of low amplitude. Subclinical evidence of dysfunction of the central motor pathways may also be documented, which is of diagnostic interest in the lower motor neuron variant of amyotrophic lateral sclerosis (ALS), in which no upper motor neuron signs are present (Schriefer et al., 1989; Cros and Chiappa, 1993). No central conduction abormalities are found in pure lower motor neuron syndromes (Triggs et al., 1992) or in pathologically proven progressive muscular atrophy (Triggs and Edgar, 1995). It is of interest to note that the marked prolongation of CCT seen in progressive lateral sclerosis (PLS) is not seen in ALS.

Transcranial magnetic stimulation also has inhibitory effects easily documented when recording from a tonically active muscle (Fuhr et al., 1991; Triggs et al., 1993; Haug et al., 1992; Haug and Kukowski, 1994) (See Section 4.8 and Fig. 13–9). The duration of this CSSP increases with the intensity of stimulation above excitation threshold and shortens with the magnitude of background contraction (Wilson et al., 1993). The first part of the CSSP is due to peripheral mechanisms, whereas the second part is due to cortical mechanisms (Shahani and Young, 1973; Fuhr et al., 1991; Triggs et al., 1992; Triggs et al., 1993). A CSSP generally follows an MEP although it is occasionally possible to evoke a CSSP using subthreshold stimuli in normal subjects (Triggs et al., 1992; Wasserman et al., 1993). In ALS, we found that the excitation and the inhibition threshold are often dissociated and that it is often possible to evoke a CSSP which is not preceded by an MEP (Triggs et al., 1992). Sequential studies in ALS patients have shown that the duration of this isolated CSSP decreases as the disease progresses (Triggs et al., 1993) (Fig. 13–11). In some patients with predominantly lower motor neuron signs or equivocal upper motor neuron dysfunction, documentation of EMG inhibition without preceding excitation is useful to confirm a diagnosis of ALS. Prout and Eisen (1994) found a linear correlation between CSSP duration and duration of the disease in definite ALS.

The firing probability of single motor units in relation to TMS can be assessed using poststimulus time histograms. In normals, two peaks of increased firing probability are seen, including an early peak corresponding to the CM volley and a late peak beginning at about 70 msec for which transcortical reflex mechanisms are invoked (Mills, 1991; 1995). An inhibition corresponding to the CSSP takes place between the peaks. These studies suggest that there is evidence for impaired initiation of the descending volley in motor neuron disease with and without upper motor neuron signs. Whether this reflects subclinical upper motor neuron involvement or supports the idea that the pathogenesis of ALS lies initially in the motor cortex is unclear at present (Eisen et al., 1992, 1993; Mills, 1995).

APB Muscle MND

Magstim Vertex
Stimulus 100%

March, 1991

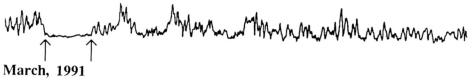

October, 1991

$200\,\mu v$

50 msec

FIG. 13–11. Inhibition elicited by maximum output vertex stimulation in a patient with ALS. Note that there is no MEP preceding the onset of the silent period. Over time as indicated the duration of the silent period decreased significantly, suggesting that the mechanisms underlying this inhibition are also affected in ALS. Recordings from the right abductor digiti minimi. The EMG was rectified and an average of 10 sweeps is presented. (From Triggs and Cros, unpublished.)

5.4. Extrapyramidal Disorders

Early studies of Parkinson's disease (PD) using transcranial stimulation [e.g., electrical stimulation (Dick et al., 1984) and magnetic stimulation (Cantello et al., 1991; Priori et al., 1992)] showed that the CCT is normal in PD, indicating that the descending motor pathways are not abnormal.

Increased amplitude of MEPs have, however, been reported in PD (Kandler et al., 1990; Cantello et al., 1991; Valls-Sole et al., 1994), which suggests that the spinal or the cortical motor neurons are more excitable in PD than in controls. This fact was further assessed using cortical threshold determinations. However, the results of such studies are variable, some authors reporting low thresholds (Cantello et al., 1991) and others increased thresholds (Davey et al., 1991), whereas thresholds were normal in other studies (Valls-Sole et al., 1994). The reasons for these discrepancies are unclear. They may involve the patient samples, methodologic differences in threshold determination (type of coil, definition of threshold), difficulty obtaining complete relaxation of the target muscles in PD patients, or any combination of these factors. Additionally, the issue of enhancement of alpha motor neuron excitability claimed by some authors (Cantello et al., 1991; Abbruzzese et al., 1985) is still unsettled.

In addition to MEPs which are readily elicited from relaxed (resting MEP) or contracting target muscles (facilitated MEPs), a silent period can be induced in a tonically active muscle. It is generally agreed that the first 50 msec of the CSSP are due to peripheral factors, whereas the later part (from 50 msec onward) involves cortical inhibitory mechanisms. Reports regarding the peripheral silent period in PD vary. Some studies showed no significant changes (Angel et al., 1966), whereas others, such as Cantello et al. (1992), found a prolonged peripheral silent period. These variable results are difficult to reconcile. In a recent study of cortical and peripheral silent periods in PD, Priori et al. (1994) found a normal peripheral silent period, the duration of which did not change with administration of levodopa (L-dopa).

Priori et al. (1994) also examined the CSSP in patients with idiopathic PD, those with extrapyramidal syndrome induced by neuroleptics, and controls. They assessed the changes in the silent period relative to pharmacologic treatment, including administration of L-dopa and of biperidin (a centrally acting antagonist of muscarinic receptors which inhibits the overactivity of cholinergic striatal interneurons). They found that the CSSP was shorter in PD than in normal subjects, confirming the finding of Cantello et al. (1992). In PD patients treated with L-dopa, the CSSP was longer in the "on" phase than in the "off" phase. Confirming again findings by Cantello et al., they found that in a patient with hemi PD, L-dopa had a more pronounced effect on the silent period on the affected side. In three patients, they found that intravenous administration of biperidin lengthened the CSSP duration. Pathologic shortening of the baseline silent period was also documented in patients with drug-induced Parkinsonism, although there was no correlation with the dose of neuroleptics, the clinical score or the duration of treatment. Administering L-dopa to controls, Priori et al. (1994) found that the CSSP was significantly lengthened relative to baseline values. They also assessed the ipsilateral CSSP in the "on" and "off" phases induced by L-dopa in PD patients and found that its duration was longer in the "on" phase. Priori and his colleagues interpret their observations in PD in light of both their investigation of the CSSP in Huntington's disease (HD) and of the pathophysiologic hypotheses delineated by DeLong (1990). In HD, they found that the CSSP was pathologically lengthened. They discussed this finding relative to DeLong's hypotheses, whereby the loss of striatal neurons in HD causes a reduced inhibitory output from the globus pallidus and the substantia nigra to the thalamus, which in turn increases the thalamocortical outflow. An increase in the excitation of intracortical inhibitory interneurons could then explain the prolongation of the CSSP seen in HD. In MPTP-treated primates, the loss of striatal dopamine increases the output of the globus pallidus and substantia nigra to the thalamus, causing excessive thalamic inhibition that results in reduction of the usually facilitatory effect of the thalamocortical outflow on the motor cortex. This in turn could result in decreased activity of intracortical inhibitory interneurons (a situation symmetric to that in HD) inducing shorter CSSPs.

Recent studies by Ridding et al. (1995) using a double-pulse paradigm suggest that there may be abnormalities of motor cortical inhibitory mechanisms in PD which are not readily detected using threshold or silent period measurent alone

L-dopa could exert its effects on the CSSP via modulation of the activity of the subcortical–cortical connections, via the basal ganglia or directly on the intracortical neurons. Two the observations made by Priori et al. (1994) suggest that modulation occurring at the level of the basal ganglia is more likely. First, the similarity in the effect on the CSSP of L-dopa and biperidin since it is known that biperidin, a muscarinic receptor antagonist, reduces striatal interneuronal activity resulting from a decreased inhibitory drive by the nigro–striatal dopaminergic pathway. Second, the similarity of CSSP abnormalities in idiopathic PD and drug-induced Parkinsonism also points to the same mechanism occurring in the basal ganglia. Although these considerations are largely speculative, it remains that CSSP studies appear to be a valid correlate of the activity of systems inhibiting the cortical motor system in PD.

In a recent paper, Valls-Sole et al. (1994) reported that the mechanisms underlying facilitation of MEPs evoked by TMS are impaired in PD. These authors found that, in six PD patients, the increase in MEP area induced by both an increase in background contraction and in cortical stimulation intensity was significantly less than in controls. This finding is in agreement with the CSSP data described above.

Cortical magnetic stimulation has also been used to investigate more complex physiologic aspects of the motor disorder characteristic of PD such as akinesia (Pascual-Leone et al., 1994a,b). Combining a simple reaction time (RT) paradigm and TMS using a figure-of-eight magnetic coil, the authors showed that a magnetic stimulus shortens the RT in PD patients and controls when delivered within −10 to +50 msec and −10 to +20 msec relative to the "go" signal, respectively. In patients, the premovement excitability build-up preceding the EMG onset is also increased in duration, this increase being partially corrected by magnetic stimulation given at the same time as the "go" signal. The authors discuss these findings relative to the physiologic basis of simple RT and the animal model of PD (see also Section 5.8).

5.5. Epilepsy

Transcranial magnetic stimulation has been investigated in epilepsy for the localization and lateralization of speech function, the determination of cortical TMS thresholds in different epileptic syndromes, the effects of anticonvulsant medications on cortical TMS thresholds, and the localization of seizure foci.

When temporal lobe surgery is being planned it is necessary to localize speech functions so that those cortical areas can be spared. This is accomplished using an intra-arterial amobarbital procedure (the Wada test), which also provides information on memory functions; speech localization is subsequently verified by intraoperative cortical stimulation. The Wada test presents procedural and interpretive difficulties beyond the scope of this text (see Rausch et al., 1993, for a review), which prompted the investigation of TMS as a tool for localization of language functions in temporal lobe neocortex. Pascual-Leone et al. (1991) used TMS at 25/sec (rTMS) delivered in trains lasting 10 seconds while the patient counted aloud and produced reproducible speech arrest from the left hemisphere in all six patients tested, in agreement with Wada testing in the same patients. However, fMRI promises to provide a more reliable and detailed mapping of language and motor functions (McCarthy et al., 1993; Rao et al., 1995; Cuenod et al., 1995), which is easily coregistered with the anatomic data. In addition, rTMS has been shown to have no effect on memory (Hufnagel et al., 1993), another function of interest in the Wada test, whereas brain regions active in memory tasks have shown activation in some fMRI paradigms (Stern et al., 1994, 1995, 1996), although this needs to be further evaluated.

Patients with various epileptic syndromes have usually shown lowered thresholds for activation of the motor cortex by TMS, and shorter latencies and higher amplitudes of the MEP (Hufnagel et al., 1990a,b; Reutens et al., 1993a,b). The addition of anticonvulsant medications reversed these effects and altered values to exceed normal levels (e.g., thresholds were higher in epileptic patients on anticonvulsant medications than in normal subjects, latencies were longer and amplitudes were lower). Hufnagel et al. (1990a,b) noted that the duration of epilepsy, the location of the epileptic focus, and the seizure type did not affect the MEPs, in agreement with the concept of a global cortical disturbance in the excitation/inhibition balance in many forms of epilepsy. In addition, cortical hyperexcitability in progressive myoclonus epilepsy produced an exaggerated effect of afferent input (Reutens et al., 1993a).

Single-pulse TMS stimulation at intervals of 1 to several seconds has never caused a seizure in a normal subject and usually does not produce clinical seizure phenomena even in patients with epilepsy. Tassinari et al. (1990) evoked no definite seizures in 58 patients with both partial and generalized epilepsies, although there were 2 patients who might have had a focal seizure triggered by the stimulation. Classen et al. (1995) reported focal seizures similar to spontaneous clinical events reliably triggered by single stimuli. Hufnagel et al. (1990a,b) produced a seizure with single pulses in only one of eight patients with temporal lobe epilepsy and concluded that TMS was not helpful in the lateralization of the primary epileptic focus during presurgical evaluation. A further series of 140 epileptic patients was reported by Hufnagel and Elger (1991a), who observed that four clinical seizures were provoked after the application of 56, 61, 78, 174, and 71 stimuli. They noted that the overall probability of inducing a seizure with TMS in epileptic patients was lower than 5%, and was enhanced by five conditions: anticonvulsants below therapeutic levels, continuous epileptiform activity prior to TMS, high frequency of spontaneous complex partial seizures of temporal lobe origin, proximity of spontaneous seizures, and stimulation over the epileptic focus. Hufnagel and Elger (1991a) monitored TMS in the region of the epileptic focus using subdural electrodes. They found excitatory, inhibitory, and no influences and could not identify a reliable practical application in this patient group.

TMS at rates of 5 to 30/sec (rTMS) can produce a seizure in normal subjects. Pascual-Leone et al. (1993) studied the safety of rTMS in nine normal subjects and produced a focal, secondarily generalized seizure in one despite the absence of risk factors. They also demonstrated an intensity- and frequency-dependent spread of excitability in the motor cortex which they considered to represent an early epileptogenic effect of rTMS. Thus, even in normal subjects the motor cortex can be stimulated to engage in epileptiform activity which can progress to a clinical seizure in a rare normal subject, much like the photoparoxysmal activity that can be produced in the occipital cortex in some subjects who have never had a clinical seizure.

Dhuna et al. (1991) investigated the effects of rapid-rate TMS on eight patients being evaluated for epilepsy surgery. They were unable to trigger seizures or induce epileptiform discharges from the epileptic focus, although a simple partial seizure was produced in one of these patients in the right hemisphere, not the site of her spontaneous seizures. They concluded that TMS does not specifically activate the epileptic focus. Schuler et al. (1993) found that magnetic stimulation was no more likely than hyperventilation to activate epileptogenic foci.

Gianelli et al. (1994) studied 20 patients with 3/sec spike–wave complexes and absence seizures, 12 of whom were receiving valproate or phenobarbital or both. The patients had higher thresholds than normals, although a correlation with anticonvulsant medication was not evident. In four patients the TMS pulse was time-locked to the different phases of the spike–wave activity; MEP size was reduced during the wave and was decreased or unchanged during the spike, consistent with the inhibitory constituency of the slow wave component.

5.6. Spinal Cord Lesions

Motor EPs using TMS are an improvement relative to the invasive technique of spinal cord motor conduction, in which activation of the descending motor tracts is obtained in the cervical region using needle electrical stimulation (Berger and Shahani, 1989). Investigation of patients with cervical spondylotic myelopathy reveals abnormalitites in the vast majority of patients (Tavy et al., 1994). Lower-extremity studies are more sensitive than those of the upper extremity, and use of tibialis anterior as a target muscle is recommended. A significant number of clinically asymptomatic motor lesions were detected.

Transcranial magnetic stimulation studies in heredodegenerative disorders affecting the spinal cord have also been reported (Claus et al., 1990; Schady et al., 1991). They may be useful in delineating subgroups of patients.

5.7. Cranial Nerve Stimulation

Cranial nerves V, VII, X, XI, and XII can be stimulated transcranially using standard magnetic stimulation equipment (Benecke et al., 1988). Schriefer et al. (1988) first reported stimulation of the intracranial portion of the facial nerve in a variety of patients. Although the latency of the motor response elicited with TMS was longer than that of the response elicited with electrical stimulation at the stylomastoid foramen, the exact locus of excitation was unclear (Schriefer et al., 1988). Indirect assessment of the site of excitation based on latency differences and estimates of intracranial conduction velocity suggested excitation of the facial motor fibers in the root exit zone segment (Seki et al., 1990). Comparison of TMS-elicited facial motor latencies and direct stimulation of the nerve at operation suggested instead that the locus of excitation was in the proximal part of the intrapetrous segment of the facial nerve (Rosler et al., 1994; Rimpilainen et al., 1994), 5 to 16 mm distal to the cerebellopontine angle (Schmid et al., 1992b).

The intracranial facial nerve is easily stimulated using a circular coil centered on a point 4 cm lateral to the vertex (Benecke et al., 1988). The motor responses evoked in facial muscles are robust, of constant latency, and relatively unaffected by changes in coil position or stimulus intensity (Schmid et al., 1992a,b). The CM pathway corresponding to facial muscles can also be activated using a circular coil centered on a point 4 cm lateral to the vertex (Benecke et al., 1988). The stimulus intensity must be precisely adjusted as supraliminar responses easily elicit stimulation of the facial nerve. The CM projection is bilateral and the MEPs so evoked can be facilitated by tonic contraction of the facial muscles (Benecke et al., 1988; Meyer et al., 1994). Two CM pathways to the lower facial muscles have been described based on poststimulus histograms of single motor unit discharges: a short latency more commonly contralateral, oligosynaptic pathway, and a bilateral, longer-latency polysynaptic pathway (Meyer et al., 1994).

In Bell's palsy, intracranial facial nerve stimulation elicits no response in a large number of cases in which stylomastoid stimulation is normal, presumably reflecting conduction block (Schriefer et al., 1988; Meyer et al., 1994). In serial studies, hypoexcitability of the intracranial facial nerve persists longer than the conduction block (Meyer et al., 1989). Two studies suggested that intracranial facial nerve stimulation is not useful as a prognostic indicator in Bell's palsy (Cocito and DeMattei, 1992; Rossler et al., 1994). Delayed facial motor latencies have been documented in demyelinating peripheral neuropathies (Schriefer et al., 1988).

Stimulation of the proximal portion of the trigeminal motor fibers using TMS has also been reported (Schmid et al., 1992a,b; Schmid et al., 1995). Thumfart and colleagues describe a large series of intracranial and cortical simulations recording from the vocalis muscle, which documented prolongation of central and peripheral latencies in recurrent neuropathies (Thumfart et al., 1992). A blink reflex can also be elicited painlessly with TMS with bilateral R1 and R2 responses (Siao et al., 1990; Bischoff et al., 1993).

5.8. Therapeutic Use of Magnetic Stimulation

Pascual-Leone et al. (1994) recently reported that repetitive, 5-Hz subthreshold TMS improved the performance of PD patients in a choice reaction time task paradigm. Reaction time (RT) and movement time (MT) were decreased in patients without concomitant increase in error rate (ER), whereas in controls RT did not change, MT decreased slightly and ER increased. The performance of PD patients in a pegboard test improved following repetitive TMS, whereas controls worsened. These observations contribute to the understanding of akinesia in PD and may provide insight into therapeutic avenues.

Nielsen et al. (1995) reported a pilot study of transspinal magnetic stimulation in the treatment of spasticity due to MS. They used a noncommercial magnetic stimulator connected to an oil-cooled coil. The patients' spinal column was stimulated at the midthoracic level at a 12 Hz frequency intermittently for 30 min. Twelve patients were evaluated before and after treatment using clinical criteria, the Ashworth's score, a self-administered functional scale, and neurophysiologic (stretch reflex EMG) and biomechanical (maximum voluntary contraction) measurements. Most parameters significantly improved from baseline to 24 hours after treatment and magnetic stimulation was well tolerated. Based on these data, a controlled study of the effect of repetitive magnetic stimulation of the spinal cord on spasticity is now under way.

It should also be noted that encouraging preliminary results have been obtained regarding treatment of major depression using repetitive TMS (George et al., 1995).

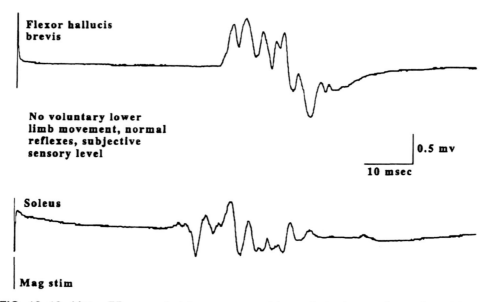

FIG. 13–12. Motor EPs recorded from upper and lower limbs in a patient referred from a prison for testing after being hit on the head with a chair by a guard and then demonstrating no voluntary leg movements. Clinical examination showed normal lower-limb reflexes and a sensory level. The CMAPs from both the upper and lower limbs are normal. The patient made a full recovery.

5.9. Functional Disorders

Lastly, TMS studies are a useful test when documenting the integrity of the upper motor neuron pathway in patients with alleged paralysis or motor somatization disorders (Fig. 13–12).

REFERENCES

Abbruzzese G, Vische M, Ratto S, Abbruzzese M, Favale E (1985): Assessment of motor neuron excitability in Parkinsonian rigidity by the F wave. *J Neurol* 232:246–249.

Amassian VE, Stewart M, Quirks GJ, Rosenthal JL (1987): Physiological basis of motor effects of transient stimulus to cerebral cortex. *Neurosurgery* 20:87–93.

Angel RW, Hoffman WW, Eppler W (1966): Silent period in patients with Parkinsonian rigidity. *Neurology* 16: 529–532.

Arac N, Sagduyu A, Binai S, Ertekin C (1994): Prognostic value of transcranial magnetic stimulation after stroke. *Stroke* 25:2183–2186.

Barker AT, Freeston IL, Jalinous R (1985): Noninvasive magnetic stimulation of human motor cortex. *Lancet* 2:1106–1107.

Barker AT, Freeston IL, Jalinous R, Jarratt JA (1987): Magnetic stimulation of the human brain and peripheral nervous system: An introduction and the results of an initial clinical evaluation. *Neurosurgery* 20:100–109.

Benecke R, Meyer BU, Schonle P, Conrad B (1988): Transcranial magnetic stimulation of the human brain: Responses in muscles supplied by the cranial nerves. *Exp Brain Res* 71:623–632.

Berardelli A, Inghilleri M, Manfredi M, Zamponi A, Cecconi V, Dolce G (1987): Cortical and cervical stimulation after hemispheric infarction. *J Neurol Neurosurg Psychiatry* 50:861–865.

Berardelli A, Inghilleri M, Cruccu G, Mercuri B, Manfredi M (1991): Electrical and magnetic transcranial stimulation in patients with corticospinal damage due to stroke or motor neurone disease. *Electroencephalogr Clin Neurophysiol* 81:389–396.

Berger AR, Shahani BT (1989): Electrophysiological evaluation of spinal cord motor conduction. *Muscle Nerve* 12:976–980.

Bischoff C, Liscic R, Meyer BU, Machetanz J, Conrad B (1993): Magnetically elicited blink reflex: an alternative to conventional electrical stimulation. *Electromyogr Clin Neurophysiol* 33:265–269.

Boniface SJ, Mills KR, Schubert M (1991): Responses of single spinal motoneurones to magnetic brain stimulation in healthy subjects and patients with multiple sclerosis. *Brain* 114:643–662.

Boniface SJ, Schubert M, Mills KR (1994): Suppression and long-latency excitation of single spinal motoneurones by transcranial magnetic stimulation in health, multiple sclerosis and stroke. *Muscle Nerve* 17:643–646.

Boyd SG, DaSilva LVK (1986): EEG and serum prolactin studies in relation to transcutaneous stimulation of central motor pathways. *J Neurol Neurosurg Psychiatry* 49:954–956.

Brasil-Neto JP, Cohen LG, Pascual-Leone A, Jabir FK, Wall RT, Hallett M (1992a): Rapid reversible modulation of human motor outputs after transient deafferentation of the forearm. *Neurology* 42:1302–1306.

Brasil-Neto JP, McShane LM, Fuhr P, Hallett M, Cohen LG (1992b): Topographic mapping of the human motor cortex with magnetic stimulation: factors affecting accuracy and reproducibility. *Electroencephalogr Clin Neurophysiol* 85:9–16.

Braune HJ, Fritz C (1995): Transcranial magnetic stimulation-evoked inhibition of voluntary muscle activity (silent period) is impaired in patients with ischemic hemispheric lesions. *Stroke* 26:550–553.

Bridgers SL, Delaney RC (1989): Transcranial magnetic stimulation: an assessment of cognitive and other cerebral effects. *Neurology* 39:417–419.

Cain DP (1979): Sensory kindling: Implications for the development of sensory prostheses. *Neurology* 29:1595–1599.

Cantello R, Gianelli M, Bettucci D, et al (1991): Parkinson's disease rigidity: magnetic motor evoked potentials in a small hand muscle. *Neurology* 41:1449–1456.

Cantello R, Gianelli M, Civardi C, Mutani R (1992): Magnetic brain stimulation: the silent period after the motor evoked potential. *Neurology* 42:1951–1959.

Catano A, Houa M, Caroyer JM, Ducarne H, Noel P (1995): Magnetic transcranial stimulation in non-haemorrhagic Sylvian strokes: Interest of facilitation in early functional prognosis. *Electroencephalogr Clin Neurophysiol* 97:349–354.

Chiappa KH, Cros D, Day B, Fang JJ, Macdonell R, Mavroudakis N (1991): Magnetic stimulation of the human motor cortex: ipsilateral and contralateral facilitation effects. *Electroencephalogr Clin Neurophysiol* Suppl 43:186–201.

Chiappa KH, Cros D, Kiers L, Triggs W, Clouston P, Fang JJ (1995): Crossed inhibition in the human motor system. *J Clin Neurophysiol* 12(1):82–96.

Chokroverty S, Flynn D, Picone MA, Chokroverty M, Belsh J (1993): Magnetic coil stimulation of the human lumbosacral vertebral column: Site of stimulation and clinical applications. *Electroencephalogr Clin Neurophysiol* 89:54–60.

Chokroverty S, Hening W, Wright D, Walczack T, Goldberg J, Burger R, Belsh J, Patel B, Flynn D, Shah S, Mero R (1995): Magnetic brain stimulation: Safety studies. *Electroencephalogr Clin Neurophysiol* 97:36–42.

Classen J, Witte OW, Schlaug G, Seitz RJ, Holthausen H, Benecke R (1995): Epileptic seizures triggered directly by focal transcranial magnetic stimulation. *Electroencephalogr Clin Neurophysiol* 94:19–25.

Claus D, Waddy HM, Harding AE, Murray NMF, Thomas PK (1990): Hereditary motor and sensory neuropathies and hereditary spastic paraplegia: A magnetic stimulation study. *Ann Neurol* 28:43–49.

Cocito D, DeMattei M (1992): Inadequacy of transcranial magnetic stimulation in the neurophysiologic assessment of Bell's palsy. *Electromyogr Clin Neurophysiol* 32:521–530.

Cohen LG, Hallett M (1987): Cortical stimulation does not cause short term changes in the electroencephalogram. *Ann Neurol* 21:512–513.

Cohen LG, Bandinelli S, Findley TW, Hallett M (1991a): Motor reorganization after upper limb amputation in man. *Brain* 114:615–627.

Cohen LG, Roth BJ, Wassermann EM, Topka H, Fuhr P, Schultz J, Hallett M (1991b): Magnetic stimulation of the human cerebral cortex, an indicator of reorganization in motor pathways in certain pathological conditions. *J Clin Neurophysiol* 8:56–65.

Counter SA, Borg E, Lofquist L, Brismar T (1990): Hearing loss from the acoustic artifact of the coil used in extracranial magnetic stimulation. *Neurology* 40:1159–1162.

Cros D, Chiappa KH (1993): Clinical applications of motor evoked potentials. *Adv Neurol* 63:179–185.

Cros D, Chiappa KH, Gominak S, Fang J, Santamaria J, King P, Shahani BT (1990): Cervical magnetic stimulation. *Neurology* 40:1751–1756.

Cuenod CA, Bookheimer SY, Hertz-Pannier L, Zeffiro TA, Theodore WH, Le Bihan D (1995): Functional MRI during word generation, using conventional equipment. *Neurology* 45:1821–1827.

Day BL, Thompson PD, Dick JP, Nakashima K, Marsden CD (1987): Different sites of action of electrical and magnetic stimulation of the human brain. *Neurosci Lett* 75:101–106.

DeLong MR (1990): Primate models of movement disorders of basal ganglia origin. *Trends Neurosci* 13:281–285.

Dhuna A, Gates J, Pascual-Leone A (1991): Transcranial magnetic stimulation in patients with epilepsy. *Neurology* 41:1067–1071.

Dick JPR, Cowan JMA, Day BL, et al (1984): The corticomotor neurone connection is normal in Parkinson's disease. *Nature* 310:407–409.

Dressler D, Voth E, Feldmann M, Benecke R (1990): Safety aspects of transcranial brain stimulation in man tested by single photon emission-computed tomography. *Neurosci Lett* 119:153–155.

Eisen AA, Shtybel W (1990): AAEM minimonograph #35: Clinical experience with transcranial magnetic stimulation. *Muscle Nerve* 1990;13:995–1011.

Eisen AA, Kim S, Pant B (1992): ALS: A phylogenetic disease of the corticomotoneuron? *Muscle Nerve* 15: 219–228.

Eisen AA, Pant B, Stewart H (1993): Cortical excitability in ALS: A clue to pathogenesis. *Can J Neurol Sci* 20:11–16.

Ferbert A, Priori A, Rothwell JC, Day BL, Colebatch JG, Marsden CD (1992): Interhemispheric inhibition of the human motor cortex. *J Physiol* 453:525–546.

Fries W, Danek A, Witt TN (1991): Motor responses after transcranial electrical stimulation of cerebral hemispheres with a degenerated pyramidal tract. *Ann Neurol* 29:646–650.

Fuhr P, Agostino R, Hallett M (1991): Spinal motor neuron excitability during the silent period after magnetic stimulation. *Electroencephalogr Clin Neurophysiol* 81:257–262.

George MS, Wasserman EM, Williams WA et al (1995): Daily repetitive transcranial magnetic stimulation improves mood in depression. *Neuroreport* 6:1853–1856.

Gianelli M, Cantello R, Civardi C, Naldi B, Bettucci D, Schiavella MP, Mutani R (1994): Idiopathic generalized epilepsy: Magnetic stimulation of motor cortex time-locked and unlocked to 3-Hz spike-and-wave discharges. *Epilepsia* 35:53–60 .

Hall EJ, Flament D, Fraser C, Lemon RN (1990): Non-invasive brain stimulation reveals reorganised cortical output in amputees. *Neurosci Lett* 116:379–386.

Haug BA, Kukowski B (1994): Latency and duration of the muscle silent period following transcranial magnetic stimulation in multiple sclerosis, cerebral ischemia and other upper motor neuron lesions. *Neurology* 44:936–940.

Haug BA, Schonle PW, Knobloch C, Kohne M (1992): Silent period measurement revived as a valuable diagnostic tool with transcranial magnetic stimulation. *Electroencephalogr Clin Neurophysiol* 85:158–160.

Heald A, Bates D, Cartlidge NEF, French JM, Miller S (1993a): Longitudinal study of central motor conduction time following stroke: 1. Natural history of central motor conduction. *Brain* 116:1355–1370.

Heald A, Bates D, Cartlidge NEF, French JM, Miller S (1993b): Longitudinal study of central motor conduction time following stroke. 2. Central motor conduction measured within 72 hours after stroke as a predictor of functional outcome at 12 months. *Brain* 116:1371–1385.

Henneman E, Somjen G, Carpenter D (1965): Functional significance of cell size in spinal motoneurons. *J Neurophysiol* 28:560–580.

Hess CW, Mills KR, Murray NMF (1987a): Responses in small hand muscles from magnetic stimulation of the human brain. *J Physiol* 388:397–420.

Hess CW, Mills KR, Murray NMF, Schriefer TN (1987b): Magnetic brain stimulation: central motor conduction studies in multiple sclerosis. *Ann Neurol* 22:744–752.

Hufnagel A, Elger CE, Marx W, Ising A (1990a): Magnetic motor-evoked potentials in epilepsy: effects of the disease and of anticonvulsant medication. *Ann Neurol* 28:680–686.

Hufnagel A, Elger CE (1991a): Induction of seizures by transcranial magnetic stimulation in epileptic patients. *J Neurol* 238:109–110.

Hufnagel A, Elger CE (1990b): Responses of the epileptic focus to transcranial magnetic stimulation. *Electroencephalogr Clin Neurophysiol* Suppl 43:86–99.

Hufnagel A, Elger CE, Klingmuller D, Zierz S, Kramer R (1990b): Activation of epileptic foci by transcranial magnetic stimulation: effects on secretion of prolactin and luteinizing hormone. *J Neurol* 237:242–246.

Hufnagel A, Claus D, Brunhoelzl C, Sudhop T (1993): Short-term memory: no evidence of effect of rapid-repetitive transcranial magnetic stimulation in healthy individuals. *J Neurol* 240:373–376.

Inghilleri M, Berardelli A, Cruccu G, Manfredi M (1993): Silent period evoked by transcranial stimulation of the human motor cortex and cervicomedullary junction. *J Physiol (Lond)* 466:521–534.

Ingram DA, Swash M (1987): Central motor conduction is abnormal in motor neuron disease. *J Neurol Neurosurg Psychiatry* 50:159–166.

Kandler RH, Jarratt JA, Sagar HJ, et al (1990): Abnormalities of central motor conduction in Parkinson's disease. *J Neurol Sci* 100:94–97.

Kandler RH, Jarratt JA, Venables GS (1991): Clinical value of magnetic stimulation in stroke. *Cerebrovasc Dis* 1:239–244.

Kiers L, Cros D, Chiappa KH, Fang J (1993): Variability of motor potentials evoked by transcranial magnetic stimulation. *Electroencephalogr Clin Neurophysiol* 89:415–423.

Kiers L, Clouston P, Chiappa KH, Cros D (1985): Assessment of Cortical motor output: compound muscle action potential versus twitch force recording. *Electroencephalogr Clin Neurophysiol* 97:131–139.

Kitagawa H, Moller AR (1994): Conduction pathways and generators of magnetic evoked spinal cord potentials: a study in monkeys. *Electroencephalogr Clin Neurophysiol* 93:57–67.

Krings T, Buchbinder BR, Butler WE, Chiappa KH, Cros D, Roy AM, Rosen BR (1997): Transcranial magnetic stimulation and functional magnetic resonance imaging: Complementary approaches in the evaluation of cortical motor function. (*Neurology*, in press)

LaJoie WJ, Reddy NM, Melvin JL (1982): Somatosensory evoked potentials: Their predictive value in right hemiplegia. *Arch Phys Med Rehabil* 63:223–226.

Levy WJ, York DH, McCaffrey M, Tanzer F (1984): Motor evoked potentials from transcranial stimulation of the motor cortex in humans. *Neurosurgery* 15:287–302.

Levy WJ, Amassian VE, Traad M, Cadwell J (1990): Focal magnetic coil stimulation reveals motor cortical system reorganized in humans after traumatic quadriplegia. *Brain Res* 510:130–134.

Liepert J, Tegenthoff M, Malin JP (1995): Changes of cortical motor area size during immobilization. *Electroencephalogr Clin Neurophysiol* 97:382–386.

Maccabee P J, Lipitz ME, Desudchit T, Golub RW, Nitti VW, Bania JP, Willer JA, Cracco RQ, Cadwell J, Hotson GC, Eberle LP, Amassian VE (1996). A new method using neuromagnetic stimulation to measure conduction time within the cauda equina. *Electroenceph Clin Neurophysiol* 101:153–166.

Macdonnell RAL, Donnan GA, Bladin PF (1989): A comparison of somatosensory evoked and motor evoked potentials in stroke. *Ann Neurol* 25:68–73.

Macdonell RAL, Cros D, Shahani BT (1992): Lumbosacral nerve root stimulation comparing electrical with surface magnetic coil techniques. *Muscle Nerve* 15:885–890.

Masur H, Papke K, Oberwittler C (1993): Suppression of visual perception by transcranial magnetic stimulation— experimental findings in healthy subjects and patients with optic neuritis. *Electroencephalogr Clin Neurophysiol* 86:259–267.

McCarthy G, Blamire AM, Rothman DL, Greutter R, Shulman RG (1993): Echo-planar magnetic resonance imaging studies of frontal cortex activation during word generation in humans. *Proc Natl Acad Sci* 90:4952–4956.

Menkes DL, Ring SR, Chiappa KH, Cros D (1994): Cortical magnetic stimulation to lower extremity muscles: Normal values and pathologic findings in 8 patients. *Neurology* 44 (suppl 2): A135 (Abstract).

Merton PA (1951): The silent period in a muscle of the human hand. *J Physiol (Lond)* 114:183–198.

Merton PA, Morton HB (1980): Stimulation of the cerebral cortex in the intact human subject. *Nature* 285:227.

Meyer B, Diehl R, Steinmetz H, Britton TC, Benecke R (1991): Magnetic stimuli applied over motor and visual cortex: influence of coil position and field polarity on motor responses, phosphenes, and eye movements. Magnetic motor stimulation: basic principles and clinical experience. *Electroencephalogr Clin Neurophysiol* 43 (Suppl).

Meyer BU, Werhahn K, Rothwell JC, Roericht S, Fauth C (1994): Functional organisation of corticonuclear pathways to motor neurones of lower facial muscles in man. *Exp Brain Res* 101:465–472.

Mills KR (1991): Magnetic brain stimulation: A tool to explore the action of the motor cortex on single human spinal motoneurones. *Trends Neurosci* 14:401–405.

Mills KR (1995): Motor neuron disease. Studies of the corticospinal excitation of single motor neurons by magnetic brain stimulation. *Brain* 118:971–982.

Mills KR, Murray NMF (1986): Electrical stimulation over the human vertebral column: Which neural elements are excited? *Electroencephalogr Clin Neurophysiol* 63:582–589.

Muller K, Homberg V, Lenard H-G (1991): Magnetic stimulation of motor cortex and nerve roots in children. Maturation of corticomotoneuronal projections. *Electroencephalogr Clin Neurophysiol* 81:63–70.

Nielsen JF (1996): Repetitive magnetic stimulation of cerebral cortex in normal subjects. *J Clin Neurophysiol* 13:69–76.

Nielsen JF, Klemar B, Hanson HJ, Sinkjaer T. (1995): A new treatment of spasticity with repetitive magnetic stimulation in multiple sclerosis. *J Neurol Neurosurg Psychiatry* 58:254–255.

Pascual-Leone A, Gates JR, Dhuna A (1991): Induction of speech arrest and counting errors with rapid-rate transcranial magnetic stimulation. *Neurology* 41:697–702.

Pascual-Leone A, Cohen LG, Shotland LI, Dang N, Pikus A, Wasserman EM, Brasil-Neto JP, Valls-Sole J, Hallett M (1992): No evidence of hearing loss in humans due to transcranial magnetic stimulation. *Neurology* 42: 647–651.

Pascual-Leone A, Houser CM, Reese K, et al (1993): Safety of rapid-rate transcranial magnetic stimulation in normal volunteers. *Electroencephalogr Clin Neurophysiol* 89:120–130.

Pascual-Leone A, Valls-Sole J, Brasil-Neto JP, et al (1994a): Akinesia in Parkinson's disease. II. Effects of subthreshold repetitive transcranial motor cortex stimulation. *Neurology* 44:892–898.

Pascual-Leone A, Valls-Sole J, Brasil-Neto JP, et al (1994b): Akinesia in Parkinson's disease. I. Shortening of simple reaction time with focal, single-pulse transcranial magnetic stimulation. *Neurology* 44:884–891.

Pascual-Leone A, Valls-Sole J, Wasserman EM, Hallett M (1994c): Responses to rapid-rate transcranial magnetic stimulation of the human motor cortex. *Brain* 117:847–858.

Priori A, Inghilleri M, Berardelli A (1992): Transcranial brain stimulation in basal ganglia disorders. In: *Clinical Applications of Transcranial Magnetic Stimulation*, edited by MA Lissens, pp 175–184. Peeters Press, Leuven.

Priori A, Berardelli A, Inghilleri M, et al (1994): Motor cortical inhibition and dopaminergic system. Pharmacological changes in the silent period after transcranial brain stimulation in normal subjects, patients with Parkinson's disease and drug-induced parkinsonism. *Brain* 117:317–323.

Prout AJ, Eisen AE (1994): The cortical silent period and amyotrophic lateral sclerosis. *Muscle Nerve* 17:217–223.

Rao SM, Binder JR, Hamoneke TA, Bandettini BS, Bobholz JA, Frost JA, Myklebust BM, Jacobson RD, Hyde JS (1995): Somatotopic mapping of the human primary motor cortex with functional magnetic resonance imaging. *Neurology* 45:919–924.

Rausch R, Silfvenius H, Wieser HG, Dodrill CB, Meador KJ, Jones-Gotman M (1993): Intraarterial amobarbital procedures. In: *Surgical Treatment of the Epilepsies*, edited by J Engel, Jr., pp 341–357. Raven Press, New York.

Ravnborg M, Liguori R, Christiansen P, Larsson H, Sorensen PS (1992): The diagnostic reliability of magnetically evoked motor potentials in multiple sclerosis. *Neurology* 42:1296–1301.

Reutens DC, Puce A, Berkovic SF (1993a): Cortical hyperexcitability in progressive myoclonus epilepsy: a study with transcranial magnetic stimulation. *Neurology* 43:186–192.

Reutens DC, Berkovic SF, Macdonell RAL, Bladin PF (1993b): Magnetic stimulation of the brain in generalized epilepsy: reversal of cortical hyperexcitability by anticonvulsants. *Ann Neurol* 34:351–355.

Ridding MC, Inzelberg R, Rothwell JC (1995): Changes in excitability of motor cortical circuitry in patients with Parkinson's disease. *Ann Neurol* 37:181–188.

Rimpilainen I (1994): Origin of the facial long latency responses elicited by magnetic stimulation. *Electroencephalogr Clin Neurophysiol* 93(2):121–30.

Rosler KM, Schmid UD, Moller AR (1994): Magnetic stimulation of the facial nerve: strong clinical and experimental evidence places the excitation site to the labyrinthine segment of the nerve (comments on technical report by Tokimura et al. published in Neurosurgery 32:114-116, 1993) [letter; comment]. *Neurosurgery* 35:1186–1188.

Rossini PM, DiStefano E, Stanzione P (1985a): Nerve impulse propagation along fast conducting central and peripheral motor and sensory pathways in man. *Electroencephalogr Clin Neurophysiol* 60:320–334.

Rossini PM, Marciani MG, Caramia MD, Roma V, Zarola F (1985b): Nervous propagation along "central" motor pathways in intact man: Characteristics of motor responses to "bifocal" and "unifocal" spine and scalp noninvasive stimulation. *Electroencephalogr Clin Neurophysiol* 61:272–286.

Rothwell JC, Thompson PD, Day BL, Dick JPR, Kachi T, Cowan JMA, Marsden CD (1987): Motor cortex stimulation in intact man: I. General characteristics of EMG responses in different muscles. *Brain* 110:1173–1190.

Sandroni P, Walker C, Starr A (1992): "Fatigue" in patients with multiple sclerosis. Motor pathway conduction and event-related potentials. *Arch Neurol* 49:517–524.

Santamaria J, King PJL, Cros D, Chiappa KH (1988): Cervical magnetic stimulation: Root or spinal nerve? *Neurology* 38 (suppl 1):199.

Schady W, Dick JPR, Sheard A, Crampton S (1991): Central motor conduction studies in hereditary spastic paraplegia. *J Neurol, Neurosurg Psychiatry* 54:775–779.

Schmid UD, Moller AR, Schmid J (1992a): The excitation site of the trigeminal nerve to transcranial magnetic stimulation varies and lies proximal or distal to the foramen ovale: an intraoperative electrophysiological study in man. *Neurosci Lett* 141:265–268.

Schmid UD, Moller AR, Schmid J (1992b): Transcranial magnetic stimulation of the facial nerve: intraoperative study on the effect of stimulus parameters on the excitation site in man. *Muscle Nerve* 15:829–836.

Schmid UD, Moller AR, Schmid J (1995): Transcranial magnetic stimulation of the trigeminal nerve: intraoperative study on stimulation characteristics in man. *Muscle Nerve* 18:487–494.

Schriefer TN, Mills KR, Murray NM, Hess CW (1988): Evaluation of proximal facial nerve conduction by transcranial magnetic stimulation. *J Neurol Neurosurg Psychiat* 51:60–66.

Schriefer TN, Hess CW, Mills KR, Murray NMF (1989): Central motor conduction studies in motor neurone diseases using magnetic brain stimulation. *Electroencephalogr Clin Neurophysiol* 74:431–437.

Schuler P, Claus D, Stefan H (1993): Hyperventilation and transcranial magnetic stimulation: two methods of activation of epileptiform EEG activity in comparison. *J Clin Neurophysiol* 10:111–115.

Seki Y, Krain L, Yamada T, Kimura J (1990): Transcranial magnetic stimulation of the facial nerve: recording technique and estimation of the stimulated site. *Neurosurgery* 26:286–290.

Shahani BT, Young RR (1993): Studies of the normal human silent period. In: *Human Reflexes. New Developments in Electromyography and Clinical Neurophysiology,* Vol 3, edited by J Desmedt, pp 589–602. Karger, Basel.

Siao P, Cros D, Shahani B (1990): Blink reflex elicited by magnetic stimulation. *Muscle Nerve* 13, 880 (Abstract).

Siao T-C P, Cros D, Chiappa K (1992): Cervical magnetic stimulation: site of stimulation. *Muscle Nerve* 15:1199 (Abstract).

Stern CE, Corkin S, Guimaraes AR, Sugiura RM, Carr CA, Baker JR, Jennings PJ, Gonzalez RG, Rosen BR (1994): A functional MRI study of long-term explicit memory in humans. *Soc Neurosci* 20(530.8):1290.

Stern CE, Corkin S, Carr CA, Sugiura RM, Guimaraes AR, Baker JR, Rosen BR, Gonzalez RG (1995): The neural substrate for working memory extends beyond prefrontal cortex. *Soc Neurosci* 21(117.5):275.

Stern CE, Corkin S, Gonzalez RG, Guimaraes AR, Carr CA, Sugiura RM, Baker JR, Vedantham V, Jennings PJ, Rosen BR (1996): The hippocampal formation participates in novel picture encoding: Evidence from functional MRI. In press.

Tassinari CA, Michelucci R, Forti A, Plasmati R, Troni W, Salvi F, Blanco M, Rubboli G (1990): Transcranial magnetic stimulation in epileptic patients: usefulness and safety. *Neurology* 40:1132–1133.

Tavy DLJ, Wagner GL, Keunen RWM, Wattendorff AR, Hekster REM, Franssen S (1994): Transcranial magnetic stimulation in patients with cervical spondylotic myelopathy: Clinical and radiological correlations. *Muscle Nerve* 17:235–241.

Triggs WJ, Edgar MA (1995): A 61-year-old man with increasing weakness and atrophy of all extemities. *N Engl J Med* 333:1406–1412.

Triggs WJ, Macdonell RAL, Cros D, Chiappa KH, Shahani B, Day BJ (1992): Motor excitation and inhibition are independent effect of magnetic cortical stimulation. *Ann Neurol* 32:345–351.

Triggs WJ, Cros D, Macdonell RAL, Chiappa KH, Day B, Fang J (1993): Cortical and spinal excitability during the cortical magnetic silent period in humans. *Brain Res* 628:39–48.

Triggs WJ, Calvanio R, Macdonell RAL, Cros D, Chiappa KH (1994): Physiological motor asymmetry in human handedness: evidence from transcranial magnetic stimulation. *Brain Res* 636:270–276.

Valls-Sole J, Pascual-Leone A, Brasil-Neto JP, et al (1994): Abnormal facilitation of the response to transcranial magnetic stimulation in patients with Parkinson's disease. *Neurology* 44:735–741.

Wasserman EM, Fuhr P, Cohen LG, Hallett M (1991): Effects of transcranial stimulation on ipsilateral muscles. *Neurology* 41:1795–1799.

Wasserman EM, Cohen LG, Flitman S, Chen R, Hallett M (1996): Seizures in healthy people with repeated "safe" trains of transcranial magnetic stimuli. *Lancet* 347:825–826.

Wilson SA, Lockwood RJ, Thickbroom GW, Mastaglia FL (1993): The muscle silent period following transcranial magnetic cortical stimulation. *J Neurol Sci* 114:216–222.

Evoked Potentials in Clinical Medicine,
3d ed., edited by Keith H. Chiappa.
Lippincott–Raven Publishers, Philadelphia © 1997.

14

Motor and Somatosensory Evoked Potentials in Spinal Cord Disorders

Lynette Kiers and °Keith H. Chiappa

Department of Neurology and Clinical Neurophysiology,
Royal Melbourne Hospital, Melbourne, Victoria, Australia 3050; and
°Department of Neurology, Harvard Medical School, and
EEG Laboratory, Massachusetts General Hospital, Boston, Massachusetts 02114

1. INTRODUCTION

Assessment of spinal cord diseases has largely been dominated by the clinical neurologic examination in combination with an imaging study. Spinal cord imaging modalities include myelography, computed tomography (CT) and magnetic resonance imaging (MRI), all of which provide *anatomic* information about the spinal cord and surrounding structures. In contrast, electrophysiologic tests such as motor and somatosensory evoked potentials provide *functional* information about the central motor and sensory pathways, and should therefore be considered complementary to the clinical examination and imaging study. The additional information provided by motor and sensory evoked potential testing depends on the etiology and pathophysiology of the spinal cord disease. The role of evoked potential testing in intraoperative monitoring of spinal cord surgery will be covered in a chapter specifically devoted to this topic (see Chapter 22).

2. MOTOR EVOKED POTENTIALS

The motor evoked potential (MEP), which is generated by stimulation of the motor cortex through the intact skull, provides the clinical neurophysiologist with a method to examine alterations in the function of central motor pathways in diseases affecting the motor system. This was initially achieved using an electrical stimulator (Merton and Morton, 1980), but for clinical purposes the more recently developed magnetic stimulator is preferable because the technique is essentially painless (Barker et al., 1985). Responses obtained by transcranial stimulation are produced primarily by activity in direct, fast-conducting corticospinal pathways (Rothwell et al., 1987; Hess et al., 1987a). Other descending pathways with monosynaptic and/or polysynaptic connections with the spinal cord, (e.g., reticulospinal tract), may be activated by the cortical stimulus and may contribute to the later phases of the compound motor action potential. Studies of single motor unit behavior (Day et al., 1987) have shown that a single cortical stimulus can produce multiple descending motor volleys in corticospinal tracts. Therefore, asynchronous activation of the population of spinal motoneurons results in complex, polyphasic electromyographic (EMG) waveforms.

By placing the magnetic or electrical stimulator over the spinal enlargements, it is also possible to activate the cervical or lumbar nerve roots. Excitation of the lower motor neurons probably occurs at or very near the emergence of their axons from the cord (Cros et al., 1990; Macdonell et al., 1992) although a number of studies have suggested that excitation occurs at the site where the nerve root exits the intervertebral foramen (Epstein et al., 1991; Maccabee et al., 1991).

It is possible to obtain estimates of central motor conduction times (CMCT) by subtracting the peripheral motor latency from spinal cord to muscle, from the latency of the MEP elicited by transcranial scalp stimulation. Peripheral motor latency can be calculated indirectly from F-wave latencies using the following formula (F + M-1)/2, where F = minimum F-latency; M = distal motor latency; and 1 msec is the estimate of F-wave turnaround time.

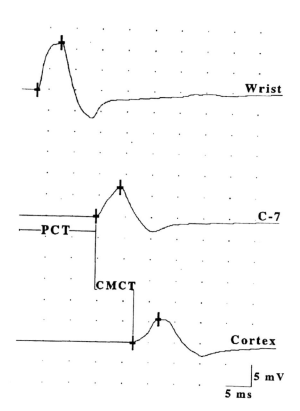

FIG. 14-1. Recordings from surface electrodes over the right abductor digiti minimi muscle in a normal subject following ulnar nerve electrical stimulation at the wrist, cervical magnetic stimulation (C7 spine level) and vertex magnetic stimulation (at rest; 100% stimulator output). PCT, peripheral conduction time, CMCT, central motor conduction time.

Alternate estimates can be obtained using cervical and/or lumbar stimulation (Fig. 14–1). Central motor conduction time reflects propagation of the impulses along fast-conducting pyramidal axons (Rothwell et al., 1987; Rossini et al., 1985; Rothwell et al., 1986). Increases in CMCT have been reported to occur in many neurologic conditions, including multiple sclerosis (Hess et al., 1986; Hess et al., 1987b; Cowan et al., 1984; Mills and Murray, 1985; Thompson et al., 1987a), motor neuron disease (Ingram and Swash, 1987; Berardelli et al., 1987; Hugon et al., 1987), cervical spondylosis (Thompson et al., 1987a; Maertens de Noordhout et al., 1991; Berardelli et al., 1988), and some types of spinocerebellar degenerations (Caramia et al., 1991; Mills et al., 1987).

Transcutaneous electrical stimulation has also been used to obtain measurement of the motor conduction velocity in the human spinal cord. Snooks and Swash (1985) stimulated the spinal cord and cauda equina at C6, L1, and L4 vertebral levels and recorded from puborectalis (S4 myotome) and tibialis anterior (L5 myotome). Latencies between C6 and L1, and between L1 and L4 represented conduction times from C6 to the conus medullaris, and rostral portion of the motor roots in the cauda equina, respectively. Measurement of the interelectrode distances allowed for calculation of motor conduction velocity, although it is recognized that the measured length of the spinal cord from C6 to T12 is some 13% less than the surface measurement of interspinous distances (Desmedt and Cheron, 1983).

2.1. Multiple Sclerosis

Multiple sclerosis (MS) may present as either an acute or a subacute myelopathy in young adults or as a chronic progressive spinal cord disease late in adult life. Multiple sclerosis has been studied extensively using both electrical and magnetic cortical and spinal stimulation.

In 1985, Mills and Murray (1985) reported marked prolongation of central conduction times in eight patients with clinically definite MS, all of whom had severe pyramidal weakness and leg spasticity. No correlation was found between the degree of central motor slowing and the degree of pyramidal motor involvement as judged on clinical grounds. Thompson et al. (1987a) studied eight patients with clinically definite MS, and noted, in addition to marked prolongation of CMCT, an increase in variability in the latency of responses from trial to trial. Caramia et al. (1988) studied 49 patients with MS and found abnormal MEPs in 51 of 94 tested arms (54%). Alterations of median nerve somatosensory evoked potentials (SEPs) were found in 36 arms (38%). In clinically unaffected arms, MEPs were abnormal in 40%, and SEPs in 27%. In a further study of 34 patients with MS (Caramia et al., 1991), CMCT prolongation, increased thresholds or absent responses, and low-amplitude, dispersed, polyphasic MEPs were found. Hess et al. (1986, 1987b) studied 83 patients with definite, probable, and possible MS and found that either the CMCTs to upper-limb muscles were prolonged or the amplitude of the response with cortical stimulation was reduced in 60 of 83 patients (72%). Central motor conduction abnormalities were seen in 7 of 39 limbs with no physical signs. In 7 of 49 sides with low-amplitude responses, CMCT was normal. In the same group of patients, pattern-shift visual evoked potentials (VEPs), median SEPs, and brain stem auditory evoked potentials (BAEPs) were abnormal in 54 of 81 cases (67%), 36 of 61 cases (59%), and 24 of 61 cases (39%), respectively. For each EP modality, some patients had abnormal central motor conduction and a normal sensory EP result. Magnetic resonance imaging findings were abnormal in 83% of patients tested. In one of the two cases in which MRI was normal, central motor conduction was abnormal.

Both Hess et al. (1987b) and Ingram et al. (1988) reported an association between prolonged CMCT and clinical findings of hyperreflexia and brisk finger flexion jerks; the latter group also found a correlation with functional motor disability in 20 patients. Increased CMCT to tibialis anterior was associated with extensor plantar responses in 16 of 17 feet.

Ravnborg et al. (1992), in a prospective study of 68 consecutive patients, evaluated the diagnostic reliability of magnetic MEPs in MS. Patients were included if they had symptoms and signs compatible with one or more demyelinating central nervous system (CNS) lesions and all were subjected to cerebrospinal fluid (CSF) analysis, MRI, VEP, BAEP, and SEP. The results were then used to categorize the patients according to the Poser criteria of MS (1983). Motor EPs were then recorded from three upper-extremity and two lower-extremity muscles in all patients. The MEP was defined as positive if the CMCT or the amplitude was abnormal in one or more muscles. Forty patients received a diagnosis of definite or probable MS. In these patients, MRI was positive in 88%, MEP in 83%, VEP in 67%, SEP in 63%, and BAEP in 42%. As to the diagnosis of MS, the reliability of a prolonged CMCT was 0.83 (0.73 to 0.93), while the reliability of a normal CMCT was 0.75 (0.61 to 0.98). Of the neurophysiologic tests, the MEP was in closest agreement with the MRI (concordance of 85%) and was considered the test of first choice in the absence of MRI.

Snooks and Swash (1985) studied motor conduction velocities in the spinal cord of 5 patients with MS, all with corticospinal signs in the legs. Transcutaneous electrical stimulation of the spinal cord and cauda equina at C6, L1, and L4 vertebral levels was performed, recording from puborectalis or tibialis anterior muscles. In four of five patients, motor conduction velocities between C6 and L1 were slowed, but cauda equina conduction was normal.

In summary, abnormalities of central motor conduction in patients with MS are characterized by markedly prolonged CMCT, slowing of spinal cord motor conduction velocity, and low-amplitude, dispersed responses to scalp stimulation. Occasionally, low-amplitude responses and increased latency variability are the only abnormalities that are seen. These abnormalities are compatible with the physiologic effects of demyelination in the CNS, namely slowing of conduction, conduction block, and temporal dispersion of descending volleys. Generally, the MEP abnormalities are well correlated with clinical deficits.

2.2. Cervical Myelopathy

Cervical spondylitic myelopathy is the most frequently observed myelopathy during and after middle age (Wilkinson, 1960). Since cervical spondylosis is very common after 50, radiologic studies may lead to overdiagnosis of the disease. Magnetic resonance imaging of the cord may show abnormalities at the level of cord compression, but gives no information on the function of the cervical cord.

Central motor conduction times are often prolonged in patients with cervical spondylosis and myelopathy, provided the recording is being done from muscles innervated by spinal motor neurons below the level of the lesion. Thompson et al. (1987a), using percutaneous electrical cortical stimulation, studied five patients with cervical spondylosis and myelographically proven cord compression at the level of C3–4 in one and C5–6 in four. Prolonged latencies to thenar muscles were found in four patients and absent responses in one. When recording was done from biceps, CMCT was prolonged in only the patient with C3–4 compression. Electromyographic responses were small and of increased duration. In all patients, peripheral conduction times were normal, implying involvement of central motor pathways. In a previous study (Thompson et al., 1987b), three patients with cervical myelopathy who had prolonged MEP latencies to thenar muscles, all had normal median SEPs; two had normal tibial SEPs.

Berardelli et al. (1988) studied seven patients with cervical spondylosis and myelographic signs of cervical cord compression. Electrical stimulation of the motor cortex was performed, recording from biceps, thenar muscles, and tibialis anterior with surface electrodes. Cortical MEPs from the upper limbs were always delayed in at least one muscle. Cortical MEPs from the tibialis anterior muscle were absent in three patients and delayed in four.

In contrast to previous studies, in which prolongation of CMCT was noted in patients with *severe* cervical spondylosis and definite spinal cord compression, Maertens de Noordhout et al. (1991) assessed the usefulness of magnetic cortical stimulation in detecting *early* dysfunction of central motor pathways. Sixty-seven patients were studied, 44 with radiologic evidence of cord compression and 23 with root compression. Thirty-four patients (51%) had upper motor neuron signs. Motor EPs to cortical stimulation were abnormal in 37 patients (84%) with radiologic signs of cord compression and in 5 (22%) of those without. Median nerve SEPs were altered in only 25% of patients. The frequency of MEP alterations correlated with upper motor neuron signs. In 5 of 44 patients (11%) with radiologic evidence of cord compression, subclinical cord compression was disclosed by cortical stimulation. The authors suggest that in some patients lesions can be detected at a preclinical stage with a sensitivity that exceeds that of SEPs. By recording responses from selected muscles, it may be possible to determine the segmental level of the cord compression.

Di Lazzaro et al. (1992) used magnetic stimulation of the motor cortex and cervical spine to study 24 patients with cervical spondylitic myelopathy documented by MRI. Compound muscle action potentials were recorded from the biceps and the thenar muscles to study central motor pathways of two different myotomes, C5–6 and C8–T1. Central motor conduction was abnormal in all 24 patients for thenar muscles and in 5 patients for biceps brachii. A significant correlation was found between CMCT abnormalities for thenar muscles and clinical signs of long motor tract involvement ($p = 0.013$, chi-square test). All patients with upper cervical cord compression (C2–4) showed an abnormal CMCT for both biceps and thenar muscles. Patients with lower cervical compression (C4–6) had abnormal thenar CMCT but normal biceps CMCT. Patients with multilevel compression of the cervical cord had abnormal CMCT for thenar muscles but normal CMCT for biceps muscles. However, the mean value of biceps CMCT was significantly greater than that in control subjects, suggesting a slight involvement of central motor pathways for proximal upper-limb muscles. The direct correlation between radiologic and electrophysiologic findings in patients with single compression levels suggests that in these cases, mechanical cord compression is the most important factor in the pathogenesis of myelopathy.

In summary, in patients with cervical myelopathy, the CMCT is usually prolonged when recording is performed from muscles innervated by spinal neurons below the level of the lesion. Low-amplitude, prolonged-duration EMG responses are often found in upper-extremity muscles and responses in lower-extremity muscles are absent or delayed. Motor EP abnormalities can identify lesions at a preclinical stage in some cases and confirm the clinical significance of radiologic abnormalities.

2.3. Motor Neuron Disease

In motor neuron disease (MND), corticospinal and corticobulbar tract degeneration is combined with varying degrees of lower motor neuron degeneration. Lower motor neuron function can be assessed using conventional EMG, but a direct neurophysiologic test has not been previously available to evaluate impairment of the corticospinal tract. Using either percutaneous electrical or magnetic cortical and spinal stimulation, a number of abnormalities have been identified. These include (1) increased thresholds or absence of response to scalp stimulation, (2) mild prolongation of CMCTs, primarily involving spinal conduction times, and (3) low-amplitude poorly defined EMG responses.

Berardelli et al. (1987) studied 20 patients with amyotrophic lateral sclerosis (ALS). In four patients, stimulation of one or both hemispheres failed to elicit cortical MEPs in both biceps and thenar muscles. In two patients, cortical MEPs were absent in the thenar muscles and delayed in the biceps muscle, and in eight patients they were delayed in at least one muscle. In 11 of 15 patients with abnormal cortical MEPs, the cervical MEPs were also delayed, which is attributed to the loss of anterior horn cells and large myelinated fibers. However, in these patients an abnormality of central motor conduction was also present because the slowing of conduction was out of proportion to the peripheral slowing. The cortical MEPs were absent in the patients with the most severe pyramidal signs, but the same patients also showed a greater degree of amyotrophy.

Ingram and Swash (1987) studied 12 patients with MND, 6 of whom had definite clinical signs of corticospinal tract involvement. In addition to electrical cortical stimulation, spinal cord motor conduction velocity was also calculated. Prominent and often asymmetrical slowing of central motor conduction was demonstrated in 7 of 12 patients with recording performed from lower-limb muscles; these findings were most marked in the spinal cord and correlated with clinical features of corticospinal involvement. Of eight patients studied with scalp stimulation with recording performed from upper-limb muscles, three had absent responses to at least one of the muscles. Evidence of subclinical involvement of central motor pathways was found in five patients. In general, it was more difficult to excite motor pathways (cortical and cervical) in the patients with MND than in control subjects.

Hugon et al. (1987) studied 13 patients with different forms of MND and found abnormal CMCTs for upper extremities in 10 patients and slowed CMCTs for lower extremities in all, even those without clinical pyramidal signs. In patients with pyramidal tract involvement, the prolongation of CMCT was generally proportional to the severity of the neurologic impairment.

Caramia et al. (1988) studied nine patients with ALS. Twelve of 18 tested arms showed an altered MEP; it was totally absent in eight arms with moderate prolongation of CMCT in the remaining four. In a further study (Caramia et al., 1991) of seven patients with ALS, CMCT was prolonged in 6 of 14 upper limbs and in 12 of 14 lower limbs. Three of four patients with primary lateral sclerosis had increased thresholds and prolonged CMCT both for upper- and lower-limb MEPs. Thompson et al. (1987a) reported small, poorly defined EMG responses following electrical cortical stimulation in four patients with MND. Estimates of central conduction times were normal or at the upper limit of the normal range. Absence of EMG responses to cortical stimulation in a particular muscle was found in three patients, despite the ability of the patient to voluntarily activate the muscle. Barker et al. (1986, 1987) found normal mean magnetic CMCT in five patients with MND. Triggs et al. (1992) studied eight patients with MND, six with clinical features of ALS and two with a syndrome suggesting primary lateral sclerosis. Elevated thresholds for magnetic cortical stimulation were found in three patients and absence of MEPs was seen in five. In six patients, silent periods could be obtained in muscles without preceding MEPs, suggesting different susceptibilities of excitatory and inhibitory pathways to pathophysiologic processes in MND.

In summary, the relative inexcitability of the central motor pathways in MND probably reflects a reduction in the size and number of excitatory postsynaptic potentials generated by the cortical stimulus as a result of motor cell loss. This finding correlates with clinical evidence of upper motor neuron involvement, but may also indicate subclinical involvement of corticospinal pathways in patients apparently presenting with "pure" lower motor neuron syndromes. The prolongation of CMCT reflects loss of large diameter fast conducting pyramidal neurons.

2.4. Traumatic Spinal Cord Lesions

In spinal cord injury, the lesions responsible for the major clinical deficit (i.e., paralysis) are inaccessible to conventional electrophysiologic tests. The spinal cord lesion at the level of the injury may be diffuse, involving all major ascending and descending tracts and neuronal systems, or it may be partial, involving only a portion of the cord. Numerous animal studies have been performed to evaluate the reproducibility and possible prognostic utility of MEPs in spinal cord injury (Levy et al., 1987; Fehlings et al., 1987; Simpson and Baskin, 1987).

Levy et al. (1987) studied the MEP elicited by transcranial electrical stimulation in a series of 30 cats subjected to a standard injury to the thoracic cord (T6) by the Allen weight drop test. The MEPs were recorded above (T3) and below (T11) the injury and from the sciatic nerves. The peripheral nerve response was the most sensitive to injury, disappearing immediately upon weight drop. The MEP spinal cord signal below the lesion showed both a latency increase and amplitude decrease after impact. In all 17 animals in whom ambulation was regained, the peripheral nerve signals returned either at or immediately before the time of ambulation. The MEP spinal cord signal below the lesion as a percentage above the lesion was a significant correlate of current ambulation recovery (r = 0.55). It was concluded that evaluation of the MEP spinal cord signals may have prognostic value in animals and perhaps in humans.

Fehlings et al. (1987) studied MEPs from normal and spinal cord-injured rats (lesion at C8) using direct cortical stimulation and recording from microelectrodes in the cord. Four rats had complete cord transection and six had clip compression injuries of varying degrees. Cord transection and severe compression injury abolished the MEP distal to the lesion, whereas the less severe compression injuries resulted in a latency shift and amplitude decrement of the MEP peaks.

Simpson and Baskin (1987) studied SEPs and MEPs following blunt spinal cord injury in the rat. Animals subjected to a 50-g/cm impact on the spinal cord showed no change in SEP waveform but all components of the MEP were greatly attenuated and accompanied by very weak or no movement to noxious stimuli. A spectrum of clinical recovery was correlated closely with the return and normalization of the amplitude of the MEP. The eventual degree of clinical and MEP improvement correlated well with the degree of histologic damage that was present.

A number of clinical studies have also been undertaken in patients with acute and chronic spinal cord injury. Gianutsos et al. (1987) studied five quadriplegic patients at 6 to 12 months following traumatic spinal cord injury (levels C3–4 to C6–7) using percutaneous electrical stimulation of the motor cortex and recording from biceps brachii and abductor pollicis brevis. In all five patients, latencies to the muscle for which innervation originated above the lesion (biceps brachii) were in the normal range, whereas latencies to the muscle for which innervation originated below the lesion (abductor pollicis brevis) were prolonged. Of particular interest was the finding in three patients that EMG responses could be obtained in muscles that showed no voluntary motor activity below the spinal cord lesion. This indicates the presence of functioning fibers that traverse the injured portion of the spinal cord, which is consistent with postmortem studies in which continuity of the white matter of the spinal cord was noted in patients who had been completely paralyzed during life, according to clinical criteria (Kakulas and Bedbrook, 1969, 1976). The prolonged latencies of the MEPs suggest transmission through slowly conducting fibers.

Thompson et al. (1987b) compared electrical stimulation of the motor cortex with cortical SEPs in three patients with cervical cord trauma. Absent, low-amplitude, or prolonged latency responses were recorded from both upper- and lower-limb muscles with segmental innervation below the level of the lesion. Furthermore, two patients had abnormal MEPs with normal cortical SEPs, demonstrating abnormal conduction in the descending motor pathways without detectable involvement of the ascending sensory pathways.

Cohen et al. (1991) studied the induction of leg paraesthesias by magnetic stimulation of the brain in seven patients with thoracic (T9–12) spinal cord injury and in four normal subjects. In three patients, all with complete lesions at T9, stimulation evoked sensations that lasted up to 10 seconds which were referred to different parts of the legs and toes. The closer the site of stimulation was to the midline the more distal the sensations were felt by the patients. It was concluded that portions of the cortical representation areas for body parts that undergo deafferentation as a result of complete spinal cord injury can remain related to those body parts for up to several years. These patients showed the lowest degree of motor reorganization in muscles proximal to the lesion.

Macdonell and Donnan (1995) studied 25 patients (16 quadriplegic, 8 paraplegic, and 1 with suspected cervical cord injury) within 6 hours of acute spinal cord injury to determine whether MEPs could be used to predict motor recovery. Motor EPs were recorded from abductor digiti minimi, biceps, flexor hallucis brevis, and tibialis anterior muscles on each side. In no patient were MEPs obtained either at rest or during contraction in any muscle, without preceding clinical or EMG evidence of voluntary activation. This was found to be the case even for muscles in which motor recovery occurred after initial paralysis. The authors concluded that magnetically evoked MEPs do not add to the clinical and EMG evaluation of the completeness of the motor injury.

Although CNS neurons are not capable of replicating, reorganization of synaptic connections has been demonstrated in animal models following peripheral nerve lesions (Wall and Cusick, 1984), amputation (Pons et al., 1991), spinal cord transections (McKinley et al., 1987) and reversible limb deafferentation (Metzler and Marks, 1979) by local anesthesia. Reorganization of the motor system in the human patient after injury has been reported by several groups. Levy et al. (1990) used a figure-of-eight magnetic coil for focal stimulation of the motor cortex of two adult paraplegics with traumatic spinal injury and three normal adults. The patients had been injured approximately 2 years previously and biceps and deltoid were the most caudally located muscles that were spared. Motor EPs were elicited from these muscles from a much wider area of scalp than in the normal subjects. Topka et al. (1991) studied magnetic MEPs in six patients with complete spinal cord injuries at low thoracic levels (2 to 20 years after injury) and eight healthy subjects. Stimuli were delivered using either a circular or figure-of-eight coil and EMG was recorded bilaterally from abdominal wall muscles at three levels using surface electrodes. Amplitudes were expressed as a percentage of the largest M-response obtained by direct (electrical or magnetic) stimulation of the ventral roots over the spine (T5–12). Magnetic stimulation at rest activated a larger fraction of the motor neuron pool and evoked MEPs with shorter latencies from a larger number of scalp positions in muscles immediately rostral to the level of the spinal cord injury than in corresponding muscles in control subjects. The MEPs associated with activation were not significantly different in the two groups. These results suggested enhanced excitability of motor pathways targeting muscles rostral to the level of spinal transection, which reflects reorganization of motor pathways either within cortical motor representation areas or at the level of the spinal cord. Possible mechanisms for such reorganization include increased efficacy of pre-existing synapses, collateral sprouting of axons, and disinhibition of longer-latency pathways secondary to reduced afferent input. Using regional anesthetic block to induce transient deafferentation of the forearm, Brasil-Neto et al. (1992) found a gradual increase in biceps MEP amplitude (the muscle immediately proximal to the block) during anesthesia and a return to preanesthetic levels within 20 minutes after anesthesia was ended. The speed of the changes described in this report, strongly suggested an unmasking of previously existing but physiologically "inactive" connections as the likely mechanism underlying motor modulation.

In summary, although studies of MEPs in animals with traumatic spinal cord injury suggested possible prognostic value, this has not been borne out in human studies of acute spinal cord injury. Furthermore, the demonstration that clinically complete lesions may not be electrophysiologically complete adds minimal prognostic data, as these remaining functioning fibers do not appear to be of clinical significance. The demonstration of motor cortical system reorganization after traumatic spinal cord injury in humans may be useful in directing the emphasis of rehabilitation programs.

2.5. Syringomyelia

Nogués et al. (1992) studied MEPs to transcranial and spinal stimulation from upper- and lower-limb muscles in 13 patients with syringomyelia. Prolonged central motor conduction times or absent motor responses in upper- or lower-limb muscles were found in 10 patients. Two of five patients undergoing surgery improved clinically and showed reduction in CMCT after surgical treatment. Caramia et al. (1988) reported prolonged CMCT with normalization after surgery in a single patient with a syringomyelic cyst that extended the entire length of the cervical spinal cord.

2.6. Miscellaneous Spinal Cord Diseases

2.6.1. Radiation Myelopathy

Snooks and Swash (1985) and Mills et al. (1987) each found central motor conduction delays in one case of radiation myelopathy.

2.6.2. Spinocerebellar Degeneration

Caramia et al. (1991) found increased threshold of thenar MEPs or absent foot responses in three patients with spinocerebellar degeneration. Mills et al. (1987) found a normal CMCT in one patient.

2.6.3. Hereditary Spastic Paraplegia

Thompson et al. (1987a) found only mildly delayed scalp to leg latencies with normal amplitude responses on one side of each of two patients with hereditary spastic paraparesis despite the presence of severe spasticity. Berardelli et al. (1988) and Mills et al. (1987) found increased latencies to upper-extremity muscles in single cases of hereditary spastic paraplegia.

Caramia et al. (1988) found prolonged CMCTs in seven patients with a variety of spinal cord lesions (foramen magnum meningioma, disk protrusions, intramedullary tumor (Fig. 14–2), anterior spinal artery infarction, syringomyelia) and in one patient with subacute combined degeneration of the spinal cord.

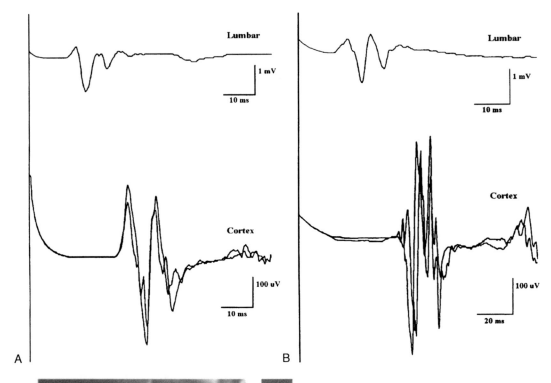

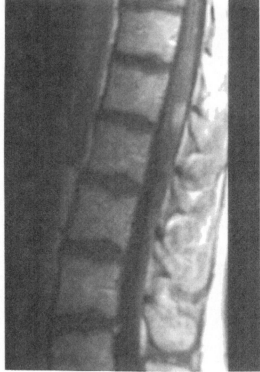

FIG. 14–2. Motor EPs and MRI in a 25-year-old woman with a 1-month history of right-leg weakness and perineal numbness. Examination revealed increased tone, hyperreflexia and pyramidal weakness in the right leg. **A.** Motor EPs from left tibialis anterior (TA) following lumbar and cortical (two replicated superimpositions) stimulation. CMCT = 16 msec. **B.** Motor EPs from right TA following lumbar and cortical stimulation. CMCT = 43 msec. Note the marked prolongation of CMCT to the clinically affected leg. **C.** The T_2-weighted MRI scan shows mild swelling of the conus and a region of increased signal extending from the T11–L1 level. Excisional biopsy revealed a histiocytoma.

3. SOMATOSENSORY EVOKED POTENTIALS

Short-latency SEPs can be recorded after electrical stimulation of peripheral sensory nerves. The close relationship between SEP waveforms and the anatomy of sensory tracts allows precise localization of conduction defects. The stimulus intensity employed excites only the largest-diameter myelinated fibers in the peripheral nerve (cutaneous and subcutaneous somaesthetic and proprioceptive fibers, and motor axons of equivalent diameter). Somatosensory EPs can reasonably be considered to be generated from volleys traversing the large-fiber sensory system (posterior columns and medial lemnisci) and possibly the spinocerebellar tracts (Chiappa, 1992). Based on results from microneurography experiments, Burke and Gandevia (1986) have suggested that the dominant afferent input for lower-limb mixed nerve SEPs are group I muscle afferents.

3.1. Multiple Sclerosis

Multiple sclerosis is a disease of the CNS characterized by multifocal areas of demyelination with relative preservation of axons and nerve cell bodies. Patients frequently present with cervical or thoracic cord syndromes. In the presence of a demyelinating process affecting sensory nerve fibers, defects in axonal conduction can be detected as delay, reduction, or absence of the SEPs. Somatosensory EPs are particularly useful for detecting subclinical spinal cord plaques in patients with suspected MS.

Small et al. (1978) studied median SEPs recorded over the cervical spine (C2, C7) in 126 patients with MS. Abnormalities of cervical N14 were found in 59% of patients, increasing to 69% of those in the definite diagnostic category. Reduction of amplitude or absence of the response was much more common than was latency prolongation. Abnormal cervical SEPs were often found in the absence of relevant clinical signs, suggesting the presence of clinically silent cervical spinal cord plaques.

Turano et al. (1991) studied 31 patients with definite or suspected MS who presented with a cervical cord syndrome. Somatosensory EPs were recorded following median and posterior tibial nerve stimulation using cephalic and noncephalic reference electrodes. Somatosensory EPs were abnormal in 67.7% of patients, whereas MRI showed cervical cord lesions in 74.2% and intracranial lesions possibly involving the somatosensory pathways in 64.5% of patients. A significant correlation was found between abnormalities of cervical (N13) and cortical (N20) potentials following median nerve stimulation and MRI abnormalities involving the ipsilateral or posterior half of the cervical cord. The N13 potential, recorded from the low cervical region, using a supraglottal reference, was most frequently abnormal in patients with MRI lesions at C6 or C7, whereas P14, recorded between the scalp and a clavicle reference, was most often affected by lesions at C1 or the cervicomedullary junction. The N9–20 interpeak latency (IPL) and the absolute P40 latency to tibial nerve stimulation were significantly correlated with the length of abnormalities in the ipsilateral cervical cord seen on MRI. No significant correlation was observed between SEP abnormalities and brain MRI lesions which were located in areas in proximity to intracranial somatosensory pathways.

In patients with MS, a peculiar SEP abnormality has been reported, consisting of absence of P/N13 with preservation of N19–P22 and a normal brachial plexus to N19 IPL (Chiappa 1992). The pathophysiology of this finding and its relation to SEP generators remain unclear.

Ropper et al. (1982) studied SEP abnormalities in 12 consecutive patients with inflammatory acute transverse myelopathy (ATM) that was not associated with other features of MS. All nine patients tested with median SEPs had normal findings, the lesions being below cervical levels mediating that response. Five of six patients tested with peroneal SEPs had abnormal findings.

In summary, upper- and lower-extremity SEPs are useful for detection of clinically silent cervical spinal cord plaques with potentials from the lower limb showing a higher abnormality rate, presumably as a result of the greater length of involved white matter. When lower-limb testing is normal, upper-limb SEPs may still be abnormal. The most frequent abnormalities are reduction or absence of the cervical N13 potential or prolongation of the Erb's point (EP)–P/N13 IPL following median nerve stimulation (Fig. 14–3), and prolongation of the N20–N/P37 IPL following tibial nerve stimulation.

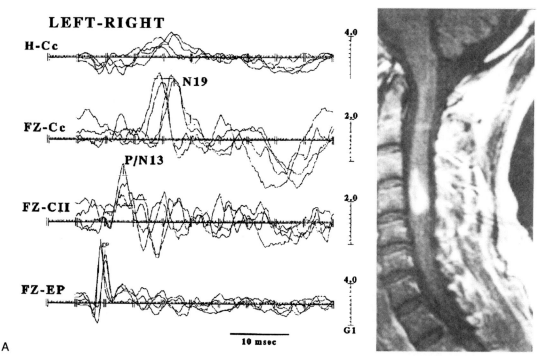

A   B

FIG. 14–3. Median nerve SEPs and MRI in a 45-year-old man with a 1-month history of progressive, bilateral hand and foot numbness and paresthesias with associated clumsiness of the hands A. Superimposed median nerve SEPs from both sides of the patient. The SEP following right median nerve stimulation shows a long-duration, low-amplitude, asynchronous P/N13, with prolongation of the EP–P/N13 IPL. The left median SEP is normal, as are both tibial SEPs (not shown). The findings suggest an abnormality of the large-fiber sensory pathways between the mid-brachial plexus and lower medulla. Cc refers to the central scalp area overlying the primary sensory cortex in the parietal lobe contralateral to the limb stimulated, H refers to hand, CII refers to the second spinous process, EP refers to Erb's point. Calibration in microvolts. Each trace is the average of 512 stimuli with two replicated superimpositions. B. The T_2-weighted MRI scan shows a bright lesion with gadolinium enhancement at the level of C4. A cranial T2-weighted MRI (*not shown*) revealed multiple bright lesions in the periventricular white matter bilaterally, consistent with demyelination. (From Kiers and Chiappa, 1995, with permission.)

3.2. Cervical Myelopathy

Few patients with cervical spondylosis have associated myelopathy and relatively little correlation exists between the severity of radiologic spondylosis and the presence or severity of myelopathy. Somatosensory EPs may, therefore, have an application in the detection of posterior column involvement.

In 1985, Yu and Jones (1985), using median, ulnar, and tibial nerve stimulation, studied 34 patients with cervical spondylosis, 15 with myelopathy, 6 with combined radiculopathy and myelopathy, 6 with radiculopathy, and 7 with nonspecific neck pain. Somatosensory EP abnormalities, particularly with lower-limb stimulation, were strongly correlated with myelopathy but not with radiculopathy. In myelopathy cases, SEPs were more sensitive to sensory pathway involvement than was clinical sensory testing. Significantly, 6 of 21 patients with clinical myelopathy had abnormal tibial SEPs but no radiologic evidence of cord compression, suggesting that ischemia may be a significant factor in the development of myelopathy. Abnormalities of at least one SEP were detected in two of six patients (33%) with radiculopathy alone; in one the abnormal SEP was consistent with subclinical posterior column involvement.

Veilleux and Daube (1987) have confirmed the high sensitivity of tibial SEPs compared with median SEPs in 37 patients with cervical myelopathy. However, they suggested that ulnar SEPs were the most sensitive, perhaps related to the fact that tibial N20–P37 IPLs were calculated in only 24 patients and 30 patients had bilateral tibial nerve stimulation which would prevent detection of interside differences. Restuccia et al. (1992a) studied 17 patients with cervical spondylitic myelopathy and found abnormal median, ulnar, and common peroneal nerve SEPs in 41%, 71%, and 100% of cases, respectively. They reported latency delay or absence of the cervical N13 or scalp far-field P14 response following upper-limb stimulation, and absence or latency delay of the P27 response following common peroneal nerve stimulation. Abnormalities of the scalp far-field P14 response evoked by upper-limb stimulation correlated with joint and touch sensation impairment, but not with radiologic findings; this may therefore be a reliable marker of dorsal column impairment.

Yiannikas et al. (1986) studied 68 patients with cervical radiculopathy and /or myelopathy. In 22 patients with clinical and radiologic features of spinal cord compression, 15 (68%) had abnormal median SEPs and 21 (95%) had abnormal tibial or peroneal studies. The abnormalities noted were a low-amplitude or absent P/N13 and N19, a prolonged EP–P/N13 conduction time, an increase in central conduction time, and low-amplitude scalp responses from the lower limb.

Restuccia et al. (1992b) have advocated use of a noncephalic reference montage (C6 to anterior cervical vertebrae) to permit selective analysis of the N13 potential which reflects the response of dorsal horn neurons to receipt of inputs from large myelinated fibers. This has been shown to uncover abnormal cervical SEPs in patients with focal cervical cord lesions and preserved dorsal column function. The researchers studied 11 patients with MRI evidence of cervical spondylosis, all of whom had clinical evidence of bilateral pyramidal tract involvement but no posterior column involvement. Normal scalp SEPs (P14, N20) were found in all patients, reflecting normal activity of the dorsal column system up to the parietal cortex, whereas segmental cervical cord dysfunction was manifested by an abnormal spinal N13 potential in 95% of radial, 90% of median, and 54% of ulnar SEPs. The abnormality consisted exclusively of an absent or reduced N13 spinal response.

In summary, in patients with cervical spondylosis, SEP abnormalities, particularly those detected after tibial nerve stimulation, are a highly sensitive indicator of myelopathy. Use of a noncephalic reference montage permits selective analysis of the N13 potential and increases diagnostic sensitivity in patients with clinically preserved dorsal column function.

3.3. Motor System Disorders

The motor system disorders (MSD) are a group of degenerative diseases with variable expression of involvement of motor neurons and their axons in cortex, brain stem, and spinal cord. Clinically they are characterized by progressive motor deficits involving the upper and lower motor neuron in the absence of sensory or autonomic involvement. A number of reports of both clinical and pathologic involvement of the sensory system have been made. Previous studies of SEPs in MSD have shown conflicting results (Cascino et al., 1988; Oh et al., 1985; Matheson et al., 1986; Subramanium and Yiannikas, 1990).

Cascino et al. (1988) found normal median SEPs in 29 of 30 patients with MSD. Care was taken to exclude patients with cervical spondylosis or other compressive lesions. Four patients were excluded on the basis of spinal cord compression on myelography and 16 further patients had normal myelograms. No statistical group tendency toward abnormalities in the EP–P/N13, P/N13–N19, and EP–N19 IPLs was manifested in patients when compared with controls. Only 1 of 18 patients had definite central conduction abnormalities following tibial stimulation. In addition, four patients had peripheral abnormalities and four had abnormalities that did not allow differentiation of central from peripheral defects. Oh et al. (1985) also reported normal median nerve cervical and cortical SEPs in 21 of 22 patients with ALS. In contrast, Matheson et al. (1986) reported abnormal median SEPs in 11 of 32 patients. However, in 8 of 11, the abnormality was only in absolute N13 latency (N19 was normal, Erb's point was not measured) and, therefore, may have been caused by peripheral lesions. Twenty of 32 patients were found to have abnormal lower-extremity SEPs, of which 13 were attributed to defects in central conduction based on normal H-reflexes (LP was not measured). The H-reflexes were performed with knee stimulation and, therefore, 30 to 40 cm of peripheral sensory nerve was not being evaluated. Other studies have not adequately distinguished central and peripheral abnormalities or excluded coexisting cervical compression or inadequate tibial nerve stimulation as the cause of apparently delayed scalp potentials.

Subramanium and Yiannikas (1990) studied 27 patients with MND. Abnormal median SEPs were found in 8 of 27 patients, all of whom had normal myelograms. The abnormalities consisted of delayed N9 potentials (one patient), prolonged N9–P/N13 (two patients) and P/N13–N19 (five patients) conduction times, as well as dispersion of the thalamocortical potential (one patient). Comparison of a group of eight patients with MND and normal myelograms with an age-matched control group showed no difference in peripheral conduction (normal N9 latency) but prolongation of N9–P/N13 and P/N13–N19 conduction was present in the group with MND. Three of 21 patients had abnormal tibial SEPs and normal myelograms. One patient had unilaterally absent N20, one had bilaterally absent N20 and delayed cortical responses, and one had bilaterally dispersed cortical potentials in the presence normal spinal potentials. Thus the conduction deficit may have been peripheral in two patients.

Caramia et al. (1988) reported abnormal median SEPs (absent cortical N20–P25 complex) in 3 of 18 tested arms of 12 patients with ALS.

In summary, the frequency of SEP abnormalities in isolated MSD remains a point of contention. However, significant SEP central conduction abnormalities are likely to be due to concurrent disease and should prompt consideration of diagnoses other than MND.

3.4. Traumatic Spinal Cord Injury

An accurate prognosis for recovery in patients with spinal cord injury is useful in planning acute management and rehabilitation. Improved imaging techniques demonstrate spinal cord compression and intrinsic spinal cord lesions, but often fail to correlate with either neurologic deficit or prognosis for recovery. Somatosensory EPs enable assessment of spinal conduction through some of the tracts traversing the level of the lesion.

A number of studies have used SEPs in spinal cord trauma (Perot and Vera, 1982; Sedgwick et al., 1980; Dorfman et al., 1980; Young, 1982; Cracco, 1973; Spielholz et al., 1979). In 377 patients who underwent median and posterior tibial SEP study a good correlation was found between the severity of the spinal cord injury and the SEP. Tibial SEPs were absent in the acute phase in patients with complete functional spinal cord transection. Median and ulnar SEPs were present or absent depending on the segmental level of the spinal cord lesion.

In patients with incomplete lesions, the presence of tibial SEPs correlated with the integrity of the posterior columns as judged by clinical examination. In some patients with apparently complete lesions, SEPs were present, suggesting some residual spinal cord function. Early persistence and progressive normalization of the SEP may antedate clinical evidence of improvement. The earliest SEP abnormality is a reduction in amplitude of the early scalp components; after several weeks, there is also latency prolongation (Young, 1982). Perot and Vera (1982) reported transient abnormalities in SEPs 3 to 6 days following injury that were inconsistently associated with clinically detectable changes in the patient's status. This was thought to be related to spinal cord edema.

Sedgwick et al. (1980) recorded spinal cord potentials (C2, C7, L1, and L4) in patients with traumatic paraplegia and quadriplegia. A normal lumbar N14 potential was found in patients with spinal cord lesions (partial or complete) several segments rostral to the generator segments (T10 or above), implying that the dorsal horn neurons were able to respond normally to an incoming volley. An unexpected finding was one of minor abnormalities in the cervical potentials in patients with lesions at T5 and below. These included an increased delay between N11 and N13 compared with that seen in controls. In high-level cervical lesions the early cervical potentials were sometimes still present but the later potentials were absent or, in partial lesions, delayed.

Dorfman et al. (1980) studied 23 patients with incomplete localized spinal cord lesions of varying etiologies. They determined a calculation for indirect spinal somatosensory conduction velocity (SSCV), based on SEP latency. The leg:arm (L:A) ratio was defined as the amplitude ratio of the cortical response following tibial nerve stimulation to that following median nerve stimulation on the same side of the body. In 8 of 46 sides, tibial SEPs were unrecordable. Of the remaining 38 sides, spinal SSCV was abnormally slow in 20 and the L:A ratio was abnormally low in 20. Serial postoperative studies in four cases documented an increase in the spinal SSCV and L:A ratio following spinal decompression.

In a subsequent study, Chen et al. (1990) examined 36 patients with cervical spinal cord injuries and obtained clinical and electrophysiologic data on the same day within 2 weeks after injury. Ulnar and tibial SEP grading was based on the presence or absence of the cortical evoked potential (CEP), the amplitude of the early cortically generated waveform (P22 or P37), and the IPL across the lesion site. Motor index score, pinprick sensory score, and joint position score were also calculated. Mean ulnar and tibial SEP grade had the strongest individual relationship with outcome ($R^2 = 0.75$, $p < 0.0001$) and mean SEP improvement over a 1-week interval during the first 3 weeks after injury was associated with motor index score improvement over a 6-month period. Somatosensory EPs had a unique role in predicting outcome for patients with neurologically incomplete injuries, because such patients with absent cortical responses had a significantly poorer outcome than did patients with responses, even though the two groups could not be differentiated on the basis of early clinical neurologic examinations.

Occasional studies have cast doubt on the ability of the SEP to predict recovery. McGarry et al. (1984), found that, of 25 spinal cord-injured patients, 9 with normal CEP latencies were paraplegic, whereas 8 with prolonged CEP latencies had "useful ambulation." York et al. (1983) found no relationship between the presence of a CEP or its wave amplitude, consistency, or latency in the early stages following injury and recovery from spinal cord injury. Both studies, however, focused on later, less reproducible CEP waveforms, including those that occurred after P22 (upper-limb stimulation) or P37 (lower-limb stimulation).

The prognostic value of performing early SEPs in patients with traumatic spinal cord lesions remains controversial. Abnormalities of median and posterior tibial SEPs correlate with the severity of spinal cord injury. In some patients, SEPs may be present despite clinically complete lesions, and progressive normalization of the SEP may antedate clinical improvement. Quantitative grading of SEP abnormalities, as performed by Chen et al. (1990), suggests that mean ulnar and tibial SEP grades are more useful in predicting outcome than are clinical motor or sensory scores, particularly in patients with incomplete lesions.

3.5. Syringomyelia

Somatosensory EP abnormalities correlate well with loss of joint and cutaneous sensations due to circumscribed lesions of the cervical cord, posterior thalamus, and parietal cortex. Traditionally they have been thought to not reflect function in the spinothalamic pathways and have therefore not been viewed as a useful investigation in patients with syringomyelia.

Veilleux and Stevens (1987) studied SEPs in 10 patients with syringomyelia; 7 patients had abnormal tibial SEPs, 3 patients had abnormal median SEPs, and 7 of 9 patients had abnormal ulnar SEPs. The authors noted that median and ulnar SEPs were usually normal in the presence of a dissociated sensory loss, and were usually abnormal (ulnar more frequently than median) when all sensory modalities were impaired; abnormalities of tibial SEPs were related to impaired proprioceptive sensation in the lower extremities.

Anderson et al. (1986) studied nine patients with syringomyelia and dissociated sensory loss. Six patients had abnormally low-amplitude or absent cervical potentials following median and ulnar nerve stimulation, with normal latencies. The abnormalities of cervical potentials were significantly asymmetrical in five of six cases, with the more abnormal findings corresponding to the side with greater clinical involvement. Six patients had abnormal central conduction times, all of whom had cerebellar herniation at the foramen magnum.

Nogués et al. (1992) studied 13 patients with syringomyelia which had been confirmed by MRI, 7 of whom had an associated Chiari type I anomaly. Eight of 13 patients had either unilateral or bilateral prolongation of central conduction time, and 4 showed abnormal latencies or an absent cervical N14 after median nerve stimulation. Three patients showed N20 abnormalities. The N40 latencies after tibial nerve stimulation were normal in four and prolonged or unobtainable in seven.

Restuccia and Mauguiére (1991) studied median nerve SEPs in 24 patients with syringomyelia documented by CT scan or MRI. Cervical N13 was recorded using a C6 anterior cervical montage, which cancels the potentials generated above the foramen magnum and enhances the amplitude of N13. Scalp far-field and early cortical SEPs were recorded using a noncephalic reference electrode. The N13/N9 amplitude ratio was used as an index to quantify N13 amplitude. Absent or reduced N13 was observed in 40 median SEPs (83%) in conjunction with normal P14 and N20 in 30 SEPs (62%). The dissociated loss of the cervical N13 was identified as the most conspicuous SEP feature in syringomyelia. A significant correlation was found between abnormal N13 and loss of pain and temperature sensations, whereas P14 abnormalities correlated well only with loss of joint and touch sensations. Posterior neck N13 negativity elicited by electrical stimulation of the median nerve is thought to have a fixed transverse generator in the lower cervical cord and reflects the response of dorsal horn neurons to non-noxious inputs. Abnormalities of N13 cervical potentials in patients with syringomyelia suggest that it is an indicator for central cervical cord lesions.

Urasaki et al. (1988) and Emerson and Pedley (1986), using a noncephalic reference and an expanded montage (including anterior cervical and lateral neck recording electrodes), identified abnormalities of spinal N13/P13 components that were not evident using a standard montage in three patients with syringomyelia.

In summary, patients with cervical cord syrinxes may show abnormalities in median nerve SEPs indicating a lesion in the upper cervical cord, with relative sparing of lower limb SEPs. The differential involvement presumably results from involvement of the lesion with the root entry zone (collateral) portion of the spinal cord rather than the dorsal columns. Detection of abnormalities of the cervical N13 response is increased by use of a noncephalic reference montage (Restuccia and Mauguiére, 1991; Urasaki et al., 1988; Emerson and Pedley, 1986).

3.6. Miscellaneous Spinal Cord Diseases

3.6.1. Friedreich's Ataxia

This autosomal recessive disorder primarily affects the spinal cord with involvement of spinocerebellar, corticospinal tracts and posterior columns. In advanced cases there is degeneration of large-diameter afferent nerve fibers.

Jones et al. (1980) studied median nerve SEPs in 22 patients with Friedreich's ataxia. They found marked attenuation of the brachial plexus potential but N9 and P/N13 latencies were normal. The N19 latency was delayed in all patients but two, in whom it could not be recognized. Peripheral nerve conduction velocities were normal, therefore providing evidence of a central conduction disturbance in the pathways mediating these SEPs. Mastaglia et al. (1978) studied eight patients, all with abnormal P/N13 and N19 components. Pederson and Trojaborg (1981) studied 10 patients, 5 with abnormal P/N13–N19 IPLs. Noel and Desmedt (1976) reported dispersed initial scalp negativity at latencies normal for N19.

3.6.2. Hereditary Spastic Paraparesis

Of seven patients with hereditary spastic paraparesis, Mastaglia et al. (1978) found abnormal P/N13 components in three and delayed, reduced-amplitude N19 latencies in two. Pederson and Trojaborg (1981) studied 13 patients with spastic paraplegia, 4 of whom had abnormal SEPs (all but 1 had normal central conduction times from the upper limb). Thomas et al. (1981) studied median SEPs in 18 patients with hereditary spastic paraplegia and normal peripheral nerve conduction studies. The P/N13 was absent in six patients and was reduced in amplitude in the remainder.

4. CONCLUSION

In patients with acute and chronic spinal cord injury, MEPs and SEPs are complementary tests that provide information regarding functional integrity of both anterolateral and posterior afferent and efferent pathways. In acute traumatic spinal cord injury, the role of EPs in predicting neurologic outcome remains controversial. Somatosensory EPs appear to be more useful than MEPs, particularly in incomplete lesions, although the number of studies with MEPs are limited. In chronic spinal cord lesions, EPs assist in lesion localization and, in contrast to imaging studies, reflect the functional integrity of spinal cord pathways. Furthermore, lesions may be detected at a subclinical stage.

REFERENCES

Anderson NE, Frith RW, Synek VM (1986): Somatosensory evoked potentials in syringomyelia. *J Neurol Neurosurg Psychiatry* 49:1407–1410.

Barker AJ, Jalinous R, Freeston IL (1985): Non-invasive stimulation of human motor cortex. *Lancet* 2:1106–1107.

Barker AT, Freeston IL, Jalinous R, Jarratt JA (1986): Clinical evaluation of conduction time measurements in central motor pathways using magnetic stimulation of human brain. *Lancet* 1:1325–1326.

Barker AT, Freeston IL, Jalinous R, Jarratt JA (1987): Magnetic stimulation of the human brain and peripheral nervous system: An introduction and the results of an initial clinical evaluation. *Neurosurgery* 20:100–109.

Berardelli A, Inghilleri M, Formisano R, Accornero N, Manfredi M (1987): Stimulation of motor tracts in motor neuron disease. *J Neurol Neurosurg Psychiatry* 50:732–737.

Berardelli A, Inghilleri M, Priori A, Accornero N, Manfredi M (1988): Electrical stimulation of motor cortex in patients with motor disturbances. In: *Neurology and Neurobiology: Non-invasive Stimulation of Brain and Spinal Cord.* edited by PM Rossini and CD Marsden, pp 219–230. Alan R Liss, New York.

Brasil-Neto JP, Cohen LG, Pascual-Leone A, Jabir FK, Wall RT, Hallett M (1992): Rapid reversible modulation of human motor outputs after transient deafferentation of the forearm: A study of transcranial magnetic stimulation. *Neurology* 42:1302–1306.

Burke D, Gandevia SC (1986): Muscle afferent contribution to the cerebral potentials of human subjects. In: *Frontiers of Clinical Neuroscience: Evoked Potentials*, edited by RQ Cracco and I Bodis-Wollner, pp 262–268. Alan R Liss, New York.

Caramia MD, Bernardi G, Zarola F, Rossini PM (1988): Neurophysiological evaluation of the central nervous impulse propagation in patients with sensorimotor disturbances. *Electroencephalogr Clin Neurophysiol* 70:16–25.

Caramia MD, Cicinelli P, Paradiso C, Mariorenzi R, Zarola F, Bernardi G, Rossini PM (1991): "Excitability" changes of muscular responses to magnetic brain stimulation in patients with central motor disorders. *Electroencephalogr Clin Neurophysiol* 81:243–250.

Cascino GD, Ring SR, King PJL, Brown RH, Chiappa KH (1988): Evoked potentials in motor system diseases. *Neurology* 38: 231–238.

Chen Li, Houlden DA, Rowed DW (1990): Somatosensory evoked potentials and neurological grades as predictors of outcome in acute spinal cord injury. *J Neurosurg* 72:600–609.

Chiappa KH, editor (1992): *Evoked Potentials in Clinical Medicine*, ed 2., Raven Press, New York.

Cohen LG, Topka H, Cole RA, Hallett M (1991): Leg paresthesias induced by magnetic brain stimulation in patients with thoracic spinal cord injury. *Neurology* 41:1283–1288.

Cowan JMA, Dick JPR, Day BL, Rothwell JC, Thompson PD, Marsden CD (1984): Abnormalities in central motor pathway conduction in multiple sclerosis. *Lancet* 2:304–307.

Cracco RQ (1973): Spinal evoked responses: Peripheral nerve stimulation in man. *Electroencephalogr Clin Neurophysiol* 35:379–386.

Cros D, Chiappa KH, Gominak S, Fang J, Santamaria J, King PJ, Shahani BT (1990): Cervical magnetic stimulation. *Neurology* 40:1751–1756.

Day BL, Rothwell JC, Thompson PD, Dick JPR, Cowan JMA, Berardelli A, Marsden CD (1987): Motor cortex stimulation in intact man. II. Multiple descending volleys. *Brain* 110:1191–1209.

Desmedt JE, Cheron G (1983): Spinal and far-field components of human somatosensory evoked potentials to posterior tibial nerve stimulation analyzed with oesophageal derivations and noncephalic reference recording. *Electroencephalogr Clin Neurophysiol* 56:635–651.

Di Lazzaro V, Restuccia D, Colosimo C, Tonali P (1992): The contribution of magnetic stimulation of the motor cortex to the diagnosis of cervical spondylotic myelopathy. Correlation of central motor conduction to distal and proximal upper limb muscles with clinical and MRI findings. *Electroencephalogr Clin Neurophysiol* 85: 311–320.

Dorfman LJ, Perkash I, Bosley TM, Cummins KL (1980): Use of cerebral evoked potentials to evaluate spinal somatosensory function in patients with traumatic and surgical myelopathies. *J Neurosurg* 52:654–660.

Emerson RG, Pedley TA (1986): Effect of cervical spinal cord lesions on early components of the median nerve somatosensory evoked potential. *Neurology* 36:20–26.

Epstein CM, Fernandez-Beer E, Weissman JD, Matsuura S (1991): Cervical magnetic stimulation: The role of the neural foramen. *Neurology* 41:677–680.

Fehlings M, Tator CH, Dean Linden R, Piper IR (1987): Motor evoked potentials recorded from normal and spinal cord-injured rats. *Neurosurgery* 20:125–130.

Gianutsos J, Eberstein A, Ma D, Holland T, Goodgold J (1987): A noninvasive technique to assess completeness of spinal cord lesions in humans. *Exp Neurol* 98:34–40.

Hess CW, Mills KR, Murray NMF (1986): Measurement of central motor conduction in multiple sclerosis by magnetic brain stimulation. *Lancet* 2:355–358.

Hess CW, Mills KR, Murray NMF (1987a): Responses in small hand muscles from magnetic stimulation of the human brain. *J Physiol* 388:397–419.

Hess CW, Mills KR, Murray NMF, Schriefer TN (1987b): Magnetic brain stimulation: central motor conduction studies in multiple sclerosis. *Ann Neurol* 22:744–760.

Hugon J, Lubeau M, Tabarand F, Chazot F, Vallar JM, Dumas M (1987): Central motor conduction in motor neuron disease. *Ann Neurol* 22:544–546.

Ingram DA, Swash M (1987): Central motor conduction is abnormal in motor neuron disease. *J Neurol Neurosurg Psychiatry* 50:159–166.

Ingram DA, Thompson AJ, Swash M (1988): Central motor conduction in multiple sclerosis: Evaluation of abnormalities revealed by transcutaneous magnetic stimulation of the brain. *J Neurol Neurosurg Psychiatry* 51:487–494.

Jones SJ, Baraitser M, Halliday AM (1980): Peripheral and central somatosensory nerve conduction defects in Friedreich's ataxia. *J Neurol Neurosurg Psychiatry* 43:495–503.

Kakulas BA, Bedbrook GM (1969): A correlative clinicopathological study of spinal cord injury. *Proc Aust Assoc Neurol* 6:123–132.

Kakulas BA, Bedbrook GM (1976): Pathology of injuries of the vertebral spinal cord—with emphasis on microscope aspects. In: *Handbook of Clinical Neurology: Injuries of the Spine and Spinal Cord,* edited by PJ Vinken and GW Bruyn, pp 27–42. Elsevier, Amsterdam.

Kiers L, Chiappa KH (1995): Motor and somatosensory evoked potentials in spinal cord disorders. In: *Diagnosis and Management of Disorders of the Spinal Cord,* edited by RR Young and RM Woolsey, pp 153–169. WB Saunders, Philadelphia.

Levy WJ, McCaffrey M, Hagichi S (1987): Motor evoked potential as a predictor of recovery in chronic spinal cord injury. *Neurosurgery* 20:138–142.

Levy WJ, Amassian VE, Traad M, Cadwell J (1990): Focal magnetic coil stimulation reveals motor cortical system reorganized in humans after traumatic quadriplegia. *Brain Res* 510:130–134.

Maccabee PJ, Amassian VE, Eberle LP, Rudell AP, Cracco RQ, Lai KS, Somasundaram M (1991): Measurement of the electric field induced into inhomogeneous volume conductors by magnetic coils: application to human spinal neurogeometry. *Electroencephalogr Clin Neurophysiol* 81:224–237.

Macdonell RAL, Cros D, Shahani BT (1992): Lumbosacral nerve root stimulation comparing electrical with surface magnetic coil techniques. *Muscle Nerve* 15:885–890.

Macdonell RAL, Donnan GA (1995): Magnetic cortical stimulation in acute spinal cord injury. *Neurology* 45:303–306.

Maertens de Noordhout A, Remade JM, Pepin JL, Born JD, Delwaide PJ (1991): Magnetic stimulation of the motor cortex in cervical spondylosis. *Neurology* 41:75–80.

Mastaglia FL, Black JL, Edis R, Collins DWK (1978): The contribution of evoked potentials in the functional assessment of the somatosensory pathway. *Clin Exp Neurol* 15:279–298.

Matheson JK, Harrington HJ, Hallett M (1986): Abnormalities of multimodality evoked potentials in amyotrophic lateral sclerosis. *Arch Neurol* 43:338–340.

McGarry J, Friedgood DL, Woolsey R, Horenstein S, Johnson C (1984): Somatosensory evoked potentials in spinal cord injuries. *Surg Neurol* 22:341–343.

McKinley PA, Jenkins WM, Smith JL, Merzenich MM (1987): Age-dependent capacity for somatosensory cortex reorganization in chronic spinal cats. *Dev Brain Res* 31:136–139.

Merton PA, Morton HB (1980): Stimulation of the cerebral cortex in the intact human subject. *Nature* 285:227.

Metzler J, Marks PS (1979): Functional changes in cat somatic sensory-motor cortex during short-term reversible epidermal blocks. *Brain Res* 177:379–383.

Mills KR, Murray NMF (1985): Corticospinal tract conduction time in multiple sclerosis. *Ann Neurol* 18:601–605.

Mills KR, Murray NMF, Hess CW (1987): Magnetic and electrical transcranial brain stimulation: Physiological mechanisms and clinical applications. *Neurosurgery* 20:164–168.

Noel P, Desmedt JE (1976): The somatosensory pathway in Freidreich's ataxia. *Acta Neurol Belg* 76:271.

Nogués MA, Pardal AM, Merello M, Miguel MA (1992): SEPS and CNS magnetic stimulation in syringomyelia. *Muscle Nerve* 15:993–1001.

Oh SJ, Sunwoo IN, Kim HS, Faught E (1985): Cervical and cortical somatosensory evoked potentials differentiate cervical spondylotic myelopathy from amyotrophic lateral sclerosis (abstract). *Neurology* 35 (suppl 1):147–148.

Pederson L, Trojaborg W (1981): Visual, auditory and somatosensory pathway involvement in hereditary cerebellar ataxia, Friedrich's ataxia and familial spastic paraplegia. *Electroencephalogr Clin Neurophysiol* 52:283–297.

Perot PL, Vera CL (1982): Scalp-recorded somatosensory evoked potentials to stimulation of nerves in the lower extremities and evaluation of patients with spinal cord trauma. *Ann NY Acad Sci* 388:359–368.

Pons TP, Garraghty PE, Ommaya AK, Kaas JH, Taub E, Mishkin M (1991): Massive cortical reorganization after sensory deafferentation in adult macaques. *Science* 252:1857–1860.

Poser CM, Paty DW, Scheinberg L, et al (1983): New diagnostic criteria for multiple sclerosis: guidelines for research protocols. *Ann Neurol* 13:227–231.

Ravnborg M, Liguori R, Christiansen P, Larsson H, Soelberg Sørensen P (1992): The diagnostic reliability of magnetically evoked motor potentials in multiple sclerosis. *Neurology* 42:1296–1301.

Restuccia D, Mauguiére F (1991): The contribution of median nerve SEPs in the functional assessment of the cervical spinal cord in syringomyelia. *Brain* 114:361–379.

Restuccia D, Di Lazzaro V, Lo Monaco M, Evoli A, Valeriani M, Tonali P (1992a): Somatosensory evoked potentials in the diagnosis of cervical spondylotic myelopathy. *Electromyogr Clin Neurophysiol* 32:389–395.

Restuccia D, Di Lazzaro V, Valeriani M, Tonali P, Mauguiére F (1992b): Segmental dysfunction of the cervical cord revealed by abnormalities of the spinal N13 potential in cervical spondylotic myelopathy. *Neurology* 42:1054–1063.

Ropper AH, Miett T, Chiappa KH (1982): Absence of evoked potential abnormalities in acute transverse myelopathy. *Neurology* 32:80–82.

Rossini PM, Di Stefano E, Stanzione P (1985): Nerve impulse propagation along central and peripheral fast conducting motor and sensory pathways in man. *Electroencephalogr Clin Neurophysiol* 60:320–334.

Rothwell JC, Thompson PD, Cowan JMA, et al (1986): A method of monitoring function in corticospinal pathways during scoliosis surgery with a note on motor conduction velocities. *J Neurol Neurosurg Psychiatry* 49:251–257.

Rothwell JC, Thompson PD, Day BL, Dick JPR, Kachi T, Cowan JMA, Marsden CD (1987): Motor cortex stimulation in intact man. I. General characteristics of EMG responses in different muscles. *Brain* 110:1173–1190.

Sedgwick EM, El-Negamy E, Frankel H (1980): Spinal cord potentials in traumatic paraplegia and quadriplegia. *J Neurol Neurosurg Psychiatry* 43:823–830.

Simpson RK, Baskin DS (1987): Corticomotor evoked potentials in acute and chronic blunt spinal cord injury in the rat: Correlation with neurological outcome and histological damage. *Neurosurgery* 20:131–137.

Small DG, Matthews WB, Small M (1978): The cervical somatosensory evoked potential (SEP) in the diagnosis of multiple sclerosis. *J Neurol Sci* 35:211–224.

Snooks SJ, Swash M (1985): Motor conduction velocity in the human spinal cord: slowed conduction in multiple sclerosis and radiation myelopathy. *J Neurol Neurosurg Psychiatry* 48:1135–1139.

Spielholz NI, Benjamin MV, Engler G, Ransohoff J (1979) *Somatosensory evoked potentials and clinical outcome in spinal cord injury.* In: *Neural Trauma,* edited by AJ Popp, pp 217–222. Raven Press, New York.

Subramanium JS, Yiannikas C (1990): Multimodality evoked potentials in motor neuron disease. *Arch Neurol* 47:989–994.

Thomas PK, Jeffreys JGR, Smith IS, Loukalis D (1981): Spinal somatosensory evoked potentials in hereditary spastic paraplegia. *J Neurol Neurosurg Psychiatry* 44:243–246.

Thompson PD, Day BL, Rothwell JC, Dick JPR, Cowan JMA, Asselman P, Griffin GB, Sheehy MP, Marsden CD (1987a): The interpretation of electromyographic responses to electrical stimulation of the motor cortex in diseases of the upper motor neuron. *J Neurol Sci* 80:91–110.

Thompson PD, Dick JPR, Asselman P, Griffin GB, Day BL, Rothwell JC, Sheehy MP, Marsden CD (1987b): Examination of motor function in lesions of the spinal cord by stimulation of the motor cortex. *Ann Neurol* 21:389–396.

Topka H, Cohen LG, Cole RA, Hallett M (1991): Reorganization of corticospinal pathways following spinal cord injury. *Neurology* 41:1276–1283.

Triggs WJ, Macdonell RAL, Cros D, Chiappa KH, Shahani B, Day BJ (1992): Motor inhibition and excitation are independent effects of magnetic cortical stimulation. *Ann Neurol* 32:345–351.

Turano G, Jones SJ, Miller DH, Du Boulay GH, Kakigi R, McDonald WI (1991): Correlation of SEP abnormalities with brain and cervical cord MRI in multiple sclerosis. *Brain* 114:663–681.

Urasaki E, Wada S, Kadoya C, Matsuzaki H, Yokota A, Matsuoka S (1988): Absence of spinal N13-P13 and normal scalp far-field P14 in a patient with syringomyelia. *Electroencephalogr Clin Neurophysiol* 71:400–404.

Veilleux M, Daube JR (1987): The value of ulnar somatosensory evoked potentials (SEPs) in cervical myelopathy. *Electroencephalogr Clin Neurophysiol* 68:415–423.

Veilleux M, Stevens C (1987): Syringomyelia: Electrophysiological aspects. *Muscle Nerve* 10:449–458.

Wall JT, Cusick CG (1984): Cutaneous responsiveness in primary somatosensory (S-1) hindpaw cortex before and after partial hindpaw deafferentation in adult rats. *J Neurosci* 4:1499–1515.

Wilkinson M (1960): The morbid anatomy of cervical spondylosis and myelopathy. *Brain* 83:589–617.

Yiannikas C, Shahani BT, Young RR (1986): Short-latency somatosensory evoked potentials from radial, median, ulnar and peroneal nerve stimulation in the assessment of cervical spondylosis. *Arch Neurol* 43:1264–1271.

York DH, Watts C, Raffensberger M et al (1983): Utilization of somatosensory evoked cortical potentials in spinal cord injury: prognostic limitations. *Spine* 8:832–839.

Young W (1982): Correlation of somatosensory evoked potentials and neurological findings in spinal cord injury. In: *Early Management of Acute Spinal Cord Injury,* edited by CH Tator, pp 153–165. Raven Press, New York.

Yu YL, Jones SJ (1985): Somatosensory evoked potentials in cervical spondylosis: correlation of median, ulnar and posterior tibial nerve responses with clinical and radiological findings. *Brain* 108:273–300.

Evoked Potentials in Clinical Medicine,
3d ed., edited by Keith H. Chiappa.
Lippincott–Raven Publishers, Philadelphia © 1997.

15

Endogenous Event-Related Potentials

Barry S. Oken

*Department of Neurology, Oregon Health Sciences University,
Portland, Oregon 97201*

1. INTRODUCTION

Long-latency evoked potentials (EPs) related to aspects of cognitive processing are referred to as *cognitive EPs* or *endogenous event-related potentials* (ERPs). The P3 (also known as the P300) is the best known of the endogenous ERPs. Others in this category include the earlier waves N1, P2, and N2, the slow wave (SW), and the contingent negative variation (CNV). These EP components as well as the movement-related potentials (e.g., *bereitschaftspotential*) are discussed here. This chapter will focus on the techniques of recording and applications in the clinical EP laboratory. Much of the psychophysiology of the cognitive EPs (e.g., Donchin, 1981), the processing or mismatch negativity (e.g., Naatanen, 1992), and the N400 (Kutas and Hillyard, 1980; Curran et al., 1993) will not be discussed. In addition, long-latency EPs are sometimes included as part of a battery of electrophysiologic tests used for diagnostic purposes (e.g., Duffy et al., 1980; John et al., 1988). Since it is often unclear whether the sensitivity of these tests is related to the electroencephalographic (EEG) or EP component and there are significant concerns about their utility (Oken and Chiappa, 1986; American Academy of Neurology, 1989), these will not be discussed further. For further review of the extensive research in the cognitive EP field refer to Hillyard and Picton (1987), Picton (1988), Rohrbaugh et al., (1990), or Brunia et al., (1991).

There are several significant differences between the endogenous ERPs and the routine short-latency EPs which are elicited by external stimuli (exogenous ERPs). Endogenous ERPs are not affected markedly by changes in physical parameters of the stimulus, such as intensity and frequency, in contrast to the short-latency EPs. Almost identical endogenous ERPs, in fact, may be elicited by stimuli of different modalities. In general, endogenous ERPs have longer latencies, greater amplitudes, and lower frequencies than routine EPs.

While the short-latency EPs can be recorded when the patient is under general anesthesia, the P3 needs to be recorded when the patient is awake and alert. The latencies and amplitudes are affected by psychologic state, including the patient's prior experience, intentions, and expectations.

2. LONG-LATENCY EPS—P3

The long-latency EPs are a series of positive and negative waves that are generated above the brain stem and have a widespread scalp distribution. There are two naming systems for these waveforms. The negative (N) or positive (P) waves can be labeled in numerical order (e.g., the third positive wave is referred to as the P3) or can be labeled by their average latency in a group of healthy subjects (the positive wave with an average latency of about 300 msec is referred to as the P300). P3 and P300 are usually used interchangeably. The major waves are the N1, P2, N2, P3, and slow wave. While all the waves can be recorded and analyzed, most clinical studies have focused on the P3 and therefore the P3 will be the focus of this discussion.

The P3 (P300) is a symmetrical positive wave, maximal over the midline central and parietal regions, with a latency that varies from 250 to 600 msec depending on stimulus and subject parameters. The P3 can be elicited with a stimulus of any modality. The most commonly used method to obtain the P3 is referred to as the "oddball" paradigm. This involves the presentation of unexpected or infrequent stimuli randomly interspersed among more frequent stimuli (Sutton et al., 1965). In most studies, the unexpected stimuli differ from the more common stimuli in terms of frequency (e.g., pitch) or intensity. The unexpected stimulus may be simply the absence of a stimulus among a train of regularly spaced stimuli (Klinke et al., 1968; Picton and Hillyard, 1974; Simson et al., 1976) or a change in the interstimulus interval among a train of regularly spaced stimuli (Ford and Hillyard, 1981; Ford et al., 1982). A method that augments the P3 and is generally used in conjunction with the "oddball" paradigm consists of attending to task-relevant target stimuli and ignoring nontarget stimuli (Chapman and Brangdon, 1964; Desmedt et al., 1965; Donchin and Cohen, 1967; Picton and Hillyard, 1974). A P3 will be seen following the target but not the nontarget stimuli (Fig. 15–1).

These two factors, stimulus infrequency or unexpectability and attention or task-relevance, operate independently. In fact, there is evidence that they produce different P3's (Squires et al., 1975; Courchesne et al., 1975). Independent of task relevance, an infrequent stimulus elicits a P3 that N. Squires and colleagues referred to as P3a. This component occurs slightly earlier and has a more frontal distribution than the parietal maximum P3b component wave, which is best elicited by attending to a task-relevant stimulus. Presumably, the routinely obtained P3 represents a sum of these two component waves.

The other long-latency EP components, N1, P2, N2, and SW, have been less useful clinically. The N2 wave may have more than one component (Renault et al., 1982; Perrault and Picton, 1984b). It is similar to the P3 component in terms of its sensitivity to attention and stimulus infrequency and its latency correlation with reaction time (e.g., Ritter et al., 1983). The N1 and P2 may also contain more than one component and are less affected by attention than the P3 (e.g., Naatanen, 1979; Knight et al., 1981; Perrault and Picton, 1984a; Woods et al., 1987).

2.1. Generator Sites

The generator site of the P3 is not known with certainty. This is in part related to the fact that neuronal activity in multiple brain regions, including inferior parietal lobule, frontal

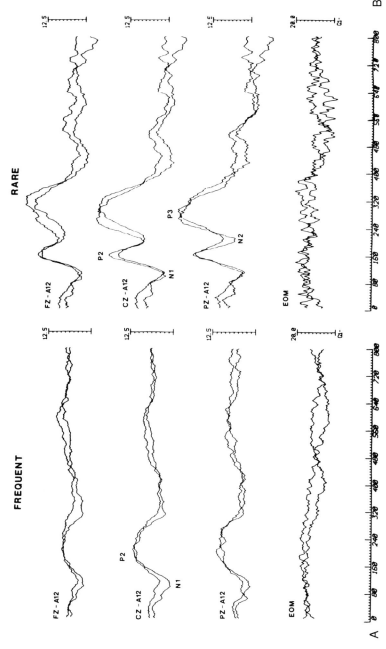

FIG. 15–1. Long-latency auditory EP recorded in a normal subject to frequent, 1,000-Hz tones (**A**), and rare, 2,000-Hz tones (**B**), with the subject instructed to raise her finger whenever hearing a rare tone. Three scalp channels are shown, all to a linked-ear reference, and one eye movement channel. Each trial consisted of 100 tones, 16% rare and 84% frequent, with two trials superimposed.

lobe, hippocampus, medial temporal lobe along with other limbic structures, and locus coeruleus, correlate to scalp recorded P3 activity (Foote et al., 1991; Kropotov and Pono-marev, 1991; Paller et al., 1992; Smith et al., 1990; Halgren et al., 1980; Smith et al., 1986). Despite some early suggestions of a medial temporal lobe origin for the P3 (Okada et al., 1983), there is not a good correlation between the medial temporal lobe potentials and the scalp-recorded P3 (Stapleton and Halgren, 1987). Additionally, the scalp-recorded P3 has not been significantly changed by temporal lobectomy for intractable epilepsy (Stapleton et al., 1987), or bilateral hippocampal or temporal lobe lesions (Onofrj et al., 1992; Polich and Squire, 1993).

Additional evidence for multiple generators comes from human lesion studies performed by Knight and colleagues. Patients with frontal lobe lesions have a significantly attenuated novelty P3 (P3a) (Knight, 1984; Yamaguchi and Knight, 1991b), while patients with tem-poroparietal junction lesions have markedly attenuated P3's to both novel and attended stimuli (P3a and P3b) (Knight et al., 1989; Yamaguchi and Knight, 1991b, 1992). Patients with lateral parietal cortex lesions have no significant change in their P3 (Knight et al., 1989; Yamaguchi and Knight, 1991b).

There is some evidence that the P3 consists of additional components besides the P3a and P3b. Using noncephalic reference recording, it has been demonstrated that there is a negative component occurring at a similar latency to the P3 recorded from nasopharyngeal and infe-rior temporal electrodes (Perrault and Picton, 1984b; Neshige and Luders, 1988; Curran et al., 1993). It is unknown whether this negative component has the same generator as the P3.

P3's or P3-like potentials have been recorded from rodents (Yamaguchi et al., 1993), cats (Wilder et al., 1981; Harrison and Buchwald, 1985), and primates (Arthur and Starr, 1984; Pineda et al., 1988; Antal et al., 1993; Glover et al., 1991; Paller et al., 1992).

2.2. Subject Parameters

There are several subject characteristics that may affect the P3. These include the age of the subject, the subject's level of attention, and the relative difficulty of the P3 task.

2.2.1. Attention and Alertness

The subject must be awake and alert to obtain the P3. There are a series of related vari-ables that affect the P3: level of attention, alertness, and response accuracy. Decreasing alertness is associated with a decrease in the amplitude of some cortical EPs (e.g., Haider et al., 1964). Drowsiness or inattention will decrease the amplitude or obliterate the P3. While an altered P3 may still be present in stage 2 sleep, it is obliterated in SW sleep (Nielson-Bohlman et al., 1991). In addition, the P3 and SW amplitudes are larger following a stimu-lus that is correctly identified than one incorrectly identified (Hillyard et al., 1971; Parasur-aman and Beatty, 1980; Ruchkin et al., 1980). Thus, an assessment of behavioral response to the stimuli is important to enable estimation of the subject's degree of attention. The sub-ject can be asked to mentally count the number of target stimuli or to respond to each target stimulus (e.g., raise a finger or push a button), which allows one to record the accuracy of response. If a motor response is used, one can average only those sweeps where a correct re-sponse was given and/or record reaction times. The P3 may be slightly different depending on whether or not the subject produces a motor response (Barrett et al., 1987), but the P3 component does not depend on the presence of a motor response. In fact, the P3 latency may be longer than the reaction time. Goodin and colleagues (1986) discuss the P3 component that can be elicited by synchronizing the EP average to the response-onset electromy-elographic (EMG) activity.

2.2.2. Task

The specific task that is given to the subject will affect the P3. In the oddball paradigm, when a subject is instructed to specifically attend to the rare stimulus, the P3 amplitude increases. An identical rare stimulus to which the subject is not told to attend will elicit a lower-amplitude response (Fig. 15–2).

The difficulty of the discrimination task used to obtain the P3 affects the latency of the P3. The P3 latency increases as a task becomes harder (Ritter et al., 1972; N Squires et al., 1977; McCarthy and Donchin, 1981; Pfefferbaum et al., 1983; Magliero et al., 1984; Polich, 1987). For example, as the pitch of the rare auditory stimulus becomes more similar to the pitch of the frequent stimulus, the task of identifying the rare stimulus becomes more difficult and the P3 latency increases.

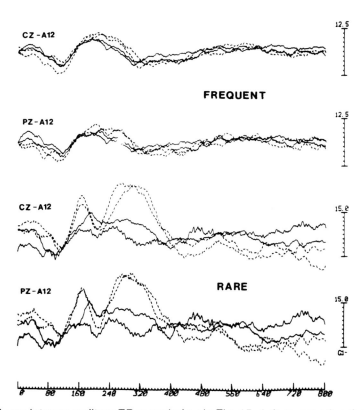

FIG. 15–2. Long-latency auditory EP recorded as in Fig. 15–1 demonstrating the effect of attention, with only CZ and PZ channels shown. Top two traces are the average EP to the frequent tones and bottom two traces to the rare tones. *Dotted line* shows EP in condition when subject was instructed to raise her finger whenever hearing the rare tone. *Solid line* shows EP to same stimuli when subject was instructed to ignore the tones. The N1–P2 complex is similar in the two conditions, while the N2–P3 complex shows enhancement in the attend condition.

2.2.3. Age

The P3 latency has a positive correlation with age for auditory (Pfefferbaum et al., 1980a,b,1984a,b; Picton et al., 1984; Goodin, 1978a; Syndulko, 1982a; Brown et al., 1983; Polich et al., 1985; Barrett et al., 1987; Oken and Kaye, 1992) (Fig. 15–3), visual (Beck et al., 1980; Mullis et al., 1985; Pfefferbaum et al., 1984a; Picton et al., 1984; Kutas et al., 1994), and somatosensory stimuli (Picton et al., 1984; Barrett et al., 1987; Yamaguchi and Knight, 1991a). There is an increase in mean latency by approximately 1 to 1.5 msec/year after age 20. The standard error of estimate (see page 572) of the age-latency regression line has ranged from 20 to 50 msec in various studies. This degree of variability is a problem if one is trying to establish a clinical test and compare patients to a normative data base. The regression line for age and P3 latency has been found by some researchers to increase in slope with increasing age (Beck et al., 1980; Brown et al., 1983; Gordon et al., 1986b), although others have not found this. Some of the variability across studies may relate to failure to control for perceptual thresholds in the elderly which may impact on the P3 (Polich, 1991b; Vesco et al., 1993) and to control for the specific task [i.e., a two-tone oddball versus a three-tone target, rare and frequent tone task (Fein and Turetsky, 1989)]. Additionally, decreased fitness levels or the presence of certain diseases (e.g., epilepsy) or medications may cause disproportionate slowing of the P3 with age (Dustman et al., 1990; Puce et al., 1989).

The correlation between adult age and P3 amplitude is uncertain because of conflicting findings (Beck et al., 1980; Pfefferbaum et al., 1980b, 1984a; Brown et al., 1983; Goodin et al., 1978a, 1978b; Picton et al., 1984), but there is an overall tendency for decreased amplitude with age, especially over 80 years (Oken and Kaye, 1992).

There is also a gradual decline of P3 latency in children, with a minimum latency being achieved between age 15 and 25 (Mullis et al., 1985; Goodin et al., 1978a; Polich et al., 1985; Martin et al., 1988) (Fig. 15–3).

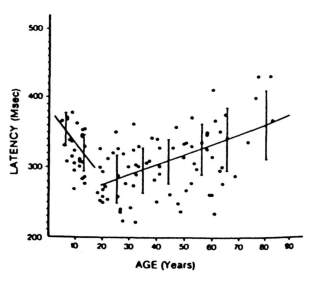

FIG. 15–3. Scattergram demonstrating the relationship in healthy subjects between age and auditory P3 latency using 160- to 1,000-Hz and 40- to 2,000-Hz tones. Regression line and standard deviations are shown. There is a decrease in P3 latency in childhood and an increase in P3 latency in adulthood. An increased standard deviation with age is also noted. (From Polich et al., 1985, with permission.)

2.2.4. Drugs

Several researchers have analyzed the relationship between the neurotransmitter-specific ascending arousal systems (e.g., Oken and Salinsky, 1992) and the P3. Anticholinergics increase the latency and decrease the amplitude of the P3 (Brandeis et al., 1992; Meador et al., 1988b) but have variable effects on N1 (Coons et al., 1981; Meador et al., 1988b). The P3 amplitude attenuation can be reversed by physostigmine, a cholinesterase inhibitor (Hammond et al., 1987). Antihistamines also prolong P3 latency (Loring and Meador, 1989; Meador et al., 1989a). Drugs increasing central monoamines (e.g., methylphenidate and amphetamine) generally have little effect on P3 latency even though reaction times are decreased (Brumaghim et al., 1987; Callaway, 1983; Fitzpatrick et al., 1988; Klorman and Brumaghim, 1991; Naylor et al., 1985). Levodopa (L-dopa) did not produce any change in the P3 in normal controls although it did decrease P3 latency in patients with Parkinson's disease (Stanzione et al., 1991). Antiserotinergic drugs also have little impact on the P3 (Meador et al., 1989b).

Meador and colleagues found no differences in P3 latency secondary to the anticonvulsants phenytoin, carbamazepine, or phenobarbital (Meador et al., 1990; Meador et al., 1991). A benzodiazepine anticonvulsant, clonazepam, also had no effect on P3 latency, although the P3 amplitude was reduced (Rockstroh et al., 1991).

2.2.5. Other

Habituation may be more prominent with longer latency EPs (Ritter et al, 1968; Picton et al., 1976). The novelty P3 or P3a may arise with any novel stimulus but it habituates (Courchesne, 1978), while the task-dependent P3 does not habituate (Courchesne, 1978; Sklare and Lynn, 1984; Polich 1986b). The P3 is not significantly affected by having the eyes open or closed (Polich, 1986a), although instructions to refrain from blinking may actually decrease the P3 amplitude (Verleger, 1991).

Polich and colleagues have evaluated the effects on the P3 of assorted other factors, including season, time of day, recency of food, menstrual cycle, and body temperature (Geisler and Polich, 1990; Polich, 1991a; Polich and Geisler, 1991). The only one with a significant effect on P3 latency was body temperature, with temperature negatively correlated with P3 latency.

2.3. Stimulus Parameters

2.3.1. Modality and Physical Properties

While most studies have used auditory or visual stimuli, somatosensory stimuli, including painful, ones can also elicit a P3 (e.g., Desmedt and Robertson, 1977; Barrett et al., 1987; Becker et al., 1993). The P3 is fairly similar following stimuli of different modalities, although there may be slight differences in latency or topography (Simson et al., 1977; Snyder et al., 1980; Barrett et al., 1987). The P3 component is also relatively independent of other physical properties of the stimulus (e.g., stimulus intensity), but slight changes in P3 latency may be seen with marked changes in stimulus intensity (Roth et al., 1982; Papanicolaou et al., 1985; Polich, 1989).

2.3.2. Stimulus Occurrence Probability

The amplitude of the P3 is affected by the probability of occurrence of the target stimulus. The probability of occurrence can be given by the probability within the global sequence of target and nontarget stimuli, the probability within the local sequence (e.g., the last five stimuli), or by the temporal probability, which is affected by the interstimulus interval as well as the sequence probability.

2.3.2.1. Global Sequence Probability

The P3 amplitude increases as the target stimulus frequency in the global sequence decreases (Tueting et al., 1971; Roth, 1973; Duncan-Johnson and Donchin, 1977; KC Squires et al., 1976,1977; Polich, 1987). An average occurrence rate below 10% to 15% does not improve test results and in clinical studies a rate of 15% to 20% has been most commonly used.

2.3.2.2. Local Sequence Probability

Another factor peculiar to the P3 is its dependence on preceding stimuli or local sequence probability (KC Squires et al., 1976,1978; Duncan-Johnson and Donchin, 1977). A target stimulus that is preceded by another target stimulus will elicit a lower-amplitude P3 than if it is preceded by a nontarget stimulus. The P3 is enhanced by increasing the number of consecutive nontarget stimuli preceding the target stimulus. For example, a target stimulus that is preceded by only one as compared to four nontarget stimuli will elicit a lower-amplitude P3 (KC Squires et al., 1976,1978; Duncan-Johnson and Donchin, 1977, Johnson and Donchin, 1980).

2.3.2.3. Interstimulus Interval

The amplitude of the P3 is increased as the temporal probability of target stimulus occurrence decreases, that is, as the interstimulus interval (ISI) is increased while the sequence probability remains unchanged (Fitzgerald and Picton, 1981; Ford et al., 1976, KC Squires et al., 1978; Polich, 1987). This factor appears to be more significant than the global sequence probability (Ford et al., 1976; Fitzgerald and Picton, 1981). In fact, omitting the frequent stimulus altogether, but presenting the target stimulus at what would be usual times in an oddball paradigm still elicits a P3 (Polich et al., 1994). A P3 may be obtained with very short ISIs, as small as 300 msec, although the latency is slightly prolonged and the amplitude mildly decreased compared to longer ISIs (Woods et al., 1980; Woods and Courchesne, 1986).

2.3.3. Stimulus Randomization

The sequence of presentation of the target and nontarget stimuli is important for a reason in addition to those listed above. If the infrequent stimuli occur at fixed intervals (e.g., every sixth stimulus in the oddball paradigm), then the rare stimulus is not unexpected and the P3 amplitude decreases. Therefore, it is important to use a random or pseudorandom sequence (Naatanen, 1970). A pseudorandom sequence contains a random sequence of targets and nontargets with conditions on the stimuli sequence (e.g., no two target stimuli appear consecutively). A pseudorandom sequence is preferred to a random sequence because of the effects of local sequence probability.

2.4. Technical Factors

2.4.1. Filters

To record the P3, 0.3- to 1-Hz high-pass and 30 to 100-Hz low-pass filters are commonly employed, although lower-frequency high-pass filters or DC amplifiers are needed to accurately measure the slow wave. Use of a high-pass filter of 1 Hz may decrease the P3 latency and the N2–P3 amplitude compared to a lower-frequency high-pass filter (Duncan-Johnson and Donchin, 1979; Ebmeier et al., 1992; Glabus et al., 1994; Goodin et al., 1992), but the best filter for clinical purposes has not been established (Goodin et al., 1992). The use of a 1 Hz high-pass filter may actually improve the sensitivity of the P3 latency despite it altering the P3 waveform (Ebmeier, 1992).

2.4.2. Channels

At least three channels of EEG activity should be recorded (Fz, Cz, Pz), in part to delineate the P3a and P3b components. The electrodes can be referenced to linked-ear, linked-mastoid electrodes, nose, or noncephalic electrodes. The ears, mastoids, and nose are somewhat active references (e.g., Wolpaw and Wood, 1982; Neshige and Luders, 1988). Brief guidelines have been proposed for some of these factors (Goodin et al., 1994).

Eye movement needs to be monitored because eye movements may be time-locked to the stimuli, especially the target (oddball) stimuli, and the field of distribution of the eye movements may include the recording electrode sites. Other sources of extracerebral artifacts, such as cranial muscle or glossokinesis, may also need to be monitored.

2.4.3. Averaging Parameters

The stimulus rate is generally about 1/sec and may be randomly varied. It is important to standardize the sequence of target and nontarget stimuli because variations in the sequence will increase the variability of the P3. The sweep duration should be 600 to 1000 msec and a prestimulus period is important in assessing the baseline for amplitude measures.

2.4.4. Intrasubject P3 Variability

The P3 is a variable response, even within a subject, and, as with other EPs, it is necessary to repeat trials to ensure reproducibility. Sklare and Lynn studied nine subjects serially and found up to an 18-msec difference between trials 1 and 2, and up to a 12-msec difference between the average of two trials performed at each of two sessions 2 to 4 weeks apart. There was a very high correlation between the two trials ($r = 0.84$) and two sessions ($r = 0.93$). Polich (1986b) studied 100 subjects and found no significant difference in P3 amplitude or latency comparing trials 1 and 2. However, correlation coefficients for P3 latency were significantly lower than those obtained by Sklare and Lynn. Another study used several different P300 latency measures and calculated test–retest correlations within a session to be about 0.7 and correlations between sessions 1 and 2 weeks apart to be about 0.5 (Fabiani et al., 1987). Two additional studies in young adults found a maximum P3 latency difference in 12 subjects tested 1 to 2 weeks apart to be 60 msec (Kileny and Kripal, 1987) and in 24 subjects tested four times each about 1 to 2 weeks apart to be 36 msec (Zamrini et al., 1991). The latter study found the 95% confidence interval for the difference between two combined sessions was 20 msec. There are limited data on the topographic stability of the P3 (Karniski and Blair, 1989).

2.4.5. Peak Detection

There is a significant problem in determining the precise P3 latency and amplitude. One cause is that the P3 is composed of two separable component peaks, P3a and P3b. Measurement of both peaks is probably the best solution (see, e.g., Polich et al., 1985), but they are not consistently seen in all subjects. Another source of error in determining the peak for P3 latency measurement is the variable morphology and broadness of the P3 (Fig. 15–4). Methods for determining the P3 latency include measuring the P3 latency as the point of maximum amplitude or as the intersection of the lines extended from the leading and trailing edges of the P3 wave (see, e.g., Goodin et al., 1978a, or as is done for P100 in Fig. 2–12 of 2nd ed., p. 57). More complex peak detection paradigms have been used for research purposes (see, e.g., Callaway et al., 1983) but have not been widely used for clinical applications. There has been an attempt to detect the P3 from a single sweep (Puce et al., 1994; Smulders et al., 1994; Suwazono et al., 1994), but these have not been used for clinical purposes.

P3 amplitude measurements may be made in comparison to a prestimulus baseline or as a peak to peak amplitude from the N2. In general, P3 amplitude decreases as latency increases (see, e.g., Polich, 1986b).

2.5. Clinical Studies

Researchers have attempted to correlate changes in cognitive EPs with clinical changes in cognitive function. In general, changes in the P3 can be seen in cognitive dysfunction but the sensitivity and specificity of the test has not been as high as for some of the earlier-latency EPs.

2.5.1. Dementia and Alzheimer's Disease

One goal of cognitive EP research has been to develop a useful tool to aid in the diagnosis of dementia. There have been many studies with differing results, which are summarized below. Initial studies combined patients with dementia secondary to different etiologies, while more recent papers have analyzed patients with only a single etiology. The research concerning nonspecific dementia cases are included with the discussion of Alzheimer's disease (AD), while dementia secondary to other diseases, such as Parkinsons' disease or multiple sclerosis, are discussed separately.

Goodin et al. (1978b) studied 27 patients with dementia of various etiologies, 26 nondemented, neurology patients, and 40 normal control subjects. The average Mini-Mental State Exam (MMSE) score of the demented subjects was 20.7, and all had scores less than 25. Eighty percent of the demented patients had P3 latencies that were more than 2 standard errors of estimate (SEE) above the age–latency regression line. There was no significant difference of the P3 latency between the nondemented patients and the normal controls. There was also no significant difference between the N1 and P2 latencies of the normals and the demented patients. On the less optimistic side, Pfefferbaum and colleagues (1984b) performed both auditory and visual P3's in 40 demented patients (mean MMSE of 22). On the average, P3 latencies in the demented patients were longer than in controls, but less than 50% had latencies longer than 2 SEE above normal. Brown and colleagues (1982) studied 18 patients with dementia (MMSE score <20), 7 patients with psychiatric diagnoses, and 26 controls. Ten of the demented patients (56%) and none of the psychiatric patients had P3 latencies significantly greater than the mean plus 2 SEE.

Studies focusing more specifically on AD have yielded similar results. Syndulko et al. (1982a) studied 12 demented patients and 45 normal controls. They also observed a prolonged (>2 SEE above normal for age) P3 latency in approximately 80% of patients with presumed AD (MMSE of 20.9, all <27). St. Clair and colleagues (1985) observed that 70% of 15 AD patients had some combination of P3 latency and amplitude abnormalities with no false positives. Polich et al. (1986) observed that only 31% of demented patients (two-thirds of whom had AD) had P3 latencies above 2 SEE from the normal P3 versus age regression line (Fig. 15–5). Later he showed that less than 50% of patients with early AD had P3 latencies greater than 2 standard deviations (SD) above the mean of the age-matched control group (Polich et al., 1990). Ito (1994) observed two-thirds of 12 AD patients (mean MMSE of 20) had P3 latencies above 2 SEE. Duffy and colleagues (1984) analyzed many topographic EP and computerized EEG frequency analysis measures in an attempt to discriminate normals from patients with AD. The P3 measures were not as good discriminants as the EEG measures. Leppler and Greenberg (1984) studied only five subjects in each of several groups, including controls, mild and moderate vascular dementia, and moderate AD. The mean P3 latency was longer than the control mean only for moderately demented patients. In addition, they noted that the behavioral counts were significantly worse for the moderately demented patients than for the controls. Another study also found a very high percentage of erroneous counts in a group of 42 demented patients, of which 34 had AD, compared to controls (Slaets and Fortgens, 1984). Only 12 of 42 gave rare tone counts within 10% of correct. This study found that although demented patients had longer P3 latencies than healthy controls, there was no significant difference in the P3 latency between demented and nondemented patients. Gordon and colleagues (1986a; 1986b) studied 55 controls and 20 demented patients, of which 14 had AD and 6 had vascular dementia. Dividing the groups into those above and below age 63, they obtained a lower false positive rate than simple linear regression and found 12 of 19 (63%) of the demented patients to have P3 latencies above 2 SEE. This group (Kraiuhin et al., 1986) also observed several single psychometric tests to be significantly more sensitive (92%) than the P3 latency in correctly identifying demented patients. Patterson and colleagues (1988) studied 12 patients with AD, 3 patients with vascular dementia, and 27 healthy controls (15 of whom were over age 57). Among the 15 demented patients (mean MMSE of 18.3), only 2 had P3 latencies more than 2 SEE above the age–latency regression line. In addition, they studied single-trial P3 latency variability. Although demented and older subjects had a greater P3 latency variability than younger controls, only four demented patients had variability measures greater than 2 SEE. Neshige et al. (1988a) observed the P3 to be prolonged in just under one-half of 13 patients with AD. While tasks more complex than the simple auditory paradigm may be more sensitive to the deficits in AD, these have not been validated (deToledo-Morrell et al., 1991; Friedman et al., 1992).

There have been several attempts to relate the alterations in P3 to cognitive function in dementia and AD. Canter et al. (1982) studied 10 patients with AD. Although they observed

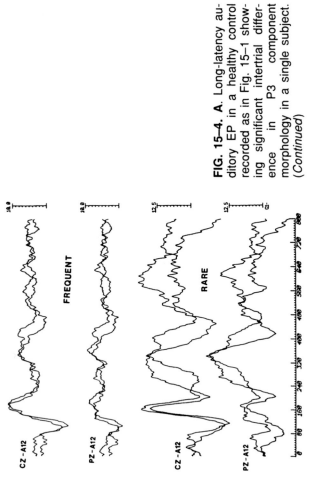

FIG. 15–4. A. Long-latency auditory EP in a healthy control recorded as in Fig. 15–1 showing significant intertrial difference in P3 component morphology in a single subject. (*Continued*)

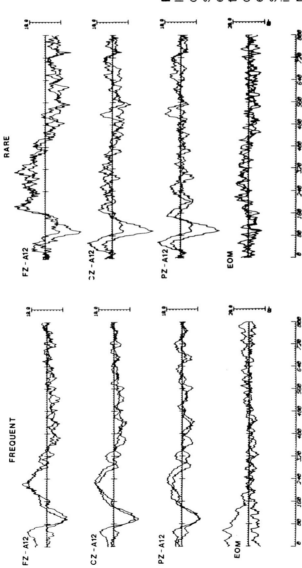

FIG. 15–4. (*Cont'd*) **B**. Long-latency EP in a healthy control demonstrating essentially no P3 component at either the CZ or PZ electrode. A poorly defined P3 component is seen at the FZ electrode. Both subjects shown were 100% accurate in their identification of the rare tones.

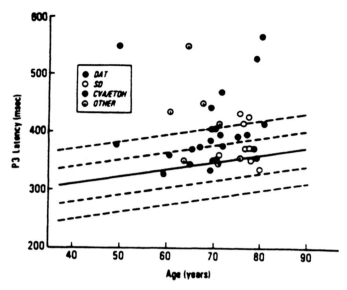

FIG. 15–5. Scattergram of P3 latency in 39 patients who met DSM-III criteria for dementia. Of the 39, 16 had dementia of the Alzheimer's type (DAT), 8 had senile dementia (SD) who would presently be considered to have DAT, 4 had alcoholic dementia (ETOH), 4 had vascular dementia (CVA), and 7 had other types of dementia (OTHER). *Solid* and *dashed lines* represent correlation line ±1 and 2 SEE lines from healthy controls. Only 31% of patients had P3 latencies above the 2 SEE. (From Polich et al., 1986, with permission.)

a significant correlation between the degree of dementia, as measured by the Blessed Dementia Scale, and the amount of delta activity in the EEG frequency analysis, there was no correlation between the degree of dementia and the P3 latency. However, others have found a correlation between the P3 latency and cognitive function, as assessed by the Global Deterioration Scale in a mixed dementia group (two-thirds with AD) (Polich et al., 1986) or with the Weschler Adult Intelligence Scale score in both AD and vascular dementia (Neshige et al., 1988a). Longitudinal studies also have shown that, on average, there is an increase in latency in the P3 with disease progression (Ball et al., 1989; St. Clair et al., 1988). There was no change in the P3 latency or the clinical assessment in 12 AD patients treated with tacrine (THA) (van Gool et al., 1991).

The above studies suggest that P3 latency in a group of patients with dementia is prolonged compared to a group of healthy controls. In addition, the P3 latency is prolonged in a percentage of individual patients with dementia. However, there are several limitations of the studies and of the potential clinical application of P3 testing in dementia. Demented patients, especially moderately to severely impaired patients as were studied by some, tend to produce more incorrect responses in the P3 testing than normal controls. This impaired response accuracy may alter the P3 latency more than the dementia itself and may be as good a screening technique as the P3 itself. In addition, the sensitivity of the test is not that high, ranging in the above studies from 13% to 80% using a cutoff of 2 SEE. Additionally, the important clinical differential diagnosis rests in cases with mild as opposed to moderate or severe dementia. It is in these mild cases that there is a greater overlap between controls and patients, especially in the older age groups. Lastly, some controls may not have a well-defined P3, thus patients with a poorly defined P3 cannot be considered to have an abnormal test result.

2.5.2. Other Degenerative Diseases

The P3 has been studied in several other degenerative diseases. Hansch et al. (1982) analyzed the P3 in 20 patients with idiopathic Parkinson's disease and 20 normal controls. The Parkinson's patients as a group had significantly longer auditory P3 latencies. Only one of five neuropsychological measures correlated strongly with the P3 latency. Goodin and Aminoff (1987) also reported prolonged latencies of P3, as well as N1 and N2, in demented compared to nondemented Parkinson's patients. Other studies have confirmed the P3 prolongation in demented Parkinson's patients both in terms of group comparisons as well as in individual classification of abnormal P3's in perhaps 50% of demented Parkinson's patients (Ebmeier, 1992; Ito, 1994; O'Mahony et al., 1993; Toda et al., 1993). The prolongation of N1 latency has not been confirmed (Ito, 1994; O'Mahony et al., 1993). One study suggested that even nondemented Parkinson's patients may show a decrease in P3 latency with L-dopa therapy (Stanzione et al., 1991). Additional evidence linking the dopamine system in Parkinson's disease with the P3 comes from a nonhuman primate study. The P3 was abolished in methyl-phenyl-tetrahydropyridine (MPTP)-treated monkeys but spontaneously recovered along with behavioral improvement 40 days after MPTP treatment (Glover et al., 1988). During the acute Parkinsonian phase administration of L-dopa did not restore the absent P3 potentials.

Twelve of 13 patients with Huntington's disease had prolonged P3 latencies on either a visual or auditory paradigm (Rosenberg et al., 1985). The authors defined prolonged as greater than mean plus 2 SEE among a control group. Increasing the cutoff to 3 SEE still produced abnormalities in 8 of 13 patients. Another study found that only slightly more than 50% of Huntington's patients had P3 latencies greater than the mean plus 2 SEE (Homberg et al., 1986).

2.5.3. Vascular Dementia

Patients with multiple lacunar infarcts without dementia have normal target P3 latencies, although they have been reported to have abnormal rare nontarget P3 latencies. The sensitivity of the P3 in vascular dementia is comparable to that in AD, with an estimated sensitivity of about 50% (Ito, 1994; Neshige et al., 1988a).

2.5.4. Multiple Sclerosis

It is well-established that patients with multiple sclerosis (MS) may have abnormal brain stem auditory (BAEPs), visual (VEPs), and somatosensory EPs (SEPs). In addition, several studies found longer P3 latencies in patients with MS than in control subjects (Honig et al., 1992; Newton et al., 1989; Polich et al., 1992). However, most patients with MS have P3 latencies that are within the normal range (Newton et al., 1989; Polich et al., 1992). There is evidence that patients with more severe disease, as assessed by MRI, or with more cognitive dysfunction, as assessed by standard neuropsychological tests, have more prolonged P3 latencies (Giesser et al., 1992; Honig et al., 1992). In fact, P3's in patients with mild MS may not even show a group difference from normal controls (Ruchkin et al., 1994). One group increased the sensitivity slightly by inputing the entire ERP waveform into a neural network classifier (Slater et al., 1994). There is conflicting evidence regarding the effect of MS on the N1 or P2 component (Giesser et al., 1992; Honig et al., 1992; Sandroni et al., 1992).

2.5.5. Human Immune Deficiency Virus Infection

Patients with human immune deficiency virus (HIV) infections may develop cognitive dysfunction, especially in later stages of the disease. In a number of studies, anywhere from 33% to 80% of patients who are symptomatic (Centers for Disease Control stages 2 to 4) have N2–P3 complex changes, including delay, amplitude reduction, and loss of waveforms (Arendt et al., 1993; Baldeweg et al., 1993; Coburn et al., 1992; Goodin et al., 1990; Messenheimer et al., 1992; Ollo et al., 1991). In addition to the loss of waveforms, there may be a more variable topography (Baldeweg et al., 1993). The sensitivity has been reported to be higher using visual compared to auditory stimuli (Baldeweg et al., 1993; Ollo et al., 1991). Abnormalities of N1 and P2 were much less commonly observed than those of N2 and P3. Asymptomatic HIV-positive patients have a much lower incidence of abnormal ERPs, with estimated P3 abnormality rates ranging from the same incidence as controls to one-third (Baldeweg et al., 1993; Goodin et al., 1990; Jabbari et al., 1993; Messenheimer et al., 1992; Ollo et al., 1991). The abnormalites of ERP components observed in HIV-positive individuals have been related to psychomotor slowing and slowed reaction time (Baldeweg et al., 1993; Jabbari et al., 1993; Ollo et al., 1991).

2.5.6. Schizophrenia

Multiple investigators have reported a lower-amplitude P3 or P3b in groups of schizophrenics compared to controls (Roth and Cannon, 1972; Shagass et al., 1977; Pfefferbaum et al., 1980c; Roth et al., 1980a, 1980b; Brecher and Begleiter, 1983; Pfefferbaum et al., 1984b; Brecher et al., 1987; Strandburg et al., 1994). Most of these studies have not reported a change in P3 latency. It has been postulated that there is an alteration of P3 topography in schizophrenia (Morstyn et al., 1983; Holinger et al., 1992). However, many patients in these studies have been on psychotropic medications and had fewer correct responses and longer reaction times in the P3 task. However, even if the differences between schizophrenics and controls are related to the pathophysiology of the disease, there is little clinical significance in the difference because there is so much overlap of the P3 amplitude between the patient and control groups.

2.5.7. Metabolic and Toxic Encephalopathies

There have been reports of changes in the P3 in metabolic and toxic encephalopathies. Goodin et al. (1983) observed a positive correlation between fluctuations of severity of various confusional states and P3 latencies in seven patients. Cohen et al. (1983) found 10 of 22 patients with chronic renal failure without clinical evidence of cognitive impairment had P3 latencies greater than 2 SEE above the normal age–latency regression line. The P3 latency was abnormal more frequently than EEG among 66 patients with hepatic encephalopathy and the sensitivity of the P3 was comparable to neuropsychological testing (Weissenborn et al., 1990).

There is some evidence that patients with alcoholism (Pfefferbaum et al., 1979; Porjesz et al., 1980; Begleiter et al., 1980) or subjects with family history of alcoholism (Begleiter et al., 1984) have altered P3's when compared with groups of controls. The P3 latency may be prolonged following exposure to hydrogen sulfide (Wasch et al., 1989) or organic solvents (Morrow et al., 1992).

2.5.8. Pediatric and Congenital Diseases

Finley and colleagues (1985) studied the utility of cognitive EP testing in 243 children with assorted neuropsychiatric diagnoses. They found a high correlation between prolonged P3 latencies (greater than 2 SEE above the age–latency regression line) and evidence of "organicity" on clinical grounds, Halstead–Reitan neuropsychological assessment, and low MMS scores. One study of mentally retarded children found altered long-latency potentials and slow potentials (Martineau et al., 1980), while another study of children with speech and language problems found only an altered ERP topography (Mason and Mellor, 1984).

NK Squires and colleagues (1979) found prolonged P3 latencies in adults with Down's syndrome compared to controls. In patients with Turner's syndrome, the P3's are abnormal on postpubertal but not prepubertal testing (Johnson et al., 1993).

Long-term survivors of childhood cancer who received cranial irradiation were found to have prolonged P3 latencies along with abnormal reaction times upon neuropsychological testing (Moore et al., 1992).

2.5.9. Other Behavioral Neurology

The P3 and other long-latency EPs have been used to investigate the pathophysiology of various neurobehavioral syndromes. These include prosopagnosia (Small, 1988), inattention following prefrontal lesions (Knight et al., 1981; Knight, 1984; Woods and Knight, 1986), visual neglect following unilateral parietal lobe lesions (Lhermitte et al., 1985), anosognosia (Mauguiere et al., 1982), "blindsight" (Shefrin et al., 1988), closed head injury (Rugg et al., 1988; Munte and Heinze, 1994), transient global amnesia (Bokura et al., 1994; Meador et al., 1988), and other memory disorders (St. Clair et al., 1985; Meador et al., 1987; Starr and Barrett, 1987). Patient's with Korskaoff's syndrome did not have any alteration in their P3 (St. Clair et al., 1988).

2.5.10. Summary

There is evidence that the endogenous ERPs may be an occasionally useful, objective, clinical adjunct to behavioral measures of cognitive processes, although this remains controversial (Goodin, 1990; Pfefferbaum et al., 1990). It is important to control for many factors, including age, medications, and behavioral performance. In addition, one needs to be aware of the high variability among normal subjects of the P3 latency and amplitude.

3. MOVEMENT-RELATED POTENTIALS

There are a series of potentials that occur in close temporal relationship with movement or motor activity that are referred to as movement-related potentials (MRPs). These potentials occur before, during, and after the motor activity. The *bereitschaftspotential* (bp) is a slow negative shift, with maximal amplitude over the vertex, that begins approximately 1 sec prior to the onset of electromyographic (EMG) activity (Kornhuber and Deecke, 1965; Gilden et al., 1966; Vaughan et al., 1968). The wave is similar in morphology to the contingent negative variation (see below). The slope of the bp increases several hundred milliseconds prior to the EMG onset. This slow potential shift with a steeper slope than the bp has been referred to by some as the negative shift (NS') (Shibasaki et al., 1980a; Barrett et al., 1986a). This wave is asymmetric, with a greater amplitude over the hemisphere contralateral to the limb performing the motor task (Fig. 15–6). Next, about 50 to 100 msec prior to EMG onset, there is a motor potential presumably related to activity in motor cortical areas that is more directly related to the motor activity. There are also a series of waves

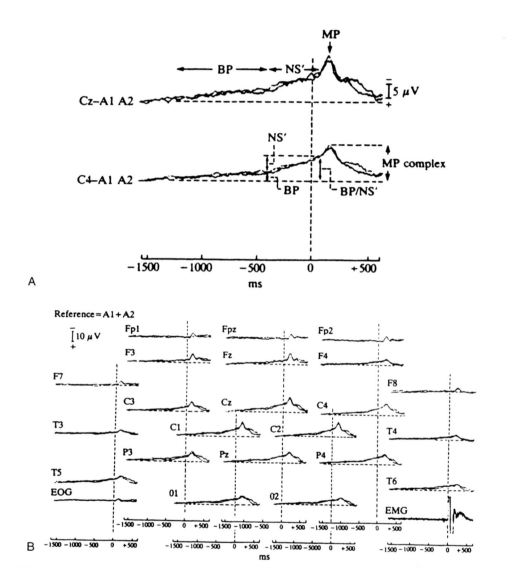

FIG. 15–6. **A.** Nomenclature for the movement-related potentials, with the Bereitschaftspotential (bp), negative slope (NS'), and motor potential (MP) with latency/duration measurement (*top*), and amplitude measurement (*bottom*). **B.** Scalp topography using linked-ear reference of the MRP in a normal subject, with two superimposed trials of 100 to 250 repetitions of self-paced, brisk, voluntary extension of the left middle finger. Averaged EOG and EMG are also shown. Sweep duration is same as in **A**. Note the central maximum and the greater amplitude over the right hemisphere. (From Neshige et al., 1988c, with permission.)

following motor activity that will not be discussed further (e.g., Shibasaki et al., 1980b; for further reviews of the movement-related potentials, see Barrett, 1992, or Hallett, 1994).

3.1. Generators

Initially, indirect evidence suggested that the bp was related to activity in the mesial supplementary motor area (Boschert et al., 1983; Deecke et al., 1978, 1987). More recent data obtained directly from intracranial recordings in humans suggest that there is significant contribution to the bp and NS' from both the sensory motor cortex and the supplementary motor area (Neshige et al., 1988b, 1988c; Ikeda et al., 1992; Rektor et al., 1994; Sakamoto et al., 1991). There may be some differences in relative amount of cortical activity contra- and ipsilateral to the movement depending on whether one analyzes foot, finger, facial, or eye movements. The intracranial recording data also confirm that the generators are quite focal despite the diffuse scalp distribution. Additionally, there is no clear difference between the bp and NS' in terms of cortical activity, and some researchers have begun using the term bp/NS' to reflect that observation. Multichannel scalp recordings have been used to calculate the dipoles that generate the scalp-recorded MRP with similar findings as the intracranial recordings, although the precise contribution of the supplementary motor area is controversial (Bocker et al., 1994; Botzel et al., 1993; Toro et al., 1993a).

There is less controversy regarding the generators of the potentials that are closer temporally to the motor activity than the bp or NS'. Using subdural electrodes, there are potentials arising from 50 to 100 msec prior to (motor potential) and up to 150 msec following the onset of hand EMG activity arising from the contralateral hand pre- and postrolandic area (Lee et al., 1986; Neshige et al., 1988c). However, activation in the supplementary motor area may also be seen during the motor potential (Ikeda et al., 1992).

The presence of a normal bp also requires some normal function in cerebellar pathways. There is no bp prior to hand movement contralateral to cerebellar dentate lesions in humans (Shibasaki et al., 1986), cerebellar outflow lesions in humans (Ikeda et al., 1994), or cerebellar hemispherectomies in monkeys (Sasaki et al., 1979). Cerebellar atrophy in humans also alters the MRPs (Wessel et al., 1994).

The MRPs are partially distinct from the EEG event-related desynchronization as assessed by EEG topography (Toro et al., 1994). The early part of the bp occurs before subjects are aware of the intention to move (Libet et al., 1983).

3.2. Technical Factors

Back-averaging is required to record the MRPs. This requires synchronizing the averager with the onset of EMG activity and averaging EEG activity prior to the onset of the EMG activity. Recording the bp requires averaging from 1 to several seconds prior to the onset of EMG activity, while the cortical potential immediately prior to the EMG activity may require back-averaging only several hundred milliseconds. The potentials related to the movement itself and the postmovement potentials may be analyzed by averaging up to several hundred milliseconds following the EMG activity.

Since the frequency of the bp is very low, the use of DC amplification or very-low-frequency high-pass filters (cutoff frequency no greater than 0.3 Hz) is required. Myoclonus-related potentials may be recorded with higher low-frequency filters (Barrett, 1992). The amplitude of the bp is 5 to 10 μV, which is significantly lower than the EMG, which is about 50 to 100 μV. The number of movements to average to obtain a reasonable signal-to-noise ratio needs to be at least 50 to 100.

3.3. Muscle and Movement Factors

Electromyographic activity used for the MRPs may be recorded with needle or surface electrodes from any muscle that produces well-defined EMG activity with a morphologically consistent onset such as middle-finger extensors (see, e.g., Shibasaki et al., 1980a; Barrett et al., 1986b), intrinsic hand muscles, foot dorsiflexors (Shibasaki et al., 1981a), or extraocular muscles (Kurtzenberg and Vaughan, 1980; Thickbroom and Mastaglia, 1985; Sakamoto et al., 1991). For jerk-locked averaging, the myoclonus or other abnormal movement must be frequent enough to obtain 50 to 100 sweeps within a reasonable time period but not so frequent that a second jerk occurs within the time sweep of the first. The EMG signal should be rectified prior to triggering the back-averaging. Since the EMG morphology may be variable, using offline analysis to manually determine the EMG onset may be more accurate than simple voltage level triggers. Alternatively, computer-assisted techniques for determining the onset of the EMG activity may be used to try to improve the averaging technique (Barrett et al., 1985). When using back-averaging to study myoclonus one needs to study at least several muscle groups to ensure one is back-averaging from the earliest contracting muscle.

The amplitude of the premotor potential is related to the force of the subsequent muscle activity (Wilke and Lansing, 1973; Kutas and Donchin, 1974; Becker and Kristeva, 1980; Hink et al., 1983). In addition, movement of more than one digit, complexity of movement, and temporal sequence of movements may alter the MRP (Benecke et al., 1985; Ikeda et al., 1993; Kitamura et al., 1993a,b; Lang et al., 1989; Simonetta et al., 1991).

3.4. Subject Parameters

The amplitude of the bp decreases with age (Barrett et al., 1986b). The amplitude of the MRPs is also related to some aspects of intention or motivation (McAdam and Seales, 1969; Hink et al., 1982, 1983).

3.5. Clinical Studies

3.5.1. Myoclonus

There are many researchers who have back-averaged the EEG activity prior to the onset of spontaneous myoclonus after the technique was first used by Shibasaki (Shibasaki and Kuroiwa, 1975; Shibasaki et al., 1981b; Hallett et al., 1977; Rothwell et al., 1984). They have found that some patients with myoclonus, who often have no obvious conventional EEG correlate to the myoclonus, have a spike, sharp-wave, slow-wave, or sinusoidal component 20 to 100 msec preceding the myoclonus using back-averaging (Fig. 15–7). Some of the myoclonus-related discharges were greater in amplitude over the hemisphere contralateral to the movement. These time-locked components have been observed in patients with generalized epileptic myoclonus (Wilkins et al., 1985), myoclonic epilepsy (Shibasaki et al., 1985; Kapoor et al., 1991), epilepsia partialis continua (Obeso et al., 1985; Chauvel et al., 1986; Celesia et al., 1994), cortical reflex myoclonus (Hallett et al., 1979; Deuschl et al., 1991; Ikeda et al., 1990; Shibasaki and Neshige, 1987; Shibasaki et al., 1994; Toro et al., 1993b), cerebellar degenerations (Obeso et al., 1985), Alzheimer's-type dementia (Wilkins et al., 1984; Ugawa et al., 1987), and Creutzfeldt–Jakob disease (Shibasaki et al., 1981b, 1985). There have been no time-locked components in patients with posthypoxic myoclonus (Hallett et al., 1977; Obeso et al., 1983a), essential myoclonus (Shibasaki et al., 1978a), myoclonus secondary to corticobasal degeneration (Thompson et al., 1994), myoclonic dystonia (Obeso et al., 1983b), myoclonus secondary to tricyclic medication (Fukuzako et al., 1989), and most myoclonus of subcortical origin (Brown et al., 1991).

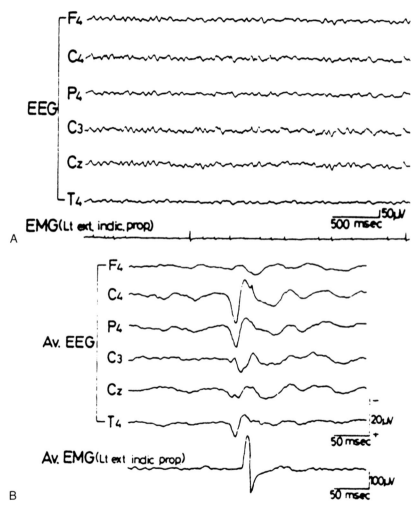

FIG. 15–7. A. Conventional EEG referenced to linked-ear electrodes in a patient with lipidosis and intermittent bilateral myoclonus that was predominantly independent on the two sides. Electromyographic channel demonstrates the myoclonus recorded from surface EMG of the left extensor indicis proprius. There are no obvious EEG correlates to the myoclonic jerks. **B.** Same patient as in **A** using back-averaging from onset of EMG activity with 100 myoclonic jerks averaged. There is a sharp wave maximal over the contralateral central region occurring 16 to 18 msec prior to the EMG onset. (From Shibasakai and Kuroiwa, 1975, with permission.)

These premovement discharges and the giant somatosensory EPs seen in patients with myoclonus (see page 429 of 2nd ed (Myoclonic Epilepsy)) share common physiologic mechanisms (Shibasaki and Kuroiwa, 1975; Shibasaki et al., 1978a; Hallett et al., 1979; Shibasaki et al., 1985; Shibasaki et al., 1994).

3.5.2. Parkinson's Disease

There is some controversy about the effect of Parkinson's disease on the premotor potentials prior to volitional movement (Shibasaki et al., 1978b, Deecke and Kornhuber, 1978; Barrett et al., 1986b; Dick et al., 1987; Dick et al., 1989; Vidailhet et al., 1993). Some of this may relate to differences in controlling for the effects of L-dopa, aging, and force of movement. It seems most likely that the onset of the bp is more gradual in Parkinsonian patients compared to controls but that the peak measured just before movement is the same.

3.5.3. Other Movement Disorders

There are limited data on the utility of the premotor potentials in studying other movement disorders, including functional movement disorders (Toro and Torres, 1986), mirror movements (Shibasaki and Nagae, 1984; Cohen et al., 1991), diagonistic dyspraxia (Yasufumi et al., 1990), and Gilles de la Tourette's syndrome (Obeso et al., 1981). There are no MRPs preceding the dyskinesias or myoclonus in restless legs syndrome (Trenkwalder et al., 1993). One group did report the amplitude of the bp was higher in schizophrenics with tardive dyskinesia compared to those without tardive dyskinesia or age-matched controls (Adler et al., 1989).

There were no premovement potentials prior to the chorea in Huntington's disease, although there was some cortical slow negativity prior to the chorea in chorea-acanthocytosis (Shibasaki et al., 1982). This suggests that the mechanisms underlying "voluntary" and some "involuntary" movements may be similar in terms of the bp.

4. CONTINGENT NEGATIVE VARIATION

The contingent negative variation (CNV) is a slow negative potential shift that was first described by Walter (Walter et al., 1964) (Fig. 15–8). This discussion will be brief because the CNV has no well-accepted clinical utility and has been the subject of several extensive reviews (Tecce, 1972; Hillyard, 1973; Tecce and Cattanach, 1993; McCallum, 1988). The experimental paradigm that most reliably elicits the CNV consists of a warning stimulus followed 1 to several seconds later by an imperative stimulus to which the subject must make a response. The duration of the interval between the warning and imperative stimulus affects the CNV (Loveless and Sanford, 1975; Klorman and Bentsen, 1975; Simons et al., 1983). The response need not be motor and, for example, could be mental counting.

The CNV begins approximately 400 msec after the warning stimulus is presented (Rebert and Knott, 1970) and terminates with the imperative stimulus presentation. The CNV has a very low frequency (<1 Hz) and is present bilaterally, with a maximum amplitude over the midline of about 15 to 20 μV. The topographic distribution of the CNV varies slightly depending on the stimulus modality (see, e.g., Poon et al., 1974).

The CNV appears to represent the summation of at least two, and probably more, component waveforms. There is a stimulus-related frontally predominant negativity, perhaps related to the orienting response, and a centrally predominant negativity thought to be related to the premotor potential associated with the motor response (Loveless and Sanford, 1974a;

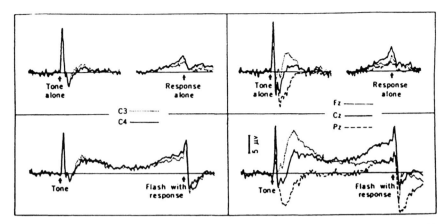

FIG. 15–8. Grand average across 14 subjects of contingent negative variation, with scalp recording C3 and C4 electrodes (*left*), and FZ, CZ, and PZ electrodes (*right*), all to a linked-ear reference. Scalp negativity is displayed as an upward deflection. Top traces show the EP to the tone alone that requires no response (*left*) and the premotor potential from a simple key press referred to as response alone (*right*). Bottom traces are the only ones to show the CNV and used a paired condition where the tone was followed 4 sec later by a light flash requiring a response with the left hand (key press). The early component of the CNV is independent of the premotor potential from the response. (From Rohrbaugh et al., 1976, with permission.)

Rohrbaugh et al., 1976, 1980; Gaillard, 1976; Sanquist et al., 1981; Morgan et al., 1992). The first portion and perhaps part of the second portion of the CNV are independent of the motor response (see, e.g., Loveless and Sanford, 1974a; Simons et al., 1983; Ruchkin et al., 1986; Brunia and Damen, 1988). Additionally, the CNV is present despite an absent bp following a cerebellar outflow lesion (Ikeda et al., 1994). There is a higher amplitude CNV during trials in which the subject has a shorter reaction time (Waszak and Obrist, 1969; Rockstroh et al., 1982). Drowsiness reduces the CNV amplitude (Naitoh et al., 1971; Yamamoto et al., 1984).

4.1. Technical Factors

The CNV should be recorded from a minimum of three scalp electrodes, FZ, CZ, and PZ, and at least one channel for electro-oculographic (EOG) monitoring. Artifacts besides EOG, such as glossokinetic and electrodermal potentials, may also need to be monitored. As with the bp, the use of DC amplification or very-low-frequency high-pass filters (cutoff frequency <0.3 Hz) is required. A warning stimulus of any modality followed by an imperative stimulus of any modality may be used. It is important to record the subject's response to the imperative stimulus since inattention will alter the response. As with other slow potential shifts, there is difficulty and imprecision in measuring the amplitude of the CNV because there is no clearly defined peak.

4.2. Clinical Studies

Aging produces change in the CNV characterized by decreased amplitude (Loveless and Sanford, 1974b; Nakamura et al., 1979; Tecce, 1978; Michalewski et al., 1980) and CNV rebound (Tecce et al., 1982). There are several reports of altered CNV using different paradigms in demented patients (O'Connor, 1980; Tecce et al., 1983; Rizzo et al., 1984).

There have been reports of alterations of CNV in various neurologic and psychiatric disorders. There is some controversy concerning these findings and some of the observed changes may represent effects impaired task performance. There are essentially no data regarding the use of the CNV in a clinical situation where one would need to classify a CNV as normal or abnormal.

Some investigators have reported changes in the CNV with various psychiatric diseases, including anxiety states, schizophrenia, depression, and psychopathic behavior (McCallum and Walter, 1968; Small and Small, 1971; Low and Swift, 1971; Timsit-Berthier et al., 1973; Knott and Irwin, 1973; van den Bosch, 1984; Rizzo et al., 1983; Proulx and Picton, 1984; Raine et al., 1990; Oke et al., 1994; Schneider et al., 1992). Patients with some neurologic disorders also have been reported to have altered CNVs compared to controls, including Gilles de la Tourette's syndrome (Van Woerkom et al., 1988), migraine headaches (Bocker et al., 1990; Gobel et al., 1993; Smits et al., 1993), dyslexia (Chayo-Dichy et al., 1990), and closed head injury (Rugg et al., 1989; Segalowitz et al., 1992). The CNV was not significantly altered in a group of chronic alcoholics (Cadaveira et al., 1991).

ACKNOWLEDGMENT

This chapter was supported in part by grants from NIH (AG08714 and AG08017). The author acknowledges Dana Jones for assistance in preparing the manuscript.

REFERENCES

Adler LE, Pecevich M, Nagamoto H (1989): Bereitschaftspotential in tardive dyskinesia. *Movement Dis* 4:105–112.

American Academy of Neurology Therapeutics and Technology Assessment Subcommittee (1989): Assessment: EEG brain mapping. *Neurology* 39:1100–1101.

Antal A, Bodis-Wollner I, Ghilardi MF, Glover A, Mylin L, Toldi J (1993): The effect of levo-acetyl-carnitine on visual cognitive evoked potentials in the behaving monkey. *Electroencephalogr Clin Neurophysiol* 86:268–274.

Arendt G, Hefter H, Jablonowski H (1993): Acoustically evoked event-related potentials in HIV-associated dementia. *Electroencephalogr Clin Neurophysiol* 86:152–160.

Arthur DL, Starr A (1984): Task-relevant late positive component of the auditory event-related potential in monkeys resembles P300 in humans. *Science* 223:186–188.

Baldeweg T, Gruzelier JH, Catalan J, et al. (1993): Auditory and visual event-related potentials in a controlled investigation of HIV infection. *Electroencephalogr Clin Neurophysiol* 88:356–368.

Ball SS, Marsh JT, Schubarth G, Brown WS, Strandburg R (1989): Longitudinal P300 latency changes in Alzheimer's disease. *J Gerontol* 44:M195–200.

Barrett G (1992): Jerk-locked averaging: technique and application. *J Clin Neurophysiol* 9:495–508.

Barrett G, Shibasaki H, Neshige R (1985): A computer-assisted method for averaging movement-related cortical potentials with respect to EMG onset. *Electroencephalogr Clin Neurophysiol* 60:276–281.

Barrett G, Shibasaki H, Neshige R (1986a): Cortical potentials preceding voluntary movement: evidence for three periods of preparation in man. *Electroencephalogr Clin Neurophysiol* 63:327–339.

Barrett G, Shibasaki H, Neshige R (1986b): Cortical potential shifts preceding voluntary movement are normal in Parkinsonism. *Electroencephalogr Clin Neurophysiol* 63:340–348.

Barrett G, Neshige R, Shibasaki H (1987): Human auditory and somatosensory event-related potentials: effects of response condition and age. *Electroencephalogr Clin Neurophysiol* 66:409–419.

Beck EC, Swanson C, Dustman RE (1980): Long latency components of the visual evoked potential in man: effects of aging. *Exp Aging Res* 6:523–545.

Becker DE, Yingling CD, Fein G (1993): Identification of pain, intensity and P300 components in the pain evoked potential. *Electroencephalogr Clin Neurophysiol* 88:290–301.

Becker W, Kristeva R (1980): Cerebral potentials prior to various force deployments. In: *Motivation, Motor and Sensory Processes of the Brain: Electrical Potentials, Behavior and Clinical Use*, edited by HH Kornhuber and L Deecke, pp 189–194. *Progress in Brain Research*, vol 54. Elsevier/North-Holland, Amsterdam.

Begleiter H, Porjesz B, Tenner M (1980): Neuroradiological and neurophysiological evidence of brain deficits in chronic alcoholics. *Acta Psychiatr Scand* 62(286):3–13.

Begleiter H, Porjesz B, Bihari B, Kissin B (1984): Event-related brain potentials in boys at risk for alcoholism. *Science* 225:1493–1496.

Benecke R, Dick JPR, Rothwell JC, Day BL, Marsden CD (1985): Increase of the bereitschaftspotential in simultaneous and sequential movements. *Neurosci Lett* 62:347–352.

Bocker KBE, Timsit-Berthier M, Schoenen J, Brunia CHM (1990): Contingent negative variation in migraine. *Headache* 30:604–609.

Bocker KBE, Brunia CHM, Cluitmans PJM (1994): A spatio-temporal dipole model of the readiness potential in humans. I. Finger movement. *Electroencephalogr Clin Neurophysiol* 91:275–285.

Bokura H, Yamaguchi S, Tsuchiya H, Yamashita K, Kobayashi S (1994): Reduction of visual P300 during transient global amnesia. *Electroencephalogr Clin Neurophysiol* 92:422–425.

Boschert J, Hink RF, Deecke L (1983): Finger movement versus toe movement-related potentials: further evidence for supplementary motor area (SMA) participation prior to voluntary action. *Brain Res* 52:73–80.

Botzel K, Plendl H, Paulus W, Scherg M (1993): Bereitschaftspotential: is there a contribution of the supplementary motor area? *Electroencephalogr Clin Neurophysiol* 89:187–196.

Brandeis D, Naylor H, Halliday R, Callaway E, Yano L (1992): Scopolamine effects on visual information processing, attention, and event-related potential map latencies. *Psychophysiology* 29:315–336.

Brecher M, Begleiter H (1983): Event-related brain potentials to high-incentive stimuli in unmedicated schizophrenic patients. *Biol Psychiatry* 18:661–674.

Brecher M, Porjesz B, Begleiter H (1987): The N2 component of the event-related potential in schizophrenic patients. *Electroencephalogr Clin Neurophysiol* 66:369–375.

Brown P, Thompson PD, Rothwell JC, Day BL, Marsden CD (1991): Axial myoclonus of propriospinal origin. *Brain* 114:197–214.

Brown WS, Marsh JT, LaRue A (1982): Event-related potentials in psychiatry: differentiating depression and dementia in the elderly. *Bull LA Neurol Soc* 47:91–107.

Brown WS, Marsh JT, LaRue A (1983): Exponential electrophysiological aging: P3 latency. *Electroencephalogr Clin Neurophysiol* 55:277–285.

Brumaghim JT, Klorman R, Strauss J, Lewine JD, Goldstein MG (1987): Does methylphenidate affect information processing? Findings from two studies on performance and P3b latency. *Psychophysiology* 24:361–373.

Brunia CHM, Damen EJP (1988): Distribution of slow brain potentials related to motor preparation and stimulus anticipation in a time estimation task. *Electroencephalogr Clin Neurophysiol* 69:234–243.

Brunia CHM, Mulder G, Verbaten MN (1991): Event-related brain research. *Electroencephalogr Clin Neurophysiology* suppl 42.

Cadaveira F, Grau C, Roso M, Sanchez-Turet M (1991): Multimodality exploration of event-related potentials in chronic alcoholics. *Alcohol Clin Exp Res* 15:607–611.

Callaway E (1983): The pharmacology of human information processing. *Psychopharmacology* 20:359–370.

Callaway E, Halliday R, Herning (1983): A comparison of methods for measuring event-related potentials. *Electroencephalogr Clin Neurophysiol* 55:227–232.

Canter NL, Hallett M, Growdon JH (1982): Lecithin does not affect EEG spectral analysis or P300 in Alzheimer's disease. *Neurology* 32:1260–1266.

Celesia GG, Parmeggiani L, Brigell M (1994): Dipole source localization in a case of epilepsia partialis continua without premyoclonic EEG spikes. *Electroencephalogr Clin Neurophysiol* 90:316–319.

Chapman RM, Bragdon HR (1964): Evoked responses to numerical and non-numerical visual stimuli while problem solving. *Nature* 203:1155–1157.

Chauvel P, Liegeois-Chauvel C, Marquis P, Bancaud J (1986): Distinction between the myoclonus-related potential and the epileptic spike in epilepsia partialis continua. *Electroencephalogr Clin Neurophysiol* 64:304–307.

Chayo-Dichy R, Ostrosky-Solis F, Meneses S, Harmony T, Guevara MA (1990): The late event related potentials CNV and PINV in normal and dyslexic subjects. *Int J Neurosci* 54:347–357.

Coburn KL, Moore NC, Katner HP, Tucker KA, Pritchard WS, Duke DW (1992): HIV and the brain: evidence of early involvement and progressive damage. *NeuroReport* 3:539–541.

Cohen LG, Meer J, Tarkka I, et al (1991): Congenital mirror movements: Abnormal organization of motor pathways in two patients. *Brain* 114:381–403.

Cohen SN, Syndulko K, Rever B, Kraut J, Coburn J, Tourtellotte WW (1983): Visual evoked potentials and long latency event-related potentials in chronic renal failure. *Neurology* 33:1219–1222.

Coons HW, Peloquin L, Klorman R, et al (1981): Effect of methylphenidate on young adults' vigilance and event-related potentials. *Electroencephalogr Clin Neurophysiol* 51:373–387.

Courchesne E (1978): Changes in P3 waves with event repetition: long-term effects on scalp distribution and amplitude. *Electroencephalogr Clin Neurophysiol* 45:754–766.

Courchesne E, Hillyard SA, Galambos R (1975): Stimulus novelty, task relevance and the visual evoked potential in man. *Electroencephalogr Clin Neurophysiol* 39:131–143.

Curran T, Tucker DM, Kutas M, Posner MI (1993): Topography of the N400: brain eletrical activity reflecting semantic expectancy. *Electroencephalogr Clin Neurophysiol* 88:188–209.

deToledo-Morrell L, Evers S, Hoeppner TJ, Morrell F, Garron DC, Fox JH (1991): A 'stress' test for memory dysfunction: Electrophysiologic manifestations of early Alzheimer's disease. *Arch Neurol* 48:605–609.

Deecke L, Kornhuber HK (1978): An electrical sign of participation of the mesial 'supplementary' motor cortex in human voluntary movement. *Brain Res* 159:473–476.

Deecke L, Lang W, Heller HJ, Hufnagl M, Kornhuber HH (1987): Bereitschaftspotential in patients with unilateral lesions of the supplementary motor area. *J Neurol Neurosurg Psychiatr* 50:1430–1434.

Desmedt JE, Robertson D (1977): Differential enhancement of early and late components of the cerebral somatosensory evoked potentials during forced-paced cognitive tasks in man. *J Physiol* 277:761–782.

Desmedt JE, Debecker J, Manil J (1965): Mise en evidence d'un signe electrique cerebral associe a la detection par le sujet d'un stimulus sensoriel tactile. *Bull Acad R Med Belg* 5:887–936.

Deuschl G, Ebner A, Hammers R, Lucking CH (1991): Differences of cortical activation in spontaneous and reflex myoclonias. *Electroencephalogr Clin Neurophysiol* 80:326–328.

Dick JPR, Cantello R, Buruma O, Gioux M, Benecke R, Day BL, Rothwell JC, Thompson PD, Marsden CD (1987): The Bereitschaftspotential, L-DOPA, and Parkinson's disease. *Electroencephalogr Clin Neurophysiol* 66:263–274.

Dick JPR, Rothwell JC, Day BL, et al (1989): The bereitschaftspontential is abnormal in Parkinson's disease. *Brain* 112:233–244.

Donchin E (1981): Surprise!..surprise? *Psychophysiology* 18:493–513.

Donchin E, Cohen L (1967): Averaged evoked potentials and intramodality selective attention. *Electroencephalogr Clin Neurophysiol* 22:537–546.

Duffy FH, Denckla MB, Bartels PH, Sandini G, Kiessling LS (1980): Dyslexia: Automated diagnosis by computerized classification of brain electrical activity. *Ann Neurol* 7:421–428.

Duffy FH, Albert MS, McAnulty G (1984): Brain electrical activity in patients with presenile and senile dementia of the Alzheimer type. *Ann Neurol* 16:439–448.

Duncan-Johnson CC, Donchin E (1977): On quantifying surprise: the variation of event-related potentials with subjective probability. *Psychophysiology* 14:456–467.

Duncan-Johnson CC, Donchin E (1979): The time constant in P300 recording. *Psychophysiology* 16:53–55.

Dustman RE, Emmerson RY, Ruhling RO, et al (1990): Age and fitness effects on EEG, ERPs, visual sensitivity, and cognition. *Neurobiol Aging* 11:193–200.

Ebmeier KP (1992): A quantitative method for the assessment of overall effects from a number of similar electrophysiological studies: description and application to event-related potentials in Parkinson's disease. *Electroencephalogr Clin Neurophysiol* 84:440–446.

Ebmeier KP, Glabus M, Potter DD, Salzen EA (1992): The effect of different high-pass filter settings on peak latencies in the event-related potentials of schizophrenics, patients with Parkinson's disease and controls. *Electroencephalogr Clin Neurophysiol* 84:280–287.

Fabiani M, Gratton G, Karis D, Donchin E (1987): Definition, identification, and reliability of measurement of the P300 component of the event-related brain potential. *Adv Psychophysiol* 2:1–78.

Fein G, Turetsky B (1989): P300 latency variability in normal elderly: effects of paradigm and measurement technique. *Electroencephalogr Clin Neurophysiol* 72:384–394.

Finley WW, Faux SF, Hutcheson J, Amstutz L (1985): Long-latency event-related potentials in the evaluation of cognitive function in children. *Neurology* 35:323–327.

Fitzgerald PG, Picton TW (1981): Temporal and sequential probability in evoked potential studies. *Can J Psychol* 35:188–200.

Fitzpatrick P, Klorman R, Brumaghim JT, Keefover RW (1988): Effects of methylphenidate on stimulus evaluation and response processes: evidence from performance and event-related potentials. *Psychophysiology* 25:292–304.

Foote SL, Berridge CW, Adams LM, Pineda JA (1991): Electrophysiological evidence for the involvement of the locus coeruleus in alerting, orienting, and attending. In: *Progress in Brain Research*, edited by CD Barnes and O Pompeiano, pp 521–532. Elsevier Science Publishers, New York.

Ford JM, Hillyard SA (1981): Event-related potentials (ERPs) to interruptions of a steady rhythm. *Psychophysiology* 322:330.

Ford JM, Roth WT, Kopell BS (1976): Auditory evoked potentials to unpredictable shifts in pitch. *Psychophysiology* 13:32–39.

Ford JM, Pfefferbaum A, Kopell BS (1982): Event-related potentials to a change of pace in a visual sequence. *Psychophysiology* 19:173–177.

Friedman D, Hamberger M, Stern Y, Marder K (1992): Event-related potentials (ERPs) during repetition priming in Alzheimer's patients and young and older controls. *J Clin Exp Neuropsychol* 14:448–462.

Fukuzako H, Hokazono Y, Tominaga H, Hirakawa K, Matsumoto K (1989): Jerk-locked averaging and somatosensory evoked potential in tricyclic-induced myoclonus: a case report. *Jpn J Psychiatr Neurol* 43:645–649.

Gaillard AWK (1976): Effects of warning-signal modality on the contingent negative variation (CNV). *Biol Psychol* 4:139–154.

Geisler MW, Polich J (1990): P300 and time of day: circadian rhythms, food intake and body temperature. *Biol Psychol* 31:117–136.

Giesser BS, Schroeder MM, LaRocca NG, et al (1992): Endogenous event-related potentials as indices of dementia in multiple sclerosis patients. *Electroencephalogr Clin Neurophysiol* 82:320–329.

Gilden L, Vaughan HG, Costa LD (1966): Summated human EEG potentials with voluntary movement. *Electroencephalogr Clin Neurophysiol* 20:433–438.

Glabus MF, Blackwood DHR, Ebmeier KP, et al (1994): Methodological considerations in measurement of the P300 component of the auditory oddball ERP in schizophrenia. *Electroencephalogr Clin Neurophysiol* 90:123–134.

Glover A, Ghilardi MF, Bodis-Wollner I, Onofrj M (1988): Alterations in event-related potentials (ERPs) of MPTP-treated monkeys. *Electroencephalogr Clin Neurophysiol* 71:461–468.

Glover A, Ghilardi MF, Bodis-Wollner I, Onofrj M, Mylin LH (1991): Visual 'cognitive' evoked potentials in the behaving monkey. *Electroencephalogr Clin Neurophysiol* 90:65–72.

Gobel H, Krapat S, Ensink FBM, Soyka D (1993): Comparison of contingent negative variation between migraine interval and migraine attack before and after treatment with sumatriptan. *Headache* 33:570–572.

Goodin DS (1990): Clinical utility of long latency 'cognitive' event-related potentials (P3): the pros. *Electroencephalogr Clin Neurophysiol* 76:2–5.

Goodin DS, Aminoff MJ (1987): Electrophysiological differences between demented and nondemented patients with Parkinson's disease. *Ann Neurol* 21:90–94.

Goodin DS, Squires KC, Henderson BH, Starr A (1978a): Age-related variations in evoked potentials to auditory stimuli in normal human subjects. *Electroencephalogr Clin Neurophysiol* 44:447–458.

Goodin DS, Squires KC, Starr A (1978b): Long latency event-related components of the auditory evoked potential in dementia. *Brain* 101:635–648.

Goodin DS, Starr A, Chippendale T, Squires KC (1983): Sequential changes in the P3 component of the auditory evoked potential in confusional states and dementing illnesses. *Neurology* 33:1215–1218.

Goodin DS, Aminoff MJ, Mantle MM (1986): Subclasses of event-related potentials: response-locked and stimulus-locked components. *Ann Neurol* 20:603–609.

Goodin DS, Aminoff MA, Chernoff DN, Hollander H (1990): Long latency event-related potentials in patients infected with human immunodeficiency virus. *Ann Neurol* 27:414–419.

Goodin DS, Aminoff MJ, Chequer RS (1992): Effect of different high-pass filters on the long-latency event-related auditory evoked potentials in normal human subjects and individuals infected with the human immunodeficiency virus. *J Clin Neurophysiol* 9:97–104.

Goodin D, Desmedt J, Maurer K, Nuwer MR (1994): IFCN recommended standards for long-latency auditory event-related potentials. Report of an IFCN committee. *Electroencephalogr Clin Neurophysiol* 91:18–20.

Gordon E, Kraiuhin C, Harris A, Meares R, Howson A (1986a): The differential diagnosis of dementia using P300 latency. *Biol Psychiatry* 21:1123–1132.

Gordon E, Kraiuhin C, Stanfield P, Meares R, Howson A (1986b): The prediction of normal P3 latency and the diagnosis of dementia. *Neuropsychologia* 24:823–830.

Haider M, Spong P, Lindsley DB (1964): Attention, vigilance, and cortical evoked-potentials in humans. *Science* 145:180–182.

Halgren E, Squires N, Wilson C, Rohrbaugh J, Babb TL, Crandall PH (1980):Endogenous potentials generated in the human hippocampal formation and amygdala by infrequent events. *Science* 210:803–805.

Hallett M (1994): Movement-related cortical potentials. *Electromyogr Clin Neurophysiol* 34:5–13.

Hallett M, Chadwick D, Marsden CD (1979): Cortical reflex myoclonus. *Neurology* 29:1107–1125.

Hallett M, Chadwick D, Adam J, Marsden CD (1977): Reticular reflex myoclonus: a physiological type of posthypoxic myoclonus. *J Neurol Neurosurg Psychiatr* 40:253–264.

Hammond EJ, Meador KJ, Aung-Din R, Wilder BJ (1987): Cholinergic modulation of human P3 event-related potentials. *Neurology* 37:346–350.

Hansch EC, Syndulko K, Cohen SN, Goldberg ZI, Potvin AR, Tourtellotte WW (1982): Cognition in Parkinson disease: an event-related potential perspective. *Ann Neurol* 11:599–607.

Harrison J, Buchwald J (1985): Aging changes in the cat P300 mimic the human. *Electroencephalogr Clin Neurophysiol* 62:227–234.

Hillyard SA (1973): The CNV and human behavior. *Electroencephalogr Clin Neurophysiol* Suppl 33:161–171.

Hillyard SA, Picton TW (1987): Electrophysiology of cognition. In: *Handbook of Physiology. Section 1. The Nervous System,* edited by VB Mountcastle. Vol V. *Higher Functions of the Brain,* edited by F Plum, pp 519–584. American Physiological Society, Bethesda, MD.

Hillyard SA, Squires KC, Bauer JW, Lindsay PH (1971): Evoked potential correlates of auditory signal detection. *Science* 172:1357–1360.

Hink RF, Kohler H, Deecke L and Kornhuber HH (1982): Risk-taking and the human bereitschaftspotential. *Electroencephalogr Clin Neurophysiol* 53:361–373.

Hink RF, Deecke L, Kornhuber HH (1983): Force uncertainty of voluntary movement and human movement-related potentials. *Biol Psychol* 16:197–210.

Holinger DP, Faux SF, Shenton ME, et al (1992): Reversed temporal region asymmetries of P300 topography in left- and right-handed schizophrenic subjects. *Electroencephalogr Clin Neurophysiol* 84:532–537.

Homberg V, Hefter H, Granseyer G, Strauss W, Lange H, Hennerici M (1986): Event-related potentials in patients with Huntington's disease and relatives at risk in relation to detailed psychometry. *Electroencephalogr Clin Neurophysiol* 63:552–569.

Honig LS, Ramsy RE, Sheremata WA (1992): Event-related potential P300 in multiple sclerosis. *Arch Neurol* 49:44–50.

Ikeda A, Kakigi R, Funai N, Neshige R, Kuroda Y, Shibasaki H (1990): Cortical tremor: a variant of cortical reflex myoclonus. *Neurology* 40:1561–1565.

Ikeda A, Luders HO, Burgess RC, Shibasaki H (1992): Movement-related potentials recorded from supplementary motor area and primary motor area. Role of supplementary motor area in voluntary movements. *Brain* 115:1017–1043.

Ikeda A, Luders HO, Burgess RC, Shibasaki H (1993): Movement-related potentials associated with single and repetitive movements recorded from human supplementary motor area. *Electroencephalogr Clin Neurophysiol* 89:269–277.

Ikeda A, Shibasaki H, Nagamine T, et al (1994): Dissociation between contingent negative variation and bereitschaftspotential in a patient with cerebellar efferent lesion. *Electroencephalogr Clin Neurophysiol* 90:359–364.

Ito J (1994): Somatosensory event-related potentials (ERPs) in patients with different types of dementia. *J Neurol Sci* 12:139–146.

Jabbari B, Coats M, Salazar A, Martin A, Scherokman B, Laws WA (1993): Longitudinal study of EEG and evoked potentials in neurologically asymptomatic HIV infected subjects. *Electroencephalogr Clin Neurophysiol* 86:145–151.

John ER, Prichep LS, Fridman J, Easton P (1988): Neurometrics: computer-assisted differential diagnosis of brain dysfunctions. *Science* 239:162–169.

Johnson R, Donchin E (1980): P300 and stimulus categorization: two plus one is not so different from one plus one. *Psychophysiology* 17:167–178.

Johnson R, Rohrbaugh JW, Ross JL (1993): Altered brain development in Turner's syndrome: an event-related potential study. *Neurology* 43:801–808.

Kapoor R, Griffin G, Barrett G, Fowler CJ (1991): Myoclonic epilepsy in an HIV positive patient: neurophysiological findings. *Electroencephalogr Clin Neurophysiol* 78:80–84.

Karniski W, Blair RC (1989): Topographical and temporal stability of the P300. *Electroencephalogr Clin Neurophysiol* 72:373–383.

Kileny PR, Kripal JP (1987): Test-retest variability of auditory event-related potentials. *Ear Hear* 110–114.

Kitamura J, Shibasaki H, Kondo T. (1993a): A cortical slow potential is larger before an isolated movement of a single finger than simultaneous movement of two fingers. *Electroencephalogr Clin Neurophysiol* 86:252–258.

Kitamura J, Shibasaki H, Takagi A, Nabeshima H, Yamaguchi A (1993b): Enhanced negative slope of cortical potentials before sequential as compared with simultaneous extensions of two fingers. *Electroencephalogr Clin Neurophysiol* 86:176–182.

Klinke R, Fruhstorfer H, Finkenzeller P (1968): Evoked responses as a function of external and stored information. *Electroencephalogr Clin Neurophysiol* 25:119–122.

Klorman R, Bentsen E (1975): Effects of warning-signal duration on the early and late components of the contingent variation. *Biol Psychol* 3:263–275.

Klorman R, Brumaghim JT (1991): Stimulant drugs and ERPs. In: *Event-Related Brain Research*, edited by CHM Brunia, G Mulder, and MN Verbaten, pp 135–141. Elsevier Science Publishers, New York.

Knight RT (1984): Decreased response to novel stimuli after prefrontal lesions in man. *Electroencephalogr Clin Neurophysiol* 59:9–20.

Knight RT, Hillyard SA, Woods DL, Neville HJ (1981): The effects of frontal cortex lesions on event-related potentials during auditory selective attention. *Electroencephalogr Clin Neurophysiol* 52:571–582.

Knight RT, Scabini D, Woods DL, Clayworth CC (1989): Contributions of temporal-parietal junction to the human auditory P3. *Brain Res* 502:109–116.

Knott JR, Irwin DA (1973): Anxiety, stress, and the contingent negative variation. *Arch Gen Psychiatry* 29: 538–541.

Kornhuber HH, Deecke L (1965): Hirnpotentialanderungen bei Willkurbewegungen und passiven Bewegungen des Menschen: Bereitschaftspotential und reafferente Potentiale. *Pflugers Arch Physiol* 284:1–17.

Kraiuhin C, Gordon E, Meares R, Howson A (1986): Psychometrics and event-related potentials in the diagnosis of dementia. *J Gerontol* 41:154–162.

Kropotov JD, Ponomarev VA (1991): Subcortical neuronal correlates of component P300 in man. *Electroencephalogr Clin Neurophysiol* 78:40–49.

Kurtzenberg D, Vaughan HG, Jr (1980): Differential topography of human eye movement potentials preceding visually triggered and self-initiated saccades. In: *Motivation, Motor and Sensory Processes of the Brain: Electrical Potentials, Behavior and Clinical Use*, edited by HH Kornhuber and L Deecke, pp 203–208. *Progress in Brain Research*, vol 54, Elsevier/North-Holland, Amsterdam.

Kutas M, Donchin E (1974): Studies of squeezing: handedness, responding hand, response force, and asymmetry of readiness potential. *Science* 186:545–547.

Kutas M, Hillyard SA (1980): Reading senseless sentences: brain potentials reflect semantic incongruity. *Science* 207:203–205.

Kutas M, Iragui V, Hillyard SA (1994): Effects of aging on event-related brain potentials (ERPs) in a visual detection task. *Electroencephalogr Clin Neurophysiol* 92:126–139.

Lang W, Zilch O, Koska C, Lindinger G, Deecke L (1989): Negative cortical DC shifts preceding and accompanying simple and complex sequential movements. *Exp Brain Res* 74:99–104.

Lee BI, Luders H, Lesser RP, Dinner DS, Morris HH (1986): Cortical potentials related to voluntary and passive finger movements recorded from subdural electrodes in humans. *Ann Neurol* 20:32–37.

Leppler JG, Greenberg HJ (1984): The P3 potential and its clinical usefulness in the objective classification of dementia. *Cortex* 20:427–433.

Lhermitte F, Turell E, LeBrigand D, Chain F (1985): Unilateral visual neglect and wave P 300. *Arch Neurol* 42:567–573.

Libet B, Gleason CA, Wright EW, Pearl DK (1983): Time of conscious intention to act in relation to onset of cerebral activity (readiness-potential). The unconscious initiation of a freely voluntary act. *Brain* 106:623–642.

Loring DW, Meador KJ (1989): Central nervous system effects of antihistamines on evoked potentials. *Ann Allergy* 63:604–608.

Loveless NE, Sanford AJ (1974a): Slow potential correlates of preparatory set. *Biol Psychol* 1:303–314.

Loveless NE, Sanford AJ (1974b): Effects of age on the contingent negative variation and preparatory set in a reaction-time task. *J Gerontol* 29:52–63.

Loveless NE, Sanford AJ (1975): The impact of warning signal intensity on reaction time and components of the contingent negative variation. *Biol Psychology* 2:217–226.

Low MD, Swift SJ (1971): The contingent negative variation and the "resting" D.C. potential of the human brain: effects of situational anxiety. *Neuropsychologia* 9:203–208.

Magliero A, Bashore TR, Coles MGH, Donchin E (1984): On the dependence of P300 latency on stimulus evaluation processes. *Psychophysiology* 21:171–186.

Martin L, Barajas JJ, Fernandez R, Torres E (1988): Auditory event-related potentials in well-characterized groups of children. *Electroencephalogr Clin Neurophysiol* 71:375–381.

Martineau J, Laffont F, Bruneau N, Roux S, Lelord G (1980): Event-related potentials evoked by sensory stimulation in normal, mentally retarded and autistic children. *Electroencephalogr Clin Neurophysiol* 48:140–153.

Mason SM, Mellor DH (1984): Brain-stem, middle latency and late cortical evoked potentials in children with speech and language disorders. *Electroencephalogr Clin Neurophysiol* 59:297–309.

Mauguiere F, Brechard S, Pernier J, Courjon J, Schott B (1982): Anosognosia with hemiplegia: auditory evoked potential studies. In: *Clinical Applications of Evoked Potentials in Neurology,* edited by J Courjon, F Mauguiere, and M Revol, pp 271–278. Raven Press, New York.

McAdam DW, Seales DM (1969). Bereitschafts potential enhancement with increased level of motivation. *Electroencephalogr Clin Neurophysiol* 27:73–75.

McCallum WC (1988): Potentials related to expectancy, preparation and motor activity. In: *Human Event-Related Potentials,* edited by TW Picton, pp 427–534. *Handbook of Electroencephalography and Clinical Neurophysiology,* revised series, vol 3. Elsevier, New York.

McCallum WC, Walter WG (1968): The effects of attention and distraction on the contingent negative variation in normal and neurotic subjects. *Electroencephalogr Clin Neurophysiol* 25:319–329.

McCarthy G, Donchin E. (1981): A metric for thought: a comparison of P300 latency and reaction time. *Science* 211:77–80.

Meador KJ, Hammond EJ, Loring DW, Allen M, Bowers D, Heilman KM (1987): Cognitive evoked potentials and disorders of recent memory. *Neurology* 37:526–529.

Meador KJ, Loring DW, King DW, Nichols FT (1988a): The P3 evoked potential and transient global amnesia. *Arch Neurol* 45:465–467.

Meador KJ, Loring DW, Lee GP, Taylor HS, Hughes DR, Feldman DS (1988b): In vivo probe of central cholinergic systems. *J Gerontol* 43:M158–M162.

Meador KJ, Loring DW, Thompson EE, Thompson WO (1989a): Differential cognitive effects of terfenadine and chlorpheniramine. *J Allergy Clin Immunol* 84:322–325.

Meador KJ, Loring DW, Davis HC, et al (1989b): Cholinergic and serotonergic effects on the P3 potential and recent memory. *J Clin Exp Neuropsychol* 11:252–260.

Meador KJ, Loring DW, Huh K, Gallagher BB, King DW (1990): Comparative cognitive effects of anticonvulsants. *Neurology* 40:391–394.

Meador KJ, Loring DW, Allen ME, et al (1991): Comparative cognitive effects of carbamazepine and phenytoin in healthy adults. *Neurology* 41:1537–1540.

Messenheimer JA, Robertson KR, Wilkins JW, Kalkowski JC, Hall CD (1992): Event-related potentials in human immunodeficiency virus infection. *Arch Neurol* 49:396–400.

Michalewski HJ, Thompson LW, Smith DBD, Patterson JV, Bowman TE, Litzelman D, Brent G (1980): Age differences in the contingent negative variation (CNV): reduced frontal activity in the elderly. *J Gerontol* 35:542–549.

Moore III BD, Copeland DR, Ried H, Levy B (1992): Neurophysiological basis of cognitive deficits in long-term survivors of childhood cancer. *Arch Neurol* 49:809–817.

Morgan JM, Wenzl M, Lang W, Lindinger G, Deecke L (1992): Frontocentral DC-potential shifts predicting behavior with or without a motor task. *Electroencephalogr Clin Neurophysiol* 83:378–388.

Morrow LA, Steinhauer SR, Hodgson MJ (1992): Delay in P300 latency in patients with organic solvent exposure. *Arch Neurol* 49:315–320.

Morstyn R, Duffy FH, McCarley RW (1983): Altered P300 topography in schizophrenia. *Arch Gen Psychiatry* 40:729–734.

Mullis RJ, Holcomb PJ, Diner BC, Dykman RA (1985): The effects of aging on the P3 component of the visual event-related potential. *Electroencephalogr Clin Neurophysiol* 62:141–149.

Munte TF, Heinze HJ (1994): Brain potentials reveal deficits of language processing after closed head injury. *Arch Neurol* 51:482–493.

Naatanen R (1970): Evoked potential, EEG and slow potential correlates of selective attention. *Acta Psychol* 33 (Suppl):178–192.

Naatanen R (1979): Early selective attention effects on the evoked potential: a critical review and reinterpretation. *Biol Psychology* 8:81–136.

Naatanen R (1992): *Attention and Brain Function*. Erlbaum, Hillsdale, NJ.

Naitoh P, Johnson LC, Lubin A (1971): Modification of surface negative slow potential (CNV) in the human brain after total sleep loss. *Electroencephalogr Clin Neurophysiol* 30:17–22.

Nakamura M, Fukui Y, Kadobayashi I, Kato N (1979): A comparison of the CNV in young and old subjects. Its relation to memory and personality. *Electroencephalogr Clin Neurophysiol* 46:337–344.

Naylor H, Halliday R, Callaway E (1985): The effect of methylphenidate on information processing. *Psychopharmacology* 86:90–95.

Neshige R, Luders H (1988): Identification of a negative bitemporal component of the event-related potentials demonstrated by noncephalic recordings. *Neurology* 38:1803–1805.

Neshige R, Barrett G, Shibasaki H (1988a): Auditory long latency event-related potentials in Alzheimer's disease and multi-infarct dementia. *J Neurol Neurosurg Psychiatry* 51:1120–1125.

Neshige R, Luders H, Friedman L, Shibaskai H (1988b): Recording of movement-related potentials from the human cortex. *Ann Neurol* 24:439–445.

Neshige R, Luders H, Shibasaki H (1988c): Recording of movement-related potentials from scalp and cortex in man. *Brain* 111:719–736.

Newton MR, Barrett G, Callanan MM, Towell AD (1989): Cognitive event-related potentials in multiple sclerosis. *Brain* 112:1637–1660.

Nielson-Bohlman L, Knight RT, Woods DL, Woodward K (1991): Differential auditory processing continues during sleep. *Electroencephalogr Clin Neurophysiol* 79:281–290.

Obeso JA, Rothwell JC, Marsden CD (1981): Simple tics in Gilles de la Tourette's syndrome are not prefaced by a normal premovement EEG potential. *J Neurol Neurosurg Psychiatry* 44:735–738.

Obeso JA, Lang AE, Rothwell JC, Marsden CD (1983a): Postanoxic symptomatic oscillatory myoclonus. *Neurology* 33:240–243.

Obeso JA, Rothwell JC, Lang AE, Marsden CD (1983b): Myoclonic dystonia. *Neurology* 33:825–830.

Obeso JA, Rothwell JC, Marsden CD (1985): The spectrum of cortical myoclonus. *Brain* 108:193–224.

O'Connor KP (1980): Slow potential correlates of attention dysfunction in senile dementia. *Biol Psychol* 11:193–202; 11:203–216.

Okada YC, Kaufman L, Williamson SJ (1983): The hippocampal formation as a source of the slow endogenous potentials. *Electroencephalogr Clin Neurophysiol* 55:417–426.

Oke S, Saatchi R, Allen E, Hudson NR, Jervis BW (1994): The contingent negative variation in positive and negative types of schizophrenia. *Am J Psychiatry* 151:432–433.

Oken BS, Chiappa KH (1986): Statistical issues concerning computerized analysis of brainwave topography. *Ann Neurol* 19:493–494.

Oken BS, Kaye JA (1992): Electrophysiologic function in the healthy, extremely old. *Neurology* 42:519–526.

Oken BS, Salinsky M (1992): Alertness and attention: basic science and electrophysiologic correlates. *J Clin Neurophysiol* 9:480–494.

Ollo C, Johnson R, Grafman J (1991): Signs of cognitive change in early HIV disease: an event-related brain potential study. *Neurology* 41:209–215.

O'Mahony D, Rowan M, Feely J, O'Neill D, Walsh JB, Coakley D (1993): Parkinson's dementia and Alzheimer's dementia: an evoked potential comparison. *Gerontology* 39:228–240.

Onofrj M, Fulgente T, Nobilio D, et al (1992): P3 recordings in patients with bilateral temporal lobe lesions. *Neurology* 42:1762–1767.

Paller KA, McCarthy G, Roessler E, Allison T, Wood CC (1992): Potentials evoked in human and monkey medial temporal lobe during auditory and visual oddball paradigms. *Electroencephalogr Clin Neurophysiol* 84:269–279.

Papanicolaou AC, Loring DW, Raz N, Eisenberg HM (1985): Relationship between stimulus intensity and the P300. *Psychophysiology* 22:326–329.

Parasuraman R, Beatty J (1980): Brain events underlying detection and recognition of weak sensory signals. *Science* 210:80–83.

Patterson JV, Michalewski HJ, Starr A (1988): Latency variability of the components of auditory event-related potentials to infrequent stimuli in aging, Alzheimer-type dementia, and depression. *Electroencephalogr Clin Neurophysiol* 71:450–460.

Perrault N, Picton TW (1984a): Event-related potentials recorded from the scalp and nasopharynx. I. N1 and P2. *Electroencephalogr Clin Neurophysiol* 59:177–194.

Perrault N, Picton TW (1984b): Event-related potentials recorded from the scalp and nasopharynx. II. N2, P3 and slow wave. *Electroencephalogr Clin Neurophysiol* 59:261–278.

Pfefferbaum A, Horvath TB, Roth WT, Kopell BS (1979): Event-related potential changes in chronic alcoholics. *Electroencephalogr Clin Neurophys* 47:637–647.

Pfefferbaum A, Ford JM, Roth WT, Kopell BS (1980a): Age differences in P3-reaction time associations. *Electroencephalogr Clin Neurophysiol* 49:257–265.

Pfefferbaum A, Ford JM, Roth WT, Kopell BS (1980b): Age-related changes in auditory event-related potentials. *Electroencephalogr Clin Neurophysiol* 49:266–276.

Pfefferbaum A, Horvath TB, Roth WT, Tinklenberg JR, Kopell BS (1980c): Auditory brain stem and cortical evoked potentials in schizophrenia. *Biol Psychiatry* 15:209–223.

Pfefferbaum A, Ford J, Johnson R, Wenegrat B, Kopell BS (1983): Manipulation of P3 latency: speed vs. accuracy instructions. *Electroencephalogr Clin Neurophysiol* 55:188–197.

Pfefferbaum A, Ford JM, Wenegrat BG, Roth WT, Kopell BS (1984a): Clinical application of the P3 component of event-related potentials. I. Normal aging. *Electroencephalogr Clin Neurophysiol* 59:85–103.

Pfefferbaum A, Wenegrat BG, Ford JM, Roth WT, Kopell BS (1984b): Clinical application of the P3 component of event-related potentials. II. Dementia, depression and schizophrenia. *Electroencephalogr Clin Neurophysiol* 59:104–124.

Pfefferbaum A, Ford JM, Kraemer HC (1990): Clinical utility of long latency 'cognitive' event-related potentials (P3): the cons. *Electroencephalogr Clin Neurophysiol* 76:6–12.

Picton TW, Hillyard SA (1974): Human auditory evoked potentials. II: effects of attention. *Electroencephalogr Clin Neurophysiol* 36:191–199.

Picton TW, Hillyard SA, Krausz HI, Galambos R (1974): Human auditory evoked potentials. I: evaluation of components. *Electroencephalogr Clin Neurophysiol* 36:179–190.

Picton TW, Hillyard SA, Galambos R (1976): Habituation and attention in the auditory system. In: *Auditory System: Clinical and Special Topics*, edited by WK Keidel and WD Neff, pp 344–389. Springer-Verlag, Berlin, Heidelberg, New York.

Picton TW, Stuss DW, Champagne SC, Nelson RF (1984): The effects of age on human event-related potentials. *Psychophysiology* 21:312–325.

Pineda JA, Foote SL, Neville HJ, Holmes TC (1988): Endogenous event-related potentials in monkey: the role of task relevance, stimulus probability, and behavioral response. *Electroencephalogr Clin Neurophysiol* 70:155–171.

Polich J (1986a): Attention, probability, and task demands as determinants of P300 latency from auditory stimuli. *Electroencephalogr Clin Neurophysiol* 63:251–259.

Polich J (1986b): Normal variation of P300 from auditory stimuli. *Electroencephalogr Clin Neurophysiol* 65:236–240.

Polich J (1987): Task difficulty, probability, and inter-stimulus interval as determinants of P300 from auditory stimuli. *Electroencephalogr Clin Neurophysiol* 68:311–320.

Polich J (1989): Frequency, intensity, and duration as determinants of P300 from auditory stimuli. *J Clin Neurophysiol* 6:277–286.

Polich J (1991a): P300 in clinical applications: meaning, method, and measurement. *Am J Electroencephalogr Technol* 31:201–231.

Polich J (1991b): P300 in the evaluation of aging and dementia. In: *Event-Related Brain Research*, edited by CHM Brunia, G Mulder, MN Verbaten, pp 304–323. Elsevier Science Publishers, New York.

Polich J, Geisler MW (1991): P300 seasonal variation. *Biol Psychol* 32:173–179.

Polich J, Squire LR (1993): P300 from amnestic patients with bilateral hippocampal lesions. *Electroencephalogr Clin Neurophysiol* 86:408–417.

Polich J, Howard L, Starr A (1985): Effects of age on the P300 component of the event-related potential from auditory stimuli: peak definition, variation, and measurement. *J Gerontol* 40:721–726.

Polich J, Ehlers CL, Otis S, Mandell AJ, Bloom FE (1986): P300 latency reflects the degree of cognitive decline in dementing illness. *Electroencephalogr Clin Neurophysiol* 63:138–144.

Polich J, Ladish C, Bloom FE (1990): P300 assessment of early Alzheimer's disease. *Electroencephalogr Clin Neurophysiol* 77:179–189.

Polich J, Romine JS, Sipe JC, Aung M, Dalessio DJ (1992): P300 in multiple sclerosis: a preliminary report. *Int J Psychophysiol* 12:155–163.

Polich J, Eischen SE, Collins GE (1994): P300 from a single auditory stimulus. *Electroencephalogr Clin Neurophysiol* 92:253–261.

Poon LW, Thompson LW, Williams, Jr. RB, Marsh GR (1974): Changes of antero-posterior distribution of CNV and late positive component as a function of information processing demands. *Psychophysiology* 11:660–673.

Porjesz B, Begleiter H, Samuelly I (1980): Cognitive deficits in chronic alcoholics and elderly subjects assessed by evoked brain potentials. *Acta Psychiatr Scand* 62(186):15–19.

Proulx GB, Picton TW (1984): The effects of anxiety and expectancy on the CNV. *Ann NY Acad Sci* 425:617–622.

Puce A, Donnan GA, Bladin PF (1989): Comparative effects of age on limbic and scalp P3. *Electroencephalogr Clin Neurophysiol* 74:385–393.

Puce A, Berkovic SF, Cadusch PJ, Bladin PF (1994): P3 latency jitter assessed using 2 techniques. I. Simulated data and surface recordings in normal subjects. *Electroencephalogr Clin Neurophysiol* 92:352–364.

Raine A, Venables PH, Williams M (1990): Relationships between N1, P300, and contingent negative variation recorded at age 15 and criminal behavior at age 24. *Psychophysiology* 27:567–574.

Rebert CS, Knott JR (1970): The vertex non-specific evoked potential and latency of contingent negative variation. *Electroencephalogr Clin Neurophysiol* 28:561–565.

Rektor I, Feve A, Buser P, Bathien N, Lamarche M (1994): Intracerebral recording of movement related readiness potentials: an exploration in epileptic patients. *Electroencephalogr Clin Neurophysiol* 90:273–283.

Renault B, Ragot R, Lesevre N, Remond A (1982): Onset and offset of brain events as indices of mental chronometry. *Science* 215:1413–1415.

Ritter W, Vaughan HG, Costa LD (1968): Orienting and habituation to auditory stimuli: a study of short term changes in average evoked responses. *Electroencephalogr Clin Neurophysiol* 25:550–556.

Ritter W, Simson R, Vaughan HG (1972): Auditory cortex potentials and reaction time in auditory discrimination. *Electroencephalogr Clin Neurophysiol* 33:547–555.

Ritter W, Simson R, Vaughan HG (1983): Event-related potential correlates of two stages of information processing in physical and semantic discrimination tasks. *Psychophysiology* 20:168–179.

Rizzo PA, Spadaro M, Albani G, Morocutti C (1983): Contingent negative variation and phobic disorders. *Neuropsychobiology* 9:73–77.

Rizzo PA, Albani G, Cicardi C, Spadaro M, Morocutti (1984): Effects of distraction on the contingent negative variation in presenile dementia and normal subjects. *Neuropsychobiology* 12:112–114.

Rockstroh B, Elbert T, Lutzenberger W, Birbaumer N (1984): The effects of slow cortical potentials on response speed. *Psychophysiology* 19:211–217.

Rockstroh B, Elbert T, Lutzenberger W, Altenmuller E (1991): Effects of the anticonvulsant benzodiazepine clonazepam on event-related brain potentials in humans. *Electroencephalogr Clin Neurophysiol* 78:142–149.

Rohrbaugh JW, Syndulko K, Lindsley DB (1976): Brain wave components of the contingent negative variation in humans. *Science* 191:1055–1057.

Rohrbaugh JW, Syndulko K, Sanquist TF, Lindsley DB (1980): Synthesis of the contingent negative variation brain potential from noncontingent stimulus and motor elements. *Science* 208:1165–1168.

Rohrbaugh JW, Parasuraman R and Johnson R (eds) (1990): *Event-Related Brain Potentials.* Oxford University Press, New York.

Rosenberg C, Nudleman K, Starr A (1985): Cognitive evoked potentials (P300) in early Huntington's disease. *Arch Neurol* 42:984–987.

Roth WT (1973): Auditory evoked responses to unpredictable stimuli. *Psychophysiology* 10:125–138.

Roth WT, Cannon EH (1972): Some features of the auditory evoked responses in schizophrenics. *Arch Gen Psychiatry* 27:466–471.

Roth WT, Horvath TB, Pfefferbaum A, Kopell BS (1980a): Event-related potentials in schizophrenics. *Electroencephalogr Clin Neurophysiol* 48:127–139.

Roth WT, Pfefferbaum A, Horvath TB, Berger, Kopell (1980b): P3 reduction in auditory evoked potentials of schizophrenics. *Electroencephalogr Clin Neurophysiol* 49:497–505.

Roth WT, Blowers GH, Doyle CM, Kopell BS (1982): Auditory stimulus intensity effects on components of the late positive complex. *Electroencephalogr Clin Neurophysiol* 54:132–146.

Rothwell JC, Obeso JA, Marsden CD (1984): On the significance of giant somatosensory evoked potentials in cortical myoclonus. *J Neurol Neurosurg Psychiatr* 47:33–42.

Ruchkin DS, Sutton S, Kietzman ML, Silver K (1980): Slow wave and P300 in signal detection. *Electroencephalogr Clin Neurophysiol* 50:35–47.

Ruchkin DS, Sutton S, Mahaffey D, Glaser J (1986): Terminal CNV in the absence of motor response. *Electroencephalogr Clin Neurophysiol* 63:445–463.

Ruchkin DS, Grafman J, Krauss GL, Johnson Jr. R, Canoune H, Ritter W (1994): Event-related brain potential evidence for a verbal working memory deficit in multiple sclerosis. *Brain* 117:289–305.

Rugg MD, Cowan CP, Nagy ME, Milner AD, Jacobson I (1988): Event related potentials from closed head injury patients in an auditory "oddball" task: evidence of dysfunction in stimulus categorisation. *J Neurol Neurosurg Psychiatr* 51:691–698.

Rugg MD, Cowan CP, Nagy ME, Milner AD, Jacobson I, Brooks DN (1989): CNV abnormalities following closed head injury. *Brain* 112:489–506.

St. Clair DM, Blackwood DHR, Christie JE (1985): P3 and other long latency auditory evoked potentials in presenile dementia Alzheimer type and alcoholic Korsakoff syndrome. *Br J Psychiatry* 147:702–706.

St. Clair D, Blackburn I, Blackwood D, Tyrer G (1988): Measuring the course of Alzheimer's disease. *Br J Psychiatr* 152:48–54.

Sakamoto A, Luders H, Burgess R (1991): Intracranial recordings of movement-related potentials to voluntary saccades. *J Clin Neurophysiol* 8:223–233.

Sandroni P, Walker C, Starr A (1992): 'Fatigue' in patients with multiple sclerosis. *Arch Neurol* 49:517–524.

Sanquist TF, Beatty JT, Lindsley DB (1981): Slow potential shifts of human brain during forewarned reaction. *Electroencephalogr Clin Neurophysiol* 51:639–649.

Sasaki K, Gemba H, Hashimoto S, Mizuno N (1979): Influences of cerebellar hemispherectomy on slow potentials in the motor cortex preceding self-paced hand movements in the monkey. *Neurosci Lett* 15:23–28.

Schneider F, Heimann H, Mattes R, Lutzenberger W, Birbaumer N (1992): Self-regulation of slow cortical potentials in psychiatric patients: depression. *Biofeedback Self-Regulation* 17:203–214.

Segalowitz SJ, Unsal A, Dywan J (1992): CNV evidence for the distinctiveness of frontal and posterior neural processes in a traumatic brain-injured population. *J Clin Exp Neuropsychol* 14:545–565.

Shagass C, Straumanis JJ, Roemer RA, Amadeo M (1977): Evoked potentials of schizophrenics in several sensory modalities. *Biol Psychiatry* 12:221–235.

Shefrin SL, Goodin DG, Aminoff MJ (1988): Visual evoked potentials in the investigation of "blindsight". *Neurology* 38:104–109.

Shibasaki H, Kuroiwa Y (1975): Electroencephalographic correlates of myoclonus. *Electroencephalogr Clin Neurophysiol* 39:455–463.

Shibasaki H, Nagae K (1984): Mirror movement: application of movement-related cortical potentials. *Ann Neurol* 15:299–302.

Shibasaki H, Neshige R (1987): Photic cortical reflex myoclonus. *Ann Neurol* 22:252–257.

Shibasaki H, Yamashita Y, Kuroiwa Y (1978a): Electroencephalographic studies of myoclonus. *Brain* 101: 447–460.

Shibasaki H, Shima F, Kuroiwa Y (1978b): Clinical studies of the movement-related cortical potential (MP) and the relationship between the dentatorubrothalamic pathway and the readiness potential (RP). *J Neurol* 219:15–25.

Shibasaki H, Barrett G, Halliday E, Halliday AM (1980a): Components of the movement-related cortical potential and their scalp topography. *Electroencephalogr Clin Neurophysiol* 49:213–226.

Shibasaki H, Barrett G, Halliday E, Halliday AM (1980b): Cortical potentials following voluntary and passive finger movements. *Electroencephalogr Clin Neurophysiol* 50:201–213.

Shibasaki H, Barrett G, Halliday E, Halliday AM (1981a): Cortical potentials associated with voluntary foot movement in man. *Electroencephalogr Clin Neurophysiol* 52:507–516.

Shibasaki H, Motomura S, Yamashita Y, Shii H, Kuroiwa Y (1981b): Periodic synchronous discharge and myoclonus in Creutzfeldt-Jakob disease: diagnostic application of jerk-locked averaging method. *Ann Neurol* 9:150–156.

Shibasaki H, Sakai T, Nishimura H, Sato Y, Goto I, Kuroiwa Y (1982): Involuntary movements in chorea-acanthocytosis: a comparison with Huntington's chorea. *Ann Neurol* 12:311–314.

Shibasaki H, Yamashita Y, Neshige R, Tobimatsu S, Fukui R (1985): Pathogenesis of giant somatosensory evoked potentials in progressive myoclonic epilepsy. *Brain* 108:225–240.

Shibasaki H, Barrett, Neshige R, Hirata I, Tomoda H (1986): Volitional movement is not preceded by cortical slow negativity in cerebellar dentate lesion in man. *Brain Res* 368:361–365.

Shibasaki H, Ikeda A, Nagamine T, et al (1994): Cortical reflex negative myoclonus. *Brain* 117:477–486.

Simonetta M, Clanet M, Rascol O (1991): Bereitschaftspotential in a simple movement or in a motor sequence starting with the same simple movement. *Electroencephalogr Clin Neurophysiol* 81:129–134.

Simons RF, Hoffman JE, Macmillan FW (1983): The component structure of event-related slow potentials: task, ISI, and warning stimulus effects on the 'E' wave. *Biol Psychol* 17:193–219.

Simson R, Vaughan HG, Ritter W (1976): The scalp topography of potentials associated with missing visual or auditory stimuli. *Electroencephalogr Clin Neurophysiol* 40:33–42.

Simson R, Vaughan HG, Ritter W (1977): The scalp topography of potentials in auditory and visual discrimination tasks. *Electroencephalogr Clin Neurophysiol* 42:528–535.

Sklare DA, Lynn GE (1984): Latency of the P3 event-related potential: normative aspects and within-subject variability. *Electroencephalogr Clin Neurophysiol* 59:420–424.

Slaets JPJ, Fortgens C (1984): On the value of P300 event-related potentials in the differential diagnosis of dementia. *Br J Psychiatr* 145:652–656.

Slater JD, Wu FY, Honig LS, Ramsay RE, Morgan R (1994): Neural network analysis of the P300 event-related potential in multiple sclerosis. *Electroencephalogr Clin Neurophysiol* 90:114–122.

Small JG, Small IF (1971): Contingent negative variation (CNV) correlation with psychiatric diagnosis. *Arch Gen Psychiatry* 25:550–554.

Small M (1988): Visual evoked potentials in a patient with prosopagnosia. *Electroencephalogr Clin Neurophysiol* 71:10–16.

Smith ME, Stapleton JM, Halgren E (1986): Human medial temporal lobe potentials evoked in memory and language tasks. *Electroencephalogr Clin Neurophysiol* 63:145–159.

Smith ME, Halgren E, Sokolik M, et al (1990): The intracranial topography of the P3 event-related potential elicited during auditory oddball. *Electroencephalogr Clin Neurophysiol* 76:235–248.

Smits MG, van der Meer YG, Pfeil JPJM, Rijnierse JJMM, Vos AJM (1993): Perimenstrual migraine: effect of Estraderm TTS and the value of contingent negative variation and exteroceptive temporalis muscle suppression test. *Headache* 34:103–106.

Smulders FTY, Kenemans JL, Kok A (1994): A comparison of different methods for estimating single-trial P300 latencies. *Electroencephalogr Clin Neurophysiol* 92:107–114.

Snyder E, Hillyard SA, Galambos R (1980): Similarities and differences among the P3 waves to detected signals in three modalities. *Psychophysiology* 17:112–122.

Squires KC, Wickens C, Squires NK, Donchin E (1976): The effect of stimulus sequence on the waveform of the cortical event-related potential. *Science* 193:1142–1146.

Squires KC, Donchin E, Herning RI, McCarthy G (1977): On the influence of task relevance and stimulus probability on event-related potential components. *Electroencephalogr Clin Neurophysiol* 42:1–14.

Squires KC, Wickens C, Squires NK, Donchin E (1978): Sequential dependencies of the waveform of the event-related potential: a preliminary report. In: *Multidisciplinary perspectives in Event-Related Brain Potential Research*, edited by D Otto, pp 215–217. US Government Printing Office, Washington, DC.

Squires NK, Squires KC, Hillyard SA (1975): Two varieties of long-latency positive waves evoked by unpredictable auditory stimuli in man. *Electroencephalogr Clin Neurophys* 38:387–401.

Squires NK, Donchin E, Squires KC (1977): Bisensory stimulation: inferring decision-related processes from the P300 component. *J Exp Psychol Hum Percept Perform* 3:299–315.

Squires NK, Galbraith GC, Aine CJ (1979): Event related potential assessment of sensory and cognitive deficits in the mentally retarded. In: *Human Evoked Potentials: Applications and Problems,* edited by D Lehmann and E Callaway, pp 397–413. Plenum Press, New York.

Stanzione P, Fattapposta F, Giunti P, et al (1991): P300 variations in Parkinsonian patients before and during dopaminergic monotherapy: a suggested dopamine component in P300. *Electroencephalogr Clin Neurophysiol* 80:446–453.

Stapleton JM, Halgren E (1987): Endogenous potentials evoked in simple cognitive tasks: depth components and task correlates. *Electroencephalogr Clin Neurophysiol* 67:44–52.

Stapleton JM, Halgren E, Moreno KA (1987): Endogenous potentials after anterior temporal lobectomy. *Neuropsychologia* 25:549–557.

Starr A, Barrett G (1987): Disordered auditory short-term memory in man and event-related potentials. *Brain* 110:935–959.

Strandburg RJ, Marsh JT, Brown WS, et al (1994): Reduced attention-related negative potentials in schizophrenic adults. *Psychophysiology* 31:272–281.

Sutton S, Braren M, Zubin J, John ER (1965): Evoked-potential correlates of stimulus uncertainty. *Science* 150:1187–1188.

Suwazono S, Shibasaki H, Nishida S, et al (1994): Automatic detection of P300 in single sweep records of auditory event-related potential. *J Clin Neurophysiol* 11:448–460.

Syndulko K, Cohen SN, Tourtellotte WW, Potvin AR (1982b): Endogenous event-related potentials: prospective applications in neuropsychology and behavioral neurology. *Bull LA Neurol Soc* 47:124–140.

Tecce JJ (1972): Contingent negative variation (CNV) and psychological processes in man. *Psychol Bull* 77:73–108.

Tecce JJ (1978): Contingent negative variation and attention functions in the aged. In: *Event-Related Brain Potentials in Man,* edited by E Callaway, P Tueting, and SH Koslow. Academic Press, New York.

Tecce JJ, Cattanach L, Yrchik DA, Meinbresse, Dessonville CL (1982): CNV rebound and aging. *Electroencephalogr Clin Neurophysiol* 54:175–186.

Tecce JJ, Cattanach L, Boehner-Davis MB, Branconnier RJ, Cole JO (1983): CNV rebound, attention performance, and Hydergine treatment in Alzheimer's patients. *Br J Clin Pract* 37:19–22.

Tecce JJ, Cattanach L (1993): Contingent negative variation. In: *Electroencephalography,* 3rd ed., edited by E Niedermeyer and F Lopes da Silva, pp 887–910. Urban & Schwarzenberg, Baltimore.

Thickbroom GW, Mastaglia FL (1985): Cerebral events preceding self-paced and visually triggered saccades. A study of presaccadic potentials. *Electroencephalogr Clin Neurophysiol* 62:277–289.

Thompson PD, Day BL, Rothwell JC, Brown P, Britton TC, Marsden CD (1994): The myoclonus in corticobasal degeneration. Evidence for two forms of cortical reflex myoclonus. *Brain* 117:1197–1207.

Timsit-Berthier M, Delaunoy J, Koninckx N, Rousseau JC (1973): Slow potential changes in psychiatry. I. Contingent negative variation. *Electroencephalogr Clin Neurophysiol* 35:355–361.

Toda K, Tachibana H, Sugita M, Konishi K (1993): P300 and reaction time in Parkinson's disease. *J Geriatr Psychiatry Neurol* 6:131–136.

Toro C, Torres F (1986): Electrophysiologic correlates of a paroxysmal movement disorder. *Ann Neurol* 20: 731–734.

Toro C, Matsumoto J, Deuschl G, Roth BJ, Hallett M (1993a): Source analysis of scalp-recorded movement-related electrical potentials. *Electroencephalogr Clin Neurophysiol* 86:167–175.

Toro C, Pascual-Leone A, Deuschl G, Tate E, Pranzatelli MR, Hallett M (1993b): Cortical tremor. A common manisfestation of cortical myoclonus. *Neurology* 43:2346–2353.

Toro C, Deuschl G, Thatcher R, Sato S, Kufta C, Hallett M (1994): Event-related desynchronization and movement-related cortical potentials on the ECoG and EEG. *Electroencephalogr Clin Neurophysiol* 93:380–389.

Trenkwalder C, Bucher SF, Oertel WH, Proeckl D, Plendl H, Paulus W (1993): Bereitschaftspotential in idiopathic and symptomatic restless legs syndrome. *Electroencephalogr Clin Neurophysiol* 89:95–103.

Tueting P, Sutton S, Zubin J (1971): Quantitative evoked potential correlates of the probability of events. *Psychophysiology* 7:385–394.

Ugawa Y, Kohara N, Hirasawa H, Kuzuhara S, Iwata M, Mannen T (1987): Myoclonus in Alzheimer's disease. *J Neurol* 233:90–94.

van den Bosch RJ (1984): Contingent negative variation: components and scalp distribution in psychiatric patients. *Biol Psychiatry* 19:963–972.

van Gool WA, Waardenburg J, Meyjes FEP, Weinstein HC, de Wilde A (1991): The effect of tetrahydroaminoacridine (THA) on P300 in Alzheimer's disease. *Biol Psychiatry* 30:953–957.

Van Woerkom TCAM, Fortgens C, Van de Wetering BJM, Martens CMC (1988): Contingent negative variation in adults with Gilles de la Tourette syndrome. *J Neurol Neurosurg Psychiatry* 51:630–634.

Vaughan HG, Costa LD, Ritter W (1968): Topography of the human motor potential. *Electroencephalogr Clin Neurophysiol* 25:1–10.

Verleger R (1991): The instruction to refrain from blinking affects auditory P3 and N1 amplitudes. *Electroencephalogr Clin Neurophysiol* 78:240–251.

Vesco KK, Bone RC, Ryan JC, Polich J (1993): P300 in young and elderly subjects: auditory frequency and intensity effects. *Electroencephalogr Clin Neurophysiol* 88:302–308.

Vidailhet M, Stocchi F, Rothwell JC, et al (1993): The bereitschaftspotential preceding simple foot movement and initiation of gait in Parkinson's disease. *Neurology* 43:1784–1788.

Walter WG, Cooper R, Aldridge VJ, McCallum WC, Winter AL (1964): Contingent negative variation: an electric sign of sensorimotor association and expectancy in the human brain. *Nature* 203:380–384.

Wasch HH, Estrin WJ, Yip P, Bowler R, Cone JE (1989): Prolongation of the P300 latency associated with hydrogen sulfide exposure. *Arch Neurol* 46:902–904.

Waszak M, Obrist WD (1969): Relationship of slow potential changes to response speed and motivation in man. *Electroencephalogr Clin Neurophysiol* 27:113–120.

Weissenborn K, Scholz M, Hinrichs H, Wiltfang J, Schmidt FW, Kunkel H (1990): Neurophysiological assessment of early heptic encephalopathy. *Electroencephalogr Clin Neurophysiol* 75:289–295.

Wessel K, Verleger R, Nazarenus D, Vieregge P, Kompf D (1994): Movement-related cortical potentials preceding sequential and goal-directed finger and arm movements in patients with cerebellar atrophy. *Electroencephalogr Clin Neurophysiol* 92:331–341.

Wilder MB, Farley GR, Starr A (1981): Endogenous late positive component of the evoked potential in cats corresponding to P300 in humans. *Science* 211:605–607.

Wilke JT, Lansing RW (1973): Variations in the motor potential with force exerted during voluntary arm movements in man. *Electroencephalogr Clin Neurophysiol* 35:259–265.

Wilkins DE, Hallett M, Berardelli A, Walshe T, Alvarez N (1984): Physiological analysis of the myoclonus of Alzheimer's disease. *Neurology* 34:898–903.

Wilkins DE, Hallett M, Erba G (1985): Primary generalised epileptic myoclonus: a frequent manifestation of minipolymyoclonus of central origin. *J Neurol Neurosurg Psychiatry* 48:506–516.

Wolpow JR, Wood CC (1982): Scalp distribution of human auditory evoked potentials. I. evaluation of reference electrode sites. *Electroencephalogr Clin Neurophysiol* 54:15–24.

Woods DL, Courchesne E (1986): The recovery functions of auditory event-related potentials during split-second discriminations. *Electroencephalogr Clin Neurophysiol* 65:304–315.

Woods DL, Knight RT (1986): Electrophysiologic evidence of increased distractibility after dorsolateral prefrontal lesions. *Neurology* 36:212–216.

Woods DL, Hillyard SA, Courchesne E, Galambos R (1980): Electrophysiological signs of split-second decision-making. *Science* 207:655–657.

Woods DL, Clayworth CC, Knight RT, Simpson GV, Naeser MA (1987): Generators of middle- and long-latency auditory evoked potentials: implications from studies of patients with bitemporal lesions. *Electroencephalogr Clin Neurophysiol* 68:132–148.

Yamaguchi S, Knight RT (1991a): Age effects on the P300 to novel somatosensory stimuli. *Electroencephalogr Clin Neurophysiol* 78:297–301.

Yamaguchi S, Knight RT (1991b): Anterior and posterior association cortex contributions to the somatosensory P300. *J Neurosci* 11:2039–2054.

Yamaguchi S, Knight RT (1992): Effects of temporal-parietal lesions on the somatosensory P3 to lower limb stimulation. *Electroencephalogr Clin Neurophysiol* 84:139–148.

Yamaguchi S, Globus H, Knight RT (1993): P3-like potential in rats. *Electroencephalogr Clin Neurophysiol* 88:151–154.

Yamamoto T, Saito Y, Endo S (1984): Effects of disturbed sleep on contingent negative variation. *Sleep* 7:331–338.

Yasufumi T, Iwasa H, Yoshida M (1990): Diagonistic dyspraxia: Case report and movement-related potentials. *Neurology* 40:657–661.

Zamrini EY, Meador KJ, Thompson WO, Lee GP (1991): Reproducibility of P3. *Int J Neurosci* 61:113–120.

Evoked Potentials in Clinical Medicine,
3d ed., edited by Keith H. Chiappa.
Lippincott–Raven Publishers, Philadelphia © 1997.

16

Statistics for Evoked Potentials

Barry S. Oken

Department of Neurology, Oregon Health Sciences University,
Portland, Oregon 97201

1. INTRODUCTION

Statistics is the science of making inferences based on observations and is extremely useful for all experimental and observational sciences. Unfortunately, in clinical medicine the statistical rules are not overtly stated. Generally, the clinician has learned the rules of inference concerning variables through education and experience (e.g., what movements of the toes and feet constitute an abnormal plantar response) without learning statistics. In the past, the relative lack of quantitative variables in clinical medicine has limited the need for the clinician to know statistics. The clinical use of evoked potentials (EPs) requires statistical knowledge because most of the clinically important parameters are quantified.

Clinical interpretation of EPs requires a decision as to whether a given test result is more likely to represent a result within the range of results of healthy persons or within the range of results of persons with some disease. While a tendency has developed to consider a test result "normal" or "abnormal," the dividing line is arbitrary and artificial and it may be better to consider a test result on a more continuous rating scale (e.g., percentiles or z scores, as explained below). In either case, it is necessary to estimate the distribution of all important test results (EP values) in the healthy and diseased population, and then compare an individual patient's results with these distributions. To do this, one needs to understand (1) why it is necessary and how to establish laboratory contols values, (2) sampling, or how to pick a group of healthy subjects for the control group, (3) distributions (normal/bell-shaped or not), (4) how to control for parameters that affect EP results (e.g., height), and (5) the problems involved in setting limits of "normality" (e.g., false positives and negatives).

2. ESTABLISHMENT OF INDIVIDUAL LABORATORY VALUES

Each clinical laboratory has its own patient population and uses its own montages, stimulus parameters, filters, recording parameters, and method of measuring peaks (e.g., point of maximum amplitude or inflection). Therefore, it is best to establish one's own laboratory control values. However, with some caveats it may be possible to do less than the ideal. For brain stem auditory EPs (BAEPs) and somatosensory EPs (SEPs), if one uses the same stimulus and recording parameters, including montage and filters, one can use control values from another laboratory. It is still mandatory to perform the tests on some number of healthy controls in order for the clinical neurophysiologist and laboratory personnel to become familiar with the equipment and the testing procedure, to fully understand the range of normality, and to make sure the control subjects have EP results that fall within the range of normal for the other reference laboratory whose values will be used in interpretations. The American EEG Society recommends this number be 20 (American EEG Society, 1994), although one may be able to use fewer. For visual EPs (VEPs), it is incorrect to use control data from another laboratory because of the uncertainty concerning the luminance of the stimulator and the resultant variability of the range of normal results. Therefore, it is mandatory that one's own VEP normative data be obtained.

3. DISTRIBUTIONS AND SAMPLING

3.1. Definitions

A distribution is a description of the probability of occurrence of all the various outcomes in the sample or population being studied (e.g., the probability that the P100 latency will be

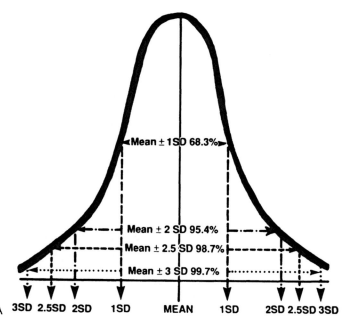

FIG. 16–1. A. The percentage of a normal distribution that has test results lying between z SD below the mean and z SD above the mean for z = 1, 2, 2.5, and 3. **B.** The percentage of a normal distribution that has test results below z SD above the mean for z = 1, 2, 2.5, and 3.

90 msec, 91 msec, 92 msec, etc.). Variables may be continuous [i.e., represented by a continuous scale (e.g., latencies)] or discrete (categorical) [i.e., represented by a finite number of levels (e.g., gender or click polarity)]. Ordinal variables are discrete variables that can be ordered or ranked (e.g., check size on a stimulator that has only several available check sizes).

Continuous variables may be further subdivided based on their distribution. A distribution may be normal, which is also referred to as Gaussian or bell-shaped, or non-normal. Some bell-shaped distributions may be non-normal if they are too peaked or too flat (see kurtosis, described below). A normal distribution describes many biologic measures, because it closely approximates measures (variables) that are the sum of many discrete variables. For example, people's height (which tends to be normally distributed) represents the sum of the influence of many different variables, genetic and environmental, each of which may only have a limited (discrete) number of possible values. This is explained by the central limit theorem, which is described in most introductory statistics books (e.g., Howell, 1987).

3.2. Parameters to Describe Distributions

A distribution may be characterized by its mean (average value), mode (most common value), and median (the value that half the population has results above and half has results below). In a normal (Gaussian) distribution the mean, the mode, and the median are equivalent. In a positively skewed distribution, the mode is less than the median, which is less than the mean. In addition, there are parameters that describe the broadness or dispersion of the distribution. The standard deviation (SD) is the most commonly used measure of broadness (see the Appendix for formula). The variance of a distribution is the standard deviation squared.

If the distribution is normal, there is a defined percentage of the population with test results lying between z SD below the mean and z SD above the mean, where z is any number (Fig. 16–1A). In clinical EPs, latencies that are at the low end of the bell curve (i.e., very short latencies) are not considered abnormal. Thus, the major concern is with the cumula-

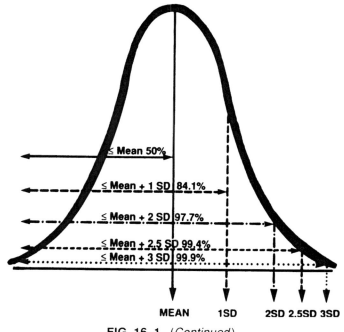

B

MEAN   1SD   2SD 2.5SD 3SD

FIG. 16–1. *(Continued)*

tive distribution, which is the percentage of the population that lies below a certain value (Fig. 16–1B). The z statistic or z score is the number of SDs away from the mean that a given observation, x, lies, calculated as z = (x − mean)/SD.

3.3. Non-normal Distributions

There are several reasons that a distribution may not be normal. The distribution may not be unimodal (i.e., not have a single peak). The distribution may be skewed (i.e., one tail of the curve is longer than the other tail). A distribution is negatively skewed when the longer

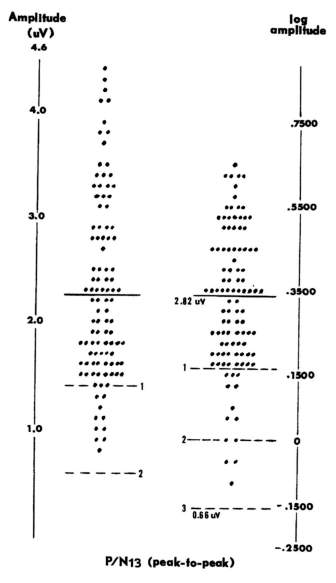

FIG. 16–2. The use of a log transform to normalize the distribution of the EP amplitudes.

tail is toward the left and positively skewed when toward the right. Many EP amplitude measurements are positively skewed, in part because the values cannot be less than zero. Kurtosis is a measure of peakedness of a distribution and is another reason for non-normality of a distribution. Further details on skewness and kurtosis may be found in statistics textbooks (e.g., Snecdor and Cochran, 1967). The mean and SD can be calculated for non-normal distributions, but have less descriptive significance than for normal distributions. The median and mode are usually not equal to the mean in non-normal distributions. For a positively skewed distribution, as commonly occurs with EP amplitude measures, the mode is less than the median, which is less than the mean.

It is best to use nonparametric (or distribution-free) statistics when describing and analyzing non-normal distributions. However, nonparametric statistics may be less powerful than parametric statistics. Thus, a transformation that converts a non-normal distribution into a normal one (e.g., logarithmic, square root) may be helpful because it allows the use of parametric statistics. An example of how a log transformation normalized an EP amplitude distribution is depicted in Fig. 16–2. If a distribution cannot be converted into a normal distribution, one can simply use the range of values or percentiles to define the spectrum of values in the sample. If one uses percentiles, it is important to realize how many control subjects may be needed [e.g., one cannot obtain a cutoff better than the 96th percentile if one tests 25 controls ($1/25 = 4\%$)]. Percentiles can also be calculated for correlated parameters (O'Brien and Dyck, 1995).

3.4. Testing for Normality

The easiest way to test for the normality of a distribution is to look at a frequency histogram to obtain a simple idea of the distribution. Obviously skewed or bimodal distributions can be identified. Statistical tests to determine the normality of a distribution include calculation of skewness, kurtosis, chi-square (for discrete ordinal variables) (Daniel, 1978), and the Kolmogrov–Smirnov test (for continuous variables) (Daniel, 1978). Grouping continuous latencies into intervals allows application of the more commonly used chi-square test.

3.5. Sampling

The process of sampling consists of using a small group or control sample to generate information about a much larger group, the entire healthy population. Sampling is susceptible to many errors if done incorrectly, and even to some errors when done correctly. The sample one chooses from the healthy population should represent the full cross-section of the population one will be testing (e.g., assorted ages, heights, and sexes). The subjects should be free of significant diseases of the nervous system and of the sensory pathway being tested (e.g., no significant ophthalmologic disease for the VEP). If the sample is biased (i.e., not representative of the entire population), then problems may result. For example, if all the healthy controls are residents or technologists under 30 years of age, there may be a high percentage of falsely abnormal tests when testing patients who are usually older. It is not advisable to use patient controls who have diseases or neurologic symptoms that may be related to dysfunction in the neural pathways involved in a particular EP modality. Whatever way one decides to actually perform the EP testing, it is imperative that patients continue to be tested in the same manner as the healthy sample was tested (e.g., one cannot change brightness or contrast of visual stimulators, recording montages, stimulus repetition rate, etc.).

3.6. Standard Error of the Mean

Even if an adequate sample is obtained, the mean of the healthy sample is not necessarily equal to the mean of the entire healthy population. The inherent error in using a sample mean to estimate a population mean is described by the standard error of the mean (SEM). The distribution of all possible sample (small group) means from the population is a normal distribution with its mean equal to the population mean and the SD equal to the SEM. The SEM is calculated as the [SD/sqrt(n)], where SD is the SD of the sample, sqrt is the square root, and n the number of subjects in the sample. The population mean has a 68% chance of lying between (the sample mean ± 1 SEM) and a 95% chance of lying between (sample mean ± 2 SEM). For example, one tests a sample of 25 healthy subjects and obtains a mean P100 latency of 100 msec and a SD of 5 msec. The SEM = 5/sqrt(25) = 1. Thus, there is a 68% chance that the actual population mean is between 99 and 101 msec, and a 95% chance the actual population mean is between 98 and 102 msec. In addition to the error in using a sample mean to estimate the population mean, there is an inherent error in using a sample SD to estimate the SD of the population. This is referred to as the standard error of the SD and equals [SD/sqrt(2n)]. Thus, using a sample containing 25 subjects, the actual population SD has a 95% chance of being between 0.7 and 1.3 times the sample SD [±2xSD/sqrt(50)].

3.7. Sample Size

In general, one should choose as large a sample as possible to minimize the SEM, but around 25 to 30 subjects is a reasonable minimum beyond which the percentage error does not decrease very rapidly with increasing numbers of subjects. It is important to emphasize that this number is the number of subjects, not the number of eyes or limbs. Since all clinically relevant parameters must be calculated for all individuals, one needs 25 subjects to determine the mean of 25 interside latency differences. In addition, there is a correlation between latencies on each side in an individual [i.e., in an individual, the right-sided latency is not independent of the left (Ederer, 1973)]. Thus, a slight underestimate of the population SD would result if both sides were pooled together. In general, it is best to calculate the SD of each side separately or average the two sides of a subject together before averaging across subjects. All measures that will be used clinically need to be calculated on the sample (e.g., absolute and interwave latencies, interside latency difference, amplitudes, and amplitude ratios).

4. CONTROLLING FOR SUBJECT PARAMETERS THAT AFFECT EPS

So far the discussion has assumed that there are no patient parameters that correlate with the EP measures. Since these parameters often exist, one needs to be able to control for them in order to make the test as sensitive as possible. Discrete parameters, such as gender (usually considered discrete), and continuous parameters, such as height, are managed differently.

4.1. Discrete Parameters

Discrete parameters can be managed by keeping the data separate when acquiring healthy controls. Once data have been gathered, the EP measures in the two groups (e.g., male and female) are compared using some statistical test to determine significance of the difference. The specific test that is most applicable depends on the two distribution types (normal or non-normal), and on whether the two groups are of the same size and have similar variances. The t-test often can be used to compare the means of two groups. The formula for calculating the t statistic is given in the Appendix, although a more complete description of the t-test can be found in most introductory statistics books (e.g., Howell, 1987). The t-test assumes the two distributions are normal and the variances are similar. However, the t-test is fairly accurate even if the distributions are non-normal and variances unequal, as long as the two samples are the same size (Boneau, 1960). If the t-test cannot be used the nonparametric tests, the Wilcoxon or Mann-Whitney, which are equivalent, can be used (Daniel, 1978). Using either parametric or nonparametric statistics, one can determine if there is a statistically significant difference between the two groups. If there is, it may be necessary to maintain two sets of normal values. Slight differences, even if statistically significant (e.g., 0.1-msec difference between males and females for the BAEPs), can probably be ignored if one uses conservative criteria for EP interpretation.

4.2. Continuous Parameters—Correlation

4.2.1. Correlation—Definition

Continuous variables need to be controlled for if there is a significant correlation between the subject factor and the EP parameter. This is most important for height in the lower-limb SEPs, although it is also of concern for age with all the EPs. Correlation is the relationship between two variables. Some variables are uncorrelated (e.g., paternal income and P100 latency). Some variables are positively correlated (e.g., as height increases the average N/P37 latency increases). Others are negatively correlated (e.g., as the conceptional age of neonates increases, the average BAEP I–V interwave latency decreases). These represent linear correlations [see (Godfrey, 1985) for a review]. Although there may be nonlinear correlations in EPs, such as an increasing slope of the EP latency–age regression line with increasing age (e.g., Brown et al., 1983), they are not currently used for routine clinical studies.

4.2.2. Correlation Coefficient

The most common method of assessing the degree of linear correlation is Pearson's correlation coefficient, r, which ranges from -1 (perfect negative correlation) to 0 (uncorrelated) to 1 (perfect positive correlation). To determine if there is a significant correlation, one needs to calculate r (see the Appendix) and refer to significance tables for r (e.g., if $r > 0.32$ in a group of 25 subjects, $p < 0.05$ that the factor does not correlate with the EP parameter). If there is a significant correlation between a subject factor and an EP parameter, one needs to establish a range of normal values for the entire range of the subject factor (e.g., height). One can do this by using regression analysis or by simply calculating control values for discrete groups (e.g., for each decade or for each 10-cm height interval).

4.2.3. Regression Analysis

The terms *correlation* and *regression* have slightly different meanings to statisticians,[1] although they will be used interchangeably here. The first step in performing a regression

---

[1]The term *regression* is used only when the independent variable (e.g., age) has been controlled by sampling or experimental design.

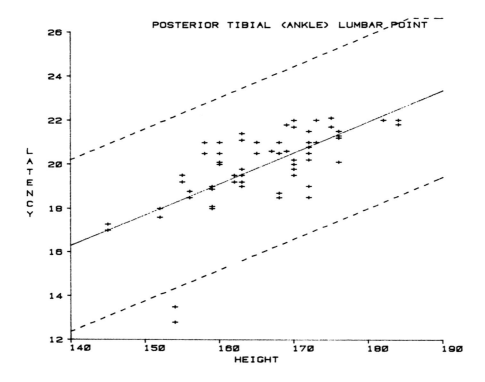

FIG. 16–3. An example of a regression line demonstrating the correlation between height and the N/P37 latency of the SEP.

analysis is to calculate the regression line, the line through the graph of all subjects' EP parameters (Fig. 16–3) that minimizes the sum of the squares of the distances from the points to the line. Next, one calculates the equivalent of a SD for the regression line, which is called the *standard error of estimate* (a line parallel to the regression line at some fixed distance). Finally, the upper limit of normal (see below) is set at some number of standard errors of estimate above the regression line. Further information on this procedure can be found in statistics books (e.g., Howell, 1987). Formulas for these measures are also given in the Appendix.

4.2.4. Sample Size

Since one is establishing a range of normal values for many different levels of the subject factor (e.g., height), the control sample needs to be larger than the 25 to 30 mentioned above, and should be at least 40 to 50. If one is planning to control adequately for age, about 10 subjects per decade is an empiric estimate for the number of subjects needed. More control subjects are also needed when using linear regression because it contains more potential errors than the sampling errors described above. There is a potential error in estimating the slope of the regression line. A potential error may arise because the correlation may not be linear and so the regression line may not be straight. An additional error may result because the SDs at each point (e.g., each age or height) may not be the same. The assumption inherent in the regression analysis is that the SD remains the same over the entire range and is referred to as *homogeneity of variance* (also called *homoscedasticity*). There is evidence that at least some electrophysiologic measures have a greater SD in taller subjects than shorter subjects (e.g., Tonzola et al., 1981) and in older subjects than younger subjects.

5. DECIDING THE UPPER LIMITS OF "NORMAL"

There are several terms that one needs to understand when deciding on the "upper limits of normal." The false negative rate, sometimes referred to as *type II error*, is the likelihood a person with a given disease has a normal test result. The false positive rate, sometimes referred to as the *type I error*, is the likelihood that a healthy person has an abnormal test result. The sensitivity of a test is the likelihood that a person with a given disease will have an abnormal test result and the specificity is the likelihood that a healthy person has a normal test result (Fig. 16–4). The false positive and false negative rates vary inversely. These measures are relatively independent of the percentages of patients and normals in the population being tested. Other measures that are more directly applicable to clinical practice, such as the positive predictive value or false alarm rate, are more dependent on the relative percentages of patients and normals in the population being tested. The predictive values are better from the clinical perspective but, unfortunately, these values are often difficult to determine precisely.

In clinical medicine there is a general tendency to err on the side of false negatives ("do no harm"). However, this depends on the specific disease being screened for, the relative likelihood it exists in the population being tested, and the outcome to a patient as a result of a false negative or positive test result. Widespread screening of asymptomatic people for easily treatable disease (e.g., early breast cancer) has a different motivation than testing patients with neurologic symptoms for Alzheimer's disease (at least at this point in time). For EP testing, it is recommended to use a cutoff of the upper limit of normal at least 2.5 SD above the mean. This is in part because of the above-stated philosophy and in part due to all the potential errors in the sampling process and establishment of laboratory norms. If there

		Disease		
		Present	Absent	
Test	Positive	a	b	a + b
	Negative	c	d	c + d
		a + c	b + d	a + b + c + d

Definitions

Sensitivity:	$\dfrac{a}{a + c}$	False negative rate:	$\dfrac{c}{a + c}$
Specificity:	$\dfrac{d}{b + d}$	False positive rate:	$\dfrac{b}{b + d}$
Predictive value positive:	$\dfrac{a}{a + b}$	False alarm rate:	$\dfrac{b}{a + b}$
Predictive value negative:	$\dfrac{d}{c + d}$	False reassurance rate:	$\dfrac{c}{c + d}$

FIG. 16–4. Definitions of commonly used terms used to evaluate clinical tests.

is a treatment for a disease only if detected early, one may want to alter this approach (e.g., in screening patients with a family history of acoustic neuroma with BAEPs). Test results between 2 and 3 SD above the mean can be described as being near or at the upper limit of normal. The inherent errors in calculating the normal limits may be partially quantified and one can generate tolerance limits which provide a confidence level for the cutoff point [e.g., a cutoff point that has a 95% chance of including 99% of healthy subjects (American EEG Society, 1994)]. Another approach to eveluting the sensitivity and specificity of a clinical test is the *receiver* (or *relative*) *operating characteristic* (ROC) plot, which basically graphs the true positive rate against the false positive rate for a range of normal cutoff values ranging from extremely strict to extremely lax criteria (Swets 1973; Somoza and Mossman, 1990). This allows one to evaluate or compare clinical tests without having to decide in advance on a specific cutoff value for normal versus abnormal. The gain in predictive value as a result of a test (the predictive positive value after a test result minus the likelihood the disease was present even before the test), also referred to as the *gain in certainty* of a diagnostic test, can be related to the sensitivity and specificity and the ROC curves (Connell and Koepsell, 1985). Alternatively, one could use the ROC curves to define an "ideal" cutoff given sufficient clinical test characteristics and the various costs of the test, including such entities as the costs and benefits to patients of false positive and false negative test results.

Also, it is important once the laboratory is set up to obtain feedback in order to assess the false positive and negative rates. In a given laboratory, one needs an estimate of how often patients who turn out to have no significant neurologic disease are considered to have abnormal EPs and how often patients who turn out to have definite disease are considered to have normal EPs.

Interpretation of test results can be made more quantitative. One can give the test results to a referring clinician in terms of the number of SDs a test result is from the mean, also known as the z score (see above) or as the percentile. Mention of these numbers in the interpretation is especially useful when the result is near (above or below) the upper limit of normal. If one knows the distribution of test results both for patients with known diseases and for the healthy population, then one can also use Bayesian inference. This is a mathematical technique that has been used in decision analysis and computer-aided diagnosis (e.g., Weinstein et al., 1980; Sox, 1986) and has been used for EP results (Blinowska et al., 1992).

6. CLINICAL SIGNIFICANCE VERSUS STATISTICAL SIGNIFICANCE

When using statistics in evaluating clinical neurophysiologic tests, it is important to differentiate statistical significance from practical significance. Test results may be statistically significantly different in two groups, but the overlap may be so great that the test would not be clinically helpful in deciding which group to assign a given patient with a given test result (Fig. 16–5). As an example, although BAEP latencies are longer in men than women, the overlap is so great it would be unwise to determine gender based on BAEP latencies. Statistically significant differences are helpful in understanding pathophysiology, but do not necessarily indicate a useful clinical test.

7. MULTIVARIATE STATISTICS

An additional complication arises when analyzing multiple variables. The false positive rate is positively correlated with the number of variables analyzed unless the upper limit of normal is changed or some technique is used that takes into account all the variables simul-

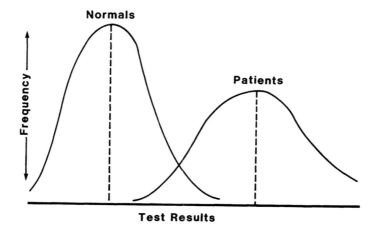

Statistically Significant and Clinically Significant

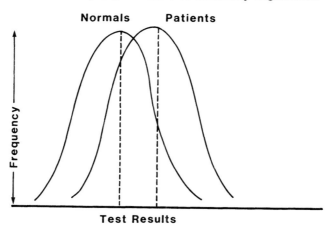

Statistically Significant but Clinically Insignificant

FIG. 16–5. Hypothetical distributions of frequency of test results that are clinically and statistically significant (*top*) and clinically insignificant but statistically significant (*bottom*).

taneously. This is both a theoretical issue as well as a practical one. Using multiple channel latency and amplitude criteria for multiple EP modalities may lead to an unacceptably high false positive rate (van Dijk et al., 1992). In general, one should limit the clinically used criteria as much as possible to include just those criteria that have high, well-established sensitivities and specificities (American EEG Society, 1994). Additionally, one can use other statistical techniques, referred to as multivariate statistics, which are specifically designed for analysis of multiple variables (Harris, 1985; Stevens 1992). The simplest multivariate technique is the Bonferroni correction or adjustment, which is unfortunately the least powerful multivariate approach to maintain the overall false positive rate. The Bonferroni adjustment lets one use standard univariate statistics when analyzing multiple variables if one divides the *p* value by the number of variables one is analyzing. It is the least powerful because it does not take into account the correlations that usually exist among the multiple variables. Other multivariate methods that may be helpful include the multivariate t-test (Hotelling's T²), multivariate analysis of variance (MANOVA), discriminant analysis, principal component analysis, and factor analysis (e.g., Harris, 1985; Stevens, 1992). John et al. (1987) have summarized some of these techniques as they are applied to electrophysiology. Neural network classifiers, which may actually be a complex implementation of discriminant or principal component analysis, have been used to classify the entire P3 waveform in patient with multiple sclerosis as normal or abnormal with slight improvements over human raters (Slater et al., 1994).

The complexities and problems with these types of multivariate analyses may be exemplified by EP topographic maps, which often consist of amplitude data for over 100 time points and at least 16 scalp locations. The 1,600 data points are highly correlated so one is analyzing far fewer independent variables. However, it still mandates great caution in analyzing the data because spurious or random results might be considered statistically significant (Oken and Chiappa, 1986) and result in erroneous diagnosis (Nuwer and Hauser, 1994). There have been some attempts to use more advanced statistical techniques to average EPs across topographic maps (e.g., John et al., 1993) but they have not yet been clinically well-validated.

ACKNOWLEDGMENT

This chapter was supported in part by grants from NIH (AG08714 and AG08017).

REFERENCES

American EEG Society (1994): Clinical evoked potential guidelines. Recommended standards for normative studies of evoked potentials, statistical analysis of results, and criteria for clinically significant abnormality. *J Clin Neurophysiol* 11:45–47.

Blinowska A, Verroust J, Malapert D (1992): Bayesian statistics as applied to multiple sclerosis diagnosis by evoked potentials. *Electromyogr Clin Neurophysiol* 32:17–25.

Boneau CA (1960): The effects of violations of assumptions underlying the t test. *Psychol Bull* 57:49–64.

Brown WS, Marsh JT, La Rue A (1983): Exponential electrophysiological aging: P3 latency. *Electroencephalogr Clin Neurophysiol* 55:277–285.

Connell FA, Koepsell TD (1985): Measures of gain in certainty from a diagnostic test. *Am J Epidemiol* 121:744–753.

Daniel WW (1978): *Applied Nonparametric Statistics*. Houghton Mifflin, Boston.

Ederer F. (1973): Shall we count the numbers of eyes or the numbers of subjects? *Arch Ophthalmol* 89:1–2.

Godfrey K (1985): Simple linear regression in medical research. *N Engl J Med* 313:1629–1636.

Harris RJ (1985): *A Primer of Multivariate Statistics*. Academic Press, Orlando.

Howell D (1987): *Statistical Methods for Psychology*. Duxbury Press, Boston.

John ER, Harmony T, Valdes-Sosa P (1987): The use of statistics in electrophysiology. In: *Methods of Analysis of Brain Electrical and Magnetic Signals*, edited by AS Gevins and A Remond, pp 497–540. *EEG Handbook* (revised series, vol 1). Elsevier Science Publishers, Amsterdam.

John ER, Easton P, Prichep LS, Friedman J (1993): Standardized varimex descriptors of event related potentials: basic considerations. *Brain Topogr* 6:143–162.

Nuwer MR, Hauser HM (1994): Erroneous diagnosis using EEG discriminant analysis. *Neurology* 44:1998–2000.

O'Brien PC, Dyck PJ (1995): Procedures for setting normal values. *Neurology* 45:17–23.

Oken B, Chiappa KH (1986): Statistical issues concerning computerized analysis of brainwave topography. *Ann Neurol* 19:493–494.

Slater JD, Wu FY, Honig LS, et al (1994): Neural network analysis of the P300 event-related potential in multiple sclerosis. *Electroencephalogr Clin Neurophysiol* 90:114–122.

Snecdor GW, Cochran WG (1967): *Statistical Methods*, 6th ed. Iowa State University Press, Ames, Iowa, pp 86–89.

Somoza E, Mossman D (1990):Utilizing REM latency as a diagnostic test for depression using receiver operating characteristic analysis and information theory. *Biol Psychiatry* 27:990–1006.

Sox HC (1986): Probability theory in the use of diagnostic tests. *Ann Intern Med* 104:60–66.

Stevens J (1992): *Applied Multivariate Statistics for the Social Sciences*, 2nd ed. Lawrence Erlbaum Associates, Hillsdale, NJ.

Swets JA (1973): The relative operating characteristic in psychology. *Science* 182:990–1000.

Tonzola RF, Ackil AA, Shahani BT, Young RR (1981): Usefulness of electrophysiological studies in the diagnosis of lumbosacral root disease. *Ann Neurol* 9:305–308.

van Dijk JG, Jennekens-Schinkel A, Caekebeke JFV, et al (1992): What is the validity of an "abnormal" evoked or event-related potential in MS? *J Neurol Sci* 109:11–17.

Weinstein MC, Fineberg HV, Elstein AS, Frazier HS, Neuhauser D, Neutra RR, McNeil BJ (1980): *Clinical Decision Analysis.* WB Saunders, Philadelphia.

APPENDIX

The following formulas are given primarily for information. For calculation, it is often easier to use statistical packages that are available for calculators and microcomputers.

I. Mean $= \overline{Y} = \dfrac{\sum\limits_i Yi}{n}$

II. Standard deviation (SD) $= \sqrt{\dfrac{\sum\limits_i (Yi - \overline{Y})^2}{n - 1}}$

$$= \sqrt{\dfrac{\sum\limits_i (Yi)^2 - (\sum\limits_i Yi)^2/n}{n - 1}}$$

III. Standard error of the mean (SEM) $= \dfrac{SD}{\sqrt{n}}$

IV. t statistic for comparing means of two independent samples, Y and Z

$$t = \dfrac{\overline{Y} - \overline{Z}}{\sqrt{\dfrac{S^2}{n_Y} + \dfrac{S^2}{n_Z}}} \quad \text{where } S^2 = \dfrac{(n_Y - 1)SD_Y^2 + (n_Z - 1)SD_Z^2}{n_Y + n_Z - 2}$$

V. Linear regression analysis

    Pearson's correlation coefficient

$$r = \dfrac{\sum\limits_i (Xi - \overline{X})(Yi - \overline{Y})}{\sqrt{\sum\limits_i (Xi - \overline{X})^2 \sum\limits_i (Yi - \overline{Y})^2}} = \dfrac{n \sum\limits_i XiYi - (\sum\limits_i Xi)(\sum\limits_i Yi)}{\sqrt{(n \sum\limits_i Xi^2 - (\sum\limits_i Xi)^2)(n \sum\limits_i Yi^2 - (\sum\limits_i Yi)^2)}}$$

    standard error of estimate

$$Syx = \sqrt{\dfrac{\sum\limits_i (Yi - YE)^2}{n - 2}}$$

$\sum_i$ the sum of the expression following, evaluated for each i
Yi, Zi   the ith subject's EP test result
Xi   the ith subject's height or age
n   the number of subjects in the sample
$\overline{X}$ the mean of the Xi's
$\overline{Y}$ the mean of the Yi's
YE   the estimated Y value calculated from the regression line

Evoked Potentials in Clinical Medicine,
3d ed., edited by Keith H. Chiappa.
Lippincott–Raven Publishers, Philadelphia © 1997.

17

Advanced Techniques of Evoked Potential Acquisition and Processing

*Joseph A. Sgro, *Ronald G. Emerson, and †Paul C. Stanton

*Department of Neurology, Columbia Presbyterian Medical Center,
Columbia University, New York, New York 10032; and
†Alacron Inc., Nashua, New Hampshire, 03060*

1. INTRODUCTION

This chapter will discuss signal processing techniques which can extend the utility and enhance the sensitivity of evoked potential (EP) testing by decreasing the time required to obtain satisfactory EP recordings, and facilitating the detection of changes in the EP signals. The techniques discussed are particularly relevant to monitoring applications in critical care settings which combine electrically "noisy" environments with the requirement for rapid detection of changes in EPs.

1.1. Noise

Evoked potential recording requires separation of the nervous system's responses from accompanying noise. The most commonly encountered noise includes myogenic electrical activity, environmental electrical noise, the electrocardiogram and the electroencephalogram (EEG). The signal-to-noise ratio (SNR) for conventional EP signals is on the order of 1:1 to 1:100 (i.e., the noise is usually much larger than the signal) (Yu and McGillem, 1983).

The power spectra of several (unaveraged) raw data trials recorded in an EP laboratory are shown in Fig. 17–1. The trials were recorded without stimulating the subject, and therefore contain only noise.

Figure 17–1A shows a "quiet" trial consisting of random noise of decreasing power with increasing frequency (i.e., *pink noise*). (By contrast, *white noise* has constant power at all frequencies.) Figure 17–1B contains sinusoidal 60-Hz contamination usually produced by

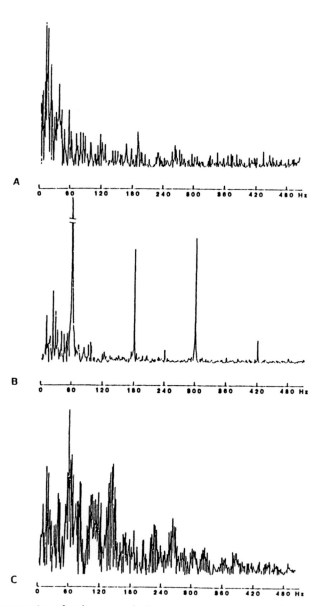

FIG. 17–1. Power spectra of noise recorded in a typical neurophysiology laboratory setting. **A.** Pink noise from relatively quite epoch. **B.** Prominent noise peaks corresponding to harmonics of 60 Hz. **C.** Abundant non-60-Hz-related noise produced by muscle activity. (From Sgro et al., 1989, with permission.)

line powered equipment. Figure 17–1C shows large amounts of non-60-Hz noise produced by muscle activity.

1.2. Averaging

The mainstay of EP signal processing is ensemble averaging. Successive trials following identical stimuli are recorded and isochronous points across trials are averaged. Implicit in the use of signal averaging is the assumption that the response of the nervous system is stable over the measurement interval and that the noise is stationary, uncorrelated to the stimulus, and zero mean. The SNR of the average will then improve in proportion to the square root of the number of trials averaged. In general 500 to several thousand trials must be averaged to obtain a satisfactory EP recording (i.e., SNR of about 10:1) (Harmony, 1984). For example, if a 1-μV EP signal is accompanied by 5 μV of noise (SNR 1:5), 2,500 trials must be averaged to obtain a SNR of 10:1, [2,500 = (10*5)^2].

Certain types of noise are poorly removed by averaging (Bendat, 1964; Childers, 1977; Ruchkin, 1965). For example, averaging has little effect on noise correlated with the stimulus (e.g., stimulus artifact, or a continuing response to a previous stimulus). Similarly, periodic noise (e.g., 60-Hz power line noise; see Fig. 17–2) is difficult, if not impossible, to remove using constant frequency stimulation (Sgro and Emerson, 1985; Evanich et al., 1972; Ackmann et al., 1980). Although individual transients are attenuated proportional to the number of trials (in contrast to the square root of the number of trials for the background random noise), high-amplitude transients can require many trials to achieve the desired SNR. For example, a single 50-μV transient, such as might be produced by subject movement, would require averaging 500 transient free trials to achieve an SNR of 10:1 with a 1-μV EP signal.

If the evoked response elicited by each stimulus is not stable (i.e., if trial-to-trial changes occur in either amplitude or latency), the resulting average will be distorted. Fig. 17–2 de-

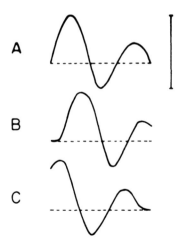

A

B

C

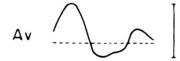

Av

FIG. 17–2. Distortion of the average waveshape produced by input waveform latency variations. Av is the average of the three signals (A, B, and C) of similar amplitude and waveform, but different latency. (From Harmony, 1984, with permission.)

picts distortion of the averaged waveform produced by latency shifts of individual responses.

Standard ensemble averaging is poorly suited to recording changeable (nonstationary) EP signals. Monitoring a changeable EP (e.g., during intraoperative monitoring) would entail comparing serially recorded independent averages of, for example, 1,000 trials each. Using this approach it could easily take several minutes to detect a change in the EP being monitored. As discussed further on, special techniques can be employed to facilitate the recording of changeable EPs.

2. LINEAR ONE-DIMENSIONAL METHODS

This section outlines several methods for filtering EP data. These methods are one dimensional (i.e., they operate on single waveforms). They are linear in that they can be applied to either the individual trials prior to averaging, or the final average waveform and produce identical results.

2.1. Standard Digital Filtering

The ability of averaging to extract the EP signal from accompanying noise is enhanced by the use of filters which eliminate noise outside the passband of the EP signal. Usually this is performed using analog filters incorporated into the amplifier. However, analog filters used in physiologic amplifiers have undesirable characteristics which can distort the signal. Fig. 17–3 shows the frequency response of a typical EP amplifier with the filters set for a passband of 30 to 3,000 Hz. Note that both the gain and the *group delay* (i.e., the time between signal input and signal output) of the system are not constant with signal frequency. These effects contribute to distortion of EP waveform morphology (Green et al., 1986). Since these adverse effects are most pronounced near the passband edges, in practice their impact is minimized by selecting wide passband settings, at the expense of reduced noise rejection. For this reason, analog filters used in physiologic amplifiers are not suited for restricted passband filtering, sometimes used to examine selected components of somatosensory EP (SEP) waveforms (Maccabee et al., 1983; Eisen et al., 1984; Yamada et al., 1988).

Digital filters perform the same function as analog filters but are implemented as software in the averaging computer, and overcome the principal limitations of analog filters. The passband of the digital filter can be made much flatter than is readily achievable using analog filters, and the group delay can be made absolutely constant (*linear phase* filters; Green et al., 1986). (Some authors use the term *zero phase* to denote constant group delay). Figure 17–4 shows the frequency response for a digital filter with passband of 30 to 3,000 Hz. Note that the gain in the passband is relatively constant and the group delay is constant across frequencies. Note also that much steeper rolloff (rate of change of gain at the edge of the passband) and greater stopband attenuation (rejection of signals outside of the passband) are achievable (compare with Fig. 17–3).

Additionally, digital filters are very stable over time, while analog filters require periodic adjustment or expensive high-stability components to retain their performance. Furthermore, because they are implemented as software, digital filter characteristics are readily changed by the operator, allowing greater selection of passband characteristics. In practice, some analog filtering is required within the amplifier to eliminate high-amplitude, low-frequency noise that would otherwise cause the amplifier to saturate, and to eliminate high-frequency noise beyond the Nyquist frequency.

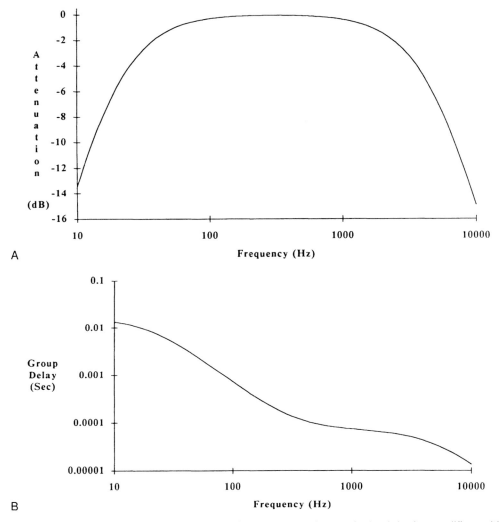

FIG. 17–3. Frequency response curves for a commonly used physiologic amplifier, with high- and low-pass filter settings of 30 and 3,000 Hz. **A.** Attenuation. **B.** Group delay. The curves were calculated using a SPICE simulation of the amplifier's circuit.

The operation of a digital filter is depicted in Fig. 17–5. The analog waveform is represented in digital form (i.e., a series of numbers as generated by an analog to digital converter). Each number in the series represents the amplitude of the waveform at successive time instances (time domain representation). The waveform is transformed by a discrete Fourier transform (DFT) into another series of complex numbers (coefficients) which represent the amplitude and phase of the separate frequency components of the original waveform (frequency domain representation). This is usually performed employing a fast Fourier transform (FFT) algorithm (Cooley and Tukey, 1965). In practice, time domain waveforms are sometimes multiplied by a window function *(windowing;* Hamming, 1983) to eliminate "leakage" of high-amplitude frequency coefficients into neighboring coefficients (*Gibbs* effect).

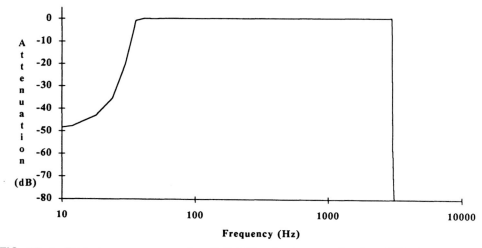

FIG. 17–4. Frequency response of a digital filter implemented using FFTs. This filter has much steeper rolloff and much flatter response in the passband than the analog filter depicted in Fig. 17–3. When comparing with Fig. 17–3, note the difference in the vertical scale. Group delay (not illustrated) is constant.

The Fourier transformation preserves all the information of the original waveform, permitting it to be reconstructed by an inverse Fourier transform. The EP signal of interest is contained in a subset of the coefficients (e.g., 30 to 3,000 Hz), while the remaining coefficients represent only noise. Filtering is accomplished by the elimination of coefficients outside the desired passband. The reduced set of coefficients is inverse Fourier transformed, using an inverse FFT (IFFT), to produce the filtered waveform. Filter rolloff may be implemented by variably attenuating coefficients at the edges of the passband.

For reasons of computational efficiency, the identical filter can be implemented in the time domain using a convolution of the unfiltered waveform with the impulse response function of the filter (Rabiner and Gold, 1975; Oppenheim and Schafer, 1975; Hamming, 1983). With the minor exception of analog-to-digital conversion noise (e.g., –72 dB for a 12-bit A/D converter; Rabiner and Gold, 1975; Oppenheim and Schafer, 1975), digital filtering is linear process. Therefore, trials may be filtered before or after averaging.

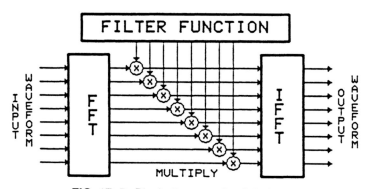

FIG. 17–5. Block diagram of a digital filter.

2.2. Wiener Filtering

Wiener filtering is sometimes used for EP applications. This method attempts to improve the SNR of the EP waveform by attenuating coefficients of low SNR more than coefficient of high SNR as shown in the equation below, where A(f) is the attenuation applied to coefficient of frequency f.

$$A (f) = \frac{\text{Signal Power(f)}}{\text{Signal Power(f)} + \text{Noise Power(f)}}$$

The utility of this method is limited by the requirement that the power spectra of the signal and the noise are known and stationary. In practice, the signal may not be known in advance of measurement, especially in clinical settings, where the EP waveform latency and morphology may deviate from normal. Similar considerations apply to advance knowledge of the noise spectrum, particularly if the noise changes during the recording. An attempt may be made to measure signal and noise spectra prior to Wiener filtering by averaging a small number of trials. However since the power spectra of the signal and noise are estimates, the filter has a large variance in areas of low SNRs—precisely the situation in which the filter is most needed (Harmony, 1984; DeWeerd, 1981; DeWeerd and Kap, 1981; Walter, 1969; Doyle, 1975).

Wiener filtering can distort the EP signal because it attenuates signal components in high-noise regions (frequencies) more than low-noise regions. This distortion is sometimes referred to as frequency *bias*. For example, if an EP waveform had a SNR of 10 at 500 Hz and 1 at 1000 Hz, the filter would attenuate the EP signal at 500 Hz by a factor of 1.1 while attenuating signal at 1,000 Hz by a factor of 2 (Carlton and Katz, 1980).

2.3. Least Mean Square Error Filters

The least mean square (LMS) error filtering is an adaptive technique in which the characteristics of a filter are continually modified to optimize detection of the EP in the presence of noise. The is accomplished by adjusting the filter to minimize the mean squared error between the input trial waveforms and a template waveform. In practice, this may be accomplished by performing FFTs on both template and trial waveforms, calculating the difference between the coefficients for each frequency bin, and using those errors to modify the coefficients of the filter by the method of steepest descent (Dentino et al., 1978; Ferrara, 1980; Ogue et al., 1983; Widrow and Hoff, 1960).

This technique suffers from the limitation that, similar to the Wiener filter, prior knowledge of the signal is required, but, in contrast to the Wiener filter, prior knowledge of the noise characteristics is not required. Operation of the LMS filter requires adjustment of a parameter which determines the rate of convergence of the filter. Selection of this parameter embodies a tradeoff between stability of the filter and the benefits to accrued by adapting the filter. This technique can introduce distortion of EP waveforms, similar to those introduced by Wiener filtering.

3. LINEAR TWO-DIMENSIONAL METHODS

Two-dimensional filtering methods operate on several EP waveforms concurrently, rather than single waveforms. The methods discussed below are linear in that they can be applied to either averaged or unaveraged data with equivalent results. These methods have particular applicability for recording changeable EP signals.

3.1. Moving Averages

A moving average is one method of recording a changeable evoked signal. The operation of a moving average is diagrammed in Fig. 17–6. An ensemble average is calculated on a continually updated set of fixed depth (i.e., a fixed number trials). As a new trial is collected, the oldest trial is discarded so that the number of trials in the average remains constant. A new moving average is calculated with each new trial, and the results may be displayed as a stacked plot of waveform for easy visual detection of change. The principal disadvantage of this method is that the average must be of sufficient depth to produce adequate noise reduction at the expense of rapid detection of change in the signal.

3.2. Two-Dimensional Fourier Filtering

Two-dimensional filtering is a method for processing changeable EP signals, which, in comparison with the moving average, provides superior detection of signal change at the expense of minimal increment in noise. Two-dimensional filtering requires no prior knowledge of the EP signal.

As illustrated in Fig. 17–7, sequential trials are stacked into a two-dimensional array, with time along the abscissa and the trial number along the ordinate. An FFT is performed on each trial in the stack, along the *time axis* (abscissa), and a standard digital filter is applied eliminating noise outside the passband of the EP signal in a manner similar to standard one-dimensional filtering (see above).

Each stack of coefficients along the *trial axis* (ordinate) represents the time evolution of a given frequency component. A second FFT is then performed on each stack of coefficients along the trial axis. The resulting two-dimensional array of "cross-trial" coefficients encodes the time evolution of the frequency spectrum of the individual EP trials. The "cross-trial" coefficients are filtered, selectively attenuating trial-to-trial variability caused by

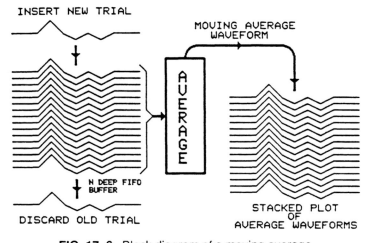

FIG. 17–6. Block diagram of a moving average.

noise, while retaining much of the variability in the signal. The modified coefficients are inverse Fourier transformed twice, once along the ordinate and again along the abscissa. Results can be presented as a stacked plot of filtered trials in which changes of the EP signal are well-demonstrated (Sgro et al., 1985). An example of the use of two-dimensional filtering to depict changes in an EP signal is shown in Fig. 17–8.

Two-dimensional filtering detects changes in the EP signal more rapidly than averaging. For the simple case of a two-dimensional filter that retains K coefficients along the ordinate (trial axis), the number of sweeps required to fully register a change in the EP signal is $N/(2K-1)$, where N is the number trials in the stack of the two-dimensional filter. Averaging required N trials to fully register a change. For two-dimensional filtering, the SNR improves as the square root of N/K, while for averaging the SNR improves with the square root of N. It is apparent that two-dimensional filtering embodies a tradeoff between elimination of noise and detection of change in the EP signal. This tradeoff is expressed in the number of coefficients retained along the trial axis (K). If a single coefficient is retained, this process is identical to a moving average. Note that one may view the moving average as

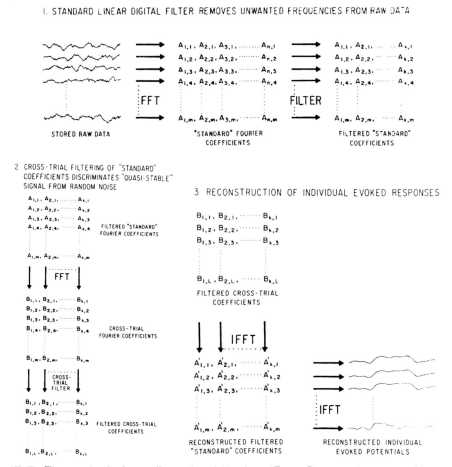

FIG. 17–7. The method of two-dimensional filtering. (From Sgro et al., 1989, with permission.)

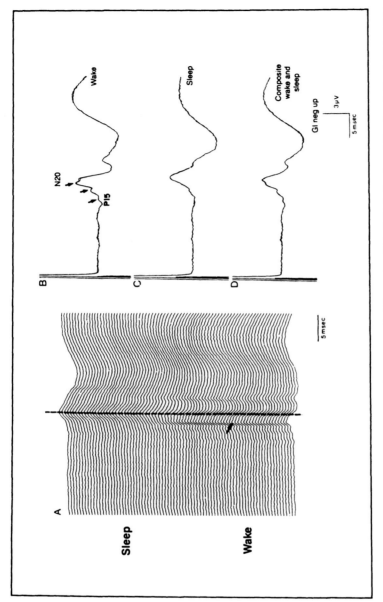

FIG. 17–8. State-dependent changes in N20, recorded from the C3'–C4' derivation following left median nerve stimulation. Sleep is accompanied by prolongation of the N20 peak latency, and loss of several inflections on initial upstroke of the N20 waveform. **A.** The transition from wake to sleep in a normal subject is illustrated using two-dimensional filtering. Each line represents the average of 32 sequential trials. **B.** Averaged N20 recorded with the subject awake. **C.** Averaged N20 recorded with the subject in stage II sleep. **D.** Averaged N20 recorded with the subject awake and in stages I and II sleep. Note that this waveform is intermediate in latency and morphology between separate wake and sleep recordings. (From Emerson et al., 1988, with permission.)

a low-pass filter along the trial axis, and that two-dimensional filtering can be viewed a wider-band low-pass filter.

4. NON-LINEAR DIGITAL METHODS

Below are described several EP processing methods which have nonlinear characteristics (i.e., the final EP waveform is a complex nonlinear function of the input trials).

4.1. Woody's Adaptive Filter

Woody devised a method for measuring the waveshape of variable-latency EPs that maintains stable morphology. An initial template is developed, either from prior knowledge of the waveform or using averaging. The trial is shifted in time to maximize the cross-correlation function with the template, and then averaged into the final output waveform. Once the average achieves a high SNR, it can be used to replace the template (Woody, 1967; Woody and Nahvi, 1973). The template is then continually adapted as more trials are processed. This technique has been extended to allow measurement of several EP peaks which may vary in relative latencies by individually cross-correlating and shifting the selected peaks (Pfurtcheller and Cooper, 1975). A method that combines LMS filtering and peak shifting has been described by McGillem and Aunon (1977).

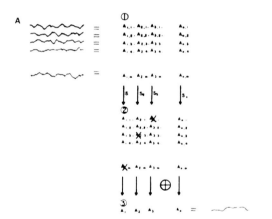

Time Domain Statistical Outlier Rejection

1. Digitized raw data is stacked as sweeps and stored.

A statistical distribution of values for each time instant across sweeps is calculated.

2. Values meeting statistical outlier criteria are eliminated.

3. For each time instant the (ensemble) average is calculated.

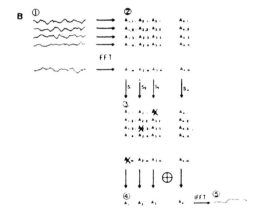

Frequency Domain Statistical Outlier Rejection

1. Raw, filtered, or subaveraged data are stored as sweeps.

2. An FFT is performed on each sweep.

A statistical distribution of Fourier coefficients is calculated for each frequency.

3. Coefficients meeting statistical outlier criteria are eliminated.

4. For each frequency the remaining coefficients are averaged.

5. An inverse FFT is performed and the filtered average is generated

FIG. 17–9. The method of statistical outlier elimination. Time and frequency domain implementations are illustrated. (From Sgro et al., 1989, with permission.)

Woody's filter method has several limitations. It is capable of generating an apparently stable output when presented with only noise as input. Furthermore, even if signal is present Woody's filter may lock on noise rather than the signal in certain circumstances (Aunon and Sencaj, 1978). It functions well only when the SNR is high (near 1:1).

4.2. Median Evoked Response

The median evoked response is calculated by taking the median value at each sample point over all the trials rather than the mean (Borda and Frost, 1968). This is advantageous in environments contaminated by bursts of high-amplitude noise because the median is less effected by outliers (points far removed from the mean or median) than the mean.

The principal disadvantage of this method is that its implementation requires large amounts of computer memory because all trials must be present in memory for them to be ranked in the process of computing the median. Additionally, this method is more susceptible to contamination by sinusoidal noise than standard averaging (Ruchin and Walter, 1975). Furthermore, the EP must be stable over the measurement interval.

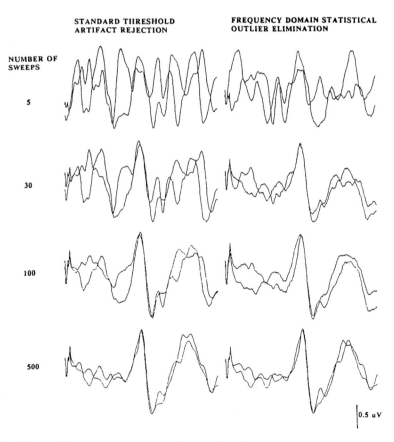

FIG. 17–10. Comparison of median nerve SEPs (C3'–C4' derivation) processed using standard threshold (entire trial) artifact rejection and statistical artifact elimination.

4.3. Statistical Outlier Elimination

Statistical outlier elimination is a process of prefiltering the population of isochronous sample points by a statistical test prior to averaging (Sgro et al., 1986). If a sample point in a trial exceeds a rejection criteria (e.g., two standard deviations from the mean for that set of isochronous sample points), the sample is excluded from the computation of the average. While conventional noise rejection techniques eliminate entire trials if they meet rejection criteria, statistical outlier elimination eliminates only individual sample points. This method can be implemented in the frequency domain as well as the time domain (Fig. 17–9). The ability of statistical outlier elimination to reduce noise in EP recordings is shown in Fig. 17–10.

Statistical outlier elimination is particularly useful when frequent bursts of impulse noise are present. Under these conditions, standard whole-trial rejection significantly prolongs the time required to obtain an acceptable EP waveform, while statistical outlier elimination allows processing to continue.

5. PHASE-SYNCHRONIZED TRIGGERING

Coherent or sinusoidal noise produced by power lines or electrical equipment is very resistant to removal by conventional averaging (Fig. 17–11) (Evanich et al., 1972). Coherent noise can be effectively eliminated by presenting the stimulus at random phase with respect to the coherent noise (Ackmann et al., 1980). More rapid elimination of coherent noise may be achieved by triggering the stimulator alternately in and out of phase with the coherent noise (Sgro et al., 1985) (Fig. 17–12). The method of phase-synchronized triggering is readily extended to eliminate coherent noise of multiple frequencies by triggering the stimulator at series of phase angles determined by the least common multiple of the frequencies to be eliminated.

Phase synchronized triggering is especially useful for the elimination of power line derived noise present in operating room and intensive care unit (ICU) settings. Coherent noise of other frequencies, such as 2-kHz noise introduced by certain monitoring equipment in ICUs, can also be removed by this phase-synchronized triggering. It should be noted phase-

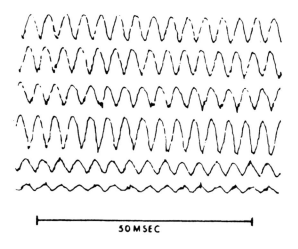

FIG. 17–11. Failure of averaging to eliminate sinusoidal noise. Each trace is the average of 64 trials containing sinusoidal noise acquired asynchronously (i.e., triggering of the averager was unrelated to the phase of the noise). (From Evanich et al., 1972, with permission.)

50 M SEC

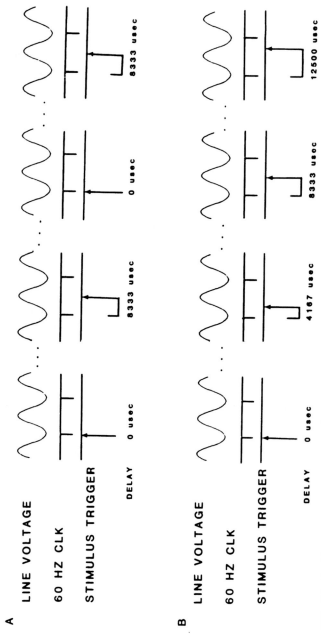

FIG. 17–12. Phase synchronized triggering. **A.** The stimulator is alternately triggered in and 180 degrees out of phase with the power line voltage to eliminate 60-Hz artifact. **B.** The stimulator is triggered at phase delays of 0, 90, 180, and 270 degrees with respect to the power line voltage to eliminate 60- and 120-Hz power line-derived artifact.

synchronized triggering is not a filtering method per se. It is a triggering technique which eliminates noise and leaves the signal entirely unaffected (Sgro et al., 1985).

6. RAPID STIMULATION

The time required to record an EP can, in principle, be reduced by increasing the stimulation rate. Using conventional recording methods, the maximum allowable stimulus rate is limited by temporal overlap of physiologic responses to sequential stimuli (Fig. 17–13). By coding stimuli with pseudorandom (rather than constant) interstimulus intervals and deconvolving the recorded response with the stimulus sequence, it is possible to separate the overlapped responses (Eysholdt and Schreiner, 1982; Sclabassi et al., 1977).

Figure 17–14 demonstrates preservation of a well-formed N20 response to median nerve stimulation at an overall rate of 344 stimuli per second with pseudorandom interstimulus intervals generated using binary M-sequences (Golomb, 1975; Simpson, 1966). Figure 17–15 illustrates a brain stem auditory EP (BAEP) recorded at rates of up to 1600 stimuli per second by the same technique, with only minimal degradation of the response.

Not only is it possible to separate overlapping responses to sequential identical stimuli, but similar techniques may be used to separate overlapping responses to physiologically different stimuli. For example, Sutter (1985) used binary M-sequences to successfully encode partial-field visual stimuli and successfully record simultaneously from multiple retinal regions.

Presentation of stimuli in rapid sequence can also disclose alterations in the nervous system's response due specifically to interactions between closely timed stimuli (Andersen et al., 1964; Winter and Frost, 1964; Wiederholt, 1978; Namerow et al., 1974; Sclabasi, 1986). For example, using pseudo-random stimulation based on a Poisson distribution, Sclabassi et al. (1977) observed that cortical activity to somatosensory stimulation (N20) showed a high degree of nonlinear interaction, primarily "occlusive" in nature, while spinal cord responses

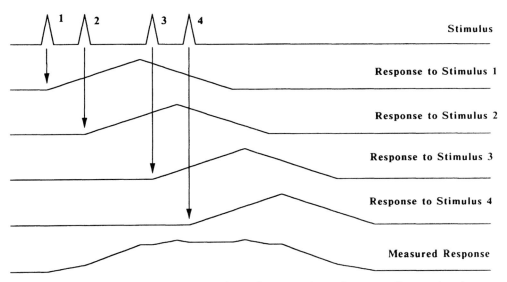

FIG. 17–13. Diagrammatic representation of summation of temporally overlapping responses.

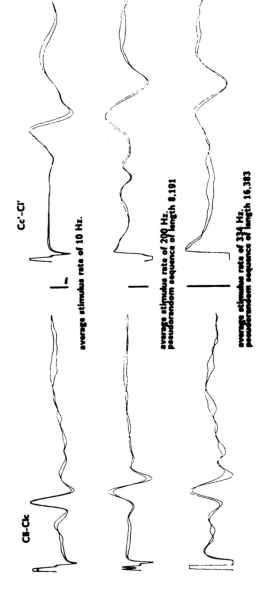

FIG. 17–14. Overlapping responses to median nerve stimulation are separated using pseudo-random stimulation based on M-sequences. Cli and Clc are Erb's point electrodes ipsilateral and contralateral to the stimulated nerve, respectively. Cc' and Ci' are electrode locations 2 cm posterior to the standard C3/C4 location, contralateral and ipsilateral to the stimulated nerve. The calibration bars represent 1 μV. Sweep duration is 40 msec. (From Sgro et al., 1989, with permission.)

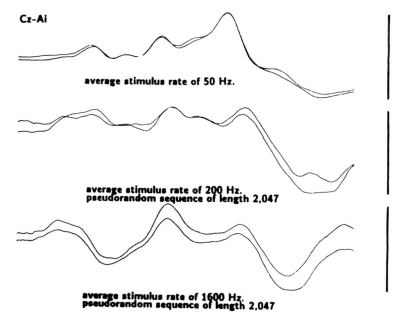

Cz-Ai

average stimulus rate of 50 Hz.

average stimulus rate of 200 Hz.
pseudorandom sequence of length 2,047

average stimulus rate of 1600 Hz.
pseudorandom sequence of length 2,047

FIG. 17–15. Overlapping BAEPs are separated using pseudo-random stimulation based on M-sequences. The calibration bars represent 1 μV. Sweep duration is 10 msec. (From Sgro et al., 1989, with permission.)

were largely linear. Interestingly, these interactions were dramatically reduced in patients with multiple sclerosis (Sclabassi et al., 1977). We believe that rapid-stimulation techniques may not only reduce the time required to obtain EP recordings, but may enhance the sensitivity of EP to certain disease states.

7. AUTOMATIC PATTERN RECOGNITION

Recently, EP monitoring has become the "standard of care" for certain neurosurgical and orthopedic procedures. Factors that make it attractive in the operating room, including the ability to detect adverse neurological events at the time when they are reversible, also apply to certain intensive care settings. However, EP monitoring is labor intensive, requiring both trained technicians and physicians. This high labor requirement makes EP monitoring costly. Evoked potential monitoring would be facilitated, and the associated costs reduced, if it were possible to automatically detect significant changes in the monitored signals.

Table 17–1 lists the major techniques that have been used for automated EP analysis. None of these techniques has achieved widespread use, reflecting, in large part, their collec-

TABLE 17–1. *Techniques used for automated EP analysis*

Methods	Disadvantages	Reference
Discriminant methods	Requires a priori definition of features	Clarson and Liang (1989)
Template methods	Requires a priori template definition	Childers et al. (1987)
Derivative methods	Extremely noise sensitive	Miskiel and Ozdamar (1987)
Rule-based methods	Very sensitive to morphology variations	Boston (1989)

tive sensitivity to artifacts and noise, and their inconsistent ability to correctly track the waveform of interest, its amplitude, or latency.

7.1. Neural Networks

"Neural networks" have recently been applied to diverse areas of computerized pattern recognition, including handwriting, voice, and visual recognition. Neural network algorithms are computationally demanding, and their use has become practical only with the recent availability of low-cost high-performance processors. In contrast to most other pattern recognition techniques, neural networks may be trained to recognize patterns in the absence of a specific heuristic method for each feature to be recognized. Rather, a neural network is trained simply by presenting it with known example patterns. It is not necessary to precisely describe the patterns to be recognized. This ability, to recognize patterns without an explicit rule, making them particularly attractive in cases where expert human recognition strategies are intuitive, or difficult to articulate (Rumelhardt and McClelland, 1987).

An essential feature of neural networks is that they are able to generalize, and adapt to distortion and noise without losing their robustness. Neural networks are capable of correctly identifying input patterns that are similar morphologically, but are not identical, to the patterns on which they were trained. This feature makes neural networks well-suited to EP analysis, which required correct identification of signals based in part on waveform morphology, often in the presence of noise.

7.1.1. Neural Network Architecture

Neural networks are based upon mathematical models of interconnected units which have the capability of "learning." The units are modeled after neurons, and their interconnections are modeled after synapses. Learning results in a functional modification of these interconnections.

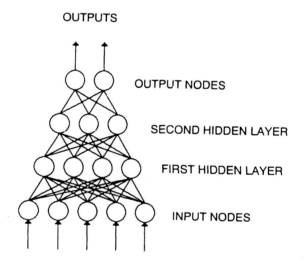

FIG. 17–16. Neural network with two hidden layers.

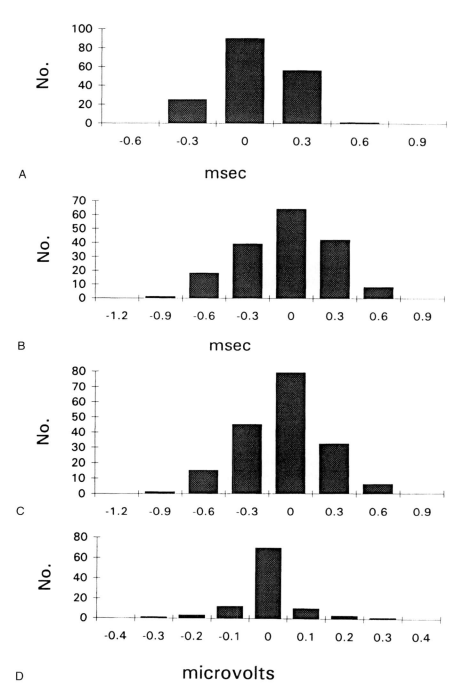

FIG. 17–17. Histograms illustrating the frequency of errors in neural network measurement of BAEP waves I (**A**), III (**B**), and V (**C**), and for the wave V amplitude (**D**).

The architecture of a feed-forward fully interconnected neural network is shown in Fig. 17–16. The network has an input layer, an output layer, and one or more hidden layers. An input pattern is presented to the input layer. Each unit in the input layer outputs to each unit in the first hidden layer with a connectivity function which determines its influence on that hidden unit. The value of each unit in the hidden layer is the sum of the products of each input times its connectivity weights. The same feed-forward relationship applies to each unit in the first hidden layer and each unit in the next hidden layer, and so on to the output layer.

Training of the network entails sequential presentation of inputs whose output are known, and determination of the networks connectivity functions. One training method, back-propagation via modified steepest descent, entails multiplication of the input values by the interconnection weights, calculation of each layer's output, propagation of those outputs forward through each successive layer of the network, and calculation of the mean square error between the output and the desired output. After all input and output pairs have been presented, the total calculated error is propagated backward, through the hidden layers, and individual weight are modified to reduce the total error (Rumelhardt and McClelland, 1987). In addition to this back-propagation architecture, other neural networks structures are available, including probablistic neural networks (PNNs) (Specht, 1990) and reduced-coulomb energy (RCE) networks (Reilly et al., 1982), which are based on radial basis functions. PNNs and RCEs require less computational overhead during training, but require more during recognition.

The composition of the set training is critical to successful training of the network. It is necessary that patterns to be recognized be adequately represented in the training set, and that the training set be "balanced," having similar numbers of examples of each type of pattern to be recognized.

7.1.2. Neural Network Results

The results in Fig. 17–17 demonstrate the ability of back-propagation neural networks to successfully "read" EPs. Separate networks were used to measure waveform latency and amplitude in BAEP recordings. Latency and amplitude data were encoded as eight-bit binary values with a granularity of 0.1 μV and 0.1 μV msec, respectively, and an output node was assigned to each bit of the binary value. The networks were trained using 197 BAEP recordings. They were tested using the "holdout" method, in which each individual BAEP recording is successively "held-out" from the training set, and used to test the networks trained on all the other BAEP recordings (Marchette and Priebe, 1987; Specht, 1990). The close agreement between latency and amplitude measurements made by back-propagation neural networks and human experts is illustrated in Fig. 17–17 (Sgro et al., 1992). We have obtained similar results using PNNs and RCEs. The optimal neural network structure for EP pattern recognition is a matter of on-going research.

ACKNOWLEDGMENT

Supported in part by grants R44 DC00391 and R44 NS30272.

REFERENCES

Ackmann JJ, Antonich FJ, Halback RE (1980): Cancellation of coherent noise in evoked potential recordings. *Med Instrum* 14:178–180.

Andersen P, Eccles JC, Oshima T, Schmidt RF (1964): Mechanisms of synaptic transmission in the cuneate nucleus. *J Neurophysiol* 27:1096–1116.

Aunon JI, Sencaj RW (1978): Comparison of different techniques for processing evoked potentials. *Med Biol Eng Comput* 16:642–650.

Bendat, JS (1964): Mathematical analysis of average response values for non-stationary data. *IEEE Trans Biomed Eng* 4:72–81.

Borda PB, Frost JD (1968): Error reduction in small sample averaging through the use of the median rather than the mean. *Electroencephalogr Clin Neurophysiol* 25:391–392.

Boston RJ (1989): Automated interpretation of brainstem auditory evoked potentials: A prototype system. *IEEE Trans Biomed Eng* 36:528–532.

Carlton EH, Katz S (1980): Is Wiener filtering an effective method of improving evoked potential estimation? *IEEE Trans Biomed Eng* 27:187–192.

Childers DG (1977): Evoked Responses: Electrogenesis, models, methodology and waveform reconstruction and tracking analysis. *IEEE Proc* 65:611–626.

Childers DG, Perry NW, Fischler IA, Boaz T, Arroyo AA (1987): Event related potentials: a critical review of methods for single trial detection. *Crit Rev Biomed Eng* 14:185–200.

Clarson VH, Liang JJ (1989): Mathematical classification of evoked potential waveforms. *IEEE Trans Sys Man Cybern* 19:68–73.

Cooley JW, Tukey JW (1965): An algorithm for the machine calculation of complex fourier series. *Math Comput* 19:297–301.

Dentino M, McCool J, Widrow B (1978): Adaptive filtering in the frequency domain. *IEEE Proc* 66:1658–1659.

DeWeerd JPC (1981): Facts and fancies about a posteriori "Wiener" filtering. *Biomed Eng* 28:252–257.

DeWeerd JPC, Kap JI (1981): A posteriori time-varying filtering of averaged evoked potentials. *Biol Cybern* 41:223–234.

Doyle DJ (1975): Some comments on the use of Wiener filtering for the estimation of evoked potentials. *Electroencephalogr Clin Neurophysiol* 38:533–534.

Eisen A, Roberts K, Low M, et al., (1984): Questions regarding the sequential neural generator theory of the somatosensory evoked potential raised by digital filtering. *Electroencephalogr Clin Neurophysiol* 59:388–395.

Emerson RG, Sgro JA, Pedley TA, Hauser WA (1988): State-dependent changes in the N20 component of the median nerve somatosensory evoked potential. *Neurology* 38:64–68.

Evanich MJ, Newberry AO, Partridge LD (1972): Some limitations on the removal of periodic noise by averaging. *J Appl Physiol* 33:535–541.

Eysholdt U, Schreiner C (1982): Maximum length sequences—A fast method for measuring brainstem evoked responses. *Audiology* 21:242–250.

Ferrara ER (1980): Fast implementation of LMS adaptive filters. *IEEE Trans Acoustics Speech Sig Proc* 28:474–475.

Golomb SW (1975): *Shift Register Sequences*. Holden-Day. San Francisco.

Green JB, Nelson AV, Michael D (1986): Digital zero-phase-shift filtering of short-latency somatosensory evoked potentials. *Electroencephalogr Clin Neurophysiol* 63:384–388.

Hamming RW (1983): *Digital Filters* 2nd ed. Prentice-Hall, Englewood Cliffs, NJ.

Harmony T (1984): *Functional Neuroscience*, vol 3: *Neurometric Assessment of Brain Dysfunction in Neurological Patients*. Lawrence Erlbaum Assoc., Hillsdale, NJ.

Maccabee PJ, Pickhasov EI, Cracco RQ (1983): Short latency somatosensory evoked potentials to median nerve stimulation: effect of low frequency filter. *Electroencephalogr Clin Neurophysiol* 55:34–44.

Marchette D, Priebe C (1987): *Proc 1987 Triservice Data Fusion Symposium* 1, 230–235.

McGillem CD, Aunon JI (1977): *IEEE Trans Biomed Eng* BME-24: 232–241.

Miskiel E, Ozdamar O (1987): Computer monitoring of auditory brainstem responses. *Comput Biol Med* 17:185–192.

Namerow NS, Sclabassi RJ, Enns NF (1974): Somatosensory responses to stimulus trains: normative data. *Electroenceph Clin Neurophysiol* 37:11–21.

Ogue JC, Saito T, Hoshiko YA (1983): Fast convergence frequency domain adaptive filter. *IEEE Trans Acoustics Speech Sig Proc* 31:312–314.

Oppenheim AV, Schafer RW (1975): *Digital Signal Processing* Prentice-Hall, Englewood Cliffs, NJ.

Pfurtscheller G, Cooper R (1975): Selective averaging in intracerebral click-evoked responses in man; an improved method of measuring latencies and amplitudes. *Electroencephalogr Clin Neurophysiol* 38:187–190.

Rabiner LR, Gold B (1975): *Theory and Applications of Digital Signal Processing* Prentice-Hall, Englewood Cliffs, NJ.

Reilly DL, Cooper LN, Elbaum C (1982): A neural model for category learning. *Biol Cybern* 45:35–41.

Ruchkin DS (1965): Analysis of average response computations based upon aperiodic stimuli. *IEEE Trans Biomed Eng* 12:87–94.

Ruchin DS, Walter DO (1975): A shortcoming of the median evoked response. *IEEE Trans Biomed Eng* BME-22:245.

Rumelhart DE, McClelland JL (1987): Parallel distributed processing. In: *Explorations in the microstructure of cognition*, vol 1: *Foundations*. The MIT Press, Cambridge, MA.

Sclabassi RJ (1986): A systems theoretic approach to the study of the somatosensory system. In: *Evoked Potentials*, edited by Cracco RQ and I Bodis-Wallner, pp 35–44.

Sclabassi RJ, Risch HA, Channing HL, Kroin JS, Nelson EF, Namerow NS (1977): Complex pattern evoked somatosensory responses in the study of multiple sclerosis. *Proc IEEE* 65:626–641.

Sgro JA, Emerson RG (1985): Phase-synchronized triggering: a method for coherent noise elimination in evoked potential recordings. *Electroencephalogr Clin Neurophysiol* 60:464–468.

Sgro JA, Emerson RG, Pedley TA (1985): Real-time reconstruction of evoked potentials using a new two-dimensional filter method. *Electroencephalogr Clin Neurophysiol* 62:372–380.

Sgro JA, Emerson RG, Pedley TA (1986): Statistical outlier elimination—a method for reduction of the noise power of the unaveraged evoked potential data. *Electroencephalogr Clin Neurophysiol* 64:41P.

Sgro JA, Emerson RG, Stanton P (1992): Neural network analysis of evoked potential waveforms. *Electroencephalogr Clin Neurophysiol* 83:86P.

Sgro JA, Emerson RG, Pedley TA (1989): Methods for steadily updating the averaged responses during neuromonitoring. In: *Neuromonitoring in Surgery*, edited by JE Desmedt. Elsevier, Amsterdam.

Simpson HR (1966): Statistical properties of a class of pseudo-random sequences. *Proc IEEE* 113:2075–2080.

Specht D (1990): *Neural Networks* 3, 109–118.

Sutter EE (1985): Multi-input VER and ERG analysis for objective perimetry. *Proceedings of the IEEE 7th Annual Conference of the Engineering in Medicine and Biology Society*, pp 414–419.

Walter DO (1969): A posteriori "Wiener filtering" of average evoked responses. *Electroencephalogr Clin Neurophysiol* Suppl 27:61–70.

Widrow B, Hoff M (1960): Adaptive switching circuits. *IRE Wescon Conv Rec* 4:96–104.

Wiederholt WDC (1978): Recovery function of short latency components of surface and depth recorded somatosensory evoked potentials in cat. *Electroencephalogr Clin Neurophysiol* 45:259–267.

Winter DL, Frost JD (1964): Recovery cycles in the lemniscal system. *Electroencephalogr Clin Neurophysiol* 16:459–469.

Woody CD (1967): Characterization of an adaptive filter for the analysis of variable latency neuroelectric signals. *Med Biol Eng* 5:539–553.

Woody CD, Nahvi MJ (1973): Application of optimum linear filter series to the detection of cortical signals preceding facial movement in cats. *Exp Brain Res* 16:455–465.

Yamada T, Kameyama S, Fuchigami Y, et al (1988): Changes of short latency somatosensory evoked potential in sleep. *Electroencephalogr Clin Neurophysiol* 70:126–136.

Yu KB, McGillem CD (1983): Optimum filters for estimating evoked potential waveforms. *IEEE Trans Biomed Eng* BME-30: 730–736.

Evoked Potentials in Clinical Medicine.
3d ed., edited by Keith H. Chiappa.
Lippincott–Raven Publishers, Philadelphia © 1997.

18

Intraoperative Evoked Potential Monitoring

R. Dean Linden, °R. Zappulla, and Christopher B. Shields

Department of Neurological Surgery, University of Louisville,
Louisville Kentucky, 40202; and °Department of Neuroscience,
Seton Hall University, Edison, New Jersey 08820

1. INTRODUCTION

Intraoperative monitoring of evoked potentials (EPs) has rapidly become a subspecialty of medicine. In addition to mastering the technology behind EP monitoring, the clinical neurophysiologist must learn a considerable amount about the tasks the other members of the surgical team are performing during surgery (Fig. 18–1). For example, he/she must become acquainted with the various surgical procedures for which monitoring is requested to ensure that the region monitored accurately assesses the component of the nervous system that may be in jeopardy. Moreover, he/she must become knowledgeable about the trigone of anesthesiology (anesthesia, muscle relaxation, amnesia), which agents are being used during the procedure, and their potential effects on the EPs. Finally he/she must collate all this information so that the surgical process can be interrupted with confidence when an adverse situation exists.

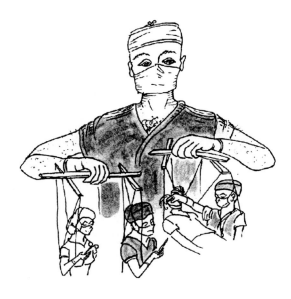

FIG. 18–1. The intraoperative clinical neurophysiologist must coordinate diverse information in order to provide effective input to the surgical team.

A close working relationship between the clinical neurophysiologist and surgeon is necessary. The surgeon should be made aware immediately of any alteration of EPs, so that appropriate measures can be implemented before irreversible neurologic changes occur. There is no place for a timid clinical neurophysiologist or overbearing surgeon in the operating room. Successful intraoperative monitoring of neurologic function can only be successful when there is mutual respect and trust among all participants of the surgical/monitoring team.

During the past decade clinical neurophysiologists have markedly improved their ability to provide technically satisfactory intraoperative EP monitoring. The operating room was once considered to be an "unfriendly and hostile" environment for monitoring purposes. Various technical obstacles had to be overcome prior to the acceptance of monitoring by the operating team. Depending upon the test performed, monitoring can improve the safety and/or the accuracy of the surgery (Table 18–1).

We consider the following to constitute a useful "primary" library for the clinical neurophysiologist:

American Electroencephalographic Society for intraoperative monitoring of sensory evoked potentials (1987): *J Clin Neurophysiol* 4:397–416.

Desmedt JE, Ed (1989): *Neuromonitoring in surgery. Clinical Neurophysiology Updates.* Elsevier, New York.

Ducker TB, Brown RH (1988): *Neurophysiology and Standards of Spinal Cord Monitoring.* Springer-Verlag, New York.

TABLE 18–1. *Intraoperative electrophysiological monitoring tests*

Safety	Accuracy
Auditory EPs	EMG
Somatosensory EPs	Compound muscle action potentials
Motor EPs	Sensory nerve action potentials
Visual EPs	

EP, evoked potential.

Moller AR (1988): *Evoked Potentials in Intraoperative Monitoring.* Williams & Wilkins, Baltimore.

Nuwer MR (1986): *Evoked Potential Monitoring in the Operating Room.* Raven Press, New York.

Schramm J, Jones SJ, Eds (1985): *Spinal Cord Monitoring.* Springer-Verlag, Berlin.

The following is meant to be an overview of intraoperative EP techniques only. Whenever possible we have directed the reader to more exhaustive reviews wherein complementary techniques are discussed.

2. BRAIN STEM AUDITORY EVOKED RESPONSE MONITORING

2.1. Introduction/History

More than 20 years of experimental and clinical experience has defined the stimulus-dependent configuration of brain stem auditory evoked response (BAEP) as well as the specific alterations in the response due to disruption of the auditory nerve and brain stem auditory pathways. Its predictability and reproducibility under fixed stimulus conditions and its stability during exposure to various anesthetic and pharmacologic agents make it the preferred method for continuous monitoring of neural activity.

Numerous published studies in both animals and humans have documented reversible alterations of the BAEP following correction of mechanical manipulation or vascular compromise of the auditory nerve or brain stem. In addition, the intraoperative changes in the BAEP have been correlated with the postoperative outcome in the vast majority of reported series. Consequently, the BAEP is considered to be a reliable way to assess neural integrity during posterior fossa surgery.

2.2. Procedures to Be Monitored

The use of the BAEP has been advocated during removal of tumors in the cerebellopontine angle (CPA), microvascular decompression of cranial nerves, vestibular nerve section (Silverstein et al., 1985) and ischemic complications subsequent to manipulation of posterior fossa circulation. The BAEP reflects injury to the cochlea, auditory nerve, and brain stem auditory pathways located between the pontomedullary junction and the superior colliculus. Consequently, brain stem lesions or vascular patterns that do not extend to adjacent auditory pathways or affect neural structures below the pons or above the superior colliculus may not be detected by the BAEP (Piatt et al., 1985; Little et al., 1987). In such cases, the use of the somatosensory evoked potential has been advocated as a complementary procedure to assess brain stem damage that may be undetected by the BAEP (Manninen et al., 1994). Operative procedures in or adjacent to the CPA carry a significant risk to the auditory nerve and brain stem. A number of specific conditions and maneuvers associated with surgery of the posterior fossa have been demonstrated to result in transient or permanent alterations in the BAEP. These include cerebellar retraction (Friedman et al., 1985; Grundy et al., 1981; Grundy et al., 1982a; Moller and Moller, 1989), manipulation of the auditory nerve (Silverstein et al., 1985), tumor dissection and debulking (Kalmanchey et al., 1986; Schramm et al., 1988; Silverstein et al., 1986; Watanabe et al., 1989), patient positioning (Friedman et al., 1985; Grundy et al., 1982b), lumbar drainage and dural opening (Kalmanchey et al., 1986), hypocarbia, hypotension, and ischemia of the cochlea (Levine et al., 1984), auditory nerve (Levine et al., 1984), or brain stem (Lam et al., 1985; Little et al.,

1983; Manninen et al., 1994). The temporal proximity of the alterations in the BAEP with these surgical maneuvers and conditions and their reversal with the correction of the inciting incident has been cited as evidence that corrective action taken in response to the BAEP changes can reduce postoperative neurologic morbidity.

2.3. BAEP Configuration

The brain stem components of the BAEP are referred to as *far-field potentials*, since they arise from dipole sources at a great distance from the recording electrodes. The features of far-field responses include low amplitude (<0.1 μV), short latency (<10 msec), high frequency, and a wide distribution over the scalp. The BAEP has a low signal-to-noise ratio (SNR) since its amplitude is much less than that of the background electroencephalographic (EEG) and electromyographic (EMG) activity. Signal averaging, used to extract the BAEP from the background activity, is done by taking advantage of both the time-locked responses of the BAEP to the stimulus onset, and the randomness of the background activity. The greater the SNR, the fewer stimulus trials that are required to obtain an adequate BAEP; consequently less time is required to evaluate a change in the BAEP. In addition, decreasing the number of stimulus trials that would have to be averaged reduces the possibility of masking peak latency changes that can occur during the time required to obtain the average. To avoid this difficulty and reduce the time required to assess auditory nerve function Moller and Jannetta (1983) have advocated recording the compound action potential directly from the eighth nerve to complement the BAEP recorded from the scalp. This technique provides instantaneous information concerning the integrity of the eighth nerve and also reduces the risk of misinterpretation, which can arise from distortion of the BAEP due to peak latency changes during the acquisition interval. Therefore, acquisition methods that increase the SNR have important implications for obtaining and maintaining an adequate response during intraoperative monitoring.

2.4. Stimulus Parameters

2.4.1. Stimulus Intensity

Auditory stimulation is delivered by a series of clicks at intensities of 60 dB SL. For patients with severe hearing loss and high auditory thresholds the intensity level for adequate stimulation must be higher. The amplitude of the BAEP, like most sensory evoked responses, can be enhanced by increasing the stimulus intensity. However, in pathologic cases the configuration and amplitude of the BAEP are frequently degraded, necessitating an increase in the number of stimulus trials to obtain a representative sample. An alternative strategy for increasing signal amplitude is the placement of intracranial recording electrodes adjacent to or on the auditory nerve or brain stem (Zappulla et al., 1984a; Silverstein et al., 1986; Moller and Jannetta, 1983). The simultaneous use of multiple recording techniques, such as the electrocochleogram (ECoG), eighth nerve compound action potential, and BAEP, has the additional value of localizing the level of neural dysfunction (Levine et al., 1984; Linden et al., 1988; Nadol et al., 1987).

2.4.2. Stimulus Rate

Similar consideration must also be given to the rate of stimulation. The more rapid the rate of stimulation the less time is required to obtain an average and the faster the feedback to the operating surgeon. However, at rapid rates of stimulation peak components of the BAEP may become indistinct. This effect may be amplified in the case of an abnormal BAEP. In such instances a compromise must be reached between the rate of acquisition and signal integrity. The rate of stimulation should be chosen to prevent time-locking the components of ambient 60-cycle interference to acquisition. This effect can be diminished by using stimulus rates (e.g., 11.3 clicks/sec) that are not exact multiples of 60 Hz.

2.4.3. Stimulus Duration

Click duration is 100 μsec. It can be delivered in rarefaction, condensation, or alternating phases. The phase of the stimulus can have differential effects on the configuration of the BAEP. Therefore, the phase should be selected to maximize the peaks of the BAEP. Alternating the clicks between the rarefaction and condensation phases reduces the stimulus artifact that is induced in the recording electrodes by the magnetic field arising from the transformer of the auditory stimulator. Alternatively, the stimulus can be delivered through an air tube positioned in the auditory canal, which places the stimulus transformer further from the patient, thereby reducing the stimulus artifact. This method introduces a delay in the stimulus onset that is proportional to the length of the tubing, which must be taken into consideration when selecting acquisition parameters.

2.4.4. Intraoperative Stimulation Precautions

Delivery of the stimulus in the operating room has unique physical considerations distinct from those in the diagnostic laboratory. The ambient sound level in the operating room is greater than in a controlled testing environment, thus increasing the stimulus threshold, and requiring an increase in stimulus intensity to elicit an adequate BAEP. This problem is exaggerated in those patients with an abnormal BAEP, as they require high levels of stimulus intensity due to an increase in the stimulus threshold. In these cases, a further increase in stimulation will augment stimulus spread via bone conduction, stimulating the opposite ear. The components of the BAEP contributed by cross-stimulation will persist in the absence of a response from the directly stimulated ear, thereby confounding interpretation. This difficulty can be addressed by appropriate sound masking of the nonstimulated ear.

Control over the operating room recording environment is restricted, consequently measures must be taken to assure constant stimulation throughout the monitoring session. Minor displacements of the auditory stimulator in the ear canal can alter the stimulus intensity, causing significant alterations in the BAEP, which can result in misleading interpretations. The stimulus device must be securely anchored in the ear canal to prevent displacement during patient prepping, positioning, and draping. Stability of the stimulus apparatus can be evaluated by repeat testing after each of the above maneuvers.

2.5. Recording Parameters

2.5.1. Electrode Placement

A representative BAEP can be obtained with three electrodes: ground, ear or mastoid on the side of stimulation, and vertex. An additional recording channel, the contralateral ear referenced to the vertex, can add additional information that can assist in peak identification. Subdermal needle electrodes or disk electrodes attached to the scalp with collodion have been found to be stable for the duration of monitoring sessions. Electrode impedances must be low (<3 kohms) in order to reduce the amplification of electrical artifacts that are endemic in the operating room environment. The placement of redundant electrodes at recording and ground sites have been used as backups when recording electrodes fail during a monitoring session.

2.5.2. Acquisition Parameters

Analog or digital filtering excludes extraneous electrophysiologic signals, and permits selective amplification of activity in the frequency band (100 to 3,000 Hz) of the BAEP. Digital filtering of the average has been shown to increase the SNR, enhance the peaks of the BAEP without shifting peak latency, and reduce sharp transients such as the stimulus artifact that can mask the early peaks of the BAEP (Moller, 1988a). The small amplitude of the BAEP, compared to other sensory evoked responses, requires high gain amplification. The amplifiers must have adequate common mode rejection (CMR) to significantly reduce or eliminate electrical noise (e.g., 60 cycles) conducted through the recording electrodes. Adequate representative sampling of the BAEP requires the use of analog to digital (A/D) converters that have sampling rates fast enough to resolve the highest-frequency component of the BAEP. Amplification of the signal should take advantage of the full voltage range of the A/D converter. The resolution of the converter (10 to 12 bits) should be adequate enough to detect small voltage differences. The number of stimulus trials can also be reduced by exclusion of trials (artifact rejection) whose voltage levels exceed the range of the BAEP before calculating the average.

2.5.3. Signal Processing

Faster microprocessors, efficient software, and on-line digital signal processors have permitted rapid signal analysis in the time and frequency domain (Moller, 1988a; Zappulla et al., 1984b). These technologies have enhanced the quality of the BAEP and expanded the information that can be extracted from the BAEP. Analysis in the frequency domain can complement visual analysis of the BAEP by producing an objective and quantitative measure of response changes (Fridman et al., 1984; Greenblatt et al., 1985; Zappulla et al., 1984b).

2.6. Anesthetic and Temperature Considerations

The BAEP is relatively resistant to anesthetic and pharmacologic manipulation (Grundy et al., 1982a). Halogenated anesthetics have been reported to increase the latency of peak V (0.1 to 0.2 msec) (Kalmanchey et al., 1986; Schramm et al., 1989). These anesthesia-induced peak latency changes have been found to be individualized, and the increases in peak V latency are not directly correlated with the concentration of the anesthetic agent. These minor anesthetic effects can be minimized by using post-induction latency values as the baseline.

While anesthetic effects may be minimal, decreases in body temperature can result in significant increases in peak and interpeak latencies (Stockard et al., 1978). These changes are linear and are seen from moderate through profound hypothermic conditions (Rosenblum et al., 1985; Sohmer et al., 1989). With the onset of significant hypothermia there is a decrease in response amplitude; the waveform is difficult to identify below 15°C. Therefore, body and irrigation fluid temperatures must be considered as potential causes of intraoperative peak latency and amplitude changes.

2.7. Interpretation of Intraoperative BAEP Changes

The BAEP is defined by a series of six vertex positive peaks occurring in the first 10 msec following stimulation. While peak amplitudes may vary between averages, peak latencies are stable across averages collected under the same stimulation and acquisition parameters. Consequently, intraoperative changes in the BAEP are frequently evaluated by comparing peak and interpeak latencies (Raudzens and Shetter, 1982) during the operative procedure with values from baseline recordings obtained with the same acquisition and stimulus parameters. However, dramatic decreases in amplitude have been reported to herald irreversible damage to brain stem auditory structures (Schramm et al., 1988). Re-establishment of baseline values is required if any change occurs in the stimulation or recording parameters during the monitoring session.

The number of peaks may vary in normal subjects, and frequently peaks may be absent or delayed in pathologic cases, even in the presence of retained hearing (Watanabe et al., 1989). Peaks I and V are the most robust and are present in pathologic cases when all other peaks are not discernable. The identification of peak V can be assisted by taking advantage of the predictable shifts in latency with changes in stimulation and the position of the recording electrode. Operative setup time can be reduced by establishing the configuration of the BAEP by preoperative testing.

The most popular method of peak identification relies on visual inspection of the waveform. The reliability of this technique is enhanced by having an experienced interpreter, a robust waveform, and favorable environmental factors. Frequently, during operative monitoring, the latter two factors may vary considerably, making even an experienced interpreter uncertain of his/her judgments. The hostile environment of the operating theater can result in electrical artifacts that can make acquisition impossible. These artifacts include large-amplitude 60-cycle interference, improper grounding, use of electrocautery devices, transducer interference from other physiologic monitors, use of ultrasonic aspirators, faulty fluorescent lighting, and synch pulses from video equipment and the operative microscope. Perhaps of more concern are low-amplitude time-locked artifacts that are below the voltage levels set for artifact rejection. These artifacts are summed with the BAEP and contribute nonphysiologic peak components to the average. In the presence of a low-amplitude BAEP, these peaks can confound interpretation. The use of no-stimulus averages is an effective strategy for addressing this problem.

2.8. Intraoperative Maneuvers and BAEP Changes

The most frequently reported reversible change in the BAEP during surgery has been associated with retractor placement (Fig. 18–2). These changes have been noted to reverse following repositioning of the retractor, although in some instances increases in peak latency have persisted throughout the surgical procedure. Alterations in the BAEP have been described during tumor debulking or dissection of the auditory nerve from the tumor capsule (Fig. 18–3). This information has been used to guide or alter the surgical manipulation and to alert the surgeon to the position of the auditory nerve, which may be difficult to visually identify due to anatomic distortions produced by the tumor (Fig. 18–4).

While the above-described changes in the BAEP have been generally accepted as indicative of a real or possible threat to the auditory system, controversy still exists regarding the magnitude of the change that should dictate a change in the surgical procedure. Several authors have proposed that changes in the latency of peak V in the range of 0.5 to 1.5 msec as being indicative of possible neural damage (Grundy et al., 1982a; Little et al., 1983; Radtke et al., 1989;

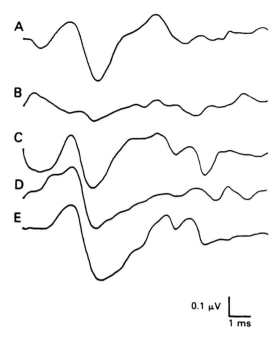

0.1 μV

1 ms

FIG. 18–2. Effects of cerebellar retraction on the BAEP. **A.** Before retractor placement. **B, D.** Depression of BAEP following placement of retractor. **C, E.** Return of BAEP following repositioning of retractor. (From Zappulla et al., 1984a, with permission.)

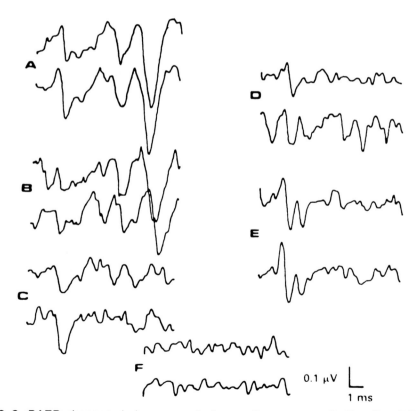

0.1 μV

1 ms

FIG. 18–3. BAEP changes during removal of acoustic neuroma. **A.** Baseline BAEP and replication. **B, C, D.** Progressive prolongation and decrease amplitude of the early and late peaks of the BAEP during tumor dissection. **E.** Recovery of the early peaks of the BAEP after tumor dissection. Sound appreciation but no speech discrimination postoperatively. **F.** No stimulus: control condition. (From Zappulla et al., 1984a, with permission.)

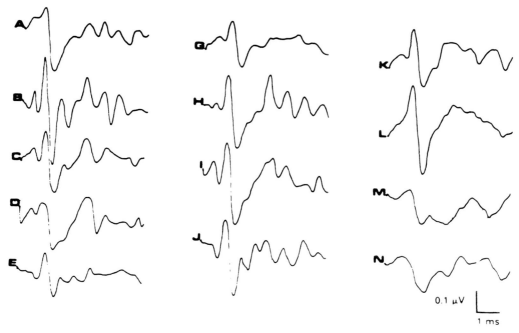

FIG. 18–4. BAEP changes during removal of acoustic neuroma. **A.** Preoperative BAEP. **B.** Dural opening. **C–G.** Decrease in peak amplitudes after cerebellar retractor placement. **H–J.** Recovery of waveform after retractor positioning. **K, L.** During tumor dissection there is a loss of the late components of the BAEP. **M, N.** Loss of all components of the BAEP after sectioning the acoustic nerve. (From Zappulla et al., 1984a, with permission.)

Raudzens and Shetter, 1982). Friedman et al. (1985) have suggested that changes in latency do not correlate with postoperative hearing status and the surgeon should be notified only if there was a complete disappearance of peak V. An alternative measure of quantifying the extent of peak latency change relies on the deviation from the baseline variance (Schramm et al., 1988).

The type, rate, and duration of BAEP changes can have heuristic value in elucidating the causes for postoperative hearing loss in the presence of an intact auditory nerve (Kveton, 1990; Levine et al., 1984). For example, several studies have attributed the intraoperative loss of the BAEP and postoperative deafness to interruption of the blood supply of the auditory nerve or cochlea by sectioning or spasm of the internal auditory artery or its branches, which may be traversing the tumor capsule (Levine et al., 1984; Nadol et al., 1987; Schramm et al., 1988). Kveton (1990) suggested that the poor blood supply and scant myelinization of the transition zone of the auditory nerve makes it susceptible to mechanical injury. He proposed that this injury is reversible and that it accounts for the cases of delayed spontaneous return (up to 2 years) of the BAEP and improvement in hearing after CPA surgery. Delayed recovery or deterioration of hearing may account for the lack of correlation between intraoperative BAEP changes and postoperative hearing status.

2.9. Prognostic Value of the BAEP

The usefulness of the BAEP in preserving hearing has been reported in a series of retrospective studies that compared patients undergoing CPA surgery with and without BAEP monitoring (Fischer et al., 1992; Harper et al., 1992; Radtke et al., 1989; Slavit et al., 1991).

In these studies there were a total of 157 and 224 patients in the monitored and nonmonitored groups, respectively. In three series there was an increase in postoperative hearing preservation in the monitored groups. The difference between the groups was significant when the comparison was limited to patients with small tumors and good preoperative hearing status. This is substantiated in other reports (Frerebeau et al., 1987; Kanzaki et al., 1989; Lenarz and Sachsenheimer, 1985). They demonstrated that small alterations in the preoperative BAEP and small tumor size were significant predictors of postoperative hearing preservation. Harper et al. (1992) and Slavit et al. (1991) demonstrated a significant beneficial effect of monitoring when the tumors were 1 cm or smaller in diameter as compared to nonmonitored patients. In a separate monitored series Nadol et al. (1987) reported 73% useful hearing postoperatively in patients with intracanalicular tumors; this percentage decreased by half with tumor extension of 1 cm into the posterior fossa. Fischer et al. (1992) argues that monitoring of larger tumors is worthwhile because useful hearing was preserved in some tumors that were 2 cm or larger. The possibility of preservation of hearing when dealing with large tumors is enhanced in those cases with minor alterations in preoperative BAEPs (Lenarz and Sachsenheimer, 1985).

The benefits of monitoring the BAEP in cases of microvascular decompression or rhizotomy, where there was no distortion of anatomic structures by a mass lesion, have been reported by Radtke et al. (1989). Seventy nonmonitored patients in this series had a 6.6% incidence of profound hearing loss compared to no instances of profound hearing loss in 70 monitored cases.

Early studies reported a very favorable predictive value of intraoperative BAEP changes for postoperative hearing status. Grundy et al. (1982a) reported hearing preservation in 32 cases with reversible alterations in the BAEP and loss of hearing in 3 cases, when the BAEP was lost following the sacrifice of the eighth nerve. Similarly, Raudzens and Shetter (1982) reported preserved hearing in a group of 34 patients with no intraoperative changes in the BAEP. In contrast, four patients with a loss of all waves subsequent to peak I had pronounced hearing loss. Seven patients with intraoperative delays in peak latency had mild or no postoperative hearing loss.

While preservation or loss of all components of the BAEP has been correlated with presence or absence of postoperative hearing, respectively, the prognostic value of less dramatic changes in the BAEP, such as the loss of selected components or prolongation of peak latencies, has been less prognostic. In a number of published series (Fischer et al., 1992; Harper et al., 1992; Slavit et al., 1991) on monitored CPA tumors, the authors reported on postoperative hearing status based on the intraoperative changes in peaks I and V. In 112 cases there was a loss of both peaks I and V at the end of the surgical procedure. Hearing was preserved in 16 cases (PTA 70 dB) with none of the cases having good hearing (SDS [speech discrimination scale] >40%). In 43 cases both peaks I and V were preserved, with 25 cases retaining hearing, 23 of which retained good hearing. Peak I was preserved in 50 cases, with 23 having hearing postoperatively; 8 of whom had good hearing. Nadol et al. (1987) reported similar findings in 69 patients monitored during the removal of CPA tumors. They concluded that hearing preservation is associated with the retention of peaks I and V. The loss of both of these peaks results in a loss of hearing postoperatively, while hearing preservation is indeterminate with just the persistence of peak I.

In a series of 31 monitored neurosurgical procedures, Schramm et al. (1988) concluded that an amplitude reduction of more than 50% for peaks I and V or the loss of one of the peaks was the best prognosticator of a postoperative hearing deficit. In contrast, an appearance of a peak intraoperatively that was absent preoperatively was a significant sign of retained postoperative hearing. No significance was attributed to transient or irreversible changes in peak latency.

2.10. Summary

Surgical intervention in the posterior fossa can threaten the integrity of brain stem and cranial nerve functions. Changes in the BAEP or auditory nerve action potential subsequent to specific operative maneuvers have been well documented. Reversal of the electrophysiologic findings following corrective action has been attributed to a reversal of neural compromise. Postoperative persistence of specific components of the BAEP has been associated with hearing preservation in the majority of cases. The lack of complete correlation between BAEP changes and hearing preservation may be attributed to a delayed reversal or deterioration of the auditory nerve.

3. SOMATOSENSORY EVOKED POTENTIALS

3.1. Introduction/History

One of the devastating complications of spine surgery is postoperative paralysis. In the 1975 report of the Scoliosis Research Society (MacEwen et al., 1975), a 0.72% incidence of spinal cord injury was associated with corrective surgery for the treatment of scoliosis. Later reviews suggest that the incidence of postoperative deficits following spine surgery may be markedly higher (King, 1984; Wilber et al., 1984). Spine surgeons have become more aggressive in their surgical approach for treating deformities. Greater degrees of correction are associated with an increased risk of postoperative neurologic deficits. Therefore, several tests have been devised for monitoring the function of the spinal cord during surgery in order to improve the safety of these procedures and reduce the incidence of these postoperative deficits.

The first test introduced for monitoring spinal cord function was the Stagnara wake-up test (Vauzelle et al., 1973). This test consists of reversing the anesthetic while the patient is on the operating table and asking him/her to move his/her legs. Many limitations are associated with this test, including both false positive and false negative results. However, the most serious limitation is that this test can measure spinal cord function only once or twice during the surgery, due to constraints imposed by the anesthetic.

The monitoring of somatosensory EPs (SEPs) was introduced as a continuous electrophysiologic test for assessing the function of the spinal cord during surgery (Fig. 18–5). Early attempts to record technically satisfactory SEPs during surgery had success rates ranging from 50% to 80% (Allen et al., 1981; Raudzens, 1982). With improved equipment, better training of monitoring personnel, and an understanding of the effects various anesthetics have on these signals, the clinical neurophysiologist is now able to provide a greater amount of useful information during surgery. Dawson et al. (1991) reviewed by questionnaire the experience of over 60,000 cases of spine surgery in which SEPs were recorded. Seventy-three percent of the postoperative neurologic deficits were accurately predicted by SEP monitoring. Further, the Nuwer et al. (1995) large multicenter survey review demonstrated that those patients monitored by experienced personnel had half as many postoperative neurologic deficits as those patients monitored by less experienced persons. This study

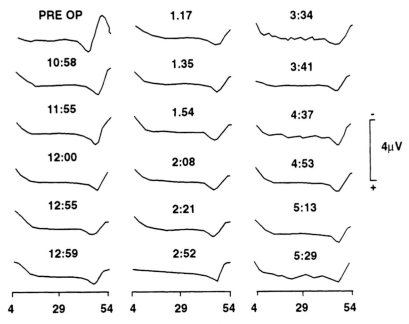

FIG. 18–5. Intraoperative monitoring of cortical SEPs during the removal of a spinal meningioma. Each tracing is the averaged response to 1,000 stimuli delivered bilaterally to the
posterior tibial nerve at the ankle. The illustrated response was recorded from CZ′referenced
to FpZ′. The preoperative (*preop*) tracing, recorded before the operation is larger and has a
shorter latency than the intraoperative tracing. (From Tator et al., 1988, with permission.)

clearly demonstrated the "clinical efficiency of experienced SEP monitoring." Epstein et al.
(1993) assessed the clinical usefulness of SEP monitoring during cervical spine decompression (posterior longitudinal ligament ossification, stenosis, disc disease, spondylosis). The
results (surgical outcome) of 218 patients who were not monitored were compared to those
100 patients who were monitored. There was a 3.7% incidence of quadriplegia and a 0.5%
incidence of death in the nonmonitored patients. There was no incidence of quadriplegia or
death in the monitored group. Given the diversity of the experience of the surgeons, the
years over which these data were assessed, and the well-recognized need for better-trained
personnel, the overall success rate is quite remarkable when intraoperative SEPs are part of
the procedure.

3.2. Procedures to Be Monitored

Table 18–2 lists the common types of surgery in which intraoperative SEP monitoring
has been performed successfully.

The clinical usefulness of SEP monitoring during spine surgery for the correction of scoliosis has been rigorously evaluated. The use of SEPs in this arena has been reviewed extensively (Desmedt, 1989; Ducker and Brown, 1988; Loftus and Traynelis, 1994; Nuwer,
1986; Salzman, 1990; Schramm and Jones, 1985). This type of monitoring is now an integral part of the surgical procedure.

TABLE 18–2. *Types of surgery in which SEP monitoring has been used*

Spine surgery
Interventional neuroradiology
Stereotactic surgery of the brain stem, thalamus, and cerebral cortex
Thalamotomy
Cortical localization
Cerebrovascular surgery
Aortic cross-clamping
Brachial plexus surgery
Pelvic fracture surgery

Several other types of spine or spinal cord surgery in which there is potential for intraoperative neurologic damage have been monitored with SEPs (e.g., spinal cord tumor, arteriovenous malformation, spine fusion, discectomy surgery). Interestingly, Kearse et al. (1993) recorded SEPs during intramedullary spinal cord surgery and demonstrated their usefulness for predicting motor outcome. Caution should be exercised in the selection of patients to be monitored. If the patient does not have recordable SEPs preoperatively, the chance of recording technically satisfactory intraoperative potentials is minimal. We are now excluding these patients from intraoperative monitoring. It is also important to realize that, in today's changing environment of health care cost containment, the surgeon may feel that the potential risk of an iatrogenic neurologic deficit is so minimal that it does not warrant the additional cost of the procedure. This decision is one for the surgeon's conscience and the medicolegal implications associated with the decision.

Berenstein et al. (1984) introduced SEP monitoring during transvascular embolization of spinal arteriovenous malformation (AVM) and spinal angiography procedures. These authors believed that SEP monitoring markedly decreased the frequency of postoperative neurologic deficits by identifying the crucial spinal cord blood supply in both normal and pathologic tissue. It was thought that SEP monitoring decreased incidence of spinal cord damage from 20% to less than 1% over an 8-year period (Young and Sakatani, 1990). One of the limitations of monitoring these procedures is the short period of time during which the neurologic damage may occur, necessitating the acquisition of a satisfactory SNR in a short period of time. Hacke (1989) recommended a moving block average technique to overcome this problem.

Other operations that are monitored at some centers include stereotactic surgery of the brain or brain stem (including tumor removal or biopsies) and hippocampectomy/amygdalectomy surgery (Harper and Daube, 1989). During thalamotomy, SEP monitoring may be used as an adjunct to bipolar microelectrode recording. Prior to applying EP methodology to a surgical event the team must carefully assess the anatomic region that they want to monitor, and then choose the most appropriate method that will meet their needs.

Direct intraoperative SEP recordings from the exposed cortex have been used by surgeons to identify landmarks during surgery. Allison et al. (1985) and Lueders et al. (1983) used these recordings to identify the precentral and postcentral gyri and the central sulcus. The median or ulnar nerves are stimulated at the wrist and large potentials are recorded from the exposed contralateral cortex. Recordings are made with ECoG electrodes. A minimum of 16 recording electrodes are recommended. Peak polarity reversal between the postcentral gyrus (N20, P30) and the precentral gyrus (P20, N30) aids in landmark identification. The signals are largest in the area of the central sulcus. Moreover, polarity inversion is clearest at the central sulcus. McCarthy et al. (1993) reported that the face and intraoral areas of the sensorimotor cortex can be identified by recording SEPs elicited by stimulating the palate, chin, lips, or tongue.

Several groups have recorded SEPs during cerebrovascular procedures in order to detect decreases in blood flow to different parts of the brain. Branston et al. (1974, 1976) introduced this application of SEP monitoring based on a series of experiments on baboons. They demonstrated that a clear relationship exists between cerebral blood flow and SEP integrity. Following middle cerebral artery occlusion, median nerve SEPs are attenuated when the blood flow is less than 16 ml/100 g per minute, and disappear at flows of less than 12 ml/100 g per minute. Hence, several teams have evaluated the usefulness of this testing during surgery when there is a possibility of a decrease in blood flow to the brain. The main procedures that have been evaluated are carotid endarterectomy, cerebral aneurysm, and hypothermic cardiopulmonary bypass surgeries.

Carotid endarterectomy surgery is commonly performed to treat obstructive vascular disease. A risk of this surgery is the potential for ischemic damage to the ipsilateral hemisphere during internal carotid artery occlusion. A variety of methods have been introduced to monitor cerebral sufficiency. They include performing the surgery under local anesthesia; recording the EEG, stump pressure, internal jugular venous oxygen pressure and saturation, and ^{133}Xe cerebral blood flow measurement (reviewed by Moorthy et al., 1982). When the carotid artery is clamped, collateral circulation through the circle of Willis is generally sufficient (approximately 90%) to adequately perfuse the ipsilateral hemisphere. If it is not sufficient, the surgeon can place a common carotid–distal internal carotid shunt, bypassing the carotid arteriotomy site. The potential problems of shunt placement are irritation of the vessel intima, increasing the time of surgery, interfering with the surgical field, and increasing the risk of emboli. Intraoperative EEG recording is the most common method for monitoring cerebral vascular insufficiency during these procedures. Both routine and processed EEG monitoring have been performed (Chiappa et al., 1979). Markand and colleagues (1984a,b) proposed SEP monitoring as an alternative to EEG testing because they assumed that EPs would be (1) easier to perform (i.e., fewer electrodes required), and (2) more resistant to changes in anesthesia and physiologic parameters of the patient, including blood pressure. Alterations in the waveform latency, amplitude, or general morphology were used as indicators of vascular insufficiency. Recordings from the contralateral, presumably normal, cerebral hemisphere provided the control. If the SEPs were preserved it was an indication of adequate perfusion.

Lindsay Symon and others have made considerable progress in applying this methodology to aneurysm surgery (Friedman et al., 1987; Symon and Murota, 1989; Symon et al., 1984). The results of these studies have demonstrated that monitoring can be helpful; however, the aneurysm or AVM must be in a location that can be mapped by the sensory pathway. The majority of experience has been during middle cerebral artery aneurysm surgery.

Measurement parameters during cerebrovascular procedures have included the central conduction time (Hume and Cant, 1978), waveform amplitude, and general morphology. Symon and Murota (1989) reported that waveform amplitude measures are too variable for accurate measurements. It is their opinion that the rate of SEP disappearance is important for predicting the functional outcome of the patient. If it takes more than 4 min for the SEPs to disappear, then the surgeon has 20 "safe" minutes of carotid and middle cerebral artery occlusion, whereas if it takes less than 4 min the window of safety from neurologic deficits narrows to 10 min. Monitoring anterior cerebral artery territory ischemia with median nerve SEPs is unsatisfactory. Posterior tibial nerve SEP recordings have been utilized for this type of monitoring (Sako et al., 1995). Schramm et al. (1990) monitored 113 operations during clipping of cerebral aneurysms. Their focus was on the electrophysiologic response observed following the clipping. This monitoring was beneficial during "temporary vessel occlusion, middle cerebral artery multilobed aneurysms, giant aneurysms, and trapping procedures." They used a 8.5-msec increase in the central conduction time as a guideline for warning the surgeon of a potential adverse event. Sako et al. (1995) used amplitude changes in the SEPs (median or posterior tibial) during the temporary occlusion. They found that if the SEPs only partially recovered following release of the clip, it suggested that new postoperative neurologic deficits would likely be present following surgery.

Intraoperative SEP recordings have been shown to be helpful in a variety of cardiovascular procedures. Several groups monitor cerebral function during cardiopulmonary bypass surgery with hypothermia (Coles et al., 1984; Kopf et al. 1985). In addition to monitoring brain ischemia, recording SEPs has been shown to decrease the incidence of brachial plexus injury following coronary artery bypass grafting (Hickey et al., 1993; Jellish et al., 1994). Guerit and his colleagues (1994) used SEPs to determine the optimal temperature for deep hypothermic circulatory arrest. Finally, vascular surgeons have used SEPs to monitor spinal cord function when they cross-clamped the aorta or for identification of crucial intercostal spinal arteries prior to ligation (reviewed by Nuwer, 1986, and Ross, 1985). Gugino et al. (1992) reported that peripheral ischemia may be a complicating factor when monitoring this type of surgery.

Electrophysiologic assessment during brachial plexus surgery includes spontaneous EMG recording, direct compound muscle action potential, sensory nerve action potentials, and SEP recordings elicited by direct nerve root stimulation. Somatosensory testing is used to make sure that avulsion of the root has not occurred (Sugioka, 1984). If these signals are present, postganglionic lesion repair would be minimal.

Because of a 50% incidence of lumbosacral plexopathy during reduction of unstable pelvic fractures, Helfet et al. (1995) proposed SEP monitoring during these procedures. It is their opinion that this type of monitoring decreased iatrogenic lumbosacral neurologic compromise. Rasmussen et al., (1994) reported that SEP monitoring was neither predictive nor helpful in preventing sciatic nerve injuries during total hip arthroplasty. Complementary spontaneous or evoked EMG myotome recordings would markedly enhance monitoring during this procedure.

3.3. Stimulus Parameters

The appropriate stimulus parameters have been reviewed by the American Electroencephalographic Society (1987).

3.3.1. Placement

The posterior tibial nerve at the ankle is stimulated when monitoring below the cervical spine. The stimulating electrodes are placed between the Achilles tendon and medial malleolus at the ankle. The benefits of this stimulus site are that it is easily accessible to the technician, and a recording electrode may be placed over the popliteal fossa to document stimulus integrity. A visible muscle twitch is not required, which allows the anesthesiologist to give the patient muscle relaxants. As an alternative site, the common peroneal nerve may be stimulated at the knee. This stimulus site is not commonly used because of the lack of an accessible site for the recording electrode to document stimulus integrity.

Upper-limb SEPs are usually recorded when the surgery is above the eighth cervical spinal cord segment. The potentials are elicited by stimulating either the median or the ulnar nerve at the wrist. Occasionally, the anesthesiologist may have placed arterial or intravenous lines in that area, thereby blocking access to either nerve. As an alternative the ulnar nerve may be stimulated at the elbow. Caution must be exercised because of the effect changing the stimulus position may have on the latency of the potentials. Stimulus integrity may be monitored by placing an electrode over the Erb's point region. O'Brien et al. (1994) recommended the concomitant recording of upper-limb SEPs during thoracic and lumbar spine deformity surgery. They suggested that this testing was 100% sensitive for detecting combined upper-limb sensory and motor deficits during these surgeries. Simply repositioning the arm can correct a potential iatrogenic deficit.

Dermatomes may be stimulated for monitoring individual nerve roots. However, these signals have several limitations (see related monitoring section of this chapter). Femoral nerve SEP monitoring has been proposed as an additional test for monitoring the midlumbar roots (Robinson et al., 1993). It is our view that myotome spontaneous EMG monitoring is a better method than dermatome somatosensory EPs for individual nerve root monitoring (Glassman et al., 1995).

3.3.2. Intensity

The recommended maximum current to apply to an anesthetized patient is 40 mA (American Electroencephalographic Society, 1987). In practice we recommend finding the minimum intensity required by titrating the intensity with the response. If possible, a preanesthetic baseline should be obtained.

3.3.3. Duration

Intraoperative SEP testing does not require conditions different from standard clinical testing. When stimulating exposed nerves, as in brachial plexus surgery, a faster duration (50 μsec) should be used to avoid stimulus artifact. Rappaport et al. (1994) reported that during nitrous oxide/isoflurane anesthesia there was no significant interaction between the intensity and duration of the stimulus. Response latency was more resistant to a change in the physical characteristics of the stimulus than was the response amplitude of the posterior tibial nerve.

3.3.4. Stimulus Rate and Average Number

The goal of monitoring is to provide immediate feedback to the surgical team about the physiologic status of the monitored component of the nervous system. When the stimulus rate is increased the response amplitude decreases, decreasing the SNR. Nuwer (1986) recommended a stimulus rate of 5 Hz. If the response is too small the stimulus presentation rate should be decreased. The number of stimuli averaged depends on the SNR. We collect our baselines with an average number of 500 and then replicate. The average number may be decreased during the procedure if the SNR is satisfactory.

3.4. Recording Parameters

3.4.1. Electrode Type

There are many types of electrodes suitable for intraoperative monitoring. Routinely, we use conventional needle electrodes. Since they can be applied quickly the set-up time is decreased. In our experience the slightly greater impedance one gets with these electrodes has little effect upon the recordings. Several companies are making disposable needle electrodes that are relatively inexpensive. We recommend their use because they do not require cleaning and disinfecting. A word of caution for the frugal practitioner: When regular needle electrodes are reused repeatedly they get worn out. This can increase the rate of needle breakage in the skin during removal. Sometimes the needle head may be removed easily with forceps; however, the broken needle head often becomes imbedded in the tissue and cannot be visualized. When this occurs you must mark its location and inform the surgeon immediately so that proper steps are taken to remove the broken electrode. Several manufacturers have proposed costly types of electrodes with configurations that are supposed to improve monitoring. Each configuration should be evaluated based on safety and cost prior to program implementation.

Epidural recording and stimulation have been proposed during spinal cord monitoring. Several groups in Japan have considerable experience with this technique (Tamaki et al., 1981). Electrodes for epidural stimulation and recording are now commercially available. Caution must be exercised on the type of electrode applied because of the sensitivity of the tissue underlying them.

3.4.2. Electrode Placement

The optimal electrode position on the scalp for recording upper- or lower-limb SEPs has been described elsewhere in this book. During surgery an electrode may be detached accidentally when the patient is repositioned. To replace the electrode the clinical neurophysiologist must then crawl under the drapes and reattach it, although optimal placement may not be possible. A new baseline should then be obtained for the new electrode location. This may result in a changed configuration of the waveform. If back-up channels of recordings are made during the initial set-up, electrode replacement will not be required.

Whenever possible a spinal EP should be recorded. These signals are more resistant to the influences of anesthesia. During thoracic and lumbar surgery we routinely place an electrode over the cervical area. We have used a number of different reference electrode positions for the cervical potentials, but routinely we use a scalp electrode. The resultant peak has been quite helpful during these procedures. Helmers et al. (1995) recommended anterior neck recordings referenced to CZ to record the spinal potentials in children when the operative site precludes posterior placement. This method is simple to use and muscle relaxants may increase the SNR (Fig. 18–6). Others have tried various elegant methods for acquiring spinal EPs during surgery. As reviewed by Nuwer (1986), epidural electrodes, screw electrodes placed in bone, and other types of electrodes placed in soft tissue have been used to record spinal EPs (Fig. 18–7).

3.4.3. System Band-Pass

The band-pass required has been reviewed in the American Electroencephalographic Society guidelines (1987). For scalp recording the high-pass filter settings should be in the

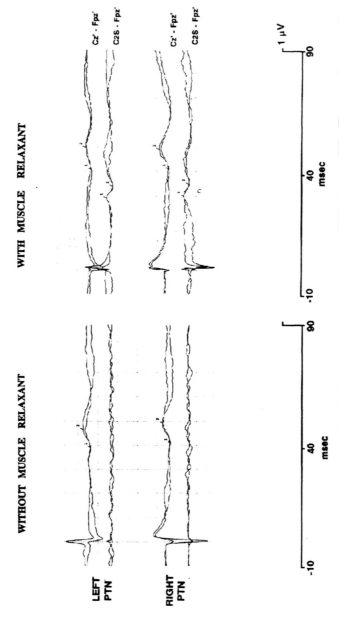

FIG. 18–6. Muscle relaxants applied during surgery may increase the SNR of spinal EPs. The waveforms on the left were recorded from a patient undergoing spinal procedure following stimulation of the posterior tibial nerve (PTN) at the ankle during surgery. The waveforms of the right were recorded from the same patient following the administration of muscle relaxants.

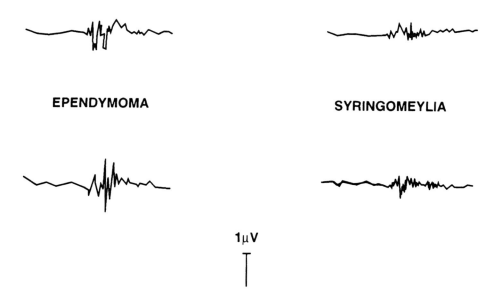

FIG. 18–7. Spinal EPs recorded with epidural bipolar electrodes. Electrodes are placed caudal and rostral to the operative site. The waveforms on the left were recorded from a patient who had an ependymoma removed from the spinal cord. The waveforms on the right were recorded from a patient who had a shunt inserted for syringomyelia. Note the variability of the response due to the varying types of myelopathy. (From Tator et al., 1988, with permission.)

1- to 30-Hz range. The low-pass filter setting should be in the 250- to 3,000-Hz range. The spinal EPs high-pass filter settings should be between 100 and 200 Hz and the low-pass filter settings should be in the 1,000- to 3,000-Hz range. The use of notch filters should be limited because they function in the frequency range of the required signal.

3.5. Anesthetic Considerations

One of the greatest problems encountered by clinical neurophysiologists in the operating room is the effect various anesthetic agents have on sensory evoked signals. A considerable effort has been made to characterize the effect various anesthetic agents have on SEPs.

Premedication agents, such as narcotic analgesics, sedatives, and antisialagogues, have been studied for their potential effect on SEPs. At premedication doses, these agents have little or no effect on the EPs. Moreover, they may enhance the SNR (Koht, 1988).

A variety of agents used for induction have been studied for their effect on SEPs (Koht, 1988). Thiopental has been studied over a wide range of doses. A decrease in the response amplitude and an increase in latency in the scalp-recorded potentials have been observed at induction doses. The cervical potentials are relatively resistant to thiopental at these doses (McPherson et al., 1986). Diazepam and narcotic agents have a similar effect on the signals.

Etomidate increases both the amplitude and latency of the cortical potentials. The amplitude of the cervical potentials decreases but the latency remains unchanged. Because of the amplitude enhancement of the cortical potentials it has been suggested that etomidate be used when the evoked signals are small. It is our experience that etomidate can induce post-operative nausea and vomiting and therefore should be used cautiously with the appropriate medication to treat these side effects. In summary, a number of different anesthetic agents are compatible with SEP monitoring during induction. Because of the different dosage required for induction and maintenance a re-establishment of the maintenance SEP baseline should be performed following induction.

Many of the agents used for induction are used for maintenance purposes but at lower doses, and therefore they have less effect on the SEPs. Often, inhalation anesthetics are delivered for maintenance purposes. Consequently, one must appreciate the effect that nitrous oxide and the halogenated agents have on the evoked responses.

It is a common misconception that nitrous oxide can be used with impunity during SEP monitoring. Indeed, McPherson et al. (1985) demonstrated that nitrous oxide at 50% concentration can be far more deleterious to scalp-recorded potentials than halogenated agents used at 0.25% to 1%. When encountering changes in the evoked signals that cannot be attributed to events related to the surgery, a decrease in the levels of the inhalation agents can often result in a return to baseline values.

The halogenated agents were, for many years, the "bad guys" in intraoperative monitoring. However, we now know that successful monitoring can be performed with the halogenated agents. What is important to understand is that a dose-related effect will be exerted upon the cortical potentials, and that the cervical potentials are far more resistant to changes in the dosage level of the halogenated agents.

Supplementary drugs and techniques may also affect the SEPs. During the course of the operation, the anesthesiologist may give the patient adjunct drugs or the surgeon may request a change in the physiologic status of the patient, such as lowering the blood pressure in order to decrease blood loss. For example, the cardiovascular drugs, such as sodium nitroprusside, result in a drop in blood pressure with a concomitant decrease in cerebral blood flow. This change in flow can effect a change in the SEPs. When a change in the evoked signals is observed, the first step for the neurophysiologist is to check for technical problems, followed by consultation with the anesthesiologist. A bolus administration of an agent can often be the cause of an electrophysiologic change.

Other physiologic manipulations that may be bothersome to the neurophysiologist are deliberate hypotension and hyperventilation. Both deliberate hypotension and hyperventilation have, as an end result, the concomitant decrease in cerebral blood flow, with a resultant change in the SEPs.

In summary, as our understanding of the complex relationship that exists between anesthesia and EPs grows, it is apparent that a number of different anesthetic protocols are suitable for monitoring purposes. Three techniques have been recommended for intraoperative SEP monitoring: narcotic/halogenated agents, narcotic/nitrous oxide, and total intravenous anesthesia (Koht, 1988). When the preoperative evoked signals have a low SNR, consultation with the anesthesiologist is a prerequisite. It is important to remember that when a change in the SEPs is observed, simply reducing the halogenated agents, followed by increasing the nitrous oxide, may be of no benefit to the monitoring team. Continuous infusions of narcotics provide stable recordings, whereas bolus injections can affect both the evoked potentials and the wake-up test (Pathak et al., 1983, 1984). For monitoring tiny signals, Kalkman et al. (1986) recommend an alfentanil–propofol anesthetic technique for signal enhancement. This may be the approach of the future because recent work has demonstrated that motor EP monitoring can be performed successfully during propofol anesthesia. This type of complementary monitoring should markedly enhance our ability to monitor the physiological integrity of the spinal cord during surgery.

3.6. Warning Criteria

When does the monitoring team inform the surgeon that a change in the electrophysiologic status of the patient has occurred? This is a difficult question to answer for there are no established criteria. Many centers consider any of the following to indicate a change in the patient's status: a 30% to 50% decrease in the amplitude of the potentials, a 2.5-msec increase in the response latency, or an increase of 5% to 10% of the response latency, or any combination of the above.

It is axiomatic that no information is better than misinformation. Selecting your patients before monitoring is important. If there are no potentials preoperatively it is highly probable that there will be no potentials intraoperatively. Further, Young and Sakatani (1990) reported that patients with pre-existing spinal cord injuries may have SEPs that are resistant to spinal cord manipulations. Educating the surgeon about these potential problems preoperatively will obviate any postoperative explanations. Young and Sakatani (1990) also stated that simple amplitude criteria for changes is not adequate. Their criteria is based on "duration" of changes. If a change lasts at least 10 min then it suggests the potential for neurologic compromise. In our institutions we take a proactive approach. Educating the surgical team as to the difficulties of performing the test and its limitations is important. If a good rapport exists within the operating room the surgeon will welcome comments from the monitoring team.

Both false negative (Lesser et al., 1986) and false positive (Tator et al., 1988) results have been reported in the literature. Figure 18–8 depicts a false positive result in which spinal epidural recordings rostral to the operative site were completely lost following biopsy during surgery to remove an ependymoma. Postoperative neurologic exami-

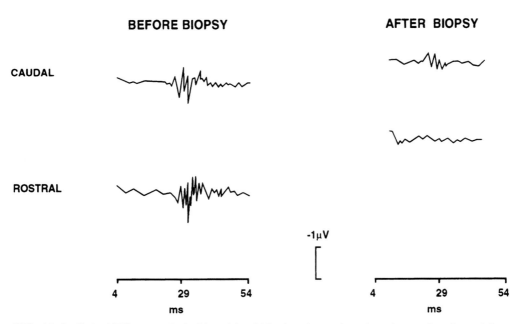

FIG. 18–8. Spinal EPs recorded with epidural bipolar electrodes placed rostral and caudal to the operative site. The tracings on the left were recorded before tumor biopsy, while those on the right were recorded after tumor biopsy, and showed absence of the rostral response. (From Tator et al., 1988, with permission.)

nation revealed minor neurologic deficits, which were completely resolved within 1 year.

Kearse et al. (1993) reported that SEP monitoring performed during intramedullary spinal cord surgery accurately predicts new postoperative motor neurologic deficits. In summary, based on the anatomic location and blood supply of the sensory tracts compared to the motor tracts, SEP monitoring has theoretical limitations for monitoring the complete physiologic integrity of the spinal cord. It is surprising, yet comforting, how few reports in the literature exist that suggest potential false positive and false negative results.

3.7. Monitoring Peripheral Nerve Function During Surgery

One of the most exciting developments in intraoperative electrophysiologic monitoring has been the development of evoked EMG testing. This technique was initially developed for monitoring facial nerve function during the removal of acoustic neuromas. Mechanical irritation of the facial nerve results in EMG activity being generated in the innervated muscle. This activity is audio-amplified, thereby providing immediate feedback to the surgical team. Other cranial motor nerves have also been monitored with this technique (Table 18–3).

In addition to mechanical irritation, monitoring can be used to identify the nerve within the operative field by intracranial stimulation. Both of these techniques have been used to avoid intraoperative damage to the cranial motor nerves. This methodology has been used recently to monitor spinal nerves during lumbar spine surgery.

When spine surgery is being performed below L1, routine monitoring with SEPs, elicited by stimulating a mixed nerve, such as the posterior tibial nerve, provides minimal information. Somatosensory EPs have been elicited by stimulating the L4, L5, and S1 dermatome region (Toleikis et al., 1993). Although the dermatome SEPs may provide information on the physiologic integrity of individual nerve roots, there are several limitations to root monitoring using this modality. First, the dermatome SEPs are small in amplitude and may require the collection of a considerable number of averages to obtain a satisfactory SNR. Second, they are more sensitive to the effects of anesthesia. Third, to monitor a number of spinal roots is time consuming. Fourth, ventral motor root function is not monitored. The intraoperative monitoring of evoked EMG activity is a better method of monitoring individual nerve roots (Glassman et al., 1995).

The principles of spinal nerve root monitoring are similar to those developed for cranial motor nerve root monitoring. Needle electrodes are inserted into muscles innervated by the

TABLE 18–3. *Cranial motor nerve monitoring*

Nerve	Muscle
Oculomotor nerve (III)	Inferior rectus
Trochlear nerve (IV)	Superior oblique
Trigeminal nerve (V)	Masseter
Abducens nerve (VI)	Lateral rectus
Facial nerve (VII)	Orbicularis oris
Glossopharyngeal nerve (IX)	Stylopharyngeal
Spinal accessory nerve (XI)	Trapezius
Hypoglossal nerve (XII)	Lateral side of tongue

TABLE 18–4. *Spinal nerve root monitoring*

Muscle	Roots
Rectus femoris	L2, L3, L4
Tibialis anterior	L4, L5
Peroneus longus	L5, S1
Gastrocnemius (medial head)	L5, S1, S2

L4, L5, and S1 roots (Table 18–4). Evoked EMG activity is monitored throughout the procedure. Whenever neurotonic discharges are observed the surgical team is informed that the nerve root is being excessively irritated.

Spinal nerve root monitoring with EMG activity has several benefits. First, immediate feedback is provided to the surgical team. Second, multiple roots can be monitored during the operation simultaneously. Third, these signals are less sensitive to anesthesia. Fourth, ventral motor root function is monitored. However, there are some limitations to this technique. First, it is unclear how much neurotonic discharge indicates that neuronal damage has occurred. Second, this technique requires that the administration of neuromuscular blocking agents be limited during the operation. Examples of neurotonic discharge activity recorded during a closing wedge osteotomy surgery are illustrated in Fig. 18–9.

Recent work in both animals (Lebwohl and Calancie, 1992) and humans (Glassman et al., 1995) has demonstrated that EMG monitoring may be enhanced by pedical screw stimulation. If the screws placed during spinal instrumentation are not positioned correctly they

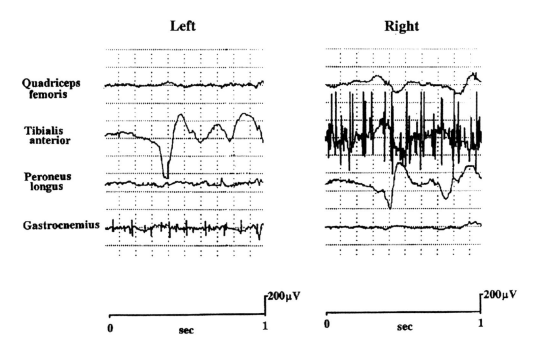

FIG. 18–9. Evoked EMG responses recorded during lumbar spinal surgery (closing wedge osteotomy) can provide real-time feedback on nerve root irritation. Note the profound neurotonic discharge activity illustrated on the right side of the figure.

may penetrate cortical bone of the pedicle and irritate the underlying nerve root, resulting in spontaneous neurotonic discharge. To determine the integrity of a screw's position, Lebwohl and Calancie (1992) connected a cathode stimulator to an awl and probed the screw placement site. If no EMG activity is elicited following stimulation with the probe (7.5 mA, 0.2 msec duration, 3 Hz) the pedicle screw is placed. To verify the safety of the screw placement the screw is then stimulated. This technique has provided a 10% detection rate of misplaced screws. This is most important if the screw has breached the medial or inferior pedicle wall, because of the immediate proximity of the adjacent spinal nerve root. If the pedicle screw breaches the superior or lateral pedical cortex, the EP may not record any abnormality because the nerve root is remote from these pedicle surfaces. Also, there is no risk of nerve root damage in these sites (superior and lateral).

4. VISUAL EVOKED POTENTIALS

"You can boast about anything if it's all you have"
John Steinbeck: East of Eden

4.1. Introduction/History

At the present time intraoperative electrophysiologic monitoring of visual evoked potentials (VEPs) is of limited use because of difficulty with the delivery of the stimulus. Outside the operating room VEPs can be recorded in a controlled environment, where the essential parameters, such as distance from the eye to the stimulator, amount of ambient light, and presenting pattern reversal stimuli, are easy to control, and normative data sets can be constructed. In the operating room few, if any, of these variables can be controlled. However, with the introduction of several innovative techniques, there may be light at the end of the tunnel. Moller (1988b) and Nuwer (1986) have reviewed this topic.

4.2. Procedures to Be Monitored

Visual EP monitoring has been performed during surgery for pituitary or cavernous sinus tumors and cerebral aneurysms.

Several groups have reported amplitude enhancement when the optic nerve was decompressed (Allen et al., 1981; Feinsod et al., 1975; Feinsod et al., 1976; Raudzens, 1982; Wilson et al., 1976). Although these findings are suggestive of the potential usefulness of this technique, it is our experience that this type of monitoring has many limitations, including an unsatisfactory number of false positive and false negative reports. Moreover the success rate for recording technically satisfactory VEPs is low.

4.3. Stimulus Parameters

4.3.1. Method

Stimulus parameters have been reviewed by the American Electroencephalographic Society (1987), but, unfortunately, all current methods of delivering the stimulus are limited in their effectiveness.

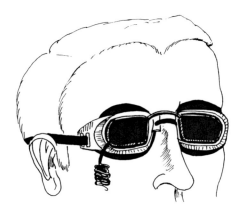

FIG. 18–10. Flash VEPs can be recorded during surgery. The stimuli are presented through goggles.

Flash visual stimuli are used to elicit the response. Early researchers used a strobe light placed 50 cm in front of the nasion (Albright and Sclabassi, 1985). Now, goggles, with light-emitting diodes in the orbit cups, are commercially available, as well as contact lenses with a light-emitting diode fastened to each lens, covering it (Figs. 18–10 and 18–11). The contact lens method probably provides a better light source. Several groups have reported success using this technique (Moller, 1988b). However, the problems that may arise with their use are corneal abrasion and/or infection. If an effective method for delivering pattern-reversal stimuli could be developed, intraoperative monitoring of VEPs may become practical. Bagolini et al. (1979) successfully recorded pattern reversal VEPs from normal subjects while they were anesthetized with enflurane.

4.3.2. Placement

Goggles are placed over both of the patient's eyes. This should be done with extreme caution, because it is easy for the surgical assistant to put pressure on the goggles during surgery, which may result in damage to the orbit. The surrounding skin can be sutured to the goggles, which should limit movement. The monitoring team should check the position of

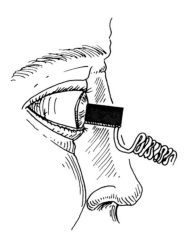

FIG. 18–11. Light-emitting diodes connected to contact lenses can be used to elicit VEPs during surgery.

the goggles throughout the procedure. The contact lenses containing light-emitting diodes should be inserted only by trained medical personnel.

4.3.3. Intensity

The actual penetrating intensity of the stimulus emitted by the goggles is difficult to measure. There is no way to increase or decrease the intensity of the stimulus given off by many of the commercially available goggles. The intensity of the stimulus given off by the contact lenses can be enhanced. In any case, the intensity level should be consistent throughout the procedure. If the intensity level is altered in any way a new baseline should be recorded.

4.3.4. Duration

The same guidelines that apply to the intensity of the stimulus should be applied to determining the duration of the stimulus.

4.3.5. Color

The color emitted by the diodes should be recorded.

4.3.6. Rate

Conventional recording of pattern-reversal VEPs consists of delivering the stimuli at a slow presentation rate (1 to 2 Hz) so that the transient potentials could be recorded. Steady-state visual potentials can be recorded by delivering the stimulus at a sufficiently fast presentation rate so that there is an overlapping of the response to subsequent stimuli. Steady-state potentials can be analyzed with frequency-based techniques (e.g., Fourier analysis). Adequate SNRs can be collected in a shorter period of time with this method compared to conventional transient EP assessment techniques. More work needs to be done in this area.

4.3.7. Stimulus

Only monocular stimuli should be delivered.

4.3.8. Pupil Size

The amount of light that reaches the retina is a function of the pupil size. Because anesthetic agents can effect the size of the pupil, mydriatic agents should be given before starting the procedure.

4.4. Recording Parameters

4.4.1. Type of Electrode

Disposable needle electrodes are used for recording scalp potentials. When recording compound nerve action potentials directly from the optic nerve cotton-wick electrodes may be used (Moller et al., 1987). This methodology improves the SNR; therefore a satisfactory signal can be recorded with a smaller number of averages. A problem with this technique is that the optic nerve must be exposed surgically before direct monitoring can be performed.

4.4.2. Electrode Placement

The scalp recording electrodes should be placed 5 cm above the inion and 12 cm above the nasion whenever the operative site permits. Other, backup, locations for the electrodes should be considered prior to the operation. The postnasion electrode may be moved behind the operative site.

4.4.3. System Band-Pass

The band-pass required for monitoring VEPs has been reviewed in the American Electroencephalographic Society guidelines (1987). The low-pass filter setting should be in the 200- to 300-Hz range. The high-pass filter setting should be in the 1- to 5-Hz range. If the SNR is too low the band-pass should be closed to 5 to 100 Hz and artifact rejection techniques should be applied.

4.4.4. Time Base and Average Number

The analysis time should be a minimum of 250 msec. The minimum number of averages required per trial in 100. Replication is a prerequisite.

4.5. Anesthetic Considerations

Flash VEPs have considerable intrasubject and intersubject variability, making it virtually impossible to evaluate the effect anesthesia has on these potentials. Early studies suggested that nitrous oxide has a minimal decremental effect on the VEP (Domino et al., 1963), whereas Sebel et al. (1984) reported a dose-related amplitude decrement and latency increase with nitrous oxide. Sebel et al. (1986) reported similar results on the VEPs with isoflurane anesthesia. Moreover, decreasing the temperature (Russ et al., 1984) and hemodilution (Nagao et al., 1978) have been shown to adversely effect the VEPs.

Interestingly, Bagolini et al. (1979) reported successful recording of pattern reversal VEPs during enflurane (Ethrane®) anesthesia. Before intraoperative recording of VEPs can be considered to be reliable, the stimulus and recording of signals must be improved, and the effect anesthesia has on reproducible signals must be determined.

4.6. Warning Criteria

If reproducible waveforms can be obtained, any deviations from the baseline should be reported to the surgical team. It is important that the surgeon be aware of the problems associated with this technique before surgery.

Currently monitoring VEPs during surgery is of limited use. However, with the development of new techniques, intraoperative VEP monitoring may become useful in the future.

5. TRIGEMINAL EVOKED POTENTIAL MONITORING

5.1. Introduction/History

It has been reported that stimulation of end organs or fibers mediating trigeminal sensation results in a series of short-latency (<10 msec) and long-latency (>10 msec) EPs that have been attributed to activation of central trigeminal pathways (Findler and Feinsod, 1982; Singh et al., 1982; Soustiel et al., 1993). The trigeminal sensory evoked response (TEP) has been advocated as being an indicator of the neural status of the peripheral (Altenmuller et al., 1990) and central trigeminal nerve pathways (Bennett and Jannetta, 1983; Bennett and Lunsford, 1984).

Considerable controversy exists concerning the exact configuration and the contribution of myogenic generators to the TEP. Studies of the TEP have reported a variability of the response between and within subjects, particularly for the longer-latency components. Stechison and Kralick (1993) have demonstrated that the long latency responses of the TEP, present in awake patients, disappeared following the induction of anesthesia irrespective of the use of neuromuscular blocking agents. Consequently, these investigators concluded that the long latency response of the TEP, due to anesthetic suppression of polysynaptic pathways, is not useful for intraoperative monitoring.

In contrast, the short-latency response, occurring in the first 3 msec following stimulation persists during anesthesia and neuromuscular blockade (Soustiel et al., 1993; Stechison, 1993). Uncertainties remain concerning the proximal location of the neural generators of these early peaks, purported to be either at the root entry zone (Stechison, 1993) or brain stem (Singh et al., 1982; Soustiel et al., 1993).

Despite these difficulties, reports indicate that alterations in the TEP reflect the integrity of trigeminal pathways (Bennett and Jannetta, 1983; Bennett and Lunsford, 1984). Intraoperative changes in the TEP have been correlated with surgical outcome during posterior fossa surgery (Soustiel et al., 1993).

5.2. Stimulation Parameters

Trigeminal EPs have been elicited following stimulation of either the upper and lower lips, gingiva, tongue, teeth, skin bordering the neural foramen, or the trigeminal nerve directly. Anode and cathode cup or needle electrodes, separated by less than a centimeter, are used to deliver the stimulus. Electrical pulses, lasting between 50 and 100 msec, are delivered at a rate of 5/sec. Alternating the stimulus polarity may be used to reduce the stimulus artifact. Stimulus intensity ranges from 5 to 15 mA.

5.3. Recording Parameters

Reliable short-latency TEPs can be obtained with the active recording electrode positioned over the mastoid ipsilateral to stimulation and referenced to FZ. Long-latency TEPs have been reported with the active electrode positioned on the scalp over the somatosensory cortex of the face. The ground electrode should be placed adjacent to the stimulating electrodes to reduce the stimulus artifact, which can block the early components of the TEP. Stechison (1993) reported that TEPs can be recorded directly from the trigeminal nerve at the root entry zone. The signals are amplified and filtered with a band-pass of 1 to 2,000 Hz. Averages are obtained from approximately 250 stimulus trials.

5.4. Intraoperative Alterations of the TEP

The use of the TEP has been reported in a series of cases undergoing posterior surgery in the proximity of the trigeminal nerve (Soustiel et al., 1993). Alterations in the waveform or peak latencies of the TEP were correlated with surgical manipulation. Retractor placement and dissection adjacent to the trigeminal nerve were identified as the major causes for these changes in the TEP. Repositioning of the retractor or a suspension of the dissection were associated with a partial or complete return to the baseline configuration. Changes in the TEP have also been reported following retrogasserian glycerol rhizotomy. These changes have been suggested as indicating the potential benefits of this procedure (Bennett and Lunsford, 1984).

6. MOTOR EVOKED POTENTIALS

6.1. Introduction/History

The monitoring of motor evoked potentials (MEPs) was one of the first electrophysiologic techniques to be used intraoperatively. Penfield and Jasper used electrophysiologic stimulation to map out the motor and sensory homunculi within the human brain during surgery (1954). A reawakening of the intraoperative application of stimulating the brain and/or spinal cord, and recording from peripheral nerves and/or muscles was generated from spinal cord monitoring. Somatosensory EP recordings during spine and spinal cord surgery monitor the motor components of the spinal cord by proxy only. Both false negative (Ginsburg et al., 1985; Lesser et al., 1986) and false positive (Tator et al., 1988) results have been reported in the literature. It would be advantageous to have techniques capable of providing complementary monitoring of both sensory and motor function.

Levy and York (1983) were the first to use MEPs for intraoperative monitoring of motor spinal cord function. The MEPs were elicited by either direct stimulation of the spinal cord or by transcranial electrical stimulation. For transcranial stimulation a scalp-to-hard palate montage was applied. As described in the following sections several modifications of this technique have been introduced.

The various types of MEP testing can be classified, based on the site and method of stimulation:

Transcranial magnetic MEPs (tcMMEPs)
Transcranial electrical MEPs (tcEMEPs)
Direct epidural spinal cord stimulation
Noninvasive spinal cord stimulation: the neurogenic MEPs

6.2. Procedures to Be Monitored

Table 18–2 lists the types of surgery in which SEP monitoring has been used. All of these procedures could also be monitored intraoperatively with MEPs.

6.3. Stimulus Parameters

6.3.1. Transcranial Magnetic MEPs

We, at the University of Louisville, use the Cadwell MES-10 magnetic stimulator to produce the stimulus. We first used the 9-cm (mean diameter) stimulating coil, but then

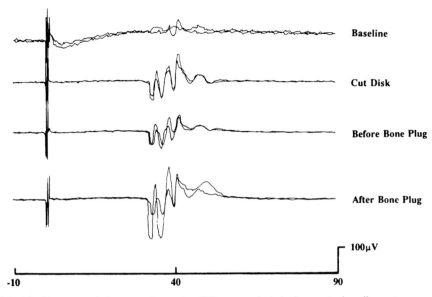

FIG. 18–12. Transcranial magnetic motor EPs recorded during anterior discectomy surgery. The signals do not require averaging and therefore a satisfactory SNR can be recorded in a shorter period of time.

switched to a skullcap coil, which increased our intraoperative success rate. The skullcap coil provides enhanced global activation of descending motor fibers (Linden et al., 1996). Figure 18–12 depicts intraoperative MEPs recorded during anterior cervical discectomy surgery. Earlier studies that reported unsatisfactory monitoring with tcM-MEPs (e.g., Taniguchi et al., 1993) should be repeated with this improved method of stimulation.

6.3.2. Transcranial Electrical MEPs

Levy and York (1983) used a scalp-to-hard palate stimulation montage. Several other groups used the digitimer stimulator (Boyd et al., 1986; Jellinek et al., 1991; Rothwell et al., 1989; Zentner, 1989). Burke et al. (1992) introduced the concomitant recording of both tcEMEPs and SEPs with bipolar electrodes placed above and below the operative site.

6.3.3. Spinal Cord Stimulation (Direct)

In 1983 Levy and York introduced this technique by directly stimulating the spinal cord following intraoperative exposure. Machida et al. (1985) refined this method by placing a pair of electrodes epidurally and recording the evoked response from peripheral muscles. Tamaki (1989) developed direct spinal cord electrical stimulation and recording techniques. Tuohy needles are inserted above and below the operative site, through which electrodes are placed. Identical electrodes are used for both stimulating and recording. Recording electrodes are placed in the subarachnoid space below the operative site. Double-pulse stimuli have been recommended to enhance the SNR through temporal stimulation (Taylor et al., 1993). Haghighi et al. (1992) demonstrated that these potentials were recordable during the removal of an intramedullary spinal tumor, while SEPs were not recordable.

6.3.4. Spinal Cord Stimulation (Indirect) (Neurogenic MEPs)

Owen et al. (1988) developed the method for monitoring neurogenic MEPs by stimulating the spinal cord outside the spinal canal. They are so named because they reflect neural activity recorded from the sciatic notch or the popliteal fossa. This technique was developed because the procedure could be performed while the patient received muscle relaxants. Moreover, since the stimulating electrodes are placed into the bone of the spinous processes, electrode migration, which could result in a change in the response or an iatrogenic-induced spinal cord injury, is reduced.

6.3.5. Intensity

To elicit a tcMMEP the maximum output of the commercially available stimulators is used (2 Tesla). When tcEMEPs are recorded epidurally, following stimulation with the Digitimer stimulator, signals can be recorded at low intensities (30% output). The first component of the waveform is an initial D-wave thought to be generated by direct stimulation of the corticospinal tracts. As the stimulation intensity is increased, the amplitude increases (supramaximal at approximately 70%), and later I-waves (indirect corticospinal activation) are observed. The maximum intensity is 700 V (peak current of 500 mA). For direct spinal cord stimulation the intensity range is 3 to 10 mA. For neurogenic MEPs the stimulation intensity is calculated by performing an intensity–output function for each patient.

6.3.6. Duration

For tcMMEP the pulse-width is 70 μsec. For tcEMEP with the Digitimer stimulator the pulse width is 50 μsec. The pulse width for Neurogenic MEPs is 200 μsec. For direct epidural stimulation the pulse width is 300 μsec.

6.3.7. Presentation Rate

Transcranial stimulus presentation rates are slow in order to decrease the potential risk of kindling. For tcMMEP the rate is 0.3/sec and for tcEMEP the interval recommended by Boyd et al. (1986) should be greater than 5/sec.

Spinal cord stimulation may be performed at a fast rate. Direct epidural stimulation presentation rates may be as high as 50 Hz. Neurogenic potentials can also be collected when the stimuli are delivered at fast presentation rates.

6.3.8. Average Number

Myogenic signals have the obvious benefit of being large, and, therefore, a satisfactory SNR can be collected with a low number of averages. Five stimuli are averaged during magnetic stimulation. The tcEMEPs recorded with bipolar electrodes do not require averaging.

6.4. Recording Parameters

6.4.1. Electrode Type

The benefits and limitations of the SEP and the MEP recording electrodes are identical (see section 3.4).

6.4.2. Electrode Placement

To record the tcMMEPs from the upper limb, electrodes are placed in the abductor pollicis brevis muscles, and for the lower limb, in the tibialis anterior muscles. The same muscles can be used for tcEMEPs. Both tcEMEPs (Zentner, 1991) and tcMMEPs (Herdman et al., 1993) have been recorded from the cauda equina during intramedullary, extramedullary, and extradural spinal tumor surgery. The false positive and false negative rates are low when using this site for recording these potentials.

Epidural recording techniques are identical to those described in section 3.4.

6.4.3. System Band-Pass

To record the MEPs a band-pass of 10 to 10,000 Hz is recommended. A narrower band-pass (10 to 2,000 Hz) is recommended when recording spinal and neurogenic potentials.

6.5. Anesthetic Considerations

Successful recording of intraoperative tcMMEPs is completely dependent upon the anesthetic regimen applied. It is clear in both human (Schmid et al., 1992; Linden et al., 1996) and animal (Haghighi et al., 1990; Stone et al., 1992; Glassman et al., 1993) studies that tcMMEPs and halogenated agents are not compatible.

Although there are probably other anesthetic regimens that would be compatible with tcMMEPs, we use the following combination. Versed® (midazolam) 1 to 2 mg IV and Robinul® (glycopyrrolate) 0.2 mg IV are the preanesthetic medications. For induction, either fentanyl citrate (3 μg/kg) or lidocaine (0.5 mg/kg) is administered with etomidate (0.3 mg/kg). A number of different agents have been used to induce muscle relaxation (e.g., succinylcholine chloride, 1 to 2 mg/kg; atracurium besylate, 250 μg/kg, vecuronium, 70 μg/kg). For maintenance of anesthesia the following combination is used: Nitrous oxide/oxygen (<60% nitrous oxide); fentanyl citrate IV infusion (1 to 3 μg/kg); atracurium or vecuronium bromide infusion (not to exceed 80% neuromuscular blockade); scopolamine hydrobromide (amnestic agent); Reglan® 10 mg (to relieve etomidate-induced nausea). If the nitrous oxide level is increased above the protocol level during the procedure the signals can be obliterated.

The tcEMEPs are more robust than the magnetic tcMMEPs. For example, several groups have demonstrated successful recording of the tcEMEPs during anesthesia, supplemented with halogenated agents (Burke et al., 1990; Calancie et al., 1991) and propofol (Jellinek et al., 1991). Adams et al. (1993) demonstrated that compound muscle action potentials could be recorded following direct spinal cord stimulation when there was 90% total neuromuscular blockade. However, the tcEMEP are not without anesthetic limitations. For example, Zentner et al. (1989) reported that nitrous oxide can have a deleterious effect on tcEMEPs.

Prior to the routine practice of recording MEPs during surgery, the exact relationship that exists between the various anesthetic techniques and agents and their effects upon these signals should be documented.

Spinal cord stimulation techniques are more resistant to the effects of anesthesia than the transcranial stimulation techniques.

6.6. Warning Criteria

Animal studies have shown that MEPs are a more sensitive indicator of potential damage to the spinal cord than SEPs (Fehlings et al., 1989). For magnetic stimulation, a 50% decrease in the size of the amplitude and a 2.5-msec increase in latency is used to alert the surgeon of a possible change in the physiologic status of the patient. Lee et al. (1995) reported that changes in amplitude are a superior criterion for monitoring evaluating neurologic status when monitoring with tcMMEPs.

The amplitude of the neurogenic MEPs is the primary variable monitored. Latency data provide auxilary information. Burke et al. (1992) use a 20% to 30% decrease in amplitude of recordings of both ascending and descending volleys to alert the surgeon of possible problems. Latency changes are considered a poor indicator of the status of the spinal cord.

Spinal cord monitoring will be enhanced when concomitant monitoring of both MEPs and SEPs become standard procedure. The optimal method for eliciting MEPs has yet to be determined. Spinal MEPs are less sensitive to the effects of anesthesia; however, in general, they require a more invasive approach in order to record them. The tcEMEPs are more robust than the tcMMEPs; however, tcMMEPs are less painful to record for preoperative baselines. The MEP techniques have the added benefit of being able to provide real-time feedback to the surgical team.

Finally, both tcMMEPs and tcEMEPs are primarily generated in the lateral corticospinal tracts, while the ventral component of the cord is responsible for ambulation (Steeves and Jordan, 1980). Evoked potentials elicited by stimulating the cerebellum have been recommended for monitoring the ventral cord (Levy, 1987).

ACKNOWLEDGMENTS

The authors wish to thank Norma B. Braver for her help in preparing and editing this manuscript; George Batik for his drawings of several of the figures; and the Alliant Health System, Louisville, Kentucky, for its support.

REFERENCES

Adams DC, Emerson RG, Heyer EJ, McCormick PC, Carmel PW, Stein BM (1994): Monitoring of intraoperative motor-invoked potentials under conditions of controlled neuromuscular blockade. *Anesth Analg* 77(5):913–918. Comments in *Anesth Analg* 1994;79(6):1206.

Albright AL, Sclabassi RJ (1985): Cavitron ultrasonic surgical aspirator and visual evoked potential monitoring for chiasmal gliomas in children: Report of two cases. *J Neurosurg* 63:138–140.

Allen A, Starr A, Nudleman K (1981): Assessment of sensory function in the operating room utilizing cerebral evoked potentials: a study of fifty-six surgically anesthetized patients. *Clin Neurosurg* 28:457–481.

Allison T, Wood CC, Spencer DD, Goff WR, McCarthy G, Williamson PD (1985): Localization of sensorimotor cortex in surgery by SEP recording. *Electroencephalogr Clin Neurophysiol* 61:S74.

Altenmuller E, Cornelius CP, Buettner UW (1990): Somatosensory evoked potentials following tongue stimulation in normal subjects and patients with lesions of the afferent trigeminal system. *Electroencephalogr Clin Neurophysiol* 77:403–415.

American Electroencephalographic Society (1984): Guidelines for clinical evoked potential studies. *J Clin Neuro-physiol* 1:3–53.

American Electroencephalographic Society (1987): Guidelines for intraoperative monitoring of sensory evoked potentials. *J Clin Neurophysiol* 4:397–416.

Bagolini B, Penne A, Fonda S, Mazzetti A (1979): Pattern reversal visually evoked potentials in general anesthesia. *Albrecht Von Graefes Arch Klin Exp Ophthalmol* 209:231–238.

Bennett MH, Jannetta PJ (1983): Evoked potentials in trigeminal neuralgia. *Neurosurgery* 13:242–247.

Bennett MH, Lunsford LD (1984): Percutaneous retrogasserian glycerol rhizotomy for tic douloureux: Part 2. Results and implications of trigeminal evoked potential studies. *Neurosurgery* 14:431–435.

Berenstein A, Young W, Ransohoff J, Benjamin V, Merkin H (1984): Somatosensory evoked potentials during spinal angiography and therapeutic transvascular embolization. *J Neurosurg* 60:777–785.

Boyd SG, Rothwell JC, Cowan JM, Webb PJ, Morley T, Asselman P, Masden CD (1986): A method of monitoring function in corticospinal pathways during scoliosis surgery with a note on motor conduction velocities. *J Neurol Neurosurg Psychiatry* 49:251–257.

Branston NM, Symon L, Crockard HA, Pasztor E (1974): Relationship between the cortical evoked potential and local cortical blood flow following acute middle cerebral artery occlusion in the baboon. *Exp Neurol* 45:195–208.

Branston NM, Symon L, Crockard HA (1976): Recovery of the cortical evoked response following temporary middle cerebral artery occlusion in baboons: relation to local blood flow and PO_2. *Stroke* 7:151–157.

Burke D, Hicks RG, Stephen JPH (1990): Corticospinal volleys evoked by anodal and cathodal stimulation of the human motor cortex. *J Physiol* 425:283–299.

Burke D, Hicks R, Stephen J, Woodforth I, Crawford M (1992): Assessment of corticospinal and somatosensory conduction simultaneously during scoliosis surgery. *Electroencephalogr Clin Neurophysiol* 85:388–396.

Calancie B, Klose KJ, Baier S, Green BA (1991): Isoflurane-induced attenuation of motor evoked potentials caused by electrical motor cortex stimulation during surgery. *J Neurosurg* 74:897–904.

Chiappa KH, Burke SR, Young RR (1979): Results of electroencephalographic monitoring during 367 carotid endarterectomies. Use of a dedicated minicomputer. *Stroke* 10:381–388.

Coles JG, Taylor MJ, Pearce JM, Lowry NJ, Stewart DJ, Trusler GA, William WG (1984): Cerebral monitoring of somatosensory evoked potentials during profoundly hypothermic circulatory arrest. *Circulation* 70(3 Pt 2):196–102.

Daube JR, Harper CM (1989): Surgical monitoring of cranial and peripheral nerves. In: *Neuromonitoring in Surgery (Clinical Neurophysiology Updates, vol. 1)*, edited by JE Desmedt, pp 115–138. Elsevier, Amsterdam.

Dawson EG, Sherman JE, Kanim LE, Nuwer MR (1991): Spinal cord monitoring. Results of the Scoliosis Research Society and the European Spinal Deformity Society survey. *Spine* 16(8 Suppl):S361–S364.

Desmedt JE, ed (1989): *Neuromonitoring in Surgery (Clinical Neurophysiology Updates, vol 1)*. Elsevier, Amsterdam.

Domino EF, Corssen G, Sweet RB (1963): Effects of various general anesthetics on the visually evoked response in man. *Anesth Analg* 42:735–747.

Ducker TB, Brown RH, eds (1988): *Neurophysiology & Standards of Spinal Cord Monitoring.* Springer-Verlag, New York.

Epstein NE, Danto J, Nardi D (1993): Evaluation of intraoperative somatosensory-evoked potential monitoring during 100 cervical operations. *Spine* 18(6):737–747.

Fehlings MG, Tator CH, Linden RD (1989): The relationships among the severity of spinal cord injury, motor and somatosensory evoked potentials and spinal cord blood flow. *Electroencephalogr Clin Neurophysiol* 74:241–259.

Feinsod M, Madey JM, Susal AL (1975): A new photostimulator for continuous recording of the visual evoked potential. *Electroencephalogr Clin Neurophysiol* 38:641–642.

Feinsod M, Selhorst JB, Hoyt WF, Wilson CB (1976): Monitoring optic nerve function during craniotomy. *J Neurosurg* 44:29–31.

Findler G, Feinsod M (1982): Sensory evoked response to electrical stimulation of the trigeminal nerve in humans. *J Neurosurg* 56:545–549.

Fischer G, Fischer C, Remond J (1992): Hearing preservation in acoustic neurinoma surgery. *J Neurosurg* 76:910–917.

Frerebeau P, Benezech J, Uziel A, Coubes P, Seqnarbieux F, Malonga M (1987): Hearing preservation after acoustic neurinoma operation. *Neurosurgery* 21:197–200.

Fridman J, Zappulla R, Bergelson M, Greenblatt E, Malis L, Morrell F, Hoeppner T (1984): Application of phase spectral analysis for brain stem auditory evoked potential detection in normal subjects and patients with posterior fossa tumors. *Audiology* 23:99–113.

Friedman WA, Kaplan BJ, Gravenstein D, Rhoton AL Jr (1985): Intraoperative brain stem auditory evoked potentials during posterior fossa microvascular decompression. *J Neurosurg* 62:552–557.

Friedman WA, Kaplan BL, Day AL, Sypert GW, Curran MT (1987): Evoked potential monitoring during aneurysm operation: observations after fifty cases. *Neurosurgery* 20:678–687.

Ginsburg HH, Shetter AG, Raudzens PA (1985): Postoperative paraplegia with preserved intraoperative somatosensory evoked potentials. Case report. *J Neurosurg* 63:296–300.

Glassman SD, Shields CB, Linden RD, Zhang YP, Nixon AR, Johnson JR (1993): Anesthetic effects of motor evoked potentials in dogs. *Spine* 18(8):1083–1089.

Glassman SD, Dimar JR, Puno RM, Johnson JR, Shields CB, Linden RD (1995): A prospective analysis of intra-operative electromyographic monitoring of pedicle screw placement with computed tomographic scan confirmation. *Spine* 20:1375–1379.

Greenblatt E, Zappulla RA, Kaye S, Fridman J (1985): Response threshold determination of the brain stem auditory evoked responses: a comparison of the phase versus magnitude derived from the fast Fourier transform. *Audiology* 24:288–296.

Grundy BL, Lina A, Procopio PT, Jannetta PJ (1981): Reversible evoked potential changes with retraction of the eighth cranial nerve. *Anesth Analg* 60(11):835–838.

Grundy BL, Jannetta PJ, Procopio PT, Lina A, Boston JR, Doyle E (1982a): Intraoperative monitoring of brain stem auditory evoked potentials. *J Neurosurg* 57:674–681.

Grundy BL, Procopio PT, Jannetta PJ, Lina A, Doyle E (1982b): Evoked potential changes produced by positioning for retromastoid craniectomy. *Neurosurgery* 10:766–770.

Guerit JM, Verhelst R, Rubay J, el Khoury G, Noirhomme P, Baele P, Dion R (1994): The use of somatosensory evoked potentials to determine the optimal degree of hypothermia during circulatory arrest. *J Card Surg* 9(5):596–603.

Gugino LD, Kraus KH, Heino R, Aglio LS, Levy WJ, Cohn L, Maddi R (1992): Peripheral ischemia as a complicating factor during somatosensory and motor evoked potential monitoring of aortic surgery. *J Cardiothorac Vasc Anesth* 6(6):715–719.

Hacke W (1989): Evoked potentials monitoring in interventional neuroradiology. In: *Neuromonitoring in Surgery (Clinical Neurophysiology Updates, vol. 1)*, edited by JE Desmedt, pp 331–342. Elsevier, Amsterdam.

Haghighi SS, Oro JJ (1989): Effects of hypovolemic hypotensive shock on somatosensory and motor evoked potentials. *Neurosurgery* 24:246–252.

Haghighi SS, Green KD, Oro JJ, Drake RK, Kracke GR (1990): Depressive effect of isoflurane anesthesia on motor evoked potentials. *Neurosurgery* 26:993–997.

Haghighi SS, York DH, Ebeling J, Gumerlock MK, Oro JJ, Gaines RW (1992): Dissociation of somatosensory and motor evoked potentials in a patient with an intramedullary spinal tumor. *Mo Med* 89(11):790–794.

Harper CM, Daube JR (1989): Surgical monitoring with evoked potentials: the Mayo Clinic experience. In: *Neuromonitoring in Surgery (Clinical Neurophysiology Updates, vol 1)*, edited by JE Desmedt, pp 275–301. Elsevier, Amsterdam.

Harper CM, Harner SG, Slavit DH, Litchy WJ, Daube JR, Beatty CW, Ebersold MJ (1992): Effect of BAEP monitoring on hearing preservation during acoustic neuroma resection. *Neurology* 42:1551–1553.

Helfet DL, Koval KJ, Hissa EA, Patterson S, DiPasquale T, Sanders R (1995): Intraoperative somatosensory evoked potential monitoring during acute pelvic fracture surgery. *J Orthop Trauma* 9(1):28–34.

Helmers SL, Carmant I, Flanigin D (1995): Anterior neck recording of intraoperative somatosensory-evoked potentials in children. *Spine* 20(7):782–786.

Herdmann J, Lumenta CB, Huse KO (1993): Magnetic stimulation for monitoring of motor pathways in spinal procedures. *Spine* 18(5):551–559.

Hickey C, Gugino LD, Aglio LS, Mark JB, Son SL, Maddi R (1993): Intraoperative somatosensory evoked potential monitoring predicts peripheral nerve injury during cardiac surgery. *Anesthesiology* 78(1):29–35. Comment in *Anesthesiology* 79(2):411,1993.

Hume AL, Cant BR (1978): Conduction time in central somatosensory pathways in man. *Electroencephalogr Clin Neurophysiol* 45:361–375.

Hurlbert RJ, Tator CH, Fehlings MG, Niznik G, Linden RD (1992): Evoked potentials from direct cerebellar stimulation for monitoring of the rodent spinal cord. *J Neurosurg* 76:280–291.

Jellinek D, Jewkes D, Symon L (1991): Noninvasive intraoperative monitoring of motor evoked potentials under propofol anesthesia: effects of spinal surgery on the amplitude and latency of motor evoked potentials. *Neurosurgery* 29:551–557.

Jellish WS, Martucci J, Blakeman R, Hudson E (1994): Somatosensory evoked potential monitoring of the brachial plexus to predict nerve injury during internal mammary artery harvest: intraoperative comparisons of the Rultract and Pittman sternal retractors. *J Cardiothorac Vasc Anesth* 8(4):398–403.

Kalkman CJ, van Rheineck-Leyssius AT, Hesselink EM, Bovill JG (1986): Effects of etomidate or midazolam on median nerve somatosensory evoked potentials. *Anesthesiology* 65(3A):A356.

Kalmanchey R, Avila A, Symon L (1986): The use of brain stem auditory evoked potentials during posterior fossa surgery as a monitor of brain stem function. *Acta Neurochir* 82:128–136.

Kanzaki J, Ogawa K, Shiobara R, Toya S (1989): Hearing preservation in acoustic neuroma surgery and postoperative audiological findings. *Acta Otolaryngol* 107:474–478.

Kearse LA Jr, Lopez-Bresnahan M, McPeck K, Tambe V (1993): Loss of somatosensory evoked potentials during intramedullary spinal cord surgery predicts postoperative neurologic deficits in motor function. *J Clin Anesth* 5(5):392–398.

King AG (1984): Complications in segmental spinal instrumentation: In: *Segmental Spinal Instrumentation*, edited by E Luque, pp 301–330. Slack, Inc., Thorofare, NJ.

Koht A (1988): Anesthesia influence on recording: summary. In: *Neurophysiology and Standards of Spinal Cord Monitoring*, edited by TB Ducker and RH Brown, pp 188–197. Springer-Verlag, New York.

Kopf GS, Hume AL, Durkin MA, Hammond GL, Hashim SW, Geha AS (1985): Measurement of central somatosensory conduction time in patients undergoing cardiopulmonary bypass: an index of neurologic function. *Am J Surg* 149:445–448.

Kveton JF (1990): Delayed spontaneous return of hearing after acoustic tumor surgery: evidence for cochlear nerve conduction block. *Laryngoscope* 100:473–476.

Lam AM, Keane JF, Manninen PH (1985): Monitoring of brainstem auditory evoked potentials during basilar artery occlusion in man. *Br J Anaesth* 57:924–928.

Lebwohl NH, Calancie B (1992): Perioperative neurologic deficit: Surgical practices and intraoperative monitoring. In: *Spine: State of the Art Reviews*, edited by RT Holt, 6(2):403–428. Hanley & Belfus, Philadelphia.

Lee WY, Hou WY, Yang LH, Lin SM (1995): Intraoperative monitoring of motor function by magnetic motor evoked potentials. *Neurosurgery* 36(3):493–500.

Lenarz T, Sachsenheimer W (1985): Prognostic factors for postsurgical hearing and facial nerve function in cases of cerebellopontine angle-tumors. The meaning of brain stem evoked response audiometry (BERA). *Acta Neurochir* 78:21–27.

Lesser RP, Raudzens P, Luders H, Nuwer MR, Goldie WD, Morris HH 3rd, Dinner DS, Klem G, Hahn JF, Shetter AG, Ginsburg HH, Gurd AR (1986): Postoperative neurological deficits may occur despite unchanged intraoperative somatosensory evoked potentials. *Ann Neurol* 19:22–25.

Levine RA, Ojemann RG, Montgomery WW, McGaffigan PM (1984): Monitoring auditory evoked potentials during acoustic neuroma surgery. *Insights into the mechanism of the hearing loss.* Ann Otol Rhinol Laryngol 93:116–123.

Levy WJ Jr (1987): Clinical experience with motor and cerebellar evoked potential monitoring. *Neurosurgery* 20:169–182.

Levy WJ Jr, York DH (1983): Evoked potentials from the motor tracts in humans. *Neurosurgery* 12:422–429.

Linden RD, Tator CH, Benedict C, Charles D, Mraz V, Bell I (1988): Electrophysiological monitoring during acoustic neuroma and other posterior fossa surgery. *Can J Neurol Sci* 15:73–81.

Linden RD, Johnson JR, Shields CB, Edmonds HL, Glassman SD. Intraoperative spinal cord monitoring with motor evoked potentials elicited by transcranial magnetic stimulation. In: *Textbook of Spinal Surgery. 2nd ed.*, edited by KH Bridwell and RL DeWald. JB Lippincott, Philadelphia. In Press.

Little JR, Lesser RP, Lueders H, Furlan AJ (1983): Brain stem auditory evoked potentials in posterior circulation surgery. *Neurosurgery* 12:496–502.

Little JR, Lesser RP, Luders H (1987): Electrophysiological monitoring during basilar aneurysm operation. *Neurosurgery* 20:421–427.

Loftus CM, Traynelis VC (1994): *Intraoperative Monitoring Techniques in Neurosurgery.* McGraw-Hill, New York.

Luders H, Lesser RP, Hahn J, Dinner DS, Klem G (1983): Cortical somatosensory evoked potentials in response to hand stimulation. *J Neurosurg* 58:885–894.

MacEwen GD, Bunnell WP, Sriram K (1975): Acute neurological complications in the treatment of scoliosis. A report of the Scoliosis Research Society. *J Bone Joint Surg* (57A):404–408.

Machida M, Weinstein SL, Yamada T, Kimura J (1985): Spinal cord monitoring. Electrophysiological measures of sensory and motor function during spinal surgery. *Spine* 10:407–413.

Manninen PH, Patterson S, Lam AM, Gelb AW, Nantau WE (1994): Evoked potential monitoring during posterior fossa aneurysm surgery: a comparison of two modalities. *Can J Anaesth* 41:92–97.

Markand ON, Dilley RS, Moorthy SS, Warren C Jr (1984a): Monitoring of somatosensory evoked responses during carotid endarterectomy. *Arch Neurol* 41:375–378.

Markand ON, Warren CH, Moorthy SS, Stoelting R, King RD (1984b): Monitoring of multimodality evoked potentials during open heart surgery under hypothermia. *Electroencephalogr Clin Neurophysiol* 59:432–440.

McCarthy G, Allison T, Spencer DD (1993): Localization of the face area of human sensorimotor cortex by intracranial recording of somatosensory evoked potentials. *J Neurosurg* 79(6):874–884.

McPherson RW, Mahla M, Johnson R, Traystman RJ (1985): Effects of enflurane, isoflurane, and nitrous oxide on somatosensory evoked potentials during fentanyl anesthesia. *Anesthesiology* 62:626–633.

McPherson RW, Sell B, Traystman RJ (1986): Effects of thiopental, fentanyl, and etomidate on upper extremity somatosensory evoked potentials in humans. *Anesthesiology* 65:584–589.

Moller AR (1988a): Use of zero-phase digital filters to enhance brain stem auditory evoked potentials (BAEPs). *Electroencephalogr Clin Neurophysiol* 71:226–232.

Moller AR (1988b): *Evoked Potentials in Intraoperative Monitoring.* Williams & Wilkins, Baltimore.

Moller AR, Jannetta PJ (1983): Monitoring auditory functions during cranial nerve microvascular decompression operations by direct recording from the eighth nerve. *J Neurosurg* 59:493–499.

Moller AR, Moller MB (1989): Does intraoperative monitoring of auditory evoked potentials reduce incidence of hearing loss as a complication of microvascular decompression of cranial nerves? *Neurosurgery* 24:257–263.

Moller AR, Burgess JE, Sekhar LN (1987): Recording compound action potentials from the optic nerve in man and monkeys. *Electroencephalogr Clin Neurophysiol* 67:549–555.

Moorthy SS, Markand ON, Dilley RS, McCammon RL, Warren CH Jr (1982): Somatosensory-evoked responses during carotid endarterectomy. *Anesth Analg* 61(10):879–883.

Nadol JB Jr, Levine R, Ojemann RG, Martuza RL, Montgomery WW, de Sandoval PK (1987): Preservation of hearing in surgical removal of acoustic neuromas of the internal auditory canal and cerebellar pontine angle. *Laryngoscope* 97:1287–1294.

Nagao S, Roccaforte P, Moody RA (1978): The effects of isovolemic hemodilution and reinfusion of packed erythrocytes on somatosensory and visual evoked potentials. *J Surg Res* 25:530–537.

Nuwer MR (1986): *Evoked Potential Monitoring in the Operating Room.* Raven Press, New York.

Nuwer MR, Dawson EG, Carlson LG, Kanim LE, Sherman JE (1995): Somatosensory evoked potential spinal cord monitoring reduces neurologic deficits after scoliosis surgery: results of a large multicenter survey. *Electroencephalogr Clin Neurophysiol* 96(1):6–11.

O'Brien MF, Lenke LG, Bridwell KH, Padberg A, Stokes M (1994): Evoked potential monitoring of the upper extremities during thoracic and lumbar spinal deformity surgery: a prospective study. *J Spinal Disord* 7(4):277–284.

Owen JH, Laschinger J, Bridwell K, Shimon S, Nielsen C, Dunlap J, Kain C (1988): Sensitivity and specificity of somatosensory and neurogenic-motor evoked potentials in animals and humans. *Spine* 13:1111–1118.

Pathak KS, Brown RH, Nash CL Jr, Cascorbi HF (1983): Continuous opioid infusion for scoliosis fusion surgery. *Anesth Analg* 62(9):841–845.

Pathak KS, Brown RH, Cascorbi HF, Nash CL Jr (1984): Effects of fentanyl and morphine on intraoperative somatosensory cortical-evoked potentials. *Anesth Analg* 63:833–837.

Penfield W, Jasper H (1954): *Epilepsy and the Functional Anatomy of the Brain.* Little, Brown, Boston.

Piatt JH Jr, Radtke RA, Erwin CW (1985): Limitations of brain stem auditory evoked potentials for intraoperative monitoring during a posterior fossa operation: case report and technical note. *Neurosurgery* 16:818–821.

Radtke RA, Erwin CW, Wilkins RH (1989): Intraoperative brainstem auditory evoked potentials: significant decrease in postoperative morbidity. *Neurology* 39, 187–191.

Rappaport M, Ruiz Portillo S, Ortiz D, Fountain SS, Kula TA Jr (1994): Effects of stimulus intensity and duration on posterior tibial nerve somatosensory-evoked potential patterns obtained under anesthesia. *Spine* 19(13): 1525–1529.

Rasmussen TJ, Black DL, Bruce RP, Reckling FW (1994): Efficacy of corticosomatosensory evoked potential monitoring in predicting and/or preventing sciatic nerve palsy during total hip arthroplasty. *J Arthroplasty* 9(1):53–61.

Raudzens PA (1982): Intraoperative monitoring of evoked potentials. *Ann NY Acad Sci* 388:308–326.

Raudzens PA, Shetter AG (1982): Intraoperative monitoring of brain-stem auditory evoked potentials. *J Neurosurg* 57:341–348.

Robinson LR, Slimp JC, Anderson PA, Stolov WC (1993): The efficacy of femoral nerve intraoperative somatosensory evoked potentials during surgical treatment of thoracolumbar fractures. *Spine* 18(13):1793–1797.

Rosenblum SM, Ruth RA, Gal TJ (1985): Brain stem auditory evoked potential monitoring during profound hypothermia and circulatory arrest. *Ann Otol Rhinol Laryngol* 94:281–283.

Ross RT (1985): Spinal cord infarction in disease and surgery of the aorta. *Can J Neurol Sci* 12:289–295.

Rothwell JC, Day BL, Thompson PD, Boyd SG, Marsden CD (1989): Motor cortical stimulation in intact man: Physiological mechanisms and application in intraoperative monitoring. In: *Neuromonitoring in Surgery (Clinical Neurophysiology Updates, vol 1)*, edited by JE Desmedt, pp 71–98. Elsevier, Amsterdam.

Russ W, Kling D, Loesevitz A, Hempelmann G (1984): Effect of hypothermia on visual evoked potentials (VEP) in humans. *Anesthesiology* 61:207–210.

Sako K, Nakai H, Takizawa K, Tokumitsu N, Satho M, Katho M (1995): Aneurysm surgery using temporary occlusion under SEP monitoring. *No Shinkei Geka — Neurol Surg* 23(1):35–41.

Salzman SK, ed (1990): *Neural Monitoring. The Prevention of Intraoperative Injury.* Humana Press, Clifton, NJ.

Schmid UD, Boll J, Liechti S, Schmid J, Hess CW (1992): Influence of some anesthetic agents on muscle responses to transcranial magnetic cortex stimulation: a pilot study in humans. *Neurosurgery* 30:85–92.

Schramm J, Jones SJ, eds. *Spinal Cord Monitoring.* Springer-Verlag, Berlin, Heidelberg.

Schramm J, Mokrusch T, Fahlbusch R, Hochstetter A (1988): Detailed analysis of intraoperative changes monitoring brain stem acoustic evoked potentials. *Neurosurgery* 22:694–702.

Schramm J, Watanabe E, Strauss C, Fahlbusch R (1989): Neurophysiologic monitoring in posterior fossa surgery. I. Technical principles, applicability, and limitations. *Acta Neurochir* 98:9–18.

Schramm J, Koht A, Schmidt G, Pechstein U, Taniguchi M, Fahlbusch R (1990): Surgical and electrophysiological observations during clipping of 134 aneurysms with evoked potentials monitoring. *Neurosurgery* 26:61–70.

Sebel PS, Flynn PJ, Ingram DA (1984): Effect of nitrous oxide on visual, auditory and somatosensory evoked potentials. *Br J Anaesth* 56:1403–1407.

Sebel PS, Ingram DA, Flynn PJ, Rutherfoord CF, Rogers H (1986): Evoked potentials during isoflurane anaesthesia. *Br J Anaesth* 58:580–585.

Silverstein H, McDaniel A, Wazen J, Norrell H (1985): Retrolabyrinthine vestibular neurectomy with simultaneous monitoring of eighth nerve and brain stem auditory evoked potentials. *Otolaryngol Head Neck Surg* 93:736–742.

Silverstein H, McDaniel A, Norrell H, Haberkamp T (1986): Hearing preservation after acoustic neuroma surgery with intraoperative direct eighth cranial nerve monitoring. Part II: A classification of results. *Otolaryngol Head Neck Surg* 95(3 Pt 1):285–291.

Singh N, Sachdev KK, Brisman R (1982): Trigeminal nerve stimulation: short latency somatosensory evoked potentials. *Neurology* 32:97–101.

Slavit DH, Harner SG, Harper CM Jr, Beatty CW (1991): Auditory monitoring during acoustic neuroma removal. *Arch Otolaryngol Head Neck Surg* 117:1153–1157.

Sohmer H, Gold S, Cahani M, Attias J (1989): Effects of hypothermia on auditory brain-stem and somatosensory evoked responses. A model of a synaptic and axonal lesion. *Electroencephalogr Clin Neurophysiol* 74:50–57.

Soustiel JF, Hafner H, Chistyakov AV, Guilburd JN, Zaaroor M, Yussim E, Feinsod M (1993): Monitoring of brain stem trigeminal evoked potentials. Clinical applications in posterior fossa surgery. *Electroencephalogr Clin Neurophysiol* 88:255–260.

Stechison MT (1993): The trigeminal evoked potential: Part II. Intraoperative recording of short-latency responses. *Neurosurgery* 33:639–644.

Stechison MT, Kralick FJ (1993): The trigeminal evoked potential: Part I. Long-latency responses in awake or anesthetized subjects. *Neurosurgery* 33:633–638.

Steeves JD, Jordan LM (1980): Localization of a descending pathway in the spinal cord which is necessary for controlled treadmill locomotion. *Neurosci Lett* 20:283–288.

Stockard JJ, Sharbrough FW, Tinker JA (1978): Effects of hypothermia on the human brainstem auditory response. *Ann Neurol* 3:368–370.

Stone JL, Ghaly RF, Levy WJ, Kartha R, Krinsky L, Roccaforte P (1992): A comparative analysis of enflurane anesthesia on primate motor and somatosensory evoked potentials. *Electroencephalogr Clin Neurophysiol* 84:180–187.

Sugioka H (1984): Evoked potentials in the investigation of traumatic lesions of the peripheral nerve and the brachial plexus. *Clin Orthop* 184:85–92.

Symon L, Murota T (1989): Intraoperative monitoring of somatosensory evoked potentials during intracranial vascular surgery. In: *Neuromonitoring in Surgery (Clinical Neurophysiology Updates, vol 1)*, edited by JE Desmedt, pp 263–274. Elsevier, Amsterdam.

Symon L, Wang AD, Costa e Silva IE, Gentili F (1984): Perioperative use of somatosensory evoked responses in aneurysm surgery. *J Neurosurg* 60:269–275.

Tamaki T (1989): Spinal cord monitoring with spinal potentials evoked by direct stimulation of the spinal cord. In: *Neuromonitoring in Surgery. (Clinical Neurophysiology Updates, vol 1)*, edited by JE Desmedt, pp 139–149. Elsevier, Amsterdam.

Tamaki T, Tsuji H, Inoue S, Kobayashi H (1981): The prevention of iatrogenic spinal cord injury utilizing the evoked spinal cord potential. *Int Orthop* 4(4):313–317.

Taniguchi M, Nadstawek J, Langenbach U, Bremer F, Schramm J (1993): Effects of four intravenous anesthetic agents on motor evoked potentials elicited by magnetic transcranial stimulation. *Neurosurgery* 33(3):407–415.

Tator CH, Linden RD, Fehlings MG, Benedict CM, Bell I (1988): Overview of fundamental and clinical aspects of monitoring the spinal cord during spinal cord surgery. In: *Neurophysiology & Standards of Spinal Cord Monitoring*, edited by TB Ducker and RH Brown, pp 368–383. Springer-Verlag, New York.

Taylor BA, Fennelly ME, Taylor A, Farrell J (1993): Temporal summation—the key to motor evoked potential spinal cord monitoring in humans. *J Neurol Neurosurg Psychiatry* 56(1):104–106.

Toleikis JR, Carlvin AO, Shapiro DE, Schafer MF (1993): The use of dermatomal evoked responses during surgical procedures that use intrapedicular fixation of the lumbosacral spine. *Spine* 18(16):2401–2407.

Vauzelle C, Stagnara P, Jouvinroux P (1973): Functional monitoring of spinal cord activity during spinal surgery. *Clin Orthop* 93:173–178.

Watanabe E, Schramm J, Strauss C, Fahlbusch R (1989): Neurophysiologic monitoring in posterior fossa surgery. II. BAEP-waves I and V and preservation of hearing. *Acta Neurochir* 98:118–128.

Wilber RG, Thompson GH, Shaffer JW, Brown RH, Nash CL Jr (1984): Post-operative neurological deficits in segmental spinal instrumentation. *J Bone Joint Surg* 66A:1178–1187.

Wilson WB, Kirsch WM, Neville H, Stears J, Feinsod M, Lehman RA (1976): Monitoring of visual function during parasellar surgery. *Surg Neurol* 5:323–329.

Young W, Sakatani K (1990): Neurophysiological mechanisms of somatosensory-evoked potential changes. In: *Neural Monitoring. The Prevention of Intraoperative Injury*, edited by SK Salzman, pp 115–148. Humana Press, Clifton, NJ.

Zappulla RA, Malis LI, Greenblatt E, Karmel BZ (1984a): Utility of brainstem auditory evoked potentials in the diagnosis and surgical treatment of tumors of the cerebellopontine angle. In: *Evoked Potentials II*, edited by RH Nodar and C Barber, pp 194–202. Butterworth-Heinemann, Newton, MA.

Zappulla R, Greenblatt E, Kaye S, Malis L (1984b): A quantitative assessment of the brain stem auditory evoked response during intraoperative monitoring. *Neurosurgery* 15:186–191.

Zentner J (1989): Noninvasive motor evoked potential monitoring during neurosurgical operations on the spinal cord. *Neurosurgery* 24:709–712.

Zentner J (1991): Motor evoked potential monitoring during neurosurgical operation on the spinal cord. *Neurosurg Rev* 14(1):29–36.

Zentner J, Kiss I, Ebner A (1989): Influence of anesthetics—nitrous oxide in particular—on electromyographic response evoked by transcranial electrical stimulation of the cortex. *Neurosurgery* 24:253–256.

Evoked Potentials in Clinical Medicine,
3d ed., edited by Keith H. Chiappa.
Lippincott–Raven Publishers, Philadelphia © 1997.

19

Electrophysiologic Monitoring During Carotid Endarterectomies

Keith H. Chiappa

*Department of Neurology, Harvard Medical School, and EEG Laboratory,
Massachusetts General Hospital, Boston, Massachusetts 02114*

1. INTRODUCTION

There are some important concepts which should be considered in the context of electrophysiologic monitoring of carotid endarterectomies (CEAs). The first is that the internal carotid artery can be cross-clamped for 30 to 45 min in the majority of patients without neurologic consequences. However, 1% to 3% of patients will suffer a major, permanent neurologic deficit if a cross-clamp is maintained for this period of time (Chiappa et al., 1979). These patients can withstand the clamp without sequelae only for less than 10 min, between 10 and 20 min they suffer varying degrees of deficit, and a cross-clamp of longer than 20 min will usually result in an immediate postoperative significant clinical deficit. Great confusion has been generated in the literature by those who do not understand this length-of-clamping principle. If the cross-clamp is maintained for less than 20 min, which is the practice in some centers, then they will see a complication of that clamping only very rarely, but their experience cannot be transferred to a center which believes that a technically adequate endarterectomy requires clamping for more than 20 min.

If the CEA cross-clamping will last longer than 10 min, a temporary bypass shunt may be used to maintain the blood flow to the brain around the length of the artery that has been clamped off for the surgical manipulations. It is believed that the shunt placement carries a finite risk related to embolic phenomena, and one would prefer to avoid shunting those patients who do not require it (Sundt et al., 1974; Marshall and Lougheed, 1969). Thus, a technique of monitoring neurologic function during the clamped period is necessary. When the surgery is performed under local anesthesia, the patient can be monitored with a clinical neurologic examination (Harris et al., 1967; Perez-Borja and Meyer, 1965). However, this operative format is not suitable for every surgeon and patient, and electrophysiologic techniques are well-suited to this task. There is a close correlation between cerebral blood flow and the electroencephalogram (EEG) (Sundt et al., 1974, 1975; Trojaborg and Boysen, 1973), and the EEG has been proven to be a reliable indicator of ischemia during CEAs (Sundt et al., 1974, 1975, 1977; Matsumoto et al., 1976; Chiappa et al., 1979).

Somatosensory evoked potentials (SEPs) have been used to monitor CEAs, with good results (Haupt and Horsch, 1992), but the signal-averaging process inserts a delay between the onset of ischemia and its demonstration as an EP change. Also, there is clinical experience which suggests that SEPs are relatively insensitive to significant levels of cerebral ischemia in some patients (Ropper, 1986; Kearse et al., 1992; Haupt et al., 1994). Since the SEP technique is somewhat more complicated than the EEG, there is no compelling reason to use it for this application.

2. METHODS

Communication with the key people in the operating room (OR) prior to starting a carotid monitoring service provides a basis for good teamwork and helps ensure efficient handling of any difficulties that may arise. The nursing supervisor should be approached to obtain dress codes and OR regulations and to give advice on how to get the EEG equipment into the OR suite and suitably placed. Electrical safety regulations have to be discussed with the OR engineer and all equipment checked for compliance with safety laws. The ground and chassis leakage currents should be checked twice per year and more frequently for instruments exposed to high-voltage cautery and rough use from transport.

A check list of EEG supplies needed for monitoring in the OR is carefully gone through before each procedure. The following items are routinely carried in a suitable container:

Tape measure
Chinagraph pencil
Pumice solution
Cotton tips
Gold cup electrodes with holes
Tubes of collodion with dispensing tip
Air gun and OR adapter
12-cc syringe with 18-gauge stub adapter
Saline gel
Impedance meter
Movement transducer
1-inch surgical tape (cloth)
Scissors
Acetone
Cotton
Pencils, ruler, screwdriver
Ink, paper packs
Spare pens
Notebook or log

A baseline recording is desirable but since most patients are admitted on the same day as the surgery this may be obtained on an outpatient basis. At least 5 min of awake baseline recording can be obtained in the OR prior to anesthetic induction, preferably without premedications. Anesthesia affects the EEG both by masking some subtle slow-wave foci and asymmetries and by revealing and enhancing others. A longer baseline recording may be necessary if a new EEG abnormality needs to be fully evaluated before proceeding with surgery.

After degreasing the skin with a pumice solution, gold cup electrodes with central holes are placed, using collodion, in the Fp1,Fp2, C3, C4, T3, T4, P3, P4, O1 and O2 positions of the International 10–20 system. A full set of electrodes is often employed to allow maximum flexibility in the choice of montages and in case of loss of electrodes since it is usually not possible to replace them during the procedure. Electrodes are placed over the C7 vertebra and on the shoulder opposite to the side of incision for electrocardiographic (ECG) recording. The skin beneath the electrodes is lightly abraded with a blunt needle tip and a saline gel is injected into the cup. Electrode impedances should be below 5,000 ohms. Other methods of electrode application such as paste-filled cups held with tape or needle insertion are generally not satisfactory as they do not have the stability required for prolonged monitoring. There has been insufficient experience with electrode caps and nets during surgical monitoring to evaluate their long-term stability under those conditions. On rare occasions, procedures have lasted as long as 9 hours and re-jellying of the cups may then be necessary. In the event of complications, follow-up recordings may be required in the recovery room.

An example of a montage that could be used on an eight-channel machine is Fp1–C3, C3–O1, Fp2–C4, C4–O2, T3–C3, T4–C4. T3 and T4 are also often recorded to a noncephalic reference such as the second cervical spinal vertebra since ischemic changes are frequently prominent there. The electrocardiogram is recorded on one channel and a movement transducer which is firmly placed with tape at the scalp line on the side of the operation is connected to the last channel. The head is then completely covered with a surgical cap, a small hole having been cut out at the center for the EEG leads. Then the headbox is attached to the underside of the OR table and the cable is taped to the floor. The EEG should be recorded without interruption from prior to induction of anesthesia until the the patient is able to respond at the end of the procedure and the surgeon confirms movement of all limbs. Sensitivity of the EEG channels is 5, μV/mm or 3 μV/mm, the latter essential for recognizing early loss of anesthetic-induced fast activity. The peak-to-peak trace excursion of the 6- to 15-Hz activity should be at least 1 cm. Initially this high gain can be disconcerting, since high-amplitude EEG activity will produce large pen excursions, but in the OR monitoring situation, where large changes in average EEG amplitude are common, the gain setting which is optimal for low-voltage activity should be used throughout the recording. It is particularly important to have an average pen deflection of at least 1 cm shortly before carotid artery clamping so that losses in amplitude will be clearly evident. It is also very important that gain changes be made as seldom as possible (and clearly marked when done) to facilitate comparisons between different portions of the record (e.g., pre- and postclamp sections).

The high-frequency setting is usually 70 Hz with the 60-Hz notch filter in operation. The low-frequency setting is around 1 Hz or lower, according to the steps available on the machine. A paper speed of 15 mm/sec or slightly slower permits easier identification of subtle slow-wave activity and saves paper. Occasionally the occipital or temporal electrodes are pulled off when supports are placed under the patient's head and in this event a montage incorporating the P3 and P4 electrodes saves the day.

Once in the OR great care should be taken in the placement of the EEG machine and cables. This is important not only for access of the surgical staff but also to lessen the chances of electrical induction artifacts during recording. Even with optimum positioning of the EEG cables and careful selection of a power outlet, electrical interference is sometimes a problem. The most common source of interference is the electrosurgical cautery units, even when they are merely powered up. Interference has been particularly worrisome when it occurs in a suite where we have not previously encountered electrical interference. The patient ground should be checked, the EEG and cautery machines should have their ground and chassis leakage currents checked, and the OR ground should be checked. Sometimes we have been able to trace the source to a piece of electrical equipment in the room which has developed a fault, such as an ECG machine or surgeon's headlight. Replacing the faulty equipment will then resolve the problem. At times when interference has been overwhelming we have recorded at a high filter setting of 35 Hz, in addition to the 60-Hz filter.

3. CLINICAL INTERPRETATION

Good communication between the anesthesiology and electrophysiology teams is imperative. The anesthesia staff need to learn what medications render the EEG less useful (e.g., any causing a burst-suppression pattern such as most inhalational agents at greater than 1%, thiopental, and propofol when given in a large bolus) so that these can be avoided at critical points in the procedure. The EEG can sometimes be useful to the anesthesiologist by alerting him/her to the fact that muscle activity has appeared on the tracing at an inappropriate time, indicating that the patient is at a very light level of anesthesia. The anesthetic level can then be adjusted before the patient's movements interfere with the surgical procedure. A sudden drop in blood pressure, manifested on the EEG by generalized high-voltage slowing, sometimes occurs outside of clamp times and the EEG changes can be helpful in early recognition and correction of this problem.

The EEG during general anesthesia is primarily a product of the anesthetic agent in use and the arterial carbon dioxide tension ($PaCO_2$) (see Stockard and Bickford, 1975, for a review of this topic). The common anesthetic agents such as halothane and fentanyl produce widespread 10- to 15-Hz activity with amplitudes of 25 to 75 μV intermixed with varying amounts of slower frequencies which are often frontally predominant. If a single anesthetic is in use and $PaCO_2$ is constant, the frequency of the EEG fast activity closely parallels anesthetic gas concentration. Although the multiplicity of agents in use usually upsets this relationship, the fast activity is still a very useful indicator of cerebral activity. Amounts and distribution of slow activity also vary depending on both the depth of anesthesia and the agents used. Asymmetries in anesthetic-induced activities may be secondary to pre-existing cortical dysfunction (e.g., prior stroke as in Fig. 9–2 in Chiappa and Hoch, 1993), although these patients are not more likely to have changes associated with carotid clamping (Chiappa et al., 1979; Kearse et al., 1995).

Attempts to correlate EEG patterns with specific medications are difficult, largely because mixtures of inhaled gases and intravenous solutions are commonly used. However, the burst-suppression pattern produced by the barbiturates used during induction of anesthesia is well-known. Enflurane sometimes produces a similar pattern, but is less dramatic and more unpredictable, so that brief episodes of suppression can occur for long periods after administration of the drug has been stopped.

The EEG patterns produced by anesthesia often change dramatically throughout a procedure. A sudden increase of bilateral slowing can be of concern, particularly when the anesthetist says that no new agent has been given. In general, the amount of fast activity intermixed with the slowing is a good indicator of whether the change is due to medication or inadequate blood flow. In the latter instance the slowing will generally be accompanied by a rapid dropout of faster frequencies, whereas with anesthesia-related changes, the fast activity is more persistent.

Fluctuating EEG amplitudes occur throughout a carotid monitor, presumably related to changes in surgical stimulation, anesthetic agent concentrations, blood gas concentrations, or blood pressure. There may be a swift overall reduction of amplitude outside of clamp time (e.g., when inhalational anesthetics are turned off). Again the presence of widespread and well-defined fast activity suggests that the amplitude loss is less likely to be significant.

The EEG interpretation presents a number of uncertainties and difficulties, ranging from unidentifiable artifacts to differentiation between anesthesia patterns and more critical changes. Most worrisome of all is the problem of whether a subtle or intermittent change during carotid artery clamping is secondary to medication or indicative of restricted cerebral blood flow and warrants alerting the surgeon. Changes related to anesthetic agents, pH, arterial oxygen and carbon dioxide tensions, and systemic blood pressure must be distinguished from changes related to cerebral anoxia. If the EEG change is generalized, especially if anteriorly predominant, then a metabolic (i.e., anesthetic or blood gas) effect is more likely. In any case, complete loss of all EEG activity (Fig. 19–1) (i.e., the traces appear flat) is a significant change and requires notification of the surgeon. As a general rule, loss of amplitude of 75% to 80% or more over less than 1 min should be treated as a complete loss of all EEG activity. Note that apparent low-voltage slow activity which may remain after all anesthetic-induced fast activity has disappeared is more artifactual (e.g., respirations, movements of the operating team) than actual cerebral electrical activity. The loss of anesthetic-induced fast activity but preservation of moderate- to high-voltage slowing, often rhythmic, indicates a borderline situation which also requires notification of the surgeon but does not carry the same prognostic significance as the loss of all activity.

A gradual loss of amplitude over 5 to 30 minutes is problematic but we consider it to be within tolerable limits as long as anesthetic-induced fast activity is still present and not less than 18 μV in amplitude.

After induction of anesthesia and placement of the endotracheal tube, the operative site is "prepped" and draped. The dissection to expose the carotid artery may take up to an hour.

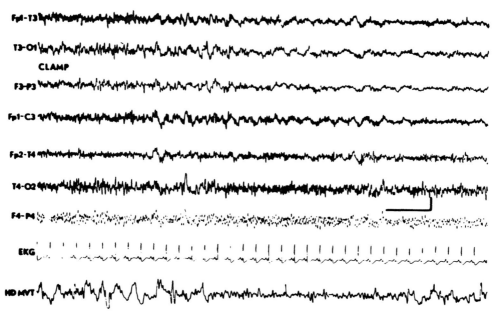

FIG. 19–1. A significant EEG change following carotid clamping—ipsilateral attenuation most obvious in the loss of anesthetic-induced 10- to 14-Hz fast-frequency activities. Left carotid clamp was applied at CLAMP. Note the presence of some slow activity although its amplitude is low. Calibration marks are 2 sec and 50 μV. (From Chiappa et al., 1979, with permission.)

The EEG should be monitored during this period of time because the trauma of the dissection sometimes causes a stenosed artery to "prematurely" occlude completely (Chiappa et al., 1979). This event may be registered by the EEG, allowing appropriate action to be taken. In addition, in patients who have not received adequate atropine and/or local anesthetic, mechanical disturbance of the carotid body, which lies at the bifurcation of the common carotid artery, can produce dramatic effects in heart rate and blood pressure. The EEG may reflect these changes and, by observation of the ECG channel, the EEG technologist may spot the problem before the anesthetist.

The greatest utility of EEG monitoring during carotid endarterectomy surgery is during the time when blood flow through the artery is stopped by clamps to allow the interior of the artery to be accessed. If the blood flow through the artery provides a critical portion of that needed by the brain, then clamping will result in possible cerebral ischemic damage. In some centers the surgery is performed under local anesthesia so that the patient's condition can be assessed by neurologic examination at any time during the procedure. Often patients and surgeons do not find this approach acceptable and general anesthesia is employed. In that circumstance a means of assessing cerebral function during the at-risk periods is needed, and the EEG can perform this task.

Surgical practices differ regarding carotid artery clamping and temporary bypass shunting. Some surgeons always shunt and use the EEG as a back-up monitor, while others shunt only if the EEG shows significant changes when the clamp is applied to the carotid artery. The time of clamping is when the EEG is most likely to show significant changes. Surprisingly, only about 10% of patients show a definite change in the EEG when the carotid is clamped (Chiappa et al., 1979) and less than 4% have a significant change (i.e., one that requires intervention by the operating team). These findings parallel the clinical experience where patients are not uncommonly found at autopsy to have one or both carotids occluded without ever having neurologic problems. Rarely, a patient is found to have all four major neck vessels occluded without problems! This is a testimony to the collateral flow capacity of the blood supply system of the brain. Patients with prior strokes are not more likely to have intraoperative EEG changes (Chiappa et al., 1979; Kearse et al., 1995).

If there is a significant change with clamping, it almost always appears within 10 or 15 sec. When the temporary bypass shunt is opened, the EEG should return to its preclamp baseline within 2 to 3 minutes. If it does not, then blood flow through the shunt is insufficient. Occasionally the shunt will occlude during a procedure, usually because of kinking, and the EEG will again demonstrate the same changes. Similarly, when the shunt is clamped for removal, the EEG changes will reoccur.

The period of carotid artery clamping (and shunting) will last for 12 min to perhaps an hour, usually 20 to 30 min, although there is a great deal of variability in this. After flow has been restored to the carotid artery, EEG monitoring should be maintained until the procedure is finished and the patient is awake enough to participate in a neurologic examination; this may be another 30 to 60 min after the carotid artery part of the surgery is finished. Electroencephalographic monitoring is continued until the patient awakens in the recovery room because sometimes the carotid artery will rethrombose at the operative site (Chiappa et al., 1979). In this instance, if the neurologic deficit is not discovered until the attempt to awaken the patient, too much time may have elapsed and the deficit may be irreversible. A significant EEG change during this stage of the procedure should result in serious consideration by the surgical team of reopening the operative site and checking the carotid artery by palpation, and possibly reopening the artery.

Thus, EEG monitoring is maintained from induction of anesthesia until the patient awakens in the recovery room, an average total time of 4 hours.

Although the EEG may show a significant change with application of the clamps, there seems to be a "safe" period during which the shunt can be placed. In our experience, this safe period may be as long as 10 min, (i.e., the EEG can demonstrate the significant change for 10 min and the patient awaken from the procedure without neurologic deficit). This is presumably because the EEG goes "flat" at a cerebral blood flow of about 12 to 15 ml/100 g per minute (Sundt et al., 1974), so that there could still be enough blood flow to maintain cell life but not enough to maintain normal electrical activity. Also, the anesthetic might provide a certain degree of protection. After 10 min duration of the significant EEG change, there is an ever-increasing likelihood that the patient will awaken with a neurologic deficit, so that by 20 min duration of the significant EEG change, there is essentially a 100% chance of such a deficit.

Perceived differences in the utility of EEG monitoring during carotid endarterectomies can largely be accounted for by differences in total clamp time relative to the above "safe" period, that is, if a surgeon routinely maintains the clamp (without shunt) for less than 20 min, he/she is much less likely to encounter postoperative neurologic deficits, especially given the low incidence (less than 4%, closer to 1% or 2%) of significant EEG changes.

Because the electrode coverage of the head is not complete, the EEG may not demonstrate changes secondary to an embolus to a branch vessel in the cortex. In this circumstance, the patient may awaken from anesthesia with a neurologic deficit without the EEG having shown any major changes. The lack of major EEG change in the presence of a definite neurologic deficit is a good indicator that the etiologic factor is an embolus. Whether or not 16 or more channels should be used to provide greater sensitivity to embolic incidents is a question without an easy answer given the difficulty of recognizing these events and the added complexity and cost. Since little can be done once an embolus has reached the cerebral convexity, the utility of the more detailed coverage may not be warranted, except that the time of occurrence might suggest changes in the surgical procedure to lessen the likelihood of embolization.

We have noted that the EEG may show little change in patients with watershed (border zone) infarcts, but presumably the state of cerebral blood flow necessary to generate this condition is attained in very few patients, so that it is not a significant problem.

Most commonly the EEG technologist is the sole EEG-trained person in the operating room. In a few hospitals the electroencephalographer (EEGer) is also present in the operating room for the entire course of the procedure. In most hospitals the EEGer will consult with the technologist and surgeon over the telephone, or, in especially difficult circumstances, will go to the operating room. The time and effort involved in the latter mitigate against this so that the threshold for such consultation may be too high. Presently there is a debate in guidelines committees concerning these matters with one point of view being that the only person who should communicate with the surgeon should be the clinical neurophysiologist. This is reasonable as a general guideline but does not take into account the expertise of excellent and highly trained technologists in some hospitals who are fully capable of providing a competent interpretation of the EEG to the surgeon in the large majority of cases.

We have taken the output of the EEG machine amplifiers and, without further electronics, piped that signal up eight floors directly into the high-level input stage of the amplifiers of another EEG machine in the EEG laboratory. A private intercom facility is maintained over the same cable. Thus, the "repeater" EEG machine in the EEG laboratory displays the same thing being viewed by the technologist in the OR. A buzzer system alerts personnel at either end to pick up their handset. We have found this very helpful in training inexperienced technologists, as well as providing a secure backup consultation facility in general.

Digital EEG machines and network technology now allow a physician to monitor the EEG in real-time from many remote locations. These systems need to be able to effectively manage the two common clinical scenarios: (1) the technologist in the OR pages the physician and informs him/her that carotid clamping will occur in a few minutes so that the physician should begin to monitor the real-time EEG from the remote location, if he/she is not already doing so; and (2) the technologist in the OR pages the physician and informs him/her that an unusual EEG event occurred a few minutes ago (at a specific stated time) and asks him/her to review it. The physician usually needs to be able to show at least two pages of EEG on the screen simultaneously, one of which will often be the real-time EEG from the OR. The use of such networked systems will allow the most efficient use of the clinical neurophysiologist's time and provide the best consultative assistance to the surgeon and the patient.

Various data reduction methods have been used to process the EEG data and present it in a variety of computer displays (see e.g., Chiappa et al., 1979; Kearse et al., 1993), but these make the recognition of spikes and sharp waves impossible, burst–suppression almost impossible, and electrographic seizure activity difficult. Although the computer output is significantly easier to understand, and trends are easier to identify, immediate access to the raw EEG data is necessary to interpret the computer output and to judge its validity. Thus, the operator still needs to be well-trained in EEG interpretation and experienced EEG consultants need to be readily available.

ACKNOWLEDGMENTS

Some of the text is taken with permission from Jenkins GM, Chiappa KH (1983): Practical aspects of EEG monitoring during carotid endarterectomies. *Am J EEG Technol* 23:191–203. Margaret Barlow, R.EEGT., CNIM, reviewed the text and contributed valuable comments and suggestions.

REFERENCES

Chiappa KH, Burke SR, Young RR (1979): Results of electroencephalographic monitoring during 367 carotid endarterectomies. *Stroke* 10:381–388.

Chiappa KH, Hoch DB (1993): Electrophysiologic monitoring. In: *Neurological and Neurosurgical Intensive Care*, 3rd ed, edited by AH Ropper, pp 147–183. Raven Press, New York.

Haupt WF, Horsch S (1992): Evoked potential monitoring in carotid surgery: a review of 994 cases. *Neurology* 42:835–838.

Haupt WF, Erasmi-Korber H, Lanfermann H (1994): Intraoperative recording of parietal SEP can miss hemodynamic infarction during carotid endarterectomy: a case study. *Electroencephalogr Clin Neurophysiol* 92:86–88.

Kearse LA Jr, Brown EN, McPeck K (1992): Somatosensory evoked potentials sensitivity relative to electroencephalography for cerebral ischemia during carotid endarterectomy. *Stroke* 23:498–505.

Kearse LA, Martin D, McPeck K, Lopez-Bresnahan M (1993): Computer-derived density spectral array in detection of mild analog electroencephalographic ischemic pattern changes during carotid endarterectomy. *J Neurosurg* 78:884–890.

Kearse LA, Lopez-Bresnahan M, McPeck K, Zaslavsky A (1995): Preoperative cerebrovascular symptoms and electroencephalographic abnormalities do not predict cerebral ischemia during carotid endarterectomy. *Stroke* 26:1210–1214.

Matsumoto GH, Baker JD, Watson CW, Gleucklich B, Callow AD (1976): EEG surveillance as a means of extending operability in high risk carotid endarterectomy. *Stroke* 7:554–559.

Ropper AH (1986): Evoked potentials in cerebral ischemia. *Stroke* 17:3–5.

Stockard JJ, Bickford RG (1975): The neurophysiology of anesthesia. In: *A Basis and Practice of Neuroanesthesia*, edited by E Gordon, pp 3–46. Excerpta Medica, Stockholm.

Sundt TM Jr, Houser OW, Sharbrough FW, Messick JM Jr (1977): Carotid endarterectomy: results, complications, and monitoring techniques. In: Thompson RH, Green JR (eds) *Advances in Neurology*. Raven Press, New York, vol 16, pp 97–119.

Sundt TM Jr, Sharbrough FW, Anderson RE, Michenfelder JD (1974): Cerebral blood flow measurements and electroencephalograms during carotid endarterectomy. *J Neurosurg* 41:310–320.

Trojaborg W, Boysen G (1973): Relation between EEG, regional cerebral blood flow and internal carotid artery pressure during carotid endarterectomy. *Electroencephalogr Clin Neurophysiol* 34:61–69.

Evoked Potentials in Clinical Medicine,
3d ed., edited by Keith H. Chiappa.
Lippincott–Raven Publishers, Philadelphia © 1997.

20

Monitoring of Spinal Cord Function Intraoperatively Using Motor and Somatosensory Evoked Potentials

°Ronald G. Emerson, †David C. Adams, and ‡Keith J. Nagle

°Department of Neurology, Columbia-Presbyterian Hospital Medical Center;
†Department of Anesthesiology, College of Physicians and Surgeons, Columbia University,
New York, New York 10032; and ‡Department of Neurology, University of Vermont,
Fletcher Allen Health Care, Burlington, Vermont 05401

1. INTRODUCTION

Over the past decade, intraoperative monitoring of spinal cord function has become an accepted means of diminishing the risk of injury to the spinal cord during surgery (Forbes et al., 1991; Nuwer et al., 1995). The principal purpose for monitoring is to identify spinal cord dysfunction in time to permit remedial action before the injury becomes permanent. Prior to electrophysiologic monitoring, the wake-up test was used for intraoperative detection of spinal cord injury (Vauzelle et al., 1973). Although sometimes viewed as a "gold-standard" for intraoperative assessment of spinal cord function, the wake-up test does not provide continuous monitoring and also entails certain risks. These include accidental extubation, dislodgment of instrumentation, and pulmonary embolism (Ben-David, 1988). Based on their experience with over 1,000 cases of scoliosis monitored at the Royal Orthopedic Hospital using SEPs, Forbes et al. conclude that SEP monitoring is much more sensitive than the wake-up test, and should probably replace it (Forbes et al., 1991).

Somatosensory (SEPs) and motor evoked potentials (MEPs) are useful monitors of spinal cord function, since graded deterioration correlating with the degree of injury occurs in both following spinal cord compression, blunt trauma, and ischemia (Baskin and Simpson Jr., 1987; Cracco and Evans, 1978; D'Angelo et al., 1973; Deecke and Tator, 1973; Ducker et al., 1978; Fehlings et al., 1989; Levy et al., 1986, 1987; Machida et al., 1988, 1989; Martin and Bloedel, 1973; Patil et al., 1985; Reuter et al., 1992; Shiau et al., 1992). Somatosensory evoked potentials are mediated primarily by the dorsal column pathways in the dorsal funiculus of the spinal cord, while MEPs depend on the integrity of the descending motor pathways in the anterior and lateral cord. Whereas the vascular supply of the posterior cord is relatively robust, the supply to the anterior and lateral portions of the spinal cord is more tenuous. These regions are supplied by the anterior spinal artery, with large watershed areas along its course. Its middle and lower portions often are narrow and supplied by few radicular branches, rendering the anterior and lateral regions of the spinal cord especially vulnerable to hypotension-induced ischemia (Szilagyi et al., 1978; Turnbull et al., 1966). It is not surprising, therefore, that intraoperative motor deficits may occur without altered SEPs (Ben-David et al., 1987; Zornow et al., 1990), and that SEPs may be preserved in patients with anterior spinal artery syndrome (Dorfman et al., 1980; Takaki and Okumura, 1985; Zornow et al., 1990). Similarly, intraoperative injury to the dorsal cord may produce loss of SEPs and position and vibration sensation in the lower extremities, while not affecting motor function (Dorfman et al., 1980; Takaki and Okumura, 1985; Zornow et al., 1990).

2. INTRAOPERATIVE RECORDING OF SEPS

Maximizing the reliability of intraoperative SEP monitoring requires adapting recording strategies to both the difficulties and the advantages presented by the operating room. In standard laboratory settings, cortical SEP components, detected using bipolar scalp–scalp derivations, are generally more easily recorded than subcortical far-field components, which require use of scalp–noncephalic electrode derivations. In the operating room, the reverse situation often applies.

The cortical components of the SEP (N20 for upper-extremity SEPs, P38 for lower-extremity SEPs) are attenuated by most general anesthetics. Halogenated inhalational agents (e.g., halothane, isoflurane) have the most potent effects, attenuating and prolonging the latency of the cortical response (Browning et al., 1992; Gravenstein et al., 1984; Perlik et al., 1992; Sebel et al., 1987). Other agents, including nitrous oxide, narcotics, benzodiazepines, and barbiturates, have similar but generally less pronounced effects (Koht, 1988; McPherson et al., 1986; Perlik et al., 1992). The attenuation of cortical SEP components by anesthetic agents is most dramatic in infants and young children (Harper and Nelson, 1992), and commonly affects lower- more than upper-extremity SEPs. In contrast, subcortical responses [P14 and N18 for upper-extremity SEPs, P31 and N34 for lower-extremity SEPs (Desmedt and Cheron, 1981; Seyal et al., 1983)] are less subject to anesthetic affects. They are much more stable in the presence of anesthetic agents, and hence are a more reliable indicator for intraoperative SEP monitoring (Sebel et al., 1987) (Fig. 20–1).

Etomidate increases the voltage of cortical SEPs, but does not effect subcortical components (Koht, 1988; McPherson et al., 1986; Samra and Sorkin, 1991). It has been suggested that an infusion of etomidate can be used as means to augment the amplitude of cortical SEPs (Sloan and D'Angell, 1992), although concern has been expressed that etomidate might mask deterioration of the SEP (McPherson et al., 1986).

Subcortical SEPs are often difficult to record in the awake patient. They are low voltage, and easily obscured by artifact. The noise susceptibility of the scalp–noncephalic electrode derivations used for recording subcortical SEPs compounds this difficulty. The most troublesome source of noise is muscle artifact, which, while difficult to suppress in the laboratory, is easily eliminated in the operating room. Figure 20–2 illustrates two intraoperative recordings obtained with the same anesthetic regimen, but before and after a bolus of vecuronium, a nondepolarizing neuromuscular blocking agent. The subcortical components are

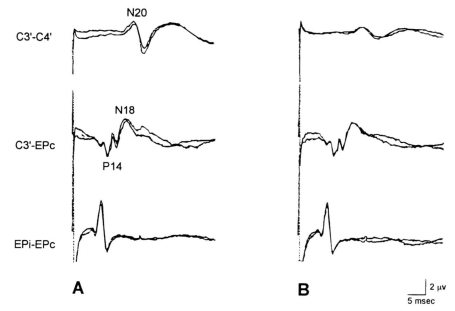

FIG. 20–1. Median SEPs recorded during nitrous oxide (70%) and isoflurane (0.5%$_{exp}$) anesthesia (**A**), and after increasing the isoflurane concentration to 1% (**B**). Increasing the isoflurane concentration produced attenuation of the cortical N20, but did not alter subcortical P14 and N18 signals.

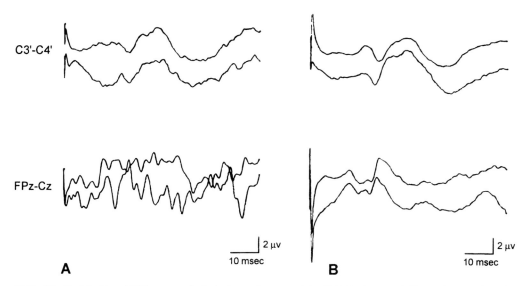

FIG. 20–2. Median SEPs recorded during nitrous oxide (70%), fentanyl (1 μg/kg per hour) and 0.7%$_{exp}$ isoflurane anesthesia, before (**A**) and after (**B**) the addition of vecuronium. Prior to administration of vecuronium, an interpretable cortical response (*top channel*) is recorded, but the subcortical response (*bottom channel*) is uninterpretable. Neuromuscular blockade reduced accompanying artifact, making the subcortical response easily interpretable.

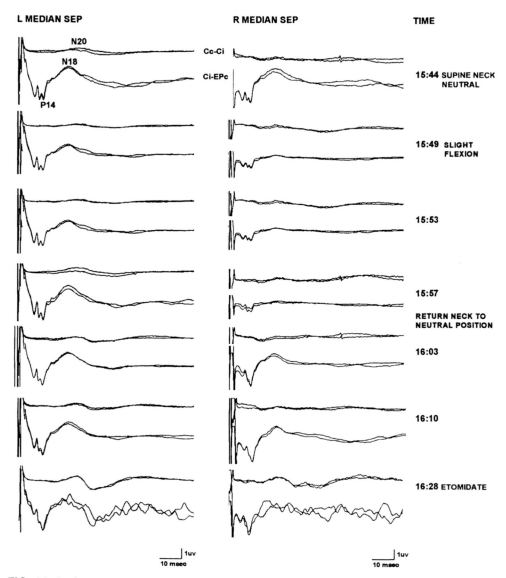

FIG. 20–3. Somatosensory EPs recorded during planned cleft palate repair in a 3-year-old patient with achondroplasia. Under halothane anesthesia by mask, with the child lying supine and the neck in a neutral position, intact subcortical SEPs were present bilaterally. Cortical SEPs were low amplitude, as expected in a young child receiving a halogenated anesthetic agent, but subcortical signals were prominent and easily recorded. Slight flexion of the neck during myringotomy resulted in loss of the N18 on the right, presumably due to cervical cord compression. The head was returned to the neutral position, and the response returned. The cleft palate repair was deferred, and etomidate (0.2 mg/kg) was administered to facilitate monitoring for the remainder of the case. The patient awoke without neurologic deficits.

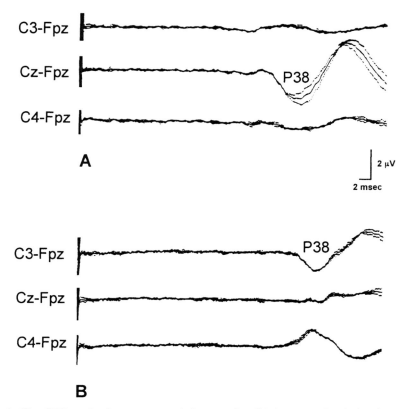

FIG. 20–4. The P38 cortical response to left posterior tibial nerve stimulation in two normal individuals. The P38 could be missed if only a C3–FpZ derivation was used in patient A, or if only a CZ–FpZ derivation was employed in patient B.

uninterpretable prior to vecuronium, and easily interpreted after pharmacologic paralysis. Monitoring of subcortical SEPs and the use of etomidate to enhance cortical SEPs are illustrated in a series of SEP recordings from a 3-year-old patient with achondroplasia undergoing a planned cleft palate repair (Fig. 20–3).

While subcortical SEPs are generally best suited for intraoperative monitoring, they are occasionally difficult to record, particularly in patients with pre-existing neurologic abnormalities. In these cases, cortical SEPs are of primary importance and it is desirable to limit the use of those anesthetics which most attenuate these responses. It is also important to employ a recording montage that accounts for the normal variability in the scalp topography of lower-extremity cortical SEPs in normals (Seyal et al., 1983). A single derivation devoted to recording the P38 cortical response for all patients is not adequate (Fig. 20–4). Two channels, for example, CZ–FpZ and C4/3$_{ipsilateral}$–FpZ, are suggested.

In some cases when scalp-recorded responses are unobtainable it is possible to monitor SEPs directly from the spinal cord. We have used this technique to monitor of SEPs following pudendal stimulation recording in children undergoing untethering of the spinal cord (Fig. 20–5).

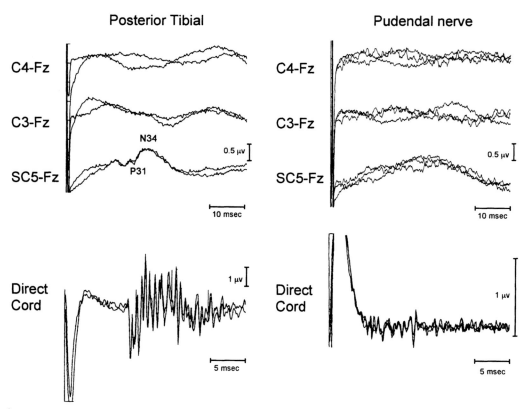

FIG. 20–5. Posterior tibial and pudendal nerve SEPs recorded from the scalp (*top panels*) and directly from the spinal cord (*bottom panels*) during untethering of the cord in a 22-month-old boy. Posterior tibial nerve stimulation produced an easily recordable scalp response, as well as large spinal cord responses. Although pudendal nerve produced no scalp recordable responses, well-formed SEPs are recorded from electrodes on the spinal cord. Direct spinal cord recordings were made using a 2-mm-diameter stainless steel disc electrode in a Silastic carrier, referred to a needle electrode in adjacent muscle.

3. INTRAOPERATIVE RECORDING OF MEPS

Motor evoked potentials may be recorded by stimulating the brain or the spinal cord. An advantage of transcranial stimulation is that the MEPs produced are mediated only by the descending motor pathways (Rothwell et al., 1994), either as a result of direct activation of pyramidal axons, or indirectly through activation of cortical interneurons which synapse on pyramidal cells. Direct pyramidal activation is thought to produce D waves, components of MEPs that precede and are more stable than the "indirect" I waves, which probably result from transynaptic activation (Amassian et al., 1987; Rothwell et al., 1994). D-waves are readily elicited by transcranial electrical stimulation, whereas transcranial magnetic stimulation generally elicits I waves (Mills, 1991). Another advantage of transcranial stimulation techniques is that the electrodes or coils are outside of the operative field, and need not be placed by the surgeon.

The principal limitation of transcranial methods of stimulation for intraoperative monitoring is that magnetically (Ghaly et al., 1990; Kalkman et al., 1992a,b) and electrically (Haghighi et al., 1990; Kalkman et al., 1991; Zentner et al., 1992) elicited transcranial MEPs (tcMMEPs) are attenuated by commonly used anesthetic regimens. In our experience, tcMMEPs are not sufficiently stable or reliable for clinical use in many patients. Although tcMMEPs are easily recorded from waking subjects, using a single-pulse magnetic stimulator (Caldwell MES-10) and a "skullcap" coil, we were able to obtain consistent tcMMEPs from the lower extremities in only 50% (8 of 16) of patients receiving nitrous oxide (70%) and fentanyl (1 to 2 μg/kg per hour) anesthesia. In some patients, tcMMEPs were obtainable only intermittently, and their amplitudes varied substantially, without apparent relationship to surgical or anesthetic variables. Often, minor, unavoidable alterations in coil position produced profound alterations in lower-extremity tcMMEPs (Fig. 20–6) (Adams et al., 1993a).

We currently monitor MEPs by electrically stimulating the spinal cord and recording compound muscle action potentials (CMAPs) from appropriate muscles. Partial neuromuscular blockade is used to permit recording of robust CMAPs, while preventing movement that would interfere with surgery (Adams et al., 1993b). A vecuronium infusion is titrated to suppress the first of four hypothenar muscle twitches (T1) elicited by a train of supramaximal ulnar nerve stimuli to 10% of baseline. Compound muscle action potentials are

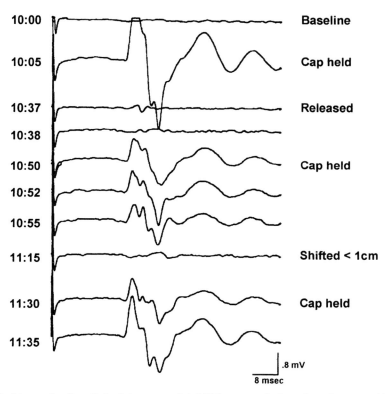

FIG. 20–6. Magnetically elicited transcranial MEPs recorded under nitrous oxide/oxygen/ opioid anesthesia using a skullcap stimulating coil. Minimal movement of the coil produced major changes in the MEP.

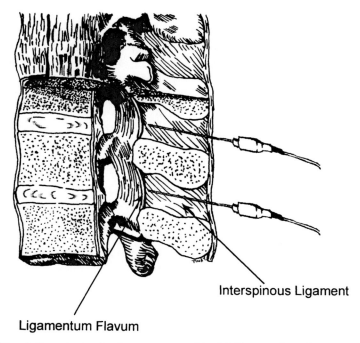

Interspinous Ligament

Ligamentum Flavum

FIG. 20–7. Stimulating electrode placement used for MEP recording. Electrodes are passed through the intraspinous ligament at two adjacent vertebral levels, and placed close to the ligamentum flavum.

recorded from surface electrodes placed over the bellies of appropriate muscles (typically quadriceps, tibialis anterior, and extensor digitorum brevis), referred to the corresponding tendons. The spinal cord is stimulated at the rostral end of the exposure using monopolar needle electrodes inserted through the intraspinous ligament at two adjacent vertebral levels, and placed close to the ligamentum flavum (Fig. 20–7). Electrodes may be placed in the surgical exposure, or positioned transcutaneously. Typically, 0.1- to 0.5-msec, 20- to 40-mA stimulating pulses delivered at a rate of 0.5 Hz are employed, adjusted to produce stable CMAPs in the monitored muscles, but with minimal or no twitch in the paraspinus muscles near the site of stimulation. Alternatively, appropriate electrodes may be placed in the epidural or subdural spaces, and corresponding lower stimulus currents employed.

We reviewed a series of 116 cases of spine or spinal cord surgery at the Columbia-Presbyterian Medical Center, during which both SEPs and MEPs were monitored . In seven patients with severe, pre-existing myelopathies, MEPs but not SEP were recordable. In two similar patients, only SEPs were recordable. Evoked potentials deteriorated in nine cases. In eight of the nine cases, both SEPs and MEPs changed. In one case of spinal cord untethering, MEPs deteriorated while SEPs remained stable (Fig. 20–8) (Nagle et al., 1996)].

Detection of intraoperative EP changes led to major alterations in surgery in 4 cases. One patient with severe kyphoscoliosis and spinal stenosis experienced loss of MEPs and SEPs during anterior spinal decompression. The change prompted termination of the procedure and delay of a planned subsequent operation. In another case, a vessel feeding an arteriovenous malformation was spared after clamping produced a loss of the MEPs (Fig. 20–9). In two additional patients, repeated attempts at correction of scoliosis produced reversible loss

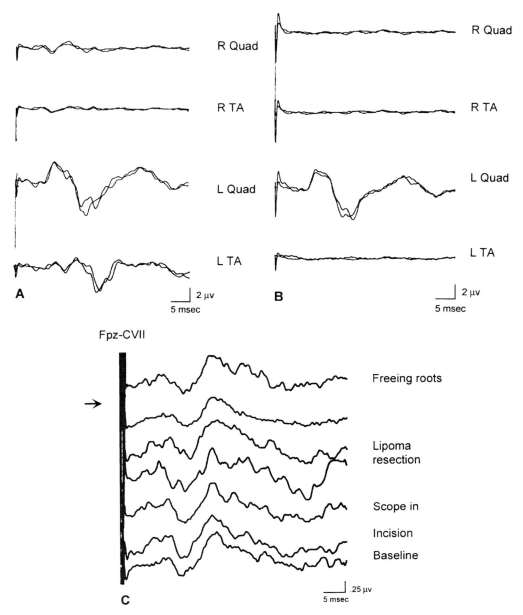

FIG. 20–8. Motor and sensory EPs recorded during untethering of the spinal cord in a 7-year-old patient. **A.** Baseline MEP. **B.** MEP recorded during lipoma resection, showing loss of responses from right and left tibialis anterior and right quadriceps muscles. **C.** Left posterior tibial SEPs revealed no change at the time that MEPs deteriorated (*arrow*). SEPs to right posterior tibial nerve stimulation were absent at baseline. L TA, R TA, L Quad, and R Quad denote left/right tibialis anterior, and left/right quadriceps muscles, respectively. CVII denotes an electrode position over the seventh cervical vertebra. (Reproduced from Nagle et al., 1996.)

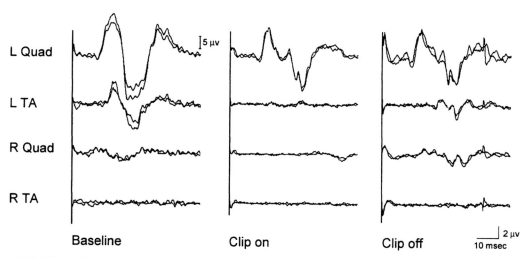

L Quad

L TA

R Quad

R TA

Baseline   Clip on   Clip off

5 µv

2 µv
10 msec

FIG. 20–9. Placement of a clip on a feeding vessel during resection of a spinal cord arterio-venous malformation resulted in almost complete loss of MEPs from left tibialis anterior and right quadriceps muscles. The responses returned when the clip was removed.

of SEP and MEP signals. In both cases, hardware was removed, and patients were placed in body casts (Fig. 20–10) (Nagle et al., 1996).

In contrast to transcranial electrical and magnetic stimulation, where intervening synapses prevent retrograde activation of descending spinal sensory pathways, direct spinal cord stimulation activates both motor and sensory pathways. Recording CMAPs eliminates confounding sensory potentials that would be recorded from spinal cord or mixed nerve (Adams et al., 1994). While it has been suggested that antidromic sensory volleys may activate motor neurons in the lumbar cord contributing to the CMAPs (Poncelet et al., 1995), a major contibution is unlikely in the presence of halogenated anesthetic agents known to suppress spinal reflexes (De Jong et al., 1968; Freund et al., 1969). A further advantage to recording CMAPs is that the gray matter of the ventral cord, especially sensitive to ischemic injury (Adams et al., 1993b; Coles et al., 1982; Levy et al., 1986), is included in the monitored system.

Motor evoked potentials recorded by our technique are generally robust, stable, and typically easy to record rapidly. Despite the use of partial neuromuscular blockade adequate to eliminate movement that would interfere with surgery, MEPs are typically an order of magnitude larger than SEP signals. Often, MEPs were visible in the raw data, and typically only 2 to 20 responses are average to produce a monitorable waveform. This contrasts with several hundred to 2,000 responses typically averaged to recording an interpretable SEP waveform.

FIG. 20–10. During correction of kyphoscoliosis in a 17-year-old patient, three attempts at tightening Luque wires resulted loss of MEPs or SEPs. On each occasion, signals returned when the wires were loosened. Instrumentation was removed, and the patient was placed in a body cast. She was paraplegic immediately postoperatively, but regained her baseline examination within 2 weeks, and was ambulatory at discharge. (Reproduced from Nagle et al., 1996.)

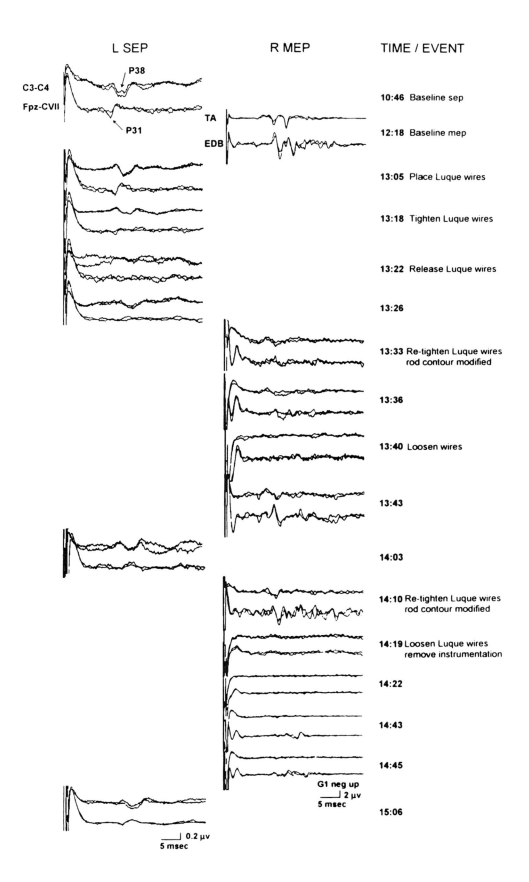

L SEP   R MEP   TIME / EVENT

C3-C4
Fpz-CVII   P38
   P31
TA
EDB

10:46 Baseline sep

12:18 Baseline mep

13:05 Place Luque wires

13:18 Tighten Luque wires

13:22 Release Luque wires

13:26

13:33 Re-tighten Luque wires
       rod contour modified

13:36

13:40 Loosen wires

13:43

14:03

14:10 Re-tighten Luque wires
       rod contour modified

14:19 Loosen Luque wires
       remove instrumentation

14:22

14:43

14:45

G1 neg up
2 µv
5 msec

15:06

0.2 µv
5 msec

4. CONCLUSION

We believe that optimal spinal cord monitoring requires recording of both motor and sensory evoked potentials, allowing detection of cases in which only motor or sensory pathways are injured intraoperatively. Of at least equal importance is that the concurrent use of both motor and sensory monitors provides the added security of redundant systems. Since, in most cases, intraoperative spinal cord injury affects both MEPs and SEPs (Nagle et al., In Press), recording both provides the neurophysiologist with independent verification of spinal cord integrity using independent, parallel systems. Intraoperative monitoring of evoked potentials is challenging technically, and even in patients with normal spinal cord function it is occasionally difficult to obtain reliable EP signals. Recording conditions deteriorate, at times, especially during protracted procedures. In these cases, concurrent monitoring of SEPs and MEPs permits continued reliable monitoring, despite technical failure of one or the other modality.

ACKNOWLEDGMENTS

The authors wish to express their appreciation to Ms. Christine Turner, Dr. Kathryn Dowling, and Mr. Edward Gallo for their technical assistance.

REFERENCES

Adams D, Emerson R, Heyer E (1994): Intraoperative monitoring of motor evoked potentials: In response. *Anesth Analg*, 79: 1206.

Adams DC, Emerson RG, Heyer EJ (1993a): Intraoperative motor tract monitoring using transcranial magnetic evoked potentials. *Neurology* 43: 426.

Adams DC, Emerson RG, Heyer EJ, McCormick PC, Stein BM, Farcy JP, Gallo E (1993b): Monitoring of intraoperative motor evoked potentials under conditions of controlled neuromuscular blockade. *Anesth Analg* 77: 913–918.

Amassian VE, Stewart M, Quirk GJ, Rosenthal JL (1987): Physiological basis of motor effects of a transient stimulus to cerebral cortex. *Neurosurgery* 20: 74–93.

Baskin DS, Simpson Jr RK (1987): Corticomotor and somatosensory evoked potential evaluation of acute spinal cord injury in the rat. *Neurosurgery* 20: 871–877.

Ben-David B (1988): Spinal cord monitoring. *Orthop Clin North Am* 19: 427–448.

Ben-David B, Haller G, Taylor P (1987): Anterior spinal fusion complicated by paraplegia. A case report of a false-negative somatosensory-evoked potential. *Spine* 12: 536–539.

Browning JL, Heizer ML, Baskin DS (1992): Variations in corticomotor and somatosensory evoked potentials: effects of temperature, halothane anesthesia, and arterial partial pressure of CO_2. *Anesth Analg* 74: 643–648.

Coles JG, Wilson GJ, Sima AF, Klement P, Tait GA (1982): Intraoperative detection of spinal cord ischemia using somatosensory cortical evoked potentials during thoracic aortic occlusion. *Ann Thorac Surg* 34: 299–306.

Cracco RQ, Evans B (1978): Spinal evoked potentials in the cat: Effects of asphyxia, strychnine, cord section and compression. *Electroencephalogr Clin Neurophysiol* 44: 187–201.

D'Angelo CM, VanGilder JC, Taub A (1973): Evoked cortical potentials in experimental spinal cord trauma. *J Neurosurg* 38: 332–336.

De Jong RH, Robles R, Corbin RW, Nace R (1968): Effect of inhalation anesthetics on monosynaptic and polysynaptic transmission in the spinal cord. *J Pharm Exp Ther* 162: 326–330.

Deecke L, Tator CH (1973): Neurophysiol assessment of afferent and efferent conduction in the injured spinal cord of monkeys. *J Neurosurg* 39: 65–74.

Desmedt JE, Cheron G (1981): Non-cephalic reference recording of early somatosensory potentials to finger stimulation in adult or aging man: Differentiation of widespread N18 and contralateral N20 from prerolandic P22 and N30 components. *Electroencephalogr Clin Neurophysiol* 52: 553–570.

Dorfman LJ, Perkash I, Bosley TM, Cummins KL (1980): Use of cerebral evoked potentials to evaluate spinal somatosensory function in patients with traumatic and surgical myelopathies. *J Neurosurg* 52: 654–660.

Ducker TB, Saleman M, Lucas JT, Garrison WB, Perot PL (1978): Experimental spinal cord trauma, II: Blood flow, tissue oxygen, evoked potentials in both paretic and plegic monkeys. *Surg Neurol* 10: 64–70.

Fehlings MG, Tator CH, Linden RD (1989): The relationships among the severity of spinal cord injury, motor and somatosensory evoked potentials and spinal cord blood flow. *Electroencephalogr Clin Neurophysiol* 74: 241–259.

Forbes HJ, Allen PW, Waller CS, Jones SJ, Edgar MA, Webb PJ, Ransford AO (1991): Spinal cord monitoring in scoliosis surgery. *J Bone Joint Surg* 73B: 487–491.

Freund FG, Martin WE, Hornbein TF (1969): The H-reflex as a measure of anesthetic potency in man. *Anesthesiology* 30: 642–647.

Ghaly RF, Stone JL, Levy WJ, Kartha R, Aldrete JA (1990): The effect of nitrous oxide on transcranial magnetic-induced electromyographic responses in the monkey. *J Neurosurg Anesthesiol* 2: 175–181.

Gravenstein MA, Sasse F, Hogan K (1984): Effects of stimulus rate and halothane dose on canine far-field somatosensory evoked potentials. *Anesthesiology* 61: A342.

Haghighi SS, Madsen R, Green KD, Oro JJ, Kracke GR (1990): Suppression of motor evoked potentials by inhalation anesthetics. *J Neurosurg Anesthesiol* 2: 73–78.

Harper CM, Nelson KR (1992): Intraoperative electrophysiological monitoring in children. *J Clin Neurophysiol* 9: 342–56.

Kalkman CJ, Drummond JC, Ribberink AA (1991): Low concentrations of isoflurane abolish motor evoked responses to transcranial electrical stimulation during nitrous oxide/opioid anesthesia in humans. *Anesth Analg* 73: 410–415.

Kalkman CJ, Drummond JC, Kennely NA, Piyush MP, Partridge BL (1992a): Intraoperative monitoring of tibialis anterior muscle motor evoked responses to transcranial electrical stimulation during partial neuromuscular blockade. *Anesth Analg* 73: 584–589.

Kalkman CJ, Drummond JC, Ribberink AA, Patel PM, Sano T, Bickford RG (1992b): Effects of propofol, etomidate, midazolam, and fentanyl on motor evoked responses to transcranial electrical or magnetic stimulation in humans. *Anesthesiology* 76: 502–509.

Koht Aea (1988): Effects of ethomicate, midazolam, and thiopental on median nerve somatosensory evoked potentilas and the additive effects of fentanyl and nitrous oxide. *Anesth Analg* 67: 435–441.

Levy W, McCaffrey M, York D (1986): Motor evoked potential in cats with acute spinal cord injury. *Neurosurgery* 19: 9–19.

Levy WJ, McCaffrey M, Hagichi S (1987): Motor evoked potential as a predictor of recovery in chronic spinal injury. *Neurosurgery* 20: 138–142.

Machida M, Weinstein SL, Yamada T, Kimura J, Toriyama S (1988): Dissociation of muscle action potentials and spinal somatosensory evoked potentials after ischemic damage of spinal cord. *Spine* 13: 1119–1124.

Machida M, Weinstein SL, Imamura Y, Usui T, Yamada T, Kimura J, Toriyama S (1989): Compound muscle action potentials and spinal evoked potentials in experimental spine maneuver. *Spine* 14: 687–91.

Martin SH, Bloedel JR (1973): Evaluation of experimental spinal cord injury using cortical potentials. *Neurosurgery* 39: 75–81.

McPherson RW, Sell B, Traystman RJ (1986): Effects of thiopental, fentanyl and etomidate on upper extremity somatosensory evoked potentials in humans. *Anesthesiology* 65: 584–589.

Mills KR (1991): Magnetic brain stimulation: a tool to explore the action of the motor cortex on single human motoneurones. *Trends Neurosci* 14: 401–405.

Nagle K, Emerson RG, Adams DA, Heyer E, Gallo E, Dowling KC, McCormick P, Roye D, Pile-Spellman J, Stein B, Weidenbaum M (1996): Intraoperative motor and somatosensory evoked potential monitoring: A review of 116 cases. *Neurology*, 47: 999–1004.

Nuwer MR, Dawson EG, Carlson LG, Kanim LEA, Sherman JE (1995): Somatosensory evoked potential spinal cord monitoring reduces neurologic deficits after scoliosis surgery: results of a large multicenter survey. *Electroencephalogr Clin Neurophysiol* 96: 6–11.

Patil A, Nagaraj MP, Mehta R (1985): Cortically evoked motor action potential in spinal cord injury research. *Neurosurgery* 16: 473–476.

Perlik SJ, VanEgeren R, Fisher MA (1992): Somatosensory evoked potential surgical monitoring. Observation during combined isoflurane-nitrous oxide anesthesia. *Spine* 17: 273–276.

Poncelet L, Michaux C, Balligand M (1995): Motor evoked potentials induced by electrical stimulation of the spine in dogs: which structures are involved? *Electroencephalogr Clin Neurophysiol* 97: 179–183.

Reuter DG, Tacker Jr WA, Badylak SF, Voorhees 3rd, WD, Konrad PE (1992): Correlation of motor-evoked potential response to ischemic spinal cord damage. *J Thorac Cardiovasc Surg* 104: 262–272.

Rothwell J, David B, Hicks R, Stephen J, Woodforth I, Crawford M (1994): Transcranial electrical stimulation of the motor cortex in man: further evidence of site of activation. *J Physiol* 481: 243–250.

Samra SK, Sorkin (1991): Enhancement of somatosensory evoked potentials by etomidate in cats: An investigation of its site of action. *Anesthesiology* 74: 499–503.

Sebel PS, Erwin CW, Neville WK (1987): Effects of halothane and enflurane on far and near-field somatosensory evoked potentials. *Br J Anaesth* 57: 1492–1496.

Seyal M, Emerson RG, Pedley TA (1983): Spinal and early scalp-recorded components of the somatosensory evoked potential following stimulation of the posterior tibial nerve. *Electroencephalog Clin Neurophysiol* 55: 320–330.

Shiau JS, Zappulla RA, Nieves J (1992): The effect of graded spinal cord injury on the extrapyramidal and pyramidal motor evoked potentials of the rat. *Neurosurgery* 30: 76–84.

Sloan T, D'Angell D (1992): Effects of halothane on cortical electric and magnetic motor evoked potentials in the monkey. *Anesthesiology* 77: A530.

Szilagyi D, Hageman JH, Smith RF, Elliott JP (1978): Spinal cord damage in surgery of the abdominal aorta. *Surgery* 83: 38–56.

Takaki O, Okumura F (1985): Application and limitation of somatosensory evoked potential monitoring during thoracic aortic aneurysm surgery. A case report. *Anesthesiology* 65: 700–703.

Turnbull I, Brieg A, Hassler O (1966): Blood supply of the cervical spinal cord in man: a microangiographic cadaver study. *J Neurosurg* 24: 951–965.

Vauzelle C, Stagnara C, Jouvinroux P (1973): Functional monitoring of spinal cord activity during spinal surgery. *Clin Orthop Rel Res* 93: 173–178.

Zentner J, Albrecht T, Heuser D (1992): Influence of halothane, enflurane, and isoflurane on motor evoked potentials. *Neurosurgery* 31: 298–305.

Zornow MH, Grafe MR, Tybor C, Swenson MR (1990): Preservation of evoked potentials in a case of anterior spinal artery syndrome. *Electroencephalogr Clin Neurophysiol* 77: 137–139.

Evoked Potentials in Clinical Medicine,
3d ed., edited by Keith H. Chiappa.
Lippincott–Raven Publishers, Philadelphia © 1997.

21

Intraoperative Neurophysiologic Monitoring in Pediatrics

Sandra L. Helmers

*Department of Neurology, Harvard Medical School, Children's Hospital,
EEG Laboratory, Boston, Massachusetts 02115*

1. INTRODUCTION

Neurophysiologic monitoring of the spinal cord and central nervous system has become quite useful in pediatrics as neurophysiologists and surgeons have gained more experience over the last several years. Intraoperative monitoring is useful in assessing functional integrity, allowing early detection of injury, identifying potential mechanisms of injury, and possibly preventing permanent damage to the spinal cord or central nervous system during procedures that carry a high risk of morbidity.

In this chapter, a review of the more common neurophysiologic techniques used in the operating room and the appropriate selection of the type of monitoring techniques will briefly be discussed. In addition, technical and patient-related problems in the pediatric age group will be discussed.

2. SPINAL CORD MONITORING

The most common type of intraoperative monitoring in children is for spinal cord integrity, using somatosensory evoked potentials (SEPs). When performing SEPs intraoperatively, posterior tibial nerves or median nerves are most commonly used. The peroneal, ulnar, and radial nerves are less commonly used because their waveforms are not as robust or reliable. When planning to monitor the somatosensory system, it is important to know at which level the surgeon is operating. Median nerve SEPs are used for the mid-cervical to rostral spinal cord, ulnar nerve SEPs are used for the lower cervical spinal cord, and posterior tibial SEPs are used for the lower lumbar and upper sacral spinal cord. Ideally, recordings are done above and below the operative site. Other important points to remember are what part of the spinal cord is being monitored and which are the posterior columns.

The techniques of stimulating and recording intraoperative SEPs are similar to those of routine laboratory SEPs except that invasive electrodes, including needle electrodes for stimulating and recording, intraesophageal recording electrodes, and epidural recording electrodes, are sometimes used. The surgeon and anesthesiologist must be comfortable with the placement and use of these types of electrodes.

The most commonly monitored procedure is corrective surgery for scoliosis using posterior tibial nerve SEPs. This type of surgery often involves instrumentation and distraction of the spine, with one of the most feared complications being paraplegia. The incidence of paraplegia with Harrington rod placement or other types of instrumentation and distraction is from 0.5% to 1.6% (MacEwen et al., 1975). Prior to the availability of intraoperative SEPs orthopedic surgeons had to use the wake-up test (Vauzelle et al., 1973; Hall et al., 1978), which involves waking the patient during surgery and telling the patient to move his/her toes, then quickly reanesthetizing the patient. The risks involved include movement of or injury from the surgical hardware, extubation, vital sign instability, and psychic trauma to the patient. In addition, the wake-up test can only be performed at most a few times during the procedure and certain patients cannot cooperate with the test. With the introduction of SEPs into the operating room, the wake-up test could be avoided in many cases.

One might argue that since only the posterior spinal cord or somatosensory pathways are being monitored, how helpful are the SEPs in predicting damage to the motor pathways (Chatrian et al., 1988; Lesser et al., 1986)? Depending upon the type of injury to the spinal cord—compression or vascular compromise, which tend to involve multiple regions of the spinal cord—there are likely to be changes in the SEPs that correspond to the injury. If a discrete area of the cord is damaged, it is unlikely to cause a change in the monitoring if the somatosensory pathways are not affected, or if the lesion is below the level of monitoring. With these limitations in mind, intraoperative evoked potential monitoring can aid the surgeon in preventing complications in many surgical procedures.

2.1. The Children's Hospital Experience

The intraoperative SEP monitoring literature has mainly dealt with the adult population (Engler et al., 1978; Lueders et al., 1982; Nuwer and Dawson, 1984; Lubicky et al., 1989; Loder et al., 1991). Therefore, the experience at Children's Hospital, Boston, between 1989 and 1991 was reviewed. Over 300 surgical procedures were monitored intraoperatively using evoked potentials, of which 95% were orthopedic cases and 5% were neurosurgical (Helmers and Hall, 1994; Helmers and Kull, 1994). Of the orthopedic cases 77.6% involved instrumentation utilizing distraction and/or rotation, and in approximately 20%, fusion without instrumentation was performed (Table 21–1). Neurosurgical procedures included cortical mapping during tumor resection or epileptic focus ablation, intramedullary and extramedullary spinal cord tumors, posterior fossa procedures for meningioma, brain stem glioma, Arnold–Chiari malformation, spinal cord lipoma with tethered cord, removal of a peripheral nerve neurofibroma, and repair of a brachial plexus injury.

The patients ranged in age from 4.5 months to 47 years (Table 21–2), with the majority being between 11 years and 19 years of age. About 20% were under 10 years of age, with 15

TABLE 21–1. *Surgical procedures monitored at Children's Hospital between 1989 and 1991*

Surgical procedure	Number of patients	Type of EP used
Orthopedic	95%	
Instrumentation + distraction	253 (77.6%)	Pt SEP
Fusion	73 (22.4%)	Pt SEP
Neurosurgical	5%	
Tethered cord with lipoma	4	Pt SEP
Cortical mapping	3	Mn SEP
Intramedullary cord tumor	3	Pt/Mn SEP
Extramedullary cord tumor	2	Pt/Mn SEP
Brain stem glioma	2	Pt/Mn SEP, BAEP
Posterior fossa meningioma	1	Pt/Mn SEP, BAEP
Arnold-Chiari malformation, type 1 decompression	1	Pt/Mn SEP, BAEP
Peripheral neurofibroma	1	Mn SEP
Brachial plexus repair	1	Mn SEP

Pt SEP, posterior tibial nerve SEP; Mn SEP, median nerve SEP.
From Helmers and Hall, 1994, with permission.

patients between the ages of 1 and 5 years, and 2 patients less than a year. Only about 10% of the patients were older than 20 years of age.

Over half of the patients had idiopathic scoliosis (63.7%), with about a third of the patients (31.2%) having neuromuscular scoliosis (Table 21–3). The most commonly associated condition was cerebral palsy. Many other conditions were seen in association with neuromuscular scoliosis, such as myelodysplasia and mental retardation. This latter group of patients is at higher risk for neurologic sequelae during corrective spinal surgery according to MacEwen and colleagues (1975), who reported an incidence of 0.72% for neurologic complications in the surgical treatment of scoliosis, with the true incidence perhaps being higher. With certain conditions, such as a pre-existing neurologic deficit, congenital scoliosis, or scoliosis of a severe degree, there is an increased risk for neurologic injury. Certain procedures also carry a higher risk for neurologic injury, such as skeletal traction, Harrington rod instrumentation, or the use of sublaminar wires (Wilber et al., 1984). Therefore, the patient most likely to benefit from intraoperative SEP monitoring is a high-risk patient undergoing a difficult procedure as defined above.

TABLE 21–2. *Age range of patients monitored intraoperatively at Children's Hospital between 1989 and 1991*

	Age Range (4.5 months to 47 years)		
	Number of patients		
Patient age	Male	Female	Total
<1 year	2	0	2
1–5 years	9	7	16
6–10 years	19	30	49
11–15 years	35	144	179
16–20 years	36	29	65
>20 years	8	24	32
Total	109	234	343

TABLE 21–3. *Type of scoliosis in patients monitored intraoperatively at Children's Hospital between 1989 and 1991*

Idiopathic scoliosis	219		
Neuromuscular scoliosis	107		
Cerebral palsy			
Myelodysplasia			
Mental retardation			
Spondylolisthesis			
Myopathy/dystrophy			
Neurofibromatosis			
Post-traumatic			
Rett's syndrome		Instrumentation and distraction	Fusion only
Tethered cord/lipoma		253	73
Marfan's syndrome			
Dwarfism			
Friedrich's ataxia			
Syringomyelia			
Peripheral sensory neuropathy			
Post-radiation			
Klippel-Trenaunay-Weber syndrome			
Other procedures	17		
Brain stem/cord neoplasm			
Cervical instability			
Arnold–Chiari malformation			
Brachial plexus injury			

Other types of procedures that employ intraoperative SEP monitoring are selective rhizotomy, surgery of selected peripheral nerves/plexus, spinal cord tumors, epilepsy, cortical/subcortical masses, carotid endarterectomy, and aortic surgery.

2.1.1. SEP Methodology

Somatosensory EPs were performed according to the guidelines of the American Electroencephalographic Society for intraoperative monitoring (1994). After marking electrode sites in accordance with the 10–20 International system (C3', C4', CZ', FpZ, FZ, A1, A2) the recording sites were prepared with a commercially available pumice-based solution. Gold cup electrodes were affixed using gauze soaked with collodion. Additional gold cup electrodes were affixed to the C2 and C3 cervical spine in the same manner. A ground electrode was placed on the left shoulder. Electrode impedances were maintained between 2,000 and 5,000 ohms.

A monophasic stimulus of 100 μsec duration and 10 to 20 mA was delivered to the posterior tibial nerve at the ankle and/or the median nerve at the wrist. The rate of stimulation was 2 Hz for posterior tibial nerve testing, and 5 Hz for the median nerve EP, delivered to each limb separately.

Posterior tibial nerve SEP recordings were obtained from the popliteal fossa (PF) referenced to an electrode located 4 cm above the popliteal fossa (PFr), upper cervical cord (CS) referenced to CZ' and ipsilateral ear, and scalp (CZ') referenced to FpZ. In some patients median nerve recordings were also obtained using electrodes placed over Erb's point (EP) referenced to the contralateral EP, mid-cervical cord (C5) referenced to CZ, and contralateral cortex (C3', C4') referenced to contralateral EP and FpZ.

Waveforms were recorded approximately every 15 to 30 min, or continuously during the critical period of instrumentation or distraction, using filter settings of 30 to 3,000 Hz with a gain of 1 K. The analysis time was 120 msec and responses were identified after 350 to 500 repetitions were averaged using a digital averaging system (Nicolet CA-2000 or Cadwell Excel). Upgoing potentials were labeled "negative." Peak latency and amplitude for all waveforms were measured using the digital cursor on the averaging system.

2.1.2. Results

There have been several patterns of change in latency and amplitude described in the literature that have correlated with postoperative outcome. It has generally been thought that if the cortical and cervical waveforms return to baseline within 15 min of an acute change there is unlikely to be postoperative sequelae. If there has been a prolonged disappearance of the evoked potentials the patient has a significant chance of neurologic impairment postoperatively. Nuwer reports that if there is a greater than 50% attenuation of the amplitude of the responses, there is perhaps a 25% chance of postoperative impairment. Less than a 50% attenuation is probably not associated with a significant risk of a deficit, although the patient should be watched very closely in the postoperative period (Nuwer, 1986). Our experience in this particular population has not been much different when interpreting intraoperative changes in children. We have used the standards that Nuwer and the Mayo Clinic (Daube, 1989) have utilized, which are a consistent increase from baseline in the latency of the responses by at least 2.0 msec, and a decrease from baseline in the amplitude of at least 50% at the neck, and scalp if it is reliable.

The outcome of our patients was reviewed, and of the orthopedic procedures monitored intraoperatively; 18 patients had changes in the cervical response that occurred gradually over a 30- to 60-min period of time (Table 21–4). The changes occurred prior to instrumentation and consisted of an increase in latency up to 2.0 msec, or a decrease in amplitude between 30% and 50% from baseline, both of which are less than the suggested parameters for significant changes (Nuwer and Dawson, 1984). Some of these changes were thought to be due to increasing hypotension, hemodilution, or hypothermia. When these factors were corrected by the anesthesiologist, the latencies and amplitudes of the waveforms returned to their baseline values.

In another nine patients, significant changes in the cervical and cortical responses (latency increase of greater than 2 msec, amplitude decrease of greater than 50%) were seen acutely during instrumentation. The surgeon was alerted and measures were taken to identify the cause and at what level it affected. Further instrumentation was halted and distrac-

TABLE 21–4. *Outcome of the patients monitored intraoperatively at Children's Hospital between 1989 and 1991*

Change in SEP	Number of patients	Outcome
Gradual	18 (5.5%)	18—No neurologic sequelae
Acute	9 (2.8%)	8—No neurologic sequelae
		1—Postop paraplegia due to cord tumor (0.2%)
No change	296 (90.8%)	293—No neurologic sequelae
	3 (0.9%)	1—Unilateral footdrop due to L5 injury. Resolved in 3 months.
		1—Urinary retention. Resolved in a week.
		1—Bilateral L4,5 weakness due to root compression from loose lamina. Resolved with correction at reoperation.

tion loosened with a return of the waveforms to baseline within 15 to 20 min. There were no changes in blood pressure, temperature, or anesthetic regimen during the time surrounding the SEP changes in all these patients. The patients were carefully monitored throughout the remainder of the operation. A wake-up test was possible in five of these patients and was satisfactory. The remaining four patients were either mentally retarded or were unable to cooperate with the wake-up test for other reasons. Postoperatively, no new neurologic sequelae were seen.

This group of nine patients illustrates one of the major differences in children with scoliosis, the associated pathologic conditions and neurologic abnormalities which are not commonly seen in adults with scoliosis. All of our monitored patients, with the exception of one, who had either a significant change during the testing, or had postoperative neurologic sequela without SEP changes were in a high-risk group due to pre-existing neurologic abnormalities or surgical procedures. Of the nine patients who had significant changes, six patients had congenital scoliosis, another had a neuroenteric cyst, and another had a myelomeningocele. Two patients had severe spondylolisthesis requiring osteotomy and correction. One additional patient had a previously resected diastomatomyelia. In addition, two of these patients were severely retarded, and one had a spastic quadriparesis. Only one patient had idiopathic scoliosis, and when significant changes were noted during the monitoring, correction was halted, with no neurologic sequelae postoperatively.

Three patients developed new neurologic deficits within 48 hours of surgery, without a change in the surgical SEP monitoring, which constitutes the group of false negatives. The first was a patient thought to have an L5 root injury which occurred intraoperatively as a result of traction of the root. As has been reported by Harper et al., (1988), lumbar radiculopathies may occur more commonly following scoliosis surgery than has been reported, and SEPs of the lower extremity are an insensitive method for detection of a radiculopathy. A second patient developed urinary retention which resolved spontaneously in a week. This may have been due to mild intraoperative trauma to several sacral nerve roots or the plexus, narcotics, or overdistention of the bladder postoperatively. The last patient was found to have suffered direct trauma to several nerve roots due to compression by a displaced lamina occurring in the immediate postoperative period after monitoring was discontinued. The problem was corrected at reoperation. Each of these patients illustrates some of the limitations of the test and the adaptations one can make to better monitor neurophysiologic function.

2.1.3. Factors to Consider When Interpreting Results of SEPs

As one can see, when interpreting significant changes intraoperatively, many factors need to be considered (Fig. 21–1). Technical problems such as stimulator failure, electrode problems, and computer failures need to be sought. The operating suite is also hostile to EP recording, and interference from other apparatus such as body warmers and electrocautery may distort the waveforms. In addition, the patient's underlying pathologic condition may contribute to absent responses. Physiologic changes also need to be considered, such as hypotension, hypothermia, and hemodilution. When these factors are ruled out or corrected, which should take no more than 5 to 10 min, and if the significant changes persist, the surgeon should be notified.

A more specific or sensitive testing modality to detect a root injury is dermatomal SEP monitoring, which has been used with variable results in adults but has been unreliable. The amplitude of the waveforms is very small as compared to the mixed nerve SEPs, and repro-

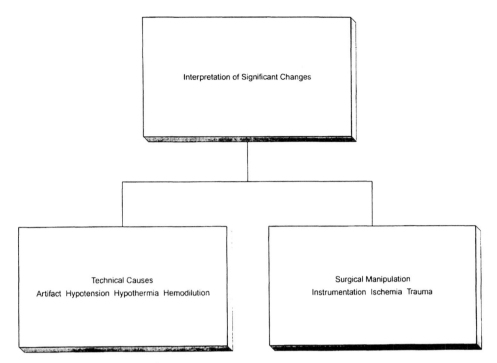

FIG. 21–1. Approach to interpretation of significant changes in intraoperative EPs.

ducibility of dermatomal responses are difficult to obtain. This technique has not been studied in children.

Another technique is electromyographic (EMG) monitoring of muscles innervated by particular lumbosacral, cervical, thoracic, and cranial nerves. Placement of wire electrodes into the specific muscles of interest allows one to monitor spontaneous muscle activity continuously. With injury to the nerve, neurotonic discharges or "injury potentials" can be heard and seen.

Electromyographic monitoring is also used in selective dorsal rhizotomy for spasticity. Using 50-Hz stimulation of dorsal rootlets, one looks for "abnormal" responses such as sustained activity or afterdischarges, lower stimulus thresholds, or spread of responses to distant muscles. Standard EMG recording settings are used in the operating room: gain of 200 to 500 μV, low-flow frequency 30 Hz, high-flow frequency 16 KHz, sweep 10 msec/cm.

A new technique has evolved over the last several years that we hope will supplement SEP monitoring. This technique involves evoking motor responses by stimulating the motor cortex or spinal cord, allowing one to monitor the anterior spinal cord. Motor evoked potentials (MEPs) can be elicited with electrical stimulation, and more recently by transcranial magnetic stimulation (Levy, 1987; Adams et al., 1993). In adults, it has been difficult to elicit MEPs consistently by magnetic stimulation because of the marked attenuation by anesthetics and neuromuscular blockade. The magnetic stimulator design also has been suboptimal. With cooperation from anesthesiologists, a regimen of anesthetics that enhance cortical excitability, and lightening of the anesthetic and neuromuscular blockade around the time of stimulation, has been more successful in evoking MEPs. This has not been studied in children at present.

2.1.4. Special Considerations in Children

In addition to the harsh recording environment of the operating room and the effects of hypothermia and hypotension, there are a number of technical and patient-related problems that we have encountered over the last few years that were specific to the pediatric age group.

Of particular concern is the small body size of the very young patient, making electrode application and stimulation difficult. With careful attention to technical detail and measurement we have had no difficulty stimulating and recording responses. To avoid stimulus artifact, we have found careful positioning of the stimulator and extremities, or use of a smaller stimulating electrode, to work well. In a number of other instances we have been unable to record responses because of the patient's underlying disease, but in a small number of these cases we have been able to use invasive electrodes to record epidurally.

Another problem is absence of all responses because of the patient's underlying disease, as stated earlier (Table 21–5). Out of all patients monitored, we were unable to obtain responses using surface recording electrodes in 18 patients because of their underlying pathologic process. We had difficulty in recording all potentials, including the popliteal fossa, from some patients with myelodysplasia and myelomenigocele or severe spastic quadriparesis with atrophy of the lower extremities. In several of these patients using epidural electrodes placed above and below the operative site by the surgeon allowed responses to be recorded. Other pathologies associated with difficulty in obtaining responses were spinal cord trauma, spinal cord tumors, myelopathy, and peripheral neuropathies.

Probably the greatest problem encountered in children is the sensitivity of their cortical response to volatile anesthetics relative to adults. Gugino and Chabot (1990) reviewed the effects of anesthetic agents on the cortical response of the SEP in adults. Almost all of the conventional inhalation agents can significantly prolong the latency and decrease the amplitude of the cortical response, with narcotics to a lesser extent also altering these responses. The usual time when one sees the most variability of the cortical potential is during induction of anesthesia or with large boluses of anesthetics, as reported by the Mayo Clinic investigators (Daube, 1989). This group looked at a group of 140 adults undergoing thoracolumbar spine surgery. During induction a mean amplitude reduction by 33% was not uncommon, and in 5% of their patients the scalp response was lost completely during induction. Through the course of the surgical procedure there was a gradual reduction (mean reduction 17%) in the amplitude and an increase in the latency (4% to 6%) of the scalp potentials. An additional 5% of their subjects lost scalp responses with continued anesthesia.

TABLE 21–5. *Underlying diseases in patients unable to be monitored intraoperatively*

Pathologic process	Number of cases
Myelodysplasia and myelomenigocele	7
Spastic quadraparesis with lower-extremity atrophy	4
Cervicothoracic spinal cord trauma	2
Severe scoliosis with myelopathy	2
Friedreich's ataxia	1
Peripheral neuropathy	1
Spinal cord tumor	1
Total	18

These effects are more profound and more common in children. In our monitored patients, 46% had unreliable cortical responses as defined by a decrease in amplitude of over 50%, an increase in latency of more than 2msec, or absence of the cortical response, with a stable cervical potential. This variability was most evident in children younger than 15 years of age and was dependent upon the anesthetic regimen used. The higher sensitivity and increased variability in young children may be related to maturational changes that take place in the somatosensory system in the first decade of life. These changes are thought to be a combination of asynchronous myelination and synaptogenesis (Gilmore et al., 1985). This inherent instability of the cortical response due to immaturity in this age group seems to be greatly increased by anesthetic agents. With the use of a single inhalation agent, with or without a narcotic, the cortical response becomes more stable and thus reliable. Isoflurane in combination with nitrous oxide most consistently abolished or reduced the cortical potentials (Fig. 21–2). With agents such as diprivan or etomidate, the latency of the cortical response remains unchanged or is only slightly prolonged, with the amplitude actually increasing. Another agent that has caused some variability in the cortical response when delivered in a bolus is lidocaine, the effect of which is short lived but must be recognized (Chaves-Vischer et al., 1994). We have found that the combination of less than 60% nitrous oxide or isoflurane (less than 0.5%) in combination with fentanyl during induction and low-dose nitrous oxide (less than 50% to 60%) or isoflurane (less than 0.6%) throughout the rest of the procedure allows for the best SEP recordings.

Because cortical responses can be so variable in children, it is imperative to add additional recording sites. In addition to recording from the popliteal fossa and scalp, additional sites to include are the posterior cervical spine and anterior neck. Unlike the cortical potential, the cervical and neck responses are more resistant to the effects of anesthesia, allowing one to monitor spinal cord integrity above the surgical level despite the absence of a scalp response (Johnson et al., 1983, Grundy, 1992). When the posterior neck recording electrode

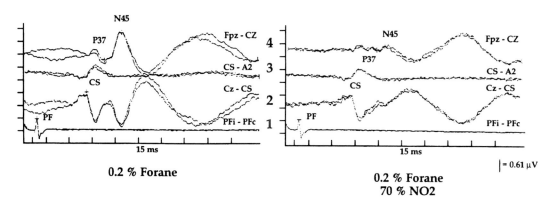

FIG. 21–2. Change in the cortical potential due to inhalation agents. Four-channel right posterior tibial nerve SEP from one patient. Recording on *left* made during the use of a small concentration of a single inhalation agent (isoflurane 0.2%). Recording on *right* made during the use of a combination of agents (isoflurane and nitrous oxide) with attenuation of the cortical potential in channel 4 and shows the cervical and popliteal fossa responses remaining stable. (Channel 1, PF–PFr = ipsilateral popliteal fossa to reference electrode. Channels 2 and 3, CZ′–CS and CS–A2, CS = cervical spine, A2 = right ear, recorded at the level of the cervical spine. Channel 4, FpZ–CZ′, is recorded from midline scalp. (From Helmers and Hall, 1994, with permission.)

lies in the operative field, one can record from the anterior neck using a surface electrode, referring to CZ' or FpZ (Helmers et al., 1994).

3. POSTERIOR FOSSA MONITORING

3.1. Intraoperative Brain Stem Auditory Evoked Potential Monitoring

With posterior fossa surgery, although not as commonly done in the pediatric patient, one can utilize several techniques to monitor brain stem function and certain cranial nerves (Raudzens and Shetter, 1982; Harper and Nelson, 1992).

Since the brain stem auditory evoked potentials (BAEPs) examine the brain stem auditory structures from the peripheral eighth nerve to the midbrain, it is useful in monitoring posterior fossa surgeries in patients at risk for loss of hearing or damage to the structures in the ventrolateral brain stem. As with routine laboratory EPs the proposed anatomic correlates of the waveform generators are:

Wave I   distal acoustic nerve
Wave II   proximal acoustic nerve or cochlear nucleus
Wave III   superior olivary nucleus (lower pons)
Wave IV   lateral lemniscus
Wave V   inferior colliculus (upper pons/lower midbrain)

Cortical and subcortical function are not generally thought to be assessed using the short-latency BAEPs.

Brain stem auditory EPs can be used in many operative procedures, including excision of acoustic neuromas, Arnold–Chiari malformations, posterior fossa meningiomas, posterior fossa microvascular decompressions, arteriovenous malformation/aneurysm of the posterior circulation, and masses of the fourth ventricle.

Techniques for stimulating and recording BAEPS intraoperatively are similar to routine laboratory tests with regard to the click features and recording parameters. The delivery of the click may be by several types of transducers, earphones and ear inserts are most commonly used, with the inserts the most stable. Additional recording techniques include direct nerve recordings with cotton wick electrodes placed on the acoustic nerve by the surgeon.

As with SEP monitoring there are several factors which can effect the BAEPs. With hypothermia (below 35°C), the latencies of the waveforms can become delayed, with wave V being the most sensitive of the responses. Wave V usually disappears below approximately 28°C.

The most important patient factor is age. As the child grows older, one sees shorter-latency, better-formed waves. This is most apparent below the age of 3 to 5 years. Wave I is the first to reach adult latency values, by about term. Wave III matures to adult values by about 12 to 18 months of age, and wave V by about 3 to 5 years.

Lastly, the medication effect on BAEPs is important. Brain stem auditory EPs are fairly resistant to barbiturates, benzodiazepines, narcotics, and nitrous oxide. The other inhalation agents (isoflurane, halothane, enflurane) have a small effect on the responses, causing a very mild delay in latency and a decrease in amplitude. As with temperature, wave V is the most sensitive to this effect.

Realizing the changes that can take place because of the above-mentioned factors, there are three types of changes that have been associated with surgical monitoring. The first is a gradual and persistent prolongation of the waveforms by 1 msec or more. The latencies may or may not return to baseline. Postoperatively, there is no clinically apparent deficit in hearing, although audiologic testing may show a mild abnormality.

The second type of change that may be observed is a sudden loss of all waveforms without return of the responses. This occurs ipsilaterally to the side of the surgery. This change is associated with postoperative hearing impairment ipsilateral to the side with changes in the BAEPs.

Lastly, one might see changes contralateral to the side of surgery intraoperatively. This usually is associated with other signs of brain stem disturbances and is associated with a poor outcome with regard to not only preservation of hearing but also surviving the surgery. Some patients with this type of change during surgery, without return of the BAEPs to baseline values, have died or survived the surgery with severe neurologic impairment.

3.2. SEP Monitoring

Monitoring of the posterior fossa can also be supplemented by the use of SEPs. Either upper- or lower-extremity SEPs can be used based upon the structures at risk for injury. The procedures, limitations, and interpretations are the same as with spinal cord monitoring.

3.3. EMG Monitoring

Recording for cranial nerve function can also be monitored, in addition to SEPs. Wire electrodes can be inserted into muscles innervated by cranial nerves III (inferior rectus), IV (superior oblique), V (masseter), VI (lateral rectus), VII (obicularis oris), IX (stylopharyngeal), X (cricothyroid, vocalis), XI (trapezius), and XII (tongue). Injury to particular nerves can be detected by neurotonic or injury potentials. Monitoring the EMG also allows one to identify nerves of interest by stimulating the nerve and monitoring the responses. Standard EMG recording settings are used in the operating room: gain of 200 to 500 μV, low-flow frequency 30 Hz, high-flow frequency 16 KHz, sweep of 10 msec/cm.

4. CORTICAL MONITORING

A number of surgical procedures involving the motor and sensory cortex may benefit from application of intraoperative neurophysiologic monitoring.

4.1. Intraoperative SEP Monitoring

For cortical localization of motor and somatosensory cortex in tumor resections or epileptic focus ablation, SEP monitoring can help localize the sensorimotor cortex. By recording from subdural strips or a grid placed over the area of interest recordings can be made one of two ways: either using a bipolar montage looking for a phase reversal or using a referential montage looking for the maximal response as compared to scalp recordings (Fig. 21–3) can help the surgeon determine to what extent the resection can be done, preserving eloquent cortex (Luders et al., 1986).

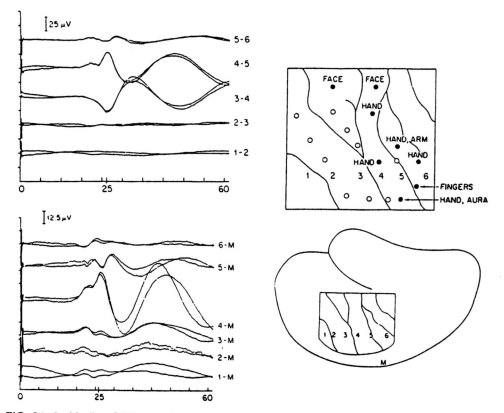

FIG. 21–3. Median SEP recorded directly from the cortex with a strip of electrodes. Comparison of two methods of recording the response. The (*top left*) recording uses a bipolar montage, showing a prominent phase reversal at 25 msec corresponding to the region under contact 4 of the strip. The (*bottom left*) recording uses a referential montage, showing a prominent positive peak at 25 msec which corresponds to contact 4. (From Nuwer, 1986, with permission.)

4.2. Intraoperative Visual Evoked Potential Monitoring

The last SEP that has been used intraoperatively is the visual evoked potential (VEP), which monitors the anterior or prechiasmal visual system. The types of procedures VEPs have been used for generally center around the sellar/suprasellar region. This would include pituitary tumors, suprasellar masses, aneurysms, optic nerve decompression, and craniopharyngiomas.

Visual testing during operations is technically very difficult to do for a number of reasons, stimulation being the first problem. Since a patient is not able to fixate upon a pattern, a flash or strobe stimulation must be used. To deliver the stimulus, light-emitting diode glasses are easiest to use since they remain out of the operative field and are not disruptive to operating personnel.

Recording has been a problem also. Because the VEP response is thought to be cortically generated, there is quite a bit of variability of the waveform intraoperatively. This is due to many factors. During hypothermia and hypotension there is a progressive fall in the amplitude and prolongation of the latency. As with the other sensory modalities, the latency is normally longer in very young patients. Another patient factor that affects the recordings is the visual acuity or impairment, both of which can affect the amplitude and latency of the VEP. Many drugs can affect the waveform, such as barbiturates and halothane, which at low doses may increase the amplitude but abolish the response at high doses. Nitrous oxide causes a dose-dependent attenuation of the response.

As one can see from the factors discussed and the random variability over time of the waveform itself, VEPs tend to have a high false positive and false negative rate. In addition, the full-field strobe is a nonspecific stimulus which can only detect defects anterior to the chiasm. Therefore, VEPs are much more difficult to interpret intraoperatively. Due to all of the technical and patient-related problems with VEPs intraoperatively, they are generally not used for monitoring intraoperatively.

REFERENCES

Adams DC, Emerson RG, Heyer EJ, McCormick PC, Carmel PW, Stein BM, Farcy JP, Gallo EJ (1993): Monitoring of intraoperative motor-evoked potentials under conditions of controlled neuromuscular blockade. *Anesth Analg* 77:913–918.

American Electroencephalographic Society (1994): Guidelines for intraoperative monitoring of sensory evoked potentials. *J Clin Neurophysiol* 11(1):77–87.

Chatrian G-E, Berger MS, Wirch AL (1988): Discrepancy between intraoperative SSEP's and postoperative function. *J Neurosurg* 69:450–454.

Chaves-Vischer V, Brustowicz R, Helmers S (1996): Effect of intravenous lidocaine on intraoperative somatosensory evoked potentials during scoliosis surgery: a report of two cases. *Anesth Anal.* In press.

Daube JR (1989): Spine surgery. In: *Mayo Clinic Course on Monitoring Neural Function During Surgery,* November 4–5, 1989.

Engler GL, Spielholz NI, Bernhard WN, Danziger F, Merkin H, Wolff T (1978): Somatosensory evoked potentials during Harrington instrumentation for scoliosis. *J Bone Joint Surg* 60 A(4):528–532.

Gilmore RL, Bass NH, Wright EA, Greathouse D, Stanback K, Norvell E (1985): Developmental assessment of spinal cord and cortical evoked potentials after tibial nerve stimulation: effects of age and stature on normative data during childhood. *Electroencephalogr Clin Neurophysiol* 62:241–251.

Grundy BL (1992): Intraoperative monitoring by evoked potential techniques. In: *Electrodiagnosis in Clinical Neurology,* third ed, edited by ML Aminoff, pp 649–682 Churchill Livingstone, New York.

Gugino V (1990): Chabot RJ. Somatosensory evoked potentials. *Int Anesth Clin* 28(3):154–164.

Hall JE, Levine CR, Sudhir KG (1978): Intraoperative awakening to monitor spinal cord function during Harrington instrumentation and spine fusion. *J Bone Joint Surg* 60A(4):533–536.

Harper CM, Daube JR, Litchy WJ, Klassen RA (1988): Lumbar radiculopathy after spinal fusion for scoliosis. *Muscle Nerve* 11:386–91.

Harper CM, Nelson KR (1992): Intraoperative electrophysiological monitoring in children. *J Clin Neurophysiol* 9(3):3423–56.

Helmers SL, Hall JE (1994): Intraoperative somatosensory evoked potential monitoring in pediatrics. *J Pediatr Orthop* 14:592–598.

Helmers SL, Kull LL (1994): Intraoperative evoked potential monitoring in pediatrics. *Am J EEG Tech* 34:75–89.

Helmers SL, Flanigin D, Carmant L (1994): Intraoperative somatosensory evoked potential monitoring using anterior neck derivations to record the cervical potential in children. *Spine* 20(7):782–786.

Johnson RM, McPherson RW, Szymanski J (1983): The effects of stimulus intensity on somatosensory evoked potentials during intraoperative monitoring. *Anesthesiology* 59(3):A365.

Lesser RP, Raudzens P, Luders H, Nuwer MR, Goldie WD, Morris HH, Dinner DS, Klem G, Hahn JF, Shetter AG, Ginsburg HH, Gurd AR (1986): Postoperative neurological deficits may occur despite unchanged intraoperative somatosensory evoked potentials. *Ann Neurol* 19:22–25.

Levy WL (1987): Clinical experience with motor and cerebellar evoked potential monitoring. *Neurosurgery* 20(1):169–182.

Loder RT, Thomson GJ, LaMont RL (1991): Spinal cord monitoring in patients with nonidiopathic spinal deformities using somatosensory evoked potentials. *Spine* 16(12):1359–1364.

Lubicky JP, Spadaro JA, Yuan HA, Fredrickson BE, Henderson N (1989): Variability of somatosensory cortical evoked potential monitoring during spinal surgery. *Spine* 14(8):790–798.

Luders H, Dinner DS, Lesser RP, Morris HH (1986): Evoked potentials in cortical localization. *J Clin Neurophysiol* 3(1):75–84.

Lueders H, Gurd A, Hahn J, Andrish J, Weiker G, Klem G (1982): A new technique for intraoperative monitoring of spinal cord function. Multichannel recording of spinal cord and subcortical evoked potentials. *Spine* 7(2):110–115.

MacEwen GD, Bunnell WP, Sriram K (1975): Acute neurological complications in the treatment of scoliosis. *J Bone Joint Surg* 57A(3):404–408.

Nuwer MR, Dawson E (1984): Intraoperative evoked potential monitoring of the spinal cord: enhanced stability of cortical recordings. *Electroencephalogr Clin Neurophysiol* 59:318–327.

Nuwer M (ed). (1986): Spinal cord monitoring. In: *Evoked Potential Monitoring in the Operating Room.* Raven Press, New York, p 126.

Raudzens PA, Shetter AG (1982): Intraoperative monitoring of brain-stem auditory evoked potentials. *J Neurosurg* 57:341–348.

Wilber RG, Thompson GH, Shaffer JW, Brown RH, Nash CL (1984): Postoperative neurological deficits in segmental spinal instrumentation. *J Bone Joint Surg* 66A(8):1178–1187.

Vauzelle C, Stagnara P, Jouvinroux P (1973): Functional monitoring of spinal cord activity during spinal surgery. *Clin Orthop Rel Res* 93:173–178.

Evoked Potentials in Clinical Medicine,
3d ed., edited by Keith H. Chiappa.
Lippincott–Raven Publishers, Philadelphia © 1997.

22

Intraoperative Monitoring with Motor and Sensory Evoked Potentials

°David J. Burke and †Richard G. Hicks

Prince of Wales Medical Research Institute and Departments of °Clinical Neurophysiology and †Neurology, The Prince Henry and Prince of Wales Hospitals, Randwick, NSW, Sydney 2031, Australia

1. INTRODUCTION

Intraoperative monitoring during scoliosis surgery has two main goals: to avoid inadvertent damage to neural structures, and to guide the surgeon on the extent of safe curve correction. The incidence of intraoperative or perioperative neurologic complications is low, but may reach 1.6% with mechanical instrumentation, particularly the Cotrel–Dubousset type (Dawson et al., 1991). Any risk is unacceptable when the majority of patients undergoing scoliosis surgery are neurologically normal and the operation is generally undertaken as much for "cosmetic" reasons as medical imperatives.

The "wake-up" test cannot adequately fulfill the requirements of a satisfactory monitoring procedure, in part because it can establish only that significant damage has already occurred, not that it is occurring. The wake-up test is performed only after the desired curve correction has been achieved and this may be some time after the onset of spinal cord dysfunction. Performing the test interrupts surgery while anesthesia is lightened and muscle relaxation reversed. The test depends on the ability of an unparalyzed waking patient to respond by moving the lower limbs to command, and this may be impossible when there is a pre-existing motor deficit regardless of whether there was additional intraoperative damage. Finally, the expected response is assessed subjectively, without documentation that can be reviewed subsequently.

These deficiencies have led to the use of somatosensory evoked potentials (SEPs) as an objective guide to the integrity of the spinal cord, but there is no unanimity on how best to measure the evoked activity. It is the authors' view that direct recordings of spinal cord volleys provide the most appropriate test of spinal cord integrity, *provided that* the volleys have a sufficiently favorable signal-to-noise ratio such that reproducible duplicate averages can be obtained relatively rapidly. Accordingly, this department has routinely used epidural electrodes, as advocated by Jones et al. (1982, 1983), for recording somatosensory volleys and resorts to less direct or more remote recordings (e.g., cortical, extraspinal) only when epidural recordings are not feasible, as in lesions in the high- or midcervical regions. Discussion of relative merits of cortical and epidural recordings of somatosensory volleys is beyond the scope of the present chapter, but some issues are summarized in Table 22–1.

The use of epidural electrodes allows the recording of corticospinal volleys set up by transcranial stimulation of the motor cortex, as was first done by Boyd et al. (1986). In addition, epidural recordings allow ascending somatosensory and descending corticospinal volleys to be recorded simultaneously using the same electrodes, as will be discussed below. Not only the integrity of a large volume of the spinal cord can be monitored but, in particular, the integrity of those pathways the loss of which would be most devastating for a patient. There is some evidence that corticospinal pathways are more vulnerable to experimental spinal cord injury (e.g., Machida et al., 1988; Owen et al., 1988; Fehlings et al., 1989). In a report by Lesser et al. (1986), six patients undergoing surgery developed neurologic deficits not detected during the procedure, even though SEPs were monitored using cerebral and extraspinal (but not epidural) recordings. The deficit was purely motor in three patients, motor and sensory in three. These findings support the view that monitoring corticospinal function may be better than monitoring only somatosensory function. In the present authors' view, it is not yet proven that human corticospinal pathways are more vulnerable to the inadvertent trauma that can occur with scoliosis surgery and, with neurosurgical operations on the brain or spinal cord, vulnerability will be determined by the proximity of pathways to the lesion. Nevertheless, paralysis is usually a functionally more devastating deficit than sensory loss and, as the cases of Lesser et al. (1986) illustrate, this may not be detected if only somatosensory function is monitored. These considerations are sufficient to prompt a search for the best technique for monitoring corticospinal function.

This chapter will discuss the preferred technique for spinal cord monitoring in the authors' unit, realizing that, with any patient, clinical conditions may dictate a departure from the preferred methodology. The described technique involves the simultaneous recording of corticospinal and somatosensory activity simultaneously at two spinal levels, and has now been used successfully in approximately 250 patients undergoing, mainly, surgery for scoliosis.

TABLE 22–1. *Somatosensory evoked potentials at cortical and spinal (epidural) levels*

The cortical potential involves transmission across at least three synapses and is sensitive to anesthesia and stimulus repetition rate.

The traveling wave recorded at spinal level contains direct and postsynaptic components but the latter involve a very secure synapse (Clarke's column and posterior spinocerebellar tract) or are of longer latency. Accordingly the volley is resistant to anesthesia, and stimulus rates of 10 to 20 Hz are optimal.

The cortical potential has a nonlinear relationship to the size of the afferent volley, saturating with moderate-high afferent inputs. As a result only a major decrease in input will produce a detectable loss of amplitude of the cerebral potential.

The traveling wave of the spinal potential is proportional to the afferent volley.

Potentials recorded at both cerebral and spinal levels require averaging, but it is 5 to 10 times quicker to acquire the requisite number of sweeps for duplicate averages with spinal recordings.

2. MONITORING TECHNIQUE

The patients lie prone (for posterior approaches to the spine), anesthetized with nitrous oxide and oxygen (70%:30%), and fentanyl, supplemented by volatile anesthetics, usually isoflurane or enflurane, with full muscle relaxation using pancuronium. Intra-arterial blood pressure, core temperature, arterial oxygen saturation, the adequacy of neuromuscular blockade, and the end-tidal concentration of volatile anesthetic are monitored throughout the operation.

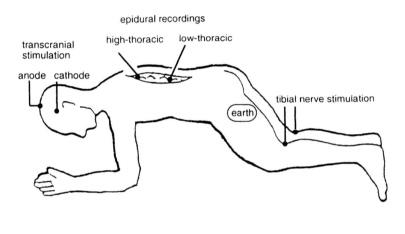

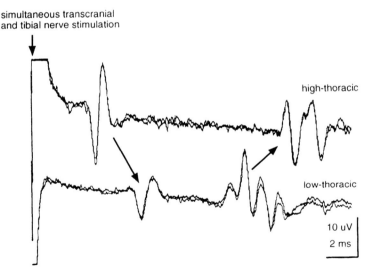

FIG. 22–1. Figurine illustrating the monitoring technique (*above*), with original data (*below*). Because bipolar electrodes were used, the negative deflections of descending motor and ascending sensory volleys are in opposite directions (downward for the motor volley and upward for the sensory volley—note that the traces in Figs. 22–3 to 22–5 have been inverted). The motor volley consists of a single D wave at both recording sites (24 μV at the rostral site and 10 μV at the caudal site) occurring at relatively short latencies (4 msec and 6.9 msec to initial negative peak, respectively). It therefore preceded and was clearly separate from the sensory potential which had latencies of 12 msec and 16.2 msec at the lower and higher recording sites, respectively. (Duplicate averages of 10 responses; female aged 14; isoflurane 2%; transcranial stimulus 525 V.) (From Burke et al., 1992, with permission.)

The motor cortex and the tibial nerves in the popliteal fossa are stimulated simultaneously once every 3 sec, so initiating descending and ascending volleys coincident with the onset of the oscilloscope sweep (Fig. 22–1). These volleys are recorded by bipolar cardiac pacing electrodes inserted by the surgeon into the epidural space at two levels, high-thoracic and low-thoracic, and advanced cephalad so that they record activity adjacent to the cervical and lumbar outflows. The leads are then secured by sutures.

Dependent on the height of the patient, the corticospinal volley reaches the high-thoracic electrode at a latency of 3 to 4 msec and the low-thoracic electrode after a further 3 to 4 msec. The somatosensory volley produces potentials at the low-thoracic electrode at a latency of 13 to 14 msec and the traveling wave reaches the high-thoracic electrode some 3 to 4 msec later. Accordingly, an oscilloscope display of four sweeps (a stored average as a template and an on-going average, from each of the two levels) with a sweep duration of 30 msec is sufficient to display an early (corticospinal) volley that increases in latency as it propagates down the cord and a later (somatosensory) volley that increases in latency as it propagates up the cord.

The evoked volleys are recorded at the two spinal levels using an input gain of 20 µV/division, sweep duration of 30 msec, and band-pass of 500 Hz to 5 or 10 kHz. Recent experience suggests that no more than 10 sweeps need be averaged to define the corticospinal volley clearly (Burke et al., 1995; see later) but, in practice, 25 sweeps are usually averaged so that the somatosensory volley can be clearly defined. The choice of filters and the reproducibility of the corticospinal volley are discussed in later sections.

3. ADDITIONAL TECHNICAL CONSIDERATIONS

Table 22–2 summarizes some of the important variables in instituting this monitoring procedure. Bipolar epidural leads are more convenient than a monopolar lead with a nearby reference because with the latter arrangement there are two leads in the surgical field and this increases the chance of one being dislodged. Cardiac pacing leads are satisfactory because they are not so flexible that insertion is difficult. In theory, the greater the interelectrode distance the better to prevent phase-cancellation of components with long wavelength. However, in practice even an interelectrode distance of 1 cm gives satisfactory recordings.

Both electrodes, particularly the low-thoracic, should be advanced in the epidural space before being secured by sutures. It has not been possible in anesthetized patients to record postsynaptic activity from the cauda equina when the low-thoracic electrode is not advanced sufficiently rostrally, though incoming sensory volleys can still be recorded (Hicks et al., 1991).

TABLE 22–2. *Technical considerations*

Recording electrodes: bipolar cardiac pacing electrodes, with recording surfaces 2 to 3 cm apart or more
Site of recording electrodes: to record from cervical and lumbar outflows, *not* over cauda equina
Stimulating electrode montage: anode at vertex; cathode laterally over one hand area
Band-pass: high-pass filter 500 Hz; low-pass filter 5–10 kHz
Stimulus repetition rate: once every 3 sec
Stimulus intensity: sufficient to produce a large simple D wave, usually 250 to 450 V (time constant 100 µsec)
Number of sweeps averaged: 10 to 25
Anesthesia and muscle relaxation: not critical

The recording bandwidth is critical for success with this technique (Fig. 22–2). Stimulus artifact and mechanical artifacts associated with the surgery are effectively controlled if the high-pass filter is 500 Hz rather than 1 Hz or 20 Hz, as other authors have used. The restricted filter setting does distort the EP waveforms, but it stabilizes the recording sweeps such that continuous recordings can usually be obtained throughout surgery on a horizontal baseline without artifact rejection. The artifact rejection facility is then triggered only by the diathermy or occasional large mechanical artifacts. The low-pass filter is less critical: 5 kHz or 10 kHz is satisfactory.

The traces in the lower panel of Fig. 22–2 were recordable only when the input gain was reduced to 50 μV/division, and even then more than 50% sweeps were rejected. This panel illustrates the baseline instability that is associated with an open band-pass. By contrast, the averages in the upper panel were obtained without rejection of any sweeps. Comparison of the upper and middle panels reveals the amplitude attenuation associated with the 500-Hz high-pass filter: it affects particularly the standing wave produced by the somatosensory

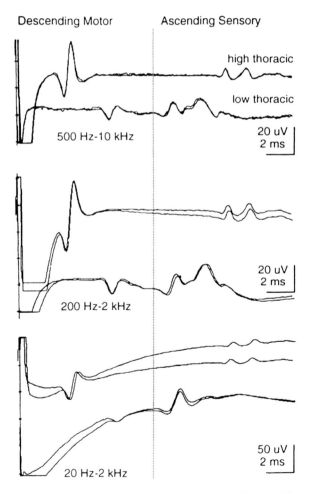

FIG. 22–2. The effects of different high-pass filters. Recordings as in Fig. 22–1. Note that, to obtain a recording, the input amplification had to be reduced when the 20-Hz high-pass filter was used. (Duplicate averages of 25 responses; female aged 19; transcranial stimulus intensity 600 V; isoflurane 2%.) (From Burke et al., 1992, with permission.)

volley at the low-thoracic electrode and has a lesser effect on the traveling waves (motor and sensory).

4. TRANSCRANIAL STIMULATION OF THE MOTOR CORTEX

With transcranial electrical stimulation, the "active" electrode is the anode (Rothwell et al., 1987), much as in animal experiments. For monitoring purposes, the motor cortex is stimulated using disposable spiral needle electrodes that are inserted into the scalp, with the anode at the vertex and the cathode 7 cm laterally over one upper-limb area. Different stimulating montages have been trialed but no other has proved superior. In particular, the montage of anode at the vertex and cathode 7 cm anterior does not allow access to motor cortex as effectively: the evoked volleys are smaller for the same absolute stimulus intensity and stimulus artifact is more prominent. The preferred montage probably activates the corticospinal projections from both leg areas at the stimulus intensities used, and for scoliosis surgery the side for the cathode is determined by convenience of access rather than deliberate choice. Clearly this would not be so for neurosurgical operations on lateralized pathology. There have been no postoperative problems with the subdermal stimulating electrodes.

In this unit, the stimulus is delivered by a Digitimer D180A stimulator, capable of delivering capacitively coupled stimuli of up to 1,500 V with a time constant of 50 μsec or 100 μsec. However, intense stimuli are undesirable because they commonly produce excessive stimulus artifact and because the D wave of the corticospinal volley becomes complex, with components initiated at a number of levels along the corticospinal tract, as deep as the pyramidal decussation (Burke et al., 1990; Rothwell et al., 1994). As discussed below, the trial-to-trial variability of the individual components of complex D waves is much greater than that of large simple D waves; the latter require stimuli of only 225 to 450 V (100 μsec time constant).

The capacitively coupled stimulus pulse delivered by the Digitimer D180 or D180A was originally introduced because it broke down skin resistance such that activation of the corticospinal system was then less painful. This factor is clearly not relevant in anesthetized patients. Whether a powerful conventional stimulator would generate the same amount of stimulus artifact for an equivalent corticospinal volley is not known. However, most stimulators associated with commercial electromyography (EMG) EP machines are not sufficiently powerful, at least for bipolar stimulation (which is more convenient than Rossini's technique using multiple cathodal plates with equal impedance, distributed around the head).

5. THE EVOKED CORTICOSPINAL VOLLEY

Threshold stimuli evoke a single descending volley (Fig. 22–3), which has a latency at the low-cervical region appropriate for direct stimulation of the corticospinal neuron or its axon close to the cell body. The evidence that the threshold D wave does not arise from a subcortical site is circumstantial but the view is supported, first, by the extreme sensitivity of the threshold D wave to changing levels of volatile anesthetics (Hicks et al., 1992a; see Fig. 22–6, lower panels), presumably due to anesthesia-induced changes in excitability of corticospinal neurons, and secondly by the fact that the threshold D wave to electrical stim-

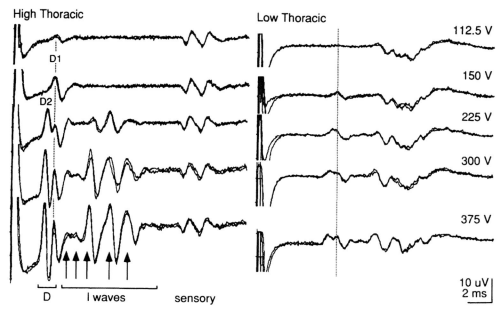

FIG. 22–3. The corticospinal volleys produced by increasingly strong transcranial electrical stimulation (after withdrawal of isoflurane). Note that traces in this figure and in Figs. 22–4 to 22–6 have been inverted compared with those in Figs. 22–1 and 22–2. With stimuli of 112.5 V and 150 V, the corticospinal volley consists of a simple D wave (D_1) with a latency to peak (indicated by the dotted vertical line) of 3.5 msec at the high-thoracic site and 6.5 msec at the low-thoracic site. At 225 V, the D wave is followed by I waves at both sites, and the D wave is becoming bifid. At 375 V, the high-threshold short-latency D_2 component occurs at 0.7 to 0.8 ms in advance of the initial low-threshold D_1 component. I waves (I_1, I_2, I_3, I_5, and I_6) are indicated by vertical arrows. At the low-thoracic site, the I waves are superimposed on the somatosensory volley. The somatosensory volley begins at 9.9 ms in the low-thoracic recording, and at 13.7 ms in the high-thoracic recording. (Duplicate averages of 25 responses; female, aged 11.) (From Hicks et al., 1992a, with permission.)

ulation has the same conduction time to the low-cervical region as the D wave produced by magnetic stimulation, which is also anesthesia-sensitive (Burke et al., 1993).

As stimulus intensity is increased there may be gradual shortening in latency of the D wave by 0.1 to 0.2 msec, presumably as more axons are activated, possibly more distally from the cell body. However, in addition, two short-latency high-threshold components (D_2, then D_3) appear, in advance of the lowest-threshold component (D_1). The D_2 component stabilizes 0.8 to 1.0 msec in advance of D_1 (Fig. 22–3), and D_3 a further 0.8 to 1.0 msec in advance of D_2 (Burke et al., 1990, 1995; Rothwell et al., 1994). With intense stimuli, the lowest-threshold component (D_1) disappears, as all axons are activated at subcortical sites, and at intensities of 750 to 1,500 V, the highest-threshold shortest-latency component (D_3) dominates the recording (Fig. 22–4). The D_3 component has the same conduction time to the low-cervical region as the volley produced by direct brainstem stimulation (Fig. 22–5), suggesting that transcranial electrical stimulation using conventional stimulating electrode placements can access corticospinal axons at the pyramidal decussation (Rothwell et al., 1994). That D_3 begins to appear with stimuli as low as 300 to

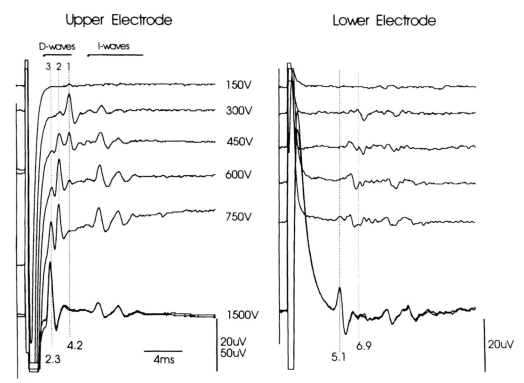

FIG. 22–4. Cortical stimulation using increasingly strong stimulus intensities. Epidural recordings from the low-cervical and low-thoracic levels (female, aged 14). Polarity as in Fig. 22–3. The stimulus artifact begins 1 msec after the start of the sweep. Two averages are superimposed for the 1,500-V stimulus. Note the gradual recruitment of earlier D-wave components as the stimulus intensity is increased, and the progressive increase in the size and number of I waves. In the recordings from the upper electrode, the 50 μV vertical calibration applies only to the responses at 1,500 V. The dotted lines indicate successive D-wave components and their respective peak latencies. In this and subsequent figures, each trace is the average of 10 responses. (From Rothwell et al., 1994, with permission.)

450 V indicates that even these stimuli may initiate activity in some corticospinal axons at the pyramidal decussation.

The site of origin of D_2 has not been established, but it is likely to be a site of preferential sensitivity, presumably associated with a bend in the corticospinal tract or some other tissue inhomogeneity. The cerebral peduncle seems a likely candidate.

Dependent on stimulus intensity and anesthetic level, several waves occur after the D wave (Figs. 22–3 and 22–4), and these have the characteristics of transsynaptically generated I waves. When they are identifiable at both recording sites, their latency after the D wave is the same at the two sites, indicating that their conduction velocity is the same as that of axons contributing to the D wave. These waves are very sensitive to the level of volatile anesthesia (Fig. 22–6), and this is so whether they are produced by electrical (Hicks et al., 1992a,b) or magnetic stimuli (Burke et al., 1993). With electrical stimuli, I waves require a higher stimulus intensity than the D wave, whether the anode is over the leg area at the vertex (Burke et al., 1990; Hicks et al., 1992a) or over the hand area (Burke et al., 1992).

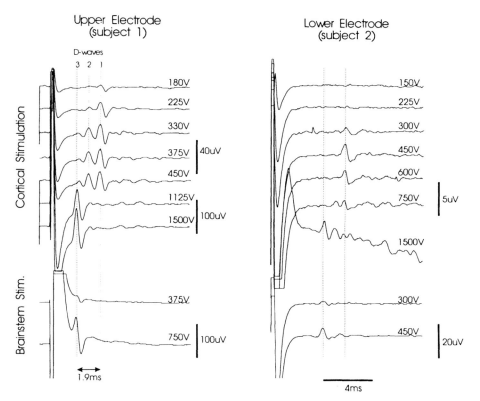

FIG. 22–5. Responses to cortical and brain stem stimulation. Averaged epidural recordings from the low-cervical and the low-thoracic levels in two subjects (subject 1: female, aged 14; subject 2: male, aged 12) in response to different stimulus intensities. Polarity as in Figs. 22–3 and 22–4. For subject 1, the stimulus was given 1 msec after the onset of the sweep; for subject 2, the stimulus occurred at the onset of the sweep. Gradually increasing intensities of cortical stimulation recruited three D-wave components (D_1, D_2, D_3) with a latency shift from D_1 to D_3 of 1.9 msec in subject 1. Brain stem stimulation evoked a volley which had the same latency as the D_3 component resulting from cortical stimulation. Note the absence of late activity with brainstem stimulation except for a small wave at 450 V in subject 2 (*bottom trace on right*). (From Rothwell et al., 1994, with permission.)

In addition, cathodal stimulation does not seem to favor the production of I waves more than anodal stimulation (Burke et al., 1992). However, magnetic stimulation does. In anesthetized subjects, following withdrawal of all volatile anesthetics, the threshold volley to magnetic stimulation using a 9-cm coil centered over the vertex may contain I waves in addition to a D wave (Burke et al., 1993), such that motor neuron discharge to such a volley would be dependent on temporal summation. D and I waves are generally of lower amplitude at the low-thoracic than the low-cervical site, generally by more than 50%, and some late (presumably I) waves may not be identifiable at the lower site. This is not surprising given that the lower electrode can detect only that part of the activity destined for the lumbar segments.

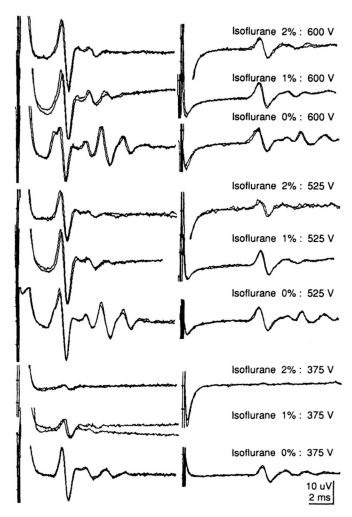

FIG. 22–6. Effects of isoflurane on corticofugal volleys evoked by vertex anodal stimulation (female, age 15). Left panels, high-thoracic recording; right panels, corresponding low-thoracic recordings. Polarity as in Figs. 22–3 to 22–5. I waves are more prominent at each stimulus intensity the lower the isoflurane concentration. Similar changes are seen with the D wave, particularly at 375 V. (From Hicks et al., 1992a, with permission.)

6. TRIAL-TO-TRIAL VARIABILITY OF THE CORTICOSPINAL VOLLEY

The variability of the different D- and I-wave components has been determined from sequences of 100 consecutive single trials, measuring consistent components of amplitude greater than 0.5 μV (Burke et al., 1995). All components have a relatively stable latency. Amplitude is highly reproducible for large simple D waves (Fig. 22–7) but not for the individual D_{1-3} components of complex D waves or for I waves (Fig. 22–8). For monitoring purposes a large simple D wave, such as in Fig. 22–1, should therefore be preferred to the more complex volleys produced by more intense stimuli (such as those in the lower traces of Fig. 22–3). Given a D wave of reasonable amplitude, I waves do not improve monitoring

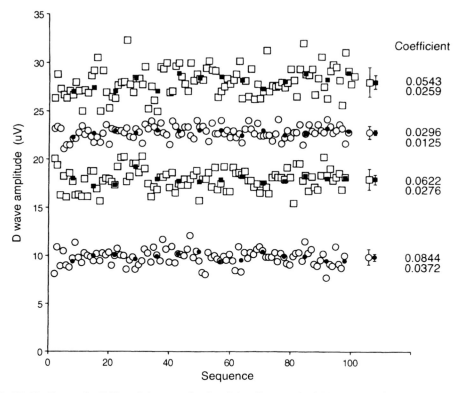

FIG. 22–7. Reproducibility of the amplitude of the D wave in 100 consecutive responses for four different subjects: from above, male aged 15, female aged 54, male aged 15, male aged 13. The filled symbols represent the average values for successive groups of 7 traces. The symbols to the right represent the mean values ±1 SD (open symbols, 100 single responses; filled symbols: 14 averages each of 7 responses). The coefficient of variation for each subject are for the 100 single trials (*upper values*) and for the 14 averages (*lower values*). (From Burke et al., 1995, with permission.)

capabilities: indeed, as is shown in Fig. 22–3, prolonged I-wave activity can overlap the somatosensory potential at the low-thoracic site, although this does not occur at the low-cervical site because of the greater latency difference. In practice I waves can be suppressed by lowering the stimulus intensity or raising the isoflurane level.

As indicated in Fig. 22–7, the coefficients of variation of the amplitude of successive D waves (i.e., standard deviation divided by mean amplitude) are low, 3% to 8%, indicating that a decrease in amplitude of 20% would be unlikely to occur by chance. If seven responses were averaged, the standard deviations would be 1% to 4% of mean amplitude, suggesting that a 10% decrease in amplitude would represent a significant change. Clearly, under the ideal conditions under which these responses were recorded, few trials need be averaged to detect significant changes in the D wave at the low-cervical region. However, the monitoring technique also relies on recording the D wave at the low-thoracic site and on recording the somatosensory volley at both sites. It is therefore usual practice to average 25 sweeps, and this has proved sufficient to define both volleys clearly at both levels, as indicated by Figs. 22–2 and 22–3.

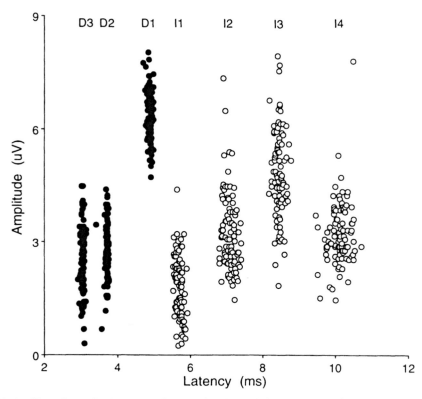

FIG. 22–8. Plot of amplitude versus latency for the individual waves of a complex volley with three D-wave components and four I waves for 100 consecutive single trials. Note the large amplitude variability for each component. (Male aged 14; isoflurane 0.2%.) (From Burke et al., 1995, with permission.)

7. EPIDURAL RECORDING OF CORTICOSPINAL VOLLEYS

Epidural recordings have three potential disadvantages. First, epidural leads can be inserted readily through the operative wound by the surgeon during posterior approaches to the spine, but anterior approaches require separate placement, not through the operative wound, perhaps performed by the anesthetist. In practice, this has proved less surgically acceptable, and in the authors' unit corticospinal function is usually monitored during anterior approaches by recording the evoked compound EMG potential rather than the evoked spinal cord volley (see later). Second, any recording lead that is within the operative field can be dislodged during the surgery. This happens frequently with the low-thoracic electrode in the technique described above, but the resultant change in the recorded waveforms can be identified readily as artifactual when two modalities (i.e., corticospinal and somatosensory) are being monitored at two levels. For example, preservation of the somatosensory volley at the rostral site indicates that deterioration at the caudal site must have been due to displacement of the caudal electrode. Third, there is a theoretical risk of spinal cord trauma from the insertion (and reinsertion) of recording electrodes into the epidural space. In practice, however, no such problems have occurred in the authors' unit; nor have they been reported by others.

TABLE 22–3. *Advantages of epidural recording of corticospinal volleys at two spinal levels*

Simple D waves do not require intense electrical stimuli and are highly reproducible from trial to trial, such that few sweeps need be averages.
The D wave is relatively impervious to the depth of anesthesia.
Full muscle relaxation can be used; indeed, it is desirable.
Somatosensory pathways can be monitored at the same time.
Monitoring should be possible in patients with lower motoneuron problems due, for example, to spina bifida.
If neither corticospinal or somatosensory volleys can be recorded, one set of epidural electrodes can be used to stimulate the cord, recording the evoked spinal cord volley using the other set.
Deficits have not resulted from the insertion and reinsertion of the epidural electrodes, that is, the recording system is safe.

The advantages of epidural recordings, and specifically epidural recordings at two spinal levels, are listed in Table 22–3. The difficulties in obtaining reproducible compound EMG potentials to transcranial stimulation of the motor cortex in an anesthetized patient are well recognized. Given the reproducibility of the epidural volleys (Burke et al., 1995; see above), the extreme variability of the evoked EMG potential presumably reflects difficulty in translating the corticospinal volley into motor neuron discharge. The small size of the resultant EMG potential suggests that only a few motor neurons of lowest threshold can be caused to discharge, and the variability suggests that the discharge involves different motor neurons of this low-threshold population each time. Clearly, anesthetic agents must be chosen with care and, of course, muscle relaxation must be titrated judiciously. In as yet unpublished studies, it has been found that small doses of volatile anesthetics (such as isoflurane 0.5%) can abolish the compound EMG potential produced by transcranial electrical stimulation completely, but that, in already-anesthetized patients, nitrous oxide probably has little additional depressant effect on the evoked EMG potential (IJ Woodforth, RG Hicks, MR Crawford, JPH Stephen, and D Burke, unpublished observations). By contrast, the large D waves of electrically evoked corticospinal volleys are relatively impervious to changes in the type or depth of anesthesia, though threshold D waves and I waves are quite sensitive to volatile anesthetics (Hicks et al., 1992a,b; see Fig. 22–6). For monitoring purposes, the goal should be to obtain large D waves which have low trial-to-trial variability (Burke et al., 1995).

8. ELECTRICAL OR MAGNETIC TRANSCRANIAL STIMULATION

Pain has been the major factor behind the growth of magnetic rather than electrical transcranial stimulation for diagnostic and research studies on the corticospinal system. There is greater variability of the amplitude of the evoked EMG potential of awake subjects with magnetic stimulation presumably because the corticospinal volley contains a relatively small D wave (Burke et al., 1993), such that motor neuron discharge is more dependent on temporal summation of the subsequent I waves. Amplitude variability may be a minor problem in diagnostic studies that rely on latency measurements, but it presents a major problem for intraoperative monitoring. It seems paradoxical that some authorities have expended a great deal of effort to make the intrinsically variable magnetic technique more suitable for intraoperative monitoring when pain is no longer a contraindication to the more reproducible electrical technique.

The corticospinal volleys evoked by modest electrical stimuli are larger and more readily defined than those using the maximal output of magnetic stimulators, at least the Magstim

200 with 9-cm round coil (Berardelli et al., 1990; Thompson et al., 1991; Burke et al., 1993). The volley evoked by magnetic stimulation contains activity due to direct stimulation of corticospinal neurons or their axons but it is still usually dominated to a greater extent than the electrically evoked volley by indirect (presumably transsynaptically generated) I waves. As discussed earlier, the trial-to-trial variability of small D-wave components and of I waves is much higher than that of large simple D waves (Burke et al., 1995), such that the spinal cord volleys produced by magnetic stimulation are less suitable for monitoring purposes.

It seems illogical to use evoked EMG potentials to transcranial magnetic stimulation as a means of monitoring corticospinal function in anesthetized patients. Such a choice implies that one has deliberately opted for the less reproducible stimulus *and* the less reproducible recording technique. In addition, the depressant effects of anesthesia are not confined to translating the evoked corticospinal volley into motoneuron discharge: the cortical response to the stimulus is very sensitive to anesthesia (and there may well be a different anesthetic sensitivity for cortical generators and the lower motoneuron).

Ultimately, magnetic stimulation activates neural tissue electrically. There is no intrinsically special feature about the magnetic stimulus other than the fact that it causes minimal discomfort in awake subjects. Accordingly, it is difficult to defend a preference for it in unconscious, anesthetized patients.

9. CRITERIA FOR ABNORMALITY

In monitoring studies, it is traditional to set an arbitrary criterion of amplitude suppression by 50%, with or without waveform degradation. Such a criterion has been based on recording a single modality (usually sensory) commonly at a single level of the neuraxis (however, see the recommendations of Harper and Daube, 1989). The criterion level is a compromise between retaining ability to detect adverse changes and not reporting artifactual or random changes ("false positives"). The present authors believe that the technique described in this chapter minimizes the reasons for "false positive" changes, first, by relying on recordings that have good signal-to-noise ratio and are highly reproducible and, secondly, by recording two different modalities at two separate levels. Accordingly, artifactual changes due to problems with one stimulator or with a recording electrode can be identified with confidence.

Coherent changes consistent with neural dysfunction must be notified to the surgeon. These could be changes in amplitude and/or waveform of the corticospinal volley at the caudal level and of the somatosensory volley at the rostral level, or of either volley (or both) at both levels. In practice, a decrease in amplitude of either volley by 20% to 30% should be viewed with caution, the change replicated, and artifactual causes eliminated. It would be imprudent to wait until an arbitrary 50% criterion was fulfilled if the waveform changes indicated neural dysfunction. By itself a latency change is of little value as an indicator of pathology.

Using these criteria, one can expect intraoperative monitoring to reveal evidence of spinal dysfunction in 7% to 10% of patients undergoing scoliosis surgery. In the authors' experience of more than 250 cases, these adverse changes respond to interruption of curve correction and elevation of blood pressure. In a few patients waveforms have improved but without complete resolution of the changes by the end of the procedure. However, so far, no patient has suffered a new postoperative deficit.

In conclusion, two additional advantages of the present monitoring technique should be highlighted. First, if the surgeon has confidence in the technique as an indicator of spinal cord integrity, the preservation of potentials can be used as a guide to the extent of safe curve correction. Second, epidural recordings allow monitoring to be undertaken in many patients with preexisting neural abnormalities. In patients with cerebral palsy, Arnold–Chiari malformation, or hydrocephalus, it may not be possible to record corticospinal volleys, but a monitoring service can then be based on epidural recording of somatosensory potentials. In patients with spina bifida and flaccid legs only corticospinal volleys may be recordable. When satisfactory recordings cannot be obtained of either volley, the spinal cord can be stimulated directly through one set of epidural electrodes, and the evoked spinal cord volley recorded using the other set (Tamaki, 1989).

REFERENCES

Berardelli A, Inghilleri M, Cruccu G, Manfredi M (1990): Descending volley after electrical and magnetic transcranial stimulation in man. *Neurosci Lett* 112, 54–58.

Boyd SG, Rothwell JC, Cowan JMA, Webb PJ, Morley T, Asselman P, Marsden CD (1986): A method of monitoring function in corticospinal pathways during scoliosis surgery with a note on motor conduction velocities. *J Neurol Neurosurg Psychiatry* 49, 251–257.

Burke D, Hicks RG, Stephen JPH (1990): Corticospinal volleys evoked by anodal and cathodal stimulation of the human motor cortex. *J Physiol* 425, 283–299.

Burke D, Hicks RG, Stephen JPH (1992): Anodal and cathodal stimulation of the upper-limb area of the human motor cortex. *Brain* 115, 1497–1508.

Burke D, Hicks R, Gandevia SC, Stephen J, Woodford I, Cawford M (1993): Direct comparison of corticospinal volleys in human subjects to transcranial magnetic and electrical stimulation. *J Physiol* 470, 383–393.

Burke D, Hicks R, Stephen J, Woodforth I, Crawford M (1995): Trial-to-trial variability of corticospinal volleys in human subjects. *Electroencephalogr Clin Neurophysiol*, 97:231–237.

Dawson EG, Sherman JE, Kanim LEA, Nuwer MR (1991): Spinal cord monitoring. *Spine* 16, S361–S364.

Fehlings MG, Tator CH, Linden RD (1989): The relationship among the severity of spinal cord injury, motor and somatosensory evoked potentials and spinal cord blood flow. *Electroencephalogr Clin Neurophysiol* 74, 241–259.

Harper CM, Daube JR (1989): Surgical monitoring with evoked potentials: the Mayo Clinic experience. In: *Clinical Neurophysiology Updates*, vol. 1. *Neuromonitoring in Surgery*, edited by JE Desmedt, pp 275–301. Elsevier, Amsterdam.

Hicks RG, Burke DJ, Stephen JPH (1991): Monitoring spinal cord function during scoliosis surgery with Cotrel-Dubousset instrumentation. *Med J Austral* 154, 82–86.

Hicks RG, Burke D, Stephen JPH, Woodforth I, Crawford M (1992a): Corticospinal volleys evoked by electrical stimulation of human motor cortex after withdrawal of volatile anaesthetics. *J Physiol* 456, 393–404.

Hicks RG, Woodforth IJ, Crawford MR, Stephen JPH, Burke DJ (1992b): Some effects of isoflurane on I waves of the motor evoked potential. *Br J Anaesth* 69, 130–136.

Jones SJ, Edgar MA, Ransford AO (1982): Sensory nerve conduction in the human spinal cord: epidural recordings made during scoliosis surgery. *J Neurol Neurosurg Psychiatry* 45, 446–451.

Jones SJ, Edgar MA, Ransford AO, Thomas NP (1983): A system for the electrophysiological monitoring of the spinal cord during operations for scoliosis. *J Bone Joint Surg* 65B, 134–139.

Lesser RP, Raudzens P, Lüders H, Nuwer MR, Goldie WD, Morris HH, Dinner DS, Kelm G, Hahn JF, Shetter AG, Ginsburg HH, Gurd AR (1986): Postoperative neurological deficits may occur despite unchanged intraoperative somatosensory evoked potentials. *Ann Neurol* 19, 22–25.

Machida M, Weinstein SL, Yamada T, Kimura J, Toriyama S (1988): Dissociation of muscle action potentials and spinal somatosensory evoked potentials after ischemic damage of spinal cord. *Spine* 13, 1119–1124.

Owen JH, Laschinger J, Bridwell K, Shimon S, Nielsen C, Dunlap J, Kain C (1988): Sensitivity and specificity of somatosensory and neurogenic-motor evoked potentials in animals and humans. *Spine* 13, 1111–1118.

Rothwell JC, Thompson PD, Day BL, Dick JPR, Kachi T, Cowan JMA, Marsden CD (1987): Motor cortex stimulation in intact man. 1. General characteristics of EMG responses in different muscles. *Brain* 110, 1173–1190.

Rothwell J, Burke D, Hicks R, Stephen J, Woodforth I, Crawford M (1994): Transcranial electrical stimulation of the motor cortex in man: further evidence for the site of activation. *J Physiol* 481, 243–250.

Tamaki T (1989): Spinal cord monitoring with spinal potentials evoked by direct stimulation of the spinal cord. In: *Clinical Neurophysiology Updates*, vol 1. *Neuromonitoring in Surgery*, edited by JE Desmedt, pp 139–149. Elsevier, Amsterdam.

Thompson PD, Day BL, Crockard HA, Calder I, Murray NMF, Rothwell JC, Marsden CD (1991): Intra-operative recording of motor tract potentials at the cervico-medullary junction following scalp electrical and magnetic stimulation the motor cortex. *J Neurol Neurosurg Psychiatry* 54, 618–623.

Subject Index

Page numbers followed by *f* indicate figures; page numbers followed by *t* indicate tables.

CPSIA information can be obtained at www.ICGtesting.com
Printed in the USA
BVOW062113150513

320843BV00007B/63/P

9 780397 516599